HIGH-ACUITY NURSING

FOURTH EDITION

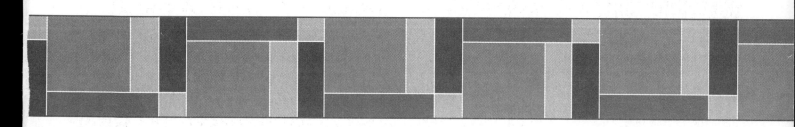

Kathleen Dorman Wagner, RN, MSN, EdD (AED)
College of Nursing
University of Kentucky
Lexington, KY

Karen L. Johnson, PhD, RN, CCRN
School of Nursing
University of Maryland
Baltimore, MD

Pamela Stinson Kidd, RN, PhD, ARNP, CEN
Formerly: Associate Dean for Research & Graduate Studies
College of Nursing
Arizona State University
Tempe, AZ

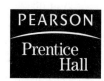
PEARSON
Prentice
Hall

Upper Saddle River, New Jersey 07458

Library of Congress Cataloging-in-Publication Data

Wagner, Kathleen Dorman.

  High-acuity nursing/ Kathleen Dorman Wagner, Karen L. Johnson,

  Pamela Stinson Kidd.—4th ed.

    p.; cm.

  Includes bibliographical references and index.

  ISBN 0–13–124508–2 (alk. paper)

  1. Intensive care nursing. I. Johnson, Karen L. II. Kidd, Pamela Stinson– III. Title.

  [DNLM: 1. Critical Care—methods. 2. Critical Illness—nursing. 3. Nursing Process. WY

  154 K46h 2006]

  RT120.I5K53 2006

  616.02'8—dc22

                                                    2005042455

Publisher: Julie Levin Alexander
Publisher's Assistant: Regina Bruno
Editor-in-Chief: Maura Connor
Acquisitions Editor: Pamela Fuller
Editorial Assistant: Eileen Monaghan/Aline Filippone
Associate Editor: Michael Giacobbe
Director of Manufacturing and Production: Bruce Johnson
Managing Production Editor: Patrick Walsh
Production Liaison: Cathy O'Connell
Production Editor: Emily Bush, Carlisle Communications
Manufacturing Manager: Ilene Sanford
Manufacturing Buyer: Pat Brown
Design Director: Maria Guglielmo
Cover and Interior Designer: Wanda España
Director of Marketing: Karen Allman
Executive Marketing Manager: Nicole Benson
Channel Marketing Manager: Rachele Strober
Marketing Assistant: Patricia Linard
Marketing Coordinator: Michael Sirinides
Media Editor: John Jordan
Media Production Manager: Amy Peltier
Media Project Manager: Tina Rudowski
Composition: Carlisle Communications
Printer/Binder: Banta Harrisonburg
Cover Printer: Coral Graphics

Pearson Prentice Hall™ is a trademark of Pearson Education, Inc.
Pearson® is a registered trademark of Pearson plc
Prentice Hall® is a registered trademark of Pearson Education, Inc.

Pearson Education Ltd.
Pearson Education Singapore, Pte., Ltd.
Pearson Education Canada, Ltd.
Pearson Education—Japan

Pearson Education Australia PTY, Limited
Pearson Education North Asia Ltd.
Pearson Educacíon de Mexico, S.A. de C.V.
Pearson Education Malaysia, Pte. Ltd.
Pearson Education Inc., Upper Saddle River, New Jersey

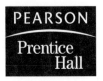

10 9 8 7 6 5 4
ISBN: 0-13-124508-2

In Memory of

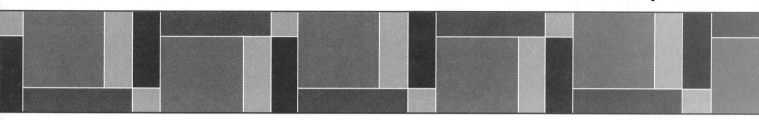

Pamela Stinson Kidd
September 16, 1957–December 25, 2002

"Pam Kidd was an internationally recognized expert in emergency nursing and injury prevention. Blessed with abundant warmth and a keen, restless intellect, she was an outstanding clinician, teacher, researcher, mentor, and friend. Pam was visionary and down to earth, unstintingly positive, yet honest to the core and never satisfied with the status quo. In all she did, she was driven by a profound commitment to making the world a better place. Pam exemplified the very best in nursing."

Mark Parshall, RN, PhD, and friend

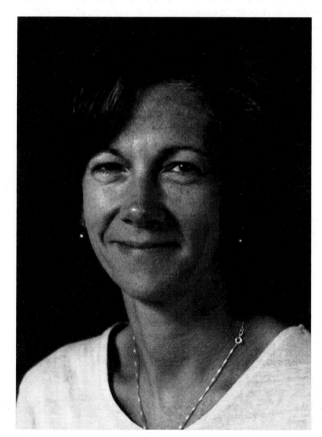

We dedicate this book to our colleague, friend, and inspiration. Pam is always with us in our hearts.

KDW & KLJ

Contents

PREFACE   vii

ABOUT THE AUTHORS   ix

ACKNOWLEDGMENTS   x

PART 1 Special Topics 1

MODULE 1 Caring for the High-Acuity Patient: Patient, Family, and Nursing Considerations   2

MODULE 2 Acute Pain in the High-Acuity Patient   24

MODULE 3 Fluid and Electrolyte Balance in the High-Acuity Patient   53

PART 2 Pulmonary Gas Exchange 79

MODULE 4 Determinants and Assessment of Pulmonary Gas Exchange   80

MODULE 5 Alterations in Pulmonary Gas Exchange   127

MODULE 6 Mechanical Ventilation   164

MODULE 7 Nursing Care of the Patient with Altered Gas Exchange   204

PART 3 Perfusion 217

MODULE 8 Determinants and Assessment of Cardiac Output   218

MODULE 9 Hemodynamic Monitoring   237

MODULE 10 Electrocardiographic Monitoring and Conduction Abnormalities   263

MODULE 11 Alterations in Myocardial Tissue Perfusion   299

MODULE 12 Alterations in Cardiac Output   324

MODULE 13 Nursing Care of the Patient with Altered Tissue Perfusion   343

PART 4 Oxygenation 353

MODULE 14 Determinants and Assessment of Oxygenation   354

MODULE 15 Shock States   369

MODULE 16 Multiple Organ Dysfunction Syndrome   384

MODULE 17 Nursing Care of the Patient with Impaired Oxygenation   394

PART 5 Neurologic 401

MODULE 18 Determinants and Assessment of Cerebral Tissue Perfusion   402

MODULE 19 Alterations in Cerebral Tissue Perfusion: Acute Brain Attack   426

MODULE 20 Decreased Adaptive Capacity: Closed-Head Injury   448

MODULE 21 Sensory Perceptual Disorders   459

MODULE 22 Nursing Care of the Patient with an Alteration in Cerebral Tissue Perfusion   484

PART 6 Metabolic   489

MODULE 23 Metabolic Responses to Stress   490

MODULE 24 Acute Hematologic Dysfunction   518

MODULE 25 Altered Immune Function   554

MODULE 26 Organ Transplantation   585

MODULE 27 Altered Glucose Metabolism   620

MODULE 28 Acute Renal Dysfunction   648

MODULE 29 Nursing Care of the Patient with Altered Metabolic Function   683

PART 7 Gastrointestinal   693

MODULE 30 Acute Gastrointestinal Dysfunction   694

MODULE 31 Acute Hepatic Dysfunction   734

MODULE 32 Acute Pancreatic Dysfunction   760

MODULE 33 Nursing Care of the Patient with Altered Gastrointestinal Function   781

PART 8 Injury   791

MODULE 34 Complex Wound Management   792

MODULE 35 Acute Burn Injury   819

MODULE 36 Trauma   849

MODULE 37 Nursing Care of the Patient with Multiple Injuries   881

INDEX   887

Preface

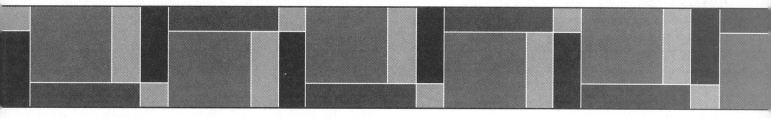

When the first edition of *High-Acuity Nursing* was published in 1992, the term *high acuity* was largely confined to leveling patient acuity for determining hospital staffing needs rather than being applied to nursing education. Today, there is a growing trend toward offering a high-acuity nursing course as part of the required undergraduate nursing curriculum. This, we believe, reflects the changing nature of the acute care adult patient population and the need to adequately prepare new nurses (and retool experienced nurses) to meet these rapidly changing needs.

The term *high acuity* refers to a level of patient problems beyond uncomplicated acute illness on a health–illness continuum. Today, high-acuity patients are increasingly found outside of critical care units or even acute care institutions. The patient population is older and sicker on entering the health care system, and hospitalized patients are being discharged earlier, often in a poorer state of health. In the home health setting, nurses are providing care to clients with mechanical ventilators, central intravenous (IV) lines, IV antibiotic therapy, and complicated injuries. Whereas critical care units are considered specialty areas within the hospital walls, much of the knowledge required to work within those specialties is generalist in nature. It is this generalist knowledge base that is needed by all nurses who work with patients experiencing complex care problems to assure competent and safe nursing practice.

Purpose of the Text

The *High-Acuity Nursing* text delivers information using learner-focused, active learning principles, and concise language and format. The format breaks down complex information into small, understandable chunks for easy understanding. Self-testing is provided throughout the text, using Pretests, short section quizzes, and Posttests. All answers are provided to give learners immediate feedback on their command of section content before proceeding to the next module section.

The self-study modules in this book focus on the relationship between pathophysiology and the nursing process with the following goals in mind:

1. To revisit and translate critical pathophysiological concepts pertaining to the high-acuity adult patient in a clinically applicable manner
2. To examine the interrelationships among physiological concepts
3. To enhance clinical decision-making skills
4. To free class time to focus on clinical application
5. To hold learners accountable for their own learning
6. To provide immediate feedback to the learner regarding assimilation of concepts and principles
7. To provide self-paced learning

Ultimately, the goal for the learner is to be able to approach patient care of the adult conceptually, so that care is given with a strong underlying understanding of its rationale.

This book is appropriate for use in multiple educational settings, for example, nursing students, novice nurses, novice critical care nurses, and home health nurses. It also serves as a review book for the experienced nurse wanting updated information about high-acuity nursing for continuing education purposes. Hospital staff development departments will find it useful as supplemental or required reading for nursing staff, or high-acuity or critical care classes. It also can be used for teaching basic pathophysiology, and as a review book for the NCLEX exam.

Organization of the Text

The book consists of eight parts: Special Topics, Pulmonary Gas Exchange, Perfusion, Oxygenation, Neurologic, Metabolic, Gastrointestinal, and Injury.

For continuity, the modules are presented in a consistent manner, using a single concept or nursing application format. The single concept modules contain an Introduction, Glossary, Abbreviation List, Objectives, Pretest, Review Questions, and Posttest. Each module is divided into sections covering one facet of the module's topic (e.g., physiology, pathophysiology, or nursing management).

Parts II through VIII conclude with a nursing care module, which uses a case study problem-solving approach to test the learner's skill in applying the information presented in each part.

Part I, "Special Topics," is composed of three modules. The topics apply to high-acuity patients in general. Module 1 addresses the psychosocial needs of high-acuity patients, their families, and the nurses who care for them. Module 2 focuses on acute pain and the unique needs of high-acuity patients in pain

assessment and management. Module 3 presents fluid and electrolyte concepts and problems.

Parts II through VIII present topics that represent the more common complex problems, assessments, and treatments associated with high-acuity patients. In each of Parts II through V, the modules are organized in a logical order. Assessment concepts comprise the initial modules, followed by one or more modules that present specific pathological problems and their management, and each part ends with a nursing application module. For example, Part II, "Pulmonary Gas Exchange;" is composed of Module 4, "Determinants and Assessment of Pulmonary Gas Exchange;" Module 5, "Alterations in Pulmonary Gas Exchange;" Module 6, "Mechanical Ventilation;" and Module 7, "Nursing Care of the Patient with Altered Pulmonary Gas Exchange." The modules in Parts VI through VIII are organized around more system-based pathological processes, with assessment and management concepts contained within each module.

New to This Edition

The fourth edition has undergone major revamping of content in Parts III and V to better address problems seen in the high-acuity population. For example, acute head injury has been added to Part V. In addition, all modules have been updated, and multiple modules have been substantially reorganized or streamlined. Test items have been revised to reflect the changes

in content. Research has been integrated throughout the content and Evidence-Based Practice boxes have been added to the majority of the modules. Because the elderly comprise a large percentage of the high-acuity patient population in most settings that provide nursing care, concepts specific to aging patients have been integrated into the modules.

Summary

This text is a series of reality-based modules that focus on concepts frequently encountered in high-acuity patients. It is not designed as a comprehensive review of pathophysiology or medical–surgical nursing. The book's format reduces learner feelings of being overwhelmed by complex information. Learners are more apt to feel in command of the concepts, giving them the confidence to proceed to the more complex concepts. The fourth edition of *High-Acuity Nursing* has maintained the look

and feel of the previous editions. Although the fourth edition has been reorganized slightly, we have not compromised on our approach. The ultimate goal of this book continues to be to enhance the preparation of nurses for practice in today's health care settings.

Kathleen Dorman Wagner
Karen L. Johnson

About the Authors

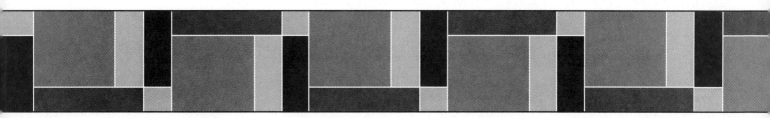

Kathleen Dorman Wagner is a lecturer in the Undergraduate Program in the College of Nursing at the University of Kentucky. Her background is as a clinical nurse specialist in adult critical care, with more than 15 years of experience in diverse critical care and high-acuity settings and 20 years as a nurse educator. As a nurse educator, she teaches pathophysiology, pathopharmacology, and high-acuity nursing at the undergraduate level. She is currently completing her dissertation for a doctoral degree in instructional systems design. Her current research interest is in case method instruction. She is the co-recipient of the AJN's Book of the Year of 1997 awards for two books: *High-Acuity Nursing, second edition,* in the emergency nursing category; and *Instructor Manual to Accompany High-Acuity Nursing, second edition,* in the critical care nursing category.

Karen L. Johnson is an assistant professor at the University of Maryland School of Nursing in Baltimore, Maryland. She teaches in the undergraduate program and in the trauma/critical care/emergency nursing master's program. She has more than 10 years experience as a critical care clinical nurse specialist at the University of Kentucky and the University of Arizona. She also taught undergraduate critical care nursing at both of these institutions. In 2000, she received the Undergraduate Excellence in Teaching Award from the University of Arizona and the "Outstanding Advanced Practice Nurse Award" from the American Association of Critical Care Nurses. She has written more than 30 book chapters in several critical care textbooks and has been writing chapters in *High-Acuity Nursing* since its first edition. Her current research interests are in physiological measurement and the effects of the physiological stress response on critical illness. Her research is published in *Critical Care Medicine,* the *American Journal of Critical Care,* and *AACN Clinical Issues.*

Acknowledgments

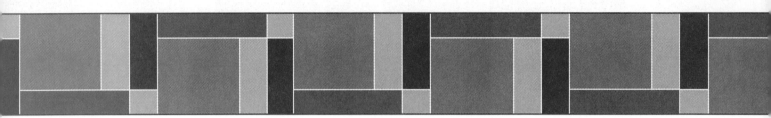

The development of each new edition presents new challenges. This edition was especially difficult with the loss of our dear friend, mentor, and colleague, Dr. Pamela Kidd, who coedited *High-Acuity Nursing* from its inception. Pam's warmth and wit are deeply missed by all who were fortunate enough to know her. My heartfelt thanks go out to my friend and colleague, Dr. Karen Johnson, for her willingness to step in and coedit the fourth edition with me. Without her energy and competence as both a writer and editor, this edition may not have come to fruition. Karen, I owe you one . . . or two . . . or three! Thanks to Deborah Wagner for her invaluable artistic contributions in developing concept art for multiple figures for this edition—I am amazed at those who can visualize and draw their vision based on the spoken word. To Don, Becky, Debby, and now Tom—my family, my joy.

KDW

To my husband Steve, for his everlasting love and support throughout my career. To my children Chris and Amy, for bringing so much joy to my life every day. In loving memory of my parents Steve and Elaine Smith, for their commitment to my education. In memory of two colleagues who died tragically and way too soon, Cheryl McGaffic, RN, PhD, CCRN, and Pam Kidd, RN, PhD, ARNP, CEN, for your passion in teaching undergraduate critical care.

KLJ

Contributors

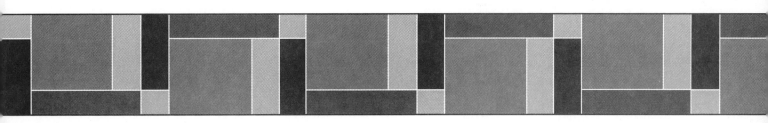

Jane Lacovara, RN-BC, MSN
University of Arizona
Tucson, AZ

Jill Arzouman, RN, MSN
University of Arizona
Tucson, AZ

Barbara L. Vanderveer, RN, MSN
University of Kentucky
Lexington, KY

Valerie K. Sabol, RN, MSN, CCRN, ACNP
University of Maryland School of Nursing
Baltimore, MD

Diana Thacker, RN, MSN, CPTC
Kentucky Organ Donor Affiliates
Lexington, KY

Connie G. Taylor, RN, BSN, CLNC
Independent Consultant
Lexington, KY

Kathleen D. Wagner, RN, EdD (AED)
University of Kentucky
Lexington, KY

Gail Priestley, RN, MS, CCRN
University of Arizona
Tucson, AZ

Conrad Gordon, RN, MS
University of Maryland School of Nursing
Ellicott City, MD

Angie Muzzy, RN, MSN, CCRN
Arizona University Medical Center
Vail, AZ

Cliff Pyne, RN, MS
Naval Medical Center
Suffolk, VA

Nancy Munro, RN, MN, CCRN, ACNP
National Institutes of Health
Bethesda, MD

Dayna Gary, RN, BSN, CWS, OTR-L
University of Maryland Hospital
Baltimore, MD

Karen Johnson, PhD, RN, CCRN
University of Maryland School of Nursing
Dayton, MD

Jean Martin, RN, MSN, CCRN
University of Arizona
Tucson, AZ

Humberto Zuniga, RN, BSN, CCRN
Naval Medical Center
Virginia Beach, VA

Amy Tarbay, RN, BSN, MSN
Naval Medical Center
Suffolk, VA

Adam DaDeppo, RN, MS, ACNP
University of Maryland
Jessup, MD

Kathy Hausman, PhD, RN
University of Maryland School of Nursing
Baltimore, MD

Susan Bohnenkamp, RN, MS, CCM
University of Arizona
Oro Valley, AZ

Diane Orr Chlebowy, PhD, RN
University of Kentucky
Lexington, KY

Melanie Hardin-Pierce, RN, MSN, APRN-BC
University of Kentucky
Lexington, KY

Catherine McDonald, RN, MSN, CS, FNP
Naval Medical Center
Chesapeake, VA

Michelle Willis, RN, MS, ACNP
University of Maryland Hospital
Baltimore, MD

Reviewers

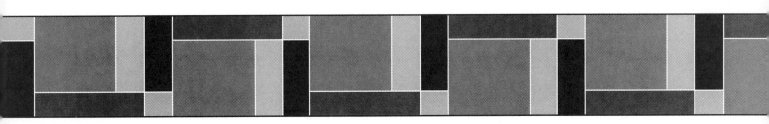

Gloria Jean Kline, MSN, RN, CNS

Stark State College of Technology
Canton, OH

Bonnie L. Kirkpatrick, RN, MS, CNS

The Ohio State University College of Nursing
Columbus, OH

Julieta Castañeda, RN, MSN

The University of Texas at El Paso, College of Health
Sciences, School of Nursing
El Paso, TX

Fran Bartholomeaux, RN, MS, CCRN

Clinical Nurse Educator/Critical Care
University Medical Center
Tucson, AZ

Mary Truelove Blankenship, MSN, RN

Anna Vaughn School of Nursing,
Oral Roberts University
Tulsa, OK

Shirley K. Woolf, RN, MSN, CCRN, CNRN, PN

Indiana University School of Nursing
Indianapolis, IN

Glenna C. McMinn, MS, RN

Thomkins Cortland Community College
Dryden, NY

Marilyn U. Cox, MS, APRN, ANP-BC

Weber State University
Ogden, UT

Lawrette Axley, PhD, RN

University of Memphis, Loewenberg School of Nursing
Memphis, TN

Anne E. Helm, RN, MSN

Owens Community College
Toledo, OH

Linda S. Dune, PhD, RN, CCRN, CEN

The University of Texas Health Science Center at Houston
School of Nursing
Houston, TX

Michelle Buchman, BSN, RNC

Springfield College
Springfield, MO

Diane Brown, MSN, RN, CCRN

The University of Akron
Akron, OH

Beverly Anderson, RN, MSN

Salt Lake Community College
S.L.C., UT

PART

1

Special Topics

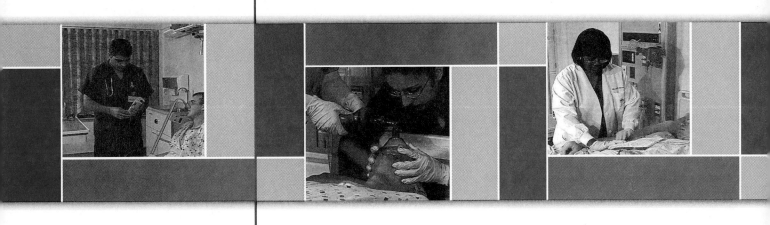

MODULE 1 Caring for the High-Acuity Patient: Patient, Family, and Nursing Considerations

MODULE 2 Acute Pain in the High-Acuity Patient

MODULE 3 Fluid and Electrolyte Balance in the High-Acuity Patient

MODULE 1

Caring for the High-Acuity Patient: Patient, Family, and Nursing Considerations

Jane Lacovara, Jill Arzouman

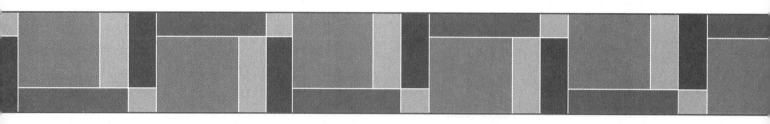

OBJECTIVES Following completion of this module, the learner will be able to

1. Discuss the various health care environments in which high-acuity patients receive care.

2. Discuss stages of illness a high-acuity patient may experience.

3. Identify ways the nurse can help high-acuity patients cope with an illness and/or injury.

4. Identify environmental stressors, their physiological impact on the high-acuity patient, and strategies to alleviate those stressors.

5. Discuss the educational needs of high-acuity patients and their families and strategies to meet these needs.

6. Discuss the rationale for visitation policies and the effects of visitation on high-acuity patients.

7. Identify work design and staffing strategies for high-acuity patients.

8. Discuss the interface between technology and caring.

9. Describe stressful and satisfying aspects of caring for acutely ill patients.

10. Describe resource allocation issues as they relate to high-acuity patients.

11. Examine personal values as they relate to the nurse's role in working with acutely ill patients.

12. Discuss end-of-life issues to be considered in caring for high-acuity patients.

This module is written at a core knowledge level for individuals who provide nursing care for high-acuity patients, regardless of the practice setting. The focus of the module is the nursing role in caring for high-acuity patients and the effect of illness or injury on the patient, family, and nurse. The module is divided into two parts: Patient and Family Considerations, and Nursing Considerations. Part I consists of five sections. Section One discusses the environments in which high-acuity patients are placed to receive care. Sections Two and Three address the stages of illness and nursing strategies to assist the patient in coping with being high-acuity. Section Four discusses the influence of the environment on the patient's psychological and physical integrity. Section Five examines the educational needs of high-acuity patients and their family. The second part, consisting of six sections, discusses the nursing role in caring for high-acuity patients. Section Six examines visitation policies and the

high-acuity patient. Section Seven discusses work design and staffing strategies for the high-acuity patient. The interface between technology and caring is discussed in Section Eight. Stressors and satisfying factors associated with nursing the high-acuity patient are addressed in Section Nine. Section Ten examines resource allocation issues, and Section Eleven encourages the learner to complete a self-assessment in order to identify potential sources of personal conflict in working with high-acuity patients and also discusses important end-of-life issues to be considered in caring for high-acuity patients. Each section includes a set of review questions to help the learner evaluate his or her understanding of the section's content before moving on to the next section. All Section Reviews and the module Pretest and Posttest include answers. It is suggested that the learner review those concepts answered incorrectly in the review questions before proceeding to the next section.

📖 PRETEST

1. High-acuity patients frequently complain about which of the following when hospitalized?
   A. lack of privacy
   B. hospital food
   C. inadequate nursing staff
   D. lack of blankets

2. Denial during acute illness
   A. can have positive effects on health outcomes
   B. increases oxygen consumption
   C. is a maladaptive coping strategy
   D. promotes false hope

3. Sensory perceptual alterations may occur because of
   A. a reduction in red blood cells related to social isolation
   B. desaturation of oxyhemoglobin
   C. an adversity to touch
   D. a state of touch deficiency

4. Who of the following is at greatest risk for developing sensory problems?
   A. an adolescent patient
   B. an unresponsive patient
   C. a female patient
   D. an elderly patient

5. A major reason that computers are being tested for use in decision making with high-acuity patients is
   A. computers are compact
   B. computers are time efficient
   C. any staff member can input available data
   D. there are large amounts of data that must be processed in order to make a decision

6. Nurses who work with high-acuity patients cite which of the following as a major stressor?
   A. overtime work
   B. nurse–patient ratio
   C. constant need to recertify skills and procedures
   D. interpersonal conflict with other health team members

7. Of the following patient populations, which population is the least vulnerable in regard to resource allocation?
   A. neonates
   B. the elderly
   C. oncology patients
   D. transplant patients

8. Which of the following factors may inhibit learning in high-acuity patients?
   A. medications
   B. previous knowledge of illness
   C. educational level
   D. gender

9. Families of high-acuity patients desire which of the following needs to be met first by the nurse?
   A. physical
   B. spiritual
   C. cognitive
   D. emotional

10. Mr. Rogers states, "I'm going to have to put up with this scar and make the best of it." This response indicates he is in which of the following states of illness?
    A. awareness
    B. resolution
    C. restitution
    D. denial

11. The purpose of imagery is to
    A. ignore the real situation
    B. replace unpleasant experiences with relaxation
    C. promote use of the senses
    D. increase neurologic stimulation

12. High-acuity patients have which of the following characteristics?
    A. have been hospitalized previously
    B. need extensive rehabilitation
    C. are physically unstable
    D. have chronic illness

13. The use of equipment in the nursing role may
    A. increase the nurse's stress level
    B. decrease nursing surveillance responsibility
    C. decrease the need for patient advocacy
    D. increase patient satisfaction

14. Which of the following is a hazard of technology?
    A. increased fragmentation of care
    B. decreased demand for nursing staff
    C. decreased competition with patient for nursing time
    D. increased patient feeling of independence

15. Which of the following may be a source of burnout?
    A. hourly nursing assessment
    B. nursing care plans
    C. continuing education requirements
    D. 1:1 nursing

16. Which of the following may be a symptom of burnout?
    A. nurse requests to work a holiday
    B. nurse assists co-workers in care
    C. nurse complains of inadequate physician standing orders
    D. nurse states that "females always give in to their pain"

17. Mr. Martin states that he has dreamed of being tortured while in the intensive care unit. The nurse recognizes that this is a symptom of
    A. sensory deprivation
    B. burnout
    C. fatigue
    D. uncontrolled pain

18. Children of high-acuity patients
    A. do not want to visit their ill parent
    B. should be given a choice to visit their parent
    C. experience emotional distress after visitation
    D. want to visit their fathers but not their mothers

19. Which of the following have nurses identified as increasing their satisfaction with their role?
   A. getting on-call pay
   B. orienting new staff
   C. working multiple shifts
   D. small nurse–patient ratio

20. All of the following have been cited to relieve stress associated with the nursing role EXCEPT
   A. discussion with co-workers
   B. self-assessment of achievements
   C. serving as unit resource person
   D. watching television

Pretest Answers:
1. A, 2. A, 3. D, 4. B, 5. D, 6. D, 7. D, 8. A, 9. C, 10. B, 11. B, 12. C, 13. A, 14. A, 15. D, 16. D, 17. A, 18. B, 19. D, 20. C

GLOSSARY

aromatherapy   Use of oils to reduce stress and anxiety.

burnout   A crisis state evolving from stress; to become exhausted by making excessive demands on energy, strength, or resources.

complementary and alternative therapies   Therapies used in lieu of, or as a complement to, standard medical treatment.

hardiness   A personality trait that enables one to feel capable of positive action in a stressful situation.

sensory perceptual alterations   The amount, character, or intensity of stimuli exceeds the person's minimum or maximum threshold of tolerance for sensory input; accompanied by a diminished, exaggerated, distorted, or impaired response.

spirituality   A sense of faith and transcendence.

sundowner's syndrome   The patient appears alert and appropriate during the day but becomes confused and agitated in the evening or at night.

ABBREVIATIONS

AACN	American Association of Critical Care Nurses	**dBA**	Decibel
ABG	Arterial blood gas	**DNR**	Do not resuscitate
ACCM	American College of Critical Care Medicine	**ICU**	Intensive care unit
AMSN	Academy of Medical Surgical Nurses	**IMC**	Intermediate care unit
ANA	American Nurses Association	**REM**	Rapid eye movement
CAT	Complementary and alternative therapies	**SIMV**	Synchronized intermittent mandatory ventilation
CISD	Critical incident stress debriefing	**SPA**	Sensory perceptual alteration
CPR	Cardiopulmonary resuscitation	**UAP**	Unlicensed assistive personnel

Patient and Family Considerations

SECTION ONE: Patient Care Areas for High-Acuity Patients

At the completion of this section, the learner will be able to discuss the various health care environments in which high-acuity patients receive care.

The nurse caring for the high-acuity patient must be able to analyze clinical situations, make decisions based on this analysis, and rapidly intervene to ensure optimal patient outcomes. Comfort with uncertainty and patient instability are required.

The nurse is instrumental in treating patients' health problems as well as their reactions to the health care environment. The nurse is the only member of the health care team who remains at the bedside and, as a result, is frequently the one who coordinates patient care.

The nurse is often the first member of the health care team to detect early signs of an impending complication. Constant surveillance by the acute care nurse involves assessing and monitoring the patient for signs of subtle changes over time. Many times subtle changes in a patient's condition are clues of a possible impending complication. Prevention of complications in the acute care patient is one of the primary goals of the acute care nurse. Evidence suggests that constant surveillance of patients by nurses reduces mortality and life-threatening complications in the hospitalized patient (Clarke & Aiken, 2003).

Intensive care units (ICUs) were first developed in the early 1960s. There were multiple reasons for their development, including (1) the implementation of cardiopulmonary resuscitation so that people might survive sudden death events; (2) better understanding of the treatment of hypovolemic shock related to recent war experiences; (3) the implementation of emergency medical services, resulting in improved transport systems; (4) the development of technologic inventions that required close observation for effective use (i.e., electrocardiographic monitoring); and (5) the initiation of renal transplant surgery. The first ICUs were recovery rooms. Patients admitted were still anesthetized. Problems resulted, however, when the volume of surgical procedures increased, and recovery rooms were full. The high-acuity patient who required extra equipment and prolonged observation was placed in the newly created ICU.

Although high-acuity patients are viewed historically as being in an acute care unit, this is no longer true because of the shortage of acute care beds. A shortage of acute care beds combined with skyrocketing costs for health care requires practitioners to make decisions about where in the hospital high-acuity patients are placed so that they receive the most efficient and cost-effective care. This may mean the patient is placed in an ICU, an intermediate care unit (IMC), or in a medical surgical acute care unit. These triage decisions require a systematic approach so that optimal outcomes and controlled costs are achieved.

The use of intermediate care, or step-down units may provide an efficient distribution of resources for the patient whose acute illness requires less use of monitoring equipment and staffing than a high-acuity ICU (American College of Critical Care Medicine [ACCM], 1998). The intermediate care unit serves as a place for the monitoring and care of patients with moderate or potentially severe physiologic instability who require technical support but not necessarily artificial life support; it is reserved for those patients requiring less-than-standard intensive care but more than that which is available from ward care (ACCM, 1998). Guidelines for the admission and discharge for adult intermediate care units are available (ACCM, 1998).

The American College of Critical Care Medicine recommends using a prioritization model to help make decisions about appropriate admission, discharge, and triage of acutely ill patients in an ICU (ACCM, 1999). The model defines which patients may benefit most from receiving care in an ICU. This prioritization model is summarized in Table 1–1. Priority 1 includes the most critically ill and Priority 4 includes those who are generally not appropriate candidates for ICU admission.

ICUs vary from hospital to hospital in terms of the services provided, the personnel, and their level of expertise. Large medical centers frequently have multiple ICUs defined by specialty area (neurosurgical ICU, trauma ICU). Small hospitals may have only one ICU designed to care for a variety of acutely ill patients with medical and/or surgical disease processes. Although the types and varieties of ICUs may differ from one hospital to the next, all ICUs have the responsibility of providing services and personnel to ensure optimal care (ACCM, 2003). The American Academy of Critical Care Medicine (2003) identified three levels of ICUs as determined by resources available to the hospital. These levels are summarized in Table 1–2.

When a patient requires more comprehensive and/or specialized care, a decision must be made to transfer the acutely ill patient to a higher level of ICU care where additional personnel and resources are available. Transporting a patient from one area of the hospital to another or from one hospital to another includes risk. The decision to transport a patient must include an assessment of the risk-to-benefit ratio. Guidelines for the transfer of critically ill patients are available to help make these important decisions (ACCM, 1993). According to these guidelines, hospitals should have policies and procedures that address

TABLE 1–1 Prioritization of Admission, Discharge, and Triage of Acutely Ill Patients in an ICU

PRIORITY FOR ICU PLACEMENT	DESCRIPTION OF PATIENT CHARACTERISTICS
Priority 1	Acutely ill, unstable, and requires intensive treatment and monitoring that cannot be provided outside of the ICU (mechanical ventilation, continuous vasoactive drug infusions). There are no limits on the extent of intended interventions. Examples of these patients may include postoperative or acute respiratory failure patients requiring mechanical ventilator support, and shock or hemodynamically unstable patients receiving invasive monitoring and/or vasoactive drugs.
Priority 2	Requires intensive monitoring, may potentially need immediate intervention. There are no limits on the extent of intended interventions. Examples include patients with chronic comorbid conditions who develop acute severe medical or surgical illness.
Priority 3	Critically ill and unstable with a reduced likelihood of recovery because of underlying disease or nature of the acute illness. May receive intensive treatment to relieve acute illness; however, limits on therapeutic efforts may be set, such as no intubation or cardiopulmonary resuscitation. Examples include patients with metastatic malignancy complicated by infection, cardiac tamponade, or airway obstruction.
Priority 4	Generally not appropriate for ICU admission. Admission should be made on an individual basis, under unusual circumstances, and at the discretion of the ICU director. Examples include patients with peripheral vascular surgery, stable diabetic ketoacidosis, conscious drug overdose, and patients with terminal and irreversible illness facing immediate death.

Source: From Task Force of the American College of Critical Care Medicine, Society of Critical Care Medicine. (1999). Guidelines for intensive care unit admission, discharge, and triage. Critical Care Medicine, *27(3):635.*

TABLE 1–2 ACCM's (2003) Definitions of ICU Levels of Care

ICU LEVEL	DESCRIPTION OF SERVICES, PERSONNEL
Level I	Hospitals with ICUs that provide comprehensive care for patients with a wide range of disorders. Sophisticated equipment is available. Units are staffed with specialized nurses and physicians with critical care training. Comprehensive support services are available and include pharmacy, respiratory therapy, nutritional support, social services, and pastoral care. These units may be located within an academic teaching hospital or may be community based.
Level II	Hospitals with ICUs that have the capability of providing comprehensive care to most critically ill patients but not to specific patient populations (neurosurgical, cardiothoracic, trauma).
Level III	Hospitals with ICUs that have the ability to provide initial stabilization of critically ill patients but are limited in ability to provide comprehensive care for all patients. Able to care for ICU patients requiring routine care and monitoring.

pretransport coordination and communication, personnel who must accompany the patient, equipment to accompany the patient, and the monitoring that will be required during the transport. It is recommended that clinicians use an algorithm (Fig. 1–1) in the decision-making process of transferring acutely ill patients to a higher level of care.

In summary, acutely ill patients often require constant surveillance by nurses to reduce morbidity and mortality. ICUs were developed in the early 1960s for these very reasons. In today's health care environment, skyrocketing costs and a shortage of acute care beds requires clinicians to make decisions about where in the hospital, or which hospital, acutely ill patients receive the most efficient and cost-effective care. Stepdown, or intermediate care, units may provide for an efficient distribution of resources for patients whose acute illness requires less monitoring equipment and staffing than a high-acuity ICU. Clinicians can use established guidelines in the priority decision-making process to determine which patients would most likely benefit from receiving care in an ICU. ICUs differ from hospital to hospital depending on services provided, the available personnel, and their levels of expertise. If a patient requires more comprehensive or more specialized care, it is important to follow established guidelines to ensure safe transition to a higher level of care.

SECTION ONE REVIEW

1. Intermediate care units
   A. are outdated and should not be used
   B. are labor intensive and are not cost effective
   C. provide an efficient distribution of resources
   D. are reserved for patients with life-threatening illnesses
2. Which of the following priority levels means that the patient is acutely ill, unstable, and requires intensive treatment and monitoring that cannot be provided outside the ICU?
   A. Priority 1
   B. Priority 2

   C. Priority 3
   D. Priority 4
3. Hospitals should have policies and procedures for transferring critically ill patients from one area to another. These policies and procedures should address
   A. pretransport coordination and communication
   B. personnel who must accompany the patient
   C. equipment to accompany the patient
   D. all of the above

Answers: 1. C, 2. A, 3. D

SECTION TWO: Stages of Illness

At the completion of this section, the learner will be able to discuss the stages of illness a high-acuity patient may experience.

High-acuity illness produces a loss of the familiar self-image and has an impact on self-esteem. The patient may need to adapt to loss of health, loss of limb, disfigurement, or a necessary change in lifestyle. Change may precipitate grieving. According to Suchman (1965), high-acuity patients may respond to these losses by experiencing certain predictable phases. Table 1–3 summarizes Suchman's stages of illness, manifestations, and nursing interventions appropriate for each stage. The first stage is shock and disbelief because the diagnosis does not have an emotional meaning. The patient may be uncooperative because he is projecting difficulties onto hospital procedures, equipment, and personnel. In this stage, a patient may worry more about the equipment being used than about the diagnosis because the diagnosis may be a threat to life. The denial stage can have positive effects. It may protect the patient against the emotional

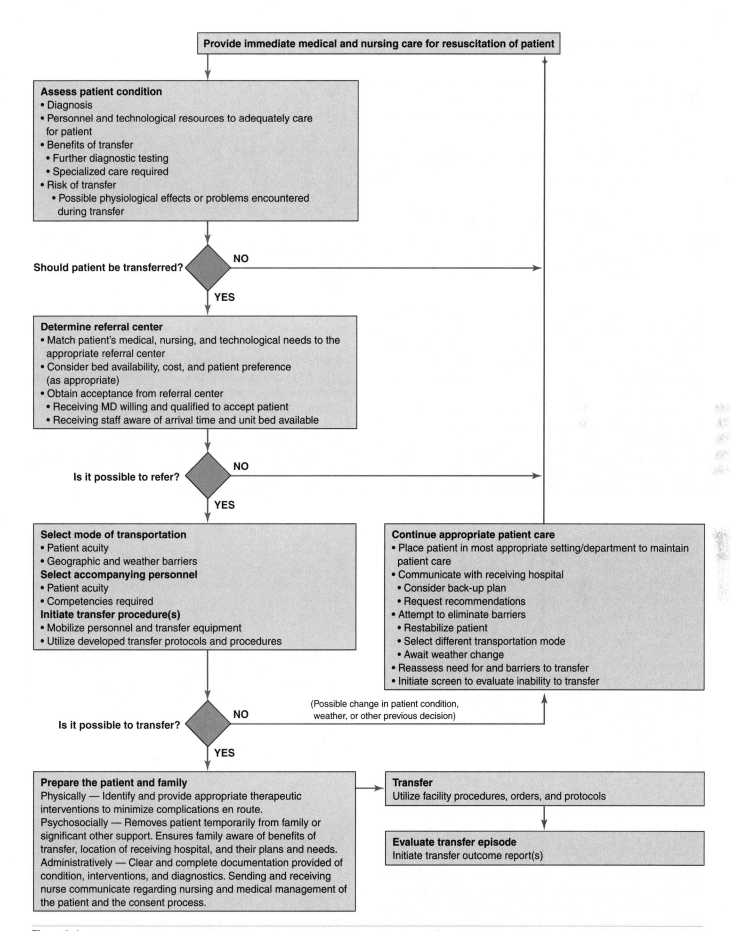

Provide immediate medical and nursing care for resuscitation of patient

Assess patient condition
- Diagnosis
- Personnel and technological resources to adequately care for patient
- Benefits of transfer
  - Further diagnostic testing
  - Specialized care required
- Risk of transfer
  - Possible physiological effects or problems encountered during transfer

Should patient be transferred? NO YES

Determine referral center
- Match patient's medical, nursing, and technological needs to the appropriate referral center
- Consider bed availability, cost, and patient preference (as appropriate)
- Obtain acceptance from referral center
  - Receiving MD willing and qualified to accept patient
  - Receiving staff aware of arrival time and unit bed available

Is it possible to refer? NO YES

Select mode of transportation
- Patient acuity
- Geographic and weather barriers

Select accompanying personnel
- Patient acuity
- Competencies required

Initiate transfer procedure(s)
- Mobilize personnel and transfer equipment
- Utilize developed transfer protocols and procedures

Continue appropriate patient care
- Place patient in most appropriate setting/department to maintain patient care
- Communicate with receiving hospital
  - Consider back-up plan
  - Request recommendations
- Attempt to eliminate barriers
  - Restabilize patient
  - Select different transportation mode
  - Await weather change
- Reassess need for and barriers to transfer
- Initiate screen to evaluate inability to transfer

Is it possible to transfer? NO YES

(Possible change in patient condition, weather, or other previous decision)

Prepare the patient and family
Physically — Identify and provide appropriate therapeutic interventions to minimize complications en route.
Psychosocially — Removes patient temporarily from family or significant other support. Ensures family aware of benefits of transfer, location of receiving hospital, and their plans and needs.
Administratively — Clear and complete documentation provided of condition, interventions, and diagnostics. Sending and receiving nurse communicate regarding nursing and medical management of the patient and the consent process.

Transfer
Utilize facility procedures, orders, and protocols

Evaluate transfer episode
Initiate transfer outcome report(s)

Figure 1–1 ■ Decision-making tree: Transferring patients to a higher level of care. *(American College of Critical Care Medicine. (1993). Guidelines for the transfer of critically ill patients. Critical Care Medicine, 21, 934. Used with permission.)*

7

TABLE 1–3 Suchman's Stages of Illness

STAGE	DEFINITION	MANIFESTATIONS	INTERVENTIONS
Shock and disbelief	Diagnosis does not have an emotional meaning	Patient may be uncooperative or worry excessively	Provide accurate information when asked
Denial	Patient rejects diagnosis	Patient may act like nothing is wrong	Nurse is noncritical; clarify statements but do not stress reality
Awareness	Attempt to regain control	Demanding and angry or quiet and withdrawn	Provide consistent nursing care; do not argue with patient
Restitution	Diagnosis is accepted	Sadness and crying; attempt to improve relationships with family and friends	Assist patient with problem solving
Resolution	Patient's identity is changed	Patient may openly participate in care	Promote self-care and independence

impact of the illness and conserve energy by removing worry. The nurse should function as a noncritical listener.

The awareness stage is characterized by an attempt to regain control. Patients may express guilt about the illness or injury as a gesture of assuming responsibility for events over which they may or may not have actual control. The patient may be demanding or exhibit signs of withdrawal. Both signs are indicative of anger toward self or others. The nurse should not argue with the patient. Consistent, dependable nursing care should be provided.

During the next stage, restitution, the patient may verbalize fears about the future. New behaviors are initiated that reflect new limitations. The patient may feel sad and have frequent crying episodes. Relationships with family and friends may be reorganized. The nurse can assist by building communication to assist with problem solving. Resolution, the final stage, involves identity change. The patient may begin to think of the illness as a growing experience. Limitations are accepted as consequences and not as defects.

These stages are not fixed but reflect a dynamic process of adjusting to an acute situation. The patient may regress to an earlier stage during periods of heightened anxiety. One aim in caring for the high-acuity patient is to foster a feeling of security. A patient may feel vulnerable because of physiological changes, such as paralysis. Emotional vulnerability may be experienced when restraints are applied. Changes in patient care routines can increase patient anxiety, even when these changes mean the patient is getting better. Examples include removing cardiac electrodes, weaning from mechanical ventilation, reducing pain medication, and increasing mobility.

The high-acuity patient cannot be considered in isolation of family members. The family is defined according to however the patient wishes to define family. The high-acuity nursing unit has evolved from a restrictive environment into a more inclusive environment for families. This change is the result of an increasing body of nursing research that demonstrates positive outcomes when family members actively participate in the recovery process of their loved one. Because of this important role, the nurse must identify and meet family needs so that they can fully participate in the care of the patient.

Nursing research has demonstrated that families frequently have the following needs: information, comfort, support, assurance, and accessibility (Counsell & Guin, 2002). Families want frequent communication about the patient's condition. They want to know why interventions are initiated. They need to be reassured frequently and honestly that the patient is receiving the best care possible. Communication must be open, honest, direct, frequent, and ongoing. Frequent meetings with the family assures healthy coping mechanisms and helps the nurse to develop a family centered plan of care (Counsell & Guin, 2002).

In summary, the high-acuity patient may progress through a series of emotional stages because of losses experienced during the illness event. The stages the patient progresses through include shock and disbelief, denial, awareness, restitution, and resolution. The nurse must be aware of manifestations and nursing interventions for each stage. Family members must be incorporated into the patient plan of care because they contribute to positive patient outcomes. Nurses should assess family needs and intervene accordingly.

SECTION TWO REVIEW

1. A major behavior of a patient in the denial stage of illness is
   A. false humor
   B. crying
   C. anger
   D. projection of difficulties onto objects and staff
2. The awareness stage of illness is characterized by all of the following EXCEPT

A. increased dependence on others
B. expression of guilt
C. withdrawal behavior
D. being demanding of caregivers

3. Mr. Abe was involved in a motor vehicle crash and sustained multiple lower extremity fractures. He will need additional surgery and prolonged physical therapy. The nurse finds Mr. Abe drawing plans for remodeling his porch to accommodate a wheelchair. This behavior reflects which stage of illness?
A. denial
B. awareness
C. restitution
D. resolution

4. When interacting with a patient in denial, the nurse should
A. reinforce reality
B. function as a noncritical listener

C. explain the current treatment plan
D. help the patient to recall the injury event

5. A patient who sustained a spinal cord injury is talking about the college football scholarship that he will need to return because of his quadriplegia. This patient exhibits behavior reflecting which stage of illness?
A. awareness
B. reconciliation
C. restitution
D. denial

6. An appropriate nursing intervention for a patient experiencing high anxiety is
A. active listening
B. providing accurate information
C. exhibiting empathy
D. acknowledging loss

Answers: 1. D, 2. A, 3. D, 4. B, 5. C, 6. B

SECTION THREE: Coping with Acute Illness

At the completion of this section, the learner will be able to identify ways the nurse can help high-acuity patients cope with an illness or injury event.

We are becoming more aware of the importance of the search for meaning in life-changing events. **Spirituality,** a sense of faith and transcendence, and a sorting out of old life views are frequently part of the experience of the patient and family after acute illness or injury. Questions such as "Why me?" "Why this?" and "Why now?" become part of the patient's and family's quest for meaning. The nurse can provide a sounding board for such questions and act as a nonjudgmental listener as patients and families sort out their answers.

Various strategies can be used with patients to help them cope with the psychological and physical stressors of an acute illness. **Complementary and alternative therapies** (CAT) may be beneficial to the high-acuity patient as a way of reducing stress. CAT may be used in lieu of, or as a complement to, standard medical treatment. It is important to remember that all patients are in need of healing, even if they cannot be cured. There are several classifications of CATs. This section is limited to therapies that focus on the mind's ability to affect the body (e.g., aromatherapy, humor, massage and therapeutic touch, and imagery/progressive relaxation). The decision to use CAT must be an informed decision. Some patients, because of personal feelings or cultural differences, may not be comfortable with massage or touch therapy. In this situation, the CAT will actually add stress and may inhibit relaxation. In addition, a complementary therapy may not be without risk. For example, massage therapy may cause tissue damage or dislodge a clot (Tracy & Lindquist, 2003).

Aromatherapy is the use of oils to reduce stress and anxiety. Aromatic plant oils such as hiba, lavender, jasmine, and others have been shown in small limited studies to reduce stress and anxiety in acutely ill patients (Richards et al., 2003). These oils may be applied topically or may be inhaled and used as an enhancement to massage therapy (Richards et al., 2003). Humor has been recognized for years as a way of relieving stress. Unlike aromatherapy, which is easy to apply, humor may be tricky to deliver by the high-acuity nurse. However, a skilled nurse may use humor as one complementary and alternative therapy (Keegan, 2003). Massage and therapeutic touch may help patients relax and promote sleep. In addition, these therapies are designed to promote circulation and a generalized sense of well-being (Keegan, 2003; Richards et al., 2003).

Imagery is a CAT that uses the patient's past positive experiences to promote a vision or fantasy that encourages relaxation. In imagery, the patient focuses on positive thoughts and experiences and blocks out negative thoughts (Tracy & Lindquist, 2003). Nurses can guide patients through imagery by asking them to place themselves in environments where they remember feeling relaxed. Many people recall the beach or ocean as having a calming effect. An example of imagery is the thought of lying on a beach on a deserted island, listening to the pounding of the surf on the shore, watching the graceful sway of the palm trees, and feeling the cool breezes, while at the same time feeling the warmth of the sun on the skin. Imagery provides an opportunity for the stressed-out patient to take a vacation or temporary mental escape from the day-to-day realities of the high-acuity environment. Imagery is a CAT that may be beneficial for patients experiencing extensive and painful dressing changes, anxiety, or pain (Richards et al., 2003). The following case study demonstrates the use of imagery. The case study is referred to again in Section Five.

■ ■ ■

Mr. T is a 79-year-old man who had an exploratory laparotomy for a perforated duodenal ulcer. He has a history of chronic airflow limitation and is steroid dependent. Mr. T's wound is healing by secondary intention. He experiences much pain during dressing changes.

The nurse prepares the environment by dimming lights and decreasing noise. She places a sign outside the patient's room indicating that an imagery session is in progress. The nurse promotes relaxation by encouraging Mr. T to imagine that each muscle is going limp starting at the top of his head. She describes it as a heavy good feeling. The nurse tells Mr. T to concentrate on each body section separately (neck, shoulders, and so on). Mr. T closes his eyes and concentrates on his body.

Nurse: As the old dressing is removed, your new tissue is getting fresh nutrients because dead skin and bacteria are being pulled away with the gauze. Imagine a tiny skin cell with hands that reach out to join another skin cell to make a firm chain. Although you are a little uncomfortable, you want the dressing to be removed because the new skin cells cannot grow underneath the debris from the old cells. As the new cells get nutrients, there is

less drainage and less discomfort. Now, imagine that the skin is completely together just like it was before surgery. There is no need for more dressing changes. Each time your dressing is changed, concentrate on this image of the skin cells joining hands to make a firm chain that is completely together and healed. Imagine the cells getting fresh air and food that make them strong.

The goal of this imagery session was to describe positive aspects of the dressing change, in order to replace Mr. T's fear with a positive image of healing.

■ ■ ■

In summary, the nurse can use several strategies to assist the high-acuity patient in coping with an illness or injury event. These strategies include instilling hope, supporting spirituality, using physical touch, promoting relaxation, and using guided imagery with progressive muscle relaxation. Regardless of what type of coping response is exhibited, the nurse can intervene to support positive coping.

SECTION THREE REVIEW

1. Complementary and alternative therapies may be used
   A. in lieu of standard medical treatment
   B. as a complement to standard medical treatment
   C. only with a physician's order
   D. A and B are correct
2. Which of the following factors influences the perception of touch as a caring behavior?
   A. environmental temperature
   B. cultural background
   C. length of the hospitalization
   D. size of caregiver's hands
3. Aromatherapy
   A. is the use of oils to reduce stress and anxiety
   B. includes plant oils that may be applied topically
   C. may be used to enhance massage therapy
   D. All of the above

Answers: 1. D, 2. B, 3. D

SECTION FOUR: Environmental Stressors

At the completion of this section, the learner will identify environmental stressors, their impact on high-acuity patients, and strategies to alleviate those stressors.

Sensory input involves all five senses: visual, auditory, olfactory, gustatory, and tactile. Individual perceptions of stimuli to the senses vary. Usually, people select stimuli that are most acceptable to them. However, during acute illness, the patient does not have control over the choice of the environment and its stimuli. Very young, very old, and postoperative or unresponsive patients are at greatest risk of experiencing **sensory perceptual alterations (SPAs).** Acutely ill patients who develop SPAs are at risk for the development of additional complications (Tracy & Linquist, 2003).

The nurse must assess whether the symptoms have a psychological or physical basis, such as hypoxia or increased intracranial pressure. Restricted movement, lack of windows, continuous light, and restricted visitation contribute to sensory deprivation.

A combination of sensory overload and deprivation can exist. The patient is deprived of normal sensory stimuli while being exposed to continuous strange stimuli. The nurse should assess what sounds are in the patient's normal environment and expose the patient to these sounds if possible (through tape recordings). Visitors can be effective by discussing familiar topics with the patient. Unresponsive patients are particularly challenging because information about the patient's normal environment must be collected through a third person. It is difficult to assess whether unresponsive patients are experiencing sensory alterations because they cannot communicate.

Sensory overload may occur when the patient is exposed to noise for continuous periods. The background environmental noise in a high-acuity unit includes annoying and frightening alarms, ringing telephones, pagers, staff conversations, loud overhead announcement systems, ventilators, cardiac monitors, the bubbling of chest tubes, and other strange and foreign sounds. However, patients report they are most disturbed by the staff's loud voices, especially at night when they interrupt sleep (Honkus, 2003). The Environmental Protection Agency recommends hospitals maintain noise levels below 45 decibels (dBA) during the day and 35 dBA at night. Because normal human conversation is usually around 60 dBA, it is important to see why keeping staff conversations to a minimum in the direct patient care areas is essential to promoting rest (Lower et al., 2002).

Sensory perceptual alterations or other physical disruptions may cause delirium in the high-acuity patient. Although most clinicians would recognize delirium as an abnormal state, it is important for the nurse to ascertain the cause of the delirium. Hypoxia, alcohol or barbiturate withdrawal, hyponatremia, drug adverse reactions, infections, and liver dysfunction can cause delirium. It is extremely important to rule out and treat any underlying causes of delirium, rather than merely medicating the patient to control behavior. Many times delirium is preceded by anxiety and restlessness that escalate to confusion and agitation and finally delirium. The night nurse may be the first person to notice a change in the patient's behavior. Night sleep cycle disturbances or sundowner's syndrome may be a warning of what is to come. In **sundowner's syndrome** the patient appears alert and appropriate during the day but becomes confused and agitated in the evening or at night (Marshall & Soucy, 2003).

Alterations in the light/dark cycle, pain, environmental noise, caregiver interruptions, and stress can contribute to the inability of hospitalized patients to get adequate sleep and rest. Interventions that contribute to the nonpharmacologic induction of sleep should be implemented. Sedative hypnotics are often the preferred method for sleep disturbances, but this method has been linked to an increase in falls, delirium, and functional decline in patients, particularly in the elderly (Nagel et al., 2003). Planned rest periods that allow for 2 hours of uninterrupted sleep are essential to promoting rapid eye movement (REM) sleep. REM sleep facilitates protein anabolism, restores the immune system, and promotes healing. Providing the patient with a few hours of REM sleep can be beneficial. Nurses should recognize this and act as a patient advocate to control the patient's environment to ensure adequate sleep and rest periods throughout the day and night. Closing and posting a sign on the patient's door is often effective. Other nursing interventions include providing relaxing music of the patient's choice, or ear plugs for those who prefer silence. Controlling pain is essential to promoting REM sleep. Care providers should place pagers on vibrate mode. Turn down (or turn off) the volume of the overhead announcement system in patient care areas. Decrease the volume of alarms on equipment. Adjust light levels and offer eye masks to patients. Encourage ancillary services, such as physical therapy or respiratory therapy, to return after the patient has rested, if appropriate. Limit visitation dur-

Evidence-Based Practice

- *Music therapy leads to reduction in psychological and physiological stress in post-MI patients (White, 2000).*
- *Music therapy leads to reduction in psychological and physiological stress in mechanically ventilated patients (Chlan, 1998; Wong et al., 2001).*
- *The most consistent psychologic effect is a reduction in anxiety after music sessions (White, 2000).*
- *The most consistent physiologic effect is decreased heart rate after music sessions (White, 2000).*

ing quiet time. Help the patient prepare mentally for quiet time through therapeutic touch or massage, guided imagery, or aromatherapy. Plan a daily schedule for the patient that includes a 2-hour quiet time everyday so the patient can look forward to a time of relaxation and rest (Lower et al., 2002).

Communicating with mechanically ventilated patients is very important to prevent SPA and promote a therapeutic nurse–patient relationship. The patient's inability to talk may cause high levels of stress, insecurity, and even panic. For many patients, the family can promote a sense of security and relaxation. However, patients and families can also become frustrated because they cannot understand lip reading. An experienced nurse is often helpful because he or she has more experience using lip reading techniques with an intubated patient. Although many nurses use nonverbal communication with their patients, most of that communication is at a very concrete level—pertaining only to physical care and including short task-oriented communication. This does not provide emotional support (Happ, 2001).

Patients use a variety of forms of nonverbal communication. Vital signs, such as an elevated heart rate or blood pressure, are one form of nonverbal communication. Facial expressions, such as smiling, grimacing, or even crying and laughing, can be valuable forms of communication. Hand gestures, such as grabbing the nurse's arm or holding hands, or even moving legs around, use movement as a method of communication. Some patients are able to write messages very clearly, whereas others attempt to write and simply become frustrated as they experience fine-motor difficulty or cannot see clearly. Large pen markers may be easier for the patient to manipulate than thin pens or pencils. Using computer keyboards or pointing to letters on alphabet boards requires gross-motor skills. A coded eye blink system may be used for patients that are unable to move anything else.

SECTION FOUR REVIEW

1. A frequently cited annoying noise among high-acuity patients is
A. an ambulance siren
B. staff's loud voices
C. television
D. equipment noise

2. REM sleep
   A. facilitates protein anabolism
   B. restores the immune system
   C. promotes healing
   D. all of the above
3. Which of the following nursing interventions would support the patient's REM sleep?

A. dimming lights during normal sleep time
B. putting a wall clock up in the patient's room
C. decreasing environmental noise
D. A and C

Answers: 1. B, 2. D, 3. D

SECTION FIVE: Educational Needs of Patients and Families

At the completion of this section, the learner will be able to identify educational needs of high-acuity patients and their families and strategies to meet these needs.

High-acuity patients have a right to know and understand what procedures are being done to and for them. Initially, when teaching high-acuity patients, the nurse must aim at decreasing stress and promoting comfort rather than increasing knowledge. The patient and family may not recall what the nurse said 10 minutes later, but the patient's blood pressure may be decreased or the pain lessened. As adult learners, high-acuity patients focus on learning in order to solve problems. Thus, the nurse must assess what the patient considers to be problematic in order to make learning meaningful. Basic questions about what the patient and family want to know will assist the nurse in focusing content. It is also helpful to identify what the patient already knows. The reduced nurse–patient ratio in high-acuity settings facilitates teaching. An interpersonal relationship allows for the patient to trust the abilities and knowledge of the nurse. For the high-acuity patient to learn, he or she must feel secure.

Several factors inhibit learning in high-acuity patients. Patients may be fatigued because of hypoxia, anemia, and hypermetabolism. Barriers to communication, such as endotracheal

tubes, many hourly procedures, and diagnostic tests interfere with teaching and learning. Pain diminishes a person's ability to concentrate; drugs may depress the central nervous system and affect memory. The nurse should assess the patient for the presence of these factors. Physiologic needs take precedence over the need to know and the need to understand (Maslow, 1970). Once the patient's condition has stabilized, however, the patient is able to concentrate on learning. Educational needs of both patients and families, according to Palazzo (2001), are summarized in Table 1–4. It is important for the nurse to incorporate adult learning theory in high-acuity areas.

■ ■ ■

Mr. T, discussed in Section Three, is improving. His blood gases have improved, and he is being weaned from the ventilator. The ventilator is in synchronized intermittent mandatory ventilation (SIMV) mode at a rate of 8. The nurse has been teaching Mr. T about his wound care, including an increased risk of a wound infection because he is also receiving steroids. Up to this point, Mr. T has been eager to learn and has asked questions using a writing board; however, this morning he appears anxious.

■ ■ ■

Before teaching Mr. T, the nurse assesses the cause of Mr. T's anxiety. Is it related to hypoxia secondary to weaning? The nurse draws blood for an arterial blood gas (ABG) measurement, and

TABLE 1–4 Educational Needs of Patients and Families

EDUCATIONAL NEEDS	NURSING CONSIDERATIONS
Current information about patient progress	Both families and high-acuity patients need daily information on the situation of the illness. Results of diagnostics and daily lab work are physiological indicators that the nurse may discuss with the patient. In general, the high-acuity environment encourages a highly motivated learner.
Informed decision making	Most adults are self-directed and want to make informed decisions themselves, not to have decisions made by someone else.
Acknowledgment of past	The adult learner has a lifetime of experiences that influence their values and opinions, and shape their decisions.
Optimal learning environment	Using the right time and environment is conducive to the learning process. Transforming the high-acuity environment into a learning environment will enhance the learning process and improve retention. Presenting the information at the appropriate time is important.
Orientation to routines and care	Teaching patients and families procedures that will improve their daily life is productive. Teaching patients and families to perform complementary and alternative therapies (CAT) to relieve pain, reduce stress, and induce sleep may be beneficial to all.
Motivation	Adults are motivated to learn something new when it will have a direct effect on their daily lives.

the results are within normal limits. Mr. T's anxiety may be related to the fear of not being able to breathe without the ventilator. On questioning, Mr. T admits he is frightened about the weaning process and the move from the ICU. The nurse explains that Mr. T will be assessed regularly to determine his ability to remain off the ventilator. Next, she explains when he will be transferred to a lower-acuity unit and how he will continue to be monitored.

The transfer from an ICU to a less acute unit may precipitate transfer anxiety in the patient or family. Transfer anxiety may be reduced by the use of a structured transfer plan. In an effort to reduce or prevent transfer anxiety, the nurse should incorporate the following strategies into the structured transfer plan: encourage patient and family questions, present the ICU as a temporary stage in the illness continuum, involve the patient and family in transfer plans, transfer during the daytime, explain any new equipment, and introduce the patient and the family to the receiving nurse before the transfer.

In summary, both high-acuity patients and their family members want to learn about their illness and the hospital environment. Multiple factors inhibit learning in high-acuity patients. A person is unable to learn if stress or anxiety levels are high. Prior to teaching high-acuity patients, the nurse must identify and address issues that provoke stress and anxiety. Transfer anxiety can be reduced by the use of a structured transfer plan.

SECTION FIVE REVIEW

Questions 1 and 2 pertain to Ms. B.

Ms. B was admitted with a diagnosis of acute myocardial infarction. Her vital signs are respiratory rate 32, heart rate 100, temperature 102°F orally, blood pressure 90/70 mm Hg. She is on a continuous nitroglycerin IV infusion for chest pain.

1. Which of the following factors would NOT interfere with Ms. B's ability to learn?
   A. pain
   B. temperature
   C. respiratory rate
   D. heart rate

2. The nurse should focus on teaching Ms. B
   A. cardiac rehabilitation plans
   B. how the heart functions
   C. why it is important to state when she is having pain
   D. rationale for the nitroglycerin

3. All of the following should be incorporated into a structured ICU transfer plan in an effort to decrease transfer anxiety EXCEPT
   A. introducing the patient to the receiving nurse
   B. transferring during daytime
   C. transferring during nighttime
   D. involving the family in the transfer plan

Answers: 1. D, 2. C, 3. C

Nursing Considerations

SECTION SIX: Visitation Policies

At the completion of this section, the learner will be able to discuss the rationale for visitation policies and the effects of visitation on high-acuity patients.

Nurses do not agree on the benefits of visitation. Some nurses view visitation as psychologically supportive to the patient but physiologically harmful. Some nurses identify family visitation as a source of job stress (Clarke & Harrison, 2001). Nurses believe long visiting hours interfere with time they need to spend with the patient (Holden et al., 2002). Hypervigilant family members may become unnerving or threatening to the staff by demanding detailed information before agreeing to treatments, requesting to examine records, and taking notes (Slota et al., 2003).

Patients also differ in their views toward visitation. The age and setting of the patient may be associated with visitation preferences. In one study, middle-aged patients (35 to 65 years old) desired frequent short visits at any time of the day, whereas elderly patients (older than 65 years) preferred 45-minute afternoon visits; patients in coronary care wanted two visits daily, whereas patients in surgical intensive care wanted more daily visits (Simpson, 1993).

As patients differ in their likes and dislikes regarding visitation, they also differ in physiologic response to visitation. Observing patient–family interactions can provide information about the nature of the patient–family relationship and clues to family needs. The more acutely ill the patient, the more urgent it becomes for family members to be at the bedside to participate in decisions about the plan of care (Holden et al., 2002).

Children are often restricted from visiting adult inpatient units because adults often believe they will be overwhelmed and unable to cope or understand. Acute illness is a source of stress and disruption for the entire family, especially children. Visiting may reassure the child that the family member is alive and has not left them permanently. It is important to use developmental psychology when discussing health and illness with children. This allows for the planning of specific nursing interventions to best meet the needs of the child (Clarke & Harrison, 2001).

Historically, family members have been restricted from visiting during invasive procedures and cardiopulmonary resuscitation (CPR). Reasons for these restrictions included fear that the family might lose control, insufficient room at the bedside, and increased risk of litigation. Many hospitals do not have written policies for family presence during CPR, yet it appears that most nurses believe families should be present (MacLean et al., 2003). Family members have stated they prefer to be present and identified the following benefits: the removal of doubt about what is happening to the patient, reduction in anxiety and fear, provision of a sense of closure, and the facilitation of grieving (Boudreaux et al., 2002).

Family centered care, a concept embraced by an increasing number of hospitals, is a care delivery model that is patient/family focused. In this care delivery model, family members are not kept away from the bedside of the acutely ill patient. Instead, they are welcomed and encouraged to be present and active in care. Nursing interventions in this care delivery model focus on humanizing the patient in the presence of advanced technology and machinery. Interventions include (1) making introductions, (2) giving the patient/family information about the routine/plan, (3) involving the family in patient care activities if they choose, and (4) encouraging the family to bring in pictures and familiar objects to promote interaction (Henneman & Cardin, 2002). Although the nurse is instrumental in making family centered care a core value in the high-acuity area, all members of the multidisciplinary team play a role in ensuring the families' needs are met.

Families may need directions in how to visit. The nurse may discuss with the family what the patient looks like prior to the family visit. It is helpful for the family to know that they should speak to the patient in a normal tone of voice, to be comfortable simply being with the patient and not speaking at all, and to ask questions away from the bedside (Twibell, 1998). Flexible visitation can be established when nurses are consistent and communicate effectively with visitors. A contract between the nursing staff and family members may be effective. Other resources can be helpful in dealing with visitors such as pastoral care, patient relations staff, social services, local support groups, physicians, and hospital administration (Slota et al., 2003). Staff must be prepared to set limits to visitation. Written hospital policies should include guidelines that define acceptable behavior and include a zero-tolerance policy that addresses unacceptable behavior, such as drug/alcohol usage, physical or verbal abuse, or the presence of weapons (Slota et al., 2003).

In summary, high-acuity patients as well as nurses differ in their opinions regarding the value and nature of visitation. Each situation should be examined and uniquely managed. Negotiations between the patient, family, and nurse may be the most effective way of facilitating visitation that is therapeutic to all involved.

SECTION SIX REVIEW

1. A.M., age 6, asks to see her father, who is comatose and receiving mechanical ventilation. The nurse should
   A. clean up the patient first
   B. grant A.M.'s request
   C. explain to A.M. that she shouldn't see her father until he gets more energy
   D. adhere to the policy that prohibits visitors under age 16
2. The physiologic effects of visitation are
   A. the same for everyone
   B. detrimental to patient stability
   C. related to patient's preference for visits
   D. positive
3. Contracting visitation policies with the family involves
   A. having the family sign in each time they visit
   B. ensuring that both the family and the nurse agree on mutually acceptable visitation times
   C. arbitration with the charge nurse
   D. developing a brochure

Answers: 1. B, 2. C, 3. B

SECTION SEVEN: Nursing Staffing Issues

At the completion of this section, the learner will be able to identify work design and staffing strategies for high-acuity patients.

Nurses willing to work with acutely ill patients are precious commodities. Decreased third-party reimbursement and managed care encouraged shorter hospital lengths of stay. As cost-reducing measures, hospitals reduced professional nursing staff positions. In the late 1990s, hospital restructuring and reengineering forced bedside nurses to accept a team concept of patient care delivery. Hospital employees, including nurses, were required to cross-train and "float" to care for patients outside their specialty areas. Unlicensed personnel were trained and supervised by nurses to complete patient care tasks. All these changes led to decreased job satisfaction, high nurse turnover rates, and nurses leaving practice in high-acuity areas (Aiken et al., 2000). Other factors have contributed to the shortage of nurses. The registered nurse (RN) workforce is rapidly aging and fewer young people are choosing nursing as a career. The nursing shortage issues are multifaceted and will continue to require comprehensive solutions (Stechmiller, 2002).

A decrease in the number of professional nurses forced hospitals to increase nurse–patient ratios. The result: One nurse cares for more patients. What is the appropriate nurse–patient ratio in high-acuity settings? The Academy of Medical Surgical Nurses (AMSN) is not in favor of establishing predetermined ratios. Rather, the needs of the patient and skill mix of the nursing staff must be considered when making decisions about staffing patterns. Adequate resources must be available to evaluate the patient/family response to treatment, education, and pharmacological interventions (AMSN, 2000a). The American Association of Critical Care Nurses' (AACN) position on this issue is that the first principle of staffing should be to provide safe and effective patient care. The patient's acuity and required intensity of their nursing care requirements should determine the nurse–patient ratio (AACN, 2000).

The reduction in professional nursing staff encouraged an upgrade of nursing assistant skills. The AMSN supports the use of unlicensed assistive personnel (UAP) to enable the professional nurse to provide nursing care (AMSN, 2000b). When UAP provide direct patient care, they are accountable to, and work under, the direct supervision of the professional nurse. The registered nurse must use leadership skills to safely and legally delegate tasks to the UAP.

One potential solution to the nursing shortage has been the magnet hospital program. This concept, originally developed in the 1980s by the American Academy of Nursing, awards hospitals a magnet designation if they are able to create working environments that are successful in recruiting and retaining professional nurses. In effect, these environments act like magnets to attract nurses. Hospitals that achieve the designation of "magnet status" have practice models that promote professional nursing. Nurses who work at magnet hospitals are more involved in decision making, report better relations with physicians, and have higher nurse–patient ratios (Stechmiller, 2002). Hospitals with magnet status report their patients have shorter ICU stays and shorter hospital stays (Stechmiller, 2002). Further studies are needed to evaluate the effects of magnet hospital status on patient outcomes.

In summary, there is a shortage of nurses to work in high-acuity units. Multiple factors contribute to this shortage. Alternate patient care delivery models have been used. The appropriate nurse–patient ratio in high acuity settings is not known. UAP enables the professional nurse to provide nursing care. Magnet hospitals are a potential solution to the nursing shortage. These hospitals have working environments that act like magnets to recruit and retain professional nurses.

SECTION SEVEN REVIEW

1. Unlicensed assistive personnel (UAP) may
   A. assist the professional nurse by providing diabetic education for a newly diagnosed diabetic
   B. work independently as long as they notify the RN at the end of their shifts
   C. perform only those tasks delegated to them by a professional nurse
   D. obtain a patient health history

2. Hospitals that achieve the designation of magnet status
   A. use UAP to deliver most nursing care
   B. have practice models that promote professional nursing
   C. indicate the hospital that has low nurse–patient ratios
   D. are not desirable places to work for professional nurses

Answers: 1. C, 2. B

SECTION EIGHT: Technology and Caring Interface

At the completion of this section, the learner will be able to describe the interface between technology and caring.

A major criticism of nurses who work with acutely ill patients is that they are strictly technologically oriented. The focus of nursing care on high-acuity patient care units is on monitoring patients for subtle physiologic changes. This monitoring requires the nurse to use multiple technologies. The patient interfaces with the staff and medical equipment in the diagnosis and management of the patient's disease process. Difficulties arise when ma-

chines, rather than individual patient needs, become the focus of care of the high-acuity patient (Benner, 2003).

There are inherent hazards to the use of technology. Technology can be so intriguing that its primary purpose—to support the well-being of the patient—is lost. Technology may create demands where no demands existed before, such as that which occurs with the fragmentation of patients into subpopulations (e.g., bone marrow transplant unit, cardiac surgery unit). Each subpopulation has its own special staff competing for hospital resources. Machines compete with the patient for nursing surveillance. It is possible that nurses become so dependent on monitoring devices that they completely trust the equipment, even when the data conflict with their own clinical assessments. Having the responsibility for multiple pieces of equipment can increase the nurse's stress level. Technical devices present mechanical impediments to touching. Little surface area may be available for physical contact and this may lead to a feeling of depersonalization. Technology may evoke fear in patients and contribute to their anxiety about their recovery process. A mechanically ventilated patient's perception of psychological and physiological stress may influence the effectiveness of optimal ventilation, weaning, or both (Thomas, 2003).

Nurses working with high-acuity patients must be capable of making critical decisions. Although decision making is viewed as somewhat artful and intuitive, computers use a scientific, programmed approach. Because of the massive amount of patient data available, nurses may be reaching a saturation point in data processing. Computer software programs are available to help diagnose patient conditions. The use of a personal digital assistant (PDA) can provide quick access to drug and diagnostic information (Jenkins, 2002). When new technologies are intro-

duced at the bedside, it is commonplace for the nurse to focus initially on the technology because she or he must be proficient in the use of this technology to support patient care. Proficiency is fostered by having the opportunity to become familiar with the technology before its use in patient care. A high degree of comfort with technology prevents it from becoming the focus of care (Milholland, 2001). Nurses are at risk for becoming overly dependent on technology for clinical decision making. It is essential that the nurse validate the technologic data with nursing assessment data. The health care practitioner, not the technology, is ultimately responsible for clinical decisions made (Milholland, 2001).

In summary, nurses who care for acutely ill patients must be able to use technology in the caring process and still recognize the limitations of technology. Equipment must be used to enhance, not take the place of, a nurse's personal knowledge, observation skills, and senses. The skilled nurse who practices in a high-acuity setting must be able to bridge the gap between complex technology and the art of caring.

SECTION EIGHT REVIEW

1. Inherent hazards to the use of technology include
   A. fragmentation of patients into subpopulations
   B. increasing the nurse's stress level
   C. allowing greater time for patient contact
   D. A and B are correct

2. Technical devices
   A. present mechanical impediments to touching
   B. lead to a feeling of depersonalization
   C. may evoke fear in patients
   D. all of the above

Answers: 1. D, 2. D

SECTION NINE: Stressors and Satisfying Factors

At the completion of this section, the learner will be able to discuss the stressful and satisfying aspects of caring for acutely ill patients.

The term **burnout** has been used to describe a crisis state evolving from stress. Nurses work in demanding situations over long periods of time. The quest to provide high-quality patient care in a work environment that has decreasing resources and increasing responsibilities creates conflict. This conflict results in burnout (Kalliath & Morris, 2002). Claus and Bailey (1980) identified sources of stress for nurses who work in high-acuity areas. The major sources of stress identified included (1) interpersonal conflict, (2) management of the patient care area, (3) nature of the direct patient care, and (4) inadequate knowledge. Maslach and Leiter (1997) attributed burnout to work overload, lack of control, insufficient rewards, unfairness, breakdown of communication, and values conflicts. The end result of burnout may be negative attitudes toward patients, decreased job performance and quality of personal life, reduced commitment to the organization, depression, and guilt (Kalliath & Morris, 2002). Symptoms indicative of burnout are summarized in Table 1–5.

TABLE 1–5   Symptoms of Burnout

Behavioral

Withdrawal	Contemplating career change
Risk taking and impulsiveness	Increased use of caffeine, alcohol, and nicotine
Ambivalence	
Decreased productivity	

Physiologic

Chronic fatigue	Appetite change
Frequent minor ailments	Sexual difficulty
Sleep changes	

Psychological

Attempt to blame others	Depression
Stereotype patients	Hostility and negativism
Nightmares	Loss of tolerance

Cognitive

Decreased ability to make decisions	Lack of initiative
Poor judgment	Forgetfulness

Patients' conditions change rapidly in high-acuity units and this may be a source of burnout for nurses who work in these areas because it requires philosophical flexibility. A patient with a poor prognosis may have a prolonged stay that involves the use of multiple technologies. Then in the middle of a shift, a decision is made to cease these efforts. The patient may improve, requiring reevaluation and escalation of care. Conversely, a patient is declared dead by brain death criteria, and immediately thereafter may become an organ donor. This requires the nurse to shift from caring for a patient, to caring for organs for another patient. It is also quite common to have a patient die and, within minutes after death, the nurse is told there is a new patient waiting to come into that very same bed. The nurse is required to grieve or mourn a death and then minutes later reinvest energy in a new patient. A significant degree of uncertainty is confronted on a daily basis. A broad-based end-of-life care curriculum may be instrumental in assisting the high-acuity nurse to cope with the daily stress of changing patient conditions (Mularski et al., 2001).

The social environment of the nursing unit plays a role in nurses' perceived levels of stress. A positive social climate, characterized by strong managerial support and cohesiveness among the staff, serves as a buffer for the negative effects of stress. Environmental uncertainty, as measured by the number of admissions, discharges, and transfers in the high-acuity area, can result in emotional exhaustion. Nurses must enhance self-awareness of personal sources of tension. Once these sources of tension are identified, strategies for alleviating stressors can be developed. Staff nurses involved in the development of unit policies, protocols, and standards of care have a greater sense of involvement in the nursing unit and are less susceptible to burnout than those who are not involved (Garrett & McDaniel, 2001). Burnout may be prevented if the nurse exhibits **hardiness**. Hardiness is a personality trait that enables a person to feel capable of positive action in a stressful situation. A strong sense of morale, increased job performance, and improved health has been linked with a high level of hardiness (Larrabee et al., 2003).

Establishing critical incident stress debriefings (CISDs) may facilitate coping with specific situations. These are structured group discussions, usually occurring 1 to 10 days postcrisis, designed to address symptoms of stress, assess the need for follow up, and provide a sense of closure (Everly & Mitchell, 2002). These sessions are a formal way of managing stress before it becomes debilitating or fosters burnout. Another strategy to prevent burnout is to assist nurses during orientation in formulating clear ideas of their professional roles and responsibilities within the high-acuity environment. Promoting a sense of community in the high-acuity care area can also provide the ability to share stresses and joys, and to seek feedback for continuing performance improvement (Taormina, 2000).

In summary, nurses who work with high-acuity patients are routinely exposed to critical incident stress. Nurses are susceptible to burnout. The symptoms of burnout may be cognitive, psychological, physiologic, and behavioral in nature. Strategies useful in limiting or buffering job-related stressors include comprehensive unit orientation, continuing education for stress reduction, and the development of strong social support groups. Establishment of CISDs accelerates recovery of health professionals who suffer painful reactions to abnormal events.

SECTION NINE REVIEW

1. High-acuity nursing
   A. produces stress because of the intensity of the nurse–patient relationship
   B. discourages collaboration among health team members
   C. prevents the nurse from reinvesting energy into a new patient after a previous patient is discharged
   D. is the preferred method of patient assignment
2. Nurses who are involved with developing policies and protocols
   A. experience greater stress
   B. have a stronger support system
   C. are more satisfied in their roles
   D. are more susceptible to burnout
3. Which of the following has been linked to burnout?
   A. a sense of control over the patient care area
   B. decreased job performance
   C. perception of change as a challenge
   D. sense of control over life

Answers: 1. A, 2. C, 3. B

SECTION TEN: Resource Allocation

At the completion of this section, the learner will be able to discuss resource allocation issues as they relate to high-acuity patients.

Decisions about allocation of resources must be made when there is a need to place patients in acute care areas (specifically in ICU or step-down), but there are no beds available. Who is in need of the greatest health care resources when they are acutely ill? The priority levels discussed in Section One (Table 1–1) of this module were developed to assist clinicians in making these tough decisions about admission, discharge, and triage in acute care areas. One could argue that intensive care resources should be used for patients who will have the greatest probability of benefiting or have a higher quality of life (Pinsky, 2003). If resource allocation were based on these principles, the actual precipitating event that created the need for resources would be irrelevant. Therefore, oncology patients, trauma patients, the young, and the old would be considered equally. Futility of treatment and informed refusal by the patient may be acceptable reasons for physicians to limit treatment. Although these issues occur daily in the care of high-acuity patients, they also occur in a larger context of society that includes ethical, economic, and legal considerations (Lanken et al., 1997).

Oncology patients are often stereotyped as not being candidates for aggressive treatment. However, they frequently become acutely ill from interventions administered by health care providers. Should these patients be denied access to resources when their conditions are induced? During a patient's final hours, high-acuity care may be deemed appropriate because intensive efforts may be required to ensure suffering is minimized during and after removal from life support (Lanken et al., 1997).

Age has been used to justify the withholding of resources from the elderly. Extended care in the ICU has been questioned because of this patient population's high mortality rate. However, studies of elderly patients have shown that they often fare as well as younger patients (Welton et al., 2002). Elderly patients appear to have similar health benefits following coronary artery bypass surgery when compared with younger patients (Conoway et al., 2003). The severity of illness episode, admitting diagnosis, and the patient's previous health status have been positively linked to health outcomes (Chelluri et al., 1993).

It is difficult to predict who will benefit from care in high-acuity areas. Severity of illness scales and probability models were developed for this purpose. The APACHE and the Injury Severity Scale are examples of severity of illness scales used in hospitals (Osler et al., 1998). However, the exclusive use of such indices has not been a completely accurate predictor of outcomes. Other factors must be taken into account. The functional capacity of the patient prior to illness has also been associated with outcome (Rockwood et al., 1993). Individual factors have been highly correlated with mortality: Presence of coma at time of ICU admission (Snyder & Colantonio, 1994) and arterial lactate levels (Tuchschmidt & Mecher, 1994) are two of these factors. Mortality may be best predicted at 24 hours postadmission (Teres & Lemeshow, 1994). Mortality is usually the outcome studied in high-acuity care. However, outcomes may also include patient comfort, well-being, functional status, and other variables in addition to living and dying (Jones, 1993). The use of tools is important to compare patient populations for research and resource allocation (Osler et al., 1998). Patients and their families consider multiple outcomes when deciding whether to withdraw life support.

As the population ages, the demand for ICU beds and the cost will only increase. Making decisions about allocation of resources is a real, but unspecified, aspect of the nursing role with high-acuity patients. These decisions force health care providers to make comparisons based on personal beliefs. Technology alone cannot provide information about who may live and die. Families play an important role in resource utilization. Family involvement in these decisions may ultimately decrease the use of technological resources and increase comfort measures during the last hours before death (Tschann et al., 2003). Patients who die in high-acuity areas consume significant resources. The value of end-of-life care is subjective and cost alone cannot be used to justify the use of health care resources (Pronovost et al., 2001). Each patient situation is different.

Do not resuscitate (DNR) orders were developed to prevent the use of CPR and advanced cardiac life-support measures. Many people have associated patients with DNR orders with a lower standard of patient care (Bains, 1998). Some high-acuity nurses are concerned that a DNR order is an effective means of emptying intensive care beds (Anderson-Shaw, 2003). Some even argue that patients with DNR orders should not be in intensive care units.

The pivotal role of the nurse is key in providing quality care and ensuring appropriate allocation of resources. The nurse must partner with the physician to provide care for the patient in addition to coordinating the consultants and ancillary care providers. He or she must notify the physician of changes in the patient's condition and ensure that interventions are consistent with standards of practice. The bedside nurse facilitates the functioning of the health care team. This multidisciplinary approach to patient management is essential to providing a high standard of care. A team of professionals from several disciplines working as a group will improve efficiency, outcomes, and the cost of caring for patients in the hospital setting (Brilli et al., 2001). When families have consistent communication with the health care team, shorter hospital stays and reduced costs have been achieved (Ahrens et al., 2003). This team approach must not be instituted as a means to financial gain. Rather, it should be instituted to ensure the wishes of high-acuity patients are honored even if death is the final outcome.

High-acuity patients often require care that balances life-prolonging interventions intended to cure with palliative care. Whenever possible, decisions about whether to use technology for life-sustaining purposes should be made by the patient. In cases in which advance decision making has not taken place, family members and other individuals requested by the patient should be involved in the process. These families require careful explanations, time to process the information, and support from hospital personnel to facilitate these ethical decisions (Ahrens et al., 2003). An ethical review committee may be used in some circumstances.

In summary, technology has produced ethical dilemmas for nurses working with acutely ill patients. Dilemmas have focused on the use of valuable acute care resources by patients with cancer, DNR orders, and the elderly. It is not the nurse's role to solve these dilemmas alone. Rather, the nurse's responsibility is to become involved in establishing guidelines for resource allocation and to represent nursing's viewpoint on ethical review committees and in hospital policy.

SECTION TEN REVIEW

1. Resource allocation for high-acuity patients may be based on all of the following EXCEPT
   A. admitting diagnosis
   B. bed availability
   C. hospital standards
   D. gender of the patient
2. Studies about the elderly patient in high-acuity areas have demonstrated that they
   A. almost always die in the ICU
   B. fare as well as younger patients
   C. suffer needlessly
   D. have no interest in life support
3. All of the following factors help predict who will benefit most from ICU care EXCEPT
   A. the person's functional status
   B. functional capacity prior to illness
   C. presence of coma at time of admission
   D. arterial lactate levels

Answers: 1. D, 2. B, 3. A

SECTION ELEVEN: Assessment of Sources of Conflict

At the completion of this section, the learner will be able to examine personal values as they relate to the nurse's role in working with acutely ill patients and discuss end-of life issues to be considered in caring for high-acuity patients.

The American Nurses Association (ANA) *Standards of Clinical Nursing Practice* states that essential components of professional nursing practice include care, cure, and coordination (ANA, 2001). The AACN position is that nurses who work with acutely ill patients should base their practice on individual professional accountability; thorough knowledge of the interrelatedness of body systems; recognition and appreciation of a person's wholeness, uniqueness, and significant social–environmental relationships; and appreciation of the collaborative role of all health team members (AACN, 2002). While working with patients in high-acuity areas, nurses are often faced with ethical dilemmas, such as those discussed in Section Ten of this module. The exposure to death and the saving of human life requires the nurse to frequently evaluate personal values. Personal values often influence decision making. It is important for the nurse to fully understand his or her personal values.

Evaluation of one's personal philosophy can improve satisfaction in working with acutely ill patients. Clarification of one's values helps to anticipate problems that may be encountered in the practice setting and supports the development of positive coping strategies. This knowledge is carried with the professional nurse throughout his or her career regardless of the practice setting or age of the patient being cared for.

The values clarification exercise shown in Table 1–6 is designed to help the learner explore personal values in relation to the profession of nursing and bioethical issues. By reflecting on personal values, we gain a better understanding of what factors may limit our ability to reason clearly and when we may not be suitable for being a patient advocate. It is important that the nurse be careful not to impose his or her own value system into

that of the patient (Robinson, 2003). There may be circumstances in which conflicts occur between the nurse's worldview and that of the patient, such as in decisions regarding withholding or withdrawing life-sustaining treatment. In these circumstances the nurse should transfer care of the patient to another qualified high-acuity nurse (ANA, 1992).

The Patient Self Determination Act, passed as part of the Omnibus Budget Reconciliation Act of 1990, requires that all patients be given information about their right to formulate advanced directives of two types: treatment directives (living wills) and appointment directives (power of attorney for health care). This has increased the role of the patient and family in making end-of-life decisions. Nurses have a primary role in ensuring that the patient makes informed decisions regarding end-of-life care (ANA, 1991). The nurse working with high-acuity patients serves as a patient advocate and intercedes for patients who cannot speak for themselves and supports the decisions of the patient or the patient's designated surrogate (AACN, 2002). Nurses are also directed to uphold the choices and values of the patient even when these wishes conflict with those of health care providers and families (ANA, 1992).

An acutely ill patient was once clearly distinguished from a terminally ill patient. Nurses and physicians focused their efforts on saving lives and not providing end-of-life care. Despite advances in technology, it is impossible to predict which patients will die in the acute care setting and which will live. There may not be a period of time when it is clear that care needs to shift from a cure-oriented to a comforted-oriented approach (Nelson & Danis, 2001). Therefore, it is incumbent on the high-acuity nurse to provide care that is comprehensive. This includes attending to comfort needs of patients and families. Patients attempting to prolong life as well as those who are at the end of life must have their pain controlled and receive ongoing communication regarding their prognosis. End-of-life care and high-acuity care must converge and not conflict (Nelson & Danis, 2001).

In summary, the ANA and AACN are two professional nursing organizations that have delineated roles of the nurse

TABLE 1–6 Values Clarification Exercise

To the left of each statement, place the number that best explains your position: 1 = mostly agree, 2 = somewhat agree, 3 = neutral, 4 = somewhat disagree, 5 = mostly disagree

___ 1. Infants with severe handicaps ought to be left to die.

___ 2. Extraordinary medical treatment is always indicated.

___ 3. My role as a nurse is to always resuscitate patients who could benefit from it, no matter what has been decided previously.

___ 4. I must follow physician's orders.

___ 5. Older patients should be allowed to die with dignity.

___ 6. Medical technology has advanced the quality of life.

___ 7. Children should not be involved in giving consent for treatments.

___ 8. Families ought to make decisions about life or death situations without involving the patient.

___ 9. Children should participate in human experimentation that is not harmful even if it has no benefit to them.

___ 10. Prisoners should participate in scientific experiments to repay society for their wrongdoings.

___ 11. Women should seek medical care from female physicians to avoid potential discrimination.

___ 12. Children whose parents refuse to have them receive medical care should be removed from their families through court action.

___ 13. Research using fetuses should be pursued vigorously.

___ 14. Life support systems should be discontinued after several days of flat electroencephalogram.

___ 15. Health professionals are a scarce resource in many parts of the country.

___ 16. Nursing is a subservient profession, especially to the medical profession.

___ 17. As a nurse, I must relinquish my personal philosophy to support the philosophies of others.

___ 18. All patients, regardless of differences, should be treated in a humanistic way.

___ 19. I should give mouth-to-mouth resuscitation to a derelict if he needs it.

___ 20. A child who is disabled has value.

___ 21. All forms of human life have value.

___ 22. I should be involved in decision making regarding ethical issues in practice.

___ 23. Committees should decide who receives scarce resources, such as kidneys.

___ 24. Patients' individual rights should be more important than the rights of society at large.

___ 25. A person has the right to make a living will.

___ 26. Underdeveloped countries should be given health and financial support from developed countries.

___ 27. I should support all the positions taken on ethical issues taken by my professional association.

___ 28. The care component of nursing practice is not as important as the cure component of medical practice.

___ 29. The nurse's primary role in decision making on ethical issues is to implement the selected alternative.

___ 30. I feel afraid when caring for a patient who is dying.

___ 31. Children who have disabilities should be institutionalized.

___ 32. Patients in mental health institutions and prisons should be given behavior modification therapy to make them conform to society.

___ 33. Personal possessions of patients should be removed to guarantee safekeeping during hospitalization.

___ 34. Patients should have access to their own health information.

___ 35. Withholding health information fosters the patient's recovery.

___ 36. A patient with kidney failure is always able to get kidney dialysis when needed.

___ 37. Society should bear the cost of extraordinary medical interventions.

___ 38. Confidentiality is an important part of the nurse's role.

___ 39. As a nurse, I should value responsibility.

___ 40. Nurses have a right to withhold information to facilitate nursing research on human subjects.

___ 41. The patient who refuses treatment should be dropped from the health supervision of an agency or professional.

___ 42. Transplantations should be done whenever needed.

Personal Application

1. Add the number of 1s, 2s, 3s, 4s, and 5s that you have.

2. How many statements do you have clear ideas (1s and 5s) about?

3. Do these outweigh the number of ambivalent (neutral) statements you listed?

4. Look at the statements that you agree with (1s and 2s). Is there a relationship between the statements that influenced your responses (e.g., age of patient, patient acuity)?

5. Look at the statements that you disagree with (4s and 5s). Is there a relationship between these statements that influenced your responses?

6. Analyze the cluster of statements below. Is there any consistency in the way that you rated these statements? What variables influenced your decision?

Cluster 5, 8, 14, 25, and 30: Relates to issues pertaining to death

Cluster 3, 4, 16, 17, 22, 27, 28, 29, and 38: Relates to the profession of nursing

Cluster 2, 6, 14, 36, 37, and 42: Relates to issues raised by advanced technology

Cluster 1, 7, 9, 12, 20, and 31: Relates to children

Cluster 9, 10, 13, and 40: Relates to human experimentation

Cluster 3, 7, 8, 11, 12, 18, 19, 21, 24, 25, 33, 34, 35, 38, and 41: Relates to patients' rights

Cluster 9, 10, 24, 26, 32, and 37: Relates to society's rights

Cluster 15, 23, and 36: Relates to allocation of resources

Cluster 3, 4, 17, 18, 19, 22, 27, 29, and 39: Relates to perceptions of obligations

Steele, S. & Harmon, V. (1983). Values clarification in nursing. *Norwalk, CT: Appleton-Century Crofts.*

caring for high-acuity patients. While caring for these patients, the exposure to death and the saving of human life requires the nurse to frequently evaluate personal values. Evaluation of a personal philosophy can improve the nurse's satisfaction in working with acutely ill patients. Clarification of the nurse's values helps to anticipate problems that may be encountered in the practice setting and supports the development of positive coping strategies. By reflecting on personal values, we gain a better understanding of what factors may limit our ability to reason clearly and when we may not be suitable for being a patient advocate. Nurses have a primary role in ensuring that the patient makes informed decisions regarding end-of-life care.

SECTION ELEVEN REVIEW

1. Nurses should reflect on their own personal values for all of the following reasons EXCEPT
   A. to teach the patient better values
   B. to gain an understanding of the factors that may limit reasoning
   C. to understand when they might not be suitable for being a patient advocate.
   D. to be careful not to impose a personal value system on that of the patient

2. The Patient Self Determination Act (1990) requires patients be given information about
   A. the right to sue hospitals
   B. the hospital bill prior to discharge
   C. the right to self-medicate
   D. the right to formulate advanced directives

Answers: 1. A, 2. D

POSTTEST

1. A patient is crying about a below-knee amputation sustained as a pedestrian in a pedestrian–vehicle crash. She expresses fears about ambulating in physical therapy. This behavior is a sign of which stage of illness?
   A. denial
   B. awareness
   C. restitution
   D. resolution

2. Which of the following groups of high-acuity patients is at greatest risk for experiencing sensory problems?
   A. middle-aged adults
   B. renal transplant patients
   C. patients in windowless patient care areas
   D. patients who have been hospitalized previously

3. Mrs. B. states she has heard her dead mother calling her. The nurse recognizes this as a symptom of
   A. sensory shutdown
   B. sensory deprivation
   C. auditory damage
   D. antibiotic toxicity

4. One of the most disturbing noises according to nurses working with high-acuity patients is
   A. a physician yelling
   B. equipment alarms
   C. ventilator cycling
   D. suction equipment

5. The more high acuity the patient, the greater the need of families to
   A. visit the patient
   B. understand the technology used in caring for the patient
   C. have a detailed explanation of procedures
   D. have a unit brochure explaining unit policies

6. Nurse–patient ratios in high-acuity areas
   A. should not be predetermined
   B. are not important
   C. should be determined by physicians
   D. are determined by the patient's level of acuity

7. The primary purpose of using technology is to
   A. support the patient's well-being
   B. decrease the patient's length of hospitalization
   C. anticipate complications of therapy
   D. decentralize patient care into specialized units

8. A hazard of technology is
   A. not trusting nursing assessment data
   B. too much touching of the patient
   C. increased nursing surveillance of the patient
   D. the demise of nursing specialty practice

9. Which of the following has been identified by nurses who work with high-acuity patients as a primary stressor?
   A. lack of pay
   B. interpersonal conflict
   C. overtime
   D. performing complex skills

10. To relieve stress associated with nursing high-acuity patients, the nurse should
    A. request a transfer
    B. drink more decaffeinated beverages
    C. work with fewer protocols
    D. attend a continuing education program for personal growth

11. Burnout is
    A. the result of sensory overload
    B. associated with ICU psychosis
    C. an automatic protective response
    D. associated with tenure as a nurse

12. Commitment to work
    A. is associated with less burnout
    B. produces greater work stress
    C. results from extensive orientation to the work area
    D. is associated with the number of years the nurse has worked in the area

13. Burnout may be manifested by all of the following EXCEPT
    A. pessimism
    B. forgetfulness
    C. tolerance
    D. nightmares
14. The decision not to use technology to sustain life should be made
    A. by the health care provider
    B. before an emergency situation
    C. based on community standards
    D. when the patient is transferred to the ICU
15. Informed refusal by the patient
    A. is an acceptable reason for limiting treatment
    B. jeopardizes the health care provider's legal status
    C. indicates that the patient did not receive adequate explanation of treatment
    D. indicates that the patient is angry
16. All of the following variables have been associated with health outcomes EXCEPT
    A. severity of illness
    B. age
    C. patient's previous health status
    D. admission diagnosis
17. Do not resuscitate orders were developed to prevent
    A. treatment for the patient
    B. use of CPR
    C. use of critical care resources
    D. patient transfer
18. An ethical review committee may
    A. decrease public scrutiny of health care providers' actions
    B. promote implementation of general standards
    C. enhance health care providers' liability
    D. increase individual responsibility for decision making
19. The essential components of professional nursing practice are all of the following EXCEPT
    A. care
    B. cure
    C. coordination
    D. culture
20. Clarification of one's values as a nurse may
    A. decrease the nurse's liability
    B. help the nurse anticipate patient care problems
    C. promote burnout
    D. decrease sensory overload

POSTTEST ANSWERS

Question	Answer	Section	Question	Answer	Section
1	C	Two	11	C	Nine
2	C	Four	12	A	Nine
3	B	Four	13	C	Nine
4	B	Four	14	B	Ten
5	A	Six	15	A	Ten
6	D	Seven	16	B	Ten
7	A	Eight	17	B	Ten
8	A	Eight	18	B	Ten
9	B	Nine	19	D	Eleven
10	D	Nine	20	B	Eleven

REFERENCES

Academy of Medical Surgical Nurses. (2000a). Position statement: Staffing standards for patient care. Available at: *http://www.medsurgnurse.org*. Accessed September 4, 2003.

Academy of Medical Surgical Nurses. (2000b). Position statement: Unlicensed assistive personnel. Available at: *http://www.medsurgnurse.org*. Accessed September 4, 2003.

Ahrens, T., Yancey, V., & Kollef, M. (2003). Improving family communications at the end of life: Implications for length of stay in the intensive care unit and resource use. *American Journal of Critical Care, 1*, 317–323.

Aiken, L., Clark, S., & Sloane, D. (2000). Hospital restructuring: Does it adversely effect care and outcomes? *Journal of Nursing Administration, 30*, 457–465.

American Association of Critical Care Nurses. (2002). Practice resources: Critical care nursing fact sheet. Available at: *http://www.aacn.org*. Accessed October 8, 2003.

American Association of Critical Care Nurses. (2000). Public policy statement maintaining patient-focused care in an environment of nursing staff shortages and financial constraints. Available at: *www.aacn.org*. Accessed September 6, 2003.

American College of Critical Care Medicine. (1993). Guidelines for the transfer of critically ill patients. *Critical Care Medicine, 21*, 931–937.

American College of Critical Care Medicine. (1998). Guidelines on admission and discharge for adult intermediate care units. *Critical Care Medicine, 26*, 608.

American College of Critical Care Medicine. (1999). Guidelines for intensive care unit admission, discharge, and triage. *Critical Care Medicine, 27*, 633–638.

American College of Critical Care Medicine. (2003). Guidelines on critical care services and personnel: Recommendations based on a system of categorization of resources: three levels of care. *Critical Care Medicine, 31*, 2677–2683.

American Nurses Association. (1991). Nursing and the patient self-determination acts. Available at: *www.nursingworld.org/readroom/position/ethics/etsdet.htm*. Accessed October 6, 2003.

American Nurses Association. (1992). Nursing care and do-not-resuscitate orders. Available at: *www.nursingworld.org/readroom/position/ethics/etdnr.html*. Accessed October 6, 2003.

American Nurses Association. (2001). *Standards of clinical nursing practice* (2nd ed). Washington, DC: American Nurses Publishing.

Anderson-Shaw, L. (2003). The unilateral DNR order—One hospital's experience. *JONAS Healthcare Law Ethics Regulations, 5,* 42–46.

Bains, J. (1998). From reviving the living to raising the dead: The making of cardiac resuscitation. *Social Science and Medicine, 47,* 1341–1349.

Benner, P. (2003). Beware of technological imperatives and commercial interests that prevent best practice. *American Journal of Critical Care, 12,* 469–471.

Boudreaux, E., Francis, J. L., & Loyacano, T. L. (2002). Family presence during invasive procedures and resuscitations in the emergency department: A critical review and suggestions for future research. *Annals of Emergency Medicine, 40,* 193–205.

Brilli, R. J., Spevetz, A., Branson, R. D., et al. (2001). Critical care delivery in the intensive care unit, Defining clinical roles and the best practice model. *Critical Care Medicine, 29,* 2007–2019.

Chelluri, L., Pinsky, M., Donohoe, M., & Grenvik, A. (1993). Long-term outcome of critically ill elderly patients requiring intensive care. *JAMA: Journal of the American Medical Association, 269,* 3119–3123.

Chlan, L. L. (1998). Effectiveness of a music therapy intervention on relaxation and anxiety for patients receiving ventilatory assistance. *Heart and Lung, 27,* 169–176.

Clarke, C. M., & Harrison, D. (2001). The needs of children visiting on adult intensive care units: A review of the literature and recommendations for practice. *Journal of Advanced Nursing, 34,* 61–68.

Clarke, S., & Aiken, L. (2003) Failure to rescue: Needless deaths are prime examples of the need for more nurses at the bedside. *American Journal of Nursing, 103,* (1), 42–47.

Claus, K., & Bailey, J. (1980). *Living with stress and promoting well being.* St. Louis: C. V. Mosby.

Conoway, D. G., House, J., Bandt, K., Hayden, L., Borlon, A. M., & Spertus, J. A. (2003). The elderly: Health status benefits and recovery of function one year after coronary artery bypass surgery. *Journal of the American College of Cardiology, 42,* 1421–1426.

Counsell, C., & Guin, P. (2002). Exploring family needs during withdrawal of life support in critically ill patients. *Critical Care Nursing Clinics of North America, 14,* 187–191.

Everly, G. S., & Mitchell, J. T. (2002) A primer on critical incident stress management (CISM). Available at http://www.icisf.org/about/cismprimer.pdf Accessed October 10, 2003.

Garrett, D., & McDaniel, A. (2001). A new look at nurse burnout: The effects of environmental uncertainty and social climate. *Journal of Nursing Administration, 31,* 91–96.

Happ, M. (2001). Communicating with mechanically ventilated patients: State of the science. *AACN Clinical Issues, 12,* 247–258.

Henneman E. A., & Cardin, S. (2002). Family centered critical care: A practical approach to making it happen. *Critical Care Nurse, 22*(6), 12–19.

Holden, J., Harrison, L., & Johnson, M. (2002). Families, nurses and intensive care patients: A review of the literature. *Journal of Clinical Nursing, 11,* 140–148.

Honkus, V. (2003). Sleep deprivation in critical care units. *Critical Care Nursing Quarterly, 26*(3), 179–189.

Jenkins, D. L. (2002). Personal digital assistants: A world of information in the palm of your hand. *Clinical Nursing Specialist, 16,* 38–39.

Jones, K. (1993). Outcomes analysis: Methods and issues. *Nursing Economics, 11,* 145–152.

Kalliath, T., & Morris, R. (2002). Job satisfaction among nurses: A predictor of burnout levels. *Journal of Nursing Administration, 32,* 648–654.

Keegan, L. (2003). Therapies to reduce stress and anxiety. *Critical Care Clinics of North America, 15,* 321–327.

Lanken, P. N., et al. (1997). Fair allocation of intensive care unit resources. *American Journal of Respiratory and Critical Care Medicine, 156,* 1282–1301.

Larrabee, J. H., et al. (2003). Predicting registered nurse job satisfaction and intent to leave. *Journal of Nursing Administration, 33,* 271–283.

Lower, J., Bonsack, C., & Guion, J. (2002). High-tech high-touch: Mission impossible? *Dimensions of Critical Care Nursing Quarterly, 21,* 201–205.

MacLean, S. L., Guzzetta, C. E., & White, C. (2003). Family presence during cardiopulmonary resuscitation and invasive procedures: Practices of critical care and emergency nurses. *Journal of Emergency Nursing, 29,* 208–221.

Marshall, M., & Soucy, M. (2003). Delirium in the intensive care unit. *Critical Care Nursing Quarterly, 26,* 172–178.

Maslach, C., & Leiter, M. P. (1997). *The truth about burnout.* San Francisco: Jossey-Bass.

Maslow, A. (1970). *Motivation and personality.* New York: Harper & Row.

Milholland, D. K. (2001). Information systems technologies: Rewards and risks. ANA Nursing Risk Management Series II. Available at: *http://www. nursingworld.org/mods/archive/mod311/cerm201.htm.* Accessed October 20, 2003.

Morrison, W., et al. (2003). Noise, stress and annoyance in a pediatric intensive care unit. *Critical Care Medicine, 31,* 113–119.

Mularski, R. A., Bascom, P., & Osborne, M. L. (2001). Educational agendas for interdisciplinary end-of-life curricula. *Critical Care Medicine, 29*(suppl), N16–N23.

Nagel, C., Markie, M., Richards, K., & Taylor, J. (2003). Sleep promotion in hospitalized elders. *Medical Surgical Nursing, 12,* 279–290.

Nelson, J. E., & Danis, M. (2001). End-of-life care in the intensive care unit: Where are we now? *Critical Care Medicine, 29*(2 suppl), N2–N9.

Osler, T. M., Rogers, F. B., Glance, L. G., Cohen, M., Rutledge, R., & Shackford, S. R. (1998). Predicting survival, length of stay and cost in the surgical ICU: Apache II versus ICISS. *Journal of Trauma Injury Infection and Critical Care, 45,* 234–238.

Palazzo, M. O., (2001). Teaching in crisis. Patient and family education in critical care. *Critical Care Clinics of North America, 13,* 83–92.

Pinsky, M. R. (2003). Genetic testing: Costs and access to intensive care unit care. *Critical Care Medicine, 31*(suppl), S411–S415.

Pronovost, P., & Angus, D. C. (2001). Economics of end-of-life care in the intensive care unit. *Critical Care Medicine, 29*(suppl), N46–N51.

Richards, K., Nagel, C., Markie, M., Elwell, J., & Barone, C. (2003). Use of complementary and alternative therapies to promote sleep in critically ill patients. *Critical Care Clinics of North America, 15,* 329–340.

Robinson, R. (2003). Ethical analysis. *Dimensions of Critical Care Nursing, 22* (2), 71–75.

Rockwood, K., et al. (1993). One year outcome of elderly and young patients admitted to intensive care units. *Critical Care Medicine, 21,* 687–691.

Simpson, T. (1993). Visit preference of middle aged versus older critically ill patients. *American Journal of Critical Care, 2,* 339–345.

Slota, M., Shearn, D., Potersnak, K., & Haas, L. (2003). Perspectives on family centered, flexible visitation in the intensive care unit setting. *Critical Care Medicine, 31*(suppl), S362–S366.

Snyder, J., & Colantonio, A. (1994). Outcome from central nervous system injury. *Critical Care Clinics, 10,* 217–228.

Stechmiller, J. K. (2002). The nursing shortage in acute and critical care settings. *AACN Clinical Issues, 13,* 577–584.

Steele, S., & Harmon, V. (1983). *Values clarification in nursing.* Norwalk, CT: Appleton-Century Crofts.

Suchman, E. (1965). Stages of illness and medical care. *Journal of Health and Human Behavior, 6,* 114.

Taormina, R. J. (2000). Approaches to preventing burnout: The effects of personal stress management and organizational socialization. *Journal of Nursing Management, 8*(2), 89–99.

Teres, D., & Lemeshow, S. (1994). Why severity models should be used with caution. *Critical Care Clinics, 10,* 93–115.

Thomas, L. (2003). Clinical management of stressors perceived by patients on mechanical ventilation. *AACN Clinical Issues, 14,* 73–81.

Tracy, M., & Lindquist, R. (2003). Nursing's role in complementary and alternative use in critical care. *Critical Care Clinics of North America, 15,* 289–294.

Tschann, J. M., Kaufman, S. R., & Micco, G. P. (2003). Family involvement in end-of-life hospital care. *Journal of the American Geriatric Society, 51,* 835–840.

Tuchschmidt, J., & Mecher, C. (1994). Predictors of outcome from critical illness. *Critical Care Clinics, 10,* 179–195.

Twibell, R. S. (1998). Family coping during critical illness. *Dimensions of Critical Care Nursing, 17*(2), 100–112.

Welton, J., Meyer, A. A., Mandelkehr, L., Fakhry, S. M., & Jarr, S. (2002). Outcomes of and resource consumption by high-cost patients in the intensive care unit. *American Journal of Critical Care, 11,* 467–473.

White, J. M. (2000). State of the science of music interventions. *Critical Care Clinics of North America, 12,* 219–225.

Wilson, L. D. (1993). Sensory perceptual alteration. Diagnosis, prediction, and intervention in the hospitalized adult. *Nursing Clinics of North America, 4,* 747–765.

Wong, H. L. C., Lopez-Nahas, V., & Molassiatis, A. (2001). Effects of music therapy on anxiety in ventilator dependent patients. *Heart and Lung, 30,* 376–387.

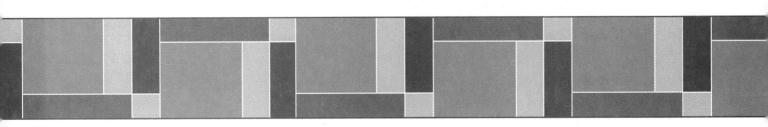

MODULE 2

Acute Pain in the High-Acuity Patient

Barbara Vanderveer, Kathleen Dorman Wagner

OBJECTIVES Following completion of this module, the learner will be able to

1. Identify the basic physiology involved in the transmission of pain.
2. Explain the multifaceted nature of pain.
3. Describe potential sources and effects of pain.
4. Discuss pain assessment.
5. Describe effective management of pain for the high-acuity patient.
6. Discuss issues related to the undertreatment of pain.
7. Identify considerations associated with pain management in special populations.

The focus of this module is on the concept of acute pain rather than chronic pain. The module is composed of seven sections. Section One provides a brief discussion of the physiology involved in the transmission of pain. Section Two defines acute pain and presents a multifaceted model of pain. Section Three discusses potential sources of pain and the effects of pain on the body. Section Four presents a variety of pain assessment tools, including unidimensional and multidimensional assessment tools. Sections Five, Six, and Seven focus on the management of pain. Information covered in these sections includes pharmacologic and nonpharmacologic approaches to pain management, reasons for undertreatment of acute pain, and special considerations regarding pain management in special patient populations. Each section includes a set of review questions to help the learner evaluate his or her understanding of the section's content before moving on to the next section. All Section Reviews and the module Pretest and Posttest include answers. It is suggested that the learner review those concepts answered incorrectly in the review questions before proceeding to the next section.

Author's Note: The Agency for Health Care Policy and Research (AHCPR) developed federal guidelines in 1992 and 1994 that remain standard policy. The agency itself, however, has been replaced by the Agency for Healthcare Research and Quality (AHRQ).

 PRETEST

1. The five types of sensory receptors include (choose all that apply)
   1. chemoreceptors
   2. nociceptors
   3. thermoreceptors
   4. odoreceptors
   A. 1, 3, and 4
   B. 2 and 3
   C. 2, 3, and 4
   D. 1, 2, and 3

2. The A nerve fibers have which of the following characteristics?
   A. myelinated
   B. primitive
   C. transmit slowly
   D. transmit aching sensations

3. Acute persistent pain is associated with
   A. a short duration
   B. a rapid healing process
   C. chronic pain conditions
   D. a distinct organic pathology

4. A second-degree burn on the arm is an example of what type of noxious stimulus?
   A. thermal
   B. physiologic
   C. chemical
   D. mechanical
5. When the stress response becomes too high, it is associated with which physiologic changes? (choose all that apply)
   1. organ hypoperfusion
   2. elevated blood endorphin levels
   3. increased vascular shunting
   4. enhanced hormone function
   A. 1 and 2
   B. 2, 3, and 4
   C. 2 and 4
   D. 1, 2, and 3
6. The clinician would anticipate a masking of the sympathetic symptoms of pain by increased parasympathetic response under which of the following circumstances?
   A. fractured ribs
   B. leg amputation
   C. injury to the bowel
   D. severe pneumonia
7. If a patient is mildly confused, the nurse should initially try to assess pain using
   A. vital signs
   B. self-report
   C. facial expression
   D. body posturing
8. A major weakness of multidimensional tools is that
   A. the nurse performs the assessment
   B. they measure only pain intensity
   C. the patient must comprehend the vocabulary
   D. they are unable to measure degree of anxiety
9. Which of the following statements is correct regarding nonopioid therapy?
   A. nonopioids have more severe side effects than opioids
   B. nonopioids are harder to access than opioids
   C. nonopioids can manage pain as effectively as opioids
   D. combining opioids with nonopioids enhances analgesia effectiveness
10. The most common route used for patient-controlled analgesia (PCA) is
    A. intramuscular
    B. intravenous
    C. subcutaneous
    D. epidural
11. Which of the following statements is correct regarding opioid use and respiratory depression?
    A. respiratory depression precedes onset of sedation
    B. respiratory depression worsens as tolerance develops
    C. sedation occurs before respiratory depression
    D. respiratory depression is a common problem in hospitalized patients
12. Accumulation of morphine metabolites in the blood secondary to renal dysfunction can cause
    A. seizures
    B. tachycardia
    C. central nervous system (CNS) stimulation
    D. severe respiratory depression
13. Elderly patients have fewer endogenous receptors and neural transmitters than younger patients. The primary clinical significance of this statement is
    A. pain relief using opioids is less effective
    B. pain relief using opioids is more unpredictable
    C. smaller doses of opioids are required to achieve pain relief
    D. larger doses of opioids are required to achieve pain relief

Pretest Answers:

1. D, 2. A, 3. D, 4. A, 5. D, 6. C, 7. B, 8. C, 9. D, 10. B, 11. C, 12. D, 13. C

GLOSSARY

acute pain   Pain that is continually changing and transient; onset is rapid and pain is of brief duration (less than 6 months).

addiction   See Psychological dependence.

epidural   Situated within the spinal canal, on or outside the dura mater (the tough membrane surrounding the spinal cord); synonyms are extradural and peridural (AHCPR, 1992).

intrathecal   Within a sheath (e.g., cerebrospinal fluid that is contained within the dura mater) (AHCPR, 1992).

nociception   The activation of pain receptors and the pain pathway by a noxious stimulus of sufficient strength to threaten tissue integrity.

nociceptors   Pain receptors.

oligoanalgesia   Treating pain with minimal drug use.

opioid pseudoaddiction   A term that has been applied to patient behaviors that mimic those associated with addiction; the behaviors result from inadequate pain management rather than psychological dependence.

opiophobia   The fear of prescribing (or consuming) adequate amounts of opiates for therapeutic results.

pain   (1) An unpleasant sensory and emotional experience associated with actual or potential tissue damage or described in terms of such damage (AHCPR, 1992, p. 95).

(2) An unpleasant phenomenon that is uniquely experienced by each individual; it cannot be adequately defined, identified, or measured by an observer (Ludwig-Beymer & Huether, 1996, pp. 319–320).

(3) Whatever the experiencing person says it is, existing whenever the experiencing person says it does (McCaffery & Pasero, 1999, p. 17).

(4) "is the perception of a noxious stimulus dependent upon events in the neurons of the spinal cord and brain stem" (Loeser & Cousins, 1990, p. 179).

pain behavior   A person's physical reaction to the conscious perception of pain.

physical dependence   A physical adaptation of the body to the presence of opioids, existing when rapid drug withdrawal produces signs and symptoms.

psychological dependence (addiction)   A pattern of compulsive drug use characterized by a continued craving for an opioid and the need to use the opioid for effects other than pain relief (or other medical indications) (AHCPR, 1994).

sedation   A state of drowsiness and clouding of mental activity that may be accompanied by impaired reasoning ability (Way et al., 2001).

tolerance   A common physiologic result of chronic opioid use; it means that a larger dose of opioid is required to maintain the same level of analgesia.

ABBREVIATIONS

AHCPR	Agency for Health Care Policy and Research	**OTC**	Over-the-counter (non-prescription)
APS	American Pain Society	**PAG**	Periaqueductal gray
ARS	Adjective Rating Scale	**PCA**	Patient-controlled analgesia
CNS	Central nervous system	**PCEA**	Patient-controlled epidural analgesia
CSF	Cerebrospinal fluid	**PO**	Oral route
IM	Intramuscular route	**PRN**	As needed
IV	Intravenous route	**SF-MPQ**	Short-form McGill Pain Questionnaire
MPQ	McGill Pain Questionnaire	**VAS**	Visual Analog Scale
NRS	Numeric Rating Scale	**WHO**	World Health Organization
NSAID	Nonsteroidal anti-inflammatory drug		

SECTION ONE: Pain Physiology—A Review

At the completion of this section, the learner will be able to identify the physiology involved in the transmission of pain.

A review of pain sensory receptors and their pathways is presented to provide a basic understanding of the assessment and management of the patient in acute pain. A description of the transmission of pain impulses is presented to provide a foundation for understanding the numerous problems involved in the effective management of pain.

The two major types of pain are *somatic pain*, which arises from stimulation of receptors in the skin, muscle, joints, and tendons; and *visceral pain*, which arises from stimulation of receptors in the viscera. Sensory stimuli, such as cold, heat, touch, and pain, are communicated to the nervous system through sensory receptors. There are five types of sensory receptors, each one with the ability to detect changes in a specific type of sensory input (Table 2–1). Sensory receptors require a certain level of excitation (called the threshold) before they will transmit input. Once the sensory threshold has been achieved, the nerve fiber is stimulated and the impulse

TABLE 2–1 Sensory Receptors

RECEPTOR	FUNCTION
Pain receptors (nociceptors)	Detection of tissue damage
Thermoreceptors	Detection of temperature changes
Electromagnetic receptors	Detection of light on eye retina
Chemoreceptors	Detection of smell, taste, concentration of arterial blood oxygen and carbon dioxide, and others
Mechanoreceptors	Detection of mechanical changes in cells adjacent to receptors (e.g., position and tactile senses)

travels the length of the associated sensory nerve (Guyton & Hall, 1997b).

Pain Nerve Fibers

The nerves that carry pain impulses are categorized in terms of their size and whether a myelin sheath is present. Nerves termed *A beta fibers* are large in diameter and have a myelin sheath. *A delta fibers* are small in diameter and are also myelinated. *C fibers* are small in diameter and are usually unmyelinated. Impulses are conducted more quickly over large, myelinated nerves in comparison to small or unmyelinated nerves (Guyton & Hall, 1997b). For example, A delta fibers conduct impulses rapidly. Sharp, pinprick-like pain is conducted along these fibers. C fibers, however, have a slow conduction rate and transmit aching, throbbing sensations (Guyton & Hall, 1997a).

Pain Transmission

Pain impulses initiated at receptor sites are transmitted to the brain along multiple pathways. A major dual pathway consists of the neospinothalamic tract and paleospinothalamic tract. An example of this dual pathway is as follows: A delta pain fibers primarily transmit thermal and mechanical pain through the neospinothalamic tract. The theory underlying the A delta route of transmission is that pain impulses travel along first-order neurons to the dorsal horn of the spinal cord, terminating primarily in the lamina marginalis. On reaching the lamina marginalis in the dorsal horn, the impulse excites second-order neurons and immediately crosses to the opposite side of the spinal cord. The impulse then ascends through the brain stem to the thalamus, where it is consciously acknowledged. From the thalamus it travels to the cerebral cortex, where analysis of pain quality takes place. The slower-transmitting C fibers travel along a cruder, more primitive pain pathway, the paleospinothalamic tract, which primarily terminates in a broad area of the brain stem, with less than a quarter of the fibers passing on through to the thalamus (Guyton & Hall, 1997a).

Endogenous Analgesia System

Although the transmission of the impulse along the spinothalamic pathways appears relatively simple and straightforward, the process is complex. Guyton and Hall (1997a) explain that the body has its own analgesia system that significantly influences how each person reacts to pain. There are three components to this system (in order of their location in the CNS): (1) the periventricular and periaqueductal gray (PAG) areas, located in the third ventricle, hypothalamus, and upper brain stem; (2) the raphe magnus nucleus, located in the brain stem; and (3) the pain inhibitory complex, located in the spinal cord's dorsal horns. Stimulation of the PAG or raphe magnus nucleus causes significant suppression of extremely strong pain signals that are coming in through the dorsal spinal roots. Pain signals that primarily stimulate the periventricular and PAG areas are suppressed but to a lesser degree. Pain signals that are blocked by the pain inhibitory complex in the spinal cord are suppressed at that level and may not be transmitted on to the brain.

The analgesia system secretes special pain-modulating neurotransmitters that influence pain impulses at various stages of transmission. These endogenously produced analgesic substances are called endogenous opioid peptides. When these substances are released, they bind to special receptor sites along the ascending pain pathway and modify the pain transmission. Three types of endogenous opioid peptides have been identified: enkephalins, beta-endorphins, and dynorphins. These substances modulate pain transmission in response to specific physiologic events, such as pain and stress (Curtis et al., 2002; Guyton & Hall, 1997a; Hawthorn & Redmond, 1998; Way et al., 2001). Table 2–2 provides a brief summary of the endogenous opioid peptides.

In addition, theorists Melzack and Wall (1965), in their classic work on pain mechanisms, contended that the substantia gelatinosa acts as a gate for pain impulses. Whether the gate is open (allowing impulses to continue along the pain pathway) or closed depends on whether large-fiber firing or small-fiber firing predominates. Large-fiber firing causes the gate to close, whereas small-fiber firing opens the gate.

TABLE 2–2 Endogenous Opiates

GROUP	PRIMARY LOCATION	COMMENTS
Enkephalins	Periaqueductal gray (PAG) in midbrain and brain stem	Most widely distributed in body Effects last minutes to hours Serotonin causes enkephalin release at dorsal horn
Beta-endorphin	Hypothalamus and pituitary gland	Hypothalamus and pituitary gland Most like morphine
Dynorphins	PAG and spinal cord	Present in minute quantities Extremely powerful (perhaps 200 times more powerful than morphine)

Data from Hawthorn, J., & Redmond, K. (1998). Pain: Causes and management. *Malden, MA: Blackwell Science; Guyton, A. C., & Hall, J. E. (1997a).* Pain, headache, and thermal sensations. In A. C. Guyton & J. E. Hall (Eds.). Human physiology and mechanisms of disease *(6th ed.). Philadelphia: W. B. Saunders; and Thelan, L. A., Urden, L. D., Lough, M. E., & Stacy, K. M. (Eds.). (1998).* Critical care nursing: Diagnosis and management *(3rd ed.). St. Louis: C. V. Mosby.*

In summary, the transmission and eventual response to pain impulses is a complex process that is not yet fully understood. Multiple pain pathways are thought to exist, including a dual pathway, consisting of the neospinothalamic tract and paleospinothalamic tract. The precise mechanisms of pain transmission cannot be described with certainty. The complexity of the process is due, in part, to known and suspected influences on the impulse as it travels along the pain pathway.

SECTION ONE REVIEW

1. The five types of sensory receptors include (choose all that apply)
    1. chemoreceptors
    2. nociceptors
    3. thermoreceptors
    4. odoreceptors
   A. 1, 3, and 4
   B. 2 and 3
   C. 2, 3, and 4
   D. 1, 2, and 3
2. Which of the following characteristics are associated with type A nerve fibers?
   A. myelinated
   B. primitive
   C. transmit slowly
   D. transmit aching sensations
3. Pain is analyzed in which part of the brain?
   A. cerebellum
   B. thalamus
   C. cerebral cortex
   D. brain stem
4. When pain is suppressed at the pain inhibitory complex, it
   A. moves on to the PAG
   B. is blocked at the spinal cord level
   C. transfers to the raphe magnus nucleus
   D. is ultimately suppressed in the hypothalamus
5. The neospinothalamic pain pathway terminates in the
   A. cerebral cortex
   B. brain stem
   C. dorsal horns
   D. substantia gelatinosa
6. The paleospinothalamic tract
   A. is the primary pain pathway
   B. terminates throughout the brain stem
   C. transmits signals to specific sensory areas
   D. transmits signals identically to the fast pathway

Answers: 1. D, 2. A, 3. C, 4. B, 5. A, 6. B

SECTION TWO: The Multifaceted Nature of Pain

At the completion of this section, the learner will be able to explain the multiple facets of pain.

A Working Definition of Acute Pain

McCaffery has defined **pain** as "whatever the experiencing person says it is, existing whenever the experiencing person says it does" (McCaffery & Pasero, 1999, p. 17). The AHCPR Guidelines (1992, p. 95) state that pain is "an unpleasant sensory and emotional experience associated with actual or potential tissue damage or described in terms of such damage."

Acute pain has been defined as pain that is continually changing and transient. It is accompanied by a high level of emotional and autonomic nervous system arousal and is usually associated with tissue pathology or surgery. It can be further divided into two types—brief acute pain (short duration, minutes to days) and acute persistent pain (longer duration, weeks to months). Acute persistent pain is primarily associated with a distinct organic pathology and a slow healing process (Chapman & Syrjala, 1990). Acute pain serves a major protective function by acting as an early warning system of impending or actual tissue injury and typically diminishes as the injury heals (Curtis et al., 2002).

A Multifaceted Model of Pain

Loeser and Cousins (1990) propose that pain is multifaceted and composed of nociception, pain, suffering, and pain behaviors. Only the outermost facet, pain behaviors, can be observed by someone other than the person experiencing the pain. The other three facets are completely personal and can only be inferred by another person. The relative contribution of each of the four facets to the pain experience is variable. Each facet is present to some degree in any pain experience. In general, the noxious stimulus and the process of nociception predominate during acute pain.

Noxious Stimuli

Noxious (pain causing) stimuli may be mechanical, thermal, or chemical, and they have the potential to excite pain receptors. These stimuli must exist in sufficient quantities to trigger the release of biochemical mediators that activate the pain response (nociception). Activation of the pain response may also be triggered

- In response to what would typically be defined as nonnoxious stimuli;
- In response to sympathetic discharge (sympathetically maintained pain); or
- Spontaneously.

The First Facet: Nociception

Nociception refers to the activation of pain receptors (**nociceptors**) and the pain pathway by a noxious stimulus of sufficient strength to threaten tissue integrity. Under normal circumstances it leads to the sensation of pain. Acute pain is primarily of nociceptive origin. Nociception does not, however, always lead to pain. Certain factors or conditions can alter or eliminate the sensation of pain even when the person is subjected to extremely noxious stimuli. Such factors include severe nerve damage (spinal cord injury, peripheral neuropathy), anesthesia, and strong analgesia therapy. Pain can also occur without nociception, such as may be found in patients with neuropathic pain and other chronic pain conditions (Loeser & Cousins, 1990).

The Second Facet: Pain

According to Loeser and Cousins (1990), pain "is the perception of a noxious stimulus dependent upon events in the neurones of the spinal cord and brain stem" (p. 179). A person can perceive pain only when transmission of the noxious stimulus terminates within the brain. It is unknown whether the patient's ability to perceive pain remains intact when cortical function is compromised or when cortical function has been chemically altered by sedative–hypnotics.

The Third Facet: Suffering

The multifaceted model describes the term *suffering* as a negative affective response that is generated in the higher nervous centers of the brain. It further states that suffering can be caused by pain or a variety of situations such as stress, anxiety, fear, loss of a loved one, and depression. The concept of suffering seems closely connected to the personal meaning of the pain. The clinician's objective assessment of suffering is restricted to observing for the presence or absence of pain behaviors. According to Loeser and Cousins (1990), suffering is particularly associated with chronic pain. The complex concept of suffering has received increased attention over the past decade and there is a growing body of literature in this area.

The Fourth Facet: Pain Behaviors

It is not coincidental that the outside circle of the multifaceted model of pain is pain behavior. **Pain behavior** refers to a person's physical reaction to the conscious perception of pain; it is what leads the observer to conclude that pain is being experienced. There are two types of pain behaviors: those that are intended to communicate pain (pain-expressing behaviors) and those that are intended to lessen or control the pain (pain-controlling behaviors). Common pain-expressing behaviors include groaning, rubbing the painful part, or lying motionless. It is often difficult for the observer to differentiate pain-controlling from pain-expressing behaviors. For example, rubbing or massaging the painful part may be a means of moderating the sensory input (pain-controlling behavior) rather than a means of communicating (expressing) the pain to others. Pain behaviors are discussed further in Section Four, "Pain Assessment."

In summary, pain can be defined in a variety of ways but is consistently viewed as a very personal, subjective experience. A multifaceted model of pain illustrates the complex nature of the pain experience. The model proposes that there are four facets of pain, including nociception, pain, suffering, and pain behaviors. The first three facets can only be inferred by anyone other than the person experiencing the pain. Only the fourth facet, pain behaviors, can be observed. Pain behaviors may be either pain-expressing or pain-controlling.

SECTION TWO REVIEW

1. Acute persistent pain is associated with
   A. a short duration
   B. a rapid healing process
   C. chronic pain conditions
   D. a distinct organic pathology
2. A second-degree burn on the arm is an example of what type of noxious stimulus?
   A. thermal
   B. physiologic
   C. chemical
   D. mechanical
3. The activation of pain receptors and the pain pathway by a noxious stimulus of sufficient strength to threaten tissue integrity is known as
   A. acute pain
   B. suffering
   C. nociception
   D. neuropathy
4. Suffering is most commonly associated with which type of pain?
   A. acute
   B. persistent acute
   C. slow chronic
   D. intermittent
5. Behaviors that are intended to communicate pain are called what type of pain behaviors?
   A. expressing
   B. heralding
   C. controlling
   D. communicating

Answers: 1. D, 2. A, 3. C, 4. C, 5. A

SECTION THREE: Acute Pain in the High-Acuity Patient

At the completion of this section, the learner will be able to discuss potential sources and effects of pain.

Potential Sources of Pain

High-acuity patients are at risk for brief acute as well as persistent acute types of pain. The initial insult requiring admission to the hospital is often linked to acute pain (e.g., traumatic injury, organ ischemia, surgical manipulation). In addition, high-acuity patients commonly have invasive lines and tubes inserted (e.g., chest tubes, intravenous lines, endotracheal and tracheostomy tubes), all of which irritate delicate tissues and cause varying degrees of pain. The patient may also be required to undergo painful procedures such as lumbar puncture or endoscopic examinations. Forced immobility because of the serious or critical nature of an illness and attachment to multiple tubes may exacerbate more chronic conditions, such as back or arthritic pain.

Acute pain is usually accompanied by some degree of anxiety, which may be further aggravated by the stress and anxiety associated with the hospital or critical care environment. High-anxiety states are associated with an increase in pain perception and may decrease pain tolerance. Pain may also be a contributor to patient confusion and inadequate sleep.

The Effects of Stress and Pain on the Body

In the high-acuity patient, pain can result from a variety of sources, such as tissue injury, ischemia, metabolic or chemical mediators, inflammation, or muscle spasm. Pain is also affected by stress. The stress response is a crucial part of self-preservation. It initiates events that increase the body's chances of survival through a life-threatening event. When the body experiences a massive insult, however, the stress response can become too high, which can cause physiological changes that are associated with poor patient outcomes. A high-stress response increases vascular shunting, resulting in hypoperfusion of vital organs. It also increases serum levels of endogenous opioid peptides, which may result in counterregulation of hormonal responses. Tissue injury is a strong stress response stimulus. The acute pain created by injured tissue initially increases both hormonal and sympathetic nervous system responses. However, if the pain becomes prolonged, the sympathetic response to pain diminishes as a result of a parasympathetic rebound effect, which results in the vital signs returning more toward normal. This is an important consideration when assessing pain in the high-acuity patient. Although the sympathetic response is important to assess, reliance on it as the sole indicator of acute pain may significantly misrepresent the intensity of pain.

Patients who are experiencing moderate to high levels of pain are often at increased risk for developing stasis-related complications because of immobility. Pain is associated with a natural limiting of activity that encourages a person to rest and, therefore, aids in the healing process. This decrease in activity, however, is also associated with negative outcomes, such as pulmonary complications and deep-vein thrombosis. Pulmonary complications, such as atelectasis and stasis pneumonia, result from splinting that decreases spontaneous ventilatory movement and oxygenation. For example, pulmonary complications are frequently noted in patients who have had thoracic surgery, abdominal surgery, or trauma, and prolonged bedrest is a significant risk factor in the development of deep-vein thrombosis. By decreasing the level of pain, patients may become more active earlier in their recovery period, thus significantly decreasing the risk of developing stasis complications.

In summary, pain is a major life-protecting sensation that is frequently accompanied by varying levels of stress and anxiety. When pain is prolonged or severe, it can have a negative physiologic impact. There are many potential sources of pain for the high-acuity patient, including those associated with the patient's admission and those associated with painful procedures, invasive lines, insertion of tubes, and imposed immobility.

SECTION THREE REVIEW

1. Which statement reflects the relationship between pain, stress, and anxiety?
   A. increased levels of stress and anxiety worsen pain
   B. increased levels of stress worsen pain but anxiety has no significant effect
   C. increased levels of anxiety worsen pain but stress has no significant effect
   D. there is no significant relationship between pain, stress, and anxiety

2. The stress response is
   A. an avoidable reaction
   B. a maladaptive response to crises
   C. a crucial part of self-preservation
   D. an unpredictable reaction to pain

3. When the stress response becomes too great, it is associated with which physiologic changes? (choose all that apply)
   1. organ hypoperfusion
   2. elevated blood endorphin levels

  3. increased vascular shunting
  4. enhanced hormone function
  A. 1 and 2
  B. 2, 3, and 4
  C. 2 and 4
  D. 1, 2, and 3

4. If acute pain is sustained for a prolonged period of time, the
  A. sympathetic response diminishes
  B. parasympathetic response diminishes
  C. pain threshold increases
  D. pain tolerance decreases

Answers: 1. A, 2. C, 3. D, 4. A

SECTION FOUR: Pain Assessment

At the completion of this section, the learner will be able to discuss pain assessment in the high-acuity patient.

Pain is a complex, subjective response that is multidimensional in nature. The patient's self-report is the most reliable indicator of the existence and intensity of adult pain, and yet it has been shown that nurses' attitudes frequently alter the assessment by subjectively interpreting the patient's self-report of pain (AHCPR, 1992; McCaffery & Pasero, 1999; Stephenson, 1994). Strict attention to applying the nursing process is crucial if acute pain is to be managed effectively because pain is an ongoing process that requires continual reassessment and reevaluation.

Pain levels vary in each individual primarily because of the biopsychological nature of pain. To manage pain effectively, it is essential to use self-report pain assessment tools whenever possible. These assessment tools help clinicians establish baseline criteria for evaluating pain and facilitate the development of appropriate comfort interventions. The ongoing challenge for caregivers and researchers is to find an effective alternative means of assessment for unconscious patients and other patients who for some reason cannot self-report their levels of pain (e.g., very confused).

Numerous studies over the past decade have described the lack of pain assessments by nurses, yet nurses are consistent in obtaining vital signs. For this reason, the American Pain Society (APS) has suggested making pain the fifth vital sign. The APS believes that by keeping the assessment of pain highly visible, it is more likely to be treated effectively (American Pain Society Quality of Care Committee, 1995).

Pain History

The pain history provides valuable information regarding the patient's preexisting pain experiences, treatment modalities, and medication history. In addition, it may also be used for obtaining information regarding the patient's usual pain behaviors and pain relief methods used at home. Having knowledge of an individual's usual pain behaviors would be of particular value if the patient should lose the ability to communicate with the health care team during hospitalization. Table 2–3 lists important information that can be obtained through a pain history.

TABLE 2–3 Pain History

Drug allergies

Prior acute pain experiences

Chronic pain problems—location? Description of pain? How often? For how long?

Activity level maintained during pain?

Any recent changes in usual pain/discomfort pattern?

How does patient express pain at home (e.g., paces, lies motionless, cries, distraction, etc.)?

How does the pain make the person feel (e.g., sad, angry, frustrated, etc.)?

Usual relief measures:

  Drug therapy—what? How much? How often? Level of relief?

  Nonpharmacologic—what? (e.g., hot water bottle, ice, heating pad, etc.) Level of relief?

The Acute Pain Assessment

Unidimensional and Multidimensional Assessment

Unidimensional pain assessment tools provide the patient with a means to rate a single pain dimension, such as pain intensity, affective distress, or the subjective meaning of the pain. When the specific cause of pain is apparent (e.g., postsurgical incisional pain), a unidimensional pain assessment tool is often considered sufficient. Unidimensional tools are especially useful in evaluating the effectiveness of the interventions used to decrease the pain. These tools are simple to use and take little time to administer. Examples of unidimensional pain assessment tools include the Visual Analog Scale (VAS); the Numeric Rating Scale (NRS); and verbal descriptor scales, such as the Adjective Rating Scale (ARS). Unidimensional tools can also be used as part of a multidimensional pain assessment.

Multidimensional pain assessment tools provide the patient with a means to express the affective and evaluative aspects of the pain experience in addition to the sensory aspect. These tools work best for patients with more complex pain such as pain of unknown origin or chronic pain. Examples of multidimensional tools include the McGill Pain Questionnaire (MPQ) and the short-form McGill Pain Questionnaire (SF-MPQ) (Wall & Melzack, 1994).

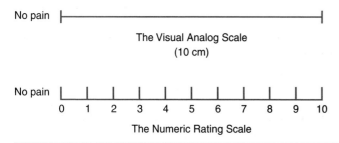

Figure 2–1 ■ Examples of unidimensional pain assessment tools.

Unidimensional Pain Assessment

Visual Analog Scale (VAS). The VAS has been shown to be an effective measurement of pain intensity. There are several variations of the VAS. The most common is a horizontal or vertical line with one end labeled "no pain" and the opposite end labeled "worst pain imaginable." The patient self-reports the level of pain is along this line. The line is usually 10 cm in length. Once the patient has indicated the point on the scale that best represents the current level of pain, a centimeter ruler is placed on the scale and a numeric rating of 0 to 10 is given. On some VAS variations, a numeric scale is present on the reverse side, with a slide rule type of device for converting the VAS to a numeric score. Figure 2–1 illustrates an example of a VAS.

Numeric Rating Scale (NRS). The NRS (Fig. 2–1) is a variation of the VAS. It uses a sequence of numbers from which the patient chooses. The most common use of the NRS is measurement of pain intensity based on a continuum of pain, with 0 being "no pain" and the extreme opposite number (5, 10, or 100) being the "worst pain imaginable." The most common and clinically proven NRS is the 0 to 10 scale. The NRS has also been used to rate numerically other dimensions of pain. An advantage of using the NRS is that the directions for using it have been translated into a variety of languages (McCaffery & Pasero, 1999).

Verbal Descriptor Scales. As a unidimensional assessment tool, a verbal descriptor scale, such as the ARS, may be used to measure any of the pain dimensions. For example, as a sensory dimension measure, the scale might include a list of adjectives, such as flickering, quivering, pulsing, throbbing, beating, pounding (from the MPQ, in Chapman & Syrjala, 1990). Using this list of words, the patient is asked to choose the adjective that best describes his or her current pain. The words should reflect

different levels of the dimension being measured. Using this type of tool has several potential disadvantages. First, careful choice of descriptor words is necessary if this type of scale is to be a useful pain assessment tool. Second, patients have a tendency to choose words from the middle of the scale rather than choosing from either end (Chapman & Syrjala, 1990).

Wong–Baker Faces Scale (Faces). The Faces Scale has been shown to be popular with both children and adults (Carey et al., 1997). It consists of six facial drawings ranging from smiling to crying. Each face is assigned a number from 0 to 5 or 0 to 10. The patient simply points to the face that represents his or her current level of pain. Directions for the Wong–Baker Faces Scale have also been translated into a variety of languages (McCaffery & Pasero, 1999). Figure 2–2 shows an example of a faces scale.

Adapting the Unidimensional Pain Assessment Tool for the Severely Ill Patient

A patient who is extremely ill or weak may be able to use unidimensional tools with the nurse's assistance. For example, the nurse can run a pencil along a VAS and have the patient nod or indicate in some way where the "point" of pain is on the scale. Sometimes, the patient may be able to point to the number on an NRS or to the location on the line of a VAS that best indicates the intensity of pain. As an alternative, the patient may be able to raise up the number of fingers that indicate the level of pain, with no fingers raised being "no pain" and 5 or 10 fingers raised being the "worst pain imaginable."

Nurses frequently assume that extreme illness, weakness, or mild confusion prevents the patient from being able to self-report pain. This is not necessarily true. Self-report methods should be attempted in this patient group even though it may require patience and flexibility on the part of the nurse. If the nurse is to be successful using these methods, brief but clear directions must be given and repeated as needed during the assessment procedure.

It has been shown that even when nurses use self-report tools, they rely more on their own nursing observations of behavioral cues in determining whether the patient is in pain (Ferrell et al., 1991). This may result in the nurse's applying a numeric value based on nursing observation and estimation of the patient's level of pain intensity (i.e., documenting a patient as rating a 5 out of 10 based strictly on nursing observation). This is an inappropriate use of the unidimensional self-report tools.

Figure 2–2 ■ Example of a faces pain scale.

TABLE 2–4 Advantages and Disadvantages of Pain Assessment Tools

UNIDIMENSIONAL TOOLS	
ADVANTAGES	DISADVANTAGES
Provide baseline data	Measure only one dimension of the pain experience
Provide a means of comparing pre- and postintervention pain intensity	Unable to measure degree of anxiety or stress accompanying the pain
Provide a standardized method for assessment of pain intensity	Require relatively high cognitive level
Can be clearly documented and reported	Require some means of communication
Adaptable for patients who cannot verbalize	
Easy to perform	
Short assessment time	

MULTIDIMENSIONAL TOOLS	
ADVANTAGES	DISADVANTAGES
Provide baseline data	Valid only if patient understands vocabulary
Provide a standardized method for assessment of pain	Long length of completion time (McGill Pain Questionnaire)
Can be clearly documented and reported	Require a high cognitive level
Assess multiple aspects of the pain experience	
Provide data for choosing nonpharmacologic interventions	
Adaptable for patients who cannot verbalize	

Both types of tools have strengths and limitations associated with their use. Table 2–4 summarizes the advantages and disadvantages of using unidimensional and multidimensional pain assessment tools. The clinician also should be aware that discrepancies may exist between the patient's self-reported level of pain and nurse-observed pain behaviors. For example, a patient may describe pain intensity as a 7 out of 10 while watching television or talking on the phone. This individual may be using coping skills that subjectively do not reflect high-pain scores. A patient's use of distraction and relaxation techniques can be misinterpreted as stoicism or exaggeration of self-reported pain levels (AHCPR, 1992).

Multidimensional Pain Assessment

The most frequently used measurement of sensory and affective pain is the MPQ. This questionnaire measures four aspects (categories) of the pain experience: sensory, affective, evaluative, and miscellaneous. Each pain category is measured using a cluster of descriptive words. The patient's choice of words assists the clinician in determining which category the pain is originating from and aids the clinician in choosing a therapeutic pain regimen that is individualized to the patient's needs. The SF-MPQ is recommended for conscious patients in the critical care area. The SF-MPQ takes 2 to 5 minutes to administer. It is more practical for many high-acuity patients, assuming that vocabulary is not a problem and that the patient is functioning at a sufficiently high cognitive level. The words are simple and are understood by most patients. Administration of SF-MPQ can be adjusted

for patients who cannot communicate verbally (e.g., intubated patients) by having them either point to desired descriptive words or, if they are too weak, use a head nod when the nurse reads the desired descriptive word. In addition to the McGill tools, the clinician can develop a simple word list using words describing emotions and sensations that would be appropriate for a particular patient or patient population.

Alternative Pain Assessment

High-acuity patients have many reasons for experiencing acute pain, and a significant number are at risk for undertreatment because of their inability to self-report pain. Many high-acuity patients have altered communication abilities for a variety of reasons, such as altered levels of consciousness and extreme weakness. Nurses must be flexible in how they assess pain in this patient population, first trying self-report whenever possible. When self-report cannot be used, the clinician can use additional data-gathering sources for obtaining information, such as the family, regarding usual expressions of pain and relief measures, and by direct nursing observations to make the determination of the presence of pain rather than trying to quantify pain intensity. Figure 2–3 is an example of an alternative pain assessment tool that has been developed by nurses for use with all patients. Figure 2–4 shows the various pain scales that accompany this tool including a 10-point behavioral pain scale, which is used for vulnerable patients, such as those in critical care settings. It is used with any adult who is unable to self-report pain level.

University of Kentucky Hospital
Chandler Medical Center
Lexington, Kentucky

PAIN ASSESSMENT/MANAGEMENT FLOW SHEET

Addressograph

Date_____   Use the following codes to document assessments of patients with c/o pain AND REASSESS these patients within a reasonable time frame following interventions.

Pain Rating Scales: 0/10   FACES   FLACC   Behavioral Other _____   Pain Management Goal: _____

Time	*Body Site (s)	*Description	*Pain Level before INTV	*Intervention(s)	*Pain Level after INTV	*Level of Arousal (S-4)	*Behavior Patterns	*SE from INTV	*Tx for SE	Comments: See Nsg Notes (Place check mark)	Nurse Initials
2400-0100											
0100-0200											
0200-0300											
0300-0400											
0400-0500											
0500-0600											
0600-0700											
0700-0800											
0800-0900											
0900-1000											
1000-1100											
1100-1200											
1200-1300											
1300-1400											
1400-1500											
1500-1600											
1600-1700											
1700-1800											
1800-1900											
1900-2000											
2000-2100											
2100-2200											
2200-2300											
2300-2400											

Codes

Body Sites
A=Abdomen   A=Arm (R or L)
C=Chest   L=Leg (R or L)
F=Face   T=Throat
H=Head   UB=Upper Back
J=Jaw   LB=Lower Back
N=Neck   Other: _____

Description
A=Ache   *Pediatrics:*
B=Burning   *O="Owie" or "boo=boo"*
D=Dull   *H="Hurt"*
P=Pressure   Other: _____
S=Sharp
St=Stabbing
T=Throbbing

Level of Arousal
S=Sleeping, Easily Aroused
1=Awake & Alert
2=Occasionally Drowsy
3=Freq. Drowsy, drifts off to sleep easily
4=Somnolent, Minimal or No Response to Stimuli

Interventions (INTV)
D=Distraction   *Pediatrics:*
GI=Guided Imagery   *C=Cuddling or holding*
H=Heat   *Mu=Music*
M=Massage   *NP=Non-pharmacologic (i.e.,*
Med=Medication (see MAR   *bubbles, pinwheel, etc.)*
of PCA sheet)   *P=Play*
R=Reposition
Rel=Relaxation
T=Teaching (i.e., PCA use)

Behavior Patterns
A=Anxious   I=Inconsolable
G=Grimacing   U=Unnoticeable
P=Peaceful, Calm, Restful   Other: _____
R=Restless, Thrashing

Side Effects (SE)   **Treatment of SE**
C=Confusion   A=Med Adjustment
I=Itching   C=In & Out Catheter
N=Nausea   F=Foley Catheter
R=Resp. Depression   Med=Medication
U=Urinary Retention S=Safety Measures
V=Vomiting   Other: _____

Signature	Initials	Signature	Initials	Signature	Initials
Signature	Initials	Signature	Initials	Signature	Initials

8/02

Figure 2–3 ■ Pain assessment/management flow sheet. *(Adapted from "Pain assessment/management flow sheet," developed by Pain Committee (2003). University Hospital, University of Kentucky.)*

Visual Analog Scale

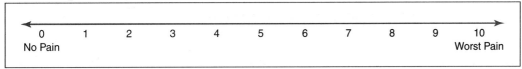

Faces Pain Rating Scale

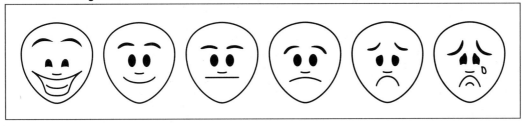

Descriptive Scale

No Pain	Mild	Moderate	Severe	Excruciating

Behavioral Observation Scale

Observed Behavior	0	1	2
Restlessness	Calm, cooperative	Slightly restless, consolable	Very restless, agitated, inconsolable
Muscle tension	Relaxed	Slight tenseness	Extreme tenseness
Facial expression	No frowning or grimacing, composed	Slight frowning or grimacing	Constant frowning or grimacing
Vocalization	Normal tone, no sound	Groans, moans, cries out in pain	Cries out, sobs
Wound guarding	No negative response to wound	Reaching/gently touching wound	Grabbing vigorously at wound

Behavioral Observation Scale Directions

- This scale can be used with very young children and patients who are unable to speak because of injury, mental status, medications, or treatment.
- Assess each of the areas identified in the Observed Behavior column, rating each behavior using the 0, 1, or 2 rating. Add the ratings together for each observed behavior.
- Assign a numerical score to the designated observations.
- Record the score on the pain assessment record or designated place on the documentation sheet.
- A low score indicates a low or acceptable level of pain and a high score (maximum score = 10) indicates the most pain.

Figure 2–4 ■ Pain assessment tools. *(Adapted from "Pain assessment tools," developed by Pain Committee (2003). University Hospital, University of Kentucky.)*

Most behavioral pain scales use patient behaviors (cues) that may indicate the presence of pain. These behaviors can be divided into three main groups: vocal, facial, and body posturing. Sympathetic nervous system response should also be considered but may become less of an indicator over time. Some scales also include compliance with ventilation instead of verbalization as an indicator of pain for intubated patients (Payen et al., 2001). Vocal behaviors are sounds, such as crying, moaning, or grunting. The primary facial cues that suggest pain are facial grimacing and a crying expression (tears may be noted). Certain body posturing behaviors are associated with the presence of pain. Typical observations include agitation or lying completely still, guarding, splinting respirations, withdrawing or localizing to invasive modalities and procedures, stiffening, and repetitive/rhythmic activity of a body part (such as rocking or tapping). Acute pain is associated with stimulation of the sympathetic nervous system response, which causes elevation of heart rate, blood pressure, and respiratory rate, and increased pallor and diaphoresis. Although it is of value in assessing short-term acute pain, the use of the sympathetic response criteria for assessing the presence of pain loses validity over time. The sympathetic response is known to adapt rapidly, within 24 hours, even in the patient experiencing severe pain.

In summary, acute pain is a subjective, multidimensional experience. The patient's self-report is the single most reliable indicator of the existence and intensity of acute pain. An effective pain manager uses patient self-report as the major pain indicator and uses nursing observations to gather additional data.

Use of self-report tools provides an effective means for measurement and documentation of pain. When patients cannot self-report their pain levels, the nurse must rely on observing for behaviors typically associated with the presence of pain and on prior history ascertained from family members and significant others. When the patient is not able to self-report, the nurse should not prematurely judge the quantity and quality of pain until appropriate pain assessment data have been collected and analyzed. Patients who cannot self-report are particularly vulnerable to inadequate pain management by nurses who either do not use alternative pain assessment methods or misinterpret patient behaviors. Therefore, it is imperative that nurses carefully assess pain when patients cannot actively participate in the assessment process.

SECTION FOUR REVIEW

1. The Numeric Rating Scale is most commonly used to measure what part of the pain experience?
   A. affective
   B. evaluative
   C. intensity
   D. coping
2. If a patient is mildly confused, the nurse should initially try to assess pain using
   A. vital signs
   B. self-report
   C. facial expression
   D. body posturing
3. A major weakness of multidimensional tools is that
   A. the patient must comprehend the vocabulary
   B. they measure only pain intensity

C. the nurse performs the assessment
D. they are unable to measure degree of anxiety
4. Examples of vocal pain behaviors include (choose all that apply)
   1. grunting
   2. moaning
   3. guarding
   4. crying
A. 1 and 2
B. 2, 3, and 4
C. 1, 2, and 4
D. 2 and 3

Answers: 1. C, 2. B, 3. A, 4. C

SECTION FIVE: Management of Acute Pain

At the completion of this section, the learner will be able to describe effective pain management for the high-acuity patient.

Organized Approach to Pain Management

Effective pain management is facilitated by use of an organized, systematic approach. The World Health Organization (WHO) Analgesic Ladder provides an example of such an approach. The ladder (Fig. 2–5) suggests general pain management choices based on the level of pain (i.e., mild, mild to moderate, or moderate to severe). In addition, it provides a step-by-step approach to adjusting the pharmacologic choices if the patient's pain is persistent or increases.

The high-acuity patient is particularly at risk for moderate to severe pain; thus, discussion will focus on management at this level of the ladder. Opioids are generally the drugs of choice for pain management at this level. In addition, the ladder recommends consideration of nonopioid and adjuvant therapies to further enhance the effects of opioid therapy.

Pharmacologic Pain Management

The pharmacologic management of pain involves modulation of pain transmission at different levels of the nervous system. For example, opioids bind with opioid receptors in such areas as the spinal cord, peripheral nervous system, and central nervous system. Nonsteroidal anti-inflammatory drugs (NSAIDs) may relieve pain by working peripherally at the site of injury, by inhibiting the formation of prostaglandins, proteolytic enzymes, and bradykinins. They may also have a CNS effect.

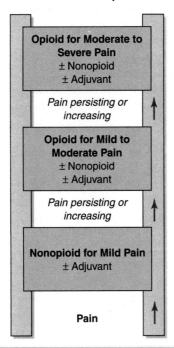

Freedom from pain

Opioid for Moderate to
Severe Pain
± Nonopioid
± Adjuvant

*Pain persisting or
increasing*

Opioid for Mild to
Moderate Pain
± Nonopioid
± Adjuvant

*Pain persisting or
increasing*

Nonopioid for Mild Pain
± Adjuvant

Pain

Figure 2–5 ■ The WHO Ladder. *(Adapted from WHO. [1996]. Cancer pain relief, (2nd ed.) Geneva, Switzerland: World Health Organization.)*

Evidence-Based Practice

- *Although nurses recorded observable pain indicators in intubated patients, they failed to record patients' self-reports of pain. The majority of the time, nurses treated pain with pharmacologic interventions rather than using nonpharmacological approaches. Nurses did not follow up pain interventions with a reassessment of the patient comfort status. The study concluded that documentation of pain in the patient's medical files is inadequate. (Gelinas, Fortier, Viens, et al., 2004).*

- *Acute pain as a result of the removal of chest tubes was significantly lower when appropriately timed analgesics were administered prior to removal. Patients received either 4 mg of IV morphine or 30 mg of IV ketorolac prior to tube removal. Following tube removal, patients scored their pain immediately and then again after 20 minutes. Use of either drug resulted in low-pain intensity and pain distress scores with no adverse effects. (Puntillo, & Ley, 2004).*

- *Postcardiac surgery patients rated levels of pain associated with a variety of activities in the following order (high to low levels of pain): coughing, moving/turning in bed, getting out of bed, use of incentive spirometry/deep breathing, and resting. Pain levels lowered significantly following removal of chest tubes. (Milgrom, Brooks, & Qi, et al., 2004).*

Nonopioid Therapy

Effective pain management can be enhanced by a combination of opioid and nonopioid therapy. A better level of analgesia is often achieved in combination than when either is administered alone. Nonopioids include such drugs as acetaminophen, as-

pirin, and, in particular, NSAIDs. Nonopioids are associated with fewer side effects than opioids.

Adjuvant Therapy

Adjuvant therapy includes drugs that can assist in reducing certain types of pain. Their assistance may be indirect (by decreasing other symptoms associated with the underlying condition) or direct, as a coanalgesic. These drugs are generally used in addition to opioid and nonopioid analgesics. Several specific examples of adjuvant drugs include corticosteroids for cancer-related pain, and antidepressants (e.g., amitriptyline [Elavil]) or anticonvulsants (e.g., gabapentin [Neurontin]) for treatment of neuropathic pain (Hawthorn & Redmond, 1998; McCaffery & Pasero, 1999).

Opioid Therapy

Therapeutic use of opioids begins with the selection of a specific opioid drug and route of administration. Once the choice of drug and route are determined, decisions are made regarding the suitable initial dose; frequency of administration; optimal doses of nonopioid analgesics, if these are to be given; and incidence and severity of side effects. The importance of careful adjustment of these medications for therapeutic effects cannot be overemphasized because dosing needs and analgesic responses vary greatly among individual patients (AHCPR, 1992).

Routes of Administration

There are many routes available for administration of analgesia. The oral, subcutaneous, intramuscular, and intravenous (IV) routes can be accessed by the nurse. Most other routes, however, require initial access by an anesthesiologist.

The oral route is most commonly used for opioids. This route is also the most inexpensive and convenient. For the high-acuity patient, however, the oral route may not be available because of a nothing-by-mouth status. Although these individuals are not able to take medications orally, many have feeding tubes that act as an alternate medication route.

AHCPR guidelines state that when IV access is not possible, the rectal or sublingual routes should be considered in preference to the traditional use of subcutaneous and intramuscular routes. Repeated use of the subcutaneous and intramuscular routes are painful to the patient and may cause tissue trauma. In addition, the lag time between injection and absorption into the circulation makes these injection routes less desirable alternatives (AHCPR, 1992).

The intravenous route can be used by the nurse or self-administered by the patient using intravenous patient-controlled analgesia (PCA). The most common method of PCA allows the patient to self-dose intravenously by pushing a button that is attached via a cord to an infusion device. The infusion device can be programmed for the patient to self-administer doses of opioid without becoming overly sedated (AHCPR, 1992). Other forms of PCA are subcutaneous, intramuscular, and epidural.

Intraspinal opioids can be administered in a variety of ways:

- Single-dose epidural or intrathecal
- Intermittent scheduled dose epidural or intrathecal
- Intermittent patient-controlled epidural (PCEA) or intrathecal
- Continuous infusion of opioid alone or in combination with local anesthetic epidural or intrathecal
- Continuous infusion plus patient-controlled opioid alone or in combination with local anesthetic (American Pain Society, 2003)

The **epidural** route requires insertion of a small catheter into the space located just before the dura mater. An opioid, or a combination of opioid and local anesthetic, is delivered using an infusion device. The opioids diffuse across the dura mater and bind at opioid receptors. The local anesthetic selectively blocks sensory nerve fibers that make up the spinal nerve roots, acting as a neural blockade. The spinal nerve roots pass through the epidural space to the spinal cord, thus making the epidural space a convenient place to infuse drugs. Combinations of opioid and local anesthetic agents are used to modulate the transmission of pain at different sites. This route requires low doses of analgesic, whether administered alone or in combination. This route also minimizes the potential for side effects. Neural blockade provides analgesia without the central nervous system effects of sedation, drowsiness, and respiratory depression that can occur when analgesics are given systemically (oral [PO], IV, or intramuscular [IM]).

The **intrathecal** route for analgesia requires the passage of a small catheter into the cerebrospinal fluid (CSF) space. Opioid flows through the CSF and rapidly binds to opioid receptors in the spinal cord. Smaller amounts of an intrathecally administered drug are required to achieve the same effects as epidural administration. This method places the spinal cord at some degree of risk, however, because of the potential for mechanical or chemical irritation or damage. There is also a higher risk of infection than with the epidural route. Many methods are available to deliver intrathecal medications, including percutaneous catheters, implanted ports, and implanted pumps. Use of the epidural or intrathecal routes requires close communication between anesthesiology and nursing staffs and careful monitoring of the patient.

Peripheral nerve blocks and pleural infusion routes also require an anesthesiologist. When a peripheral nerve block is performed, the peripheral nerve path that is transmitting the pain is located, and local anesthetic is injected medial to the point of pain origin. The sites most frequently used for peripheral nerve blocking are the intercostal nerves medial to the insertion site of chest tubes. The duration of the analgesia depends on the half-life of the local anesthetic that has been injected.

The pleural infusion route primarily is used when multiple rib fractures are present. A small catheter is placed into the pleural space (between the visceral and parietal pleura) and a local anesthetic is injected. By administering a local anesthetic via this route, multiple intercostal nerves can be blocked at one time without repeated needlesticks to the skin.

Whenever local anesthetics are administered, it is important for the health care provider to monitor the patient for systemic anesthetic toxicity. Signs and symptoms of this complication include a 25 percent drop in baseline heart rate, tinnitus, slurred speech or thick tongue, and mental confusion. Table 2–5 provides a comparison of pharmacologic pain interventions.

Nonpharmacologic (Complementary) Interventions

Nonpharmacologic therapies, often referred to as complementary therapies, can be used concurrently with medications to manage pain. The role of the clinician is to assist the patient in identifying effective alternative interventions to be systematically incorporated into the care plan. All clinicians involved in the patient's care have a role in providing the necessary support for utilization of these therapies as outlined in the care plan. Guidelines for choice of nonpharmacologic interventions include pain problem identification, effectiveness for a specific patient, and the skill of the clinician. Table 2–6 lists examples of nonpharmacologic interventions for the management of pain.

The AHCPR (1992) guidelines support use of nonpharmacologic interventions in patients who

- Find such an intervention appealing
- May benefit from avoiding or reducing drug therapy (e.g., history of adverse reactions; fear of or physiologic reason to avoid oversedation)
- Have incomplete pain relief following appropriate pharmacologic intervention
- Are likely to experience and need to cope with a prolonged period of postoperative pain, particularly if punctuated by recurrent episodes of intense treatment or procedure-related pain
- Express anxiety or fear, as long as the anxiety is not incapacitating or secondary to a medical or psychiatric condition that has a more specific treatment

The last three guidelines could apply to many high-acuity patients; thus, nonpharmacologic interventions should be seriously considered in this patient population.

In summary, effective pain management requires the use of pharmacologic as well as nonpharmacologic interventions. To increase effectiveness of the analgesic response, medications can be given by a variety of routes and in combination with other medications. The use of nonpharmacologic interventions can also modulate the analgesic response. Health care providers are encouraged to explore which interventions (both pharmacologic and nonpharmacologic) have been used by the patient in the past when formulating a plan of care for decreasing pain.

TABLE 2–5 Pharmacologic Interventions

INTERVENTION	COMMENTS
Nonsteroidal Anti-inflammatory Drugs (NSAIDs)	
Oral (alone)	Effective for mild-to-moderate pain. Begin preoperatively. Relatively contraindicated in patients with renal disease and risk of or actual coagulopathy. May mask fever.
Oral (adjunct to opioid)	Potentiating effect resulting in opioid sparing.
	Begin preop. Cautions as above.
Parenteral (ketoralac)	Effective for moderate to severe pain. Expensive. Useful where opioids contraindicated, especially to avoid respiratory depression and sedation. Advance to opioid.
Opioids	
Oral	As effective as parenteral in appropriate doses. Use as soon as oral medication tolerated. Route of choice.
Intramuscular	Has been the standard parenteral route, but injections painful and absorption unreliable. Hence, avoid this route when possible.
Subcutaneous	Preferable to intramuscular when a low-volume continuous infusion is needed and intravenous access is difficult to maintain. Injections painful and absorption unreliable. Avoid this route for long-term repetitive dosing.
Intravenous	Parenteral route of choice after major surgery. Suitable for titrated bolus or continuous administration (including PCA), but requires monitoring. Significant risk of respiratory depression with inappropriate dosing.
PCA (systemic)	Can be used for intravenous, subcutaneous, and epidural routes. Good steady level of analgesia. Popular with patients but requires special infusion pumps and staff education.
Epidural and intrathecal	When suitable, provides good analgesia. Requires careful monitoring. Use of infusion pumps requires additional equipment and staff education.
Local Anesthetics	
Epidural and intrathecal	Effective regional analgesia. Opioid sparing. Addition of opioid to local anesthetic may improve analgesia. Risks of hypotension, weakness, numbness. Requires careful monitoring. Use of infusion pump requires additional equipment and staff education.
Peripheral nerve block	Limited indications and duration of action. Effective regional analgesia. Opioid sparing. May be used as a one-time injection or with a continuous infusion through a catheter.

Adapted from AHCPR. (1992). Acute pain management: Operative or medical procedures and trauma. Clinical practice guideline. *Rockville, MD: Agency for Health Care Policy and Research, Public Health Service, U.S. Department of Health and Human Services. ACHPR Pub. No. 92–0032.*

TABLE 2–6 Nonpharmacologic Interventions

Simple Relaxation (begin preoperatively)	
Interventions:	Jaw relaxation, progressive muscle relaxation, and simple imagery
Comments:	Effective in reducing mild to moderate pain and as an adjunct to analgesic drugs for severe pain. Use when patients express an interest in relaxation. Requires 3 to 5 minutes of staff time for instructions.
Intervention:	Music
Comments:	Effective for reduction of mild to moderate pain. Requires skilled personnel.
Complex Relaxation (begin postoperatively)	
Intervention:	Biofeedback
Comments:	Effective in reducing mild to moderate pain and operative site muscle tension. Requires skilled personnel and special equipment.
Intervention:	Imagery
Comments:	Effective for reduction of mild to moderate pain. Requires skilled personnel.
Education/Instruction (begin preoperatively)	
Comments:	Effective for reduction of pain. Should include sensory and procedural information and instruction aimed at reducing activity-related pain. Requires 5 to 15 minutes of staff time.
TENS (transcutaneous electrical nerve stimulation)	
Comments:	Effective in reducing pain and improving physical function. Requires skilled personnel and special equipment. May be useful as an adjunct to drug therapy.

Adapted from AHCPR. (1992). Acute pain management: Operative or medical procedures and trauma. Clinical practice guideline. *Rockville, MD: Agency for Health Care Policy and Research, Public Health Service, U.S. Department of Health and Human Services. ACHPR Pub. No. 92–0032.*

SECTION FIVE REVIEW

1. The World Health Organization (WHO) Analgesic Ladder provides the clinician with
   A. general pain management choices based on level of pain
   B. nonpharmacologic interventions based on level of pain
   C. specific pain management choices based on severity of pain
   D. pharmacologic and nonpharmacologic pain management choices
2. Which of the following statements is correct regarding nonopioid therapy?
   A. nonopioids have more severe side effects than opioids
   B. nonopioids are harder to access than opioids
   C. nonopioids can manage pain as effectively as opioids
   D. combining opioids and nonopioids enhances analgesia effectiveness
3. The most common route used for PCA is
   A. intramuscular
   B. intravenous

C. subcutaneous
D. epidural
4. A major advantage of using the epidural route for analgesia is that it
   A. can be accessed by the nurse
   B. uses only nonopioid analgesics
   C. blocks a specific peripheral nerve path
   D. provides analgesia without CNS side effects
5. The guidelines for choosing appropriate nonpharmacologic interventions include (choose all that apply)
   1. skill of clinician
   2. effectiveness for patient
   3. type of opioid being used
   4. pain problem identification
   A. 1, 2, and 3
   B. 2 and 4
   C. 1, 2, and 4
   D. 2 and 3

Answers: 1. A, 2. D, 3. B, 4. D, 5. C

SECTION SIX: Issues in Inadequate Treatment of Acute Pain

At the completion of this section, the learner will be able to discuss issues related to the undertreatment of pain.

Definitions

It is important to differentiate among tolerance, dependence, and addiction, terms that are misused and have potentially negative connotations. These terms are defined as follows:

- **Tolerance.** A common physiologic result of chronic opioid use; it means that a larger dose of opioid is required to maintain the same level of analgesia (AHCPR, 1994)
- **Physical dependence.** A physical adaptation of the body to the presence of opioids, existing when rapid drug withdrawal produces signs and symptoms (Hawthorn & Redmond, 1998)
- **Psychological dependence (addiction).** A pattern of compulsive drug use characterized by a continued craving for an opioid and the need to use the opioid for effects other than pain relief (or other medical indications) (AHCPR, 1994)
- **Opioid pseudoaddiction.** A term applied to patients who develop behaviors that mimic those associated with addiction. The individual may be labeled as drug craving or drug seeking. Pseudoaddiction, however, results from inadequate

pain management, not psychological dependence. A variety of responses are noted in patients who experience unrelieved pain, from acceptable drug-seeking to pathologic behaviors. Unfortunately, it is often extremely difficult for nurses and physicians to discriminate between these two types of behaviors, particularly in situations in which patient–physician/ nurse contact is limited, such as in the emergency department. Behaviors that suggest undertreatment of pain but are frequently misread as drug seeking rather than pain relief seeking include demands for different or more pain medications that escalates, clock watching, preoccupation with obtaining pain medications, anger, and others (ASAM, 2001; ASPMN, 2002). Pseudoaddiction results in a patient's distrust and suspicion of staff and avoidance of the patient by staff (ASPMN, 2002). Pseudoaddiction is distinguishable from actual addiction by resolution of aberrant behaviors when pain is relieved (ASAM, 2001).

Reasons for Opioid Undertreatment of Pain

Inadequate treatment of pain is a complex problem that is based on misconceptions widely held by physicians, nurses, and patients. The practice of treating pain with minimal drug use is known as **oligoanalgesia** (Kurtz, 2003). Physicians underprescribe opioids by two methods: prescribing subtherapeutic doses and prescribing time intervals for drug doses that are less than the pharmacologic duration of action. Nurses undertreat pain by administering less than what the patient can receive per physician orders and administering opioids at longer intervals than prescribed. Minimal drug use for the treatment of pain is called oligoanalgesia. Patients often contribute to their own undertreatment of pain by not requesting as needed (PRN) pain medications, taking medication at longer-than-ordered intervals, taking less than the amount prescribed, or refusing to take the drug at all (McCaffery & Pasero, 1999).

There are four common misconceptions regarding opioid use that contribute to inadequate treatment: fear of addiction, physical dependence, tolerance, and respiratory depression.

Fear of Addiction (Psychological Dependence)

Fear of addiction is probably the major cause of undertreatment of pain. The term **opiophobia** has been used to describe the irrational fear of prescribing (or consuming) adequate amounts of opiates for therapeutic results. In fact, very few hospitalized patients who receive opioids become addicted; as the pain subsides, so does the use of the opioids. The term **addiction** should be used with extreme caution. The indiscriminate labeling of a person who uses drugs as being an addict carries a strong social stigma that may label an individual negatively (McCaffery & Pasero, 1999). The National Institute of Drug Abuse (NIDA) in its Research Report Series, has this to say regarding use of opioids in treating pain:

> Most patients who are prescribed opioids for pain, even those undergoing long-term therapy, do not become addicted to the drugs. The few patients who do develop rapid and marked tolerance for and addiction to opioids usually have a history of psychological problems or prior substance abuse. In fact, studies have shown that abuse potential of opioid medications is generally low in healthy, nondrug-abusing volunteers. One study found that only 4 out of about 12,000 patients who were given opioids for acute pain became addicted. In a study of 38 chronic pain patients, most of whom received opioids for 4 to 7 years, only 2 patients became addicted, and both had a history of drug abuse. (NIDA, 2002)

Fear of Physical Dependence

Some of the fear associated with physical dependence is generated from the belief that opioid withdrawal is life-threatening, the symptoms associated with physical dependence are difficult to control, and the presence of symptoms of physical dependence prevent decreases in opioid doses as the pain decreases. In addition, many people believe that addiction is the natural progression of physical dependence. It is true that any patient who receives repeated doses of opioids is at risk for some degree of withdrawal symptoms if the opioid is suddenly stopped. These symptoms, however, can be effectively managed by gradual reduction in opioid dosage as the patient's pain subsides (McCaffery & Pasero, 1999).

Fear of Tolerance

Fear of tolerance is usually seen in patients with long-term pain associated with either a disease process or painful treatments (e.g., patients with burns, cancer, or life-threatening illnesses). Patients, physicians, and nurses have expressed fear that opioids lose their effectiveness over time and may not work when really needed. A part of this fear is the belief in an imaginary dose ceiling, beyond which the patient cannot be taken. In fact, this feared dose ceiling does not seem to exist. As tolerance to an opioid develops, so does the patient's tolerance to the side effects of sedation and respiratory depression. Tolerance is treated by decreasing the dose interval or increasing the dose. Nursing management should focus on patient education about the concept of tolerance, and monitoring for the therapeutic and nontherapeutic effects of the adjusted dosage (McCaffery & Pasero, 1999).

Fear of Respiratory Depression

Physicians and nurses are particularly sensitive to the fear of respiratory depression. All opioids have the capability of causing respiratory depression, yet it need not be a life-threatening problem and should not prevent therapeutic opioid use. In the majority of hospitalized patients, respiratory depression has not been shown to be a significant problem. Nursing management should focus on close observation of the patient's response. **Sedation** develops before respiratory depression; therefore, the nurse should observe and document the patient's sedation level (e.g., wide awake, drowsy, dozing intermittently, mostly sleeping, or awakens only when aroused). Respiratory depression is dose related, and low doses are generally considered safe. It is impossible, however, to know what dose of an opioid will cause respiratory depression in any given patient. It is more important to watch the individual's response, especially to the first dose (McCaffery & Pasero, 1999).

Nursing Approach in Acute Pain Management

The way in which an analgesic is used is probably more important than which drug is used (McCaffery & Pasero, 1999). In the acute care setting, the nurse maintains significant control over how analgesics are used. Nursing activities that have an impact on therapeutic pain management include the following:

- Selecting an appropriate opioid or nonopioid from the analgesics ordered
- Evaluating when to administer the analgesic
- Evaluating how much analgesic to administer
- Obtaining a change in prescription when required

Effective pain management requires objective assessment skills and specific knowledge of opioids and nonopioids. In addition, the nurse must individualize the care plan to best meet the patient's individual comfort needs.

There are two major approaches to effective pain management: the preventive and the titration approaches.

Preventive

Using the preventive approach, analgesics are administered before the patient complains of pain. For example, when pain is occurring consistently over a 24-hour period, administering analgesics on a regular around-the-clock (ATC) schedule is more effective than administering them as needed (PRN). This method helps to maintain a consistent therapeutic level of analgesic in the bloodstream. Administering pain medication on a PRN basis can cause prolonged delays in treating the patient's pain. If PRN analgesia is to be used, it is important for the clinician to know the half-life and effectiveness of the medication being administered in order to predict when the patient is likely to need another dose. Maintaining awareness of pain by offering pain medication on a routine basis is more effective for pain control than requiring the patient to ask for medication (PRN). The patient may wait for the pain to become severe before requesting analgesia, or the clinician may be delayed in getting the drug to the patient. Either situation makes adequate pain relief more difficult to obtain.

There are times when PRN administration is an acceptable option, for example, changing to PRN late in the postoperative course to help decrease side effects; or when the pain is incidental, intermittent, or unpredictable (AHCPR, 1992; McCaffery & Pasero, 1999). In addition, PRN analgesics may be used as supplemental doses to regularly scheduled analgesics, primarily when a certain known activity causes pain (i.e., ambulation, sitting up in a chair, coughing, and deep breathing).

As the patient's advocate, it is recommended that the nurse be alert to the patient's comfort status and be proactive in consulting with the physician regarding changing the PRN order to ATC if a more effective analgesia schedule is required. The nurse also has an important role in educating the patient and family regarding effective analgesia scheduling.

Titration

The titration approach calls for adjusting and individualizing therapy based on the effects the drug is having on the patient rather than the milligrams being administered. The goal is to gain the desired level of pain relief with minimum side effects. When using this approach, the clinician should consider the following:

- **Dose.** Analgesic potency helps provide a rational basis for choosing the appropriate starting dose (AHCPR, 1992).
- **Interval between doses.** Assess the patient regarding the amount of time it takes for the pain to increase. For example, if the nurse is administering an analgesic every 4 hours and the patient notices that the pain increases quickly after 3 hours, the interval should be changed to 3 hours.
- **Route of administration.** Use a conversion chart for equal analgesic dosing when switching from one route to another (see Table 2–7). Dosing conversion factors based on relative potency estimates may differ between patients (AHCPR, 1992).
- **Choice of drug.** Opioids are classified as full (pure) opioid agonists, partial agonists, or mixed agonist–antagonists. Full agonists are more potent than partial agonists. Agonist–antagonists activate one type of opioid receptor and at the same time block another type (AHCPR, 1992). Withdrawal-like symptoms can occur when switching a patient from a pure agonist to an agonist–antagonist.

In summary, undertreatment of pain results from misconceptions regarding addiction, physical dependence, tolerance, and respiratory depression. These misconceptions may be held by physicians and nurses, as well as by patients. Effective pain management can be approached using two methods: the preventive and titration approaches. The preventive approach focuses on "staying on top" of the pain, whereas the titration approach emphasizes the patient's response to therapy rather than dose and interval between doses. The PRN approach for pain management is not recommended except in specific situations.

TABLE 2–7   Equianalgesic Doses of Selected Opioids

DRUG	TRADE NAME	ROUTES	EQUIANALGESIC DOSE (MG)	DURATION (HOURS)
Morphine	Generic	IM/IV	10	4–6 (IM)
		PO/R	60	4–7
Hydromorphone	Generic; Dilaudid	IM/IV	1.5	4–5 (IM)
		PO/R	7.5	4–6
Codeine	Generic; 2 APAP; Tylenol 3, etc.	IM/IV	130	4–6 (IM)
		PO	200[a]	4–6
Oxycodone	Generic; w/APA; Percocet w/ASA; Percodan	PO	30	3–5
Fentanyl	Generic; Sublimaze; Duragesic	IM/IV	0.1	1–2
		Topical		
Oxymorphone	Numorphan	IM	1	4–6
		R	10	4–6
Meperidine[b]	Generic; Demerol	IM/IV	75	4–5 (IM)
		PO	300	4–6

[a]The dose of codeine may be lowered when administered as a combination product containing aspirin or acetaminophen, which work synergistically.
[b]Meperidine has very limited use, as the toxic metabolite, normeperidine, builds to unacceptable levels in the CNS.

SECTION SIX REVIEW

1. A common physiologic consequence of chronic opioid use that results in a person's requiring an increasing dose of opioids to maintain the same level of analgesia is the definition of
   A. pseudoaddiction
   B. tolerance
   C. psychologic dependence
   D. physical dependence
2. Which of the following statements is correct regarding opioid use and respiratory depression?
   A. respiratory depression precedes the onset of sedation
   B. respiratory depression worsens as tolerance develops
   C. sedation occurs before respiratory depression
   D. respiratory depression is a common problem in hospitalized patients
3. PRN analgesics are appropriately used in which situations? (choose all that apply)
   1. when pain is intermittent

   2. when pain is consistent
   3. when pain is unpredictable
   4. when used as a supplement to scheduled doses
   A. 2, 3, and 4
   B. 1, 3, and 4
   C. 2 and 3
   D. 1, 2, and 3
4. When the titration approach to pain management is used, the emphasis is on
   A. the patient's analgesic response
   B. total milligrams per day
   C. physical dependence
   D. psychological dependence

Answers: 1. B, 2. C, 3. B, 4. A

SECTION SEVEN: Pain Management in Special Patient Populations

At the completion of this section, the learner will be able to identify considerations associated with pain management in special populations.

Several important patient-focused factors influence acute pain management. These factors include age, concurrent medical disorders, and history of substance abuse. A basic understanding of these factors helps to facilitate effective pain management.

Pharmacology and Aging

The relationship that exists between aging and adverse drug reactions is much more ambigious and complex than once thought (Gurwitz & Avorn, 2001). Chronologic age does not have a direct relationship with deterioration of organ function; thus aging individuals vary greatly in their capacity to absorb, metabolize, and excrete drugs. It can be stated, however, that as a group, older adults are at higher risk for drug toxicity than younger adults for a variety of reasons (Fig. 2–6). Drug reactions may be dose related or the result of the drug's interaction at the cellular level. Older adults tend to take more drugs, including analgesics, on a long-term basis often related to the presence of chronic illnesses that require drug therapy. These medications may interact, producing symptoms. Older adults tend to have less body water and increased body fat. Less body water causes high blood levels of water-soluble drugs because of decreased distribution volume. Increased body fat causes prolonged effects of fat-soluble drugs because of increased distribution volume in fat tissue. Other complicating factors that increase the risk of adverse reactions or subtherapeutic dosing include the fact that short-term memory impairment may cause a person to take incorrect dosages, miss doses, or take multiple doses. Impaired vision may lead to overdosage. Impaired agility in opening containers may encourage a patient to miss a dose. Financial factors as well as limited transportation may keep the patient from filling prescriptions.

In obtaining a medication history, the nurse should ask about prescription and over-the-counter (OTC) preparations, OTC supplements, alcohol, caffeine, and tobacco use; and home remedies. The nurse should be aware that certain drugs often prescribed for older adults, such as diuretics, anticholinergics, and sedatives, have a great number of undesirable side effects in this patient population. In assessing the older adult, symptoms suggesting drug toxicity frequently include delirium, depression, worsening dementia, orthostatic hypotension, falls, and incontinence, rather than the more commonly seen nausea, vomiting, diarrhea, and rash.

According to Katzung (2001), opioid use in the older adult is associated with variable alterations in pharmacokinetics. This patient population is particularly at risk for respiratory depression; thus opioids should be initiated with caution until sensitivity is determined. Studies have shown that opioids are underutilized in older patients who could significantly benefit from their use. Katzung suggests that there is no justification for this underutilization if opioids are administered according to an appropriate pain management plan.

Box 2-1   Pain Cultural Considerations

Cultural Group	Expressions of Pain and Nursing Considerations
American Indians/ Native Americans	*Expressions of pain:* Understated; often general (e.g., "I don't feel so good"); if verbalizes discomfort but does not get pain relief, may not speak of discomfort again. May speak of pain to close family or friends who can relay message to staff.
	Nursing Consideration: Follow up with patient who makes general statements of discomfort and intervene accordingly. Consider asking family or close friends about patient's comfort level.
Black/African Americans	*Expressions of pain:* Often overt; pain scales can be effective measure of pain levels.
	Nursing Considerations: May be disinclined to use analgesics because of fear of addiction.
Chinese Americans	*Expressions of pain:* Understated; may not verbalize complaints of pain.
	Nursing Considerations: Observe patient closely for presence of nonverbal cues suggesting pain. Offer analgesia rather than waiting for patient request.
Mexican Americans	*Expressions of pain:* Understated; may not verbalize complaints of pain. In men, verbalization of pain may be viewed as a weakness. Women may express pain but are frequently stoic.
	Nursing Considerations: Observe patient closely for presence of nonverbal cues suggesting pain.
Arab Americans	*Expressions of pain:* Overt, particularly with close family or friends. Pain is feared and to be avoided. May speak of pain in metaphors (e.g., knives, fire).
	Nursing Consideration: Explain benefits of tests and procedures. High pain tolerance for procedures when knowledgeable about benefits. Often prefer analgesic injections rather than oral medications.

Data from Lipson, J. G., Dibble, S. L., & Minarik, P. A. (2002). Culture & nursing care: A pocket guide. *San Francisco: UCSF Nursing Press.*

Patients with Concurrent Medical Disorders

High-acuity patients frequently have more than one dysfunctioning organ at any single time. Impaired function of the liver and kidneys has serious implications for analgesic therapy. Analgesics are primarily metabolized in the liver, with a small percentage being excreted unchanged. The kidneys have the major responsibility for opioid excretion. When either of these organs has decreased functioning, serum drug levels increase, placing the patient at increasing risk for the development of adverse effects.

Certain opioids (e.g., morphine) are converted into polar glucuronidated metabolites in the liver and then excreted through the kidneys. The glucuronidated metabolites maintain analgesic capabilities that may be stronger than the actual opioid. If kidney function is significantly impaired, these metabolites may accumulate in the blood, resulting in prolonged and deeper analgesia. This can compromise the patient by precipitating severe respiratory depression, deep sedation, or intractable nausea. Meperidine, a synthetic opioid, may also accumulate in the presence of renal dysfunction or when high doses are used. Normeperidine, the metabolite of meperidine, is associated with CNS stimulation, which can precipitate tachycardia and seizure activity. The risk of seizures increases as normeperidine levels increase (Way et al., 2001). The half-life of normeperidine is 15 to 20 hours, which is significantly longer than that of the parent compound meperidine (3 to 8 hours); thus, adverse effects caused by elevated levels of normeperidine can remain for a prolonged period in patients with liver or kidney dysfunction (Deglin & Vallerand, 2002). When kidney or liver impairment is present, doses of most opioids must be reduced and the patient monitored closely for the development of accumulative effects.

Patients who have been receiving long-term opioid therapy for chronic pain are at risk for undertreatment of acute pain as a result of opioid drug tolerance. In such cases, the opioid dose requirements may be significantly higher than what is usually recommended (or needed) to reach a satisfactory level of analgesia. A thorough pain history provides valuable information regarding the potentially altered dose requirements of this patient population.

The Known Active or Recovering Substance Abuser as Patient

Pain management of the high-acuity patient who is either an active or recovering substance abuser has important nursing implications. Substance abusers experience traumatic injuries and a variety of health problems more often than the general popu-

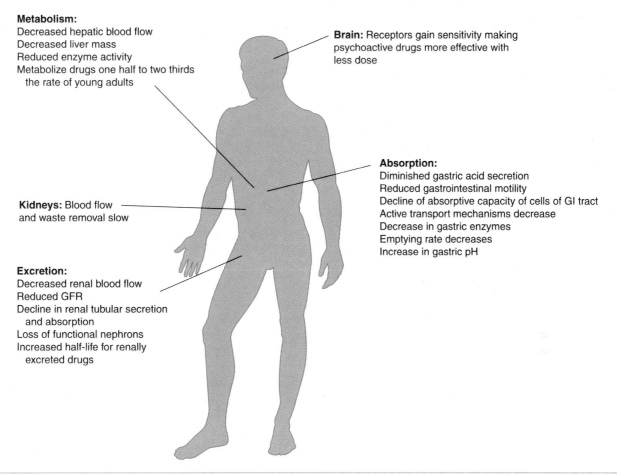

Metabolism:
Decreased hepatic blood flow
Decreased liver mass
Reduced enzyme activity
Metabolize drugs one half to two thirds
   the rate of young adults

Brain: Receptors gain sensitivity making
psychoactive drugs more effective with
less dose

Absorption:
Diminished gastric acid secretion
Reduced gastrointestinal motility
Decline of absorptive capacity of cells of GI tract
Active transport mechanisms decrease
Decrease in gastric enzymes
Emptying rate decreases
Increase in gastric pH

Kidneys: Blood flow
and waste removal slow

Excretion:
Decreased renal blood flow
Reduced GFR
Decline in renal tubular secretion
   and absorption
Loss of functional nephrons
Increased half-life for renally
   excreted drugs

Figure 2–6 ■ Pharmacologic-related alterations in the aging body.

lation (AHCPR, 1992). Pain management of the substance abuser constitutes a challenge for physicians and nurses. This section presents a brief overview of some of the issues and nursing implications related to dealing with pain in the substance-abusing patient.

An Ethical Dilemma

The American Society of Pain Management Nurses (ASPMN, 2002) views addiction as a treatable disease that is chronic and relapsing. It is characterized by uncontrolled, compulsive use and overconsumption of substances despite known harmful effects. Treating pain in this population poses a dilemma that is largely attributable to the medical maxim, "do no harm." Can and should pain in addicted patients be treated using substances that are in themselves addicting, thereby potentially contributing to the addiction? Experts in the fields of pain and addiction answer "yes" to this question. All people, regardless of whether they are substances abusers, have the right to have their pain relieved; thus relief of pain temporarily overrides the problem of addiction (ASAM, 2001; ASPMN, 2002; NCI, 2003; Prater et al., 2002).

Drug-Seeking and Pain Relief-Seeking Behaviors

It can be extremely difficult to evaluate whether a person's behaviors are drug seeking or pain relief seeking, particularly in health care settings where there is often limited assessment and evaluation time involved, such as walk-in clinics and emergency departments (Kurtz, 2003). However, it is also true that pain relief-seeking and drug-seeking behaviors are often interchangeable when pain is not adequately relieved, regardless of whether a person is an active substance abuser.

Health care providers should be aware of maladaptive behaviors that suggest active addiction. Table 2–8 lists some of the more common maladaptive behaviors. The problem of discriminating between pseudoaddiction and addiction-driven behaviors may become even more difficult if the person has previously experienced inadequate pain relief when seeking medical help (Prater et al., 2002). Previous negative pain relief-seeking experiences tend to foster more maladaptive behaviors that can be misconstrued by the health care team and perpetuate suspicion and distrust, and encourage the practice of oligoanalgesia. One way to differentiate between drug-seeking and pain relief-seeking behaviors is that

TABLE 2–8 Maladaptive Behaviors Suggestive of Active Addiction

Individual Actions

Drug hoarding during periods of reduced symptoms

Injecting oral medications

Unapproved use of other psychotropic drugs during opioid therapy

Concurrent abuse of alcohol

Evidence of use of illegal drugs (cocaine, marijuana, heroin)

Risk-taking behaviors while using psychotropic medications

Frequent signs of intoxication: significant impairment of physical, mental, or social skills

Social Interactions

Selling drugs

Stealing or borrowing drugs from others

Continued dosing in spite of significant side effects or consequences that are due to the drug and not to the pain or the condition causing the pain (e.g., alienation of friends or family, inability to work)

Physician/Nurse Interactions

Requesting specific drugs

Losing medication

Looking for pain medication at first visit to a new physician

Seeking medication for new sources of pain or unapproved use of the drug to treat other symptoms

Unwillingness to comply with full treatment plan (e.g., utilization of nonopioid pain management techniques)

Overwhelming concerns about the continued availability of the opioid being used

Unsanctioned dose escalation

Prescription Related

Prescription forgery

Using multiple pharmacies

Obtaining prescription drugs from nonmedical sources

From Prater, C. D., Zylstra, R. G., & Miller, K. E. (2002). *Successful pain management for the recovering addicted patient.* Journal of Clinical Psychiatry, *4(4):125–131.* Copyright 2002, Physicians Postgraduate Press. Adapted by permission.

pseudoaddiction behaviors cease when pain relief is achieved, whereas addiction behaviors continue when the primary motivation is drug seeking rather than pain relief (Kurtz, 2003; Prater et al., 2002). It is crucial then, to closely observe and document changes in behavior prior to and during pain relief interventions.

Major Considerations in Pain Management

Kurtz (2003) emphasizes the importance of not confusing physical dependence with the addiction when considering how best to manage pain in the active or the recovering addict. Although treatment may renew physical dependence, it does not necessarily foster a relapse to active addiction (Heit, 2002). In fact, failure to relieve pain increases the likelihood of relapse (Kurtz, 2003). Stress is known to increase substance craving and inadequate pain relief often increases stress, which may result in an escalation of substance use in the acute abuser or relapse in the recovering abuser. Although managing pain in this population may be difficult, it is not impossible. Employing recommendations of experts, such as those developed by the ASPMN, can be useful in guiding medical and nursing pain interventions in this population. Table 2–9 provides a list of recommendations based on ASPMN's position paper, *Pain Management in the Patient with Addictive Disease.*

Clinical Management Considerations

NCI (2003) offers guidelines that can be applied to pain treatment of the high-acuity patient with a history of substance abuse:

- Involve a multidisciplinary team
  - Substance abuse is complex and requires interdisciplinary care, such as pain expert physicians, nurses, social workers and, if available, an addiction medicine expert.
- Set realistic goals for therapy
  - The risk of relapse increases with the heightened stress associated with life-threatening disease. Prevention of relapse may be impossible, requiring altered goal setting for management to include structured therapy, support, and limit setting.
- Evaluate and treat comorbid psychiatric disorders
  - The substance abuser is at extreme risk for anxiety, personality disorders, and depression. Presence of these disorders may require treatment during acute disease states.
- Prevent or minimize withdrawal symptoms
  - Obtain a complete drug history, keeping in mind that many patients abuse multiple drugs. Laboratory drug screening tests can provide a baseline of currently abused substances. Health care professionals should be familiar with the manifestations of commonly abused substances (see Table 2–10).

TABLE 2–9   Recommendations of the ASPMN

Recommendations for all patients with addictive disease:

- Identify and use resources available to assist in the diagnosis and treatment of both addiction and pain.
- Encourage the patient to use support systems, such as family, significant others, or a rehabilitation sponsor; offer additional resources, such as an addiction counselor.
- Involve the patient in pain management planning and, with the patient's consent, include family and significant others.
- Provide the patient with verbal and written information on the pain management plan, including what the patient can expect from caregivers and what the patient's responsibilities are.
- Ensure consistency in the implementation of the pain management plan.
- Educate the patient, family, and significant others on the differences among addiction, physical dependence, and tolerance.
- Help the patient make informed choices regarding medications by educating the patient, family, and significant others on medication options.
- Select and titrate analgesics based on pain assessment, side effects, and function, as well as sleep and mood.
- Be prepared to titrate opioid analgesics and benzodiazepines to doses higher than usual. The patient may have developed tolerance to some medications, or drug use may have caused sensitivity to pain.
- Benzodiazepines, phenothiazines, or other sedating medications that do not relieve pain should not be used as substitutes for analgesics.
- If pain is present most of the time, provide analgesics around the clock.
- Use the oral route and long-acting analgesics when possible.
- Consider the use of IV or epidural patient-controlled analgesia for acute pain management.
- Record and discuss with the patient any behavior suggestive of inappropriate medication use, especially of controlled substances.
- When opioids, benzodiazepines, or other medications with a potential for physical dependence are no longer needed, taper them very slowly to minimize withdrawal symptoms.
- Consider nonpharmacologic methods of treatment for pain, but do not use them in place of appropriate pharmacologic approaches.

Recommendations for patients who are actively using alcohol or other drugs, in addition to the recommendations for all patients with addictive disease:

- Distinguish between pseudoaddiction (an iatrogenic syndrome created by the undertreatment of pain, characterized by behaviors such as anger and escalating demands for more or different medications; distinguished from true addiction in that the behaviors resolve when pain is effectively treated) and addiction. This may be difficult in the presence of unrelieved pain.
- Assess for and treat symptoms of withdrawal from alcohol or other drugs.
- If the patient acknowledges inappropriate use of prescribed medications or nonprescribed substances, openly discuss this and encourage the patient to express any fear of how this may affect pain management and treatment by staff.
- Assess for psychiatric comorbidity, such as anxiety and depression, and obtain treatment if needed.
- If the patient is physically dependent on morphine-like opioids, do not treat pain with opioid agonist–antagonists, such as nalbuphine, butorphanol, buprenorphine, or pentazocine, because it will precipitate acute withdrawal.
- Once pain is controlled, provide information on options for treatment of addictive disease.

Recommendations for patients in recovery, in addition to the recommendations for all patients with addictive disease:

- Explain any intent to use opioids or other psychoactive medications.
- Explain the health risks associated with unrelieved pain, including increased risk of relapse.
- Encourage the patient, family, and significant others to discuss concerns about relapse, and offer assistance.
- Respect the patient's decision about whether to use opioids or other psychoactive medications. Reassure the patient that other methods of pain relief, such as nonsteroidal anti-inflammatory drugs and regional or local anesthetics, can be used if the patient prefers not to use opioid analgesics.
- Encourage a therapeutic plan in case relapse occurs.
- If relapse occurs, intensify recovery efforts; do not terminate pain care.

Recommendations for patients on methadone maintenance treatment, in addition to the recommendations for all patients with addictive disease:

- Initiate and continue regular discussions of the pain management plan with methadone treatment providers.
- Methadone doses used for methadone maintenance in the treatment of opioid addiction should be continued but not relied on for analgesia. When opioid analgesics are appropriate for pain management, two options are available:
  1. Add another opioid on an around-the-clock basis, or
  2. Give additional methadone doses. Methadone given for analgesia must be given more than once a day.

Visit the ASPMN Web site for tools for assessing withdrawal, protocols for treatment of withdrawal, the risks of unrelieved pain, treatment options for addictive disease, and therapeutic plans in case of relapse.

Adapted with permission of the American Society of Pain Management Nurses.

TABLE 2–10   Commonly Abused Substances and Withdrawal Manifestations

SUBSTANCE	COMMON EXAMPLES	COMMON STREET NAMES	WITHDRAWAL ONSET AND MANIFESTATIONS
Opiates (CNS depressant)	Codeine, hydromorphone (Dilaudid), morphine, oxycodone (Percodan), others Heroin, opium	Morphine: morph, M Dilaudid: little D, dillies, lords Percodan: percs Heroin: horse, smack, H Opium: hop, tar	**Onset:** 4–6 hours following last dose **Manifestations:** Mild initially and becoming more severe; dilated pupils, runny nose, diarrhea, abdominal pain, chills, gooseflesh, insomnia, aching joints and muscles, nausea and vomiting, muscle twitching and tremors (may become severe), mental depression
Alcohol (CNS depressant)	Many	Liquor, beer, booze, wine	**Onset:** 12–48 hours **Manifestations:** Headache, anxiety, depression, nervousness, shakiness, irritability, depression, fatigue, clouded thinking, emotionally labile; GI: nausea, vomiting, anorexia; CV: heart palpitations; EENT: enlarged, dilated pupils; skin: clammy, pale, sweaty palms; musculoskel: tremors, abnormal movements **Severe (complicated) withdrawal:** Rapid muscle tremors, seizures, tachycardia, cardiac dysrhythmias, profuse sweating, hallucinations, others
Barbiturates (CNS depressant)	Phenobarbital, pentobarbital	Barbs, red devils, goof balls, yellow jackets, downers	**Onset:** 12–20 hours following last dose **Manifestations:** Similar to alcohol withdrawal in the absence of alcohol; other mental changes: blank facial expression, slurred speech, flat affect; severe withdrawal can result in respiratory and heart failure, seizures, and death
Cocaine (CNS stimulant)	None	Coke, blow, snow, nose candy	**Onset:** 4–8 hours **Manifestations:** Few physical withdrawal symptoms; strong psychological symptoms, including rapid onset of depression, fatigue/sleepiness, strong craving for more cocaine, loss of pleasure; may also experience paranoia, agitation
Amphetamines (CNS stimulant)	Methylphenidate (Ritalin), pemoline (Cylert)	Speed, uppers, dexies, crank, meth, ice, crystal	**Onset:** 4–8 hours **Manifestations:** Depression, severe craving, mental confusion, insomnia, restlessness, paranoia, possible psychosis

From Prater, C. D., et al. (2002). Successful pain management for the recovering addicted patient. Journal of Clinical Psychiatry, 4(4): 125–131. Copyright 2002, Physicians Postgraduate Press. Adapted by permission.

- Consider the impact of tolerance
  - Substance abusers may require significantly higher doses (one-and-a-half times or more) of analgesia to achieve the same level of pain relief as a nonabuser (Kurtz, 2003). This varies widely among individuals.
- Apply appropriate pharmacologic principles to treat chronic pain
  - Analgesic dose individualization is an important principle; focusing on dose size rather than pain relief achievement may result in pain undertreatment and subsequent development of pseudoaddiction behaviors.
- Recognize specific drug abuse behaviors (see Table 2–8)
- Use nondrug approaches as appropriate
  - These may include further patient education, relaxation and coping techniques, and other complementary pain relieving interventions.

Other clinical pain management suggestions include the following:

- Avoid (if possible) analgesics that have the same pharmacologic basis as the abused drug. For example, heroin is a form of opiate.
- Choose extended-release and long-acting analgesics (e.g., fentanyl and methadone) rather then short-acting ones and restrict short-acting opiates for breakthrough pain (Kurtz, 2003).
- Avoid naloxone (Narcan) unless life-threatening toxic effects are present because use of naloxone will precipitate immediate opiate withdrawal (Kurtz, 2003)
- Administer analgesics orally rather than intravenously when possible

In summary, certain patient populations need special consideration when managing the analgesic response. To manage pain effectively in the older adult, the clinician must consider the possible physiologic changes associated with aging. Medication doses must often be adjusted on the basis of metabolic and analgesic responses. Concurrent medical problems complicate pain management, particularly the presence of impaired liver or kidney function. Finally, treatment of pain in the known substance abuser requires special consideration to be able to differentiate between drug-seeking and pain-avoidance behaviors. Guidelines are available for better assurance of positive outcomes in treatment of pain in the patient with a history of substance abuse.

SECTION SEVEN REVIEW

1. Older patients have fewer endogenous receptors and neurotransmitters than younger patients. The primary clinical significance of this statement is
   A. larger doses of opioids are required to achieve pain relief
   B. pain relief using opioids is more unpredictable
   C. smaller doses of opioids are required to achieve pain relief
   D. pain relief using opioids is less effective

2. Accumulation of morphine metabolites in the blood because of renal dysfunction can cause
   A. severe respiratory depression
   B. seizures
   C. tachycardia
   D. CNS stimulation

3. Accumulation of the metabolite of meperidine (normeperidine) in the blood can result in
   A. severe sedation
   B. bradycardia
   C. severe respiratory depression
   D. seizures

4. The known substance abuser who is hospitalized
   A. should receive no opioids
   B. may require higher-than-usual opioid dose ranges
   C. should receive only one type of opioid
   D. may require lower-than-usual opioid dose ranges

5. True or False: Substance abusers may require significantly higher doses of analgesia to achieve the same level of pain relief as a nonabuser.

6. Amphetamine withdrawal is associated with which manifestation?
   A. depression
   B. nausea and vomiting
   C. severe headache
   D. muscle twitching

Answers: 1. C, 2. A, 3. D, 4. B, 5. True, 6. A

POSTTEST

The following posttest is constructed in a case study format. A patient is presented, and questions are asked based on available data. New data are presented as the case study progresses.

Marcos M, 32 years old, was involved in a pedestrian–car crash in which he sustained multiple injuries. It is now 4 days after open reduction of his left femur and left humerus; a splenectomy was also necessary. He is complaining of severe sharp pain at his abdominal incision site.

1. His sharp pain is transmitted through
   A. A fibers
   B. B fibers
   C. C fibers
   D. D fibers

2. Marcos's acute pain sensation is transmitted up the spinal cord and terminates in the
   A. thalamus
   B. substantial gelatinosa
   C. cerebral cortex
   D. brainstem

It is now 1 week postinjury. Marcos's wounds are healing well, but he continues to require pain management.

3. The type of pain that Marcos is most likely experiencing at this time is
   A. brief acute
   B. acute persistent
   C. chronic
   D. chronic intermittent

4. Which of the following statements is correct regarding suffering?
   A. it is related to the personal meaning of pain
   B. it is measurable
   C. it is associated with acute pain
   D. it bears no relationship to stress and anxiety

The nurse notes that Marcos continues to be in a high-anxiety state and continues to require analgesia at regular intervals.

5. The relationship between pain and anxiety is
   A. anxiety increases pain tolerance
   B. anxiety decreases pain complaints
   C. anxiety decreases pain-related stress
   D. anxiety increases pain perception

6. If Marcos's stress response becomes too high, it can result in (choose all that apply)
     1. counterregulation of hormone responses
     2. decreased vascular shunting
     3. hypoperfusion of vital organs
     4. elevated levels of blood endorphins
   A. 2, 3, and 4
   B. 1, 3, and 4
   C. 2 and 3
   D. 1, 2, and 3

The nurse notes that Marcos is becoming increasingly agitated, and he has begun rhythmically hitting his right foot on the rail of the bed.

7. The nurse's initial intervention should consist of
   A. administering his ordered analgesic
   B. contacting the physician
   C. having him indicate his pain level on a VAS
   D. documenting his new behaviors
8. The best method of assessing Marcos for pain is by
   A. self-report
   B. facial cues
   C. vital sign changes
   D. body posturing behaviors

Marcos is bilingual, with Spanish as his first language. His understanding of spoken English is only fair and he states that he does not read English well.

9. Based on Marcos's language status, which of the following assessment approaches would be most valid (assuming all assessments are written in English)?
   A. Short-Form McGill
   B. VAS/NRS
   C. McGill Pain Questionnaire
   D. nurse observation
10. Marcos describes his pain as being severe and sharp. He is grimacing and continues to tap his foot on the bed rail. The nurse assigns him a pain intensity score of 8/10 (8 out of a possible 10). This method of assigning a score is
   A. probably accurate in reflecting his pain level
   B. an acceptable alternative pain assessment tool
   C. acceptable only under special circumstances
   D. an inappropriate use of a unidimensional tool

Marcos is complaining of pain at a level of 7/10. The nurse notes that his vital signs are normal and he is watching television. He is requesting pain medication.

11. Based on this new information, the nurse should
   A. contact the physician
   B. wait for 1 hour and recheck his vital signs
   C. administer his ordered analgesic
   D. suspect that he is exaggerating

Marcos has the following pain management orders: morphine 10 mg (IM) every 3 to 4 hours PRN; ibuprofen 400 mg (PO) every 6 hours.

12. Marcos's combination pain therapy is ordered for which primary purpose?
   A. to enhance the level of analgesia
   B. to increase sedation effects
   C. to decrease respiratory depressive effects
   D. to significantly reduce opioid dose

Marcos is switched to intravenous PCA.

13. The primary advantage for switching Marcos from injections to intravenous PCA is that PCA
   A. decreases the number of painful injections
   B. allows Marcos to gain some control over his analgesia
   C. decreases the frequency of patient assessment
   D. reduces the risk of severe respiratory depression
14. If the epidural route for analgesia had been chosen, the nurse would focus the pain assessment on the degree of
   A. sedation
   B. respiratory depression
   C. pulse decrease
   D. pain relief

Marcos indicates that he is interested in trying some nonpharmacologic interventions.

15. The AHCPR guidelines support use of nonpharmacologic interventions in patients who (choose all that apply)
     1. are comatose
     2. have prolonged pain
     3. express anxiety or fear
     4. would benefit from reducing drug therapy
   A. 2, 3, and 4
   B. 1, 2, and 3
   C. 2 and 3
   D. 1, 3, and 4

Marcos has been receiving morphine on a regular basis for several weeks. He is now complaining that the usual dose he has been receiving is no longer relieving his pain as effectively.

16. Assuming nothing has changed in Marcos's condition, the nurse would suspect that Marcos is
   A. exaggerating his level of pain
   B. becoming psychologically dependent
   C. developing tolerance to the morphine
   D. needing to have the morphine discontinued
17. The term *pseudoaddiction* refers to behaviors that mimic those associated with addiction but are motivated by
   A. drug craving
   B. drug tolerance
   C. PRN drug administration
   D. pain undertreatment
18. Marcos is refusing to take any more morphine because he is afraid he will stop breathing. The nurse teaches Marcos about opioid therapy based on which facts? (choose all that apply)
     1. opioid use places him at high risk for respiratory depression
     2. sedation occurs before respiratory depression

3. respiratory depression is dose related
4. his level of sedation and respiratory rate will be closely monitored

A. 2, 3, and 4
B. 1, 2, and 3
C. 2 and 3
D. 1, 3, and 4

19. If Marcos develops renal function impairment while receiving morphine, he will need to be monitored closely for

A. tachycardia
B. severe tachypnea
C. seizure activities
D. severe respiratory depression

POSTTEST ANSWERS

Question	Answer	Chapter Section	Question	Answer	Chapter Section
1	A	One	11	C	Four
2	C	One	12	A	Five
3	B	Two	13	B	Five
4	A	Two	14	D	Five
5	D	Three	15	A	Five
6	B	One	16	C	Six
7	C	Four	17	D	Six
8	A	Four	18	A	Six
9	B	Four	19	D	Seven
10	D	Four			

REFERENCES

AHCPR [Agency for Health Care Policy and Research]. (1992). *Acute pain management: Operative or medical procedures and trauma. Clinical Practice Guideline No. 1.* Rockville, MD: U.S. Department of Health and Human Services. [AHCPR Publication No. 92-0032.]

AHCPR [Agency for Health Care Policy and Research]. (1994). *Management of cancer pain. Clinical Practice Guideline No. 9.* Rockville, MD: U.S. Department of Health and Human Services. [AHCPR Publication No. 94-0592.]

American Pain Society. (2003). *Principles of analgesic use in the treatment of acute pain and cancer pain* (5th ed.). Glenview, IL: Author.

American Pain Society Quality of Care Committee. (1995). Quality improvement guidelines for treatment of acute pain and cancer pain. *JAMA: Journal of the American Medical Association, 274*(23), 1874–1880.

ASAM (2001). American Academy of Pain Medicine. Public Policy of ASAM: Definitions related to use of opioids in pain treatment. Available at: *www.asam.org/ppol/paindef.htm.* Accessed February 11, 2004.

ASPMN [American Society of Pain Management Nurses]. (2002). ASPMN position statement: Pain management in patients with addictive disease. Available at: *www.aspmn.org/html/PSaddiction.htm.* Accessed February 11, 2004.

Carey, S. J., Turpin, C., Smith, J., et al. (1997). Improving pain management in an acute care setting. *Journal of Orthopedic Nursing, 16*(4), 29–36.

Chapman, C. R., & Syrjala, K. L. (1990). Measurement of pain. In J. J. Bonica (Ed.), *The management of pain, Vol. 1* (2nd ed., pp. 480–594). Philadelphia: Lea & Febiger.

Curtis, S., Kolotylo, C., & Broome, M. E. (2002). Somatosensory function and pain. In C. M. Porth (Ed.), *Pathophysiology: Concepts of altered health states* (6th ed., pp. 1091–1122). Philadelphia: J. B. Lippincott.

Deglin, J. H., & Vallerand, A. H. (2002). *Davis's drug guide for nurses* (7th ed.). Philadelphia: F. A. Davis.

Ferrell, B. R., McCaffery, M., & Grant, M. (1991). Clinical decision making and pain. *Behavior Research and Therapy, 30*(1), 71–73.

Gelinas, C., Fortier, M., Viens, C. et al. (2004). Pain assessment and management in critically ill intubated patients: A retrospective study. *American Journal of Critical Care, 13*(2), 126–135.

Gurwitz, J. H., & Avorn, J. (2001). The ambiguous relation between aging and adverse drug reactions. *Annals of Internal Medicine, 114*(11), 956–966.

Guyton, A. C., & Hall, J. E. (1997a). Pain, headache, and thermal sensations. In A. C. Guyton & J. E. Hall (Eds.), *Human physiology and mechanisms of disease* (6th ed., pp. 392–399). Philadelphia: W. B. Saunders.

Guyton, A. C., & Hall, J. E. (1997b). Sensory receptors; neuronal circuits for processing information; tactile and position senses. In A. C. Guyton & J. E. Hall (Eds.), *Human physiology and mechanisms of disease* (6th ed., pp. 376–391). Philadelphia: W. B. Saunders.

Hawthorn, J., & Redmond, K. (1998). *Pain: Causes and management.* Malden, MA: Blackwell Science.

Heit, H. A. (2002, December). The best methods of managing pain in the recovering patient. *Counselor, 3*(6), 28–32.

Katzung, B. G. (2001). Special aspects of geriatric pharmacology. In B. G. Katzung (Ed.), *Basic & clinical pharmacology* (8th ed., pp. 1025–1035). New York: McGraw Hill/Appleton & Lange.

Kurtz, D. R. (2003). Managing acute pain in admitted or suspected substance abusers. *Physician Assistant, 27*(7), 36–44.

Loeser, J. D., & Cousins, M. J. (1990). Contemporary pain management. *The Medical Journal of Australia, 153,* 208–212, 216.

Ludwig-Beymer, P., & Huether, S. (1996). Pain, temperature, sleep, and sensory function. In S. E. Huether & K. L. McCance (Eds.). *Understanding pathophysiology,* (pp. 319–345). St. Louis: Mosby.

McCaffery, M., & Pasero, C. (1999). *Pain: Clinical manual for nursing practice* (2nd ed.). St. Louis: C. V. Mosby.

Melzack, R., & Wall, P. (1965). Pain mechanisms: A new theory. *Science, 150*(699), 971–979.

Milgrom, L. B., Brooks J. A., & Qi, R., et al. (2004). Pain levels experienced with activities after cardiac surgery. *Amerian Journal of Critical Care, 13,* 116–125.

NCI [National Cancer Institute]. (2003). Cancer.gov-Substance abuse issues in cancer (PDQ®). Available at: *www.cancer.gov/cancerinfo/pdq/supportivecare/substanceabuse/patient.* Accessed February 11, 2004.

NIDA [National Institute on Drug Abuse]. (2002). Research report series—Prescription drugs: Abuse and addiction. Pain and opiophobia. National Institute on Drug Abuse, National Institutes of Health. Available at: *www.drugabuse.gov/ResearchReports/Prescription/Prescription6a.html.* Accessed August 8, 2004.

Payen, J. F., Bru, M. D., Bosson, J. L., et al. (2001). Assessing pain in critically ill sedated patients by using a behavioral pain scale. *Critical Care Medicine, 29*(12), 2258–2263.

Prater, C. D., Zylstra, R. G., & Miller, K. E. (2002). Successful pain management for the recovering addicted patient. *Journal of Clinical Psychiatry, 4*(4), 125–131.

Puntillo, K., & Ley, S. J. (2004). Appropriately timed analgesics control pain due to chest tube removal. *American Journal of Critical Care, 13*(4), 292–304.

Stephenson, N. A. (1994, September/October). A comparison of nurse and patient perceptions of postsurgical pain. *Journal of Intravenous Nursing, 17,* 235–239.

Wall, P. D., & Melzack, R. (Eds.). (1994). *Textbook of pain* (3rd ed.). New York: Churchill Livingstone.

Way, W. L., Fields, H. L., & Schumacher, M. A. (2001). Opioid analgesics and antagonists. In B. G. Katzung (Ed.), *Basic and clinical pharmacology* (8th ed., pp. 512–531). New York: McGraw Hill/Appleton & Lange.

World Health Organization. (1996). *Cancer pain relief* (2nd ed.). Geneva, Switzerland: Author.

ADDITIONAL READINGS

Cohen, I. L., Gallagher, T., James, M. D., Pohlman, A. S., Dasta, J. F., et al. Management of the agitated intensive care unit patient. (2002). *Critical Care Medicine, 30*(1)(suppl), S97–S123.

Joint Commission on Accreditation of Healthcare Organizations (JCAHO). (2001). *Pain: Current understanding of assessment management and treatments.* Oakbrook Terrace, Illinois: Joint Commission Resources, Inc.

Joint Commission on Accreditation of Healthcare Organizations (JCAHO). (2003). *Improving the quality of pain management through measurement and action.* Oakbrook Terrace, Illinois: Joint Commission Resources, Inc.

Kahn, D. L., & Steeves, R. H. (1986). The experience of suffering: Conceptual clarifications and theoretical definition. *Journal of Advanced Nursing, 11,* 623–631.

Nichols, R. (2003). Pain management in patients with addictive disease. *American Journal of Nursing, 103*(3), 87–90.

Salmore, R. (2002). Development of a new pain scale: Colorado behavioral numerical pain scale for sedated adult patients undergoing gastrointestinal procedures. *Gastroenterology Nursing, 25*(6), 257–262.

MODULE 3

Fluid and Electrolyte Balance in the High-Acuity Patient

Valerie Sabol, Kathleen Dorman Wagner

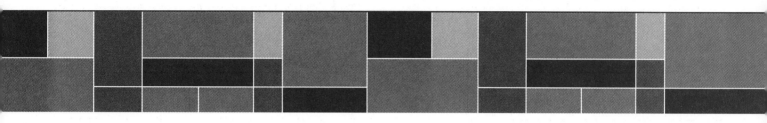

OBJECTIVES Following the completion of this module, the learner will be able to

1. Discuss the distribution of body fluids.
2. Describe the regulation of fluid balance.
3. Discuss fluid imbalance, including edema, third spacing, fluid volume deficit, and fluid volume excess.
4. Discuss the nursing implications associated with fluid imbalances.
5. Discuss the extracellular compartment electrolyte, sodium.
6. Describe the extracellular compartment electrolyte, chloride.
7. Discuss the extracellular compartment electrolyte, calcium.
8. Discuss the intracellular compartment electrolyte, potassium.
9. Describe the intracellular compartment electrolyte, magnesium.
10. Discuss the intracellular compartment electrolyte, phosphorus (phosphate).

The focus of this module is on the physiologic and pathologic processes involved in fluid and electrolyte balance. Maintenance of fluid and electrolyte balance is a major goal in improving the outcomes of patients with diverse health problems. Therefore, in many of the text's modules, fluid and electrolyte balance is addressed as it applies to specific module topics.

This module is composed of 10 distinct sections. Sections One and Two present the concepts of body fluid distribution and fluid balance regulation. Section Three focuses on fluid imbalances, including edema, third spacing, and fluid volume deficit and excess. Section Four describes nursing implications associated with fluid imbalance problems. In Sections Five

through Seven, specific extracellular electrolytes are discussed: sodium, chloride, and calcium. Sections Eight through Ten address three major intracellular electrolytes: potassium, magnesium, and phosphorus. Discussion of each electrolyte includes major functions, causes, and clinical manifestations of imbalances.

Each section includes a set of review questions to assist the learner in evaluating his or her understanding of the section's content before moving on to the next section. All Section Reviews and the module Pretest and Posttest include answers. It is suggested that the learner review those concepts answered incorrectly in the review questions before proceeding to the next section.

PRETEST

1. Two thirds of total body fluid is in which of the following compartments?
   A. intracellular
   B. extracellular
   C. intravascular
   D. interstitial

2. The elderly patient is at increased risk for developing a fluid volume problem related to
   A. high metabolic rate
   B. diminished renal function
   C. inability to concentrate urine
   D. greater ratio of surface area to volume

3. Which of the following electrolytes are found predominantly in the extracellular fluid?
   A. potassium
   B. magnesium
   C. phosphate
   D. sodium

4. Which of the following is the primary regulator of water intake?
   A. nervous system
   B. endocrine system
   C. renal system
   D. hypothalamus

5. The sympathetic nervous system responds to decreased volume by producing
   A. antidiuretic hormone (ADH)
   B. adrenocorticotropic hormone (ACTH)
   C. vasoconstriction
   D. aldosterone

6. When the hypothalamus senses a decrease in serum sodium or potassium, it responds by stimulating the pituitary to release
   A. renin
   B. aldosterone
   C. ADH
   D. ACTH

7. A low serum osmolality may suggest
   A. fluid volume deficit
   B. fluid volume overload
   C. dehydration
   D. isotonic balance

8. The most common cause of edema resulting from increased capillary hydrostatic pressure is
   A. liver failure
   B. congestive heart failure
   C. immune reactions
   D. burn injury

9. Nursing assessment data found in the patient with fluid volume excess would include
   A. low pulmonary artery wedge pressure (PAWP)
   B. increased hematocrit
   C. moist crackles
   D. decreased blood pressure

10. Which of the following intravenous solutions closely approximates serum osmolality?
    A. 0.45 percent normal saline
    B. 5 percent dextrose in normal saline
    C. lactated Ringer's
    D. 3 percent normal saline

11. Signs and symptoms of hypernatremia include
    A. diarrhea
    B. muscle twitching
    C. stomach cramps
    D. decreased muscle tone

12. Hyponatremia is associated with which of the following symptoms?

A. edema
B. hyperreflexia
C. lethargy
D. restlessness

13. Chloride levels closely follow the levels of which of the following electrolytes?
    A. potassium
    B. sodium
    C. calcium
    D. magnesium

14. Calcium is absorbed in the intestines under the influence of
    A. phosphorus
    B. vitamin D
    C. sodium
    D. vitamin C

15. Hypocalcemia is associated with which of the following clinical findings?
    A. tingling and numbness
    B. constipation
    C. lethargy
    D. shortened QT interval

16. The presence of hypokalemia alters renal excretion of potassium in which of the following ways?
    A. urine output increases
    B. potassium excretion increases
    C. potassium is reabsorbed
    D. potassium excretion does not change

17. The normal range of serum magnesium is
    A. 1.5 to 2.5 mEq/L
    B. 3.5 to 5.3 mEq/L
    C. 4.5 to 5.5 mEq/L
    D. 135 to 145 mEq/L

18. The symptoms of hypomagnesemia reflect
    A. central nervous system (CNS) hypoactivity
    B. fluid compartment shifts
    C. cardiac depressant effects
    D. neuromuscular and CNS hyperactivity

19. Hypophosphatemia is associated with which of the following conditions?
    A. malnourished state
    B. metabolic alkalosis
    C. hypocalcemia
    D. hyperthyroidism

20. Severe hypophosphatemia is associated with which of the following symptoms?
    A. joint pain
    B. muscle cramping
    C. respiratory arrest
    D. peptic ulcer disease

Pretest Answers:
1. A, 2. B, 3. D, 4. D, 5. C, 6. D, 7. B, 8. B, 9. C, 10. C,
11. B, 12. C, 13. B, 14. B, 15. A, 16. D, 17. A, 18. D, 19. A,
20. C

GLOSSARY

anions   Negatively charged ions.

atrial natriuretic peptide (ANP)   An amino acid produced and stored in the myocytes of the atria. ANP is released from the myocytes under certain conditions, such as atrial distension. Elevated serum levels result from congestive heart failure (CHF) and hypervolemic states.

baroreceptors   Pressure receptors located in the arch of the aorta and carotid sinus that detect arterial pressure changes.

cations   Positively charged ions.

dilutional effect   Net gain of water in the extracellular spaces.

electrolytes   Electrically charged microsolutes found in body fluids.

extracellular   Fluid compartment within the body composed of plasma and interstitial fluid.

hypertonic   A high-osmolarity state in which the concentration of particles is greater on one side of a membrane than the other side of the membrane; in the body, the solution has a higher osmolarity than exists inside of the cells.

hypervolemia   Excess volume of circulating fluids.

hypotonic   A low-osmolarity state in which the concentration of particles in a solution is greater on one side of a membrane than the other side of the membrane; in the body, the solution has a lower osmolality than exists inside of the cells

hypovolemia   Decreased volume of circulating fluids.

intracellular   Fluid compartment within the body's cells; composes approximately two thirds of the total body water.

intravascular   Fluid compartment in the blood vessels; fluid is available for exchange of nutrients and oxygen.

isotonic   The concentration of particles in a solution on one side of a membrane is the same as it is on the other side of the membrane; in the body, it closely approximates normal serum plasma osmolality.

osmosis   The net diffusion of water from an area of greater concentration to an area of lesser concentration across the cell membrane; occurs as the result of osmotic pressure.

osmolality   The solute concentration per volume of a solution (refers to body fluids).

osmolarity   The solute concentration per volume of a solution (refers to outside of body).

serous cavity   A body cavity that is lined with serous membrane (e.g., pericardial sac, pleural, peritoneal).

tonicity   Osmolarity of an intravenous fluid.

ABBREVIATIONS

ACTH	Adrenocorticotropic hormone	**ICF**	Intracellular fluid
ADH	Antidiuretic hormone	**IV**	Intravenous
ATP	Adenosine triphosphate	**K**	Potassium
BUN	Blood urea nitrogen	**Mg**	Magnesium
Ca	Calcium	**mOsm**	Milliosmole
Cl	Chloride	**Na**	Sodium
CNS	Central nervous system	**PAWP**	Pulmonary artery wedge pressure
CVP	Central venous pressure	**PO$_4$**	Phosphate
DKA	Diabetic ketoacidosis	**PTH**	Parathyroid hormone
ECF	Extracellular fluid	**SIADH**	Syndrome of inappropriate antidiuretic hormone

SECTION ONE: Body Fluid Distribution

At the completion of this section, the learner will be able to discuss the distribution of body fluid.

Body fluids compose about 60 percent of the body weight in the average adult male and about 50 percent in the average female. The composition of body fluids is primarily water with various electrolytes, glucose, urea, and creatinine. These fluids provide both an internal and external environment for the cells, playing crucial roles as a medium for metabolic reactions, a cushion to protect body parts from injury, and an influence on regulation of body heat.

Age as a Variable Affecting Body Fluid Content

The percentage of body water diminishes as one grows older (Lemone & Burke, 2004). Greater percentages of body fluids are found in individuals with a small body surface area; thus, infants have a larger fluid reserve. Infants, however, are predisposed to serious, rapid fluid volume deficit because of their limited ability to concentrate urine, their proportionately greater ratio of surface area to volume, and their higher metabolic rate. Individuals over the age of 20 have a reduction in total fluid body weight (Metheny, 2000). The elderly patient's fluid balance is affected by alterations in thirst and nutritional intake, diminished renal function, chronic illness, and medications. The elderly are predisposed to developing fluid volume deficit related to decreased muscle mass, increased fat stores, and a reduction in percentage of body fluids.

Fluid Compartments

Body fluids are primarily found in two compartments: the **intracellular** compartment (within the cells) and the **extracellular** compartment (all other body fluids) (Fig. 3–1). About two thirds of total body fluid is intracellular and the remaining one third is extracellular. Table 3–1 summarizes water distribution in the adult.

Intracellular Compartment

The intracellular fluids (ICFs) are rich in potassium, phosphate, and protein and contain moderate amounts of magnesium and sulfate ions. Intracellular fluids provide the cells with nutrients and assist in cellular metabolism. Porth (2002) explains that ICF volume is regulated by several important mechanisms. First, the

TABLE 3–1 Water Distribution in the Body (Adult)[a]

COMPARTMENTS/ SUBCOMPARTMENTS	% BODY WEIGHT	VOLUME (LITERS)
Intracellular	40	25
Extracellular		
Interstitial	14	11
Plasma	5	3
Transcellular	1	2
TOTAL	60	41

[a]Approximate

presence of nondiffusible intracellular protein attracts fluid into the cells. Second, negatively charged ions within the cells attract positively charged ions, such as sodium (Na) and potassium (K). These two activities draw fluid into the cells, causing cellular expansion. Without the counterregulating forces provided by the Na^+/K^+ pump, the cells would rupture and die. The Na^+/K^+ pump is an active transport mechanism that exchanges Na^+ ions for K^+ ions at a ratio of 3:2; thus, more Na^+ ions are moved out of the cells than K^+ ions. Because water is attracted to Na^+ ions, more water accumulates in the extracellular compartment and ICF balance is maintained. Certain pathologic situations harm the Na^+/K^+ pump, including hypoxia and cell expansion associated with excess Na^+ ions within the cells (e.g., overload of a hypotonic saline IV fluid).

Extracellular Compartment

All body fluid outside of the cells exists in the extracellular compartment and is referred to as extracellular fluid (ECF). The major components of the ECF are plasma (**intravascular** compartment) and interstitial fluid (interstitial compartment). Plasma is the fluid portion of the blood and is composed of water (about 90 percent), plasma proteins (about 7 percent), and other substances (Gaspard, 2002). According to Porth (2002), interstitial fluid functions as a transport medium for shuttling nutrients, gases, waste products, and other substances between the blood and the body cells. It also acts as a backup fluid reservoir that can rapidly provide fluid during situations in which there is vascular fluid loss (e.g., hemorrhage). The interstitial compartment contains a spongelike substance called *tissue gel* that helps distribute interstitial fluid evenly. The gel is held together with collagen fibers. Tissue gel exerts force against the capillaries, which helps maintain fluids inside the capillaries. It also keeps free water from accumulating in the interstitial spaces. Transcellular fluid normally comprises about 1 percent of total ECF. It is located in joints, connective tissue, bones, body cavities, cerebrospinal fluid (CSF), and other tissues (Porth, 2002; Woods, 1998). A minor but potentially significant ECF component is transcellular fluid (transcellular compartment). Transcellular fluid has the potential to increase significantly when fluids become abnormally sequestered in body cavities and tissues, as occurs with third spacing.

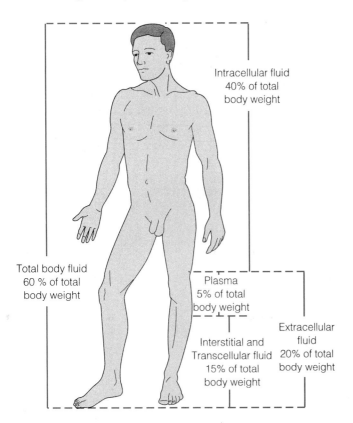

Intracellular fluid
40% of total
body weight

Total body fluid
60 % of total
body weight

Plasma
5% of total
body weight

Interstitial and
Transcellular fluid
15% of total
body weight

Extracellular
fluid
20% of total
body weight

Figure 3–1 ■ Water distribution in the adult body.

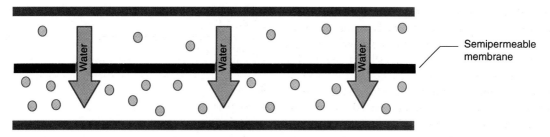

Figure 3–2 ■ Osmosis. Fluid moves across a semipermeable membrane from an area of low concentration to an area of higher concentration.

Intercompartmental Movement of Fluids

To understand intercompartmental fluid movement, it is crucial to first understand the concepts of osmosis and osmolality. The principle of **osmosis** explains the net diffusion or movement of water across the cell membrane (Fig. 3–2). Water moves across a semipermeable (or selectively permeable) cell membrane from an area of lesser concentration of solutes to an area of greater concentration of solutes. Osmosis is a passive process, requiring no expenditure of energy. Its purpose is to maintain fluid equilibrium between the fluid compartments. Water moves freely between the various fluid compartments; therefore, an alteration in one compartment produces a shift in body fluids in another compartment.

Osmolality refers to the concentration of solute in body water and reflects a patient's hydration status. The **osmolarity** of a solution is the solute (or particle) concentration per volume of water. Although osmolality is the correct term to use when referring to body fluids, osmolarity is often used because it is another way to measure concentration. However, instead of representing the number of particles per liter of water, osmolarity instead represents the number of particles per liter of solution (Porth, 2002). Measurement of the serum osmolality can be used as an approximation of the extracellular fluid volume. According to Kee (2002), osmolality is expressed in milliosmoles (mOsm), with normal serum osmolality in an adult being 280 to 300 mOsm/kg. Serum values of less than 240 mOsm/kg or more than 320 mOsm/kg are considered critically abnormal. A low serum osmolality suggests fluid volume excess or hemodilution, meaning there is more fluid than solute in the serum. A high serum osmolality suggests fluid volume deficit or hemoconcentration, meaning there is less fluid than solute in the serum. Kee (2002) suggests the following formula for determining serum osmolality:

$$\text{Serum Osm/L} = (\text{serum Na} \times 2) + \frac{\text{BUN}}{3} + \frac{\text{Glucose}}{18}$$

[For example: Given that a patient's sodium (Na) is 140 mEq/L, blood urea nitrogen (BUN) is 20 mg/dL, glucose is 250 mg/dL, using the preceding formula, it can be calculated that the serum osmolality is 301 Osm/L. This indicates that there are more particles than fluid in this patient's serum. This osmolality is slightly high, which suggests fluid volume deficit.]

Clinically, serum osmolality can be used to determine the need for fluid replacement in the high-acuity patient.

Serum osmolality may be increased or decreased in various diseases. Hyperglycemia, diabetes insipidus, and hypernatremia produce an increased serum osmolality, whereas syndrome of inappropriate antidiuretic hormone (SIADH) and certain antidiuretic hormone (ADH)-secreting carcinomas of the lung can produce a low serum osmolality. The clinical manifestations of decreased serum osmolality (fluid volume excess) are similar to those of hyponatremia and those of increased serum osmolality (fluid volume deficit) are similar to those of hypernatremia.

Through the processes of osmosis and diffusion, body fluids move freely between the interstitial and intravascular compartments. According to Porth (2002), there are four forces, called *Starling forces*, that control this movement (Fig. 3–3). The

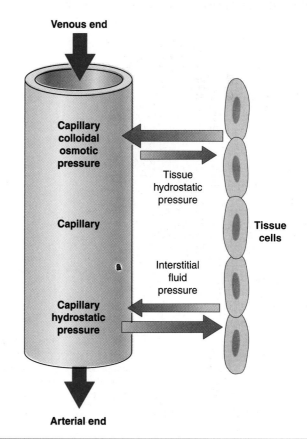

Figure 3–3 ■ Intracompartmental fluid movement.

forces include capillary hydrostatic (or filtration) pressure, capillary colloidal osmotic pressure, tissue hydrostatic pressure, and tissue fluid pressure. *Capillary hydrostatic (filtration) pressure* is the pressure exerted by fluid moving through the capillaries to push fluid out of the capillary into the interstitial space. The majority of this movement occurs at the arterial end of the capillary, where the pressure is greatest (30 to 40 mm Hg). The venous end of the capillary has a much lower pressure (10 to 15 mm Hg), and fluid is reabsorbed back into the capillary at this end. *Capillary colloidal osmotic pressure* is the pressure exerted by plasma proteins as they flow through the capillary to draw fluid into the capillary. *Interstitial fluid pressure* is the pressure exerted by fluid in the interstitial space that pushes against the capillaries, opposing shifts of fluid out of the capillaries. *Tissue hydrostatic pressure* is pressure exerted by the small amount of proteins located in the interstitial space, which attracts fluid out of the capillaries and into the interstitium. As can be seen, the opposing forces found in the capillaries and the interstitial spaces cause fluids to shift in and out of the capillaries, maintaining fluid balance between compartments and preventing excess fluid buildup in the interstitial spaces. In high-acuity patients, these forces can become unbalanced, causing abnormal fluid shifts or trapping of intravascular fluid into the interstitium, otherwise known as third spacing.

In summary, body fluids compose more than 60 percent of total body weight. Age can influence total fluid volume. Infants and the elderly are both at increased risk for imbalances in fluid volume. Two thirds of the body's fluids are found in the intracellular fluid and one third exists in the extracellular fluid compartments. Each compartment has its own functions and major electrolytes. The processes of osmosis and diffusion allow intercompartmental shifting of fluids. Fluid shifts alter serum osmolality, which is a measure of the solute concentration in body water. There are two major fluid compartments—intracellular and extracellular. The extracellular compartment can be further divided into the interstitial and intravascular compartments. The transcellular compartment is a small part of the extracellular compartment and has normally an insignificant volume of fluid but has the potential to expand under pathologic circumstances. Fluid shifts out of the intravascular compartment can disrupt homeostasis, resulting in decreased circulating volume.

SECTION ONE REVIEW

1. Two thirds of total body fluid is in which of the following compartments?
   A. intracellular
   B. extracellular
   C. intravascular
   D. interstitial
2. The elderly patient is at increased risk for developing a fluid volume problem related to
   A. high metabolic rate
   B. diminished renal function
   C. inability to concentrate urine
   D. greater ratio of surface area to volume
3. Which of the following electrolytes are found predominantly in the extracellular fluid?
   A. potassium
   B. magnesium
   C. phosphate
   D. sodium
4. The major function of tissue gel in the interstitial compartment is to
   A. shift fluid out of capillaries
   B. provide a source of electrolytes
   C. distribute fluid evenly
   D. dispose of cellular waste products
5. Which of the following statements is correct regarding a low serum osmolality?
   A. it reflects fluid volume deficit
   B. it reflects fluid volume excess
   C. it is associated with dehydration
   D. it is associated with hypernatremia
6. Capillary hydrostatic pressure is the pressure exerted by
   A. plasma proteins in the capillaries
   B. fluid in the interstitial spaces
   C. plasma proteins in the interstitial spaces
   D. fluid moving through the capillaries

Answers: 1. A, 2. B, 3. D, 4. C, 5. B, 6. D

SECTION TWO: Regulation of Fluid Balance

At the completion of this section, the learner will be able to describe the regulation of fluid balance.

Nervous System Regulation

Hypothalamus

According to Guyton and Hall (2000), the lateral area of the hypothalamus regulates body water, especially thirst and renal excretion of excess water. Cells located in the hypothalamus are sensitive to body fluid concentration (serum osmolality). Thirst is activated by an increase in serum osmolality, decreased arterial blood pressure or circulating blood volume, increased secretion of angiotensin II, and mouth dryness. Thirst is decreased by a lower-than-normal serum osmolality, decreased angiotensin II, increased circulating blood volume or arterial blood pressure, and distention of the stomach. When thirst is triggered, the conscious person responds by drinking fluids. Clinical conditions that decrease the sense of thirst or the individual's ability to respond to thirst can decrease the circulating extracellular volume. The unconscious or high-acuity patient often cannot respond to thirst signals. For this reason, in the clinical setting, the nurse needs to closely evaluate the patient's fluid status using objective data obtained through physical assessment, and urine and serum lab analysis data.

Arterial Baroreceptors

Arterial **baroreceptors** (pressure receptors) located in the arch of the aorta and carotid sinus detect arterial pressure changes. When baroreceptors sense a decrease in arterial blood pressure, they send a message to the autonomic nervous system. The sympathetic nervous system responds to this message by causing peripheral vasoconstriction. Vasoconstriction of renal arteries decreases glomerular filtration, which reduces urine output in an attempt to increase circulating blood volume. The baroreceptors trigger opposite actions if they detect increased arterial blood pressure, causing vasodilation.

Renal and Endocrine Regulation

Adrenocorticotropic Hormone

The renal and endocrine systems work synergistically to regulate blood volume. When the hypothalamus senses a decrease in serum sodium or an increase in serum potassium, it sends a message to the pituitary to release adrenocorticotropic hormone (ACTH). In response, the ACTH stimulates the adrenal cortex to release aldosterone. Aldosterone is the most potent of the mineralocorticoids and is sometimes referred to as the salt-regulating hormone. It regulates water balance by facilitating sodium reabsorption in the renal distal tubules, the collecting tubules, and collecting duct (Guyton & Hall, 2000). As sodium is reabsorbed, potassium is excreted by the kidneys. The sodium reabsorption increases circulating blood volume by increasing water reabsorption. In this way, circulating blood volume and arterial blood pressure increase.

Antidiuretic Hormone

When the hypothalamus detects a change in the concentration of body fluid, it also sends a message to the posterior pituitary to either decrease or increase the release of antidiuretic hormone (ADH), which is also called vasopressin. For example, when serum osmolality increases, ADH increases permeability of the renal distal tubules and collecting ducts, which allows a large volume of water to be reabsorbed. This results in expansion of the ECF, decreases serum osmolality, and improves arterial blood pressure and perfusion. (The ADH-regulating mechanism is further described in Module 15: Shock States.)

Renin–Angiotensin System

When sodium concentration in the ECF is decreased or blood flow through the kidneys is diminished, the kidneys release renin, a protein enzyme. In response to a drop in arterial blood pressure, renin acts on a plasma protein (renin substrate) to release angiotensin I. Angiotensin I ultimately converts to angiotensin II, a powerful vasoconstrictor. Angiotensin II also causes retention of sodium and water by the kidneys. The combination of actions results in a rapid increase in blood pressure, which improves perfusion. The renin, aldosterone, and ADH mechanisms are three endocrine responses to decreased circulating blood volume.

In summary, the nervous, renal, and endocrine systems work synergistically to maintain fluid balance. Aldosterone, ADH, and the renin–angiotensin–aldosterone cycle regulate fluid balance. When these physiologic mechanisms fail or when conditions exist that affects fluid elimination, a fluid volume imbalance occurs.

SECTION TWO REVIEW

1. Which of the following is the primary regulator of water intake?
   A. nervous system
   B. endocrine system
   C. renal system
   D. hypothalamus

2. The sympathetic nervous system responds to decreased volume by producing
   A. ADH
   B. ACTH
   C. vasoconstriction
   D. aldosterone

---

3. When the hypothalamus senses a decrease in serum sodium or potassium, it responds by stimulating the pituitary to release
   A. ACTH
   B. ADH
   C. aldosterone
   D. renin
4. When the hypothalamus senses a change in serum osmolality, it stimulates the posterior pituitary to release
   A. renin
   B. aldosterone

   C. ADH
   D. ACTH
5. Angiotensin II is a powerful
   A. diuretic
   B. vasoconstrictor
   C. thirst trigger
   D. sodium waster

Answers: 1. D, 2. C, 3. A, 4. C, 5. B

SECTION THREE: Fluid Imbalance

At the completion of this section, the learner will be able to discuss fluid imbalance, including edema, third spacing, fluid volume deficit, and fluid volume excess.

Edema

Edema refers to an accumulation of fluid in the interstitial tissues. It most commonly occurs in the extracellular compartment but can occur intracellularly if the active transport Na^+/K^+ pump fails. Edema is not a disease; rather, it is an important manifestation of some underlying problem. The mechanisms that lead to edema are interrelated and include (1) an imbalance in one or more Starling forces and/or (2) an obstruction in the lymphatic system.

Problems of Starling Forces

Increased Capillary Hydrostatic Pressure. As described in Section One, capillary hydrostatic pressure exerts force against the capillary walls, which shifts fluid out of the capillaries and into the interstitium at the arterial end of the capillary. The fluid is then reabsorbed at the venous end of the capillary (low capillary hydrostatic pressure) or is taken up by the lymphatic system. Under normal conditions, these activities maintain fluid balance. With certain pathologic conditions, the capillary hydrostatic pressure becomes abnormally increased and the fluid cannot be reabsorbed back into the capillaries at the venous end. This usually results in a localized form of edema. The most common cause of increased capillary hydrostatic pressure is congestive heart failure (CHF) as a result of increased blood volume and increased systemic venous pressure. Other causes include renal failure, prolonged standing, hepatic obstruction (portal hypertension), and decreased venous circulation (e.g., thrombophlebitis) (Mulvey & Bullock, 2000).

Decreased Capillary Colloidal Osmotic Pressure. Plasma proteins (primarily albumin) within the capillaries exert a force that draws fluid into the capillaries, counterbalancing the outward fluid movement caused by capillary hydrostatic forces. When plasma proteins are decreased, the capillary hydrostatic pressure pushes fluid out of the capillaries faster than it can be drawn in, causing generalized edema and decreased intravascular fluid volume. Examples of pathologic conditions associated with decreased plasma proteins include liver failure, starvation and protein malnutrition, and burn injury (Mulvey & Bullock, 2000).

Increased Capillary Permeability. Under certain circumstances, the capillaries develop increased permeability, which allows more fluid, plasma proteins, and other active particles to escape into the interstitial spaces (Mulvey & Bullock, 2000; Porth, 2002). This can result from loss of capillary wall integrity through injury or enlargement of capillary pores (e.g., problems causing vasodilatation) (Porth, 2002). The edema resulting from increased capillary permeability can be either localized or generalized, depending on how widespread the underlying problem is. Edema is further increased as plasma proteins escape into the interstitial spaces and begin exerting increased tissue colloidal osmotic pressure, which attracts more fluid into the area. Examples of conditions associated with increased capillary permeability include burns, inflammation, direct trauma, immune reactions, bacterial infections, and certain toxins (Guyton & Hall, 2000; Mulvey & Bullock, 2000).

Lymphatic Obstruction

Normally, the lymphatics pick up excess fluid and plasma proteins that have leaked out of the capillaries and return them to the circulation. If the lymphatics become obstructed, however, fluid and plasma proteins accumulate in the affected interstitial spaces. According to Mulvey and Bullock (2000), the most common cause of lymphatic obstruction is the surgical removal of lymph nodes as part of cancer treatment. Other pathologic conditions associated with lymphatic obstruction include lymphoma (cancer involving the lymphatic structures), and a rare parasitic disorder of the lymph vessels called filariasis (filaria nematodes) (Guyton & Hall, 2000; Mulvey & Bullock, 2000).

Regardless of the mechanism that precipitates the development of edema, fluid accumulates in the interstitial spaces in the body. As fluid shifts out of the intravascular compartment, the intravascular volume becomes depleted, causing a decrease in arterial blood pressure. When the blood pressure drops significantly, the renin–angiotensin system is activated. Sodium and water are conserved and arterioles vasoconstrict, resulting in an increase in the arterial blood pressure. In addition to accumulating in the interstitial spaces, fluid can also accumulate in the transcellular spaces, causing third spacing.

Third Spacing

According to Porth (2002), third spacing is the shift of fluid from the intravascular compartment into a "third" (transcellular) space—usually a **serous cavity**. Normally, there is no accumulation of serosal fluid in a serous cavity. The cavities usually remain empty because of balanced Starling forces and the presence of a rich lymphatic network. If, however, any of the Starling forces become imbalanced or lymphatic drainage becomes obstructed or inadequate, a significant volume of serous fluid or exudate can rapidly accumulate. As fluid fills the cavity, pressure is exerted on the soft structures in the cavity, which can result in compression of those structures (e.g., cardiac tamponade). Fluids that are sequestered in a third space are unavailable for physiologic use by the body and may accumulate rapidly because of protein-rich contents, which causes increased tissue colloidal osmotic pressure, attracting more fluids. Third spacing may occur in the peritoneal cavity, pleural cavity, and pericardial sac and is associated with underlying problems such as intestinal obstruction, liver or renal failure, and peritonitis. Clinically, third spacing manifests itself as ascites, pericardial and pleural effusions, and other conditions.

Fluid Volume Deficit

Extracellular fluid volume deficit exists when there is an abnormally low volume of body fluid in the intravascular (**hypovolemia**) or interstitial compartments. It produces a state of extracellular dehydration associated with serum hyperosmolality that can lead to intracellular dehydration as fluid shifts out of the cells to increase extracellular volume. It is a common and potentially serious problem in the high-acuity patient. Many factors can cause or contribute to development of fluid volume deficit. These factors are summarized in Table 3–2. The clinical manifestations of ECF volume deficit are presented in Section Four. Fluid volume deficit in elderly patients is exacerbated by a decreased thirst sensation, a reduction in responsiveness to ADH and kidney concentrating ability (because of decreased glomerular filtration rate), decreased serum concentrations of renin and aldosterone, and increased serum **atrial natriuretic peptide (ANP)** levels.

TABLE 3–2 Factors That Produce Fluid Volume Deficit

SOURCE OF FLUID LOSS	RELATED FACTORS
Gastrointestinal	Diarrhea, vomiting, nasogastric suction, fistulas
Urinary	Drug therapy (e.g., diuretics), uncontrolled diabetes, diabetes insipidus, diuretic phase of acute tubular necrosis (ATN)
Integumentary	Burns, diaphoresis, increased capillary permeability
Insensible	Hyperventilation, fever, hypermetabolism, tachypnea, mechanical ventilation
Other	Wound drainage

TABLE 3–3 Factors That Produce Fluid Volume Excess

SOURCE OF FLUID GAIN	RELATED FACTORS
Cardiovascular	Heart failure
Urinary	Renal failure (acute or chronic)
Hepatic	Cirrhosis
	Liver failure
Other	Cancer
	Thrombus
	Peripheral vascular disease
	Drug therapy (e.g., corticosteroids)
	High sodium intake
	Protein malnutrition

Fluid Volume Excess

Extracellular fluid volume excess, also called fluid overload, produces a state of overhydration in the intravascular (**hypervolemia**), interstitial, or transcellular compartments. It is associated with fewer contributing factors than are seen with fluid volume deficit. These factors are summarized in Table 3–3. The clinical manifestations associated with ECF volume excess are presented in Section Four.

In summary, edema is an accumulation of fluid in the interstitial spaces. It is caused by imbalances in Starling forces or lymphatic obstruction. Third spacing of fluids occurs when intravascular fluids shift into the transcellular compartment, usually a serous body cavity. Third spacing results in the development of ascites and pleural or pericardial effusions. Third spacing can occur in the presence of edema. *ECF volume deficit* is a term used to describe dehydration in the interstitial or intravascular compartments. It is associated with conditions in which there is a fluid loss in excess of fluid gain. ECF volume deficit can eventually lead to intracellular dehydration. *ECF volume excess* (fluid overload) describes a state of overhydration in the intravascular, interstitial, and, possibly, the transcellular compartments. It commonly results in edema or third spacing.

Fluid volume excess is associated with pathologic conditions in which there is a net fluid gain in relation to fluid loss.

SECTION THREE REVIEW

1. The most common cause of edema resulting from increased capillary hydrostatic pressure is
   A. liver failure
   B. burn injury
   C. immune reactions
   D. congestive heart failure
2. When capillary plasma protein levels are lower than normal, it results in
   A. increased intracellular fluid volume
   B. decreased intravascular fluid volume
   C. increased intravascular fluid volume
   D. decreased interstitial fluid volume
3. Edema resulting from escape of fluid and plasma proteins through enlarged pores in the capillary walls is caused by
   A. increased capillary permeability
   B. decreased capillary permeability
   C. increased colloidal osmotic pressure
   D. decreased tissue colloidal osmotic pressure
4. The most common cause of edema due to lymphatic obstruction is
   A. lymphatic cancer
   B. filariasis parasitic infection

C. surgical removal of lymph nodes
D. tumor compression on lymph nodes
5. Which of the following is an example of third-spaced fluids?
   A. pericardial effusion
   B. wound swelling
   C. dependent edema
   D. peripheral edema
6. Third spacing of fluids is most commonly located in
   A. joints
   B. a serous cavity
   C. the cranial vault
   D. interstitial fluid
7. Which statement is correct regarding ECF volume deficit?
   A. it can lead to transcellular expansion
   B. it can lead to intracellular expansion
   C. it is associated with low serum osmolality
   D. it is associated with high serum osmolality

Answers: 1. D, 2. B, 3. A, 4. C, 5. A, 6. B, 7. D

SECTION FOUR: Nursing Implications

At the completion of this section, the learner will be able to describe the nursing implications associated with fluid imbalances.

Clinical Manifestations of Edema and Third Spacing

If a hemodynamically significant volume of fluid escapes from the intravascular compartment into the interstitial or transcellular spaces, the high-acuity patient is at high risk for developing clinical manifestations consistent with hypovolemia or hypovolemic shock. (Hypovolemia and hypovolemic shock are discussed in detail in Module 15: Shock States.) Edema and third spacing can be described in terms of certain characteristics, including location, whether it is pitting or nonpitting, and amount of fluid weight gain.

Location

Determining whether the edema is localized or generalized gives important clues as to its possible origin because pathologic conditions are usually associated with one or the other. Generalized edema is present all over the body and is primarily seen in the presence of decreased plasma proteins resulting from severe protein malnutrition. Localized edema results from a more localized pathologic condition, for example, local inflammation and infection. Sometimes, however, generalized edema develops secondary to a localized process that has expanded, causing widespread damage to the capillary endothelium and generalized edema. Examples of severe conditions in which this form of secondary generalized edema can occur are septic and anaphylactic shock.

Localized edema is confined to areas in which the causative condition is affecting the capillaries or lymph tissues (e.g., the area of inflammation, obstruction, or high capillary hydrostatic pressure). The edema associated with congestive heart failure is considered localized because it is confined to the gravity-dependent body areas (e.g., feet, lower legs, and sacrum).

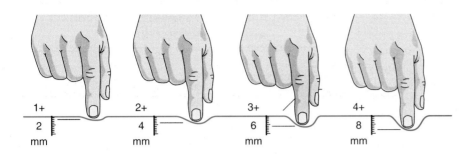

Figure 3–4■ Assessment for pitting edema. *(Reprinted from Seidel et al. (2003).* Mosby's Guide to Physical Examination, *(5th ed.),* Figure 14-15, *Copyright 2003 with permission from Elsevier.)*

Pulmonary edema caused by left-sided heart failure is localized edema created by increased capillary hydrostatic pressure in the lungs as a result of elevated left heart pressures.

The exact clinical manifestations associated with edema and third spacing depend on their location. For example, a patient with pulmonary edema or pleural effusion is at risk for developing pulmonary gas exchange problems, usually hypoxemia. A patient with cerebral edema is at risk for cerebral herniation, which is a life-threatening complication that clinically presents as a rapid deterioration of the patient's level of consciousness, visual, motor, and respiratory status. Edema around a joint reduces range of motion or immobilizes the joint. Severe edema can compress capillary blood flow, causing tissue ischemia and pain. A patient with ascites may develop problems with gas exchange as fluid in the peritoneal cavity begins to displace the diaphragm upward or impede diaphragmatic movement. A patient with pericardial effusion may develop signs of circulatory shock in the presence of cardiac tamponade.

Pitting or Nonpitting Edema

Pitting edema develops when the accumulation of fluid exceeds what can be absorbed by the interstitial tissue gel (Porth, 2002). Firm pressure applied to the edematous area displaces the interstitial fluid, causing a temporary pitting (Fig. 3–4). It can be measured on a scale of 1 to 4 based on the depth and the length of time it takes for the indentation to disappear.

- +1: 2 mm indentation, disappears rapidly;
- +2: 4 mm indentation, disappears in 10 to 15 seconds;
- +3: 6 mm indentation, disappears within 1 to 2 minutes;
- +4: 8 mm indentation; disappears in 2 to 5 minutes (Porth, 2002; Timby, 2004)

Body Weight

In the adult, peripheral edema develops when 5 L or more of fluid have accumulated in the interstitial spaces, and pitting edema develops with an accumulation of 10 L or more of interstitial fluid. Clinically, a weight gain or loss of 1 kg (2.2 lbs) represents a fluid gain or loss of about 1 L (Larocca & Otto, 1997). Evaluating daily weight trends provides valuable information on fluid status.

Assessment of third-spaced fluids is more difficult because the serous cavities are deep structures, particularly the pericar-

dial sac and pleural cavity. A thorough evaluation is necessary and may include a comprehensive physical examination, chest or abdominal radiography, electrocardiogram, echocardiogram, and others. Ascites can involve fluid shifts that are hemodynamically significant. For this reason, close evaluation of arterial blood pressure and serum albumin is important. In addition, daily weights and abdominal girth measurements provide valuable trending data.

Assessment of Fluid Volume Deficit

Assessing the high-acuity patient for the presence of fluid volume deficit is an important part of the daily nursing assessment. Table 3–4 summarizes common clinical assessments. High-acuity patients with fluid volume deficit require close monitoring and additional fluids to achieve and maintain a balanced intake and output.

TABLE 3–4 Nursing Assessment of a Patient with Fluid Volume Deficit

ASSESSMENT	DATA
Physical assessment	Mental status changes Weight loss Poor skin turgor Dry mucous membranes Flattened neck veins
Vital signs	Orthostatic changes Decreased blood pressure Rapid, weak, thready pulse Rapid, shallow respirations Temperature may be elevated Low CVP and PAWP Decreased cardiac output
Laboratory data	Elevated hematocrit Elevated BUN (normal creatinine) High serum osmolality
Urine	Increased osmolality Increased specific gravity Decreased volume

Nursing interventions may include measures to decrease vomiting, diarrhea, or fever; increasing oral fluid intake or administration of intravenous solutions; and monitoring of fluid and electrolyte status. Desired patient outcomes include pulse, blood pressure, central venous pressure (CVP), and pulmonary artery wedge pressure (PAWP) within acceptable ranges for the patient; normal serum osmolality; increased urine output with normal specific gravity; improved skin turgor; balanced intake and output; stable weight; moist mucous membranes; hematocrit and blood urea nitrogen (BUN) within acceptable limits; and absence of other dehydration manifestations.

Older patients may experience fluid volume deficit from high-acuity problems, such as pneumonia and urinary tract infections. Excessive water loss from fever, sweating, and tachypnea may occur more readily because younger patients are better protected by a normal thirst response. However, mobility restrictions and even the use of restraints (e.g., for safety) may limit access to fluids. Additionally, older patients may suffer fluid losses because of self-restriction of fluids to prevent incontinence and overuse of laxatives to prevent constipation.

Assessment of Fluid Volume Excess

ECF volume excess can be generalized or localized. The assessment procedures are essentially the same as those used for assessing for fluid volume deficit. The findings, however, are almost in complete opposition, with the exception of urinary output. A low urine output can be indicative of either a deficit or an excess. For example, a low urine output (less than 30 mL/hr) may be indicative of dehydration or renal failure. Decreased urinary output in the patient with dehydration is actually a protective mechanism for the body to reserve volume. Decreased urinary output in the patient with renal failure, however, causes fluid volume excess. Nursing assessment of the patient for fluid volume excess is summarized in Table 3–5.

Nursing interventions may include fluid or salt restrictions; administration of diuretics; or dialysis. The desired patient outcomes for intravascular fluid excess include pulse, blood pressure, CVP, and PAWP within acceptable ranges for the patient; lung sounds clear to auscultation; balanced intake and output; weight loss and resolution of edema; and hematocrit and BUN within acceptable limits.

Use of Intravenous Fluids to Manage Fluid Volume Imbalances

High-acuity patients frequently require fluid or electrolyte support through use of intravenous (IV) fluid administration. IV fluids are classified according to their osmolarity or tonicity. **Tonicity** refers to the effect the solution has on the ECF and ICF compartments (see Fig. 3–5). Intravenous solutions are classified as isotonic, hypotonic, or hypertonic. Table 3–6 provides examples of common intravenous solutions classified by tonicity.

TABLE 3–5 Nursing Assessment of the Patient with Fluid Volume Excess

ASSESSMENT	DATA
Physical assessment	Mental status changes
	Weight gain
	Distended neck veins
	Periorbital edema, pitting edema over body processes
	Adventitious lung sounds, moist crackles
	Shortness of breath
	Generalized or dependent edema
Vital signs	Elevated blood pressure
	High CVP and PAWP
	Increased cardiac output
Laboratory data	Decreased hematocrit (dilutional)
	Low serum osmolality
	Radiography: pulmonary vascular congestion, pleural effusion, pericardial effusion, ascites
	Low urine-specific gravity (decreased concentration)

Isotonic Solutions

The term **isotonic** means that the osmolarity of the solution on one side of a membrane is the same as the osmolarity on the other side of the membrane. The osmolarity of isotonic fluid closely approximates normal serum plasma osmolality (280 to 300 mOsm/L) (Kee, 2002). For this reason, a steady osmolar state is maintained between the ICF and ECF. Isotonic fluids are used when rapid ECF expansion is needed (Metheny, 2000). The most common reason for administration of isotonic solutions is intravascular dehydration (intravascular fluid volume deficit). In the high-acuity patient, intravascular dehydration can result from hemorrhage, massive gastrointestinal bleeding, or dehydration.

Hypotonic Solutions

Hypotonic solutions contain a lower concentration of particles than exists in the ICF and ECF, giving them a low osmolarity. The low osmolarity shifts fluid from the intravascular compartment into the intracellular compartments. Hypotonic fluids are primarily used for treatment of cellular dehydration because they expand the intracellular volume. Hypotonic solutions are useful for prevention of dehydration or for hydration. Hypotonic solutions are used with caution, however, because their overuse causes cells (including blood cells) to expand and burst, resulting in cellular destruction (Porth, 2002). For example, it is of particular importance to avoid hypotonic solutions in patients with neurological problems, particularly those with increased intracranial pressure. Cellular overexpansion from hypotonic solutions will result in increased intracranial pressure and mental status deterioration.

A.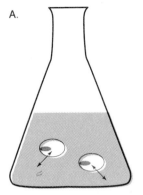
B.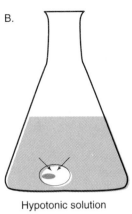
C.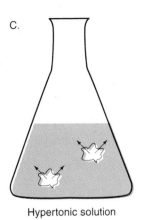

Isotonic solution

Hypotonic solution

Hypertonic solution

Figure 3–5 ■ Tonicity. *A* Isotonic solution—Intracellular osmolality is same as solution; no change in cell size. *B* Hypotonic solution—Intracellular osmolality is lower than solution. Fluid moves into cells, enlarging them. *C Hypertonic solution*—Intracellular osmolality is higher than solution. Fluid moves out of cells, shrinking them.

TABLE 3–6   Common Intravenous Solutions Classified by Tonicity

SOLUTION TYPE	SOLUTION EXAMPLES	COMMENTS
Isotonic	5% dextrose in water 0.9% normal saline (NS) Lactated Ringer's	Solution osmolarity approximates serum osmolality Expands intravascular volume Used for dehydration, shock states
Hypotonic	0.45% normal saline 0.2% normal saline 2.5% dextrose	Low solution osmolarity in relation to serum osmolality Fluid shifts into intracellular compartment Used for replacement of hypotonic fluid deficit (e.g., intracellular dehydration)
Hypertonic	5% dextrose in 0.45% normal saline 10% dextrose in water 3% normal saline	High solution osmolarity in relation to serum osmolality Fluid shifts from intracellular to extracellular compartments Used for treatment of water intoxication, symptomatic hyponatremia

Hypertonic Solutions

Hypertonic solutions have a high osmolarity because they contain a higher concentration of particles than exists in the ICF and ECF. The high osmolarity of the hypertonic solutions shifts fluids from the ICF and ECF into the intravascular compartment, expanding blood volume. Kee and Paulanka (2000) explain that hypertonic solutions are used in the treatment of water intoxication (intracellular fluid volume excess). In the high-acuity patient, water intoxication can be caused by administration of large amounts of electrolyte-free water, overuse of hypotonic solutions (e.g., 0.45 percent sodium chloride), elevated ADH secretion, or renal failure. In addition, overuse of 5 percent dextrose and water (an isotonic solution) can result in water intoxication because of the rapid metabolizing of glucose, which then leaves a hypotonic water solution remaining in the intravascular compartment.

In summary, assessment of the patient with fluid imbalances should include a physical assessment, vital signs, and laboratory data. Clinical assessment of edema and third-spaced fluids includes evaluation based on the specific location. Edema is further evaluated as to whether it is pitting or nonpitting. Body weight changes can provide important clues regarding net fluid gain or loss. Evaluation of third-spaced fluid is more difficult because of the deep locations of some of the serous cavities and usually requires an evaluation that is more complex. Nursing diagnoses for alterations in fluid balance may include *fluid volume deficit* or *fluid volume excess*. The assessment procedures of these two diagnoses are similar, but the findings are opposite.

SECTION FOUR REVIEW

1. A weight gain of 10 kg indicates what volume of fluid volume excess?
   A. 5 L
   B. 10 L
   C. 15 L
   D. 20 L

2. An example of a patient problem in which the patient develops generalized edema stemming from a problem that usually causes localized edema is
   A. sepsis
   B. congestive heart failure
   C. pulmonary edema
   D. burns

3. Which complication is specifically associated with third spacing of fluid into the pericardial sac?
   A. pulmonary edema
   B. peripheral edema
   C. right heart failure
   D. cardiac tamponade
4. The nurse charts that a patient has "+3 pitting edema." Which assessment best fits this notation?
   A. indentation was 8 mm and disappeared within 20 to 30 seconds
   B. indentation was 4 mm and disappeared rapidly
   C. indentation was 2 mm and disappeared within 10 to 15 seconds
   D. indentation was 6 mm and disappeared within 1 to 2 minutes

5. Nursing assessment data found in the patient with fluid volume excess would include
   A. low PAWP
   B. increased hematocrit
   C. moist crackles
   D. decreased blood pressure
6. Which intravenous solution closely approximates serum osmolality?
   A. 0.45 percent normal saline
   B. 5 percent dextrose in normal saline
   C. lactated Ringer's
   D. 3 percent normal saline

Answers: 1. B, 2. A, 3. D, 4. D, 5. C, 6. C

SECTION FIVE: Sodium

At the completion of this section, the learner will be able to discuss the extracellular compartment electrolyte, sodium.

Electrolytes are electrically charged microsolutes found in body fluids. There are two types of electrolytes: **cations** (positively charged ions) and **anions** (negatively charged ions). Electrolytes play a vital role in many physiologic activities, including enzyme activities, muscle contraction, and metabolism. There are three major extracellular electrolytes—sodium (Na), chloride (Cl), and calcium (Ca)—and three major intracellular electrolytes—potassium (K), magnesium (Mg), and phosphorus (PO_4). Sections Five through Ten present an overview of these six major electrolytes. Table 3–7 lists the normal serum electrolyte ranges as well as the panic, or life-threatening, levels.

Normal serum sodium is 135 to 145 mEq/L (Kee, 2002). It is the most abundant cation in the extracellular fluid. Sodium is responsible for shifts in body water and the amount of water retained or excreted by the kidneys. It is required for normal transmission of impulses across muscle and nerve cells through the sodium pump mechanism. It helps maintain acid–base balance by combining with chloride or bicarbonate to increase or decrease serum pH.

Sodium and Water Balance

Changes in sodium levels alter water balance; thus, the clinical manifestations of sodium alterations also reflect symptoms of water imbalance. Because water is drawn to sodium, an excess sodium level in the extracellular fluid pulls water from the intracellular spaces. This results in shrinking of the intracellular fluid compartment and expansion of the extracellular compartment. Such expansion may precipitate congestive heart failure and pulmonary edema in patients whose renal or cardiovascular systems cannot tolerate such fluid shifts.

When serum levels of sodium are low, water moves from an area of low-sodium concentration (extracellular) to an area of high-sodium concentration (intracellular). This causes excess

TABLE 3–7 Serum Electrolytes and Osmolality Normal Ranges and Critical Abnormal Values

ELECTROLYTE	NORMAL RANGE	CRITICAL ABNORMALS
Sodium (Na$^+$)	135–145 mEq/L (or mmol/L)	
Chloride (Cl$^-$)	95–105 mEq/L (or mmol/L)	
Calcium (Ca^{++})	4.5–5.5 mEq/L (9–11 mg/dL)	> 14 mg/dL
Potassium (K$^+$)	3.5–5.3 mEq/L (or mmol/L)	< 2.5 mEq/L or > 7 mEq/L
Magnesium (Mg^{++})	1.5–2.5 mEq/L (1.8–3.0 mg/dL)	< 1.0 mEq/L or > 10 mEq/L
Phosphate (PO$_4^-$)	1.7–2.6 mEq/L (2.5–4.5 mg/dL)	< 0.5 mEq/L
Serum osmolality	280–300 mOsm/kg	< 240 or > 320

Values from Kee, J. L. (2002). Laboratory diagnostic tests with nursing implications, *(6th ed.) Upper Saddle River, NJ: Prentice Hall; Kee, J. L., & Paulanka, B. J. (2000).* Handbook of fluid, electrolyte and acid–base imbalances. *Albany, NY: Delmar Publishers.*

volume in the intracellular compartment and fluid volume deficit in the extracellular compartment.

The amount of sodium in the diet varies widely because the supply is abundant in many (particularly processed) foods. When sodium intake is excessive, fluid volume in the intravascular compartment increases. In response, the kidneys increase urinary excretion of sodium through enhanced filtering from the blood; inhibition of ADH prevents reabsorption of sodium by the kidneys; and aldosterone release is suppressed, enhancing urinary excretion of sodium. When sodium intake is excessively low, plasma volume is decreased. The kidneys sense the decreased volume, triggering the renin–angiotensin–aldosterone system, which causes increased sodium reabsorption, thus decreasing urine output and increasing fluid volume.

Hypernatremia

Serum sodium levels above 145 mEq/L can result from excessive sodium intake or excess water loss. In the high-acuity patient, excessive sodium intake can occur from the overadministration of hypertonic intravenous fluid or sodium bicarbonate, or from overconsumption of dietary sodium. High-serum sodium pulls water from the ICF compartment into the intravascular compartment. The cells shrink and shrivel because of cellular dehydration, whereas the ECF becomes overloaded with water.

Hypernatremia caused by excess water loss can result from renal dysfunction, profuse diaphoresis, or increased ACTH secretion (e.g., Cushing's syndrome) (Kee & Paulanka, 2000). Excess fluid loss can also develop from gastrointestinal loss if fluid loss exceeds electrolyte loss (e.g., severe vomiting or diarrhea and excessive nasogastric tube drainage loss). Diabetes insipidus and administration of osmotic diuretics can cause a significant loss of body water without equivalent loss of sodium, which drives up the serum sodium concentration.

Hyponatremia

Hyponatremia occurs when the serum sodium levels fall below 135 mEq/L. It can result from excessive sodium loss, or water gain, which produces a **dilutional effect.**

Excessive Sodium Loss

In high-acuity patients, major sources of sodium loss are through the gastrointestinal tract and kidneys. Gastrointestinal-related losses occur when electrolyte loss is in excess of fluid loss and may result from severe diarrhea, vomiting, or nasogastric suction. Renal loss of sodium is usually a result of diuretic therapy or severe renal dysfunction. Severe diaphoresis can lead to significant loss of sodium through the skin. Excessive sodium loss also results from hyperglycemic osmotic diuresis, as seen with diabetic ketoacidosis (DKA). Persistent sodium excretion

can occur with consistent release of ADH from the pituitary or ectopic production of ADH. This unregulated production of ADH is associated with SIADH, which can result from cerebral trauma, narcotic use, lung cancer, and certain drugs.

Dilutional Effect

Hyponatremia can result from a net gain of water in the ECF compartment. This occurs when water moves into an area without an equivalent increase in sodium. For example, when a patient develops DKA, excessively high-serum glucose levels cause a shift of water from the ICF and other compartments into the intravascular compartment to dilute the glucose and regain equilibrium.

Clinical Manifestations of Sodium Imbalances

The clinical manifestations of hypernatremia are predominantly neurologic because brain cells are especially sensitive to sodium levels. If hypernatremia develops rapidly, cellular shrinkage also contributes to the neurologic symptoms. Hyponatremia is associated with early changes in muscle tone because sodium plays a role in transmission of neuromuscular impulses. If sodium levels continue to fall (less than 120 mEq/L), intracellular edema occurs, producing further neurologic deterioration. The clinical manifestations of hypernatremia and hyponatremia are summarized in Table 3–8.

In summary, sodium is the major extracellular cation. It is crucial to regulation of body fluids. It also plays an important role in nerve impulse transmission. Hypernatremia primarily results from excessive sodium intake or excess water loss. Hyponatremia usually results from excessive sodium loss or the dilutional effect. The clinical manifestations of sodium imbalances are predominantly neurologic because of the sodium sensitivity of brain cells.

TABLE 3–8 Clinical Manifestations of Sodium Imbalances

Hypernatremia (> 145 mEq/L)	*Moderate:* Confusion, thirst *Severe:* Cardiovascular: hypertension, tachycardia Neurologic: restlessness, seizures, coma Neuromuscular: hyperreflexia, muscle twitching Gastrointestinal: nausea and vomiting
Hyponatremia (< 135 mEq/L)	Cardiovascular: hypotension Neurologic: confusion, headache, lethargy, seizures Neuromuscular: decreased muscle tone, muscle twitching, tremors Gastrointestinal: vomiting, diarrhea, cramping

SECTION FIVE REVIEW

1. The normal range of serum sodium is
   A. 1.5 to 2.2 mEq/L
   B. 3.5 to 5.5 mEq/L
   C. 8.5 to 10.5 mg/dL
   D. 135 to 145 mEq/L
2. Hypernatremia can be caused by
   A. diabetes insipidus
   B. hyperglycemia
   C. SIADH
   D. DKA
3. Signs and symptoms of hypernatremia include
   A. diarrhea
   B. muscle twitching
   C. stomach cramps
   D. decreased muscle tone
4. Hyponatremia is associated with which symptom?
   A. edema
   B. hyperreflexia
   C. lethargy
   D. restlessness
5. The major function of sodium is
   A. carbohydrate metabolism
   B. tissue oxygenation
   C. blood coagulation
   D. fluid balance

Answers: 1. D, 2. A, 3. B, 4. C, 5. D

SECTION SIX: Chloride

At the completion of this section, the learner will be able to describe the extracellular compartment electrolyte, chloride.

Chloride (Cl) is the most abundant anion in the ECF. The normal serum chloride range is 95 to 105 mEq/L (Kee, 2002). Chloride works with sodium in regulation of body fluids by its influence on osmotic pressures within the interstitial and intravascular compartments. Serum chloride levels tend to closely follow sodium levels because chloride normally follows sodium in the body. Aldosterone regulates chloride levels indirectly by stimulating reabsorption of sodium in the kidney. Chloride assists in maintaining the resting membrane potential of cells and, with sodium, maintains osmolality of the extracellular fluid space.

The extracellular fluid acid–base status requires a balance between the total number of anions and cations within the fluid. Thus, the major cation (sodium) must be in balance with the two major extracellular anions (chloride and bicarbonate). To regulate this balance, chloride and bicarbonate maintain an inverse relationship, competing for sodium ions. For example, if a patient receives an excessive dose of sodium bicarbonate to treat metabolic acidosis, the presence of excess bicarbonate ions in the serum results in the excretion of chloride ions, precipitating hypochloremia.

Hyperchloremia

Hyperchloremia is defined as a serum chloride of more than 105 mEq/L. Hyperchloremia is associated with excessive loss of bicarbonate and normal anion gap metabolic acidosis. Normal anion gap metabolic acidosis is most commonly caused by loss of bicarbonate ions through either renal or gastrointestinal loss (e.g., diarrhea). As bicarbonate is lost, chloride is reabsorbed to maintain the acid–base balance.

Hypochloremia

Hypochloremia is defined as a serum chloride of less than 95 mEq/L. Hypochloremia can result from metabolic alkalosis or hypokalemia. Excessive use of loop diuretics, such as furosemide, enhances the loss of chloride and sodium in the urine. When chloride levels are low, the kidneys sense the need for more anions to maintain electrical neutrality and bicarbonate is reabsorbed.

Clinical Manifestations of Chloride Imbalances

The signs and symptoms of chloride imbalance reflect the manifestations of the associated acid–base imbalance. Neurologic, musculoskeletal, respiratory dysfunction, and the symptoms of a concurrent sodium imbalance are also associated with chloride imbalances. The clinical manifestations of chloride imbalances are listed in Table 3–9.

TABLE 3–9   Clinical Manifestations of Chloride Imbalances

Hyperchloremia (> 105 mEq/L)	Musculoskeletal: muscle weakness
	Respiratory: rapid, deep respirations
	Neurologic: headache, lethargy, decreasing level of consciousness
	Symptoms of hypernatremia and fluid volume deficit
Hypochloremia (< 95 mEq/L)	Neurologic: irritability, tetany, agitation
	Respiratory: shallow breathing, bradypnea
	Musculoskeletal: muscle weakness
	Symptoms of hyponatremia

In summary, chloride is the major extracellular anion. It maintains a direct relationship with sodium and an inverse relationship with bicarbonate. Chloride is important in fluid regulation and acid–base balance. Hyperchloremia is associated with loss of bicarbonate ions and metabolic acidosis (normal anion gap). Hypochloremia is associated with loss of sodium or potassium ions and metabolic alkalosis.

SECTION SIX REVIEW

1. Chloride levels closely follow the levels of which electrolyte?
   A. potassium
   B. sodium
   C. calcium
   D. magnesium
2. Hypochloremia is associated with which symptom?
   A. tetany
   B. headache
   C. lethargy
   D. rapid, deep respirations
3. The normal serum chloride range is
   A. 3.5 to 5.3 mEq/L
   B. 4.5 to 5.5 mEq/L
   C. 95 to 105 mEq/L
   D. 135 to 145 mEq/L

4. Hyperchloremia is associated with which problem?
   A. metabolic acidosis (normal anion gap)
   B. metabolic acidosis (high anion gap)
   C. metabolic alkalosis (normal anion gap)
   D. metabolic alkalosis (high anion gap)
5. Which substance indirectly regulates serum chloride levels?
   A. parathyroid hormone
   B. calcitonin
   C. renin
   D. aldosterone

Answers: 1. B, 2. A, 3. C, 4. A, 5. D

SECTION SEVEN: Calcium

At the completion of this section, the learner will be able to discuss the extracellular compartment electrolyte, calcium.

Almost all of the body's calcium is located within bone, with a small amount existing in the ECF and soft tissues. Calcium is required for blood coagulation, neuromuscular contraction, enzymatic activities, and for bone integrity.

Calcium regulation is under the influence of parathyroid hormone (PTH), calcitonin, and calcitriol. Serum calcium levels are maintained by calcium excretion from the kidneys, absorption of calcium from the gastrointestinal tract, and mobilization of calcium from the bone. Calcium is absorbed in the intestines only under the influence of vitamin D, which is activated in the kidneys. It is reabsorbed in the proximal renal tubules after being filtered by the glomerulus and is excreted by the kidneys. Renal disease prevents activation of vitamin D, thus reducing the body's ability to absorb calcium.

Calcitonin and parathyroid hormone work in opposition to regulate calcium levels. When calcium levels are low, PTH is released by the parathyroid gland, stimulating the conversion of calcitriol (the active form of vitamin D), which causes the small intestines to absorb more calcium. PTH also stimulates release of calcium from bony tissues into the blood. When calcium levels are high, PTH secretion is suppressed and calcitonin is secreted by the thyroid, inhibiting the release of calcium from bone into the blood.

Serum calcium can be measured in two different ways: as total calcium and as ionized calcium. These two measurements evaluate body calcium in two different states:

- **Total calcium.** Normal levels: 4.5 to 5.5 mEq/L or 9 to 11 mg/dL (Kee, 2002). Total calcium reflects calcium that is bound to proteins (primarily albumin) in the serum. Total calcium levels are influenced by the patient's nutritional state. Therefore, if a patient's serum albumin level is low (e.g., from malnutrition, liver dysfunction), serum calcium levels will also be low.
- **Ionized calcium.** Normal levels: 2.2 to 2.5 mEq/L or 4.25 to 5.25 mg/dL (Kee, 2002). Approximately 50 percent of serum calcium exists in an ionized state. Ionized calcium represents the calcium that is used in the physiologic activities and is crucial for neuromuscular activity. Ionized calcium levels may remain normal even when total calcium (and serum albumin) levels are low.

Hypercalcemia

Hypercalcemia is defined as a serum calcium level above 5.5 mEq/L (11 mg/dL). Hypercalcemia results from mobilization of calcium from bone. Malignancy is a common cause of hypercalcemia, usually through destruction of bone (from bone metastasis). Another malignancy-related mechanism for hypercalcemia is the presence of PTH-secreting tumors. Malignancies

TABLE 3–10   **Clinical Manifestation of Calcium Imbalances**

Hypercalcemia (> 5.5 mEq/L or 9–11 mg/dL) (Severe = > 14 mg/dL)	Gastrointestinal: anorexia, constipation, peptic ulcer disease Neurologic: lethargy, depression, fatigue; if severe: confusion, coma Cardiovascular: cardiac dysrhythmias, heart block, shortened QT interval, decreased ST segment Skeletal: pathologic bone fractures, bone thinning Other: renal stones
Hypocalcemia (< 4.5 mEq/L or 9 mg/dL)	Musculoskeletal: cramps (abdominal and extremities); tingling and numbness; severe: positive Chvostek's or Trousseau's sign, tetany Neurologic: irritability, reduced cognitive ability, seizures Cardiovascular: electrocardiographic changes: prolonged QT interval, long ST segment, decreased blood pressure and myocardial contractility Skeletal: bone fractures possible Hematologic: abnormal clotting

that are most commonly associated with development of hypercalcemia include pulmonary, breast, ovarian, and others (Kee & Paulanka, 2000). Hypercalcemia also develops from prolonged immobility, hyperparathyroidism, thyrotoxicosis, and thiazide diuretics. Excessive ingestion of vitamin D or calcium and altered renal tubular absorption of calcium also elevate serum calcium levels. Gastrointestinal and renal absorption of calcium decrease the reabsorption of phosphorus; therefore, hypercalcemia accompanies hypophosphatemia because calcium and phosphorus levels shift in opposite directions.

Hypocalcemia

Hypocalcemia is defined as a serum level below 4.5 mEq/L (9 mg/dL). In the high-acuity patient, the most common cause of hypocalcemia is depressed function or surgical removal of the parathyroid gland following thyroid surgery. It is also associated with hypomagnesemia and hyperphosphatemia, which can cause diminished vitamin D synthesis by the kidneys. Hypocalcemia can be induced by the administration of large amounts of stored blood because stored blood is preserved with citrate. When citrate is administered, it binds with calcium, which lowers serum calcium. In older patients, causes of low calcium levels include decreased oral intake of calcium, lower serum albumin levels, and decreased vitamin D intake or activation. Additionally, many medications that are administered during periods of high-acuity illness (e.g., certain antibiotics, heparin, and insulin) may impair calcium reabsorption (Kee, 2002).

Clinical Manifestations of Calcium Imbalances

The signs and symptoms of hypercalcemia primarily reflect dysfunction of the gastrointestinal and musculoskeletal systems. The signs and symptoms of hypophosphatemia can accompany hypercalcemia. Hypocalcemia becomes symptomatic when ionized calcium levels fall to below normal limits. Symptomatic hypocalcemia affects the musculoskeletal, neurologic, and cardiovascular systems. The clinical manifestations associated with hypercalcemia and hypocalcemia are presented in Table 3–10.

In summary, calcium plays an important part in blood coagulation and is the major component of bone tissue. It is regulated by PTH, calcitonin, and calcitriol. Calcium is measured in its protein-bound state (total calcium) and its ionized state (ionized calcium). Hypercalcemia results from movement of calcium from the bone. Hypocalcemia is associated with depressed parathyroid function. Calcium imbalances are particularly associated with neuromuscular and cardiac dysfunction.

SECTION SEVEN REVIEW

1. The normal range of total serum calcium is
   A. 1.5 to 2.5 mEq/L
   B. 3.5 to 5.3 mEq/L
   C. 4.5 to 5.5 mEq/L
   D. 135 to 145 mEq/L

2. Calcium is absorbed in the intestines under the influence of
   A. phosphorus
   B. vitamin D
   C. sodium
   D. vitamin C

3. Hypocalcemia is associated with which of the following?
   A. tingling and numbness
   B. constipation
   C. lethargy
   D. shortened QT interval on ECG
4. Calcium regulation is under the influence of all of the following EXCEPT
   A. calcitriol
   B. calcitonin
   C. PTH
   D. aldosterone

5. Which of the following statements is correct regarding serum total calcium?
   A. it may remain normal even if ionized calcium is abnormal
   B. it represents calcium that is physiologically active
   C. it is influenced by the patient's nutritional state
   D. it measures calcium that is not bound to protein

Answers: 1. C, 2. B, 3. A, 4. D, 5. C

SECTION EIGHT: Potassium

At the completion of this section, the learner will be able to discuss the intracellular compartment electrolyte, potassium.

The normal serum potassium level is 3.5 to 5.3 mEq/L (Kee, 2002). Potassium is the major intracellular cation, with almost all potassium being located within the cells. Although the concentration in the plasma is small, monitoring serum potassium is very important because the body is intolerant of abnormal serum levels. Potassium is readily found in many foods; thus, we normally consume sufficient quantities of potassium to meet daily requirements. Excess potassium is eliminated in the urine by the kidneys, and about 40 mEq/L of potassium is excreted daily in the urine (Kee, 2002).

Potassium is vital in maintaining normal cardiac and neuromuscular function because it affects muscle contraction. Potassium also influences nerve impulse conduction; therefore, abnormal serum potassium levels can produce potentially lethal cardiac conduction abnormalities, which could result in cardiac arrest. Potassium is vital to carbohydrate metabolism and plays an important role in normal cell membrane function. It is important in maintaining acid–base balance because hydrogen ions exchange with potassium ions.

Hyperkalemia

Hyperkalemia is defined as a potassium level above 5.3 mEq/L. Hyperkalemia can result from a variety of situations. In the high-acuity patient, administration of potassium supplements, either oral or IV, can cause hyperkalemia, particularly in the presence of reduced urinary output (e.g., renal dysfunction). Significant quantities of intracellular potassium are released into the extracellular space in response to injury, stress, acidosis, or a catabolic state. Acidosis contributes to hyperkalemia because excess hydrogen ions shift into the cells, forcing potassium out into the serum (Kee & Paulanka, 2000). Additionally, sodium depletion results in hyperkalemia as potassium is exchanged for sodium across the proximal renal tubule.

Hypokalemia

Hypokalemia is defined as a serum potassium below 3.5 mEq/L. Hypokalemia can result from the following:

- A loss of gastrointestinal secretions (e.g., vomiting, diarrhea, excessive nasogastric suction fluid loss, and fistulas)
- Excessive renal excretion of potassium
- Movement of potassium into the cells (e.g., diabetic ketoacidosis)
- Prolonged fluid administration without potassium supplementation
- Excessive use of potassium-wasting diuretics without adequate potassium supplementation

When hypokalemia occurs, the body does not attempt to retain or reabsorb potassium. The kidneys continue to excrete it regardless of the existing potassium state. If it is allowed to continue, the hypokalemia becomes increasingly severe, causing a steady deterioration in the patient's condition. Because the body does not compensate for potassium loss, it is essential that hypokalemia be rapidly detected and corrected through appropriate potassium supplementation. The body is intolerant of abnormal serum potassium levels. According to Kee and Paulanka (2000), potassium levels that are less than 2.5 mEq/L or more than 7 mEq/L are critically deranged and can result in cardiac arrest. Hypokalemia is common in the older patient (Beers & Berkow, 2000–2005). Common causes include decreased potassium intake during periods of high-acuity illness, nausea and vomiting, and use of diuretics.

Clinical Manifestations of Potassium Imbalances

Because potassium is important in nerve impulse conduction, muscle contraction, and cell membrane function, the signs and symptoms of imbalances reflect interference with these activities. The clinical manifestations of potassium imbalances are summarized in Table 3–11.

TABLE 3–11 Clinical Manifestations of Potassium Imbalances

Hyperkalemia (> 5.3 mEq/L)	Musculoskeletal: weakness, muscle cramps
	Gastrointestinal: nausea, vomiting, abdominal cramping, diarrhea
	Cardiovascular: electrocardiographic changes: progression from tachycardia to bradycardia to cardiac arrest is possible; prolonged P-R interval; flat or absent P wave; slurring of QRS; tall peaked T wave; ST segment depression
	Acid–base effect: metabolic acidosis
Hypokalemia (< 3.5 mEq/L)	Musculoskeletal: skeletal muscle weakness; decreased smooth muscle function; decreased deep tendon reflexes
	Cardiovascular: hypotension, electrocardiogram: ST segment depression; U waves; T wave inversion, flattening, or depression; cardiac arrest if severe
	Gastrointestinal: nausea and vomiting, paralytic ileus, diarrhea
	Acid–base effect: metabolic alkalosis
	Neurologic: depression, confusion

In summary, potassium is the major intracellular cation. It is vital in maintaining normal cardiac and neuromuscular function. Hyperkalemia results from excessive potassium intake, renal failure, or use of potassium-sparing diuretics. Hypokalemia results from excessive loss of potassium through the gastrointestinal tract or urine, shifting of potassium into the cells, or excessive administration of potassium-free intravenous fluids. The clinical manifestations of potassium imbalances reflect dysfunctions in nerve impulse conduction, muscle contraction, and cell membrane activities.

SECTION EIGHT REVIEW

1. The normal range of serum potassium is
   A. 1.5 to 2.2 mEq/L
   B. 3.5 to 5.3 mEq/L
   C. 4.5 to 5.5 mEq/L
   D. 135 to 145 mEq/L
2. Hyperkalemia can be caused by
   A. renal failure
   B. potassium-wasting diuretics
   C. metabolic alkalosis
   D. severe diarrhea
3. The clinical findings of hyperkalemia include
   A. muscle weakness, T wave inversion on ECG
   B. muscle twitching, ST segment depression on ECG

C. vomiting, peaked T wave on ECG
D. diarrhea, presence of U wave on ECG
4. The presence of hypokalemia alters renal excretion of potassium in which way?
   A. urine output increases
   B. potassium excretion increases
   C. potassium is reabsorbed
   D. potassium excretion does not change

Answers: 1. B, 2. A, 3. C, 4. D

SECTION NINE: Magnesium

At the completion of this section, the learner will be able to describe the intracellular compartment electrolyte, magnesium.

Magnesium is an intracellular electrolyte with a distribution similar to potassium. The normal serum magnesium level is 1.5 to 2.5 mEq/L (Kee, 2002). Magnesium ensures sodium and potassium transportation across cell membranes. It is needed for activation of certain enzymes required for normal protein and carbohydrate metabolism. Magnesium is crucial to many biochemical reactions and plays a significant role in nerve cell conduction. It is important in transmitting CNS messages and maintaining neuromuscular activity.

Magnesium is predominantly excreted in feces, but a small amount is excreted in the urine. The kidneys, however, have a remarkable ability to conserve magnesium. Magnesium balance is closely related to potassium and calcium balance.

Hypermagnesemia

Hypermagnesemia results when magnesium levels rise above 2.5 mEq/L. This abnormality is rare but can occur with diminished renal excretion as seen in renal dysfunction, or excessive magnesium intake. Consumption of large quantities of magnesium-containing antacids or laxatives can be a source of excessive intake.

TABLE 3–12 Clinical Manifestations of Magnesium Imbalances

Hypermagnesemia (> 2.5 mEq/L or 3.0 mg/dL)	Neuromuscular: absent deep tendon reflexes, lethargy, drowsiness
	Cardiovascular: hypotension, bradycardia, cardiac arrest; electrocardiogram: prolonged P-R intervals, complete heart block, wide QRs complex
	Respiratory: depression
Hypomagnesemia (< 1.5 mEq/L or 1.8 mg/dL)	Neuromuscular: tremors, tetany, positive Chvostek's and Trousseau's signs
	Cardiovascular: premature ventricular contractions, ventricular tachycardia and/or fibrillation; T wave flattening, decreased ST segment

Hypomagnesemia

Hypomagnesemia is defined as a serum magnesium of less than 1.5 mEq/L. It can result from decreased intake or decreased absorption of magnesium, or excessive loss through urinary or bowel elimination. Magnesium deficiency can be caused by many disorders, including acute pancreatitis, starvation, malabsorption syndrome, chronic alcoholism, burns, and prolonged hyperalimentation without adequate magnesium replacement. Hypoparathyroidism, with resultant hypocalcemia, can also cause hypomagnesemia because the regulatory mechanisms of magnesium and calcium are closely related.

Clinical Manifestations of Magnesium Imbalances

The signs and symptoms of magnesium and calcium imbalances are similar. Because magnesium is important in maintaining normal CNS and neuromuscular function, magnesium imbalances can cause dysfunction of these activities. Hypermagnesemia has a depressant effect, and hypomagnesemia is associated with hyperactivity. The clinical manifestations associated with hypermagnesemia and hypomagnesemia are presented in Table 3–12.

In summary, magnesium is primarily an intracellular cation with a distribution similar to potassium. Magnesium has many functions, including assisting in transport of sodium and potassium across the cell membrane, and transference of energy. Hypermagnesemia is rare and is primarily caused by either excessive intake of magnesium-containing drugs, or renal failure. Hypomagnesemia can result from decreased intake or excessive loss of magnesium. The clinical manifestations of magnesium imbalances primarily reflect CNS and neuromuscular dysfunction.

SECTION NINE REVIEW

1. The normal range of serum magnesium is
   A. 1.5 to 2.5 mEq/L
   B. 3.5 to 5.3 mEq/L
   C. 4.5 to 5.5 mEq/L
   D. 135 to 145 mEq/L

2. Magnesium balance is closely related to which other two electrolytes?
   A. potassium and phosphorus
   B. calcium and sodium
   C. sodium and phosphorus
   D. calcium and potassium

3. The symptoms of hypomagnesemia reflect
   A. CNS hypoactivity
   B. fluid compartment shifts
   C. cardiac depressant effects
   D. neuromuscular and CNS hyperactivity

4. Hypermagnesemia is associated with which symptom?
   A. tetany
   B. lethargy
   C. tremors
   D. positive Chvostek's sign

5. Magnesium plays an active part in which physiologic functions (choose all that apply)?
   1. sodium and potassium transport
   2. nerve cell conduction
   3. fluid regulation
   4. transference of energy
   A. 2 and 4
   B. 1, 2, and 3
   C. 1, 2, and 4
   D. 2, 3, and 4

Answers: 1. A, 2. D, 3. D, 4. B, 5. C

TABLE 3–13 Clinical Manifestations of Phosphate Imbalances

Hyperphosphatemia (> 2.6 mEq/L or 4.5 mg/dL)	Musculoskeletal: muscle cramping and weakness Cardiac: tachycardia Gastrointestinal: diarrhea, nausea, abdominal cramping *Note:* Many other symptoms are those of hypocalcemia
Hypophosphatemia (< 1.7 mEq/L or 2.5 mg/dL)	Musculoskeletal: weakness, numbness, and tingling; pathologic fractures Cardiac: diminished myocardial function Gastrointestinal: nausea and vomiting, anorexia Neurologic: disorientation, irritability, seizures, coma *Severe hypophosphatemia:* severe myocardial, respiratory, and nervous system dysfunction; hemolysis, white blood cell and platelet dysfunction

SECTION TEN: Phosphorus/Phosphate

At the completion of this section, the learner will be able to discuss the intracellular compartment electrolyte, phosphorus/phosphate.

Phosphorus is an intracellular mineral commonly found in many foods. According to Kee and Paulanka (2000), the normal serum level of inorganic phosphorus is 1.7 to 2.6 mEq/L or 2.5 to 4.5 mg/dL. In the body, it predominantly exists as phosphate (PO_4). Phosphorus plays an essential part in the development of teeth and bones. It is vital for normal neuromuscular function and is required for energy in the production of adenosine triphosphate (ATP). It also contributes to protein, fat, and carbohydrate metabolism and assists in the maintenance of acid–base balance.

The serum phosphate level is under the influence of PTH and maintains an inverse relationship to calcium. The kidneys are essential to phosphorus regulation through reabsorption and excretion. When glomerular filtration is decreased, phosphorus reabsorption increases, causing an elevation in serum levels. As glomerular filtration increases, phosphorus reabsorption diminishes and more phosphorus is excreted by the kidneys, reducing the serum phosphate level. Age-related changes in parathyroid function, along with decreased intake and impaired intestinal absorption, make mild hypophosphatemia common in the elderly high-acuity patient (Beers & Berkow, 2000–2005).

Hyperphosphatemia

Hyperphosphatemia is defined as a serum level above 2.6 mEq/L (4.5 mg/dL). Hyperphosphatemia is not as common in the high-acuity patient as hypophosphatemia. It is predominantly associated with chronic renal failure. Other causes include hyperthyroidism, hypoparathyroidism, severe catabolic states, and conditions causing hypocalcemia.

Hypophosphatemia

Hypophosphatemia is defined as a serum phosphorus level below 1.7 mEq/L (2.5 mg/dL). This condition is associated with malnourished states and is a relatively common imbalance in the high-acuity patient. Other conditions that can cause hypophosphatemia include hyperparathyroidism, certain renal tubular defects, metabolic acidosis (including DKA), and disorders that cause hypercalcemia.

Clinical Manifestations of Phosphate Imbalances

Hypophosphatemia depresses cellular function, particularly of the hematologic and cardiovascular systems. This results in symptoms of impaired heart function and poor tissue oxygenation. Because phosphorus is essential in providing energy for ATP, muscle fatigue develops. The clinical manifestations associated with hyperphosphatemia and hypophosphatemia are presented in Table 3–13.

In summary, phosphorus, which exists in the serum as phosphate, works closely with calcium and is important in tissue oxygenation and energy production. Hyperphosphatemia is most commonly associated with chronic renal failure. Hypophosphatemia most commonly results from malnourished states. The clinical manifestations of phosphate imbalances primarily reflect dysfunction of the hematologic, cardiovascular, and neuromuscular systems.

SECTION TEN REVIEW

1. The normal range of serum phosphorus is
   A. 1.7 to 2.6 mEq/L
   B. 3.5 to 5.3 mEq/L
   C. 4.5 to 5.5 mEq/L
   D. 135 to 145 mEq/L

2. Hypophosphatemia is associated with which condition?
   A. malnourished state
   B. metabolic alkalosis
   C. hypocalcemia
   D. hyperthyroidism
3. Severe hypophosphatemia is associated with which symptom?
   A. joint pain
   B. muscle cramping
   C. respiratory arrest
   D. peptic ulcer disease
4. Phosphorus is important for which functions? (choose all that apply)
   1. tissue oxygenation
   2. sodium transport
   3. calcium regulation
   4. production of ATP
   A. 1 and 3
   B. 1, 3, and 4
   C. 2 and 4
   D. 1, 2, and 3
5. The clinical picture of hyperphosphatemia frequently reflects which other electrolyte abnormality?
   A. hypercalcemia
   B. hypochloremia
   C. hypernatremia
   D. hypocalcemia

Answers: 1. A, 2. A, 3. C, 4. B, 5. D

POSTTEST

The following Posttest is constructed in a case study format. A patient is presented, and questions are asked based on available data. New data are presented as the case study progresses.

Donald R, 75 years old, was admitted to the hospital with severe dyspnea. He has a history of chronic alcohol abuse and cirrhosis. On admission, the nurse assesses the following: Thin, chronically ill-appearing male. Blood pressure, 108/62; pulse, 118/min; RR, 26/min; temperature, 97.8°F (36.6°C). 3+ pitting generalized edema is noted. His abdomen is distended and tight. He is orthopneic and complains of shortness of breath. Mr. R states that he has been confined to his chair or couch for the past two weeks because of his breathing difficulty and general weakness.

1. Mr. R's age and poor physical condition place him at risk for development of
   A. hypertension
   B. dehydration
   C. acute renal failure
   D. congestive heart failure
2. Mr. R's edema is an example of fluid located in which space?
   A. intracellular
   B. intravascular
   C. interstitial
   D. transcellular
3. Assuming Mr. R's abdominal distention is ascites, the shift of intravascular fluid into his peritoneal cavity is referred to as
   A. third spacing
   B. congestive failure
   C. edema
   D. peritonitis
4. As Mr R's blood pressure decreases, the baroreceptors will trigger
   A. renal vasodilation
   B. increased heart rate
   C. suppression of ACTH release
   D. peripheral vasoconstriction

Mr. R's urine output has been 25 mL/hr for the past 2 hours. His most current serum osmolality is 315 mOsm/L. He is complaining of extreme thirst.

5. Based on the available data, his urine output and serum osmolality are most likely because of
   A. renal failure
   B. peripheral edema
   C. suppressed ADH release
   D. intravascular fluid deficit
6. His thirst is activated by
   A. hemodilution
   B. release of aldosterone
   C. increased osmolality
   D. ADH release

Mr. R has a serum albumin drawn. The results show a significantly low albumin level.

7. A low serum albumin directly alters the Starling forces in which way?
   A. fluids escape out of the capillaries
   B. fluids are drawn into the capillaries
   C. fluids escape out of the interstitial spaces
   D. fluids are drawn into the interstitial spaces

It is decided that Mr. R requires intravenous fluids.

8. The decision of which type of IV fluid is best for Mr. R is based on osmolarity. A solution's osmolarity refers to its _____ concentration in relation to the ICF and ECF.
   A. particle
   B. protein
   C. glucose
   D. anion

9. Which type of IV solution would be best for treating intravascular fluid deficit?
   A. hypertonic solutions
   B. isotonic solutions
   C. hypotonic solutions
   D. colloid solutions

10. Mr. R receives an IV fluid to increase his intravascular volume and increase his arterial blood pressure. The best IV fluid(s) to accomplish this goal is/are (select all that apply)
    A. 5 percent dextrose in normal saline
    B. 0.45 percent normal saline
    C. 0.9 percent normal saline
    D. 0.2 percent normal saline

Mr. R has received a large volume of IV fluids. His serum electrolytes are drawn. The results are

Sodium: 128 mEq/L
Chloride: 90 mEq/L
Total calcium: 5.8 mEq/L
Potassium: 5.2 mEq/L
Magnesium: 2.7 mEq/L
Phosphate: 1.5 mEq/L

11. Mr. R's serum sodium can cause body water to shift from the
    A. extracellular into the intravascular compartment
    B. interstitial into the intravascular compartment
    C. extracellular into the intracellular compartment
    D. intracellular into the extracellular compartment

12. If Mr. R's chloride level continues to fall, he will need to be assessed for
    A. rapid, deep respirations
    B. muscle weakness
    C. depressed breathing
    D. lethargy

13. Mr. R's total calcium level is 4.0 mEq/L. This level is most likely caused by his
    A. renal status
    B. nutritional status
    C. chloride status
    D. immobilized status

14. Should Mr. R's serum potassium level approach 7 mEq/L, the nurse would be MOST concerned about changes in which body system?
    A. cardiovascular
    B. respiratory
    C. neurologic
    D. renal

15. If Mr. R's chloride level dropped significantly, the nurse would need to monitor him for development of which of the following primary acid–base problems?
    A. metabolic acidosis
    B. metabolic alkalosis
    C. respiratory acidosis
    D. respiratory alkalosis

16. Hypomagnesemia, such as Mr. R has, can be caused by all of the following problems EXCEPT
    A. hypercalcemia
    B. chronic alcoholism
    C. starvation
    D. acute pancreatitis

17. Mr. R's hypophosphatemia can affect his musculoskeletal system in which way?
    A. muscle spasm
    B. joint pain
    C. muscle weakness
    D. muscle cramping

POSTTEST ANSWERS

Question	Answer	Chapter Section
1	B	One
2	C	One
3	A	Three
4	D	Two
5	D	One
6	C	One
7	A	One, Three
8	A	Four
9	B	Four

Question	Answer	Chapter Section
10	A, C	Four
11	C	Five
12	C	Six
13	B	Seven
14	A	Eight
15	B	Six
16	A	Nine
17	C	Ten

REFERENCES

Beers, M., & Berkow, R. (Eds.), (2000). *The Merck manual of geriatrics* (3rd ed.). Pennsylvania: Merck & Co.

Beers, M. H., & Berkow, R. (Eds.) (2000–2005). Metabolic and endocrine disorders: Disorders of water and electrolyte balance. In M. H. Beers & R. Berkow (Eds.). Merck manual of geriatrics. Accessed February 03, 2005 @ *http://www.merck.com/mrkshared/mm_ geriatrics/home.jsp*.

Bickley, L. S. (2003). The peripheral vascular system. In L. S. Bickley & P. G. Szilagyi *Bates guide to physical examination and history taking* (8th ed., pp. 441–464). Philadelphia: Lippincott, Williams & Wilkens.

Gaspard, K. J. (2002). Blood cells and the hematopoietic system. In C. M. Porth (Ed.), *Pathophysiology: Concepts of altered health states* (6th ed., pp. 251–257). Philadelphia: J. B. Lippincott.

Guyton, A. C., & Hall, J. E. (2000). The body fluid compartments: Extracellular and intracellular fluids; interstitial fluid and edema. In A. C. Guyton & J. E. Hall (Eds.). *Human physiology and mechanisms of disease* (10th ed., pp. 264–278). Philadelphia: W. B. Saunders.

Kee, J. L., (2002). *Laboratory diagnostic tests with nursing implications* (6th ed.). Upper Saddle River, NJ: Prentice Hall.

Kee, J. L., & Paulanka, B. J. (2000). *Handbook of fluid, electrolyte and acid–base imbalances.* Albany, NY: Delmar Publishers.

Larocca, J. C., & Otto, S. E. (Eds.), (1997). *Pocket guide series: Intravenous therapy* (3rd ed.). St. Louis: C. V. Mosby.

Lemone, P., & Burke, K. (2004). Nursing care of clients with altered fluid, electrolyte, or acid–base balance. In P. Lemone & K. Burke, *Medical-surgical nursing: Critical thinking in client care* (3rd ed., pp. 76–135). Upper Saddle River, NJ: Pearson/Prentice Hall

Metheny, N. M. (2000). *Fluid & electrolyte balance: Nursing considerations* (4th ed.). Philadelphia: J. B. Lippincott.

Mulvey, M., & Bullock, B. L. (2000). Fluid, electrolyte, and acid–base balance. In B. L. Bullock & R. L. Henze (Eds.), *Focus on pathophysiology.* Philadelphia: J. B. Lippincott.

Porth, C. M. (2002). Alteration in fluid and electrolytes. In C. M. Porth (Ed.), *Pathophysiology: Concepts of altered health states* (6th ed., pp. 693–734). Philadelphia: J. B. Lippincott.

Timby, B. K. (2004). Physical assessment. In B. K. Timby (Ed.), *Fundamental nursing skills and concepts* (8th ed., pp. 185–208). Philadelphia: Lippincott, Williams & Wilkins.

Tripp, T. R. (2000). Laboratory and diagnostic tests. In A. G. Lueckenotte (Ed.), *Gerontologic nursing* (2nd ed., pp. 405–424). St. Louis: C. V. Mosby.

Whalen, D. A., & Kelleher, R. M. (1998). Cardiovascular patient assessment. In M. R. Kinney, S. B. Dunbar, J. A. Brooks-Brunn, N. Molter, & J. M. Vitello-Cicciu (Eds.), *AACN's clinical reference for critical care nursing* (4th ed., pp. 277–318). St. Louis: C. V. Mosby.

Woods, S. (1998). Fluid and electrolyte homeostasis. In M. R. Kinney, S. B. Dunbar, J. A. Brooks-Brunn, N. Molter, & J. M. Vitello-Cicciu (Eds.), *AACN's clinical reference for critical care nursing* (4th ed., pp. 113–133). St. Louis: C. V. Mosby.

PART

2

Pulmonary Gas Exchange

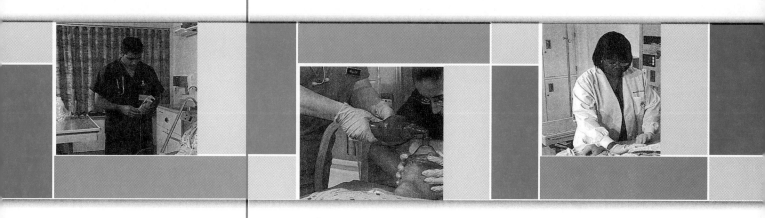

MODULE 4 Determinants and Assessment of Pulmonary Gas Exchange

MODULE 5 Alterations in Pulmonary Gas Exchange

MODULE 6 Mechanical Ventilation

MODULE 7 Nursing Care of the Patient with Altered Gas Exchange

4 Determinants and Assessment of Pulmonary Gas Exchange

Kathleen Dorman Wagner

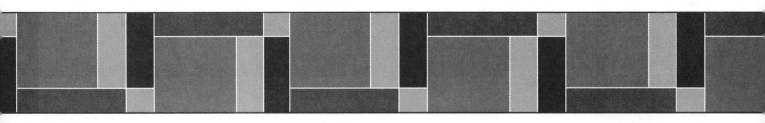

OBJECTIVES   Following completion of this module, the learner will be able to

Part One: *"Determinants of Pulmonary Gas Exchange"*

1. Explain the conducting airway and the concept of ventilation.

2. Discuss external respiration and pulmonary gas diffusion.

3. Discuss pulmonary perfusion.

4. Identify mechanisms that the body uses to compensate for acid–base imbalances, and differentiate between respiratory acidosis and alkalosis, and metabolic acidosis and alkalosis.

Part Two: *"Assessment of Pulmonary Gas Exchange"*

5. Discuss a respiratory nursing assessment.

6. Describe various tests used to evaluate pulmonary function.

7. Identify normal values for and interpret arterial blood gases.

8. Recognize mixed acid–base disorders.

9. Discuss noninvasive methods of monitoring gas exchange and applications.

10. Perform selected respiratory calculations.

Module 4 is divided into two distinct parts. Part One, "Determinants of Pulmonary Gas Exchange," is composed of four sections. Sections One through Three discuss the underlying principles involved in the respiratory process, including the mechanics of breathing—ventilation, external respiration and pulmonary diffusion, and pulmonary perfusion. Section Four describes acid–base physiology and disturbances, including respiratory and metabolic alkalosis and acidosis.

Part Two, "Assessment of Pulmonary Gas Exchange," is divided into six sections, all of which describe various ways in which a high-acuity patient's oxygenation and ventilation status is evaluated. Section Five focuses on collection of nursing history and physical assessment data as they apply to the high-acuity patient. Section Six describes a variety of common pulmonary function tests that evaluate ventilatory status. Sec-

tion Seven provides a systematic approach to interpretation of arterial blood gases. Section Eight introduces the advanced concept of mixed acid–base disorders and provides basic instruction on the interpretation of more complex arterial blood gases. Section Nine provides an overview of two common noninvasive monitoring methods, including pulse oximetry and end-tidal carbon dioxide monitoring. Finally, Section Ten introduces the reader to the essentials of respiratory calculations that evaluate oxygenation status.

Each section includes a set of review questions or exercises to help the learner evaluate basic understanding of each section before moving on to the next. All Section Reviews and the Pretest and Posttest in the module include answers. It is suggested that the learner review those concepts answered incorrectly in the review questions before proceeding to the next section.

GLOSSARY

absolute shunt   The sum of anatomic shunt and capillary shunt.

accessory muscles   Muscles not normally used during quiet breathing that are available for assisting either inspiration or expiration during times of increased work of breathing.

acids   Substances that dissociate or lose ions.

acute respiratory distress syndrome (ARDS)   A type of respiratory failure caused by diffuse injury to the alveolar–capillary membrane, resulting in noncardiogenic pulmonary edema.

anatomic shunt   Movement of blood from the right heart and back into the left heart without coming into contact with alveoli.

bases   Substances capable of accepting ions.

base excess   A measure of the amount of buffer required to return the blood to a normal pH state. It is used in reference to metabolic acid–base states. A person can develop a base excess (metabolic alkalosis) or a base deficit (metabolic acidosis).

buffer   A substance reacting with acids and bases to maintain a neutral environment of stable pH.

capillary shunt   Normal flow of blood past completely unventilated alveoli.

capnogram   Graphic representation of carbon dioxide levels during respiration.

capnometry   Measurement of carbon dioxide in expired gas.

carina   The junction of the Y formed by the two primary bronchial branches.

compensated   A state in which the pH is within normal limits with the acid–base imbalance being neutralized but not corrected.

compliance (C_L)   Measurement of the relative ease with which the lungs accept a volume of air; reflects relative stiffness of lungs.

cor pulmonale   Right ventricular hypertrophy and dilation secondary to pulmonary disease.

corrected   A state in which all acid–base parameters have returned to normal ranges after a state of acid–base imbalance.

crackles (rales)   Adventitious breath sounds associated with fluid or secretions or both in small airways or alveoli.

diffusion   Movement of gases down a pressure gradient from an area of high pressure to an area of low pressure.

dyspnea   Difficulty breathing.

end-tidal carbon dioxide ($P_{ET}CO_2$ or $ETCO_2$)   Concentration of carbon dioxide at the end of exhalation.

external respiration   Movement of gases across the alveolar–capillary membrane.

forced expiratory volumes (FEVs)   Measure of how rapidly a person can forcefully exhale air after a maximal inhalation; a measurement of dynamic lung function.

hemoptysis   Expectoration of bloody secretions.

internal respiration   Movement of gases across systemic capillary–cell membrane in the tissues.

minute ventilation ($\dot{V}E$)   The total volume of expired air in one minute.

nonvolatile acids   Metabolic acids that cannot be converted to a gas, requiring excretion through the kidneys.

oxyhemoglobin dissociation curve   A graphic representation of the relationship between oxygen saturation of hemoglobin (SaO_2) and the partial pressure of oxygen (PaO_2) in the plasma.

parietal pleura   The moist membrane that adheres to the thoracic walls, diaphragm, and mediastinum.

paroxysmal nocturnal dyspnea (PND)   A symptom usually associated with transient pulmonary edema secondary to heart failure; patient awakens from sleep with severe orthopnea.

partial pressure   Pressure each gas exerts in a total volume of gases.

partially compensated   A state in which the pH is abnormal but the body buffers and regulatory mechanisms have started to respond to the imbalance.

perfusion   The pumping or flow of blood into tissues and organs.

pH   Represents free hydrogen ion concentration.

pleural rub   Adventitious breath sound caused by inflammation of the pleural membrane.

pleurisy (pleuritis)   Pain caused by inflammation of the parietal pleura.

pressure gradient   Difference between the partial pressures of a gas; influences rate of diffusion.

pulmonary shunt   The percentage of cardiac output that flows from the right heart and back into the left heart without undergoing pulmonary gas exchange or not achieving normal levels of PaO_2 because of abnormal alveolar functioning.

pulmonary vascular resistance (PVR)   Measures the resistance to blood flow in the pulmonary vascular system, which is a low-resistance system.

pulse oximetry   Noninvasive technique for monitoring arterial capillary hemoglobin saturation.

respiration   The process by which the body's cells are supplied with oxygen and carbon dioxide is eliminated from the body.

rhonchi   Adventitious breath sounds associated with an accumulation of fluid or secretions in the larger airways.

shuntlike effect   Effect created by an excess of perfusion in relation to alveolar ventilation.

surfactant   A lipoprotein produced by type II alveolar cells that reduces the surface tension of the alveolar fluid lining.

tidal volume (TV or VT)   The amount of air that moves in and out of the lungs with each normal breath.

total lung capacity (TLC)   The amount of gas present in the lungs after maximal inspiration.

true shunt   Flow of blood from the right heart, through the lungs, and on into the left heart without taking part in alveolar–capillary diffusion.

uncompensated   An acid–base state in which the pH is abnormal because other buffer and regulatory mechanisms have not begun to correct the imbalance.

V̇/Q̇ ratio   A ratio expressing the relationship of ventilation to perfusion.

venous admixture   The effect that a physiologic shunt has on the oxygen content of the blood as it drains into the left heart.

ventilation   The mechanical movement of airflow to and from the atmosphere and the alveoli.

visceral pleura   The moist membrane that adheres to the lung parenchyma and is adjacent to the parietal pleura.

vital capacity (VC)   The maximum amount of air expired after a maximal inspiration; a measurement of lung capacity.

volatile acids   Acids that can convert to a gas form for excretion.

wheeze   Adventitious breath sound caused by air passing through constricted airways.

ABBREVIATIONS

ABG	Arterial blood gas
ARDS	Acute respiratory distress syndrome
BE	Base excess
C_L	Lung compliance, expressed in cm H_2O/mL
CO	Cardiac output
CO_2	Carbon dioxide
COPD	Chronic obstructive pulmonary disease
CVP	Central venous pressure
DKA	Diabetic ketoacidosis
ERV	Expiratory reserve volume
f	Frequency, rate of breathing, expressed in breaths per minute
FEV	Forced expiratory volume
F_{IO_2}	Fraction of inspired oxygen
FRC	Functional residual capacity
H^+	Hydrogen ion
H_2CO_3	Carbonic acid
HCO_3	Bicarbonate
Hgb (Hb)	Hemoglobin
HR	Heart rate
IPPB	Intermittent positive pressure breathing
IRV	Inspiratory reserve volume
MAP	Mean arterial pressure
mcm	micrometers
mEq/L	Milliequivalents per liter
mm Hg	Millimeters of mercury
MODS	Multiple organ dysfunction syndrome
O_2	Oxygen
P_{CO_2}	Partial pressure of carbon dioxide or carbon dioxide tension, expressed in mm Hg; variations:
	$P_{A_{CO_2}}$ Specifies alveolar carbon dioxide tension
	Pa_{CO_2} Specifies arterial carbon dioxide tension
	Pv_{CO_2} Specifies venous carbon dioxide tension
PEEP	Positive end–expiratory pressure
$P_{ET_{CO_2}}$	Partial pressure of end-tidal carbon dioxide
pH	Free hydrogen ion concentration
PND	Paroxysmal nocturnal dyspnea
P_{O_2}	Partial pressure of oxygen or oxygen tension, expressed in mm Hg; variations:
	$P_{A_{O_2}}$ Specifies alveolar oxygen tension
	Pa_{O_2} Specifies arterial oxygen tension
	Pv_{O_2} Specifies venous oxygen tension
PFT	Pulmonary function tests
PVR	Pulmonary vascular resistance
Q̇	Pulmonary capillary perfusion
RV	Residual volume
Sa_{O_2}	Saturation of arterial oxygen, measured in percentage
Sp_{O_2}	Saturation of arterial capillary hemoglobin determined by pulse oximetry, measured in percentage
SV	Stroke volume
TLC	Total lung volume
V̇	Ventilation
V̇E	Minute ventilation
V̇/Q̇ ratio	Ventilation–perfusion ratio
VC	Vital capacity
VT (TV)	Tidal volume, expressed in milliliters (mL) or liters (L)

PRETEST

1. Ventilation is best defined as
   A. movement of gases across the alveolar–capillary membrane
   B. mechanical movement of gases in and out of the lungs
   C. transport of gases through the blood to and from the tissues
   D. movement of gases down a pressure gradient

2. During inspiration, air is drawn into the lungs because intrapulmonary pressure is
   A. below atmospheric pressure
   B. equal to intra-abdominal pressure
   C. above alveolar–capillary pressure
   D. above intrathoracic pressure

3. Which of the following factors affect pulmonary diffusion? (choose all that apply)
   1. gradient
   2. thickness
   3. surface area
   4. barometric pressure
   A. 2, 3, and 4
   B. 1, 2, and 4
   C. 2 and 3
   D. 1, 2, and 3

4. If the ventilation–perfusion $\dot{V}/\dot{Q}$ ratio is low, it will affect arterial blood gases in which way?
   A. decreased Pa_{O_2}
   B. decreased Pa_{CO_2}
   C. increased Pa_{O_2}
   D. increased pH

5. Pulmonary shunt refers to
   A. blood that bypasses the heart
   B. blood that bypasses the lungs
   C. blood that does not take part in gas exchange
   D. blood that does not release carbon dioxide

6. Normal tidal volume in an average-sized adult male would be how many mL/kg?
   A. 3 to 4
   B. 4 to 5
   C. 5 to 7
   D. 7 to 9

7. Common factors affecting gas exchange include (choose all that apply)
   1. partial pressure
   2. oxyhemoglobin dissociation
   3. mixed venous saturation
   4. diffusion
   A. 1, 3, and 4
   B. 2 and 4
   C. 1, 2, and 4
   D. 1 and 4

8. Which partial statement reflects the natural movement of gas diffusion?
   A. from low to high pressure
   B. from high to low pressure
   C. from equal to unequal pressure
   D. from negative to positive pressure

9. The body compensates for acid–base imbalances by which mechanisms? (choose all that apply)
   1. buffering
   2. hepatic compensation
   3. respiratory compensation
   4. excretion of bicarbonate
   A. 1, 2, and 3
   B. 1, 3, and 4
   C. 2, 3, and 4
   D. 1 and 3

10. Respiratory compensation involves excretion or retention of
    A. CO_2
    B. HCO_3
    C. H_2O
    D. K^+

11. Normal values for arterial blood gases (ABGs) include
    A. pH 7.5
    B. Pa_{CO_2} 20 mm Hg
    C. HCO_3 26 mm Hg
    D. Sa_{O_2} 75 mm Hg

12. According to the oxyhemoglobin dissociation curve, at a Pa_{O_2} of less than 60 mm Hg, a large decrease in Pa_{O_2} should produce what in the Sa_{O_2}?
    A. a small increase
    B. a large increase
    C. a small decrease
    D. a large decrease

13. Respiratory acidosis is caused by
    A. alveolar hypoventilation
    B. alveolar hyperventilation
    C. mechanical ventilation
    D. inadequate perfusion

14. Patient situations associated with respiratory alkalosis include
    A. sedation
    B. anxiety
    C. pulmonary edema
    D. neuromuscular blockade

15. Metabolic disturbances are reflected by changes in
    A. HCO_3, Sa_{O_2}
    B. Pa_{O_2}, base excess
    C. base excess, HCO_3
    D. HCO_3, Pa_{O_2}

16. Metabolic acidosis results in
   A. increased Pa_{CO_2}
   B. decreased pH
   C. increased base excess
   D. increased HCO_3

17. A patient has the following ABG results: pH 7.48, Pa_{CO_2} 38 mm Hg, HCO_3 30 mEq/L. The correct acid–base interpretation of this ABG is
   A. uncompensated respiratory alkalosis
   B. partially compensated respiratory acidosis
   C. uncompensated metabolic alkalosis
   D. partially compensated metabolic acidosis

18. A patient has the following ABG results: pH 7.48, Pa_{CO_2} 33 mm Hg, HCO_3 26 mEq/L, Pa_{O_2} 68 mm Hg. The correct interpretation of this ABG is
   A. acute respiratory alkalosis with hypoxemia
   B. uncompensated respiratory acidosis with normal oxygenation status
   C. acute metabolic alkalosis with normal oxygenation status
   D. partially compensated metabolic acidosis with hypoxemia

19. Which statement most accurately describes a mixed acid–base disorder?
   A. it can have a nullifying effect on the pH
   B. it has no predictable effect on the pH
   C. it is primarily associated with respiratory disorders
   D. it has a respiratory as well as a metabolic acid–base component

20. The key to recognizing mixed acid–base disorders on an arterial blood gas is
   A. looking for pH extremes
   B. recognizing abnormal base excess levels
   C. knowing the predicted compensation relationships
   D. the presence of abnormal HCO_3 with a normal pH

21. Pulse oximetry measures
   A. mixed venous saturation
   B. transcutaneous oxygen saturation
   C. venous oxygen capillary hemoglobin saturation
   D. arterial oxygen capillary hemoglobin saturation

22. The end-tidal CO_2 is an indicator of alveolar
   A. ventilation
   B. acid–base state
   C. oxygenation
   D. compensation

Pretest Answers:

1. B, 2. A, 3. D, 4. A, 5. C, 6. D, 7. C, 8. B, 9. B, 10. A,
11. C, 12. D, 13. A, 14. B, 15. C, 16. B, 17. C, 18. A, 19. A,
20. C, 21. D, 22. A

Part One
Determinants of Pulmonary Gas Exchange

SECTION ONE: Mechanics of Breathing— Ventilation

At the completion of this section, the learner will be able to explain the conducting airway and the concept of ventilation.

The respiratory process has three vital components: ventilation, diffusion, and perfusion. The next three sections of this module discuss each of these concepts and their importance to the entire respiratory process. This section provides an overview of ventilation.

The Conducting Airway

The respiratory tract can be divided into the conducting and respiratory airways. The conducting airways consist of the nasal passages, mouth, pharynx, larynx, trachea, bronchi, and bronchioles. These airways serve as an air conduit to move air to and from the atmosphere and alveoli. They also provide important protective functions by humidifying, filtering, and warming air passing through them. In addition, much of the conducting airway contains a mucociliary system that removes pathogens and foreign materials by capturing them on the mucus layer and removing them through ciliary movement that transports foreign particles toward the pharynx where they can be swallowed and destroyed in the stomach. In high-acuity patients who require an artificial airway (e.g., tracheostomy or endo-/nasotracheal tube), the initial conducting airway is bypassed, which significantly reduces the protective functions. In such cases, the protective functions are artificially replaced using special equipment that provides humidity, warmth, and possibly filtering services.

The tracheobronchial tree consists of the trachea, which branches into the right and left bronchi. It may be helpful to think of the trachea as being the base of the tree and the alveoli as being the tiny terminal fruit clusters of the tree. At the junction of the "Y" formed by the two primary bronchial branches is the **carina.** This structure is heavily enervated and extremely sensitive to stimulation. The carina becomes clinically significant when touched by a suction catheter (or other device), which can trigger bronchospasm or severe coughing. The right bronchus is shorter, larger in diameter than the left bronchus, and is at almost a straight angle with the trachea. The left bronchus is longer, smaller in diameter, and at a more acute angle than the right bronchus. The bronchial anatomic structure has clinical significance because the size and positioning of the right bronchus makes it more vulnerable to the introduction of pathogens and foreign particles as well as for the misplacement of an endotracheal tube. The trachea and bronchial walls contain a C-shaped cartilage structure, which is present down to the bronchiole level. The cartilage gives structure and protection to the larger airways.

Toward the terminal end of the bronchial tree are the bronchioles, which are surrounded by smooth muscle but lack cartilage. Martini and Bartholomew (2003) state that, "Bronchioles are to the respiratory system what arterioles are to the circulatory system" (p. 463). By this statement, they are referring to the fact that bronchioles (like arterioles) have the ability to regulate resistance to flow by causing constriction or dilation, thus controlling airflow distribution. However, arterioles control blood flow via vasoconstriction and vasodilation, whereas the bronchioles control airflow through bronchoconstriction and bronchodilation. Figure 4–1 provides an illustration of the anatomy of the respiratory system.

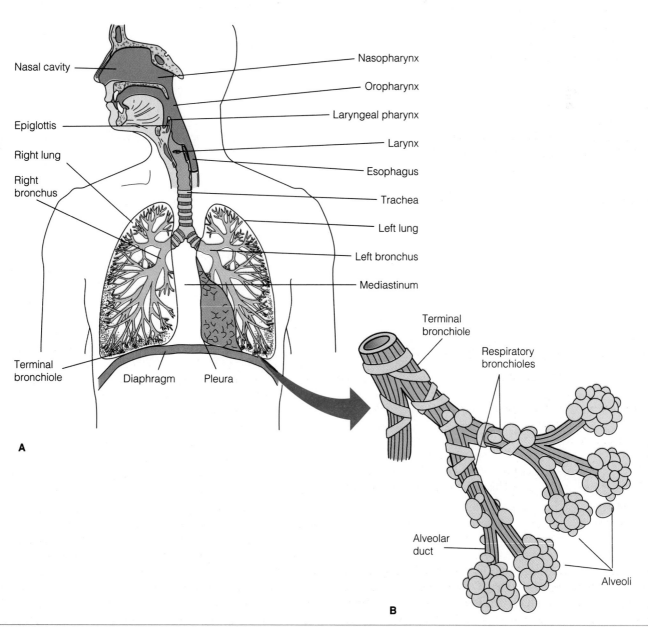

Figure 4–1 ■ Anatomy of the respiratory system.

Ventilation

Ventilation is the first of the three components of the respiratory process and is defined as the mechanical movement of airflow to and from the atmosphere and the alveoli. Ventilation involves the actual work of breathing and requires nervous system control and adequate functioning of the lungs and conducting airways, thorax, and ventilatory muscles. Decreased functioning of any one of these factors will affect the body's ability to ventilate properly.

Ventilation is accomplished through a bellows-like action. Air is able to move in and out of the lungs as a result of the changing size of the thorax caused by ventilatory muscle activity. When the thorax enlarges, the intrapulmonary pressure drops to below atmospheric pressure. Air then moves from the area of higher pressure to the area of lower pressure, resulting in air flowing into the lungs (inspiration) until the pressure in the lungs becomes slightly higher than atmospheric pressure. At this point, air flows back out of the lungs (expiration) until once again pressures are equalized.

Lung tissue has a constant tendency to collapse because of several important properties. First, the fluid lining of the alveoli has a naturally high surface tension, creating a tendency for the alveolar walls to collapse. To prevent this, special cells (type II cells) in the alveoli secrete a lipoprotein called **surfactant.** Surfactant has a detergent-like action that reduces the surface tension of the fluid lining the alveolar sacs, thereby decreasing the tendency toward collapse. Second, the lungs are composed of elastic fibers. The elastic force of these fibers constantly seeks to return to a resting state (i.e., collapsed lungs). To maintain the lungs in an inflated state, the elastic forces must constantly be overcome by opposing forces (Fig. 4–2).

The thorax is the primary opposing force that maintains the lungs in an expanded state. The thoracic bony structure provides a cagelike framework that maintains the lungs in a baseline inflated state even at rest because of the attraction that exists between the visceral and parietal pleura. The pleura are slick-surfaced moist membranes. The **parietal pleura** adheres to the thoracic walls, diaphragm, and mediastinum; and the **visceral pleura** adheres to the lung parenchyma. To understand the pleural attraction, it may help to think of placing two moistened sheets of smooth glass together. Although it would be relatively easy to glide one sheet over the other in a parallel fashion, it would be very difficult to pull them directly apart at a 180° angle. The glass sheets represent the two pleurae. Under normal circumstances (a negative intrapleural state), the parietal and visceral pleura act as one membrane. Therefore, as the thorax increases and decreases in size, so will the lungs increase and decrease in volume.

Lung Compliance

The ease with which the lungs are able to be expanded is measured in terms of lung compliance. For example, it is much more difficult to blow up a small balloon than a large balloon. To

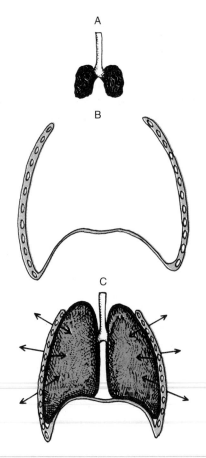

Figure 4–2■ Opposing elastic forces of lungs and thorax. *A.* The resting state of normal lungs when removed from the chest cavity. Elasticity causes total collapse. *B.* Resting state of normal chest wall and diaphragm when apex is open to the atmosphere, and the thoracic contents are removed. *C.* End expiration in the normal, intact thorax. Note that the elastic forces of the lung and chest wall are in opposite directions. The pleural surfaces link these two opposing forces. *(From Shapiro, B. A., et al. [1991]. Clinical application of respiratory care (4th ed.) [p. 22]. St. Louis: Mosby-Year Book.)*

inflate the small balloon, you would need to blow harder (exert more pressure force) to obtain the same volume that you would be able to obtain with less force in the large balloon. The small balloon is less compliant than the large balloon. **Compliance (C_L)** is defined in terms of lung volume (mL) and pressure (cm H_2O) as

$$C_L = \Delta V / \Delta P$$

where C_L is lung compliance, ΔV is change in volume (mL), and ΔP is change in pressure (cm H_2O).

Like a bag of assorted-sized balloons, alveoli also come in many sizes. Each size of alveolus has a certain filling capacity beyond which it becomes overexpanded and may even burst. As the alveoli approach their filling capacity, they become less compliant; that is, it takes more force to completely expand the alveoli and even greater force to hyperexpand them. For example, patients with acute respiratory distress syndrome (ARDS) require moderate to high levels of positive end–expiratory pressure (PEEP) to open, expand, or hyperexpand alveoli that have become significantly noncompliant because of the disease process. Use of PEEP ideally increases lung compliance. However, if too much PEEP (measured in cm H_2O pressure) is used, alveoli become so hyperexpanded that compliance decreases dramatically and the alveoli are at risk of rupture, causing pneumothorax. PEEP is explained in detail in the mechanical ventilation module.

Many pulmonary and extrapulmonary problems influence compliance. Compliance is very sensitive to any condition that affects the lung's tissues, particularly if the disorder causes a reduction in pulmonary surfactant, which is crucial to maintenance of functional alveoli. When there is a deficiency of surfactant, compliance is decreased. Decreased compliance is sometimes referred to as "stiff lungs," meaning that it now takes more force (pressure) to increase lung volume. For example, whereas a person with normal lungs can inhale 50 to 100 mL of air for every 1.0 cm H_2O of pressure exerted, a person with decreased compliance might be able to inhale 30 to 40 mL/cm H_2O of pressure. Decreased compliance increases the work of breathing and causes a decreased tidal volume. The breathing rate increases to compensate for the decreased tidal volume. Pulmonary problems causing decreased compliance are called restrictive pulmonary disorders. (Examples of conditions associated with decreased lung compliance can be found in Module 5, Table 5–1.)

Effects of Aging on Ventilation

As a person ages, the diaphragm flattens, the chest wall becomes more rigid, the respiratory muscles weaken, and the anterior–posterior diameter of the chest increases. All of these factors contribute to decreased lung compliance, altered pulmonary mechanics, and air trapping. The lung's functional ability reduces roughly about 5 to 20 percent per decade of life (Ross, n.d.). A person who has never smoked and who has maintained normal lungs throughout life may exhibit little if any clinically significant changes in ventilation through aging. In contrast, the aging person who has a history of smoking with some degree of lung damage tends to become increasingly symptomatic with aging and is at increased risk for developing respiratory complications (Beers & Berkow, 2004).

In summary, the respiratory system can be divided into the conducting and respiratory airways. The conducting airways act as a conduit for airflow. They provide protective functions of humidification, filtration, and warming of air passing through. The tracheobronchial tree begins at the trachea and continuously branches down to the tiny terminal bronchioles. Most of the tree contains cartilage, which provides structure and protection. The tiny bronchioles are important in regulating airflow distribution because they can constrict and dilate. Ventilation involves the actual work of breathing through mechanical movement of the thorax and diaphragm. The respiratory process has two major components: respiration and ventilation. Lung tissue has to constantly overcome the tendency to collapse. The substance surfactant is crucial in maintaining the alveoli in an open state. Lung compliance is decreased by many intrapulmonary and extrapulmonary disorders affecting the volume of air moved in and out of the lungs. As a person ages, lung compliance decreases and anterior-posterior diameter of the chest increases. The aging person who has healthy lung tissue will maintain good ventilatory capacity throughout life.

SECTION ONE REVIEW

1. The conducting airways serve what major functions? (choose all that apply)
   1. gas exchange
   2. filtering
   3. immune
   4. humidifying
   5. warming
   A. 1, 2, and 4
   B. 2, 3, and 5
   C. 1, 3, and 4
   D. 2, 4, and 5
2. The elastic force of lung tissue seeks to
   A. keep lungs expanded
   B. collapse the lungs
   C. flatten the diaphragm
   D. decrease thorax size

3. During expiration, air flows out of the lungs because the intrapulmonary pressure
   A. increases to above atmospheric pressure
   B. is equal to perfusion pressure
   C. drops to below atmospheric pressure
   D. is equal to alveolar pressure
4. The purpose of surfactant is to
   A. decrease lung compliance
   B. increase alveolar surface tension
   C. cleanse the alveoli
   D. decrease alveolar surface tension
5. The lungs adhere to the thoracic walls because of
   A. elastic forces
   B. pulmonary surfactant
   C. pleural attraction
   D. lung compliance

6. As alveoli near their filling capacity, they become
   A. less compliant
   B. less elastic
   C. more compliant
   D. hyperexpanded

7. The primary function of the type II alveolar cells is
   A. filtration
   B. gas exchange
   C. immune protection
   D. surfactant production

Answers: 1. D, 2. B, 3. A, 4. D, 5. C, 6. A, 7. D

SECTION TWO: Pulmonary Gas Exchange— Respiration and Diffusion

At the completion of this section, the learner will be able to discuss external respiration and pulmonary gas diffusion.

The Cardiopulmonary Circuit and Respiration

Respiration is the process by which the body's cells are supplied with oxygen and carbon dioxide (cellular waste product) is eliminated from the body. Respiration can be further divided into internal and external respiration. **Internal respiration** refers to the movement of gases across systemic capillary–cell membranes in the tissues. Internal respiration is presented in detail in Module 14, "Oxygenation." **External respiration** refers to the movement of gases across the alveolar–capillary membrane (i.e., pulmonary gas exchange). External respiration is the focus of this module. Both external and internal respiration use diffusion as their means of exchanging gases. To understand diffusion, it is helpful to first understand the concept of partial pressure and the oxyhemoglobin dissociation curve. Figure 4–3 illustrates the cardiopulmonary circuit and respiration.

Figure 4–3 ■ Cardiopulmonary circuit and respiration.

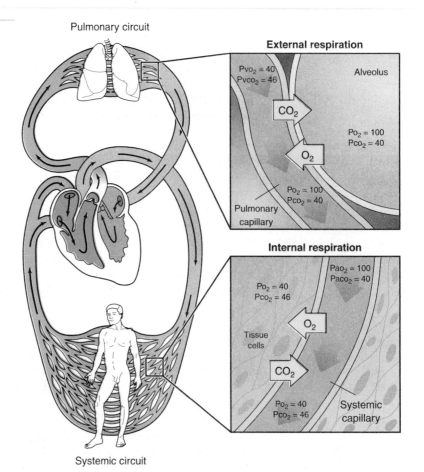

Pulmonary circuit

External respiration

$Pvo_2 = 40$
$Pvco_2 = 46$

Alveolus

CO_2

$Po_2 = 100$
$Pco_2 = 40$

O_2

$Po_2 = 100$
$Pco_2 = 40$

Pulmonary capillary

Internal respiration

$Pao_2 = 100$
$Paco_2 = 40$

$Po_2 = 40$
$Pco_2 = 46$

O_2

Tissue cells

CO_2

$Po_2 = 40$
$Pco_2 = 46$

Systemic capillary

Systemic circuit

Diffusion

Diffusion is the second of the three components of the respiratory process. Oxygenation of tissues is dependent on the process of diffusion as the vital mechanism for both external and internal respiration. Diffusion is the movement of gases down a pressure gradient from an area of high pressure to an area of low pressure. The alveolar–capillary membrane is very thin (0.5 mcm), offering little resistance to diffusion in normal circumstances. The membrane can thicken when pulmonary pathologic processes exist, reducing diffusion (e.g., pulmonary edema, acute respiratory distress syndrome). Because carbon dioxide diffuses 20 times faster than oxygen, the carbon dioxide tension may remain at normal levels initially, but the oxygen tension decreases. There are four factors that affect diffusion through the alveolar–capillary membrane: partial pressures and gradient, surface area, thickness, and length of exposure. In addition, the oxyhemoglobin dissociation curve plays an important role in determining the affinity of oxygen to hemoglobin, which directly affects diffusion.

Partial Pressures and Gradient

Atmospheric air is composed of molecules of nitrogen, oxygen, carbon dioxide, and water vapor. The combination of all of these gases exerts about 760 mm Hg of pressure at sea level. The respiratory process, however, does not actively involve the use of the water vapor or nitrogen. It is concerned with exchange of oxygen and carbon dioxide.

Oxygen and carbon dioxide both exert a certain percentage of the total air pressure. Oxygen in the alveoli exerts approximately 100 mm Hg pressure, and this partial pressure of oxygen is called P_{O_2}, or oxygen tension. When the P_{O_2} refers to oxygen in the alveoli, it is more precisely referred to as $P_{A}O_2$. When it refers to arterial blood, it is abbreviated as $P_{a}O_2$, and when it refers to venous blood, it is specified as $P_{v}O_2$. Carbon dioxide in the alveoli exerts approximately 40 mm Hg of pressure. This partial pressure is called P_{CO_2}. The abbreviation alterations of A, a, and v used for describing P_{O_2} also apply to P_{CO_2}.

Venous blood returning to the lungs from the tissues is oxygen poor ($P_{v}O_2$ less than 40 mm Hg) because the blood has dropped off its load of oxygen for use by the tissues. Venous blood is rich in carbon dioxide ($P_{v}CO_2$ greater than 45 mm Hg) because of transport of the cellular waste product, carbon dioxide (CO_2), for removal from the lungs.

The differences in gas partial pressures between the alveoli and pulmonary capillary blood and the systemic capillary blood and the tissues dictate which direction each gas will flow based on the law of diffusion (i.e., from an area of higher pressure to an area of lower pressure). For example, if alveolar oxygen ($P_{A}O_2$) is 100 mm Hg and mixed venous oxygen ($P_{v}O_2$) is 40 mm Hg, alveolar oxygen will diffuse across the alveolar-capillary membrane into the capillary blood to equalize the partial pressures. Figure 4–4 shows the movement of gases during diffusion.

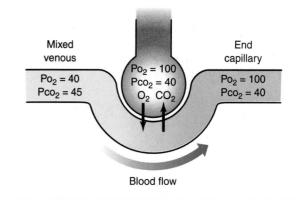

Figure 4–4 ▪ Gas distribution.

Henry's law states that when a gas is exposed to liquid, some of it will dissolve in the liquid. The partial pressure of the gas and its solubility determine the amount of gas that dissolves. Oxygen is not very soluble in plasma. Only 3 percent of the total oxygen content dissolves in blood. It is the partial pressure of gases (oxygen and carbon dioxide) flowing in the arterial system that is measured in an arterial blood gas sample (see Figure 4–5).

The difference between the partial pressures is called the **pressure gradient.** In external respiration, a pressure gradient (difference) exists between the atmosphere and the alveoli and between the alveoli and the pulmonary capillaries. The greater the pressure difference, the more rapid the flow of gases. Multiple factors can increase the gradient; for example, exercise, positive pressure mechanical ventilation, and intermittent positive pressure breathing (IPPB). Air enters the alveoli from the atmosphere because the atmospheric air pressure is slightly higher than alveolar pressure, which creates a pressure gradient.

In external respiration, a pressure gradient exists between the alveoli and the pulmonary capillaries, causing flow of gases across the alveolar–capillary membrane. For example, Patient X has a $P_{v}O_2$ (oxygen–poor blood returning to the heart) of 45 mm Hg and a $P_{v}CO_2$ of 55 mm Hg, whereas his alveolar P_{O_2} ($P_{A}O_2$) is 100 mm Hg and $P_{A}CO_2$ is 25. Because the oxygen tension in the alveolus is much higher than in the capillary, oxygen will diffuse down the gradient from the alveolus into the blood passing by. The carbon dioxide tension, however, is lower in the alveolus than it is in the blood, causing a pressure gradient that will move CO_2 out of the blood and into the alveolus.

In internal respiration, the process is reversed. The arterial blood is rich (high) in oxygen and poor (low) in carbon dioxide, whereas the cells are poor in oxygen and rich in carbon dioxide. The pressure differences between the $P_{a}O_2$ and $P_{a}CO_2$ in the blood and cells cause oxygen to move from the circulating hemoglobin into the cells. The cells release carbon dioxide into the bloodstream for transport back to the lungs for excretion.

Figure 4–5 ■ Partial pressure—atmosphere and alveoli.

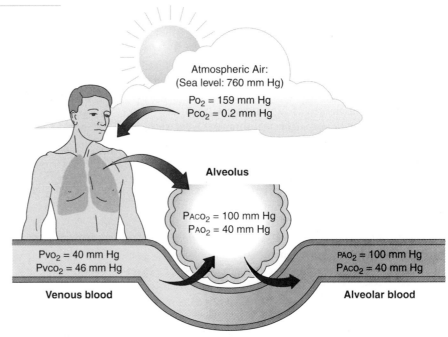

A handy rule to remember is that gradients seek to equalize by flowing from an area of high pressure to an area of low pressure.

Surface Area

The total surface area of the lung is very large. The greater the available alveolar–capillary membrane surface area, the greater the amount of oxygen and carbon dioxide that can diffuse across it during a specific time period. Emphysema is a major pulmonary disorder that destroys the alveolar–capillary membrane. This greatly reduces surface area and consequently impairs gas exchange. Many pulmonary conditions, including severe pneumonia, lung tumors, pneumothorax, and pneumonectomy, can reduce functioning surface area significantly.

Thickness

The thickness of the alveolar–capillary membrane is of major importance—the thinner the membrane, the more rapid the rate of diffusion of gases. Several conditions can increase membrane thickness, thereby decreasing the rate of diffusion:

- Fluid in the alveoli or interstitial spaces or both (e.g., pulmonary edema)
- An inflammatory process involving the alveoli (e.g., pneumonia)
- Lung conditions that cause fibrosis (e.g., ARDS or pneumoconiosis)

Length of Exposure

During periods of rest, blood flows through the alveolar–capillary system in approximately 0.75 second. Diffusion of oxygen and carbon dioxide requires about 0.25 second to reach equilibrium (the balance between alveolar and capillary gas levels). During periods of high cardiac output, such as occurs with heavy exercise or stress, blood flow is faster through the alveolar–capillary system. Under these circumstances, diffusion takes place during a shortened exposure time. In healthy lungs, oxygen exchange is usually not impaired with high cardiac output states; however, hypoxemia may result if diffusion abnormalities are present, such as pulmonary edema, alveolar consolidation (e.g., pneumonia), or alveolar fibrosis.

Oxyhemoglobin Dissociation Curve

Hemoglobin is the primary carrier of oxygen in the blood. It has an affinity or attraction for oxygen molecules. In the pulmonary capillaries, oxygen binds loosely and reversibly to hemoglobin, forming oxyhemoglobin for transport to the tissues where it can be released. The amount of oxygen that loads onto hemoglobin is expressed as a percentage of hemoglobin saturation by oxygen (percent SaO_2). The affinity of hemoglobin for oxygen varies, depending on certain physiologic factors. The **oxyhemoglobin dissociation curve** represents the relationship of the partial pressure of arterial oxygen (PaO_2) and hemoglobin saturation (SaO_2). The curve (Fig. 4–6) is depicted as an S-curve rather than a straight line, showing that the percentage saturation of hemoglobin does not maintain a direct relationship with the PaO_2.

The top portion of the curve (PaO_2 greater than 60 mm Hg) is flattened into a horizontal position. In this portion of the curve, a large alteration in PaO_2 produces only small alterations in the percentage of hemoglobin saturation. For example, note that a 10 mm Hg decrease of a patient's PaO_2 from 80 mm Hg to 70 mm Hg would produce very little change in SaO_2

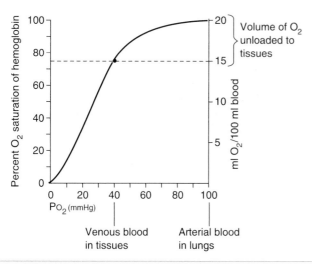

Figure 4–6 ■ Oxyhemoglobin dissociation curve.

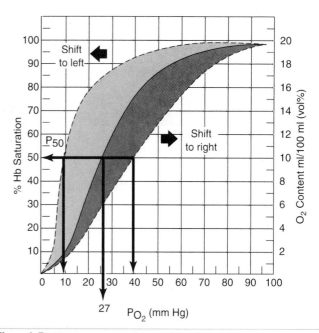

Figure 4–7 ■ The P_{50} represents the partial pressure at which hemoglobin is 50 percent saturated with oxygen. When the oxygen dissociation curve shifts to the right, the P_{50} increases. When the oxygen dissociation curve shifts to the left, the P_{50} decreases. (*From* Cardiopulmonary Anatomy and Physiology, *2nd ed. by J. R. Des Jardins © 1993. Reprinted with permission of Delmar, a division of Thomson Learning. Fax [800] 730-2215.*)

(see Fig. 4–6). Clinically, this means that although administering supplemental oxygen may significantly increase the patient's PaO_2, the resulting SaO_2 increase will be small in proportion. The patient's oxygenation status is better protected at the top of the curve.

The bottom portion of the curve (PaO_2 less than 60 mm Hg) is steep. In this portion, any alteration in PaO_2 yields a large change in percentage of hemoglobin saturation (SaO_2). For example, a 10 mm Hg decrease in PaO_2 from 60 mm Hg to 50 mm Hg decreases the SaO_2 from about 85 percent to about 75 percent (a decrease of approximately 10). Clinically, this means that administration of supplemental oxygen sufficient to increase the PaO_2 should yield large increases in SaO_2. However, abnormalities in the ventilation–perfusion relationship may exist, interfering with reoxygenation.

Low PaO_2 at the tissue level stimulates oxygen release from hemoglobin to the tissue. High PaO_2 at the pulmonary capillary level stimulates hemoglobin to bind with more oxygen. Other factors can change the curve, shifting it to the right or the left (Fig. 4–7). A right shift prevents hemoglobin from binding as readily with oxygen, although oxygen is able to be released at the tissue level more readily. A left shift causes hemoglobin to bind more readily with oxygen in the lungs, but inhibits release at the tissue level. Factors that shift the curve to the right and left are listed in Table 4–1. Slight shifts are adaptive. For example, an increased body temperature increases oxygen demand, causing a slight right shift, which increases release of oxygen to the tissues to meet increasing tissue oxygen demand. Severe or rapid shifts, however, can produce life-threatening tissue hypoxia.

The Effects of Aging on Diffusion

As a person ages, total lung surface area decreases, the alveolar–capillary membrane thickness increases, and alveoli are destroyed because of aging processes. These changes result in decreased diffusion across the alveolar–capillary membrane, altering the

TABLE 4–1 Factors Affecting the Oxyhemoglobin Dissociation Curve

RIGHT SHIFT	LEFT SHIFT
Acidosis	Alkalosis
Hyperthermia	Hypothermia
Hypercarbia	Hypocarbia
Increased 2,3-DPG[a]	Decreased 2,3-DPG

[a]2,3-DPG = 2,3-diphosphoglycerate.

ventilation–perfusion relationship. Overall, gas exchange becomes less efficient, placing the high-acuity aging patient at risk for hypoxemia and/or hypercapnia problems. Additionally, over time, the airways become larger, increasing dead space ventilation and terminal airways lose supportive structures, which can result in airtrapping. Both of these physiologic changes can lead to carbon dioxide retention.

In summary, external respiration is the movement of gases across the alveolar–capillary membrane by the process of diffusion. This section described diffusion through examination of the factors that affect it, including the partial pressure of gases (e.g., PO_2 and PCO_2) and, more indirectly, the oxyhemoglobin dissociation curve. An understanding of these concepts assists in determining alternatives for clinical interventions. Diffusion is the process by which gases are exchanged in the lungs and in the tissues. The factors of gradient, surface area, thickness, and length of exposure all greatly influence the ef-

fectiveness of diffusion. Should a pulmonary disorder cause a problem with any one of these factors, gas exchange becomes impaired, which may result in an increase in arterial carbon dioxide levels, a decrease in arterial oxygen levels, or both.

SECTION TWO REVIEW

1. Pressure gradient affects diffusion of gases in which of the following ways?
   A. the more rapid the ventilatory rate, the greater the gradient
   B. the greater the difference, the more rapid the gas flow
   C. the less rapid the ventilatory rate, the greater the gradient
   D. the smaller the difference, the more rapid the gas flow
2. Which factor increases the diffusion pressure gradient?
   A. increased exercise
   B. decreased activity
   C. negative pressure ventilation
   D. amount of lung surface area
3. The normal partial pressure of alveolar oxygen is approximately
   A. 60 mm Hg
   B. 80 mm Hg
   C. 100 mm Hg
   D. 110 mm Hg
4. Surface area as a factor affecting diffusion refers to the
   A. size of the alveoli
   B. conducting airways
   C. functional capillary perfusion
   D. functional alveoli and surrounding capillaries
5. An example of a disease process that would increase the thickness of the alveolar–capillary membrane is
   A. pneumothorax
   B. pneumonia

C. lung tumor
D. pneumonectomy
6. Which statement regarding diffusion is correct?
   A. diffusion refers to capillary pressure
   B. diffusion refers to alveolar pressure
   C. gas flows up a pressure gradient
   D. gas flows down a pressure gradient
7. Which statement is correct regarding the normal relationship between oxygen and hemoglobin?
   A. oxygen binds loosely and reversibly to hemoglobin
   B. hemoglobin is attracted to oxygen molecules
   C. the affinity of hemoglobin to oxygen is constant
   D. the relationship is expressed in mm Hg (pressure)
8. True or False: On the oxyhemoglobin dissociation curve, at a PaO_2 less than 60 mm Hg, any change in PaO_2 yields a large change in SaO_2.
9. External respiration refers to
   A. movement of air from the atmosphere to the alveoli
   B. diffusion of gases across the alveolar–capillary membrane
   C. movement of air from the alveoli to the atmosphere
   D. diffusion of gases across the tissue–capillary membranes

Answers: 1. B, 2. A, 3. C, 4. D, 5. B, 6. D, 7. A, 8. True; this is why it is so important to maintain the PaO_2 above 60 mm Hg, 9. B

SECTION THREE: Pulmonary Gas Exchange— Perfusion

At the completion of this section, the learner will be able to discuss pulmonary perfusion.

Perfusion is the third and final component of the respiratory process. For the purposes of this chapter, **perfusion** refers to the pumping or flow of blood into tissues and organs. Perfusion can be divided into two circulatory systems: the systemic system and the pulmonary system. The *systemic system* is vast, running from the aorta through the right atrium of the heart. The *pulmonary system* is much smaller, running from pulmonary artery through the left atrium (Des Jardins, 2002). The pulmonary system is dependent on adequate perfusion in the

systemic system and adequate perfusion in both systems is required for oxygenation of the tissues in the entire body. Both of these perfusion systems are composed of a complex network of blood vessels of varying sizes and functions (Fig. 4–8).

Pulmonary perfusion depends on three factors: cardiac output (CO), gravity, and pulmonary vascular resistance (PVR).

Cardiac Output

Cardiac output (CO) is a function of stroke volume (SV) and heart rate (HR)—$CO = SV \times HR$. Normal cardiac output is between 4 and 8 liters per minute. Stroke volume is a function of ventricular preload, afterload, and contractility. A common measurement that is used clinically to reflect adequacy of perfu-

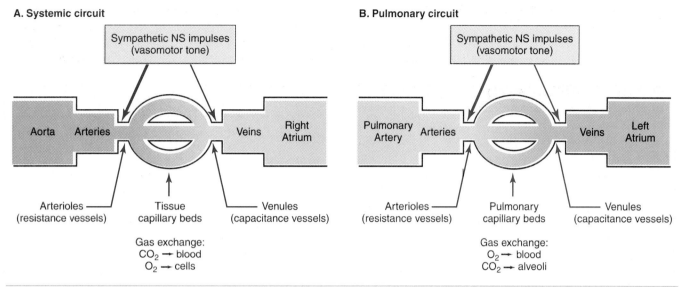

A. Systemic circuit

Sympathetic NS impulses
(vasomotor tone)

Aorta   Arteries

Veins   Right Atrium

Arterioles
(resistance vessels)

Tissue
capillary beds

Venules
(capacitance vessels)

Gas exchange:
$CO_2 \rightarrow$ blood
$O_2 \rightarrow$ cells

B. Pulmonary circuit

Sympathetic NS impulses
(vasomotor tone)

Pulmonary
Artery   Arteries

Veins   Left Atrium

Arterioles
(resistance vessels)

Pulmonary
capillary beds

Venules
(capacitance vessels)

Gas exchange:
$O_2 \rightarrow$ blood
$CO_2 \rightarrow$ alveoli

Figure 4–8 ▪ Two perfusion systems: **A.** systemic and **B.** pulmonary.

sion is the mean arterial pressure (MAP). This can be approximated using the equation: $MAP = [2(P_{dias}) + P_{sys}]/3$, where P_{dias} is diastolic blood pressure and P_{sys} is systolic blood pressure. Ideally, the MAP is maintained between 70 and 110 mmHg. It is known that a MAP of less than 60 mmHg is inadequate for perfusing major organs, such as the brain, heart, and kidneys. Typically, the clinical goal is to maintain the MAP at 70 or above to prevent organ hypoperfusion, which can then lead to organ ischemia and multiple organ dysfunction syndrome (MODS). Systemic perfusion, including cardiac output and mean arterial pressure, are presented in detail in Module 8, "Determinants and Assessment of Cardiac Output."

Gravity

The effects of gravity on blood are an important consideration in pulmonary gas exchange. Because blood has weight, it is gravity dependent; thus it naturally flows toward (and is greatest) in dependent areas of the body. Gravity has a major influence on the relationship that ventilation maintains with pulmonary perfusion.

Ventilation–Perfusion Relationship

Normal diffusion of gases requires a certain balance of alveolar ventilation (movement of gas into the alveoli) and pulmonary perfusion (blood flow through the pulmonary capillaries). Should a significant imbalance in this relationship develop, normal gas exchange cannot take place in the affected areas. For this reason, it is important to gain a basic understanding of the relationship of ventilation ($\dot{V}$) to perfusion ($\dot{Q}$). This relationship is expressed as a ratio of alveolar ventilation to pulmonary capillary perfusion (**$\dot{V}/\dot{Q}$ ratio**). For ideal gas exchange to occur, we

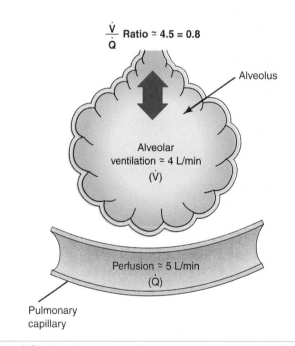

$\dfrac{\dot{V}}{\dot{Q}}$ **Ratio ≈ 4.5 = 0.8**

Alveolus

Alveolar
ventilation ≈ 4 L/min
($\dot{V}$)

Perfusion ≈ 5 L/min
($\dot{Q}$)

Pulmonary
capillary

Figure 4–9 ▪ The relationship of ventilation to perfusion. The normal ventilation–perfusion ratio ($\dot{V}/\dot{Q}$ ratio) is about 0.8. (*From* Cardiopulmonary Anatomy and Physiology (2nd *ed.*), by J. R. Des Jardins © 1993. *Reprinted with permission of Delmar, a division of Thomson Learning. Fax [800] 730-2215.*)

might expect that for every liter of fresh air coming into the alveoli, 1 L of blood would flow past it, creating a 1:1 ratio of ventilation to perfusion. In reality, for approximately every 4 L of air flowing into the alveoli, about 5 L of blood flows past (an average ratio of 4:5, or 0.8) (Fig. 4–9).

The balance of ventilation to perfusion is greatly affected by the P_{AO_2} and P_{ACO_2}. This balance depends on adequate diffusion of oxygen and carbon dioxide across the alveolar–capillary membrane, and movement of oxygen into and carbon dioxide out of the alveoli.

Although normal values are given for P_{AO_2} (100 mm Hg) and P_{ACO_2} (40 mm Hg), these numbers only express an average. The actual partial pressures of oxygen and carbon dioxide vary throughout the lungs because ventilation is not distributed evenly because of gravity-dependent factors. In an upright person, alveolar ventilation is moderate in the apices of the lungs because of increased negative pleural pressures in the apices in relation to the lung bases. This makes the alveoli in the lung apices more resistant to airflow during inspiration. When breathing spontaneously, airflow naturally moves toward the diaphragm, which results in more air movement into the bases and peripheral lung during inspiration (airflow follows the path of least resistance). Pulmonary capillary perfusion is gravity dependent, making perfusion greatest in the dependent areas of the lungs (the bases in an upright person). Consequently, because ventilation and perfusion are both greatest in the bases of the lungs, the greatest amount of gas exchange occurs in this portion of the lung fields.

In the upper lungs, there is moderate alveolar ventilation and significantly reduced perfusion, making an excess of ventilation to available perfusion. This results in a "high" $\dot{V}/\dot{Q}$ ratio; that is, a $\dot{V}/\dot{Q}$ ratio that is higher than the average of 0.8. In the lower lungs, there is a moderate increase in ventilation with a great increase in perfusion. This results in a "low" $\dot{V}/\dot{Q}$ ratio (lower than the average of 0.8) because there is a relatively moderate increase in ventilation associated with a significant increase in perfusion.

The clinical significance of ventilation–perfusion balance becomes apparent when considering its implications in high-acuity patients. This patient population generally requires prolonged bedrest, usually in a relatively horizontal position. Because blood is gravity dependent, it will shift from the lung bases to whichever lung area is now in the dependent position; however, air continues to be drawn toward the diaphragm (Fig. 4–10).

Keeping the principles of $\dot{V}/\dot{Q}$ ratio in mind, what could happen if a patient is positioned on the right side when there is significant pneumonia in the right lung fields? Because the patient is lying on the right side, maximum pulmonary capillary perfusion will be on the right. Pneumonia is associated with secretions and other factors that cause obstruction to airflow into the affected right lung alveoli. Therefore, because airflow follows the path of least resistance, it will avoid the diseased right lung area. This combination of a significant decrease in ventilation in the presence of normal-to-increased perfusion causes a mismatching of ventilation to perfusion, creating a low $\dot{V}/\dot{Q}$ ratio. If sufficient mismatching occurs, Pa_{O_2} and oxygen saturation levels can decrease significantly. Positioning this patient on the left side may be tolerated better because $\dot{V}/\dot{Q}$ matching would be improved. This, then, is one reason why some high-acuity patients tolerate being turned on one side more than another. Table 4–2 compares high and low $\dot{V}/\dot{Q}$ ratios.

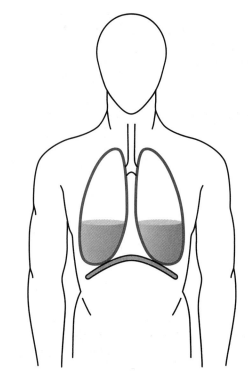

A. Upright position—Air moves towards diaphragm and blood gravitates to bases. Best $\dot{V}/\dot{Q}$ match

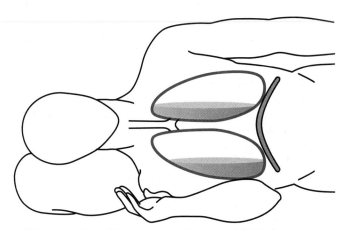

B. Side lying position—Air moves towards diaphragm while blood gravitates to lateral dependent lung fields.

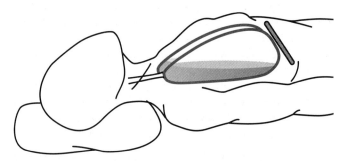

C. Supine position—Air moves towards diaphragm while blood gravitates to posterior dependent lung fields.

Figure 4–10 ■ Positioning and ventilation-to-perfusion relationship.

TABLE 4–2 Comparison of High and Low V̇/Q̇ Ratios

HIGH V̇/Q̇ RATIO	LOW V̇/Q̇ RATIO
Normal to increased alveolar ventilation associated with decreased perfusion	Decreased alveolar ventilation associated with normal to increased perfusion
Alveolar gas effect	**Alveolar gas effect**
Increased cardiac output	Decreased oxygen in alveoli
Decreased alveolar CO_2	Increased carbon dioxide in alveoli
Normally exists in upper lung fields	Normally exists in lower lung fields
Abnormally present with	**Abnormally present with**
Decreased cardiac output	Hypoventilation
Pulmonary emboli	Obstructive lung diseases
Pneumothorax	Restrictive lung diseases
Destruction of pulmonary capillaries	
Arterial blood gas effects	**Arterial blood gas effects**
Increased Pa_{O_2}	Decreased Pa_{O_2}
Decreased Pa_{CO_2}	Increased Pa_{CO_2}
Increased pH	Decreased pH

Pulmonary Shunt

The term **pulmonary shunt** refers to the percentage of cardiac output that flows from the right heart and back into the left heart without undergoing pulmonary gas exchange (**true shunt, or physiologic shunt**) or not achieving normal levels of Pa_{O_2} ("shuntlike effect") because of abnormal alveolar functioning. Pulmonary shunting is a major cause of hypoxemia in high-acuity patients. It also helps explain how problems in ventilation and perfusion originate. There are two types of true shunts—anatomic shunt and capillary shunt (Fig. 4–11).

Anatomic Shunt. Not all blood that flows through the lungs participates in gas exchange. **Anatomic shunt** refers to blood that moves from the right heart and back into the left heart without coming into contact with alveoli. Normally, this is approximately 2 to 5 percent of blood flow. Normal anatomic shunting occurs as a result of emptying of the bronchial and several other veins into the lung's own venous system. Abnormal anatomic shunting can occur because of heart or lung problems. For example, a ventricular septal defect, in the presence of pulmonary hypertension, shunts venous blood from the right heart directly into the arterial blood in the left heart. Traumatic injury to pulmonary blood vessels and tissues and certain types of lung tumors also can cause abnormal anatomic shunting.

Capillary Shunt. **Capillary shunt** is the normal flow of blood past completely unventilated alveoli. Capillary shunt results from such conditions as consolidation or collapse of alveoli, atelectasis, or fluid in the alveoli.

The combined amount of anatomic shunt and capillary shunt is called **absolute shunt.** The total percentage of cardiac output involved in absolute shunt has important clinical implications. Lung tissue that is affected by absolute shunt is unaffected by oxygen therapy because it involves nonfunctioning alveoli. No matter how much oxygen is administered, diffusion cannot take place if alveoli are completely bypassed or nonfunctioning. Shunting of more than 15 percent of cardiac output can be noted in severe respiratory failure. In fact, patients with **acute respiratory distress syndrome (ARDS)** generally have an absolute shunt of more than 20 percent of their cardiac output. The hallmark of ARDS is refractory hypoxemia (hypoxemia that is not significantly affected by administration of increasing levels of oxygen), which is consistent with the clinical picture of absolute shunt. Estimates of the amount of shunt can be made using relatively easy calculations. These are presented in Section Ten.

Shuntlike Effect. **Shuntlike effect** is not a true shunt because the shunting is not complete. Shuntlike effect exists when there is an excess of perfusion in relation to alveolar ventilation–in other words, when alveolar ventilation is reduced but not totally absent. Common causes include bronchospasm, hypoventilation, or pooling of secretions. Fortunately, because the alveoli are still functioning to some extent, hypoxemia secondary to shuntlike effect is very responsive to oxygen therapy.

Venous Admixture. **Venous admixture** refers to the effect that pulmonary shunt has on the contents of the blood as it drains into the left heart and out into the system as arterial blood. Beyond the shunted areas, the fully reoxygenated blood (from normal alveolar units) mixes with the completely or relatively unoxygenated blood (from true or shuntlike effect alveolar units). The oxygen molecules remix in the combined blood to establish a new balance, resulting in a Pa_{O_2} that is higher than that which existed in blood affected by shunt but lower than what it would be if the alveoli were normal (Fig. 4–12).

Pulmonary Vascular Resistance

Pulmonary vascular resistance (PVR) measures the resistance to blood flow in the pulmonary vascular system, which is a low-resistance system. In effect, it represents right ventricular afterload in much the same way that systemic vascular resistance represents left ventricular afterload (a high-resistance system). The right ventricle pumps oxygen-poor blood into the pulmonary capillaries by way of the pulmonary artery. The amount of right ventricular force required to pump the blood into the lungs depends on the resistance to flow present in the pulmonary vascular system. This resistance to flow is called *pulmonary vascular resistance.*

Three main factors determine the amount of pulmonary resistance: the length and radius of the vessels and the viscosity of the blood. Of these factors, the major determinant of pulmonary vascular resistance is vessel radius (caliber).

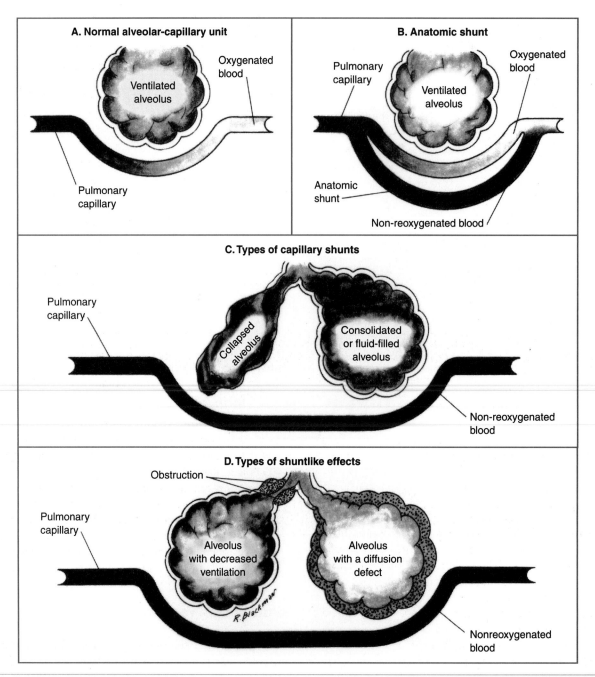

Figure 4–11 ■ Types of physiologic shunt. *A.* Normal alveolar–capillary unit. *B.* Anatomic shunt. *C.* Types of capillary shunts. *D.* Types of shuntlike effects. *(From* Cardiopulmonary Anatomy and Physiology *(2nd ed.), by J. R. Des Jardins © 1993. Reprinted with permission of Delmar, a division of Thomson Learning. Fax [800] 730-2215.)*

Vessel Radius Determinants

Vessel radius refers to the diameter (caliber) of the vessels. Vessel radius is altered by

■ The volume of blood in the pulmonary vascular system
■ The amount of vasoconstriction
■ The degree of lung inflation

Factors related to the volume of blood in the pulmonary vascular system include capillary recruitment and distention. Of these factors, recruitment is the most influential. The small pulmonary capillaries open up (are recruited) in response to an increase in blood flow. Under circumstances in which pulmonary blood flow is low (e.g., shock), the smaller capillaries may receive so little blood that they collapse. The concept of pul-

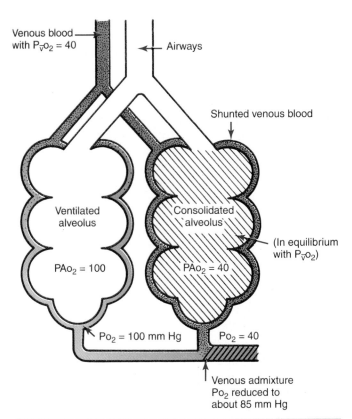

Figure 4–12 ■ Venous admixture. Venous admixture occurs when reoxygenated blood mixes with nonreoxygenated blood distal to the alveoli. *(From Des Jardins, T. R. [1990]. Clinical manifestations of respiratory disease, 2nd ed. [p. 22]. Chicago: Year Book Medical Publishers.)*

TABLE 4–3 Pulmonary Vascular Resistance (PVR)

EQUATION	$PVR = (\overline{PAP} - PCWP) \times \dfrac{80}{CO}$
Components	$\overline{PAP}$ = mean pulmonary artery pressure
	PCWP = pulmonary capillary wedge pressure
	CO = cardiac output
	80 = conversion factor
Normal values	50–150 dynes · sec · cm^{-5}
Example	A patient has a $\overline{PAP}$ of 22 mm Hg, a PCWP of 9 mm Hg, and a CO of 4.5 L/min
	$PVR = 22 - 9 \times \dfrac{80}{4.5}$
	$PVR = 13 \times 17.78$
	$PVR = 231.14$
Factors associated with increased PVR	Decreased PaO_2, decreased pH, increased $PaCO_2$; mechanical ventilation, positive end expiratory pressure (PEEP); pulmonary emboli, scleroderma, emphysema, pneumo- and hemothorax; histamine, prostaglandin, angiotensin

Data from Des Jardins, T. R. (1998). Cardiopulmonary anatomy and physiology: Essentials for respiratory care (3rd ed.). Albany, NY: Delmar Publishers; and Chang, D.W. (1998). Respiratory care calculations. (2nd ed.) Albany, NY: Delmar Publishers.

monary capillary recruitment is similar to the recruitment and collapse of alveoli based on volume of airflow. The second factor, distention, occurs in response to increased cardiac output or increased intravascular fluid volume. By distending, the capillaries are able to accommodate the increased flow. Distention of the capillaries decreases PVR.

Pulmonary vasoconstriction occurs in response to hypoxia, hypercapnia, and acidosis. Vasoconstriction is a major cause of increased PVR in the high-acuity patient, and hypoxia is the strongest stimulant for pulmonary vasoconstriction. When an area of the lung becomes hypoxic, such as is seen in shunt, vasoconstriction is triggered. This response effectively diverts blood flow to more functional areas of the lungs and results in a reduction in the impact of shunt. Unfortunately, in cases involving a generalized pulmonary disease process (e.g., late-stage emphysema), pulmonary vasoconstriction becomes global and PVR increases significantly. The elevated PVR requires the right heart to work against elevated pressures. In response to this increased workload, the right heart hypertrophies and cor pulmonale develops.

The degree of lung inflation also has an impact on the diameter of the pulmonary capillaries. As the lung inflates, capillaries become stretched. In states of high lung inflation, capillaries become compressed, which decreases their diameter and thus increases PVR. The opposite is also true: Lower lung volumes are associated with decreased PVR.

Calculating pulmonary vascular resistance requires the presence of a flow-directed pulmonary artery catheter. The calculation measures resistance, which is a function of pressure and flow. Pressure is determined by the mean pulmonary artery pressure and the pulmonary capillary wedge pressure. Flow is measured as the cardiac output. Table 4–3 summarizes the calculation of pulmonary vascular resistance.

Cor Pulmonale

Cor pulmonale refers to right ventricular hypertrophy and dilation secondary to pulmonary disease. It is a complication of both restrictive and obstructive pulmonary diseases. Cor pulmonale can cause right heart failure and is a major cause of death in the chronic obstructive pulmonary disease (COPD) patient. It is the result of a sequence of events precipitated by pulmonary hypertension. Pulmonary vessels normally function in a low-pressure system. Many pulmonary conditions cause pressures to increase in the vascular bed, creating a state of pulmonary hypertension. When this occurs, PVR increases. Pressure in the pulmonary artery is increased, making it more difficult to push blood out of the right heart during systole. The right heart becomes congested because less blood is moved out with each contraction. Over time, this congestion causes the right heart chambers to dilate. The right heart muscle

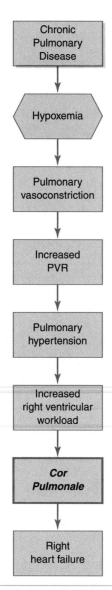

```
┌─────────────┐
│   Chronic   │
│  Pulmonary  │
│   Disease   │
└─────────────┘
       │
       ▼
  ⬡ Hypoxemia ⬡
       │
       ▼
┌─────────────┐
│  Pulmonary  │
│vasoconstric-│
│    tion     │
└─────────────┘
       │
       ▼
┌─────────────┐
│  Increased  │
│     PVR     │
└─────────────┘
       │
       ▼
┌─────────────┐
│  Pulmonary  │
│hypertension │
└─────────────┘
       │
       ▼
┌─────────────┐
│  Increased  │
│ right ven-  │
│tricular     │
│ workload    │
└─────────────┘
       │
       ▼
┌─────────────┐
│    Cor      │
│  Pulmonale  │
└─────────────┘
       │
       ▼
┌─────────────┐
│    Right    │
│heart failure│
└─────────────┘
```

Figure 4–13 ■ Cor pulmonale. Severe chronic pulmonary diseases are associated with a pattern of increasing hypoxemia that causes the lungs to vasoconstrict. The pulmonary vascular vasoconstriction increases PVR, which results in pulmonary hypertension. The right heart is required to work harder to pump blood into the pulmonary vascular system, and, over time, the right ventricle dilates and hypertrophies in response to the increased PVR. The adaptation of the right ventricle is called *cor pulmonale*.

hypertrophies to compensate for the required increased work of contraction. Figure 4–13 shows how the heart is affected by pulmonary hypertension.

In summary, the circulatory system can be divided into two circuits: the systemic and the pulmonary. These systems are interdependent; thus, if one circuit develops problems, the other eventually will become stressed. Pulmonary perfusion depends on three factors: cardiac output, gravity, and pulmonary vascular resistance. The relationship of ventilation to perfusion ($\dot{V}/\dot{Q}$ ratio) varies throughout the lung, based on the effects of gravity on blood. An overall balance in this relationship must be maintained to optimize proper diffusion of gases. Pulmonary disorders may create a mismatching of ventilation and perfusion, with either a high $\dot{V}/\dot{Q}$ ratio or low $\dot{V}/\dot{Q}$ ratio, either of which can result in hypoxemia. Oxygenation is greatly affected by the amount of blood that does not take part in gas exchange in the lungs. Shunt helps explain how hypoxemia develops. There are two types of shunt, true (anatomic and capillary) and shuntlike effect. The combination of anatomic and capillary shunt is called absolute shunt, which is refractory to oxygen therapy because it involves nonfunctioning alveoli. Shuntlike effect, however, is at least partially treatable using oxygen therapy because the alveoli are still functioning to some extent. The end result of shunting is called venous admixture, which represents the final oxygen content of the blood as it moves into arterial circulation. It is composed of the blending of the reoxygenated and unoxygenated (shunted) blood. An arterial blood gas (ABG) specimen gives a representative sample of venous admixture blood. Pulmonary vascular resistance (PVR) measures the resistance to blood flow in the pulmonary vascular system. Three main factors determine the amount of pulmonary resistance: the length and radius of the vessels and the viscosity of the blood. Of these factors, the major determinant of pulmonary vascular resistance is vessel radius (caliber). Chronically elevated PVR results in right ventricular hypertrophy, which eventually results in cor pulmonale. Calculating PVR requires a flow-directed pulmonary artery (PA) catheter.

SECTION THREE REVIEW

1. Which statement is true regarding the relationship of ventilation to perfusion in an upright person?
   A. it varies throughout the lung
   B. ventilation is best in the apices
   C. perfusion is best in peripheral lung areas
   D. it maintains a 1:1 relationship

2. During spontaneous breathing, air flows toward
   A. the apices
   B. the diaphragm
   C. the higher-pressure gradient
   D. higher-resistance areas

3. Mr. M has left lower lobe pneumonia. His remaining lung fields are clear. It is time to reposition Mr. M in bed. Of the following positions, which is most likely to optimize the ventilation–perfusion relationship?
   A. place him on his right side
   B. place him on his back
   C. place him on his left side
   D. place him flat in the bed

4. When ventilation–perfusion mismatching occurs, it can be detected by which parameter?
   A. hemoglobin (Hgb) level
   B. oxygen saturation level (SaO_2)
   C. partial pressure of arterial carbon dioxide ($PaCO_2$)
   D. arterial sodium bicarbonate level (HCO_3)

5. A decrease of airflow to the apices of the lungs is caused by increased
   A. natural airflow toward lung periphery
   B. negative pleural pressure in bases
   C. negative pleural pressure in apices
   D. positive pleural pressure in apices

6. Which statement best describes the term *true shunt*?
   A. alveoli that have no airflow
   B. alveoli that have air trapped in them
   C. blood that does not take part in pulmonary gas exchange
   D. blood entering the right heart without being oxygenated

7. The normal percentage of cardiac output as a result of anatomic shunt is
   A. 0 to 5 percent
   B. 2 to 5 percent
   C. 10 to 30 percent
   D. 20 to 40 percent

8. Anatomic shunt would be most increased with which disorder?
   A. pneumonia
   B. pulmonary edema
   C. tuberculosis
   D. ventricular septal defect

9. Normal blood flow past completely unventilated alveoli is the definition of
   A. physiologic shunt
   B. anatomic shunt
   C. capillary shunt
   D. venous admixture

10. Oxygen therapy is most effective in treating
    A. shuntlike effect
    B. anatomic shunt
    C. capillary shunt
    D. absolute shunt

11. The nurse is calculating a patient's pulmonary vascular resistance (PVR). The latest hemodynamic values are PAP, 30 mm Hg; PAWP, 15 mm Hg; CO 5.2 L/min. What is the PVR and what is its significance? (fill in the blanks)

    PVR = _____

    Significance: _____

Answers: 1. A, 2. B, 3. A, 4. B, 5. C, 6. C, 7. B, 8. D, 9. C, 10. A, 11. PVR = 230.7; significance = abnormally high PVR

SECTION FOUR: Acid–Base Physiology and Disturbances

At the completion of this section, the learner will be able to identify mechanisms that the body uses to compensate for acid–base imbalances, and differentiate between respiratory acidosis and alkalosis, and metabolic acidosis and alkalosis.

The acid–base status is another type of determinant of gas exchange because the lungs are heavily invested in maintaining acid–base homeostasis and they are also the source of severe acid–base imbalances in the presence of certain pulmonary disease states. This section provides an overview of acid–base physiology and disturbances. In Part Two of this module, interpretation of acid–base status through arterial blood gas interpretation is presented.

Acid–Base Physiology

Acid–base balance is crucial to the effective functioning of the body systems. Severe imbalances can be lethal to the patient. The body contains many acid and base substances. **Acids** are substances that dissociate or lose ions. **Bases** are substances capable of accepting ions. A **buffer** is a substance that reacts with acids and bases to maintain a neutral environment of stable pH. The **pH** represents the free hydrogen ion (H^+) concentration. An increase in H^+ concentration lowers pH and increases acidity. A decrease in H^+ concentration increases pH and increases alkalinity.

The body's acids include volatile acids and nonvolatile acids. **Volatile acids** can convert to a gas form for excretion (carbonic acid). Carbonic acid rapidly converts to carbon dioxide for excretion from the lungs. The lungs excrete a very large

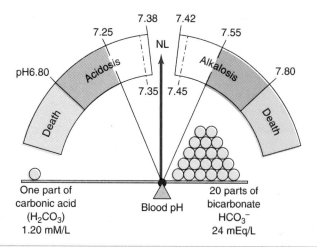

Figure 4–14 ■ Normal blood pH is 7.40 ± 0.02 (1 SD) or ± 0.05 (2 SD). Acid–base balance occurs when the ratio of bicarbonate to carbonic acid is 20:1. Any change in this ratio tips the balance and swings the pointer to the acidosis or alkalosis side. A pH <7.25 or > 7.55 is life threatening, and the extremes of 6.8 or 7.8 cause death. *(From Price, S. A., & Wilson, L. M. [1992].* Pathophysiology: Clinical concepts of disease processes, *(4th ed., p. 260). St. Louis: C.V. Mosby.)*

amount of acid each day in this manner. **Nonvolatile (metabolic) acids** cannot be converted to gas, so they must be excreted through the kidneys. Examples of nonvolatile acids include lactic acid and ketones. Unlike the lungs, the kidneys are capable of excreting only a small amount of acid each day and respond slowly to changes. Hydrogen ions are excreted in the proximal and distal tubules of the kidneys in exchange for sodium.

Maintaining Acid–Base Balance: Buffer Systems and Compensation

Buffer Systems

The body is intolerant of wide changes in pH and works constantly to maintain the pH range between 7.35 and 7.45 (Fig. 4–14). A normal pH is maintained if the ratio of bicarbonate (HCO_3) to carbon dioxide (CO_2) remains at approximately a 20:1 (HCO_3/CO_2) ratio. The body has three mechanisms to maintain acid–base balance: the buffering mechanism, the respiratory compensation mechanism, and the metabolic or renal compensation mechanism.

Buffering Mechanisms. The buffering mechanisms represent chemical reactions between acids and bases to maintain a neutral environment. Bases react with excess hydrogen ions (H^+) and acids react with excess HCO_3 to prevent shifts in pH. The buffering mechanisms are triggered quickly in response to any change in pH.

Compensation

Compensation is the process whereby an abnormal pH is returned to within normal limits through counterbalancing acid-base activities. Compensation occurs over time; thus, it is referred to in terms of the degree (or level) to which the body has achieved compensation. There are four levels of compensation: uncompensated (acute), partially compensated, compensated (chronic), or corrected. An **uncompensated** (acute) acid-base state is one in which the pH is abnormal because other buffer and regulatory mechanisms have not begun to correct the balance. A **partially compensated** acid-base state is one in which the pH is abnormal; however, the body buffers and regulatory mechanisms have begun to respond to the imbalance. A compensated acid-base state is one in which the pH has returned to within normal limits, with the acid-base imbalance being neutralized but not corrected. Finally, a **corrected** acid-base state is one in which all acid-base parameters have returned to normal ranges after a state of acid-base imbalance. Table 4–4 summarizes the characteristics and provides examples of the levels of compensation.

TABLE 4–4 Levels of Compensation

LEVEL OF COMPENSATION	CHARACTERISTICS	EXAMPLE
Uncompensated (acute)	Abnormal pH with one abnormal value and one normal value.	pH 7.20, $Paco_2$ 60 mm Hg, HCO_3 24 mEq/L. *Interpretation:* The pH and $Paco_2$ match (acid). HCO_3 is normal. No compensation is occurring. An uncompensated (acute) acidosis state exists.
Partially compensated	Abnormal pH with two abnormal values ($Paco_2$ and HCO_3 are moving in opposite directions).	pH 7.30, $Paco_2$ 60 mm Hg, HCO_3 30 mEq/L. *Interpretation:* The pH and $Paco_2$ match (acid). HCO_3 is alkaline or moving in the opposite direction from the $Paco_2$. The pH is still abnormal. A partially compensated acidosis state exists.
Compensated (chronic)	Normal pH plus two abnormal values ($Paco_2$ and HCO_3 are moving in opposite directions).	pH 7.38, $Paco_2$ 50 mm Hg, HCO_3 30 mEq/L. *Interpretation:* The pH and $Paco_2$ match (acid). HCO_3 is alkaline (opposite of $Paco_2$). pH is normal. A (chronic) compensated acidosis state exists.
Corrected	Normal pH and two normal values. No acid–base disturbance currently exists.	pH 7.36, $Paco_2$ 43 mm Hg, HCO_3, 26 mEq/L. *Interpretation:* A normal acid-base state in a person who, until recently, had an acid-base disturbance.

Respiratory (Pulmonary) Compensation Mechanism. The respiratory buffer system is the rapid-response compensatory mechanism for metabolic acid–base disturbances. It responds within minutes of development of a metabolic acid-base disturbance. The lungs have two ways in which they compensate: (1) alveolar hypoventilation in response to metabolic alkalosis and (2) alveolar hyperventilation in response to metabolic acidosis. Hypoventilation (slow and/or shallow breathing) retains CO_2, which is then available to shift the carbonic acid equation toward the left (see the preceding discussion), resulting in shifting the pH toward acid. Hyperventilation (rapid and/or deep breathing) blows off CO_2, which then shifts the carbonic acid equation back toward the right, resulting in driving the pH up, toward alkaline.

Metabolic (Renal) Compensation Mechanism. The bicarbonate buffer system is the major buffering system in the body. Its components are regulated by the lungs (CO_2) and kidneys (HCO_3). The following reversible reaction (carbonic acid equation) represents the shifts that occur as carbonic acid (H_2CO_3) is shifted depending on body needs (left shift makes pH more acid and right shift makes pH more alkaline):

$$H^+ + HCO_3 \longleftrightarrow H_2CO_3 \longleftrightarrow CO_2 + H_2O$$

Additional nonbicarbonate buffers include hemoglobin, serum proteins, and the phosphate system, the latter of which is mainly a function of the kidneys. The bicarbonate system is a relatively slowly responding system, taking hours to days to respond to acid–base disturbances.

The metabolic compensation mechanism controls the rate of elimination or reabsorption of hydrogen and bicarbonate ions in the kidney. In situations of increased acid loads (acidosis), H^+ elimination and bicarbonate reabsorption are increased. In alkalosis, H^+ is reabsorbed and HCO_3^- is excreted.

Metabolic compensation is slow. It begins in hours but takes days to reach maximum compensation.

Respiratory Acid–Base Disturbances

Primary respiratory disturbances are reflected by changes in the $Paco_2$, being either above normal as in respiratory acidosis, or below normal as in respiratory alkalosis.

Respiratory Acidosis

Respiratory acidosis occurs when the $Paco_2$ moves above 45 mm Hg and the pH drops below 7.35. The elevated carbon dioxide (CO_2) indicates alveolar hypoventilation. The lungs are not blowing off enough carbon dioxide, causing a carbonic acid excess. Carbon dioxide is considered an acid because it combines with water to form carbonic acid. It is essential to determine the cause of hypoventilation and then to correct it when possible. Table 4–5 lists some of the major causes of acute respiratory acidosis.

A "chronic" abnormal acid–base state means that a state of compensation exists. Chronic respiratory acidosis usually is associated with a chronic obstructive pulmonary disease, such as chronic bronchitis or emphysema. The elevation of carbon dioxide occurs gradually over many years; thus, the body is able to compensate to maintain a normal pH by elevating the bicarbonate. Because these individuals have little respiratory reserve, additional stressors can cause decompensation, which produces respiratory failure. Table 4–6 compares the effects of acute and chronic acidosis on ABG levels. (Respiratory failure is discussed in depth in Module 5.)

Respiratory Alkalosis

Respiratory alkalosis occurs when the $Paco_2$ falls below 35 mm Hg with a corresponding rise in pH to greater than 7.45. The decreased carbon dioxide indicates alveolar hyperventilation. The lungs are eliminating too much carbon dioxide, creating a carbonic acid deficit. In the presence of respiratory alkalosis, there is insufficient carbon dioxide available to combine with water to form carbonic acid (H_2CO_3). The key to effective treatment of respiratory alkalosis is to determine the cause of the hyperventilation and provide the intervention necessary to

TABLE 4–5 Common Causes of Acute Respiratory Acidosis

Alveolar hypoventilation, caused by
  Respiratory depression
    Oversedation
    Overdose
    Head injury
  Decreased ventilation
    Respiratory muscle fatigue
    Neuromuscular diseases
    Mechanical ventilation (underventilation)
  Altered diffusion/ventilation–perfusion mismatch
    Pulmonary edema
    Severe atelectasis
    Pneumonia
    Severe bronchospasm

TABLE 4–6 Comparison of Acute and Chronic Respiratory Acidosis

| PARAMETER | UNCOMPENSATED | COMPENSATED | |
	ACUTE	PARTIAL	CHRONIC
pH	↓	↓	Normal
$Paco_2$	↑	↑	↑
HCO_3	Normal	↑	↑

TABLE 4–7 Common Causes of Acute Respiratory Alkalosis

Alveolar hyperventilation, caused by
  Anxiety, fear
  Pain
  Hypoxia
  Head injury
  Fever
  Mechanical ventilation (overventilation)

correct the problem. Common causes of acute respiratory alkalosis are listed in Table 4–7.

Chronic respiratory alkalosis is uncommon. The same factors causing acute respiratory alkalosis could cause a chronic state if the problem remained uncorrected. Table 4–8 compares the effects of acute and chronic respiratory alkalosis on ABG levels.

Metabolic Acid–Base Disturbances

Primary metabolic disturbances are reflected by changes in bicarbonate (HCO_3) levels and abnormal base excess (BE) levels (either less than −2, "base deficit" or greater than +2, base excess). Metabolic acidosis and anion gap (another measure of metabolic disorders) are further described in Module 27, "Altered Glucose Metabolism."

Metabolic Acidosis

Metabolic acidosis can be defined clinically as HCO_3 less than 22 mEq/L, pH less than 7.35, with a base deficit (less than −2). Metabolic acidosis can be caused by an increase in metabolic acids or excessive loss of base.

Examples of conditions that can cause an increase in hydrogen ion (H^+) concentration include

- Diabetic acidosis as a result of elevated ketones (sometimes referred to as 'anion gap' acidosis)
- Uremia associated with increased levels of phosphates and sulfates

- Ingestion of acidic drugs, such as aspirin (salicylate) overdose
- Lactic acidosis caused by increased lactic acid production

Examples of conditions that precipitate a decrease in bicarbonate (HCO_3) levels include

- Diarrhea, which causes loss of alkaline substances
- Gastrointestinal fistulas leading to loss of alkaline substances
- Loss of body fluids from drains below the umbilicus (except urinary catheter) causing loss of alkaline fluids
- Drugs causing loss of alkali, such as laxative overuse
- Hyperaldosteronism, which causes increased renal loss

Lactic Acidosis

Currently, there is increased clinical interest in evaluating metabolic acidosis that is precipitated by elevated lactate levels. Acid metabolites, such as lactic acid (lactate), result from cellular breakdown and anaerobic metabolism. The normal range for serum lactate is 0.5 to 2.0 mEq/L. High-acuity patients are at particular risk for developing elevated levels of lactate because lactic acidosis is closely associated with shock and other severe physiologic insults. During a shock episode, cellular hypoxia drives serum lactate levels up rapidly, usually greater than 5 mEq/L. This rise often precedes decompensatory signs, such as decreased urine output and decreased blood pressure, and thus may be an indicator of impending shock. Other conditions that can cause lactic acidosis include severe dehydration, severe infection, severe trauma, diabetic ketoacidosis, and hepatic failure (Kee, 2002).

Table 4–9 compares the effects of acute and chronic metabolic acidosis on arterial blood gases.

Metabolic Alkalosis

Metabolic alkalosis can be defined clinically as a bicarbonate (HCO_3) level greater than 26 mEq/L, pH greater than 7.45, and a base excess (greater than +2). Metabolic alkalosis occurs when the amount of alkali (base) increases or excessive loss of acid occurs.

TABLE 4–8 Comparison of Acute and Chronic Respiratory Alkalosis

PARAMETER	UNCOMPENSATED ACUTE	COMPENSATED PARTIAL	CHRONIC
pH	↑	↑	Normal
$Paco_2$	↓	↓	↓
HCO_3	Normal	↓	↓

TABLE 4–9 Comparison of Acute and Chronic Metabolic Acidosis

PARAMETER	UNCOMPENSATED ACUTE	COMPENSATED PARTIAL	CHRONIC
pH	↓	↓	Normal
$Paco_2$	Normal	↓	↓
HCO_3	↓	↓	↓

A common cause of increased alkali is ingestion of alkaline drugs associated with the overuse of antacids or overadministration of sodium bicarbonate during a cardiac arrest emergency. Examples of conditions that result in a decrease in acid include:

- Loss of gastric fluids from vomiting or nasogastric suction
- Treatment with steroids, especially those with mineralocorticoid effects
- Diuretic therapy with certain drugs, such as furosemide (Lasix), causing loss of potassium
- Binge–purge syndrome

Table 4–10 compares the effects of acute and chronic metabolic alkalosis on arterial blood gases.

In summary, to differentiate between primary metabolic acidosis or alkalosis, the bicarbonate and pH must be evaluated. Base excess provides additional data. Conditions that cause each acid–base disturbance have been presented. Compensation of a metabolic acid–base disturbance requires evaluation of the $Paco_2$. The body attempts to maintain pH within a narrow range. Compensatory mechanisms include buffering, excretion

TABLE 4–10 Comparison of Acute and Chronic Metabolic Alkalosis

| PARAMETER | UNCOMPENSATED | COMPENSATED | |
	ACUTE	PARTIAL	CHRONIC
pH	↑	↑	Normal
$Paco_2$	Normal	↑	↑
HCO_3	↑	↑	↑

or retention of carbon dioxide (respiratory), and excretion or retention of H^+/HCO_3^- (metabolic). To differentiate between primary respiratory acidosis and alkalosis, the $Paco_2$ and pH must be evaluated. The cause of respiratory acidosis is alveolar hypoventilation, and the cause of respiratory alkalosis is alveolar hyperventilation. Compensation of respiratory acid–base disturbances requires evaluation of changes in bicarbonate. Treatment includes correction of the underlying problem.

SECTION FOUR REVIEW

1. The body compensates for acid–base imbalance with which mechanisms? (Choose all that apply)
    1. buffering
    2. hepatic compensation
    3. respiratory compensation
    4. excretion of bicarbonate
   A. 1, 2, and 3
   B. 1, 3, and 4
   C. 2, 3, and 4
   D. 1 and 3
2. Respiratory compensation involves excretion or retention of
   A. CO_2
   B. HCO_3
   C. H_2O
   D. K^+
3. Metabolic compensation involves changes in renal excretion or reabsorption of
   A. H^+, CO_2
   B. HCO_3, H^+
   C. glucose, HCO_3
   D. CO_2, HCO_3
4. The body's buffering system continually works toward maintenance of a bicarbonate/carbon dioxide ratio of
   A. 1:5
   B. 1:20
   C. 5:1
   D. 20:1

5. Respiratory acidosis is caused by
   A. alveolar hyperventilation
   B. alveolar hypoventilation
   C. mechanical ventilation
   D. inadequate perfusion
6. Which parameter change occurs as a result of acute respiratory acidosis?
   A. pH increases
   B. pH decreases
   C. CO_2 decreases
   D. HCO_3 decreases
7. Respiratory alkalosis can result from which problem?
   A. alveolar hyperventilation
   B. alveolar hypoventilation
   C. metabolic alkalosis
   D. inadequate perfusion
8. Patient situations associated with respiratory alkalosis include
   A. sedation
   B. neuromuscular blockade
   C. pulmonary edema
   D. anxiety
9. Metabolic disturbances are reflected by changes in
   A. HCO_3, Fio_2
   B. Pao_2, Sao_2
   C. HCO_3, BE
   D. BE, Pao_2

10. Metabolic acidosis results in
    A. increased Pa_{CO_2}
    B. decreased BE
    C. increased pH
    D. increased HCO_3
11. A condition that may cause metabolic acidosis because of decrease in bicarbonate levels is
    A. diarrhea
    B. uremia
    C. aspirin ingestion
    D. diabetic ketoacidosis

12. Metabolic alkalosis is caused by a (an) _____ in acid or a (an) _____ in base.
    A. increase, increase
    B. decrease, decrease
    C. decrease, increase
    D. increase, decrease

Answers: 1. B, 2. B, 3. B, 4. D, 5. B, 6. B, 7. A, 8. D, 9. C, 10. B, 11. A, 12. C

Part Two
Assessment of Pulmonary Gas Exchange

SECTION FIVE: Respiratory Nursing Assessment

Upon completion of this section, the learner will be able to discuss a respiratory nursing assessment.

Nursing History

When a patient is admitted to the hospital in acute distress, the nurse initially assesses airway, breathing, and circulation (ABCs), and immediately takes appropriate action based on those assessments. As soon as is feasible, information regarding the immediate events leading to admission should be obtained. A recent history gives important clues as to the etiology and chain of events related to the current problem.

The presence of severe respiratory distress limits the amount of health history information a patient is able to relate. Minimize questions directed to the patient to reduce the stress on breathing, stating all inquiries in such a way that they require very brief answers.

Historical data of particular importance to assess in the patient with pulmonary problems include the following.

Social History

Assess tobacco and alcohol use. Tobacco use is associated with many pulmonary diseases, and current use may further aggravate acute pulmonary problems. Alcohol use in association with prescribed drug therapy may adversely affect the patient's respiratory condition. Problems with alcohol withdrawal can complicate the cardiopulmonary status should delirium tremens develop.

Nutritional History

The nutritional state of a pulmonary patient is crucial to assess because malnutrition is contributory to the development of respiratory failure. There are several ways in which this can happen. First, a protein–calorie deficit weakens muscles, including the respiratory muscles. Second, malnutrition is associated with a weakened immune system, which increases susceptibility to infection and makes it harder to fight against existing infections. The increased stress associated with an acute infection can precipitate acute respiratory failure. Third, a high-carbohydrate diet increases the overall carbon dioxide load in the body. This may lead to ventilatory complications in certain patients.

Cardiopulmonary History

The lungs, heart, and blood vessels comprise a common circuit. For this reason, factors that alter any part of the circuit can cause a subsequent alteration in other parts. It is often difficult to differentiate between problems of pulmonary and cardiovascular etiology. Because of this, obtaining sufficient data regarding the cardiovascular system will be invaluable in planning the management of the patient. Of particular importance is data concerning preexisting cardiovascular or pulmonary problems and prehospitalization activity tolerance levels.

Elimination History

Urinary elimination is not directly affected by pulmonary function. It can, however, be indirectly affected when the patient experiences a severe hypoxic episode. If the kidneys sustain an acute hypoperfusion/hypoxic episode, acute tubular necrosis/acute renal failure could result.

Bowel elimination can negatively affect pulmonary status when constipation occurs. A full, extended bowel can push abdominal contents against the diaphragm, restricting expansion of the lungs. Oxygen consumption can increase when the patient strains to evacuate a hard stool, further compromising oxygen levels in patients with marginal or poor arterial blood gases. Patients with pulmonary disorders often experience constipation because of decreased activity levels and decreased intake of fluids and appropriate foods.

Sleep–Rest History

Pulmonary problems frequently interfere with sleep and rest for a variety of reasons. If the respiratory problem is severe enough to cause hypoxia, the patient often exhibits restlessness associated with inadequate oxygenation of the brain. Pulmonary disorders often increase the work of breathing, which can interfere with rest and sleep. Patients in respiratory distress may sleep poorly because they fear that they will cease to breathe when they are unaware. Others cannot sleep because of their level of general discomfort. Dyspnea and air hunger are anxiety-producing and threatening experiences for pulmonary patients.

Common Complaints Associated with Pulmonary Disorders

If a respiratory problem is suspected, the nurse should focus on obtaining information concerning the most common respiratory complaints: dyspnea, chest pain, cough, sputum, and hemoptysis. This can be accomplished by interviewing the patient and/or family (subjective data) and by performing a nursing assessment (objective data). Regular assessment of the common respiratory symptoms is also important in monitoring the patient for acute changes in respiratory status.

Dyspnea

Subjective Data. **Dyspnea** is a subjective (patient-based) symptom. It refers to the feeling of difficult breathing or shortness of breath. Physiologically, dyspnea is associated with increased work of breathing—a supply-and-demand imbalance. Increased work of breathing occurs when ventilatory demands go beyond the body's ability to respond. Progressive dyspnea is noted commonly in both restrictive and obstructive pulmonary disorders.

Orthopnea is a type of dyspnea closely associated with cardiac problems or severe pulmonary disease. It refers to a state in which the patient assumes a head-up position to relieve dyspnea. Orthopnea may be mild (the patient may need several pillows to sleep comfortably in bed), or it may be severe (the patient may need to sit upright in a chair or in bed).

One type of dyspnea is of particular interest in differentiating cardiac from pulmonary disorders. **Paroxysmal nocturnal dyspnea (PND)** is associated with left heart failure. The typical patient report is that of waking during the night, after being asleep for several hours, with a sudden onset of severe dyspnea. On sitting up or getting out of bed, the dyspnea is relieved, and the patient is able to resume sleep. Paroxysmal nocturnal dyspnea is a form of transient mild pulmonary edema. It is believed that fluids that have been congested in the lower extremities during the day because of gravity drainage shift to the heart and lungs, causing a fluid volume overload when the person becomes horizontal (as in sleep) for several hours.

Objective Data. Objectively, the nurse may note tachypnea, nasal flaring, use of **accessory muscles,** or abnormal arterial blood gases. The patient may voluntarily assume a high-Fowler sitting position secondary to orthopnea. Severe tachypnea, a respiratory rate of more than 30 breaths per minute, significantly increases the work of breathing. If allowed to continue for a prolonged period of time, respiratory muscle fatigue can occur, which may ultimately cause acute respiratory failure.

Chest Pain

Subjective Data. The type of chest pain the patient describes can be helpful in differentiating cardiogenic (originating from the heart) from pleuritic (originating from the pleura) pain. Cardiogenic pain generally is described as dull, pressure like discomfort often radiating to the jaw, back, or left arm. If asked to point to the painful area, the patient often uses the palm of the hand, indicating a somewhat general area. Cardiogenic pain is unaffected by breathing.

Pleuritic pain frequently is described as sharp and knifelike, and the patient is able to point to the pain focal area with one finger. When the patient is between breaths or the breath is held, pain decreases or ceases. The pain increases with deep breathing. A pleural friction rub may sometimes be auscultated at the focal pain point.

Most pulmonary disorders affecting only the lung parenchyma (lung tissue) are not associated with chest pain as an early symptom because the parenchyma is insensitive to pain. For example, lung cancer frequently goes undetected until a routine chest x-ray is taken or the tumor impinges on innervated thoracic structures, causing deep pain. Like lung tissue, the attached visceral pleura is insensitive. The parietal pleura, however, is well innervated, and when inflammation (called **pleurisy** or **pleuritis**) occurs, it can trigger the sharp pain as previously described.

Objective Data. Objective data the nurse may note include splinting, shallow respirations, tachypnea, facial changes associated with pain, and increased blood pressure and pulse.

Cough

Subjective Data. Coughing is an important reflex activity that assists the mucociliary escalator in removing secretions and foreign particles from the lower airway. It is triggered by irritation, the presence of foreign particles, or obstruction of the airway. The patient should be asked to provide the following information about cough: frequency, character, duration, triggers, and pattern of occurrence.

Objective Data. The nurse can observe the strength, character, and frequency of the cough.

Sputum

Subjective Data. It is important to obtain a description of sputum production in a pulmonary patient. If the patient has a disease that is associated with chronic production of sputum, he or she should be asked to describe the usual quantity, characteristics, and color. It is important to get the patient to describe any changes in sputum associated with the current pulmonary problem.

Objective Data. Sputum may consist of a variety of substances, such as mucus, pus, bacteria, or blood. Sputum should be monitored on a regular basis for quantity, characteristics (thin, thick, tenacious), color, and odor. Careful attention to sputum changes should be noted and documented because they may reflect a change in the patient's pulmonary status. Normal secretions are thin and clear. Sputum color varies depending on the underlying problem (Table 4–11).

If a sputum specimen is ordered for laboratory studies, it is best to obtain the specimen in the early morning on awakening because secretions pool during sleep. To ensure that the specimen is not composed of upper airway secretions, instruct the patient to take several large breaths and then cough forcefully from the diaphragm. If the patient's cough is weak and nonproductive, deep tracheal suctioning may be necessary, collecting the specimen in a special suction trap device, such as the Lukens tube. The sputum specimen should be obtained before initiation of antibiotic therapy.

Hemoptysis

Subjective Data. **Hemoptysis** refers to expectoration of bloody secretions. It is important to determine the source of the bleeding, which may be from the upper airway (e.g., the oral cavity) or the lower airway (e.g., the lungs). In patients who are experiencing respiratory problems, the presence of hemoptysis can be a significant finding and may be of cardiovascular or pulmonary origin.

Common causes of cardiovascular-related hemoptysis include pulmonary embolism and cardiogenic pulmonary edema secondary to left heart failure. The most common source of hemoptysis, however, is lung disease, particularly as a result of infection and neoplasms. Lung diseases associated with hemoptysis include bronchitis, bronchiectasis, pneumonia, tuberculosis, fungal and parasitic infections, and lung tumors. Information to obtain concerning hemoptysis includes color, consistency and quantity, and frequency and duration.

Objective Data. When hemoptysis is noted, it should be assessed for color, consistency, and quantity. The frequency and duration also should be noted and documented.

Respiratory Physical Assessment

The initial general nursing assessment focuses on all body systems in detail. Once the initial assessment is completed and baseline data are documented, the nurse conducts more specific shift assessments. These frequent bedside assessments often are focused on organ systems (or functional patterns) that have the potential for changing rapidly, indicating a status change in actual or potential patient problems.

Vital Signs and Hemodynamic Values

Vital signs and hemodynamic values give crucial baseline data and are important indicators of changing patient status when trended over time. Vital signs include arterial blood pressure, pulse, respirations, and temperature. If a pulmonary artery catheter is in place, important hemodynamic monitoring assessments include central venous pressure (CVP), pulmonary artery pressure, pulmonary artery wedge pressure, mean arterial pressure, and cardiac output. Hemodynamic monitoring generally is initiated when cardiac involvement is suspected or fluid status is questioned. If the patient's condition is purely pulmonary in nature, data collected from hemodynamic monitoring may be of insufficient use to warrant such an invasive procedure. The presence of pulmonary hypertension can alter hemodynamic measurements. Hemodynamic monitoring is presented in detail in Module 9.

Inspection and Palpation

Skin coloring should be inspected closely for cyanosis. Observe the lips, earlobes, and beneath the tongue for central cyanosis, which may indicate prolonged hypoxia. In patients with dark skin tones, cyanosis can be observed on the lips and tongue, which will appear ashen-gray. Cyanosis is not a reliable indicator of hypoxia because it is dependent on the amount of reduced hemoglobin present. Its value, therefore, is as supportive rather than diagnostic data. Observe chest movement for symmetry of expansion and the rate, depth, and pattern of breathing. If the

TABLE 4–11 Sputum Color and Consistency and Underlying Problems

COLOR AND CONSISTENCY	UNDERLYING PROBLEM
Yellow-green	Bacterial infection
White, tenacious, mucoid	Acute asthma
Rust colored/blood-tinged	Trauma of coughing, pneumonia, pulmonary infarction
Frothy, pink-tinged	Pulmonary edema

TABLE 4–12 Normal Breath Sounds

BREATH SOUND	NORMAL LOCATION	DESCRIPTION
Vesicular	Peripheral lung fields	Whispering, rustling quality; quiet and low pitched; inspiratory phase is longer than expiratory phase; no distinct pause between inspiration and expiration
Bronchial (tubular)	Over the trachea	High-pitched, loud sound; pause heard between inspiratory and expiratory phases; expiration phase is longer than inspiration (abnormal if heard in peripheral lung; may indicate a consolidation, such as pneumonia)
Bronchovesicular	In all lobes near major airways	Sound is between vesicular and bronchial

patient has sustained chest trauma or has chest tubes in place, the chest should be observed for changes in appearance and palpated for subcutaneous emphysema and areas of tenderness.

Percussion

Percussion is an assessment skill that often is not used on a regular shift-by-shift basis in the acute care setting. It can be used to detect the presence of air, fluid, or consolidation under the area being percussed.

Auscultation

Auscultation is one of the most important pulmonary assessments. The diaphragm of the stethoscope is best for hearing most breath sounds, auscultating in a pattern that allows comparison of one lung to the other.

Normal Breath Sounds. There are three types of normal breath sounds: vesicular, bronchial (tubular), and bronchovesicular. Table 4–12 differentiates the various normal sounds.

Abnormal Breath Sounds. The chest should be auscultated routinely for diminished or absent sounds in any field. The presence of abnormal breath sounds is associated with a change in lung status, such as partial or complete obstruction of a part of the airway by secretions or fluid.

Adventitious breath sounds are heard on top of other breath sounds. They are never considered normal. Adventitious sounds may be caused by fluid or secretions in the airways or alveoli, by alveoli opening or collapsing, or by bronchoconstriction. Adventitious sounds are classified as crackles, rhonchi, wheeze, and rub.

Crackles (previously called **rales**) are heard as relatively discrete, delicate popping sounds of short duration. They are associated with either fluid or secretions in the small airways or alveoli, or opening of alveoli from a collapsed state. Crackles are heard most commonly during inspiration. Crackles may be described as fine or coarse. Fine crackles are delicate and high pitched and are of short duration. Conditions such as atelectasis and pneumonia are associated with fine crackles. Coarse or loud crackles are louder, lower-pitched sounds of longer duration than fine crackles. They are heard in conditions such as bronchitis and pulmonary edema. The classic description of crackles is that they sound similar to the noise that can be made by rubbing hair between the fingers next to the ear.

Rhonchi are heard as coarse, "bubbly" sounds. They are most commonly present during expiration and are auscultated over the larger airways. Rhonchi are associated with an accumulation of fluid or secretions in the larger airways.

Wheeze is caused by air passing through constricted airways. The constriction may be caused by bronchospasm, fluid, secretions, edema obstructing the airway, or the presence of an obstructing tumor or foreign body. Wheeze has a musical quality that may be high pitched or low pitched. It may be heard on inspiration or expiration and is of long duration.

Pleural rub is caused by an inflammation of the pleural linings (membranes). When inflammation occurs, the linings become resistant to free movement. The characteristic sound is heard during breathing and ceases between breaths or with breath holding. It has been described as sounding like leather rubbing together or creaking.

Focused Respiratory Assessment

The onset of acute respiratory distress can be rapid and severe. The nurse should be alert to changes from previously assessed baseline data and data trends. Rapid respiratory assessment should focus on the following data that strongly suggest an acute alteration in respiratory function.

- Suddenly increased restlessness and agitation (hypoxia)
- Suddenly decreased level of responsiveness, increased lethargy (hypercapnia)
- Significant change in pattern of breathing:
    Respiratory rate less than 10/min or greater than 30/min
    Shallow or erratic breathing
- Increased cyanosis or duskiness
- Increased use of accessory muscles
- Increased dyspnea or orthopnea
- Increase in adventitious breath sounds or development of abnormal breath sounds
- Changing trends noted in vital signs (blood pressure, pulse, respirations):
    Increasing trends indicate that compensation is occurring
    Decreasing trends indicate that decompensation activities may be occurring
- Presence of pain

In summary, the most common respiratory-related complaints are dyspnea, chest pain, cough, sputum, and hemoptysis. The nursing history and assessment should include careful data collection focusing on these common complaints. The database can be helpful in differentiating an underlying pulmonary problem from one of cardiac origin. The bedside-focused respiratory assessment includes vital signs, inspection of skin coloring, chest movement and pattern of breathing, and auscultation for the presence of adventitious breath sounds (e.g., crackles, rhonchi, wheeze, or pleural rub).

SECTION FIVE REVIEW

1. When a patient is admitted in acute respiratory distress, the initial history should focus on which priority?
   A. smoking history
   B. events leading to current admission
   C. nutritional history
   D. events leading to previous admissions
2. The most common complaints associated with pulmonary disease include: (choose all that apply)
   1. cough
   2. sputum
   3. dyspnea
   4. pleural pain
   A. 1, 3, and 4
   B. 2 and 3
   C. 2, 3, and 4
   D. 1, 2, and 3
3. Chest pain that is typical of pleuritic pain can be best characterized as
   A. sharp
   B. pressurelike
   C. radiating
   D. dull

4. Normal sputum should appear
   A. white and tenacious
   B. yellow-green
   C. clear and thin
   D. frothy and pink-tinged
5. Breath sounds that are auscultated in the peripheral lung fields and have a whispery, rustling quality are
   A. vesicular
   B. bronchovesicular
   C. bronchial
   D. wheezes
6. Crackles are caused by
   A. secretions in the large airways
   B. an inflammation of the pleural linings
   C. air passing through constricted airways
   D. fluid or secretions in the small airways or alveoli

Answers: 1. B, 2. D, 3. A, 4. C, 5. A, 6. D

SECTION SIX: Pulmonary Function Evaluation

At the completion of this section, the learner will be able to briefly describe various tests used to evaluate pulmonary function.

The medical team generally initiates orders for pulmonary function testing to assist in diagnosing a pulmonary problem or updating or evaluating a patient's pulmonary status. Actual implementation and interpretation of the tests often becomes an interdisciplinary undertaking.

Pulmonary Function Tests

Ventilation is measured in a variety of ways using pulmonary function tests (PFTs). These tests provide baseline data and also provide a means to monitor the progress of functional impairments associated with pulmonary diseases. They help differentiate a restrictive pulmonary problem from an obstructive problem. In addition, PFTs are useful for monitoring the effectiveness of therapeutic interventions (see Figure 4–15).

Total Lung Capacity

Total lung capacity (TLC) is the amount (volume) of gas present in the lungs after maximal inspiration, which is equal to about 6,000 mL in an adult. Total lung capacity is composed of four separate volumes, each of which can be measured separately. These volumes are called inspiratory reserve volume (IRV), tidal volume (TV), expiratory reserve volume (ERV), and residual volume (RV). Volumes also can be measured in combinations called lung capacities. Lung capacities include inspiratory capacity (IC), vital capacity (VC), functional residual capacity (FRC), and TLC.

Bedside Pulmonary Function Measurements

High-acuity patients with or without direct pulmonary involvement are at risk of developing pulmonary complications associated with immobility and respiratory muscle fatigue. Pulmonary function may be monitored in patients who are at particular risk for ventilatory decompensation. Of partic-

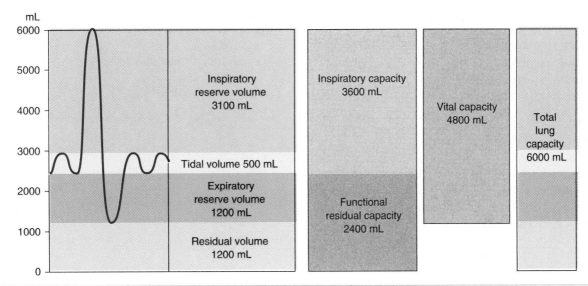

Figure 4–15 ■ Pulmonary function tests lung volumes and capacities.

ular interest are tidal volume, vital capacity, and minute ventilation.

Tidal volume (TV or V$_T$) is the amount of air that moves in and out of the lungs with each normal breath. Normal TV is approximately 7 to 9 mL/kg, about 500 mL in the average-sized man. When TV drops below 4 mL/kg, a state of alveolar hypoventilation develops. Acute respiratory failure results when hypoventilation becomes too severe.

Vital capacity (VC) is the maximum amount of air expired after a maximal inspiration. Normal VC is approximately 4,800 mL in the average-sized man. Both TV and VC help monitor respiratory muscle strength. As the patient experiences respiratory muscle fatigue, these values will decrease. Both of these PFTs can be measured using a respiratory spirometer.

Minute ventilation (V̇$_E$) is the total volume of expired air in 1 minute. It is used as a rapid method of measuring total lung ventilation changes, but it is not considered to be an accurate measure of alveolar ventilation. Minute ventilation is not a direct measurement but a simple calculation,

$$\dot{V}_E = TV \times f$$

where f = frequency, breaths per minute. Normal minute ventilation is 5 to 10 L/min. When it increases to greater than 10 L/min, the work of breathing is significantly increased. Minute ventilation less than 5 L/min indicates that the patient is at risk for problems associated with hypoventilation.

Forced Expiratory Volumes

Forced expiratory volumes (FEVs) are important diagnostic measurements that help differentiate restrictive pulmonary problems from obstructive problems and measure airway resistance. FEVs measure how rapidly a person can forcefully exhale air after a maximal inhalation, measuring volume (in liters) over time (in seconds). Patients who have a restrictive airway problem will be able to push air forcefully out of their lungs at a normal rate, whereas persons who have an obstructive disorder will have a delayed emptying rate (a reduced rate of expiratory air flow).

In summary, there are a variety of methods by which pulmonary function can be evaluated. Pulmonary function tests, such as tidal volume, vital capacity, and total lung capacity, help measure the effects of a disease process on ventilation. Table 4–13 shows normal pulmonary function values.

TABLE 4–13 Pulmonary Function Measurements

MEASUREMENT	NORMAL ADULT RANGE/VALUE
Total lung capacity (TLC)	6,000 mL
Tidal volume (TV, V$_T$)	7–9 mL/kg
Vital capacity (VC)	4,800 mL (average male)
Minute ventilation (V̇$_E$) (V̇$_E$ = V$_T$ × f)	5–10 mL/min

SECTION SIX REVIEW

1. In the acutely ill patient, pulmonary function testing helps monitor for
   A. impending ventilatory failure
   B. acute hypoxemia
   C. acute metabolic acidosis
   D. impending oxygenation failure

2. Minute ventilation (V̇$_E$) is calculated as
   A. (V̇$_E$) = V̇C × f
   B. (V̇$_E$) = TV/f

C. $(\dot{V}_E) = \dot{V}C \times TV$
D. $(\dot{V}_E) = TV \times f$

3. Patients who have obstructive pulmonary disease will have which pattern of FEVs?
   A. increased FEVs
   B. delayed FEVs
   C. normal FEVs
   D. variable FEVs

4. Total lung capacity is defined as the
   A. rate at which air can be forcefully exhaled after a maximal inspiration
   B. amount of air that moves in and out of the lungs with each normal breath

C. volume of gas present in the lungs after a maximal inspiration
D. maximum amount of air expired after a maximal inspiration

5. Normal tidal volume in an average-sized adult male would be _____ mL/kg
   A. 3 to 4
   B. 4 to 5
   C. 5 to 7
   D. 7 to 9

Answers: 1. A, 2. D, 3. B, 4. C, 5. D

SECTION SEVEN: Arterial Blood Gases

At the completion of this section, the learner will be able to identify normal values for and interpret arterial blood gases.

Determinants of Acid–Base Status

pH

The pH represents the amount of free H^+ available in the blood (normal value 7.35 to 7.45). The body's normal state is slightly alkaline, and the body strives to maintain this range. Extreme deviation for long periods of time is incompatible with survival. pH reflects the body's total acid–base balance. It is shifted by changes in hydrogen (H^+) or bicarbonate (HCO_3) ion concentration. Gain of acid or loss of base shifts the acid–base balance to the acid side. Loss of acid or gain of base or both shift the balance to the alkaline side.

$Paco_2$

The $Paco_2$ is the **partial pressure** of carbon dioxide in arterial blood (normal value 35 to 45 mm Hg). $Paco_2$ represents the respiratory component of the arterial blood gases (ABGs). The lungs control the excretion or retention of carbon dioxide through alveolar ventilation. Elevated $Paco_2$ indicates hypoventilation of the alveoli. Decreased $Paco_2$ represents alveolar hyperventilation.

HCO_3

HCO_3 represents the concentration of bicarbonate in the blood (normal value 22 to 26 mEq/L). HCO_3 represents the renal or metabolic component of the arterial blood gases. It is influenced by metabolic processes.

Base Excess

Base excess (BE) is a measure of the amount of buffer required to return the blood to a normal pH state. The normal range is

± 2 mEq/L. Base excess is considered a purely nonrespiratory measurement because it is not affected by carbonic acid concentrations. A base excess is present if the BE is greater than +2 mEq/L, reflecting either an excess of base or a deficit of fixed acids. It signals the presence of a metabolic alkalosis state. A base deficit is present if BE is less than −2 mEq/L, reflecting an excess of fixed acids or a deficit in base in the blood. It signals the presence of a metabolic acidosis state. Base excess measurement is not considered an essential step in basic ABG interpretation.

Determinants of Oxygenation Status

Pao_2

Pao_2 represents the partial pressure of the oxygen dissolved in arterial blood (3 percent of total oxygen) (normal value 80 to 100 mm Hg), not the total amount of oxygen available. Though it accounts for only a small percentage of total oxygen in the blood, it is an important indicator of oxygenation because Pao_2 and oxygen saturation (Sao_2) maintain a relationship. This relationship is reflected in the oxyhemoglobin dissociation curve, which was discussed in Section 2.

Sao_2

Oxygen saturation (Sao_2) is the measure of the percentage of oxygen combined with hemoglobin compared with the total amount it could carry (normal value greater than 95 percent). The degree of saturation is important in determining the amount of oxygen available for delivery to the tissues.

Hemoglobin

Hemoglobin (Hgb or Hb) is the major component of red blood cells (normal values 12 to 15 g/dL in women, 13.5 to 17 g/dL in men). It is composed of protein and heme, which contains iron. Oxygen binds to the iron atoms located on the four heme groups of each hemoglobin molecule. Hemoglobin is the major carrier of oxygen in the blood and is, therefore, an important factor in tissue oxygenation.

Arterial Blood Gas

Arterial blood gas (ABG) normal values typically are reported as normal at sea level (760 mm Hg) partial pressures, room air (21 percent oxygen), and a blood temperature of 37°C (98.6°F). Changes in these factors need to be considered during interpretation. Age also affects the normal values. Newborns have a lower PaO_2 (40 to 70 mm Hg), as do elderly people, whose PaO_2 decreases approximately 10 mm Hg per decade (in the 60- to 90-year age range). Normal ABG values are ranges for normal, healthy adults. It is important to establish a baseline for the individual because abnormal values become "normal" for some individuals. A patient with chronic lung disease may have a PaO_2 of 60 mm Hg with a $PaCO_2$ of 50 mm Hg as a normal baseline. Attempts to return ABG values to those of a normal, healthy individual would have serious consequences.

A person receiving supplemental oxygen also can be evaluated without determining room air gas. The PaO_2 should rise approximately 50 mm Hg for each 10 percent rise in oxygen concentration. A simple way to estimate what the PaO_2 should be is to multiply five times the percent of oxygen. If the PaO_2 is less than this value, the patient would probably be inadequately oxygenated on room air. For example, $5 \times 50\% \ O_2 = 250$ mm Hg PaO_2.

Arterial Blood Gas Interpretation

A single ABG measurement represents only a single point in time. Arterial blood gases are most valuable when trends are evaluated over time, correlated with other values, and incorporated into the overall clinical picture. Interpretation of ABGs includes determination of acid–base state, level of compensation, and oxygenation status. The oxygenation status reflects alveolar ventilation, the amount of oxygen available in arterial blood for possible tissue use, oxygen-carrying capacity, and oxygen transport. The severity of hypoxemia is frequently referred to in terms of being mild, moderate, or severe; however, the exact associated PaO_2 levels are somewhat arbitrary and vary between experts. For the purposes of this chapter, the levels of hypoxemia are defined as:

- Mild hypoxemia: PaO_2 60 to 75 mm Hg
- Moderate hypoxemia: PaO_2 45 to 59 mm Hg
- Severe hypoxemia: PaO_2 of less than 45 mm Hg

A step-by-step process for ABG interpretation evaluates each component to determine acid–base balance and oxygenation status (Table 4–14). Although acid–base balance determination is presented first, oxygenation status often is analyzed

TABLE 4–14   Steps in Determining Acid–Base and Oxygenation Status

STEP	NORMAL VALUES	QUESTIONS
Acid-Base Interpretation		
Step 1: Evaluate pH	pH = 7.35 to 7.45; midpoint = 7.40. If less than 7.40 = acid. If greater than 7.40 = alkaline.	Ask: ∎ Is the pH within normal range? ∎ Is pH on acid or alkaline side of 7.40?
Step 2: Evaluate $PaCO_2$	$PaCO_2$ = 35 to 45 mm Hg. If less than 35 mm Hg = alkaline. If greater than 45 mm Hg = acid.	Ask: ∎ Is $PaCO_2$ within normal range? ∎ If not, does it deviate to acid or alkaline side?
Step 3: Evaluate HCO_3	HCO_3 = 22 to 26 mEq/L. If less than 22 mEq/L = acid. If greater than 26 mEq/L = alkaline.	Ask: ∎ Is HCO_3 within normal range? ∎ If not, does it deviate to alkaline or acid side?
Step 4: Determine Acid–Base Status	The acid–base status has now been determined for the individual components of $PaCO_2$ and HCO_3.	Ask: ∎ Which individual component matches the pH acid–base state? ∎ The match determines the *primary* acid–base disturbance.
Oxygenation Status Interpretation		
Step 5: Evaluate PaO_2	PaO_2 = 80 to 100 mm Hg.	Ask: ∎ Is it within normal range? ∎ What is this person's baseline? ∎ Is it within acceptable range for this person? ∎ If not, is it too low or too high?
Step 6: Evaluate SaO_2	SaO_2 = greater than 95 percent.	Ask: ∎ Is it within acceptable range?
Step 7: Evaluate Hgb	Hgb = 12 to 15 g/dL (females) and 13.5 to 17 g/dL (males).	Ask: ∎ Are there enough oxygen carriers?
Step 8: Evaluate patient	Although ABG interpretation is an important adjunct to assessing a patient's status, it cannot take the place of direct evaluation of the patient.	Ask: ∎ Does patient's clinical picture match the acid–base and oxygen interpretation? ∎ Does the patient have a chronic disorder that is associated with long-term alterations in ABGs? ∎ Are there any acute processes occurring that need to be taken into consideration? ∎ Does the patient have a fever?

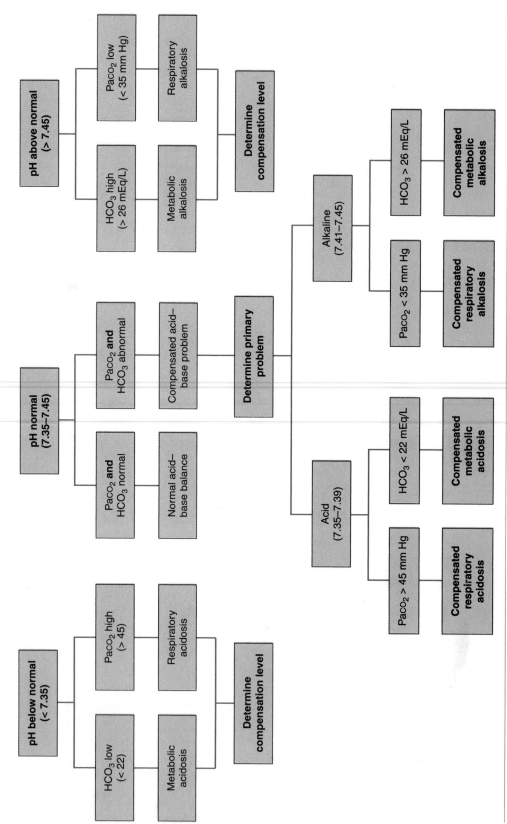

Figure 4–16 ■ Algorithm for interpreting primary acid-base disturbances.

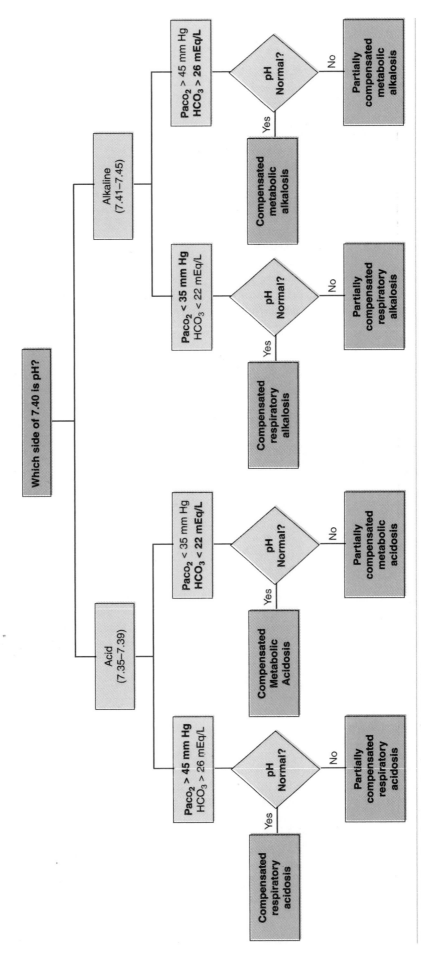

Figure 4–17 ■ Algorithm for interpreting degree of compensation.

first, based on the needs of the patient and the preference of the person performing the analysis. In addition, Figures 4–16 and 4–17 provide algorithms for interpreting primary acid–base disturbances and level of compensation.

In summary, indicators of acid–base and oxygenation states have been presented. Included in the discussion were normal values and a brief description of each indicator. The concept of arterial blood gases was presented in regards to the basis of normal values, gas considerations, and alterations in normal blood gas values associated with the pathophysiologic changes of chronic obstructive pulmonary disease. Table 4–15 summarizes normal arterial blood gas values. ABG analysis is a step-by-step process. Each component is evaluated individually and then in relationship to other components. Although acid–base state, compensation, and oxygenation status are important factors, the most important step is applying the results to the individual patient and the particular clinical situation.

TABLE 4–15 Normal Arterial Blood Gas Values

	RANGE
Acid–base	
pH	7.35–7.45
$Paco_2$	35–45 mm Hg
HCO_3	22–26 mEq/L
BE	± 2 mEq/L
Oxygenation Status	
Pao_2	80–100 mm Hg
Sao_2	95–100%
Hgb*	13.5–17 g/dL (males)
	12–15 g/dL (females)

*From Kee, J. L. (2002). Laboratory and diagnostic tests with nursing implications, (6th ed.) Upper Saddle River, NJ: Prentice Hall.

SECTION SEVEN REVIEW

1. Normal values for arterial blood gases include
   A. pH 7.5
   B. $Paco_2$ 20 mm Hg
   C. HCO_3 26 mm Hg
   D. Sao_2 75 mm Hg
2. An increase in bicarbonate would cause the pH to become more
   A. acidic
   B. alkaline
   C. neutral
   D. no change
3. $Paco_2$ is the _____ component, and HCO_3 is the _____ component.
   A. oxygenation, metabolic
   B. respiratory, metabolic
   C. metabolic, respiratory
   D. hepatic, oxygenation

4. In people over the age of 60, Pao_2 decreases about _____ mm Hg per decade.
   A. 4
   B. 6
   C. 8
   D. 10
5. What factor must you always evaluate to place ABGs in the proper context?
   A. laboratory values
   B. oxygen supplemental therapy
   C. mode of ventilation
   D. patient

Answers: 1. C, 2. B, 3. B, 4. D, 5. D

SUPPLEMENTAL ABG EXERCISES

Take time to practice determining acid–base state and oxygenation status using the steps and algorithms provided in this section. Interpret the acid–base status as normal, metabolic or respiratory, alkalosis or acidosis. Indicate the state of compensation as being uncompensated (acute state), partially compensated, or compensated (chronic state). Indicate the oxygenation status as adequate or inadequate, when indicated.

1. pH 7.58, $Paco_2$ 38 mm Hg, HCO_3 30 mEq/L
   Interpretation:

   Compensation:

2. pH 7.20, $Paco_2$ 60 mm Hg, HCO_3 26 mEq/L
   Interpretation:

   Compensation:

3. pH 7.39, $Paco_2$ 43 mm Hg, HCO_3 24 mEq/L
   Interpretation:

   Compensation:

4. pH 7.32, $Paco_2$ 60 mm Hg, HCO_3 30 mEq/L
   Interpretation:

   Compensation:

5. pH 7.5, $Paco_2$ 50 mm Hg, HCO_3 38 mEq/L

   Interpretation:
   Compensation:

6. pH 7.45, $Paco_2$ 30 mm Hg, HCO_3 20 mEq/L

   Interpretation:
   Compensation:

7. pH 7.40, $Paco_2$ 40 mm Hg, HCO_3 24 mEq/L

   Interpretation:
   Compensation:

8. pH 7.37, $Paco_2$ 48 mm Hg, HCO_3 29 mEq/L, Pao_2 80 mm Hg, Sao_2 95 percent

   Acid–base state:
   Oxygenation status:

9. pH 7.48, $Paco_2$ 30 mm Hg, HCO_3 24 mEq/L, Pao_2 90 mm

Hg, Sao_2 98 percent

Acid–base state:
Oxygenation status:

10. pH 7.48, $Paco_2$ 33 mm Hg, HCO_3 25 mEq/L, Pao_2 68 mm Hg, Sao_2 98 percent

   Acid–base state:
   Oxygenation status:

11. pH 7.38, $Paco_2$ 38 mm Hg, HCO_3 24 mEq/L, Pao_2 269 mm Hg, Sao_2 100 percent

   Acid–base state:
   Oxygenation status:

12. pH 7.17, $Paco_2$ 18 mm Hg, HCO_3 7 mEq/L, Pao_2 100 mm Hg, Sao_2 99 percent

   Acid–base state:
   Oxygenation status:

ANSWERS

1. pH 7.58 (alkaline) and HCO_3 30 mEq/L (alkaline) match. $Paco_2$ 38 mm Hg (normal). Interpretation: metabolic alkalosis. Compensation: uncompensated.

2. pH 7.20 (acid) and $Paco_2$ 60 mm Hg (acid) match. HCO_3 26 mEq/L (normal). Interpretation: respiratory acidosis. Compensation: uncompensated.

3. pH 7.39 (normal, slightly to acid side of 7.4) and $Paco_2$ 43 mm Hg (normal). HCO_3 24 (normal). Interpretation: normal. Compensation: none required.

4. pH 7.32 (acid) and $Paco_2$ 60 mm Hg (acid) match. HCO_3 30 mEq/L (alkaline). Interpretation: respiratory acidosis. Compensation: partial compensation.

5. pH 7.5 (alkaline) and HCO_3 38 mEq/L (alkaline) match. $Paco_2$ 50 mm Hg (acid). Interpretation: metabolic alkalosis. Compensation: partial compensation.

6. pH 7.45 (normal, alkaline side) and $Paco_2$ 30 mm Hg (alkaline) match. HCO_3 20 mEq/L (acid). Interpretation: respiratory alkalosis. Compensation: full compensation.

7. pH, $Paco_2$, and HCO_3 are all normal. Interpretation: normal. Compensation: none required.

8. pH 7.37 (normal range, acid) and $Paco_2$ 48 mm Hg (acid) match. HCO_3 29 mEq/L (alkaline) is opposite. Pao_2 80 mm Hg and Sao_2 95 percent both are low normal. Acid–base state: compensated respiratory acidosis (pH normal). Oxygenation status: adequate. The Hgb is not known, but the relationship between Pao_2 and Sao_2 appears normal. Assessing trends is important. Is the $Paco_2$ continuing to increase and PaO_2 continuing to decrease? Continue to monitor.

9. pH 7.48 (alkaline) and $Paco_2$ 30 mm Hg (alkaline) match, HCO_3 24 mEq/L, Pao_2 90 mm Hg, and Sao_2 98 percent are all normal. Acid–base state: acute respiratory alkalosis (uncompensated). Oxygenation status: within normal limits and seems adequate. Look at your patient.

10. pH 7.48 (alkaline) and $Paco_2$ 33 mm Hg (alkaline) match. HCO_3 25 mEq/L is normal. Pao_2 68 mm Hg (low) and Sao_2 98 percent (normal). Acid–base state: acute respiratory alkalosis. Oxygenation status: low oxygen with high saturation. Hemoglobin is carrying a full load but needs more carriers. What is this patient's hemoglobin? Nursing interventions may focus on decreasing oxygen demand. Is this patient tachypneic? Is supplemental oxygen available? Is a transfusion ordered?

11. pH 7.38, $Paco_2$ 38 mm Hg, HCO_3 24 mEq/L are all normal. Pao_2 269 mm Hg is high, and Sao_2 100 percent is high normal. Acid–base state: normal. Oxygenation status: too high! What oxygen percentage is this patient on? Oxygenation supplement needs to be decreased.

12. pH 7.17 (acid) and HCO_3 7 mEq/L (acid) match. $Paco_2$ 18 mm Hg (alkaline) is opposite. Pao_2 100 mm Hg is high, and Sao_2 99 percent is high normal. Acid–base state: severe metabolic acidosis with partial compensation. Oxygenation status: adequate oxygen provided, but it is doubtful that the patient can use what is available efficiently because of the state of severe acidosis. Cellular metabolism is compromised and cannot function efficiently in the acid environment. Cardiovascular status is very likely compromised. The reactivity and effectiveness of many drugs are altered severely in an acidic environment such as this.

SECTION EIGHT: Advanced Interpretation: Mixed Acid–Base Disorders

At the completion of this section, the learner will be able to recognize mixed acid–base disorders.

It is not always clear whether the patient is experiencing a simple acid–base disorder with compensation or a mixed acid–base disorder. Recognition and analysis of mixed acid–base disorders is a more complex skill than basic blood gas analysis. This section focuses on the basic concepts involved in recognition of mixed acid–base disorders and provides four rules that help differentiate mixed acid–base disorders from simple (single) disorders with compensation.

The majority of acid–base disturbances have one primary origin with a single secondary acid–base compensatory response. The high-acuity patient, however, is at increased risk for more complex acid–base disorders and may have several different primary acid–base disturbances at the same time. For example, a patient with diabetic ketoacidosis (DKA), a primary metabolic acidosis, might also develop respiratory failure, a primary respiratory acidosis. This situation represents a mixed acid–base disorder. Mixed disorders can have an additive effect, such as is seen with the preceding example (two forms of acidosis), which results in a major derangement in pH. Mixed disorders can also have a nullifying effect (e.g., a primary metabolic alkalosis in the presence of a primary respiratory acidosis), which may rebalance the pH. Table 4–16 lists some complex health problems that are frequently involved in mixed acid–base disorders.

Identifying a Mixed Acid–Base Disorder

Initial Recognition

Before the nurse can attempt to analyze an ABG for the presence of a mixed acid–base disorder, she or he must first recognize the characteristics of a mixed disorder. When either the $PaCO_2$ or the HCO_3 value appears to be out of the ordinary boundaries, a mixed disorder should be suspected. The following rule summarizes the initial recognition:

RULE: A mixed acid–base disorder is present when either the $PaCO_2$ or the HCO_3 value is

1. In a direction opposite to its predicted direction, or
2. Not close to the predicted value, during normal compensatory activity (see Table 4–17).

For example, a patient with DKA has an ABG drawn, which shows a pH of 7.05 and an HCO_3 of 16. In this instance, both the pH and the HCO_3 are acidotic. Depending on the level of compensation, one would predict that the $PaCO_2$ level should be either normal or predictably alkaline, as a secondary acid–base response to this situation. If, however, the same DKA patient develops ventilatory failure (hypercapnia), the $PaCO_2$ will also be acidotic (indicating respiratory acidosis), which is not a predicted alteration. The presence of both an acid HCO_3 and $PaCO_2$ is an example of an additive type of mixed acid–base problem, which would drop the pH significantly.

A second example is one that presents a situation in which a nullifying mixed acid–base problem might develop. Assume that the same acute DKA patient develops severe vomiting or diarrhea, causing metabolic alkalosis. This patient, then, will have metabolic acidosis (caused by DKA) plus metabolic alkalosis (caused by vomiting or diarrhea). The opposing metabolic disturbances represent a nullifying mixed acid–base problem. In this situation, the pH will lean toward the predominant problem, but it will not be as severely deranged as one would predict based on the patient's DKA status. As a result of these opposing metabolic derangements, the patient's $PaCO_2$ compensatory changes will reflect the predominant acid–base disorder. The degree of $PaCO_2$ compensation, however, will not be as would be predicted for either metabolic disturbance existing alone. In this complex clinical situation, evaluation of the patient's condition must be an integral part of the acid–base assessment. In addition, the base excess and anion gap can be obtained to assist in the analysis of the situation. This type of complex interpretation is generally beyond the nurse's responsibility. It is more important that the nurse (1) recognizes that the patient's clinical picture does not coincide with the ABG results and (2) contacts the physician to report the concern.

The key is learning how to predict the "normal" compensation relationships between $PaCO_2$, HCO_3, and pH so that you can recognize when the relationships are abnormal.

Systematic Evaluation

Once a mixed acid–base problem is suspected, a systematic approach should be used to interpret the disorder. The first two steps are common to all blood gas analyses. It is at Step 3 that mixed acid–base analysis begins. Table 4–18 summarizes a four-step interpretation approach.

TABLE 4–16 Examples of Clinical Problems Associated with Mixed Acid–Base Disorders

CLINICAL PROBLEM	ASSOCIATED MIXED DISORDERS
Cardiac arrest	Metabolic acidosis and respiratory acidosis
Salicylate toxicity	Metabolic acidosis and respiratory alkalosis
Renal failure with vomiting	Metabolic acidosis and metabolic alkalosis
Vomiting with chronic obstructive pulmonary disease	Metabolic alkalosis and respiratory acidosis

From Czekaj, L. A. (1998). Promoting acid–base balance. In M. R. Kinney, S. B. Dunbar, J. A. Brooks-Brunn, N. Molter, & J. M. Vitello-Cicciu (Eds.), AACN clinical reference for critical care nursing, *(4th ed.) (pp. 135–144). St. Louis: C.V. Mosby.*

TABLE 4–17 A Comparison of Mixed Acid–Base Disorders[a]

PARAMETER	MIXED DISORDERS				
	MATCHING DERANGEMENTS		OPPOSITE DERANGEMENTS		
	Metabolic acidosis + Respiratory acidosis	Metabolic alkalosis + Respiratory alkalosis	Metabolic acidosis + Respiratory alkalosis	Metabolic alkalosis + Respiratory acidosis	Metabolic acidosis + Metabolic alkalosis
pH	$\downarrow\downarrow$	$\uparrow\uparrow$	NL, $\downarrow$, or $\uparrow$	NL, $\downarrow$, or $\uparrow$	NL, $\downarrow$, or $\uparrow$
$Paco_2$	$\uparrow$	$\downarrow$	$\downarrow$	$\uparrow$	$\downarrow$, or $\uparrow$
HCO_3	$\downarrow$	$\uparrow$	$\downarrow$	$\uparrow$	NL, $\downarrow$, or $\uparrow$

[a]The columns on the left, Matching Derangements, illustrate the direction of the value trends when both primary disorders are the same (acidotic or alkalotic). This situation results in a severely deranged pH (as shown by two arrows). The three columns on the right, Opposite Derangements, illustrate the direction of value trends when the primary disorders are the opposite of each other (one is acidotic and the other is alkalotic). When opposite primary derangements coexist, they may fully or partially nullify the impact of the pH. If one disorder is predominant, the pH will lean toward the pH associated with that disorder, but to a lesser degree (as shown by single arrows). NL = normal.

Expected Compensatory Responses

Three pairs of relationships require analysis when seeking to differentiate the nature of a mixed acid–base disorder: (1) pH to HCO_3, (2) pH to $Paco_2$, and (3) $Paco_2$ to HCO_3.

Each pair is accompanied by a rule that defines the relationship. If the calculated (predicted) values are similar to the actual values, a simple acid–base disturbance with compensation is present. If, however, the calculated (predicted) values are not similar to the actual values, a mixed disorder is present.

The pH to HCO_3 Relationship.   If a metabolic disturbance is present, the pH and HCO_3 should maintain a stable relationship.

RULE: If the acid–base problem is purely metabolic, a pH change of 0.15 will result in a corresponding change in HCO_3 of approximately 10 mEq/L (Pilbeam, 1998).

Example 1: Max W had an ABG drawn revealing a pH of 7.55 and an HCO_3 of 34 mEq/L. The pH difference between the initial standard of 7.40 and Max's ABG pH of 7.55 is 0.15. The HCO_3 difference between the initial

TABLE 4–18 Interpretation of Mixed Blood Gases. The First Two Steps Are Common to all Blood Gas Analyses. Step 3 Begins Mixed Acid–Base Analysis.

STEP	QUESTIONS	EXAMPLES/DISCUSSION
Step 1: Identification of primary disorder	Ask: ■ Does pH indicate acidosis or alkalosis? ■ To which side of 7.40 does pH lean?	pH less than 7.40? ■ Acid side of normal pH greater than 7.40? ■ Alkaline side of normal
Step 2: Identification of primary disorder	Ask: ■ Which value ($Paco_2$ or HCO_3) matches the acid–base state of pH? ■ Discussion: If both values match the pH, a mixed acid–base disturbance is present. Several primary disorders are at work.	pH less than 7.30, $Paco_2$ greater than 50 mm Hg, HCO_3 less than 20 mEq/L. All three indicators are acidotic; thus, the problem is a mixed acid–base disorder.
Step 3: Estimate expected compensatory responses using appropriate rule[a]	Ask: ■ Is the relationship between pH and $Paco_2$ (respiratory component) as predicted? ■ Is the relationship between pH and HCO_3 (metabolic component) as predicted? ■ Is the relationship between $Paco_2$ and HCO_3 as predicted? ■ If the relationships are not as predicted, has there been sufficient time for compensation to have taken place?	Use the appropriate rule related to one of the three blood gas relationships: ■ pH to HCO_3 relationship ■ pH to $Paco_2$ relationship ■ $Paco_2$ to HCO_3 relationship See examples in text.
Step 4: Compare ABG with patient's clinical status	Ask: Is the patient at risk for ■ Alveolar hyper- or hypoventilation? ■ Lactic acidosis? ■ Ketoacidosis? ■ Loss of bicarbonate?	Knowledge of patient's clinical status and risk factors for possible metabolic and respiratory disorders is essential when attempting to interpret mixed acid–base problems.

[a] See text, "Expected compensatory responses"

standard of 24 mEq/L and Max's HCO_3 is 10 mEq/L. Therefore, because Max's pH and HCO_3 altered within the parameters of the rule, the relationship has been maintained, indicating that a pure metabolic acidosis is present.

The pH and $PaCO_2$ Relationship.   If the acid–base problem may have a primary respiratory origin, the relationship of pH to $PaCO_2$ can be estimated.

RULE: For every 20 mm Hg increase in $PaCO_2$ above 40, the pH will decrease by 0.10 unit. For every 10 mm Hg decrease in $PaCO_2$ below 40, the pH will increase by 0.10 unit. pH decreases as $PaCO_2$ increases; pH increases as $PaCO_2$ decreases (Pilbeam, 1998).

Example 2: Jill B's $PaCO_2$ is 60 mm Hg, which is 20 mm Hg above the standard of 40 mm Hg. In response, her pH should predictably decrease by 0.10 unit, dropping from 7.40 to 7.30.

Example 3: Lee C's $PaCO_2$ is 30 mm Hg, which is 10 mm Hg below the standard of 40 mm Hg. In response, his pH should increase to 7.50 (an increase of 0.10 unit).

Example 4: Eva T has a $PaCO_2$ of 60 mm Hg, which is 20 mm Hg above the standard of 40 mm Hg, and a pH of 7.20. Her pH is NOT close to the predicted pH value of 7.30. Assuming that there has been sufficient time for compensatory mechanisms to take effect, a mixed disorder is present.

The $PaCO_2$ to HCO_3 Relationship.   Under normal conditions the $PaCO_2$ and HCO_3 maintain a stable relationship.

RULE: For every increase of 10 mm Hg in $PaCO_2$, there is a corresponding increase of 1.0 mEq/L of HCO_3. For every decrease of 10 mm Hg in $PaCO_2$, there is corresponding decrease of 1.5 mEq/L of HCO_3 (Pilbeam, 1998).

Example 5. Richard C has an ABG drawn. The $PaCO_2$ was 60 mm Hg and the HCO_3 was 31.2 mEq/L. The difference between his $PaCO_2$ (60 mm Hg) and the standard of 40 mm Hg is 20 mm Hg. The predicted HCO_3 is 26 mEq/L. Richard's actual HCO_3 compensatory response level is 31.2 mEq/L, which is significantly different from the predicted answer. Assuming that his compensatory mechanisms have had sufficient time to take effect, a mixed disorder is present.

Example 6: Joseph B has an ABG drawn. The $PaCO_2$ was 35 mm Hg and the HCO_3 was 26 mEq/L. The difference between Joseph's $PaCO_2$ (35 mm Hg) and the standard is 5 mm Hg. This means that for a $PaCO_2$ of 35 mm Hg, the predicted HCO_3 compensatory response level would be approximately 25 mEq/L. Joseph's HCO_3 is close to the predicted level. The appropriate level of compensation suggests a simple acid–base disorder.

In summary, high-acuity patients may develop mixed acid–base disorders. These complex derangements can be recognized and broadly differentiated by answering a series of questions and estimating expected predicted responses. Three rules of normal compensatory relationships have been presented, including pH to HCO_3, pH to $PaCO_2$, and $PaCO_2$ to HCO_3. A four-step mixed-gas interpretation approach provides a systematic method for identifying a mixed acid–base disorder. Once estimations have been made and relationships have been analyzed, data must be compared with the patient's clinical situation. For many nurses, the major responsibility as regards mixed acid–base disorders is recognizing ABG values that are not congruent with predicted results, while taking the patient's clinical status into consideration. This recognition should then be followed up in a timely manner by contacting the physician.

SECTION EIGHT REVIEW

1. A mixed acid-base disorder should be suspected when either the $PaCO_2$ or the HCO_3 value is
   A. in a direction opposite of its predicted direction.
   B. close to the predicted value during normal compensatory activity.
   C. either significantly alkalotic or acidotic.
   D. impossible to interpret.
2. Mixed acid-base disorders may have what two effects on the pH? (short answer)
   1.
   2.
3. When evaluating a possible mixed acid-base problem, it is crucial to
   A. obtain a second arterial blood gas.
   B. contact the physician immediately.

   C. assess patient's current clinical picture.
   D. initiate oxygen therapy.
4. The relationship between pH and HCO_3 is best reflected in which statement?
   A. A pH change of 0.15 will result in an opposite change in HCO_3 of about 10 mEq.
   B. A 10 mEq increase in HCO_3 will result in approximately 0.15 increase in pH.
   C. A pH decrease of 0.30 will result from a HCO_3 decrease of about 10 mEq.
   D. The relationship is unpredictable.
5. Which statement is correct regarding the relationship between pH and $PaCO_2$?
   A. There is no predictable relationship.
   B. If a patient's $PaCO_2$ increases from 41 to 61, the pH will increase 0.10 units (e.g., from 7.39 to 7.49).

SECTION NINE: Noninvasive Monitoring of Gas Exchange

At the completion of this section, the learner will be able to discuss noninvasive methods of monitoring gas exchange and applications.

Pulse Oximetry

Pulse oximetry is a noninvasive technique for monitoring arterial capillary hemoglobin saturation (SpO_2) and pulse rate. It uses light wavelengths to determine oxyhemoglobin saturation. It also detects pulsatile flow to differentiate between venous and arterial blood. A sensor is placed on a finger, nose, or ear, and an oximeter provides a constant assessment of arterial oxygen saturation. Pulse oximetry is best used as an adjunct to a variety of assessment modalities in providing continuous information for evaluation of oxygenation status. Ideally, the continuous arterial oxygen saturation readings reflect the patient's oxygenation status and alert the clinician to subtle or sudden changes. In some patients, use of oximetry may decrease the frequency of invasive ABG measurements if acid–base and ventilation are not problems.

Many factors can alter the accuracy of pulse oximetry in high-acuity patients. In general, these factors can be divided into problems of technical (mechanical) origin and those of physiologic origin. Technical problems include external light sources and improper sensor placement. Bright light sources within the patient's immediate environment can compete with the pulse oximetry sensor light source. When this is a problem, the sensor must be covered up to protect it from the external lighting. An improperly placed sensor may not be able to register arterial pulsations because of lack of sufficient arterial flow. An additional technical problem is excessive patient movement, which can cause the sensor to misinterpret body movement as arterial pulsations. Mechanical problems are generally easy to correct once they are recognized.

Physiologic factors that alter the accuracy of SpO_2 to predict blood oxygen content (and ultimately delivery of oxygen to the tissues) include hemoglobin level, acid–base imbalance, and vasoconstrictive situations (e.g., peripheral vascular disease, hypothermia, shock, hypovolemia, and vasopressors in high doses). The level of hemoglobin greatly affects the oxygen content of the blood. When a patient is severely anemic, the SpO_2 may remain high, indicating sufficient oxygen saturation of available hemoglobin. The actual oxygen content of the blood, however, may be inadequate to meet tissue oxygenation needs, thus increasing the risk of tissue hypoxia. Hemoglobin levels should be monitored and taken into consideration when analyzing SpO_2 measurements.

When an acid–base imbalance exists, acidosis may cause a lower saturation reading and alkalosis may cause a higher reading because of shifts in the oxyhemoglobin dissociation curve. Severe peripheral vasoconstriction creates a low-flow arterial state in which the pulsatile force is too weak to be accurately read by pulse oximetry. When severe vasoconstriction is present, the sensor may read more accurately if it is removed from distal sites (fingers, toes) and attached to a more central location, such as the bridge of the nose or the ear lobe. The hypothermic patient generally requires warming to normothermic levels before pulse oximetry can be used. In addition, patients who have abnormal levels of carboxyhemoglobin (carbon dioxide and carbon monoxide) may have a high SpO_2 even though the oxyhemoglobin level is very low. This false reading occurs because pulse oximetry cannot differentiate carboxyhemoglobin from oxyhemoglobin.

End-Tidal Carbon Dioxide Monitoring

Capnometry is the noninvasive measurement of carbon dioxide (CO_2) concentration in expired gas. It results in a single value measurement called the $PETCO_2$ (partial pressure of end-tidal CO_2). Continuous bedside monitoring of CO_2 is accomplished using infrared light absorption or mass spectrometry (Anderson & Breen, 2000). Infrared analyzers measure carbon dioxide based on its strong absorption band at a distinctive wavelength. A **capnogram** displays the capnometry measurements as a continuous waveform that can be read throughout the breathing cycle.

CO_2 can be sampled using either sidestream or mainstream techniques. When a sidestream analyzer is used, a small volume of exhaled gas is diverted from the main airway circuit through a small tube and is analyzed in a special chamber apart from the airway circuit. This causes a time delay between the carbon dioxide sampling and the display of data. Using this technique, the capnogram is averaged and the PETCO$_2$ can be underestimated, particularly if breathing rates are rapid or the sampling catheter is long (Anderson & Breen, 2000). The small tubing may become obstructed with secretions or water. Sidestream analysis devices can be applied to nonintubated patients as well as those who are intubated. Mainstream infrared analyzers use a technology that is similar to sidestream analyzers. Mainstream analyzers, however, are placed in-line as part of the airway circuit, and PETCO$_2$ analysis occurs in-line. Their major advantage is that they provide rapid response readings. Mainstream devices are relatively heavy and cumbersome additions to the artificial airway circuit that increases dead space. In addition, there is a slight risk of burning because of heating of the analyzer. This type of analyzer is primarily used on intubated patients (Anderson & Breen, 2000).

The normal capnogram shows a PETCO$_2$ within several mm Hg of arterial PaCO$_2$ at the end of the plateau phase (the end-tidal CO$_2$). In a normal capnogram, the carbon dioxide concentration is zero at the beginning of expiration, gradually rising until it reaches a plateau. The end-tidal carbon dioxide is the highest concentration at the end of exhalation. **End-tidal carbon dioxide (PETCO$_2$)** monitoring is used in the clinical setting as a noninvasive indirect method of measuring PaCO$_2$. In a normal person, PETCO$_2$ is typically 4 to 6 mm Hg below PaCO$_2$ (Pilbeam, 1998).

End-tidal carbon dioxide monitoring may be used to assess ventilatory status to provide an early warning of changes in ventilation. An abnormally low PETCO$_2$ (less than 36 mm Hg) most commonly is associated with hyperventilation. Increased PETCO$_2$ (greater than 44 mm Hg) is associated with increased production of carbon dioxide or problems causing hypoventilation (e.g., respiratory center depression, neuromuscular diseases, COPD). Use of the capnogram may help detect improper intubation, ventilation patterns, mechanical problems, or failure in ventilators. Certain capnographic patterns are associated with hyperventilation, incomplete exhalation, and a variety of disease states. Anesthesiologists frequently use capnography in the operating room, and new applications continue to be explored in critical care, emergency care, and outpatient care.

In patients with ventilation–perfusion abnormalities, the PETCO$_2$ may not accurately reflect PaCO$_2$. However, it still may be helpful if a correlation between PaCO$_2$ and PETCO$_2$ can be established and used for trending. Unfortunately, high-acuity patients commonly have ventilation–perfusion abnormalities, which may limit the usefulness of PETCO$_2$ monitoring.

In summary, pulse oximetry and PETCO$_2$ monitoring are noninvasive tools to assist in monitoring oxygenation and ventilation parameters. They can be used singly, but dual use provides information on capillary arterial oxygen saturation (oxygenation) and PaCO$_2$ (ventilation). Advantages of use include continuous readings to trend conditions and less invasive procedures.

SECTION NINE REVIEW

1. Pulse oximetry measures
   A. mixed venous saturation
   B. transcutaneous oxygen saturation
   C. venous oxygen capillary hemoglobin saturation
   D. arterial oxygen capillary hemoglobin saturation
2. Conditions that impair the accuracy of pulse oximetry include (choose all that apply)
   1. excessive movement
   2. vasodilation
   3. hypothermia
   4. improper sensor placement
   A. 1, 2, and 3
   B. 1, 3, and 4
   C. 2, 3, and 4
   D. 3 and 4

3. PETCO$_2$ is used as a reflection of
   A. arterial carbon dioxide
   B. $\dot{V}/\dot{Q}$ ratio
   C. oxygenation status
   D. venous carbon dioxide
4. PETCO$_2$ is an indicator of alveolar
   A. acid–base state
   B. compensation
   C. oxygenation
   D. ventilation

Answers: 1. D, 2. B, 3. A, 4. D

SECTION TEN: Respiratory Calculations

At the completion of this section, the learner will be able to perform selected respiratory calculations.

A variety of simple calculations can provide significant information regarding the oxygenation status of the high-acuity patient. Increasingly, nurses who take care of this patient population are expected to have a basic understanding of these calculations and their significance. This section presents several of the more uncomplicated but clinically useful equations that can estimate the degree of intrapulmonary shunt (e.g., A–a gradient, a/A ratio, and PaO$_2$/FIO$_2$ ratio).

Ideal Alveolar Gas Equation

The more simple measurements of shunt require two oxygen-derived variables, PAO_2 and PaO_2. The laws of diffusion state that gases will flow from higher concentration to lower concentration until a state of equilibrium exists. This means that the partial pressure of alveolar oxygen (PAO_2) should approximate the partial pressure of arterial oxygen (PaO_2). As a general clinical guideline, the maximum acceptable range for PaO_2 is 60 to 100 mm Hg, and the maximum acceptable difference between PAO_2 and PaO_2 is 40 mm Hg (Ahrens & Rutherford, 1993). A difference of greater than 40 mm Hg suggests abnormal intrapulmonary shunt.

Several respiratory calculations (e.g., a/A ratio, and A–a gradient) require an estimate of the PAO_2 level. Unlike its arterial counterpart (PaO_2), alveolar oxygen is not measured directly. It is derived from an equation called the ideal alveolar gas equation (or alveolar air equation). At first sight, the equation appears complicated. In fact, it is quite simple to perform because many of the calculation components are constants that are plugged into the equation.

To work the equation, the following bits of data must be obtained: current $PaCO_2$ and FIO_2 (the concentration of oxygen being breathed). The barometric pressure (PB) should be determined based on the altitude of the local area. This often can be obtained from the respiratory therapy department. Once barometric pressure is determined, it can be used as a constant for your institution. Table 4–19 explains the equation and provides a method for estimating barometric pressure based on the altitude of a general location.

Alveolar–Arterial Pressure Gradient (A–a Gradient)

A–a gradient (also called $P[A–a]O_2$) is useful for estimating the degree of physiologic shunt and hypoxemia. Although the PAO_2 and PaO_2 should approximate each other during gas exchange, in reality, the level of alveolar oxygen is normally slightly higher (about 104 mm Hg) than the level of arterial oxygen (about 95 mm Hg) while breathing room air. The difference between these two levels is called the Alveolar–arterial pressure gradient (A–a gradient) and is attributable to physiologic shunt. Certain factors are associated with a high A–a gradient, including normal aging and diffusion abnormalities such as shunt and $\dot{V}/\dot{Q}$ mismatch.

TABLE 4–19 Ideal Alveolar Gas Equation

EQUATION	$PaO_2 = [P_B - P_{H_2O}]FIO_2 - PaCO_2(1.25)$	
Components	$PaO_2 =$	Partial pressure of alveolar oxygen (mm Hg)
	$P_B =$	Barometric pressure (mm Hg)[a] (750 mm Hg is sometimes used as a constant)
	$P_{H_2O} =$	Water vapor constant (mm Hg) (47 mm Hg)
	$FIO_2 =$	Fraction of inspired oxygen (O_2 concentration) (decimal)
	$PaCO_2 =$	Partial pressure of arterial carbon dioxide (mm Hg)
	$1.25 =$	A number derived from the respiratory exchange ratio
Example	A patient is receiving oxygen at an FIO_2 of 0.40. Her latest ABG showed a $PaCO_2$ of 45 mm Hg. The barometric pressure (P_B) is 750 mm Hg.	
	$PaO_2 = [750 - 47]0.40 - 45(1.25)$	
	$PaO_2 = [703]0.40 - 56.25$	
	$PaO_2 = 281.2 - 56.25$	
	$PaO_2 = 224.95$	

[a]Estimating barometric pressure (see the following examples)

Near the earth's surface, pressure decreases with altitude at a rate of approximately 2.63 mm Hg for every 100 feet (30 m). To calculate:

$$760 \text{ mm Hg} - \frac{\text{(Local altitude)}}{100 \text{ feet}}\, 2.63 = \text{estimated barometric pressure}$$

1. Estimate the altitude of your city (for example, Denver is about 5,280 feet above sea level)
2. Divide the local altitude by 100 feet
3. Multiply the number derived in Step 2 by 2.63
4. Subtract the number derived in Step 3 from 760 mm Hg

Examples of barometric pressures by altitude:
Sea level = 760 mm Hg
500 feet above sea level = 747 mm Hg estimated P_B
1,000 feet above sea level = 734 mm Hg estimated P_B
1,500 feet above sea level = 721 mm Hg estimated P_B
2,000 feet above sea level = 707 mm Hg estimated P_B

TABLE 4–20 A–a Gradient (P(A–a)O$_2$)

EQUATION:[a]	A–a gradient = P_{AO_2} − Pa_{O_2}
Components	P_{AO_2} = partial pressure of alveolar oxygen (mm Hg)
	Pa_{O_2} = partial pressure of arterial oxygen (mm Hg)
Normal values (age dependent)	On room air:
	1. Calculate the normal for the person's age: < 4 mm Hg for every decade of life
	2. Compare the actual A–a gradient to the answer obtained in Step 1. Normal is any number less than the answer to Step 1.
	On 100 percent F_{IO_2}:
	1. Estimate 2 percent shunt for each 50 mm Hg difference in A–a gradient
Examples	On room air:
	A 40-year-old patient is breathing room air. The patient's P_{AO_2} is 100 mm Hg. An ABG is drawn with the Pa_{O_2} being 89 mm Hg.
	100 mm Hg − 89 mm Hg = 11 mm Hg.
	Normal A–a gradient in a 40-year-old would be less than 16 mm Hg.
	The A–a gradient is less than 16 and therefore is within normal range.
	On 100% oxygen:
	A 42-year-old patient is receiving 100 percent oxygen. She has a P_{AO_2} of 632 mm Hg. Her Pa_{O_2} is 89 mm Hg.
	A–a gradient = 632 mm Hg − 89 mm Hg
	A–a gradient = 543 mm Hg
	Estimating shunt:
	$\dfrac{543}{50} = 10.86 = 11$ (rounded)
	$11 \times 2\% = 22\%$ estimated shunt is present

Data from Chang, D. W. (1998). Respiratory care calculations, (2nd ed.) Albany, NY: Delmar Publishing; and Des Jardins, T. R. (1998). Cardiopulmonary anatomy and physiology: Essentials for respiratory care, (3rd ed.) Albany, NY: Delmar Publishing.

[a]This formula is best used as a rough estimate only. It is not sensitive to changes in oxygen concentration and can give false data regarding the presence and degree of shunt.

Normal Aging

As a person ages, diffusion becomes less efficient. The A–a gradient should be less than 4 mm Hg for every decade (10 years) of life (Chang, 1998). For example, in a 50-year-old patient, the A–a gradient should be less than 20 mm Hg (4 mm Hg × 5 decades = 20 mm Hg). When the difference is too high (greater than 4 mm Hg for every decade) an abnormal process is present that can cause hypoxemia. Caution must be used when interpreting data obtained from evaluation of A–a gradient because it is not sensitive to changing oxygen concentration (F_{IO_2}) levels. As the oxygen concentration is increased, the A–a gradient normally increases and, therefore, does not necessarily reflect intrapulmonary shunt. This measurement then is of use at the bedside for a quick estimate but should not be relied on as an accurate measurement of shunt. Table 4–20 explains how to calculate A–a gradient.

a/A Ratio and Pa$_{O_2}$/F$_{IO_2}$ Ratio

Like a–A gradient, arterial/Alveolar (a/A) and Pa$_{O_2}$/F$_{IO_2}$ ratio are simple equations that can indicate the presence of intrapul-monary shunt, $\dot{V}/\dot{Q}$ mismatch, or a diffusion abnormality. These two measurements are more accurate estimates of intrapulmonary shunt than A–a gradient because they are more sensitive to changes in oxygen concentration.

The a/A ratio is a commonly used measurement. It is a simple calculation, but requires calculation of P_{AO_2} first. The equation takes into consideration changes in F_{IO_2} and Pa_{CO_2}. The a/A ratio is the preferred shunt estimate when the patient's Pa_{CO_2} is unstable. Table 4–21 summarizes how to derive the a/A ratio. Pa$_{O_2}$/F$_{IO_2}$ ratio is the simplest way to estimate intrapulmonary shunt. It is best used when the patient's Pa_{CO_2} is stable because it is not sensitive to changes in that value. Table 4–22 provides a summary on calculating Pa$_{O_2}$/F$_{IO_2}$ ratio.

In summary, a variety of respiratory calculations can assist the nurse in determining the oxygenation status of a patient. Several equations were presented that help estimate the degree of intrapulmonary shunt (e.g., A–a gradient, a/A ratio, and Pa$_{O_2}$/F$_{IO_2}$ ratio).

TABLE 4–21 a/A Ratio

EQUATION[a]	$\dfrac{Pa_{O_2}}{P_{A_{O_2}}}$
Components	Pa_{O_2} = partial pressure of arterial oxygen
	$P_{A_{O_2}}$ = partial pressure of alveolar oxygen (derived from ideal alveolar gas equation)
Normal values	> 0.60—no supplemental oxygen is needed
	< 0.60—shunt is becoming worse
	An inverse relationship is present: as the a/A ratio value drops, intrapulmonary shunt worsens
Example	A patient's $P_{A_{O_2}}$ is currently 350 mm Hg. His Pa_{O_2} is 88 mm Hg.
	$\dfrac{88}{350} = 0.25$
	A significant intrapulmonary shunt is present.

[a]This formula is best used when Pa_{CO_2} is not stable.
Data from Chang, D. W. (1998). Respiratory care calculations, (2nd ed.) Albany, NY: Delmar Publishing.

TABLE 4–22 Pa_{O_2}/F_{IO_2} Ratio

EQUATION[a]	$\dfrac{Pa_{O_2}}{F_{IO_2}}$
Components	Pa_{O_2} = partial pressure of arterial oxygen (mm Hg)
	F_{IO_2} = fraction of inspired oxygen (O_2 concentration) (decimal)
Normal values	> 350
	Minimum clinically acceptable level = 286
	Inverse relationship: The lower the ratio value drops below normal, the more intrapulmonary shunt worsens
Example	A patient has a Pa_{O_2} of 92 mm Hg on a F_{IO_2} of 0.60
	$\dfrac{92}{0.60} = 153$
	This is below the minimum acceptable level.

[a]This formula is best used when Pa_{CO_2} is stable.

SECTION TEN REVIEW

Juan M, 30 years old, is admitted in respiratory distress. His arterial blood gases are as follows: pH 7.32, Pa_{CO_2} 50 mm Hg, Pa_{O_2} 79 mm Hg. The barometric pressure is 750 mm Hg. He is currently breathing oxygen at 0.28 F_{IO_2}.

1. Based on the data available regarding Juan, what is his $P_{A_{O_2}}$?

2. If Juan's $P_{A_{O_2}}$ is 100 mm Hg and his Pa_{O_2} is 80 mm Hg, what would his A–a gradient be?

   Answer:
   Significance:

3. Given that Juan's $P_{A_{O_2}}$ is 110 mm Hg and his Pa_{O_2} is 80 mm Hg, what is his a/A ratio?

   Answer:
   Significance:

4. Juan's status has changed. The nurse performs two sequential calculations of his a/A ratio, 1 hour apart. The first is 0.58 and the second is 0.56. What is the significance of this change?

   Significance:

5. The nurse is considering calculating Juan's shunt by using the Pa_{O_2}/F_{IO_2} ratio. This calculation is best used when
   A. Pa_{CO_2} is unstable
   B. Pa_{O_2} is unstable
   C. Pa_{CO_2} is stable
   D. Pa_{O_2} is stable

Answers: 1. 134.34 mm Hg; 2. 20 mm Hg, significance: abnormally high A–a gradient; 3. 0.73, significance: greater than 0.60 suggests no significant shunt; 4. shunt is worsening; 5. C

POSTTEST

The following Posttest is constructed in a case study format. A patient is presented, and questions are asked based on available data. New data are presented as the case study progresses.

James Smith is a 55-year-old construction worker. He is active and considers himself fairly healthy. He has a history of smoking one pack of cigarettes per day for 35 years.

1. When Mr. Smith inhales, air moves into his lungs because
   A. intrapulmonary pressure has dropped below atmospheric pressure
   B. intrapleural pressure has dropped below atmospheric pressure

C. intrapulmonary pressure has risen above atmospheric pressure

D. intrapleural pressure has risen above atmospheric pressure

2. If his surfactant production would cease, how would it affect the alveoli?
A. alveoli would hyperinflate
B. alveoli would be destroyed
C. alveoli would collapse
D. alveoli would have decreased surface tension

3. Should Mr. Smith develop a pulmonary problem that decreases his lung compliance, it would
A. increase his tidal volume
B. increase his work of breathing
C. decrease his oxygen consumption
D. decrease his carbon dioxide level

Mr. Smith becomes ill. He develops a cough and fever and is producing greenish sputum. He is diagnosed as having right middle lobe pneumonia. He also has an underlying chronic obstructive pulmonary disorder.

4. His pneumonia can affect pulmonary diffusion by increasing membrane thickness as a result of
A. atelectasis
B. inflammation
C. bronchial secretions
D. surfactant deficiency

5. Ventilation will decrease in his affected lung area because
A. pressure gradient is increased
B. gas moves from low-pressure to high-pressure areas
C. decreased perfusion causes decreased ventilation
D. gas follows the path of least resistance

6. Mr. Smith has a low $\dot{V}/\dot{Q}$ ratio. This means that there is
A. decreased ventilation in relation to perfusion
B. increased ventilation with decreased perfusion
C. decreased ventilation with decreased perfusion
D. increased ventilation in relation to perfusion

7. Mr. Smith has developed a pulmonary shunt of 20 percent. As a result, one would anticipate which type of clinical manifestations?
A. hypercarbia
B. infection
C. hypoxemia
D. pleuritis

Mr. Smith's shunt is a capillary shunt. Oxygen therapy has been initiated per Venti-mask.

8. Considering his type of shunt, the nurse can anticipate that his hypoxemia will
A. remain the same
B. worsen
C. be relieved
D. initially improve and then worsen

Mr. Smith has pulmonary mechanics tests performed. Both his tidal volume and vital capacity are below normal.

9. Inadequate volumes of tidal volume and vital capacity most likely indicate
A. respiratory muscle fatigue
B. increased atelectasis
C. loss of pulmonary surfactant
D. worsening of his pneumonia

10. If Mr. Smith develops heart failure secondary to cor pulmonale, he will most likely experience
A. pulmonary edema
B. left ventricular enlargement
C. low blood pressure
D. dependent edema

11. Based on Mr. Smith's diagnosis of cor pulmonale, the nurse can anticipate that his pulmonary vascular resistance (PVR) will be
A. low
B. unchanged
C. high
D. vacillating

12. Pulmonary vascular resistance (PVR) increases in response to
A. hypercapnia
B. alkalosis
C. hypoxemia
D. low lung volumes

[end of Mr. Smith scenario]

Una W, a 21-year-old college student, is admitted to the hospital with complaints of severe chest pain and dyspnea. She has an oral temperature of 101°F.

13. When a pulmonary disorder is suspected, obtaining a nutritional history is important for which reason?
A. hypoglycemia weakens respiratory muscles
B. high-carbohydrate diets decrease carbon dioxide levels
C. high-fat intake decreases respiratory rate and depth
D. poor nutritional status increases susceptibility to infection

14. Una continues to complain of feeling dyspneic. The nurse will need to monitor her closely for other major indicators of respiratory fatigue including (choose all that apply)
1. heart rate of 100
2. respiratory rate greater than 30/min
3. shallow respirations
4. use of accessory muscles
A. 2, 3, and 4
B. 1, 2, and 3
C. 2 and 4
D. 1, 3, and 4

The nurse has noted the following acute changes in Una's condition: increased restlessness and confusion, respiratory rate 32/min and shallow, increased use of accessory muscles, increased blood pressure and heart rate.

15. Based only on these changes in Una's status, the nurse would hypothesize that Una is most likely experiencing
    A. a pneumothorax
    B. pneumonia
    C. a pulmonary embolus
    D. an acute alteration in respiratory function

While receiving oxygen at an FIO_2 of 0.40, Una has two ABGs drawn, 1 hour apart. (Assume that barometric pressure is 750 mm Hg.) The results are

1. 10:00 A.M.: pH 7.47, $PaCO_2$ 34 mm Hg, PaO_2 90 mm Hg
2. 11:00 A.M.: pH 7.49, $PaCO_2$ 32 mm Hg, PaO_2 86 mm Hg

16. The nurse calculates Una's $P[a/A]O_2$ ratios based on ABGs 1 and 2. (fill in the blanks)
    A. a/A ratio on 1 ABG is _____
    B. a/A ratio on 2 ABG is _____
17. Based on the $P[a/A]O_2$ ratios calculated in question 16, what can be stated regarding the degree of shunt? (short answer)

[end of Una scenario]

Juanita M, 32 years old, was admitted to the hospital last night with a diagnosis of pneumonia. She is receiving oxygen and mist through an aerosol face tent.

18. Juanita's febrile state would cause the oxyhemoglobin dissociation curve to shift away from the normal curve. Based on the direction of the shift associated with fever, which statement is correct?
    A. oxygen binds rapidly to hemoglobin
    B. carbon dioxide binds rapidly to hemoglobin
    C. hemoglobin readily releases its oxygen to tissues
    D. hemoglobin is prevented from releasing its oxygen to tissues
19. Juanita has another arterial blood gas drawn. The nurse makes the following comment regarding the results: "The pH is abnormal, but the body buffers and regulatory mechanisms have begun to respond to the imbalance." This statement describes which level of acid–base compensation?
    A. uncompensated
    B. partially compensated
    C. compensated
    D. corrected
20. Juanita's normal bicarbonate–carbon dioxide ratio should remain at approximately
    A. 5:1
    B. 10:1
    C. 15:1
    D. 20:1
21. On the original arterial blood gas, Juanita's base excess (BE) was +1.5. Which statement is correct regarding base excess?
    A. it reflects only her metabolic status
    B. any value that is outside a BE of ±1 is abnormal
    C. it reflects only her respiratory status
    D. any value that is outside a BE of ±2.5 is abnormal

Juanita has a complete blood count (CBC) and ABG drawn. Her Hgb is currently 10 g/dL. Her latest temperature was 102.4°F (39.1°C). The ABG has the following results: pH 7.47, $PaCO_2$ 32 mm Hg, HCO_3 25 mEq/L, BE ±1.5, PaO_2 74 mm Hg, SaO_2 89 percent. She is started on 40 percent oxygen.

22. If Juanita has normal gas exchange, her predicted response to initiation of 40 percent oxygen therapy would be an increased PaO_2 to about
    A. 100 mm Hg
    B. 150 mm Hg
    C. 200 mm Hg
    D. 250 mm Hg
23. The underlying problem associated with Juanita's acid–base status is
    A. pulmonary edema
    B. alveolar hyperventilation
    C. atelectasis
    D. alveolar hypoventilation
24. Juanita's body is beginning to compensate for her $PaCO_2$ of 32 mm Hg. The predicted compensation for her respiratory situation is
    A. increased $PaCO_2$
    B. increased HCO_3
    C. decreased $PaCO_2$
    D. decreased HCO_3

[end of Juanita scenario]

Thomas J, a 46-year-old type I diabetic, is admitted to the hospital with a serum glucose of 650 mg/dL and positive serum ketones. He is diagnosed with DKA. He has blood gases drawn with the following results: pH 7.25, $PaCO_2$ 36 mm Hg, HCO_3 14 mEq/L.

25. Thomas's current pH is most likely due to
    A. accumulating ketones
    B. lactic acidosis
    C. severe diarrhea
    D. severe hyperglycemia
26. If Thomas's acid–base status becomes fully compensated, the nurse would anticipate seeing which acid–base trends?
    A. normal range of pH, normal HCO_3
    B. elevated pH, low HCO_3
    C. low pH, high $PaCO_2$
    D. normal range of pH, low $PaCO_2$
27. The nurse would correctly interpret Thomas's arterial blood gas as
    A. acute metabolic acidosis
    B. partially compensated metabolic acidosis
    C. compensated metabolic acidosis
    D. corrected metabolic acidosis

[end of Thomas scenario]

28. Joshua K has the following arterial blood gas results: pH 7.50, $PaCO_2$ 30 mm Hg, HCO_3, 20 mEq/L, PaO_2

88 mm Hg, Sa_{O_2} 98%. The nurse would correctly interpret this ABG as

- **A.** compensated metabolic alkalosis
- **B.** partially compensated metabolic acidosis
- **C.** partially compensated respiratory alkalosis
- **D.** compensated respiratory acidosis

29. Carrie D has the following ABG results: pH 6.83, Pa_{CO_2} 50 mm Hg, HCO_3, 20 mEq/L. The nurse would correctly conclude that these results are

- **A.** suspicious of a mixed disorder
- **B.** typical of acute metabolic acidosis
- **C.** an impossible combination
- **D.** within ordinary compensatory boundaries

30. The nurse believes that Wendell Q has a mixed acid–base disorder. When this type of acid–base disorder is suspected, it is crucial that the clinician obtain a

- **A.** computer analysis
- **B.** second sample of arterial blood
- **C.** mixed venous blood sample
- **D.** summary of the patient's medical status

31. Adam D is in hypovolemic shock secondary to a massive gastrointestinal bleed. The nurse is preparing to place him on pulse oximetry. Based on the provided data, the best location for the pulse oximetry sensor would be a (an)

- **A.** toe
- **B.** earlobe
- **C.** fingertip
- **D.** forearm

32. Beverly P has been in a critical care unit for a week. She has Pet_{CO_2} monitoring attached to her mechanical ventilator circuit. This type of monitoring is primarily used to assess

- **A.** early tissue metabolic changes
- **A.** oxygenation failure
- **C.** early changes in ventilation
- **D.** ventilator dependency

POSTTEST ANSWERS

Question	Answer	Section	Question	Answer	Section
1	A	One	17	Shunt is worsening	Ten
2	C	One	18	C	Two
3	B	One	19	B	Four
4	B	Two	20	D	Four
5	D	Two	21	A	Four
6	A	Three	22	C	Four
7	C	Three	23	B	Four
8	B	Three	24	D	Four
9	A	Six	25	A	Four
10	D	Three	26	D	Four
11	C	Three	27	A	Seven
12	C	Three	28	C	Seven
13	D	Five	29	A	Eight
14	A	Five	30	D	Eight
15	D	Five	31	B	Nine
16	A. 0.38; B. 0.36	Ten	32	C	Nine

REFERENCES

Ahrens, T., & Rutherford, K. (1993). *Essentials of oxygenation.* Boston: Jones & Bartlett.

Anderson, C. T., & Breen, P. H. (2000). Carbon dioxide kinetics and capnography during critical care. *Critical Care, 4,* 207–215.

Beers, M. H., & Berkow, R. (Eds.). (2004). Aging and the lungs (pp. 753–757). *The Merck manual of geriatrics.* Available at: *www.merck.com/mrkshared/mm_geriatrics/sec10/ch75.jsp#ind10-075-4966.* Accessed May 19, 2004.

Chang, D. W. (1998). *Respiratory care calculations* (2nd ed.). Albany, NY: Delmar Publishers.

Des Jardins, T. R. (2002). *Cardiopulmonary anatomy & physiology: Essentials for respiratory care* (4th ed.). Albany, NY: Delmar Publishers.

Kee, J. L. (2002). *Laboratory and diagnostic tests with nursing implications* (6th ed.). Upper Saddle River, NJ: Prentice Hall.

Martini, F. H., & Bartholomew, E. F. (2003). *Essentials of anatomy & physiology* (3rd ed.). Upper Saddle River, NJ: Prentice Hall Pearson Education.

Pilbeam, S. P. (1998). *Mechanical ventilation: Physiological and clinical applications* (3rd ed.). St. Louis: C.V. Mosby.

Ross, B. K. (n.d.). Aging and the respiratory system. American Society of Anesthesiologists. Available at: *www.asahq.org/clinical/geriatrics/aging.htm.* Accessed May 19, 2004.

Alterations in Pulmonary Gas Exchange

Kathleen Dorman Wagner

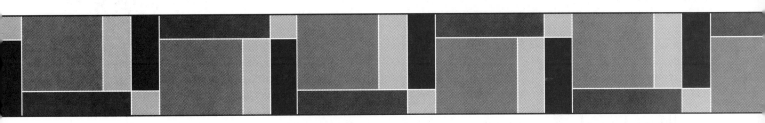

OBJECTIVES Following completion of this module, the learner will be able to

1. Explain the basic difference between restrictive and obstructive pulmonary diseases.

2. Discuss the pathophysiologic basis of respiratory failure.

3. Describe acute lung injury (ALI)/acute respiratory distress syndrome (ARDS).

4. Explain acute pulmonary embolism.

5. Explain severe acute respiratory syndrome (SARS).

6. Describe the principles and management of chest drainage.

7. Develop a plan of care for a patient with altered respiratory function.

This module focuses on pulmonary disorders of interest to the high-acuity patient population. The module is composed of seven sections. Section One differentiates pulmonary diseases on the basis of restrictive versus obstructive processes. Section Two describes the pathophysiologic basis of acute respiratory failure. Section Three provides an in-depth discussion of acute lung injury (ALI)/acute respiratory distress syndrome (ARDS). Section Four discusses acute pulmonary embolism, with a particular emphasis on thromboembolism. Section Five presents information on severe acute respiratory syndrome (SARS), including clinical features and

management. Section Six provides an overview of the management of the patient who requires a chest tube. Finally, Section Seven describes respiratory-focused nursing diagnoses and how they apply to patients with restrictive and obstructive pulmonary disorders. Each section includes a set of review questions to help the learner evaluate his or her understanding of the section's content before moving on to the next section. All Section Reviews and the module Pretest and Posttest include answers. It is suggested that the learner review those concepts answered incorrectly in the review questions before proceeding to the next section.

PRETEST

1. The primary ventilatory problem associated with obstructive pulmonary disease is
   A. delay of airflow out of the lungs
   B. obstruction to perfusion
   C. decreased diffusion of gases
   D. inability to achieve normal tidal volumes

2. Restrictive pulmonary diseases are associated with
   A. increased lung expansion
   B. increased lung compliance

   C. decreased lung expansion
   D. decreased airflow into lungs

3. Lung compliance is increased with which disorder?
   A. chest burns
   B. pneumonia
   C. pneumothorax
   D. emphysema

4. The nurse would expect a person who has respiratory insufficiency to have which of the following blood gas conditions?
   A. pH below normal
   B. Pa_{CO_2} below normal
   C. pH normal
   D. Pa_{CO_2} normal

5. Classic symptoms associated with hypercapnia would include
   A. weak, thready pulse
   B. flushed, wet skin
   C. hypotension
   D. slow, shallow breathing

6. The most common indirect predisposing disorder of ALI/ARDS is:
   A. sepsis
   B. severe trauma
   C. gastric aspiration
   D. pneumonia

7. The pulmonary edema associated with ALI/ARDS is caused by
   A. capillary microembolism
   B. left ventricular failure
   C. loss of surfactant
   D. injured alveolar–capillary membrane

8. Which clinical finding is typically present with ALI/ARDS?
   A. decreased Pa_{O_2}/F_{IO_2} ratio
   B. increased lung compliance
   C. decreased airway resistance
   D. increased functional residual capacity

9. Which type of embolism manifests itself as dyspnea, tachypnea, neurological symptoms, AND petechiae?
   A. venous air
   B. fat
   C. thrombus
   D. amniotic

10. Venous (endothelial) injury is one of three major factors that causes formation of deep vein thrombosis. This type of injury can result from
    A. immobility
    B. sepsis
    C. surgery
    D. varicose veins

11. The definitive test to diagnose a pulmonary embolism is
    A. angiography
    B. $\dot{V}/\dot{Q}$ scan
    C. D-dimer
    D. compression ultrasound

12. The pathogen that causes SARS is a unique form of which virus?
    A. hantavirus
    B. coronavirus
    C. rhinovirus
    D. influenza-A virus

13. Which statement is correct regarding the clinical features of the SARS virus?
    A. a persistent dry cough is present
    B. the chest radiograph is usually normal
    C. the patient has been experiencing hemoptysis
    D. the incubation period is 10 days to 2 weeks

14. The SARS virus is known to be transmitted by
    A. contaminated feces
    B. blood contact
    C. tears
    D. airborne droplet

15. Pneumothorax caused by positive end expiratory pressure (PEEP) represents which type of injury?
    A. procedural rupture
    B. chest contusion
    C. spontaneous bleb rupture
    D. barotrauma induced

16. Common clinical findings associated with pneumothorax include (choose all that apply)
    1. tachypnea
    2. bradycardia
    3. respiratory acidosis
    4. shortness of breath
    5. decreased Pa_{O_2}
    A. 1, 4, and 5
    B. 2, 3, and 4
    C. 1, 3, and 5
    D. 1 and 5

17. The purpose of the water-seal chamber in a three-chamber chest drainage system is to
    A. facilitate drainage from the chest tube
    B. prevent airflow back into the patient
    C. facilitate control of level of negative suction
    D. prevent fluid from draining into the suction chamber

18. Nursing interventions that would assist in maintaining effective airway clearance would include
    A. restrict fluids to 1 L/day
    B. cough and deep breathe every 1 to 2 hours
    C. minimize use of opioid analgesics
    D. restrict activities

Pretest Answers: 1. A, 2. C, 3. D, 4. C, 5. B, 6. A, 7. D, 8. A, 9. B, 10. C, 11. A, 12. B, 13. A, 14. D, 15. D, 16. A, 17. B, 18. B

GLOSSARY

acute lung injury (ALI)/acute respiratory distress syndrome (ARDS) ALI and ARDS are "syndromes with a spectrum of increas-ing severity of lung injury defined by physiologic and radiographic criteria in which widespread damage to cells and structures of the alveolar capillary membrane occurs within hours to days of a predisposing insult" (Matthay et al., 2003, p. 1027).

acute respiratory distress syndrome (ARDS)   ARDS is "a devastating, often fatal, inflammatory disease of the lung characterized by the sudden onset of pulmonary edema and respiratory failure, usually in the setting of other acute medical conditions resulting from local (e.g., pneumonia) or distant (e.g., multiple trauma) injury" (ARDS Network, nd).

bleb   A type of cyst (or blister) of gas that develops in the visceral pleura of the lung.

chronic bronchitis   A chronic obstructive pulmonary disease of the larger airways that is defined clinically as the presence of chronic productive cough that occurs daily for at least 3 months per year for at least 2 years in succession.

chronic obstructive pulmonary disease (COPD)   (chronic airflow limitation disease). A group of pulmonary diseases that cause obstruction to expiratory airflow.

CO_2 narcosis   A state of hypercapnic encephalopathy caused by toxic levels of $PaCO_2$ that produces drowsiness, stupor, or coma.

compliance (C_L)   Measurement of the relative ease with which the lungs accept a volume of air; reflects relative stiffness of lungs.

cor pulmonale   Right ventricular hypertrophy and dilation secondary to pulmonary disease.

emphysema   A pathologic pulmonary process characterized by enlargement of alveoli and destruction of alveoli and surrounding capillary beds.

empyema   Abnormal accumulation of purulent fluid in the intrapleural space as a result of inflammation or infection.

forced expiratory volume (FEV)   Measure of how rapidly a person can forcefully exhale air after a maximal inhalation; a measurement of dynamic lung function.

hemopneumothorax   Abnormal accumulation of air and blood in the intrapleural space.

hemothorax   Abnormal accumulation of blood in the intrapleural space.

obstructive pulmonary disorders   Pulmonary disorders that are associated with decreased or delayed airflow during expiration.

oxygenation failure   A respiratory crisis in which the primary problem is one of hypoxemia; clinically, it is defined as a PaO_2 of less than 60 mm Hg.

pleural effusion   Abnormal accumulation of fluid in the intrapleural space.

pneumothorax   Abnormal accumulation of air in the intrapleural space.

pulmonary embolism   Blockage of a pulmonary vessel caused by lodging of a thromboembolism or other blood borne material.

respiratory failure   A state of pulmonary decompensation in which the body is no longer able to maintain normal gas exchange; it can be expressed as PaO_2 less than 60 mm Hg or $PaCO_2$ greater than 50 mm Hg at pH less than 7.30.

respiratory insufficiency   A state of pulmonary compensation in which a normal blood pH is maintained only at the expense of the cardiopulmonary system.

restrictive disorders   Pulmonary disorders associated with a decrease in lung volume.

sepsis   A pathologic state in which microorganisms, or their toxins, are present in the bloodstream.

severe acute respiratory syndrome (SARS)   An atypical pneumonia caused by a novel form of coronavirus called SARS-CoV.

surfactant   A lipoprotein produced by type II alveolar cells that reduces the surface tension of the alveolar fluid lining.

tidal volume (TV or V_T)   The amount of air that moves in and out of the lungs with each normal breath.

total lung capacity (TLC)   The amount of gas present in the lungs after maximal inspiration.

ventilatory failure   A condition caused by alveolar hypoventilation; clinically, it is called acute respiratory acidosis.

$\dot{V}/\dot{Q}$ ratio   A ratio expressing the relationship of ventilation to perfusion.

ABBREVIATIONS

ABG	Arterial blood gas
ALI/ARDS	Acute lung injury/acute respiratory distress syndrome
ARDS	Acute respiratory distress syndrome
C_L	Lung compliance, expressed in cm H_2O/mL
COPD	Chronic obstructive pulmonary disease
FEV	Forced expiratory volume
IPPB	Intermittent positive pressure breathing
NANDA	North American Nursing Diagnosis Association
$PaCO_2$	Specifies arterial carbon dioxide tension
PaO_2.	Specifies arterial oxygen tension
PE	Pulmonary embolism, pulmonary embolus
PEEP	Positive end expiratory pressure
SARS	Severe acute respiratory syndrome
VAE	Venous air embolism
$\dot{V}/\dot{Q}$ ratio	Ventilation–perfusion ratio

SECTION ONE: A Review of Restrictive and Obstructive Pulmonary Disorders

At the completion of this section, the learner will be able to explain the basic differences between restrictive and obstructive pulmonary diseases.

Pulmonary diseases may be divided into acute and chronic problems. Acute problems have a rapid onset, are episodic, and frequently are confined to the lungs. In contrast, chronic problems usually have a slow, often insidious onset, and the pulmonary impairment either does not change or slowly worsens over an extended period. Chronic pulmonary problems generally involve other organs as part of the disease process. Patients with chronic pulmonary problems, such as emphysema, may develop an acute problem (e.g., pneumonia) that may further stress their pulmonary status.

Pulmonary diseases may be divided further into problems of inflow of air (restrictive) and problems of outflow of air (obstructive). By being able to differentiate between obstructive and restrictive pulmonary diseases, the nurse can apply appropriate nursing diagnoses regardless of the medical diagnosis of the specific pulmonary disease process.

Restrictive Pulmonary Disorders

Restrictive disorders are associated with decreased lung compliance (CL) and decreased lung expansion. They may be caused by internal problems, such as a decrease in the number of functioning alveoli (e.g., atelectasis or pneumonia) or lung tissue loss (e.g., pneumonectomy or lung tumors), or by external problems (e.g., chest burns or morbid obesity). Table 5–1 provides a more complete listing of restrictive disorders.

Restrictive disorders are problems of volume (the amount of air measured in mL or L that flows in and out of the lungs) rather than airflow (the rate or speed at which air moves into or out of the lungs). In other words, the volume of air that is inhaled can be exhaled at a normal rate of flow. The patient with a restrictive disorder will have a reduced **tidal volume** and **total lung capacity (TLC).** Air cannot move into the alveoli as readily as it should because of limited expansion (decreased lung compliance), which can lead to alveolar hypoventilation. Hypoxemia will result if alveolar oxygen diffuses into the blood at a faster rate than it is replaced by ventilation. When this occurs, the PaO_2 falls at approximately the same rate as the $PaCO_2$ rises, assuming that diffusion is normal.

Restrictive pulmonary problems often disturb the relationship of ventilation to perfusion ($\dot{V}/\dot{Q}$ ratio). In mild-to-moderate restrictive disease, the $\dot{V}/\dot{Q}$ ratio may stay normal because both ventilation and perfusion may be fairly equally disturbed. In many acute restrictive diseases, perfusion becomes diminished because of edema that results from an inflammatory process. Perfusion can also become reduced by compression or blockage of the pulmonary vasculature. In severe disease, a low $\dot{V}/\dot{Q}$ ratio may develop because ventilation is greatly diminished, whereas perfusion may be fairly normal or moderately disturbed. A low $\dot{V}/\dot{Q}$ ratio is associated with hypoxemia with a decreasing pH and increasing $PaCO_2$. Table 5–2 lists the typical signs and symptoms associated with restrictive pulmonary disorders.

Obstructive Pulmonary Disorders

Chronic obstructive pulmonary disease (COPD) is the term commonly applied in the clinical setting to pulmonary disorders that hinder expiratory airflow. The more accurate and preferred term for these disorders, however, is *chronic airflow limitation.* Currently, these two terms are often used interchangeably. Some of the major obstructive disorders include

- **Emphysema**
- **Chronic bronchitis**
- Asthma
- Cystic fibrosis

Asthma differs from the other diseases in that airflow obstruction is episodic rather than continuous.

In **obstructive pulmonary disorders,** air is able to flow into the lungs but then becomes trapped, making it difficult to rid

TABLE 5–1 Common Restrictive Pulmonary Disorders

EXTERNAL PROBLEMS	INTERNAL (PARENCHYMAL) PROBLEMS
Obesity	Pneumonia
Extensive chest burns	Atelectasis
Flail chest	Congestive heart failure
Neuromuscular diseases	Pulmonary edema
Myasthenia gravis	Pulmonary fibrosis
Muscular dystrophy	Pulmonary tumors
Guillain–Barré syndrome	Pneumothorax
Spinal cord trauma	

TABLE 5–2 Signs and Symptoms of Restrictive Pulmonary Disorders

Increased respiratory rate
Decreased tidal volume (TV)
Normal to decreased PaO_2
Shortness of breath
Cough
Chest pain or discomfort
Fatigue
History of weight loss

the lungs of the inhaled air. The inability to exhale rapidly causes a prolongation of expiratory time. If expiratory time becomes significantly prolonged, the alveoli are unable to empty before the person inhales again, trapping CO_2 within them. Expiratory times are measured using **forced expiratory volume (FEV)** testing (see Module 4).

Obstructive problems may be caused by airway narrowing, such as bronchospasm and bronchoconstriction; or by airway obstruction, such as is seen with pooling of secretions or destruction of bronchioles and alveoli. Obstructive disorders are associated with increased lung **compliance** (hyperinflated lungs) accompanied by a loss of elastic recoil. The $\dot{V}/\dot{Q}$ ratio also may be disturbed with this group of disorders. In disease processes that do not destroy alveoli (e.g., chronic bronchitis), a low $\dot{V}/\dot{Q}$ ratio may exist (i.e., ventilation is reduced, whereas perfusion remains normal). If lung tissue is actually destroyed (e.g., emphysema), the $\dot{V}/\dot{Q}$ ratio may remain normal because both ventilation and perfusion are equally impaired. A normal $\dot{V}/\dot{Q}$ ratio does not necessarily indicate healthy lungs. It indicates only that a balance exists between ventilation and blood flow. Table 5–3 lists the typical clinical manifestations associated with obstructive pulmonary disorders.

In summary, restrictive diseases are those that interfere with lung expansion. They cause a decrease in lung volumes while expiratory airflow remains normal. They are associated with decreased lung compliance. Restrictive diseases can be measured by pulmonary function tests, particularly TLC. Obstructive diseases are those that interfere with expiratory air-flow. Airflow is reduced or delayed, whereas lung volume remains normal. Obstructive diseases are associated with increased lung compliance and air trapping. They can be evaluated by measuring FEV flow rates. Table 5–4 compares these two disease processes.

TABLE 5–4   Comparison of Restrictive and Obstructive Pulmonary Diseases

RESTRICTIVE DISORDERS	OBSTRUCTIVE DISORDERS
Characteristics	
Decreased lung expansion	Increased lung expansion
Decreased lung compliance	Increased lung compliance
Normal airflow	Decreased expiratory airflow; prolonged expiratory time
Pulmonary Function Testing	
Decreased TLC	Decreased FEVs
Decreased tidal volume	
Pathologic Disturbances	
Internal Problems	
Decreased functioning alveoli	Bronchoconstriction
Loss of pulmonary tissue	Bronchospasm
	Airway obstruction
	Airway collapse
	Pooling of copious secretions
External Problems	
Disorders that decrease lung compliance external to the lungs	
Associated Blood Gas Disturbances	
Decreased Pa_{O_2}	Increased Pa_{CO_2}
Normal to low $\dot{V}/\dot{Q}$ ratio	Decreased pH (if not compensated)
Increased intrapulmonary shunt	Normal to decreased Pa_{O_2} (may stay stable until severe disease state)
Increased Pa_{CO_2} and decreased pH if ventilatory pump failure is present	
Associated Lung Sounds	
Crackles (most common)	Wheezes (most common)
Rhonchi, if secretions build up in large airways	Rhonchi, if secretions build up in large airways
	Crackles (particularly associated with cor pulmonale)

TABLE 5–3   Clinical Manifestations of Obstructive Pulmonary Disorders

Mucus hypersecretion (except with pure emphysema)
Wheezes, rhonchi
Dyspnea (episodic or progressive)
Diminished breath and heart sounds
Barrel chest (increased AP diameter)
Progressive hypercapnia and respiratory acidosis
Progressive or episodic hypoxemia (particularly in later stages)
Cor pulmonale
Accessory muscle use
Increased expiratory time (expiration time longer than inspiration time)
PFTs: Normal to increased TLC, increased FRC, decreased FEV, decreased VC

SECTION ONE REVIEW

1. Restrictive pulmonary diseases are associated with
   A. increased lung expansion
   B. increased lung compliance
   C. decreased lung expansion
   D. decreased airflow into lungs

2. Which pulmonary disorder is considered a restrictive disease?
   A. pneumonia
   B. asthma
   C. emphysema
   D. chronic bronchitis
3. Obstructive pulmonary diseases are associated with decreased
   A. lung expansion
   B. lung compliance
   C. airflow into lungs
   D. expiratory airflow
4. An example of an obstructive pulmonary disorder is
   A. multiple sclerosis
   B. asthma
   C. tuberculosis
   D. pneumonia
5. Lung compliance is increased with which disorder?
   A. emphysema
   B. pneumonia
   C. pneumothorax
   D. chest burns
6. A patient who has cor pulmonale will have
   A. left heart dilation
   B. right heart hypertrophy
   C. pulmonary fibrosis
   D. left ventricular hyperplasia

Answers: 1. C, 2. A, 3. D, 4. B, 5. A, 6. B

SECTION TWO: Acute Respiratory Failure

At the completion of this section, the learner will be able to discuss the basis of respiratory failure.

Cardiopulmonary System

In Module 4, perfusion was divided into two circuits—pulmonary and systemic. For the purposes of this module, it is helpful to reconsider these circuits in a slightly different manner. That is, view the heart and lungs as a complex integrated cardiopulmonary system that shares volume and pressure with the rest of the systemic circulation (see Fig. 4–3, Module 4)—whatever affects one part of the system potentially affects the whole. The cardiopulmonary system is very sensitive to pressure changes within it, requiring compensatory adjustments to maintain homeostasis. Primary problems of cardiac origin can create secondary pulmonary problems. For example, left heart failure can cause cardiogenic pulmonary edema. The opposite is true as well. Pulmonary problems can affect cardiac status, for example, cor pulmonale. If a pulmonary disorder decreases the ability of the lungs to maintain adequate acid–base balance and oxygenation, the patient's heart must work harder to make more blood available for diffusion, causing a compensatory increase in vital signs (increased blood pressure and pulse). The patient's lungs work harder by altering the breathing by increasing rate (tachypnea) and depth (hyperventilation).

Respiratory Insufficiency and Failure

Respiratory disorders vary greatly in the way in which they affect lung function. The amount of diffusion surface area that becomes impaired is a major factor in altering gas exchange. The extent of impairment coupled with the rate of disease onset contributes greatly to the ability of the body to cope adequately through compensatory mechanisms. The terms *chronic respiratory insufficiency* and *acute respiratory failure* are used to differentiate the level of compensation.

Chronic Respiratory Insufficiency

Respiratory insufficiency is a state in which an acceptable level of gas exchange is maintained only through cardiopulmonary compensatory mechanisms. Chronic pulmonary problems have a slow onset and often are progressive in nature. The body has time to compensate for growing pulmonary deficits, thereby maintaining an adequate level of oxygenation and acid–base balance. A person can lead a relatively normal life in a state of chronic respiratory insufficiency. Arterial blood gases typically noted when chronic respiratory insufficiency exists include a normal pH, an elevated Pa_{CO_2}, accompanied by an elevated HCO_3 (a compensated respiratory acidosis), and a normal to low Pa_{O_2}. This compensated state, however, is not normal. A person in chronic respiratory insufficiency is always in a state of impending respiratory failure. Should a new stress overtax the body's ability to meet a greater demand, the person may eventually decompensate and develop acute respiratory failure.

Acute Respiratory Failure

Respiratory failure is a life-threatening state in which the cardiopulmonary system is unable to maintain adequate gas exchange. The clinical definition and manifestations of acute respiratory failure are given in Table 5–5. Acute respiratory failure is caused by an imbalance in supply and demand. Normally, the cardiopulmonary system is able to meet the demands of the body by increasing its work to supply adequate oxygen and ridding the body of carbon dioxide. If the body's demands become higher than the cardiopulmonary system can supply, the system will fail, precipitating acute respiratory failure.

TABLE 5–5   Acute Respiratory Failure and Its Components

TYPE OF FAILURE	CLINICAL DEFINITION	CLINICAL MANIFESTATIONS
Acute respiratory failure	$Paco_2$ greater than 50 mm Hg with a pH less than 7.30 and/or Pao_2 less than 60 mm Hg	See below
Oxygenation failure	Pao_2 less than 60 mm Hg	Pulmonary: dyspnea, tachypnea, increased pulmonary vascular resistance Cardiovascular: increased blood pressure, heart rate, cardiac dysrhythmias, cyanosis; weak, thready pulse Central nervous system: altered level of responsiveness; restlessness, confusion
Ventilation failure	$Paco_2$ greater than 50 mm Hg with a pH less than 7.30 (acute respiratory acidosis)	Pulmonary: tachypnea Vascular: headache; flushed, wet skin Cardiovascular: bounding pulse, increased blood pressure and heart rate Central nervous system: anesthetic effects of carbon dioxide: lethargy, drowsiness, coma (CO_2 narcosis)

Components of Acute Respiratory Failure. The term *acute respiratory failure* is a general one that pertains to both gas exchange gases: oxygen and carbon dioxide. To better understand and clarify respiratory failure, it is helpful to break it down into its two component parts, failure of oxygenation and failure of ventilation. Sometimes, both failure components are present initially; however, more commonly, a failure of one or the other system occurs initially, causing respiratory failure. For this reason, it is important to be able to differentiate the two failure components.

Failure of Oxygenation. When a state of **oxygenation failure** exists, the primary problem is one of hypoxemia. Carbon dioxide (CO_2) is able to diffuse across the alveolar–capillary membrane approximately 20 times more rapidly than is oxygen. For this reason, CO_2 levels may remain normal when diffusion is interfered with, even though the patient is showing signs of moderate to severe hypoxemia. Conditions that can cause oxygenation failure are frequently restrictive pulmonary disorders, such as acute respiratory distress syndrome and pneumonia. Should these conditions worsen or should the patient fatigue, the ventilatory component can be initiated. Hypoxemia is accompanied by multiple compensatory mechanisms that work to regain an adequate oxygenation state. Clinically, it is important to maintain the Pao_2 at 60 mm Hg or above because of oxygen's decreased affinity to hemoglobin at a Pao_2 less than 60 mm Hg. At this crucial point, any further drop in Pao_2 will result in a large decrease in hemoglobin saturation (Sao_2). The clinical manifestations and clinical definition of oxygenation failure are presented in Table 5–5.

Failure of Ventilation. **Ventilatory failure** (acute respiratory acidosis) is caused by alveolar hypoventilation; that is, the inability to move air adequately out of the alveoli, allowing a buildup of carbon dioxide. Ventilatory failure can be caused by any problem that interferes with adequate movement of airflow (e.g., neuromuscular disorders, respiratory muscle fatigue, and COPD).

Clinical manifestations of ventilatory failure reflect hypercapnia (elevated carbon dioxide). Most of the symptoms associated with hypercapnia are the result of the strong vasodilator effect of carbon dioxide. The term **CO_2 narcosis** is sometimes used to describe ventilatory failure based on its anesthetic effects. The clinical manifestations and clinical definition of ventilatory failure are presented in Table 5–5.

Complications of Respiratory Failure. Acute respiratory failure can affect virtually all body systems by causing organ hypoxia. If the respiratory failure is coupled with decreased cardiac output, the patient is at particular risk for development of hypoperfusion/hypoxic organ shock complications, such as those seen with multiple organ dysfunction syndrome (MODS), including ALI/ARDS. The presence of hypercapnia, with its accompanying respiratory acidosis and vasodilation states, adds an additional pathophysiologic burden on the body because cellular function rapidly becomes impaired in acidotic states. In addition, the generalized vasodilatory effects can increase intracranial pressure and decrease cardiac output and systemic vascular resistance. As a general rule, ventilation failure is considered a more serious problem than oxygenation failure. Acute respiratory acidosis can quickly deteriorate to systemic acidosis, which is poorly tolerated by the body. Oxygenation failure, however, is associated with better compensatory mechanisms and, therefore, is better tolerated.

Pathogenesis of Respiratory Failure

The sequence of events that leads to the development of respiratory failure is a complicated one. It is initiated by the presence of a disease process that either directly (e.g., pneumonia) or indirectly (e.g., Guillain-Barré syndrome) interferes with normal lung function. As pulmonary function deteriorates, the patient develops $\dot{V}/\dot{Q}$ ratio abnormalities and decreasing Pao_2. The body recognizes increased oxygen demand and responds by increasing the rate and depth of respirations to move more air into and out of the alveoli (compensation). This compensatory mechanism increases the PaO$_2$ and decreases the PaCO$_2$ to regain an adequate level of oxygenation and acid–base balance. Compensatory mechanisms (including increased work of breathing) require more energy; thus, the body's metabolic rate increases. As the metabolic rate increases, more oxygen is consumed by the tissues and more carbon dioxide is produced, as an end product of metabolism. The overall effect of the sequence is a progressive increase in arterial carbon dioxide and a decrease in arterial oxygen. A state of acute respiratory failure exists when the patient meets the clinical criteria (i.e., PaCO$_2$ greater than 50 mm Hg with a pH of less than 7.30 and/or a PaO$_2$ of less than 60 mm Hg).

Should the sequence of events that precipitated the acute respiratory failure not be corrected adequately, the level of respiratory failure worsens, causing a further increase in the work of breathing. As the work of breathing increases, the patient de-

velops respiratory muscle fatigue, which can eventually lead to respiratory muscle failure and decompensation with worsening of both ventilation and oxygenation. If this sequence of events is allowed to continue, arterial blood gas concentrations steadily deteriorate, leading to death of the patient.

In summary, respiratory failure is a potential complication of respiratory insufficiency. Although respiratory insufficiency is compatible with life, respiratory failure is not, and it is considered a medical emergency. Acute respiratory failure can be divided into two components: failure to oxygenate and failure to ventilate. Although they can occur simultaneously, one is often the primary trigger. Ventilation failure is considered more serious than oxygenation failure because of the presence of respiratory acidosis, which can have severe tissue consequences. Respiratory failure can cause dysfunction of all organs as a result of tissue hypoxia, possibly leading to multiple organ dysfunction syndrome (MODS).

SECTION TWO REVIEW

1. Which arterial blood gas pH results would the nurse most commonly note with respiratory insufficiency?
   A. pH within normal limits
   B. pH above normal range
   C. pH below normal range
   D. variable pH

2. Which arterial blood gas pH results, when noted by the nurse, would be most suspicious of acute respiratory failure?
   A. normal pH
   B. pH higher than normal
   C. pH lower than normal
   D. variable pH

3. Failure to oxygenate refers to which of the following primary problems?
   A. ventilation
   B. hypoxemia
   C. arterial pH
   D. carbon dioxide

4. Which symptom, if noted by the nurse, would suggest that the patient is experiencing failure to oxygenate?
   A. bounding pulse
   B. headache

C. flushed skin
   D. restlessness

5. The primary problem associated with failure to ventilate is
   A. alveolar hypoventilation
   B. capillary hypoperfusion
   C. alveolar hyperventilation
   D. capillary hyperperfusion

6. Many of the common clinical manifestations that are typically noted in patients with ventilatory failure are primarily the result of
   A. vasoconstriction
   B. hypoxemia
   C. vasodilation
   D. acidosis

7. The result of increased metabolic demand is
   A. decreased oxygen consumption
   B. decreased carbon dioxide production
   C. increased oxygen consumption
   D. increased carbon dioxide consumption

Answers: 1. A, 2. C, 3. B, 4. D, 5. A, 6. C, 7. C

SECTION THREE: Acute Lung Injury/Acute Respiratory Distress Syndrome

At the completion of this section, the learner will be able to discuss acute lung injury and acute respiratory distress syndrome.

Adult respiratory distress syndrome (ARDS) was first described in 1967 as a respiratory failure syndrome characterized

by bilateral pulmonary filtrates (Ashbaugh et al., 1967). Until recently it was referred to as "adult" RDS to differentiate it from infant hyaline membrane disease. As the disorder became better understood, the word *adult* was replaced by *acute* to acknowledge the similarities between the adult and child versions of the disorder. Currently, **acute respiratory distress syndrome** is conceptualized as the most severe expression of **acute lung injury** (ALI); thus, it is frequently referred to as ALI/ARDS. Acute lung injury can be viewed as a continuum of severity from mild, subclinical injury at one end of the continuum to severe injury (ARDS) at the opposite end. ALI and ARDS are "syndromes with a spectrum of increasing severity of lung injury defined by physiologic and radiographic criteria in which widespread damage to cells and structures of the alveolar capillary membrane occurs within hours to days of a predisposing insult" (Matthay et al., 2003, p. 1027). The ARDS Network (n.d.) further defines ARDS as, "a devastating, often fatal, inflammatory disease of the lung characterized by the sudden onset of pulmonary edema and respiratory failure, usually in the setting of other acute medical conditions resulting from local (e.g., pneumonia) or distant (e.g., multiple trauma) injury."

Etiologic Factors

ARDS is predominantly a complication of systemic disease processes (Matthay et al., 2003). As the ARDS Network definition implies, ARDS can be precipitated by a variety of direct or indirect pulmonary injuries. Table 5–6 provides a list of some of the more common predisposing factors. Predisposing factors have one thing in common—all of them are known to trigger a systemic inflammatory response that, if sufficiently strong, may involve the lungs, leading to diffuse lung injury (Crouser & Fahy, 2003). Currently, there is no explanation as to why, in similar pathologic conditions, a few people develop ARDS when most do not. Crouser and Fahy suggest that the determination of who actually develops ARDS depends to some extent on the characteristics and severity of the primary injury, and the presence of coexisting risk factors.

> gastric aspiration and septic shock (sepsis with hypotension) are associated with a greater than 25% risk of development of ARDS, whereas use of multiple transfusions carries a risk of ARDS of less than 5%. The risk for development of ARDS also appears to be additive when multiple risk factors are present. (Crouser & Fahy, 2003, p. 539)

In addition, it is suspected that there are other, yet unknown, factors that influence who develops ARDS—some of which may be genetic (Matthay et al., 2003).

Diagnosis

Defining ARDS and differentiating it from other acute pulmonary disorders has been a difficult task since it was first described. In 1992, the American–European Consensus Conference on ARDS defined ALI/ARDS on the basis of clinical criteria (often referred to as "ARDS consensus criteria"). Using the consensus criteria, ALI is differentiated from ARDS based on the ratio of PaO_2 to FIO_2 (see Table 5–7). These criteria are still commonly used in clinically defining and diagnosing ALI/ARDS. Differentiating the pulmonary edema of ARDS from that of congestive heart failure (CHF) can be difficult because both cause pulmonary edema. It is important, however, to make this differentiation because therapy differs between the two distinct disease states. There are several criteria that assist in making a differential diagnosis:

1. **Pulmonary artery wedge pressure (PAWP).** A PAWP of 18 or greater is suggestive of CHF, whereas a PAWP of less than 18 is suggestive of ARDS.
2. **Bronchoalveolar lavage (BAL) fluid.** Bronchoalveolar fluid is obtained during a bronchoscopic examination into a lung lobe. BAL fluid present in CHF (hydrostatic pulmonary edema) is protein poor and lacks inflammatory cells, whereas BAL fluid present in ARDS pulmonary edema is protein rich and contains inflammatory cells (Crouser & Fahy, 2003).
3. **Chest radiography.** Heart enlargement is typically noted in CHF, whereas it is not typically noted in ARDS. Pulmonary infiltrates noted in CHF are typically greatest in the dependent lung fields, whereas pulmonary infiltrates noted in ARDS are more diffuse (throughout the lung fields). Pulmonary effusions may be noted in CHF, whereas they are not common in ARDS.

TABLE 5–6   Common Predisposing Disorders of ALI/ARDS

DIRECT	INDIRECT
Pneumonia[a]	Sepsis[a]
Gastric aspiration[b]	Severe traumatic injury with shock requiring massive blood transfusions[b] (Each factor alone [traumatic injury, shock, massive blood transfusions] can lead to ALI/ARDS; the combination increases the risk significantly)
Near drowning	Severe head injury
Direct severe chest contusion	Acute pancreatitis
	Drug overdose

[a]Most common predisposing disorders.
[b]Common predisposing disorders.

TABLE 5–7   1992 American–European Consensus Conference on ARDS Definition of ALI/ARDS

ARDS Consensus Criteria

Acute onset

Bilateral infiltrates on chest x-ray (frontal view)

Pulmonary artery wedge pressure (PAWP) 18 mm Hg or less and/or no left atrial hypertension (CHF)

Oxygenation status measured as PaO_2/FIO_2 ratio (regardless of PEEP level)

   ALI = 300 mm Hg or less

   ARDS = 200 mm Hg or less

There is also investigational interest in finding a serum molecular marker that measures acute lung injury similar to measuring serum CPK-MB for myocardial cell injury. Newman and colleagues (2000) studied alveolar type I cell-specific protein (HTI_{56}) as an alveolar-specific marker for alveolar type I cell damage in humans. Their results are encouraging but more extensive research is required before its usefulness can be determined.

ALI/ARDS has also been diagnosed using the Modified Lung Injury Score. The Modified Lung Injury Score clinically defines ARDS as the presence of bilateral infiltrates by chest x-ray with a decreased PaO_2/FIO_2 ratio of less than 175 mm Hg. The Modified Lung Injury Score and the American–European Consensus Conference on ARDS clinical criteria are both considered highly predictive of ARDS (Vollman & Aulbach, 1998).

Pathogenesis

ALI/ARDS is not a disease but a pattern of pathophysiological lung changes resulting in a corresponding pattern of clinical manifestations (i.e., a syndrome). It is a distinct type of acute lung injury resulting in severe respiratory failure. ALI/ARDS is caused by diffuse inflammatory injury to the alveolar–capillary membrane, resulting in disruption of both the pulmonary capillary endothelium and the alveolar epithelium. Invasion of lung tissue by neutrophils (PMNs), which activate a variety of inflammatory by-products, is believed to be central to the inflammatory response related injury. Disruption of the pulmonary capillary endothelium allows plasma proteins and fluid to escape into the pulmonary interstitial spaces. Injured alveolar epithelial linings permit fluid and plasma proteins to flood into the alveoli, resulting in nonhydrostatic pulmonary edema (Crouser & Fahy, 2003; Matthay et al., 2003). Figure 5–1 provides a graphic map of one possible explanation of the pathogenesis of this form of pulmonary edema.

The hydrostatic pulmonary edema of CHF has a different pathogenesis. Crouser and Fahy (2003) explain that, normally, hydrostatic pressure in the alveoli is greater than the pressure in the pulmonary interstitium, which protects the alveoli from abnormal inflow of interstitial fluid. In situations where left heart pressures create an elevated backup pressure into the pulmonary veins (as seen in CHF), the resulting elevated hydrostatic capillary pressure causes increased flow out of the capillaries into the interstitium because fluid passes through a semipermeable membrane (alveolar-capillary membrane) from greater pressure to lower pressure. Eventually, if interstitial pressures become sufficiently elevated, the alveoli can begin to take

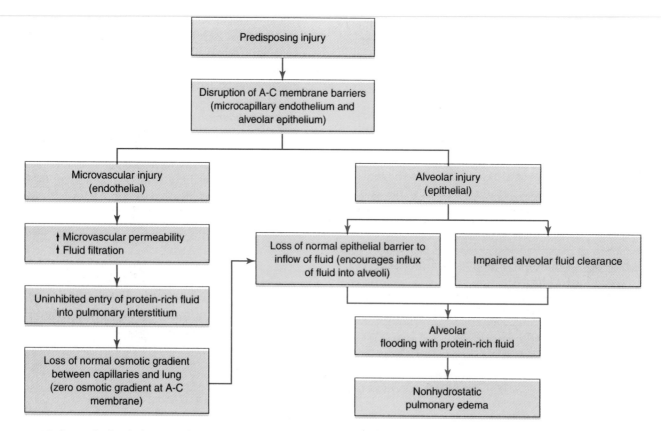

Figure 5–1 ■ Pathogenesis of nonhydrostatic pulmonary edema. This simplified diagram illustrates one explanation of the origin of nonhydrostatic (noncardiogenic) pulmonary edema noted in ARDS. A major function of the alveolar epithelium (type I pneumocytes) is as a selective barrier to fluids. Damage to these cells results in failure of the fluid barrier, allowing alveolar flooding. (Data from Crouser, E. D., & Fahy, R. J. [2003]. Acute lung injury, pulmonary edema, and multiple system organ failure. In R. L. Wilkins, J. K. Stoller, & C. L. Scanlan, *Egan's Fundamentals of Respiratory Care*, [8th ed., pp. 537–556] St. Louis: Mosby.)

in fluid as well (the mechanism for this form of alveolar flooding is not fully understood).

ARDS can be triggered either from a local (pulmonary) inflammatory problem or from a distant systemic problem (particularly sepsis or systemic inflammatory response syndrome—SIRS). ARDS is the lung's expression of this widespread inflammatory event. No matter what initial direct or indirect insult triggers the onset of ALI/ARDS, the subsequent sequence of events remains relatively predictable. Figure 5–2 provides a theoretical pathogenesis pathway of ARDS. The pathogenesis of SIRS is discussed in detail in Module 16.

Crouser and Fahy (2003) describe two phases of ARDS, the exudative phase and the fibroproliferative phase. These phases reflect the early phase of acute injury followed by a phase of lung repair. These phases are summarized in Table 5–8.

Clinical Presentation

There are two patterns of clinical presentation based on the pre-existing health state of the individual and time of ARDS diagnosis. These patterns impact prognosis and thus should be taken into consideration. Vollman and Aulbach (1998) suggest that in an otherwise healthy person onset of ALI/ARDS usually occurs rapidly, often only a few hours following the triggering insult. In persons who have chronic illnesses or comorbid pathologic

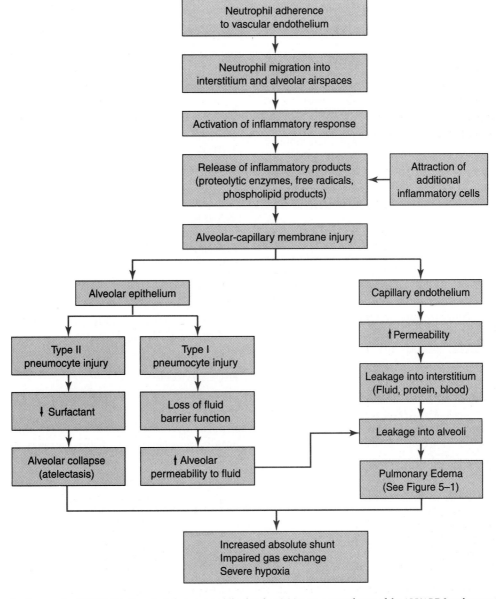

Figure 5–2 ■ Theory of pathogenesis of ARDS. It is theorized that neutrophil-related activities are a central part of the ALI/ARDS pathogenesis.
(Data from Porth, C. M. [2002]. *Pathophysiology: Concepts of altered health states,* (6th ed.), Philadelphia: J. B. Lippincott; and Carpenter, C. C. J., Griggs, R. C., & Los Calzo, J. (Ed.). [2001]. *Cecil essentials of medicine,* (5th ed.) Philadelphia: W. B. Saunders.)

TABLE 5–8   Phases of ARDS

PHASE	CHARACTERISTICS	PATHOLOGY
Exudative phase (1 to 3 days)	Diffuse microvascular injury and alveolar damage Invasion of inflammatory cells into interstitium Development of hyaline membranes [a] in alveolar spaces	Destruction of type I pneumocytes

Fibroproliferative phase (3 to 7 days)	Lung repair period
	Degree of recovery is dependent on
	  1. Severity of primary lung injury
	  2. Influence of secondary forms of injury (e.g., baro-trauma, nosocomial infection, oxygen toxicity)
		Hyperplasia of type II pneumocytes
		Proliferation of fibroblasts in basement membrane of alveoli
		  Development of intra-alveolar and interstitial fibrosis[b]
		Lung remodeling
		  Degree of lung repair is variable
		    Full repair of lung architecture
		    Return to normal compliance and gas exchange over 6- to 12-month period
		    Permanent damage to lung architecture
		Occurs if basement membrane becomes disrupted—cannot repair correctly

[a]Hyaline membranes consist of plasma proteins and cellular debris.
[b]Severity of pulmonary disability in survivors of ARDS depends on extent of fibrosis.
Data from Crouser, E. D., & Fahy, R. J. (2003). Acute lung injury, pulmonary edema, and multiple system organ failure. In R. L. Wilkins, J. K. Stoller, & C. L. Scanlan, Egan's Fundamentals of Respiratory Care, (8th ed., pp. 537–556). St. Louis: C. V. Mosby.

conditions, the presenting clinical findings are often more insidious, being initially hidden by other concurrent health problems. In the latter group, ALI/ARDS becomes apparent within 24 to 48 hours after the initial insult. Croce and colleagues (1999) noted that in posttrauma victims, there were two distinct forms of ARDS, early and late. Characteristics of early ARDS included diagnosis of ARDS within the first 48 hours of admission, the presence of hemorrhagic shock, and death most commonly from hemorrhagic shock. Characteristics of late ARDS included diagnosis after 48 hours of admission, presence of pneumonia prior to ARDS onset, multiple organ involvement, and death from complications of multiple organ dysfunction syndrome(MODS).

As ARDS progresses, cyanosis and accessory muscle use may be noted. A cough develops, frequently producing sputum that is typical of pulmonary edema. Arterial blood gas findings show a pattern of increasing hypoxemia that is refractory to increasing concentrations of oxygen. The refractory nature of the hypoxemia is largely a result of increasing capillary shunt as alveolar units collapse and become dysfunctional. Pulmonary function tests will be consistent with lung restriction, including decreased lung compliance (CL) and decreased functional residual capacity (FRC). Table 5–9 provides a summary of the typical clinical presentation of ALI/ARDS.

Treatment

Treatment of ALI/ARDS varies widely and is continuously being researched and improved. Management is a collaborative effort between medicine and nursing and requires multidisciplinary planning and interventions. Medical therapy centers on pro-

TABLE 5–9   Common Clinical Presentation of ARDS

Early Onset

Onset: Within first 24 to 48 hours postadmission

Chest radiograph: Initially normal

Increasing respiratory distress, tachypnea, and dyspnea

Initial ABGs: Respiratory alkalosis (secondary to hyperventilation); Pao_2 normal or mild hypoxemia

Late Onset

Onset: After 24 to 48 hours postadmission

Chest radiograph: May show evidence of pneumonia

Labs: Reflect multiple body system dysfunction

Rate of onset: May be insidious (related to overall poor condition)

Progressive Manifestations

Cyanosis

Cough (productive)

Increasing use of accessory muscles

ABGs: Pattern of increasing hypoxemia (refractory to oxygen therapy)

Pulmonary function tests: Increasing pulmonary restriction (e.g., decreasing lung compliance, decreasing FRC)

moting oxygenation, maintaining adequate hemodynamics, and promoting healing. Nursing plays a crucial role in the care of the ALI/ARDS patient, focusing on implementing supportive measures to maintain the patient until the alveolar–capillary membrane regains its integrity and the syndrome resolves; and monitoring the patient's status, the therapeutic and nontherapeutic effects of medical therapy; and monitoring for possible

TABLE 5–10   Supportive Care of Patients with ALI/ARDS

1. Identify and manage underlying cause of ARDS
2. Avoid secondary (iatrogenic or nosocomial) lung injury
   a. O_2 toxicity
   b. Aspiration
   c. Barotrauma, volume trauma
   d. Identify and manage nosocomial infection and pneumonia
   e. Extubate as soon as is feasible
3. Maintain adequate Do_2 to systemic organs
   a. Minimize demand by reducing metabolic rate
      (1) Control fever
      (2) Control anxiety and pain
   b. Support cardiovascular system with intravenous fluids and vasopressor agents, as necessary, to:
      (1) Prevent hypotension (SBP greater than 90 mm Hg; MAP greater than 70 mm Hg)
      (2) Reverse lactic acidosis
      (3) Maintain adequate urine output
4. Provide nutritional support

Key: Do_2: oxygen delivery; SBP: systolic blood pressure; MAP: mean arterial pressure
From Crouser, E. D., & Fahy, R. J. (2003). Acute lung injury, pulmonary edema, and multiple system organ failure. In R. L. Wilkins, J. K. Stoller, & C. L. Scanlan. Egan's Fundamentals of Respiratory Care, (8th ed., p. 546). St. Louis: C. V. Mosby.

multiple system complications. No specific therapies have been found that directly heal the lungs, thus, historically, treatment of ALI/ARDS has been primarily supportive and anticipatory in nature. The patient must have all needs met for adequate lung healing, and complications must be anticipated and either prevented or aggressively treated. Regardless of the precipitating event, the management for ALI/ARDS is similar and includes mechanical ventilation with PEEP, patient positioning strategies, drug therapy, and other interventions based on the complex nature of the disease and its detrimental effect on other body systems. Table 5–10 summarizes supportive management of ALI/ARDS.

Mechanical Ventilation and PEEP

Two mainstays of ALI/ARDS therapy have been positive pressure mechanical ventilation and positive end expiratory pressure (PEEP) to adequately overcome low lung compliance and refractory hypoxemia.

Protective Ventilation.   Until recently, high tidal volume (10 to 15 mL/kg body weight) was recommended for treatment of ALI/ARDS. Unfortunately, high tidal volumes are known to cause ventilator associated lung injury (VALI) (ARDS Network, 2000; Moloney & Griffiths, 2004). Current research suggests that using a low tidal volume (6 mL/kg body weight) with a plateau pressure of 30 cm H_2O or less significantly reduces mortality as

well as ventilator days in ALI/ARDS patients regardless of the precipitating cause (ARDS Network, 2000; Eisner et al., 2001).

Positive End Expiratory Pressure (PEEP).   A major complicating factor in ALI/ARDS is the massive collapse of alveoli, which causes a significant shunt, decreased lung compliance, and severe hypoxemia. This explains the refractory nature of ALI/ARDS to conventional oxygen therapy. Recall that atelectasis is a type of capillary shunt, which is absolute in nature. Regardless of the oxygen concentration delivered, the gas never enters into the affected alveoli for gas exchange. Until positive end expiratory pressure (PEEP) became available there was no way to force alveoli open once they had collapsed.

PEEP applies positive pressure into the patient's airway at the end of expiration such that the alveoli are prevented from closing. PEEP maintains the alveoli in an open state throughout the breathing cycle, which increases gas diffusion time, thus increasing gas exchange. PEEP also reduces shunt by recruiting collapsed alveoli (popping them open). The goal in using PEEP is to achieve an adequate PaO_2 (usually at least 60 mm Hg) while reducing the inspired oxygen concentration (FIO_2) to less than 0.6 (60 percent) because high concentrations of oxygen eventually cause oxygen toxicity. The level of desired PEEP is individually evaluated. Usually the "optimal" level is between 8 and 15 cm H_2O (Crouser & Fahy, 2003). Although PEEP has been invaluable for treatment of ALI/ARDS, it is not without hazards, including decreased cardiac output and overdistention of alveoli, among others. PEEP is further described in Module 6, "Mechanical Ventilation." Table 5–11 summarizes mechanical ventilation settings that strive to support oxygen exchange while protecting the lungs.

Alternative mechanical ventilation options may be initiated when conventional therapy has not been effective in attaining adequate gas exchange. Some of the more common alternatives include pressure control ventilation, inverse I-E ratio, and high-frequency ventilation.

Patient Positioning Strategies

There has been increasing interest in the effects of various types of patient positioning in improving patient outcomes. Two major types of therapy, continuous lateral rotation therapy and prone positioning, are briefly described here.

Continuous Lateral Rotation Therapy (CLRT).   Beds that provide CLRT (also called Kinetic Therapy™ or oscillation therapy) continuously rotate the patient's body from side to side (with brief pauses), thus shifting pressure and fluid. Martin (2001) explains that, for many years, patients on prolonged bedrest were manually turned from side to side primarily to prevent the formation of decubitus ulcers. Beginning in the 1980s, research began linking prolonged immobility with a variety of serious complications, such as pneumonia, pulmonary embolus, and deep vein thrombosis. CLRT is commonly employed in critical care units as an alternative to manual turning for the purpose of reducing stasis of fluid and gas-related complications.

TABLE 5–11   Supporting Gas Exchange and Protecting the Lungs

INTERVENTION	RATIONALE
Mechanical ventilation	These settings reduce ventilator associated lung injury (VALI)
■ Tidal volume: 5 to 10 mL/kg	■ Low tidal volumes prevent alveolar overexpansion.
■ Least PEEP: Sufficient for SaO_2 90% or higher at FiO_2 of 0.6 (60%) or less	■ Least PEEP applies minimum of pressure necessary to attain the goals. FiO_2 greater than 0.6 for more than 24 hours leads to oxygen toxicity, which worsens ARDS and lung injury.
■ Permissive hypercapnia: Maintain peak airway pressure (PAP) less than 40 to 45 cm H_2O [a]	■ Allowing some degree of hypercapnia lowers the peak airway and plateau pressures, which reduces lung trauma.
■ Mean airway pressure: 35 cm H_2O or less	■ Prevents/minimizes barotrauma.

[a]Permissive hypercapnia is contraindicated in patients with unstable intracranial pressure or hemodynamic status.
Data from Crouser, E. D., & Fahy, R. J. (2003). Acute lung injury, pulmonary edema, and multiple system organ failure. In R. L. Wilkins, J. K. Stoller, & C. L. Scanlan. Egan's Fundamentals of Respiratory Care, (8th ed., pp. 537–556). St. Louis: C. V. Mosby.

Evidence supports use of CLRT to mobilize pulmonary secretions, and reduce pulmonary complications, such as pneumonia and atelectasis, and it may decrease length of stay in ICU (Davis et al., 2001; Martin, 2001). Figure 5–3 shows an example of a CLRT bed.

Prone Position Therapy. Prone positioning ("proning") is the periodic placement of a patient in a face-down (prone) position for the purpose of increasing oxygenation while potentially reducing oxygen therapy concentration (Curley, 1999). The exact mechanism for improved oxygenation is unknown, but it is theorized that prone positioning increases the homogeneity of pulmonary blood flow (Breiburg et al., 2000), which

reduces ventilation-to-perfusion mismatch and decreases right-to-left shunt (Miller et al., 2004; Murray & Patterson, 2002). A major advantage of prone positioning is that improved oxygenation can be achieved using a noninvasive, relatively simple procedure. Evidence suggests that there is a window of opportunity in which prone positioning is therapeutic in ALI/ARDS patients, effectiveness being limited to the early phase of the disease, with up to 70 percent of patients benefiting (Gattinoni et al., 2001). Although oxygenation may improve rather dramatically, there is as yet no clear evidence that use of prone position improves survival (Gattinoni et al., 2001). Not all patients can tolerate being placed in prone position and may develop worsening oxygenation or hemodynamic instability. Proning is contraindicated in some patients, for example, those with unstable hemodynamic status, intracranial pressure, or spinal injury (Breiburg et al., 2000). Complications associated with turning patients into the prone position include possible accidental extubation or loss of venous access, and problems with monitoring or CPR.

When prone positioning is first initiated, a trial period of 2 hours may be used to watch for improvement in oxygenation. Ideally, an increased PaO_2 of 10 mm Hg or increased PaO_2/FiO_2 ratio greater than 20 percent is noted during the trial period (Curley, 1999). If no significant improvement is noted during the trial period, the patient is considered a "nonresponder" and is returned to supine position and can be retested again daily to evaluate for a possible positive response.

Drug Therapy

Pharmacologic-based treatment of ARDS has failed to significantly improve ALI/ARDS patient outcomes (Meduri et al., 1998). Currently, there are several therapies that warrant description.

Corticosteroids. The use of corticosteroids as a treatment for ALI/ARDS remains controversial and is based on the inflammatory nature of the disease pathology. Inflammation and lung injury from the by-products of inflammation are a major source of lung destruction in the ALI/ARDS pathogenesis. As the sever-

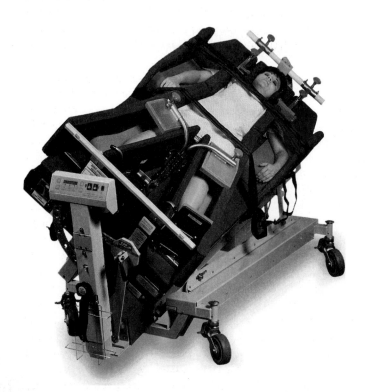

Figure 5–3 ■ RotoRest bed. A form of CLRT therapy. *(Courtesy KCI.)*

ity of pulmonary inflammation and fibrotic activities increase, patient prognosis worsens and mortality increases (Crouser & Fahy, 2003; Meduri et al., 1998). Clinical trials investigating patient outcomes following corticosteroid therapy have had promising results in reducing permanent lung damage and mortality. Research continues in this area to determine the optimal dosage level, length of treatment, and timing for initiation of corticosteroid therapy. Early research findings suggest that high dose, prolonged corticosteroid therapy (longer than 48 hours) may reduce lung injury scores and mortality when initiated before the fibroproliferative phase of ALI/ARDS begins (Crouser & Fahy, 2003; Meduri et al., 1998).

Inhaled Nitric Oxide (iNO). Nitric oxide should not be confused with nitrous oxide (N_2O, "laughing gas"), which is used for mild anesthesia. Nitric oxide, a potent vasodilator, is normally produced by the body and plays an important role in pulmonary blood flow regulation. The pathology of ALI/ARDS includes acute pulmonary hypertension as a result of pulmonary vasoconstriction in early ALI/ARDS (Gerlach et al., 1999). Inhalation of low doses of nitric oxide increases PaO_2 by redistributing pulmonary blood flow to working alveoli (Bigatello & Hellman, 2003). Research to date has not shown long-term clinical benefits from use of NO in ALI/ARDS patients. It may reduce ventilator association lung injury (VALI) by increasing PaO_2 using lower oxygen concentrations, which reduces problems with oxygen toxicity (Hite & Morris, 2001).

Surfactant Replacement Therapy. Use of surfactant therapy in treating infant distress syndrome is a well-known, highly successful therapy. Use of exogenous surfactant in adults with ALI/ARDS has not met with the same success because of the complexity of the pathology of ARDS in adults with loss of surfactant being only one part of the disease process (Crouse & Fahy, 2003). Hite and Morris (2001) maintain that one major problem with surfactant therapy is that it requires large doses for an extensive period of time, which becomes a significant product resource and cost issue. Clinical trials are ongoing to determine what role, if any, surfactant replacement therapy has in treatment of ARDS. Early studies have had mixed results, some suggesting that surfactant therapy may decrease lung injury, increase oxygenation, and possibly decrease mortality. Research continues on cost effectiveness, exogenous surfactant composition, best delivery route, and timing (Hite & Morris, 2001).

Partial Liquid Ventilation. Partial liquid ventilation is the introduction of perfluorocarbon liquid into the lungs. Perfluorocarbons are carbon-based molecules that readily dissolve oxygen and carbon dioxide. Perfluorocarbons are able to flow into the terminal airways where they enhance gas exchange, thus improving oxygenation. Partial liquid ventilation seems to be tolerated better than full liquid ventilation. Early studies have been promising, suggesting that this therapy may result in reduction of the inflammatory response and lung injury and may enhance oxygenation and improve lung mechanics (Crouser & Fahy, 2003).

Prognosis

The mortality rate associated with ARDS varies widely depending on its etiology and comorbidity factors, and ranges from estimates of about 30 percent to more than 85 percent. Until recently, the general estimate of mortality was about 50 percent regardless of advances in therapy. In general, patients who show improvement within the first week of treatment have outcomes that are more successful. Two relatively new interventions, however, have reduced the mortality rates, including low (protective) tidal volumes using mechanical ventilation, and use of activated protein C for treatment of **sepsis** (the major cause of ARDS) (Matthay et al., 2003). Mortality rates highly correlate with the severity of lung injury at 72 hours postonset (Vollman & Aulbach, 1998).

Currently, there is research interest in finding a feasible method to more effectively evaluate the degree of lung injury in the critically ill as a predictor of prognosis. Sakka and colleagues (2002) investigated the use of extravascular lung water (EVLW) for determining severity of degree of lung injury. EVLW represents the amount of fluid that has leaked out of permeable pulmonary capillaries causing pulmonary edema. Their results suggest that the higher the degree of EVLW, the worse the prognosis, as survivors of ARDS had lower levels of EVLW.

For those who survive, lung repair occurs slowly and terminates by about 6 months following the onset of ARDS. Although about 50 percent of survivors ultimately have no significant permanent lung damage (Vollman & Aulbach, 1998), many ARDS survivors have a significantly reduced health-related quality of life (HRQL) that can be attributed solely to ARDS (Davidson et al., 1999). The lower HRQL is primarily noted in physical functioning and continuing pulmonary problems (e.g., dyspnea, cough).

In summary, ALI/ARDS is a severe inflammatory lung disorder characterized by nonhydrostatic pulmonary edema and refractory hypoxemia. It can be triggered by local or distant predisposing factors. Thus far, there is no way to predict who will develop ALI/ARDS; however, the most common predisposing factors include sepsis, pneumonia, gastric aspiration, and posttrauma injury with shock. Diagnosis is usually based on the ARDS consensus criteria or the Modified Lung Injury Score. Clinical presentation is fairly predictable regardless of predisposing event. Pathogenesis involves injury to the pulmonary alveolar–capillary membrane associated with inflammatory cells with their products. Treatment continues primarily to be supportive, centering on improving gas exchange through mechanical ventilation. Mortality remains high, although some reduction has been noted using protective ventilation and through a breakthrough in treating sepsis, the major cause of ALI/ARDS. Positioning therapy improves oxygenation by decreasing $\dot{V}/\dot{Q}$ mismatch and shunt. Drug therapy may include corticosteroids or inhaled nitric oxide. Research is continuing on corticosteroid therapy, surfactant replacement therapy, and partial liquid ventilation.

SECTION THREE REVIEW

1. The most common indirect predisposing disorder of ALI/ARDS is:
   A. gastric aspiration
   B. severe trauma
   C. sepsis
   D. pneumonia

2. The pulmonary edema associated with ALI/ARDS is caused by
   A. capillary microembolism
   B. left ventricular failure
   C. loss of surfactant
   D. injured alveolar–capillary membrane

3. Which clinical finding is typically present with ALI/ARDS?
   A. decreased PaO_2/FIO_2 ratio
   B. increased lung compliance
   C. decreased airway resistance
   D. increased functional residual capacity

4. The refractory (resistant) nature of ARDS to oxygen therapy is based on the amount of
   A. anatomic shunt
   B. venous admixture
   C. capillary shunt
   D. shuntlike effect

5. The pulmonary edema of ALI/ARDS differs from pulmonary edema of CHF in which way?
   A. in CHF, PAWP is less than 18
   B. in CHF, bronchoalveolar lavage (BAL) fluid is protein rich
   C. in ARDS, heart enlargement is typically noted
   D. in ARDS, BAL fluid contains inflammatory cells

6. According to the ARDS consensus criteria, a diagnosis of ARDS requires a PaO_2/FIO_2 ratio of less than _____ mm Hg.
   A. 175
   B. 200
   C. 225
   D. 300

7. Which type of inflammatory cell is believed to be the major cause of lung injury?
   A. neutrophils
   B. lymphocytes
   C. eosinophils
   D. basophils

8. The nurse would expect to see which ABG trend in an ALI/ARDS patient?
   A. low pH
   B. low PaO_2
   C. high $PaCO_2$
   D. high HCO_3

9. Protective ventilation uses tidal volumes of _____ mL/kg.
   A. 4
   B. 6
   C. 8
   D. 10

10. The term *permissive hypercapnia* refers to
    A. reducing peak airway pressures by allowing some increase in $PaCO_2$
    B. controlling $PaCO_2$ level at 45 to 50 mm Hg
    C. enhancing gas exchange by allowing some increase in $PaCO_2$
    D. controlling PaO_2 level by allowing hypercapnia

11. Optimal PEEP level is usually between
    A. 5 and 10 cm H_2O
    B. 6 and 12 cm H_2O
    C. 8 and 15 cm H_2O
    D. 10 and 18 cm H_2O

12. Which statement is correct regarding the primary purpose of CLRT?
    A. it prevents pneumonia
    B. it saves manual turning time
    C. it prevents decubitus ulcers
    D. it prevents reduced stasis of fluid and gas

13. When initiating prone positioning, the nurse would monitor the patient for a significant improvement in
    A. PaO_2
    B. $PaCO_2$
    C. breathing pattern
    D. level of consciousness

14. Inhaled nitric oxide is sometimes ordered because of which physiologic effect?
    A. vasoconstriction
    B. vasodilation
    C. anesthetic
    D. analgesic

15. Corticosteroid therapy may be used for the ALI/ARDS patient because of which ALI/ARDS characteristic?
    A. atelectasis
    B. pulmonary edema
    C. loss of surfactant
    D. diffuse inflammation

Answers: 1. C, 2. D, 3. A, 4. C, 5. D, 6. B, 7. A, 8. B, 9. B, 10. A, 11. C, 12. D, 13. A, 14. B, 15. D

SECTION FOUR: Pulmonary Embolism

Pulmonary embolism accounts for about 250,000 hospitalizations in the United States per year and 50,000 deaths annually (Porth, 2002), and has a high mortality rate if untreated (Chunilal et al., 2003). Although many pulmonary emboli are asymptomatic, others lead to rapid death. This section provides an overview of the types, causes, signs and symptoms, and treatment of pulmonary emboli but focuses on thromboembolism. At the completion of this section, the learner will be able to explain pulmonary embolism and its treatment.

Pulmonary embolism is blockage of a pulmonary blood vessel caused by lodging of a thromboembolism or other blood-borne material that has passed through the venous system, into the right side of the heart and into the pulmonary artery. Emboli become lodged in the lungs because of the natural blood flow of the venous system into the lungs for gas exchange through a decreasing-size pulmonary vascular system that begins at the pulmonary artery trunk and ends in the microvasculature of the pulmonary capillary system. This system makes the lungs act as a filtering organ, stopping any material that is too large to squeeze through the tiny microvasculature (Awtry & Loscalzo, 2001). Therefore, a variety of blood-borne material can flow through the system until it can no longer move forward, lodging and obstructing flow distal to the obstruction.

Types and Causes of Emboli

There are four types of pulmonary emboli: thrombus, fat, amniotic, and venous air.

Thromboembolism

A thrombus or blood clot comprises almost all pulmonary emboli. The major source of thromboembolism is deep vein thrombosis (DVT) in the lower extremities, usually in the thigh or pelvis areas. Thromboembolism is discussed in detail later in this section.

Fat Embolism

Fat embolism occurs when fat gains access into the venous circulation. Fat embolism is quite rare and usually results from long bone trauma or orthopedic surgery. Fat emboli are often small and may go undetected. When symptoms are present, they usually appear within 12 to 36 hours after the predisposing event. Major criteria for fat embolism syndrome include petechiae, dyspnea and tachypnea, hemoptysis, neurologic symptoms (e.g., confusion, drowsiness, or coma), and diffuse bilateral shadowing on chest radiography (Mellor & Soni, 2001). A person experiencing this form of embolus may also exhibit a fever, tachycardia, and a variety of other signs and symptoms.

Amniotic Embolism

Normally, the fetal membranes prevent amniotic fluid from gaining access to the maternal circulation (Davies, 2001). Amniotic emboli can develop during the birthing process when amnionic fluid mixes with maternal blood. Normally, during the labor and delivery process, uterine contractions collapse endometrial vessels; however, sometimes, the vessels do not collapse completely, allowing access of amniotic fluid into maternal circulation. It is theorized that the amniotic fluid embolus causes a mechanical obstruction that leads to obstruction of pulmonary vessels and neurohumoral obstruction resulting in vasospasm of the pulmonary vessels. These two events create pulmonary hypertension and hypoxemia, which then can result in spontaneous resolution, left ventricular failure, or death.

Venous Air Embolism

Venous air embolus (VAE) results from a bolus of air being introduced into the venous circulation. VAE is a rare, but potentially lethal, complication usually of iatrogenic procedures or trauma. Common predisposing factors for development of air embolism include venous or arterial intravenous catheters, cardiac pacemaker placement, or penetrating chest trauma. Conrad (2002) explains that central venous cannulization (e.g., subclavian) and pressurized IV infusion systems carry the greatest risk. The exact volume required for a lethal air bolus is unknown but volumes of 3 to 8 mL/kg can cause right heart outflow obstruction, subsequent cardiovascular collapse, and death. For example, a lethal dose in a 150-pound (68-kg) adult male would be a bolus of 204 to 544 mL of air. Smaller volumes of air can move from the right heart into the pulmonary artery system, causing pulmonary vascular injury (e.g., vasoconstriction, pulmonary hypertension, injury to the capillary endothelium, and pulmonary edema). Mortality rate, as a result of an air bolus following a central venous cannulization procedure, is about 30 percent. The clinical manifestations of VAE are similar to thromboembolism.

Predisposing Factors of Thromboembolism

More than 80 percent of pulmonary emboli (PE) originate as deep-vein thromboses (DVT) in lower extremity deep veins. Many high-acuity patients are at increased risk for development of DVT and, therefore, for development of PE. There are three major factors (called Virchow's triad) that place a person at risk for development of DVT:

- **Venous stasis.** Venous stasis refers to slowing of blood flow. It most commonly results from significantly reduced mobility, such as is seen with prolonged bedrest, severe illness, or major surgery; or immobility states, such as limb casts or paralysis. It can also develop when vein valves in the extremities are incompetent, for example, in severe varicose veins. People with polycythemia vera can also develop venous stasis because of a thickening of the blood (hyperviscosity) from a significantly elevated red blood cell count.

■ **Hypercoagulability.** Hypercoagulability refers to an abnormal tendency to form thrombi that can be inherited or acquired. Acquired causes include such conditions as cancer, oral contraceptives, sepsis, and others.

■ **Venous (endothelial) injury.** Endothelial injury can occur either directly or indirectly. It can result from such predisposing events as surgery or trauma, infection, and central venous catheters.

Table 5–12 lists the most common predisposing factors for development of thromboembolism.

TABLE 5–12   Most Common Predisposing Factors for Thromboembolism. Listed in Order of Frequency.

■ Immobilization (within past 3 months)[a]
■ Surgery (within past 3 months)
■ History of coronary artery disease
■ History of thrombophlebitis
■ Malignancy

[a]54 percent of confirmed acute pulmonary emboli.
Data from Quinlan, D. J., McQuillan, A., & Eikelboom, J. W. (2004). Low-molecular-weight heparin compared with intravenous unfractionated heparin for treatment of pulmonary embolism. Annals of Internal Medicine 140(3),175–183.

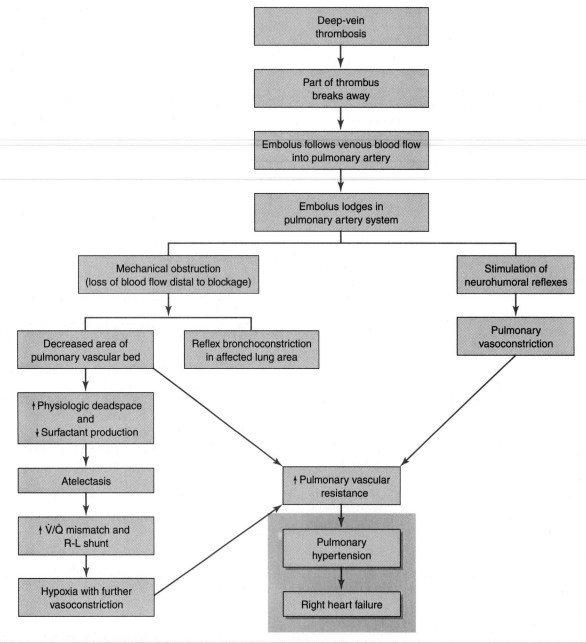

Figure 5–4 ■ Pathophysiology of pulmonary embolus.

Pathophysiology of Pulmonary Embolism

The severity of pulmonary embolism depends on the degree of obstruction and location of the embolus. More than half of pulmonary emboli lodge in the main or lobar pulmonary arteries and about 36 percent lodge in the segmental branches (Quinlan et al., 2004). Figure 5–4 illustrates some of the major pathophysiologic events associated with pulmonary embolism. Pulmonary embolism creates a decreased pulmonary vascular bed area and is a major etiology of secondary pulmonary hypertension (Jassal et al., 2004).

Signs and Symptoms of Pulmonary Embolism

Pulmonary embolism is often a hidden killer because only about 30 percent of patients who die (directly or indirectly from PE) are diagnosed prior to their death (Quinlan et al., 2004), and approximately one third of patients experiencing PE die within 2.5 hours of onset (Stein & Henry, 1997). Pulmonary embolism often is not easy to recognize or diagnose, particularly when the patient's health status is deteriorating rapidly. Although the presenting manifestations of PE are frequently described in general terms (see Table 5–13), not all episodes of pulmonary embolism present in the same way. Stein and Henry (1997) identified three presenting syndromes that suggest the degree of severity of PE. The syndromes are seen in patients who survive long enough to be evaluated and diagnosed. Stein and Henry, however, also found that patients who have a history of cardiopulmonary diseases may either hide or mimic any of the syndromes. Table 5–14 summarizes three syndromes of pulmonary embolus.

TABLE 5–13　Common Signs and Symptoms of Pulmonary Embolism in Order of Frequency

Dyspnea	Tachypnea
Pleural pain	Crackles (rales)
Tachycardia	Cough
Unilateral leg swelling and pain[a]	

[a] DVT findings (present in only one-third of PE cases)

Data from Quinlan, D. J., McQuillan, A., & Eikelboom, J. W. (2004). Low-molecular-weight heparin compared with intravenous unfractionated heparin for treatment of pulmonary embolism. Annals of Internal Medicine 140*(3),175–183.*

TABLE 5–14　Three Syndromes of Pulmonary Embolus Presentation.

NAME	FREQUENCY/SEVERITY[a]	PRESENTING DEFINING CHARACTERISTICS	OTHER SUPPORTIVE DATA
Pulmonary infarction syndrome	Frequency: 65% Severity: Mild	Pleuritic pain Crackles (rales)	Tachypnea, dyspnea, hemoptysis may be present. Absence of tachycardia ECG: Normal reading is more likely seen than in isolated dyspnea syndrome Chest radiograph: May show atelectasis or lung tissue abnormality and pleural effusion (more commonly noted than in isolated dyspnea syndrome) $\dot{V}/\dot{Q}$ scan probability:[b] Usually intermediate but may be low
Isolated dyspnea syndrome	Frequency: 22% Severity: Moderate	Dyspnea Absence of pleuritic pain and hemoptysis	Tachycardia (greater than 120/min) ECG: T= wave or ST= segment changes may be present or may be normal Chest radiograph: May show atelectasis or lung tissue abnormality and pleural effusion may be present $\dot{V}/\dot{Q}$ scan probability: Usually high but may be intermediate
Circulatory collapse syndrome	Frequency: 8% Severity: Severe	Tachycardia Hypotension or loss of consciousness Complete right bundle branch block Cardiomegaly Absence of pleural effusion	ECG: Likely to show T-wave or ST-segment changes Chest radiograph: May be normal $\dot{V}/\dot{Q}$ scan probability: High

The defining characteristics of each syndrome were made based on percentage of presence or absence of characteristic

[a]Frequency is the percentage of occurrence in the study.
[b] $\dot{V}/\dot{Q}$ scan probability: The probability of a positive PE reading on $\dot{V}/\dot{Q}$ scan.
Data from Stein, P. D., & Henry, J. W. (1997). Clinical characteristics of patients with acute pulmonary embolism stratified according to their presenting syndromes. Chest, 112*(4),974–979.*

Diagnosis

Diagnosis of pulmonary embolism frequently is not made until autopsy. The presenting manifestations may not be recognized or may be misinterpreted and there are few tests available for making a definitive diagnosis. Diagnostic testing generally is initiated based on clinical suspicion, such as a positive history and presenting signs and symptoms. A variety of tests are recommended to aid in diagnosis.

D-dimer

A preliminary D-dimer assay is often performed to eliminate pulmonary embolism as a diagnosis. A D-dimer level of less than 1.0 mcg/mL is highly predictive for exclusion of pulmonary embolism as a diagnosis (Abcarian et al., 2003). D-dimer is a specific type of fibrin degradation product (i.e., a product of fibrin clot breakdown) that increases in the blood following any thrombotic event in the body (e.g., pulmonary embolus, venous thrombosis, or myocardial infarction). An elevated (positive) D-dimer level is indicative of the presence of thrombolytic activity but the test is too non-specific to indicate a location. A normal (negative) D-dimer level strongly suggests that the patient has no detectable thrombolytic activity present in the body; therefore, no active pulmonary embolism.

Ventilation–Perfusion ($\dot{V}/\dot{Q}$) Scan

A $\dot{V}/\dot{Q}$ scan may be ordered if the D-dimer assay is positive for thrombolytic activity. The $\dot{V}/\dot{Q}$ scan provides information on ventilation and perfusion relationships in areas of the lung. An intermediate- or high-probability abnormal $\dot{V}/\dot{Q}$ scan result supports a diagnosis of PE but is not specific to this diagnosis.

Compression Ultrasound

Ultrasound of both lower extremities may be ordered to rule out deep-vein thrombosis. This is often done if the $\dot{V}/\dot{Q}$ scan is non-diagnostic. A positive result suggestive of DVT occurs when the vein cannot be fully compressed. This test, in conjunction with unilateral lower extremity swelling, tenderness, redness, and a positive Homan's sign, are strongly suggestive of DVT. Evaluating the patient for DVT is important because of the high percentage of PE being attributed to DVT.

Chest Radiography

Chest x-rays are frequently normal early in the course of a pulmonary embolus and, depending on the severity of the PE, they may remain normal. Atelectasis, pleural effusions, or pulmonary tissue abnormalities may be noted but are nonspecific for PE. For these reasons, chest radiographs are not considered a good diagnostic tool but may be helpful when accompanied by other tests.

ECG

Electrocardiograms (ECG) are often normal and may only indicate sinus tachycardia. The ECG may show certain abnormalities that can be used to support a diagnosis of PE but are not diagnostic in themselves.

Pulmonary Angiography

The angiogram is considered the definitive diagnostic test for pulmonary embolus because it can pinpoint the blockage(s). However, angiography is invasive, carries serious risks of its own, and is expensive. It is not considered a legitimate test if other tests (i.e., $\dot{V}/\dot{Q}$ scan and DVT testing) have been negative (low probability). Angiogram is contraindicated if the patient has already received a thrombolytic agent and is generally reserved for patients with low cardiopulmonary reserve (Quinlin et al., 2004).

Arterial Blood Gases

Abnormal arterial blood gas (ABG) results typical of PE (low PaO_2 and $PaCO_2$, and elevated $P[A-a]O_2$) are nonspecific for pulmonary embolus. A normal PaO_2 cannot exclude the patient from a diagnosis of PE. However, ABG results are helpful in assessing the level of hypoxia present, and severe hypoxemia accompanied by a negative chest x-ray is considered suspicious of PE (Quinlin et al., 2004).

Treatment

On diagnosis of pulmonary embolus, a variety of therapy options become available. Table 5–15 summarizes the typical medical treatment options of pulmonary embolism.

Nursing Considerations

The primary nursing diagnoses that are typically appropriate in care of the patient with pulmonary embolism include

- Immobility
- Risk for ineffective peripheral tissue perfusion
- Impaired gas exchange
- Ineffective breathing pattern
- Chest pain
- Fear/anxiety
- Knowledge deficit (Carpenito-Moyet, 2004; Ulrich & Canale, 2001).

Pulmonary embolism is a potential complication (PC) rather than a nursing diagnosis; thus, it requires a collaborative practice model. This means that, in addition to addressing any appropriate nursing diagnoses, the nurse also focuses on administering treatments as ordered by the physician or the ad-

TABLE 5–15   Summary of Medical Treatment Options for Pulmonary Embolism

MEDICAL THERAPY	TREATMENT/COMMENTS
General	Hospitalization recommended for anyone suspected of pulmonary embolism
	Oxygen therapy and airway management (as required)
	Management of shock (as required)
Anticoagulant therapy	Time of Initiation: Immediately when diagnosis of pulmonary embolism is established
	Type
	■ Heparin (either UH or LMWH)
	○ Usually administered for 5 to 6 days. Discontinued when INR has been therapeutic for 2 days consecutively
	○ Loading dose followed by continuous IV drip.
	○ May be ordered for home management (subcutaneously)
	■ Unfractionated Heparin (UH)
	○ First 24 hours—use sliding scale dose based on APTT
	○ Draw APTT every 6 hours for first 24 hours then once daily
	■ Low-molecular-weight heparin (LMWH)
	○ Routine lab monitoring may not be required
	■ Warfarin
	○ May also be initiated at same time as heparin therapy
	○ Goal: Maintain prothrombin time at INR 2.0–3.0
	○ May be ordered for 3 to 6 months or indefinitely
Thrombolytic therapy	Indication: Circulatory collapse; emergency situation
Surgical embolectomy	Indication: If emergency thrombolytic therapy is not successful, requires cardiopulmonary bypass; often used as a last resort to save patient; associated with high mortality

Key: UH – Unfractionated Heparin; LMWH – Low-molecular-weight Heparin; INR – International Normalized Ratio; APTT – Activated Partial thromboplastin time.
Data from Quinlan, D. J., McQuillan, A., & Eikelboom, J. W. (2004). Low-molecular-weight heparin compared with intravenous unfractionated heparin for treatment of pulmonary embolism. Annals of Internal Medicine 140*(3):175–183.*

vanced practice nurse, monitoring for status changes, and monitoring for the therapeutic and nontherapeutic effects of prescribed treatments.

Carpenito-Moyet (2004) suggests the following interventions for PC: Pulmonary embolism (not including potential interventions unique to air or fat embolism):

- Monitor for signs and symptoms of pulmonary embolism
- Initiate shock protocols if manifestations of PE develop
- Initiate O_2 therapy and monitor SpO_2 or SaO_2
- Monitor labs: ABG, CBC, Electrolytes, BUN
- Initiate thrombolytic therapy as ordered
- Initiate and monitor heparin therapy as ordered following thrombolytic therapy
- Monitor clotting times
- Monitor closely for abnormal bleeding when patient is receiving thrombolytics or anticoagulant therapy

In summary, this section has provided an overview of pulmonary embolism. There are four major types of embolism, including thrombus, fat, amniotic, and venous air. In addition, other blood-borne substances such as vegetative bacterial growths or sloughing dead tissue can become emboli. Thromboembolism is by far the major cause of pulmonary emboli;

and deep-vein thrombosis is the major source of thromboembolism. Predisposing factors for deep-vein thrombosis include Virchow's triad (venous stasis; hypercoagulability; and endothelial injury, either direct or indirect). Signs and symptoms of pulmonary embolism were discussed and three syndromes of PE by presentation were provided. Many people experiencing PE, particularly those who are elderly or who have preexisting cardiopulmonary conditions, may exhibit a variety of different manifestations that either mask or redirect pulmonary embolism as a diagnosis. Pulmonary embolism is most often diagnosed postmortem because of the clinician's inability to recognize it. There are a variety of tests that can help in making the diagnosis of PE, including D-dimer assay, $\dot{V}/\dot{Q}$ scan, compression ultrasound of the lower extremities, chest radiography, and ECG. The pulmonary angiogram is considered the definitive test for PE but it should not be ordered to rule out PE when other, less invasive and less expensive tests have been negative. Treatment of PE is focused on fibrinolytic therapy followed by anticoagulant therapy. Oxygen therapy is commonly used. Other care is supportive in nature, based on the severity of the PE. Most patients with a severe PE die within 2.5 hours of admission, making timely recognition and aggressive intervention crucial.

SECTION FOUR REVIEW

1. The most common type of pulmonary embolism is
   A. venous air
   B. amniotic
   C. thrombus
   D. fat

2. Which type of embolism manifests itself as dyspnea, tachypnea, neurological symptoms, AND petechiae?
   A. venous air
   B. amniotic
   C. thrombus
   D. fat

3. Venous (endothelial) injury is one of three major factors that causes formation of deep-vein thrombosis. This type of injury can result from
   A. immobility
   B. sepsis
   C. surgery
   D. varicose veins

4. Which factor determines the severity of a pulmonary embolus?
   A. type of embolus
   B. degree of obstruction
   C. speed of onset
   D. general health of patient

5. The most common predisposing factor for development of thromboembolism is
   A. immobility
   B. postsurgery status
   C. malignancy
   D. coronary artery disease

6. Mechanical obstruction of a pulmonary vessel results in
   A. vasodilation
   B. atelectasis
   C. decreased vascular resistance
   D. left heart failure

7. Common signs and symptoms of pulmonary embolism include
   A. rhonchi
   B. pneumothorax
   C. dyspnea
   D. bradycardia

8. The most common clinical presentation of someone with a pulmonary embolism is seen with pulmonary infarction syndrome. The defining characteristics of the syndrome include
   A. absence of pleuritic pain
   B. pleuritic pain
   C. hypotension
   D. hemoptysis

9. Under what circumstances is surgical embolectomy usually done?
   A. if heparin therapy is unsuccessful
   B. if symptoms are severe
   C. if patient is unconscious
   D. if thrombolytic therapy is unsuccessful

10. The definitive test to diagnose a pulmonary embolism is
    A. angiography
    B. $\dot{V}/\dot{Q}$ scan
    C. D-dimer
    D. compression ultrasound

11. The major initial treatment for pulmonary embolism is
    A. thrombolytic therapy
    B. surgical embolectomy
    C. oxygen therapy
    D. anticoagulant therapy

Answers: 1. C, 2. D, 3. C, 4. B, 5. A, 6. B, 7. C, 8. B, 9. D, 10. A, 11. D

SECTION FIVE: Severe Acute Respiratory Syndrome (SARS)

On completion of this section, the learner will be able to describe **severe acute respiratory syndrome** (SARS).

Author note: SARS is the "new kid on the block" in potentially lethal communicable diseases. At the time of this writing, information is based primarily on clinical reporting from physicians who have treated it in their hospitals, scientists who are studying the virus, and the Centers for Disease Control (CDC) and World Health Organization (WHO). For this reason, although the information in this section is current at the time of this writing, it cannot be considered the "final" word on SARS.

It is included here because available information on this disease is essential for future recognition, management, and protection.

In March of 2003, Dr. Carlo Urbani died of SARS. Although his name is unfamiliar to many of us, it is not without significance. Dr. Urbani was "the WHO scientist who first alerted the world to the existence of SARS in Hanoi, Vietnam" (WHO, 2003). Ironically, he died 1 month before the SARS virus was identified.

SARS was first described in March 2003 and first called an atypical pneumonia. At that time, the CDC could describe the condition but the pathogen remained unknown. In April of 2003, the WHO announced that it had isolated the virus—a new virus never before seen in humans. This is a novel form of coronavirus, a major cause of the common cold worldwide, and usually affects the upper respiratory tract. The origin of the new SARS-associated coronavirus (referred to as SARS-CoV) remains unknown, but it is suspected that it originated as a nonhuman virus that jumped to humans (Holmes, 2003). The CDC reports that from November 2002 through May 2003, 28 countries reported a total of 7,956 cases of SARS (MMWR, 2003).

Clinical Features of SARS

Unlike the regular coronavirus, the SARS-CoV concentrates in the lungs. The key features of SARS are

- Incubation period of 2 to 10 days (median of 4 to 6 days)
- Early systemic symptoms followed within 2 to 7 days by dry cough or shortness of breath, often without upper respiratory symptoms
- Development of radiographically confirmed pneumonia by day 7 to 10 of illness
- Lymphopenia in most cases (CDC, 2004)

Transmission

Transmission of SARS-CoV is by airborne droplet (e.g., cough, secretions) or aerosol (e.g., humidifier) in close person-to-person contact. It is believed that the virus may live up to 24 hours in the environment. It spreads rapidly through an unprotected population, as demonstrated in the Toronto 2003 outbreak when 77 percent of the cases of SARS were contracted while in the hospital and almost 25 percent of the cases were in unprotected health care workers who were exposed before the hazard was recognized (SARS Scientific Committee, 2003).

Clinical Presentation and Course

The most common presenting symptoms include fever (greater than 100°F or 37.8°C), myalgias (severe), extreme weakness, mild headache, and a dry cough. Other, less common manifestations include dyspnea, arthralgias, nausea, chills, chest pain, dizziness, sore throat, and anxiety (Avendano et al., 2003). Most patients are able to be discharged without complications by day 14 postadmission. The typical clinical course of the disease runs 7 to 14 days, however, Lapinsky and Hawryluck (2003) reported that some patients demonstrated a biphasic disease course, that is, onset of illness, improvement, deterioration.

Lew and colleagues (2003) reported that about 25 percent of SARS patients in their study progressed to ALI/ARDS. Approximately 10 percent of the SARS patients who developed ALI/ARDS died within the first 28 days postadmission. Early deaths (within first 7 days) were attributed primarily to single organ complications (e.g., heart, lungs), whereas late deaths (after seven days) were usually a result of systemic complications such as sepsis, thromboembolic problems, and MODS. Age was a strong factor in increased mortality, with patients 60 years of age or older having a mortality rate of more than 43 percent.

Diagnosing SARS

Diagnosing SARS has been difficult because it initially presents as an atypical pneumonia. For this reason, the CDC (2004) makes this statement regarding case detection:

> Severe respiratory illness in the context of a documented exposure risk is the key to diagnosing SARS-CoV disease. Providers should therefore consider SARS-CoV disease in patients requiring hospitalization for:

- Radiographically confirmed pneumonia or acute respiratory distress syndrome of unknown etiology, AND
- One of the following risk factors in the 10 days before illness onset:
  - Travel to mainland China, Hong Kong or Taiwan, or close contact with an ill person with a history of recent travel to one of these areas, OR
  - Employment in an occupation associated with a risk for SARS-CoV exposure (e.g., health care worker with direct patient contact, worker in a laboratory that contains live SARS-CoV), OR
  - Part of a cluster of cases of atypical pneumonia without an alternative diagnosis

Infection control practitioners and other health care personnel should be alert for clusters of pneumonia among two or more health care workers who work in the same facility.

Diagnosis

Diagnosis is based on clinical presentation, history of possible exposure (major criterion), and laboratory testing. Suspicious cases should have initial testing performed, some of which help in ruling out other pathogens:

- Chest radiograph
- Pulse oximetry
- CBC with differential
- Blood cultures
- Sputum Gram stain and culture
- Testing for viral respiratory pathogens, notably influenza A and B and respiratory syncytial virus
- Specimens for Legionella and pneumococcal urinary antigen testing (CDC, 2004)

When other pathogens are ruled out, SARS-CoV is tested for, including antibody testing (enzyme immunoassay); and RT-PCR tests (reverse transcription polymerase chain reaction) of stool, blood, and respiratory specimens. The CDC cautions that without confirmation of exposure to SARS-CoV, the predictive value of these tests is very low and may lead to false positive diagnoses. Diagnostic laboratory tests are to be sent to the local or state public health department (CDC, 2004). Currently, scientists are exploring better SARS-specific diagnostic methods.

Infection Control

If SARS is suspected, strict droplet precautions should be initiated immediately. The patient should wear a mask to protect others in the environment prior to being placed in isolation. Ideally, a patient with active SARS-CoV is placed in a single room with negative air pressure and a two-door anteroom system. The air in the room should discharge directly out of doors or a special filtering system should be in place. The room should have only necessary equipment in it. Staff protective attire should include hair cover, fluid resistant gown, N96 or equivalent mask, protective eyewear, and fluid resistant gown (SARS Scientific Committee, 2003). Should the SARS patient require intubation, there is increased risk of health care worker exposure because of the large viral burden being shed during intubation (Cooper et al., 2003). It is recommended that only the required personnel directly involved in intubation be present in the room for the procedure while backup personnel wait outside of the room, entering only as necessary. Deep sedation without use of topical or nebulized local anesthesia is recommended. Both of these recommendations are based on the need to minimize cough stimulation during the procedure, thereby significantly decreasing droplet exposure probability.

Medical Management

At this time, there is no definitive medical therapy to treat SARS. The recommended pharmacotherapy currently includes:

- **Antibiotic therapy.** Respiratory fluoroquinolone or macrolide
- **Antiviral therapy.** Ribavirin, 400 mg IV every 8 hours for 3 days followed by 1,200 mg orally every 12 hours for 7 days. The efficacy of Ribavirin has not been established for use in SARS and side effects are significant and potentially severe (e.g., hemolytic anemia and electrolyte disturbances).
- **Corticosteroid therapy.** Methylprednisolone 40 mg IV every 12 hours for 3 days followed by prednisone orally per day for 7 days (Lapinsky & Hawryluck, 2003)

Lapinsky and Hawryluck (2003) pose that there are certain respiratory-related procedures that place the staff at higher risk of exposure, including the following:

- Use of a bag-valve (Ambu) bag with mask with a poor seal. Recommendation—Limit use.
- Disconnections from a mechanical ventilator may spray contaminated droplets. Recommendation—Avoid disconnections; always place ventilator on "standby" prior to disconnection.
- During suctioning, coughing may spray contaminated droplets. Recommendation—Use in-line suctioning system

In summary, this section has presented a brief overview of current knowledge about severe acute respiratory syndrome (SARS). The first SARS outbreak occurred in late 2002 and was formally described in early 2003. A novel coronavirus, SARS-CoV, is a distinct variant of a common cold virus, which prior to the SARS outbreak had never been identified in humans. SARS-CoV is extremely communicable via droplet spread and may survive outside of the body for up to 24 hours. Currently, there is no specific diagnostic test to differentiate SARS-CoV, but research is moving toward this end. Exposed people become symptomatic by approximately 4 days after exposure and the virus has a course of 7 to 14 days. Approximately 10 percent develop ALI/ARDS. Specific suggestions for prevention of infection spread in hospitals are provided and focus on minimizing spraying of airway secretion droplets.

SECTION FIVE REVIEW

1. The pathogen that causes SARS is a unique form of which virus?
   A. hantavirus
   B. coronavirus
   C. rhinovirus
   D. influenza–A virus
2. Which statement is correct regarding the clinical features of the SARS virus?
   A. a persistent dry cough is present
   B. the chest radiograph is usually normal
   C. the patient has been experiencing hemoptysis
   D. the incubation period is 10 days to 2 weeks
3. The SARS virus is known to be transmitted by
   A. contaminated feces
   B. blood contact

   C. tears
   D. airborne droplets
4. A common presenting clinical manifestation of SARS is
   A. fever greater than 102°F (38.9°C)
   B. petechiae
   C. severe myalgias
   D. confusion
5. The CDC recommends that SARS should be suspected in anyone who presents with confirmed pneumonia or ARDS of unknown etiology AND
   A. travel to South Africa within the past 2 weeks
   B. travel to China, Hong Kong, or Taiwan within the past 10 days
   C. travel to South America within the past 2 weeks
   D. travel to Canada within the past 10 days

6. At what point in suspecting SARS is actual testing for the virus performed?
   A. when the patient first presents to the health care system
   B. when a sputum culture comes back positive for the SARS virus
   C. when the patient develops acute respiratory distress syndrome (ARDS)
   D. when other, more common causes of viral pneumonia are ruled out
7. True or False: There is no definitive test that diagnoses the SARS virus.
8. Intubation of a SARS patient is considered a high-risk period for health care workers because _____. (fill in blank)
9. Suctioning the airway of a SARS patient is considered a high-risk procedure for spread of the virus. What is recommended to reduce this risk?

A. minimize suctioning
B. use in-line suctioning system
C. use the unique SARS suctioning system
D. use regular suctioning system, but wear protective face gear

10. Which statement correctly reflects the pharmacotherapy regimen for SARS?
    A. antibiotic therapy is not recommended
    B. corticosteroid therapy is not recommended
    C. ribavirin has been found to be effective against the SARS virus
    D. the efficacy of ribavirin has not yet been established for SARS

Answers: 1. B, 2. A, 3. D, 4. C, 5. B, 6. D, 7. True, 8. Viral burden is high because of shedding and coughing during the procedure, 9. B, 10. D

SECTION SIX: Chest Drainage Management

Upon completion of this section, the learner will be able to describe principles and management of chest drainage.

This section provides an overview of chest drainage principles and management. The anatomy and physiology of the lungs is available for review in Module 4, "Determinants and Assessment of Pulmonary Gas Exchange." Trauma aspects of pneumo- and hemothorax, and tension pneumothorax are presented in Module 36, "Trauma," and are not presented here.

CASE 1

Nineteen-year-old TJ was thrown from his motorcycle onto the hood of a vehicle approaching from the opposite direction. He was stabilized at the scene by the rescue squad and rapidly transferred to a nearby hospital emergency department (ED). On arrival at the ED, a rapid assessment revealed the following: TJ was oriented and complaining of severe left chest pain. Chest contusions were noted on the left upper chest. He was tachypneic with circumoral cyanosis noted. Chest auscultation revealed positive breath sounds on the right but negative breath sounds in the left upper lung field. A portable chest x-ray showed multiple left rib fractures and left hemopneumothorax—preparations were made for immediate chest tube placement.

CASE 2

MT, a 55-year-old woman, was admitted to the hospital with a diagnosis of "exacerbation of COPD." She has been receiving intermittent positive pressure breathing (IPPB) therapy, oxygen at 2 L per nasal cannula, and a bronchodilator drug. This afternoon, MT suddenly developed sharp right side chest pain and increased shortness of breath. Her nurse was unable to auscultate breath sounds in the right upper anterior lung field during a rapid focused respiratory assessment. A portable chest x-ray was taken, showing a right upper lobe pneumothorax. Chest drainage was initiated with one chest tube being inserted on the right side of MT's chest.

Chest Drainage

Chest drainage is the active or passive removal of air or fluid from the intrapleural space of the lungs or from the mediastinal compartment. Chest drainage may be a short term or intermittent therapy (e.g., aspiration of intrapleural air or fluid using a needle and syringe); or it may be relatively long-term therapy (e.g., treatment of pneumothorax or hemothorax resulting from chest trauma).

Who Requires Chest Drainage?

Both TJ and MT required chest drainage but for different reasons. Chest drainage is used to treat thoracic problems that may be external or internal in origin. External origins include blunt chest trauma, traumatic or surgical entry into the intrapleural or mediastinal spaces, resulting in pneumothorax or hemothorax. **Pneumothorax** (sometimes referred to as "pneumo") refers to the abnormal presence of air in the intrapleural space, whereas **hemothorax** refers to the abnormal presence of blood in the intrapleural space. Frequently both pneumothorax and hemothorax exist simultaneously (**hemopneumothorax**). TJ's case is an example of an external origin problem. Internal origins of pneumothorax include spontaneous rupture of a pulmonary **bleb,** procedural rupture of the visceral pleura, or barotrauma. Bleb rupture is most commonly found in patients

TABLE 5–16   Origins of Pneumothorax

EXTERNAL ORIGINS	INTERNAL ORIGINS
Thoracic surgery (e.g., open heart surgery)	Spontaneous bleb rupture
Penetrating chest trauma (e.g., knife or bullets)	Procedural rupture of visceral pleura (e.g., lung tissue biopsy)
Unintentional catheter entry into intrapleural space during central line placement	Barotrauma (e.g., mechanical ventilation, positive end expiratory pressure)
Chest contusion	

TABLE 5–17   Summary of Common Clinical Findings of Pneumothorax

Signs of chest trauma (external origin)

Tachypnea, tachycardia (with possible onset of dysrhythmias)

Shortness of breath

Diminished or absent breath sounds on one side (or one area of lung)

ABG: Decreased Pao_2 and Sao_2, respiratory alkalosis

May complain of sharp chest pain on one side of chest (may not be present initially)

Positive chest x-ray for pneumothorax

with chronic lung diseases. Barotrauma-induced pneumothorax results from therapies that increase airway pressure and hyperinflate the alveoli. MT's case is an example of an internal origin. Common external and internal origins of pneumothorax are listed in Table 5–16. In addition to treating pneumo- or hemothorax, chest tubes may be inserted to drain severe **pleural effusion** or **empyema** if either condition is causing significant compression of lung tissue.

Pathogenesis of a Collapsed Lung

The mechanics of normal ventilation can be reviewed in Section One of Module 4. The thorax and lungs exist as opposing forces (i.e., the thorax's natural state is expansion, whereas the lungs' natural state is collapsed). Normal lung inflation depends on the intactness of the two pleural linings, which act as a single unit because of a state of negative intrapleural pressure; thus, as the thorax expands during inhalation, the lungs expand with it. Loss of negative intrapleural pressure, either of external or internal origin, results in rapid collapse (atelectasis) of the affected lung tissue because the two pleura separate, allowing the opposing forces to come into play. The size of lung collapse depends on how much of the intrapleural space loses negative pressure.

Size of the pneumothorax is an important consideration in making the decision whether chest drainage is required. Pneumothorax can be classified by the percentage of collapsed tissue—small (less than 15 percent), medium (15 to 60 percent), or large (greater than 60 percent). A small pneumothorax does not require insertion of a chest tube, whereas a medium-to-large pneumothorax does require chest tube insertion and drainage (Lynn-McHale & Carlson, 2001).

■ ■ ■

TJ's chest trauma with rib fractures is the probable cause of his left-sided hemopneumothorax. In MT's case, her history of COPD suggests that a pulmonary bleb has probably ruptured, causing a pneumothorax in the right upper lung field.

■ ■ ■

Common Clinical Findings

Although TJ's case greatly differs from MT's in etiology, their clinical presentation related to pneumothorax may be similar, dependent on the size of the pneumothorax. Many of the typical clinical findings are those noted with an acute hypoxia episode and reflect normal compensatory mechanisms, including tachypnea, tachycardia, agitation, and confusion. If chest pain is present, shallow respirations with splinting may be noted. In addition, the presence of tachypnea is frequently associated with initial respiratory alkalosis. Table 5–17 provides a summary of common clinical findings.

Chest Tube Insertion

The nurse frequently assists with insertion of chest tubes; thus, a brief description of necessary equipment and procedure are provided here. The *AACN Procedure Manual for Critical Care* lists the following equipment for chest tube insertion:

- Chest tube thoracotomy tray and drainage system
- Antiseptic solution
- Protective eyewear
- Local anesthetic (1 percent lidocaine)
- Sterile gowns, gloves, masks, caps, and drapes (Lynn-McHale & Carlson, 2001)

Depending on the size of the pneumothorax and other circumstances, preparation for insertion may need to be rapid. It is important to prepare the patient for the procedure as thoroughly as possible based on the patient's condition and the need for speed. The nurse's role in assisting with the procedure varies but often centers on obtaining (and possibly preparing) the necessary equipment, supporting the patient, and maintaining the patient in the appropriate position during the procedure. Table 5–18 summarizes common nursing activities in preparation for and during chest tube insertion.

The Procedure

If a pneumothorax is present, the chest tube typically is inserted anteriorly at the level of the second intercostal space, which ap-

TABLE 5–18   Nursing Considerations for Chest Tube Insertion

Patient Preparation

Assure that the patient understands the reason for the procedure and what to expect during and following the procedure

Assure that written consent has been obtained

Acquire and administer ordered sedation or analgesic prior to the procedure, timing the administration for the peak effect during the procedure

Assist the patient into the appropriate position (pneumothorax—lateral or supine; hemothorax—semi-Fowler)

Remind the patient not to move during the procedure (nurse may have to hold the patient in correct position)

Nurse's Role during Procedure

Pouring the antiseptic

Swabbing off lidocaine vial top with alcohol and holding vial for solution withdrawal

Supporting patient and maintaining correct patient position during procedure

Data from Lynn-McHale, D., & Carlson, K. (eds). (2001). AACN procedure manual for critical care, (4th ed.). Philadelphia: W. B. Saunders.

proximates the lung apex; and if a hemothorax (or fluid) is present, the chest tube typically is inserted midaxillary at the fourth or fifth intercostal space to drain the base of the lung field (Lynn-McHale & Carlson, 2001). Once the chest tube has been inserted, it is quickly connected to a special extension tubing that joins with the collection chamber of the chest drainage system. The chest tube is then sutured to the patient to prevent unintentional removal. An occlusive dressing (Fig. 5–5) is applied and all connections are properly taped or otherwise secured (Fig. 5–6) to prevent unintentional disconnection. The chest drainage system is placed and maintained below heart level at all times to assure proper drainage. A chest x-ray is ordered immediately following the procedure to assure correct tube placement.

■■■

TJ, with a hemopneumothorax, had two chest tubes inserted—an upper anterior tube to drain air (his pneumothorax) and a midaxillary tube to drain blood (his hemothorax). To facilitate chest drainage, the head of the bed should be elevated to enhance reduction of the pneumothorax, and he should be routinely turned to his affected (hemothorax) side to improve drainage of blood. Because MT had a simple pneumothorax, she required only one upper anterior tube to drain air. MT's head should be elevated to encourage air removal.

■■■

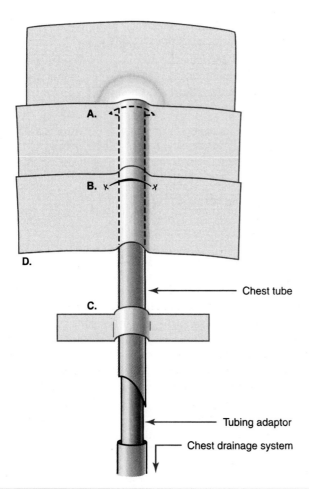

Figure 5–5 ■ Securing the chest tube. *A)* Incision site. *B)* Tube sutured to patient. *C)* Tube stabilized with tape. *D)* Occlusive dressing.

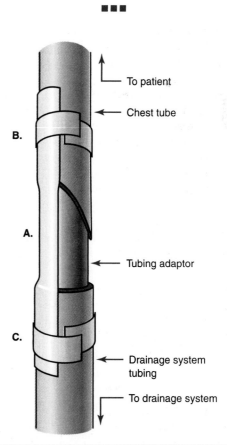

Figure 5–6 ■ *A)* Strip of cloth tape overlaps connection points along vertical axis. *B and C)* Strip of tape placed horizontally, overlapping vertical axis tape on both sides of connection.

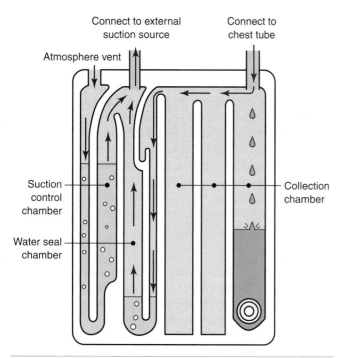

Figure 5-7 ■ Disposable self-contained chest drainage system.

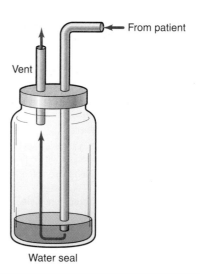

Figure 5-8 ■ Single-chamber (one-bottle) chest drainage system.

Chest Drainage System

Although there are a variety of chest drainage systems available, the most common is the disposable self-contained system such as is seen in Figure 5–7. This type of drainage system is sometimes referred to as a "three-chamber system," which includes the collection, water-seal, and suction chambers.

Collection Chamber. The collection chamber accepts air or fluid coming into the system through extension tubing directly attached to the patient's chest tube. The collection chamber is composed of several interconnected vertical towers that are marked in mL for ease of fluid volume measurement.

Water-Seal Chamber. The water-seal (or air-leak) chamber is located in the center of a three-chamber system. Its purpose is to act as a one-way valve to prevent airflow back into the patient. Prior to initial use, the water-seal chamber is filled with sterile water to the 2 cm mark.

The design of the water-seal chamber is simple but effective, being based on the one-bottle chest tube drainage system. To understand how the water-seal works, it may help to visualize a bottle filled with 2 cm (about 0.8 in.) of water (Fig. 5–8). The bottle is sealed with a tight lid with two holes punched into it. A long tube is inserted into the bottle through one of the holes such that the distal tip is under water (a water-seal). The bottle is placed on the floor and the proximal end of the tube is kept at bed height. Air is drawn into the bottle through the tube because of negative gravity pull. As the air is pulled through the distal end of the tube, it bubbles through the water and escapes through the second hole in the lid. Air left in the bottle, how-

ever, cannot move back into the tube because of the presence of the water-seal and negative gravity pull. Although it is not used commonly anymore in the United States, the one-bottle system is an effective method of managing simple pneumothorax.

Bubbling in the water-seal chamber indicates one of two things: (1) intermittent bubbling noted with pneumothorax suggests that air continues to be present in the intrapleural space, or (2) constant or vigorous bubbling may indicate an air leak in the system. If the patient's chest tube drainage system is not attached to external suction, the water level in the water-seal chamber should move up and down with breathing. This is a normal phenomenon called "tidling." Tidling ceases when the lung has reinflated.

Suction Chamber. The suction chamber regulates the amount of negative suction pressure being exerted on the intrapleural space. The amount of negative pressure is determined by the volume of water in the suction chamber. Typically, it is set at 20 cm H_2O in the adult. The suction chamber does not require attachment to external suction (e.g., wall suction) to work, but it is commonly added to make the system more effective. In the absence of external suction, the suction chamber does not bubble; however, if additional vacuum suction is used, continuous bubbling should be present. Vigorous bubbling in the suction chamber has no advantage and results in rapid evaporation, which requires more frequent refilling by the nurse. Gentle bubbling is all that is required.

Assessment of the Patient with a Chest Tube in Place

Assessing the patient with a chest tube includes assessment of the patient as well as assessment of the chest tube and drainage system. In assessing the patient's status, vital signs and respiratory status are closely monitored, including chest auscultation and oxygenation status (e.g., level of consciousness, ABG, pulse oximetry (SpO_2), skin/mucous membrane coloring, and respiratory effort). Chest radiographs may be ordered to monitor the status of the pneumothorax. Chest tube–related pain is common and should be assessed frequently with appropriate administration of analgesia.

Assessment of the chest tube and drainage system includes the dressing and site, position and patency of the extension tubing, type and amount of output draining into the collection chamber, and assessment of fluid levels and activities in the water-seal and suction chambers. Table 5–19 provides a summary of the assessment of the patient with a chest tube and drainage system.

Related Nursing Diagnoses

There are multiple nursing diagnoses and potential complications (PC) that frequently are applicable to the patient who requires a chest tube, including

- Anxiety
- Impaired gas exchange
- Ineffective breathing pattern
- Knowledge deficit
- Chest pain
- Risk for infection
- PC: hemorrhage
- PC: pneumothorax

TABLE 5–19   Assessment of the Patient with a Chest Tube Drainage System

Patient assessment	Vital signs
	Respiratory and oxygenation status (chest auscultation, level of consciousness, ABG, SpO_2, skin/mucous membrane coloring, and respiratory effort)
	Level of pain
Chest tube insertion site	Dressing should be occlusive, dry, and intact—reinforce as necessary (dressings may or may not be initially changed by the nurse based on hospital policy or physician or advanced practitioner orders)
	If dressing is changed, note appearance of tube insertion and suture sites
	Monitor for excessive bleeding through the dressing
	Palpate around dressing site for subcutaneous emphysema
	If affected area is enlarging, mark edge of area with pen to further evaluate rate and size of spread
Chest drainage system tube	**Extension tubing**
	Check all tubing connections to assure that they are secured to avoid unintentional disconnection
	Loop extension tubing horizontally on the bed to avoid excessive dependent looping, which may decrease drainage flow
	Collection chamber
	Routinely check blood or fluid output in the collection chamber
	Assess volume and appearance (sanguineous, serosanguineous, serous, purulent, etc.)
	Be aware of expected volume of bleeding for the first 24 hours following surgery and be alert for drainage above acceptable volume; a reverse appearance of drainage (serous → serosanguineous → sanguineous) as potential hemorrhage complication
	If clots are present, gently milk[a] the tubing to facilitate movement of clots into collection chamber
	Do not "strip" tubing[b]
	Routinely mark the volume on the outside of the collection chamber, indicating the time and date of the marking
	Water-seal chamber
	Assess for the presence of abnormal bubbling as an indication of a system leak
	Check water level to assure that it is at 2-cm level and refill if necessary
	Suction chamber
	Check level of water in chamber to assure that it is at 20-cm H_2O or other prescribed level and refill to prescribed level as required (to stop bubbling, temporarily pinch off the tubing that connects the drainage system to the external suction equipment)
	Check degree of bubbling in chamber and decrease level of external suction as needed to create gentle bubbling action
Documentation	If charting by exception, document abnormal vital signs and respiratory/oxygenation parameter; site appearance, excessive bleeding; presence of subcutaneous emphysema; abnormal chest output, such as excessive volume or change in drainage appearance (e.g., reversal of drainage appearance, or other abnormal characteristics)

[a]*Milking* refers to repeatedly squeezing the extension tubing without using a pulling motion. This is usually done starting at the proximal end (chest tube connection) and working down toward the collection chamber to encourage movement of clots.

[b]*Stripping* is a vigorous squeezing/pulling motion on extension tubing to move an obstructing clot. Stripping can create excessive negative intrapleural pressure that damages the pleura.

In summary, chest tube insertion is often required when the integrity of the pleural linings has been compromised, causing a loss of negative intrapleural pressure. Pneumothorax or hemothorax may result from an internal or external insult. Chest tube insertion is indicated when the percentage of lung collapse is 15 percent or greater. The nurse frequently assists with the chest tube insertion procedure in a variety of ways. The location of the chest tube insertion depends on the type of problem. A pneumothorax tube is placed high on the anterior chest to facilitate removal of air, whereas a hemothorax tube is placed lower on the chest near the midaxillary line to drain the lower lung field. The most common chest tube system is based on the three-bottle system. It is a disposable three-chamber unit containing the collection, water-seal, and suction chambers. Nursing diagnoses and collaborative potential complications guide the nurse in managing the care of the patient requiring a chest tube.

SECTION SIX REVIEW

1. Examples of internal origin problems that may require chest tube insertion include (choose all that apply)
   1. barotrauma
   2. penetrating chest trauma
   3. procedural rupture of visceral pleura
   4. chest contusion
   5. bleb rupture
   A. 1, 4, and 5
   B. 2, 3, and 4
   C. 1, 3, and 5
   D. 2, 4, and 5
2. Pneumothorax caused by positive end expiratory pressure (PEEP) represents which type of injury?
   A. procedural rupture
   B. chest contusion
   C. spontaneous bleb rupture
   D. barotrauma induced
3. Lung tissue collapses under which set of circumstances?
   A. increased pulmonary interstitial fluid pressure
   B. loss of negative intrapleural pressure
   C. increased pulmonary vascular resistance
   D. loss of capillary endothelium integrity
4. Common clinical findings associated with pneumothorax include (choose all that apply)
   1. tachypnea
   2. bradycardia
   3. respiratory acidosis
   4. shortness of breath
   5. decreased PaO_2
   A. 1, 4, and 5
   B. 2, 3, and 4
   C. 1, 3, and 5
   D. 1 and 5
5. The patient with a pneumothorax would most likely have a chest tube inserted at which location?
   A. midaxillary line, second intercostal space
   B. anterior chest, fourth intercostal space
   C. midaxillary line, fourth or fifth intercostal space
   D. anterior chest, second intercostal space
6. Immediately following the chest tube insertion procedure, correct placement is confirmed by
   A. arterial blood gas
   B. auscultation
   C. chest x-ray
   D. ultrasonography
7. The purpose of the water-seal chamber in a three-chamber chest drainage system is to
   A. facilitate drainage from the chest tube
   B. prevent airflow back into the patient
   C. facilitate control of level of negative suction
   D. prevent fluid from draining into the suction chamber
8. Vigorous bubbling in the water-seal chamber suggests that
   A. an air leak is present
   B. pneumothorax is still present
   C. wall suction pressure is too high
   D. the system is working correctly
9. The collection chamber is routinely assessed for (choose all that apply)
   1. fluid volume
   2. rate of volume increase
   3. drainage characteristics
   4. degree of bubbling
   A. 1, 2, and 4
   B. 2, 3, and 4
   C. 1, 2, and 3
   D. 1 and 2

Answers: 1. C, 2. D, 3. B, 4. A, 5. D, 6. C, 7. B, 8. A, 9. C

SECTION SEVEN: Developing a Pulmonary Plan of Care

Upon completion of this section, the learner will be able to develop a plan of care for a patient with altered respiratory function.

This section presents a standard respiratory plan of care based on the three approved nursing diagnoses, from the North American Nursing Diagnosis Association (NANDA), that focus on respiratory function. Each nursing diagnosis is defined, major patient outcomes are listed, and some of the major independent nursing interventions are provided. Patient outcomes reflect the relative nature of "normal" parameters, as they apply to the high-acuity patient population, who often has chronic respiratory disorders in addition to the current acute health problem.

Evidence-Based Practice

- *Morphine 4 mg (IV) administered 20 minutes prior to chest tube removal or ketorolac 30 mg (IV) administered 30 minutes prior to chest tube removal significantly reduced the pain associated with chest tube removal without causing adverse effects (Puntillo, Ley, 2004).*

- *Intratracheal instillation of a water-soluble vitamin E derivative may reduce the degree of injury of Gm-negative bacteria-induced acute lung injury (ALI) (Uchiyama, Takano, Yanagisawa, Inoue, et al., 2004).*

- *In patients with ALI/ARDS, prone positioning improved lung function, but not long-term survival (Gattinoni, Tognoni, Pesenti, et al., 2001).*

- *Use of a 0.12 percent chlorhexidine gluconate (Peridex) oral rinse was found to significantly reduce the incidence of nosocomial pneumonia in heart surgery patients who required intubation for more than 24 hours when compared to Listerine oral rinse (Houston, Hougland, Anderson, et al., 2002).*

- *ICU nurses' exposure to nitric oxide and its product nitrogen dioxide during nitric oxide therapy did not seem to pose a danger to nurses at concentrations up to 20 ppm. (Qureshi, Shah, Hemmen, et al., 2003).*

The Standard Respiratory Plan of Care

The three NANDA-approved respiratory nursing diagnoses are

- Breathing pattern, ineffective
- Gas exchange, impaired
- Airway clearance, ineffective

All three of the pulmonary-related nursing diagnoses may apply to high-acuity patients during a single illness. For this reason, the nurse may consider using an alternative that joins all three NANDA diagnoses, *impaired respiratory function* (Ulrich & Canale, 2001).

Breathing Pattern, Ineffective

Ineffective breathing pattern is defined as "[i]nspiration and/or expiration that does not provide adequate ventilation" (Ulrich & Canale, 2001, p. 19).

Desired Patient Outcomes. Maintenance of an effective breathing pattern is evidenced by

1. Normal respiratory rate, depth, and rhythm
2. ABGs and/or SpO_2 within normal limits for patient
3. Bilateral chest excursion
4. No dyspnea

Independent Nursing Interventions

1. Assess for ineffective breathing patterns (report abnormals)
   A. Respirations less than 8/min or greater than 30/min
   B. Increasingly shallow, labored breathing
   C. Increasing dyspnea
   D. Increasingly abnormal ABGs or pulse oximetry results
   E. Increasingly irregular breathing pattern
   F. Increasing use of accessory muscles
2. Monitor for abdominal or chest pain
3. Reduce level of abdominal or chest pain
   A. Regular administration of pain medication (observe for respiratory depression)
   B. Splint chest or abdomen with pillow or arms for coughing and deep-breathing exercises
4. Implement respiratory muscle strengthening exercises
5. Encourage incentive spirometer use every 1 to 2 hours
6. Encourage slow, deep breaths (as appropriate)
7. Elevate head of bed to 45 degrees or level of comfort
8. Turn (self or assisted) every 2 hours

Gas Exchange, Impaired

Impaired gas exchange is defined as "[e]xcess or deficit in oxygenation and/or carbon dioxide elimination at the alveolar–capillary membrane" (Ulrich & Canale, 2001, p. 35).

Desired Patient Outcomes. Maintenance of normal gas exchange is evidenced by

1. ABGs within normal (acceptable) limits for patient
2. Usual mental status
3. Breathing unlabored (or baseline for patient)
4. Respiratory rate 12 to 20/min (or usual rate for patient)
5. No use (or decreased use) of accessory respiratory muscles

Independent Nursing Interventions

1. Assess for impaired gas exchange (report abnormals)
   A. Change in mental status
      1. Increased lethargy
      2. Increased restlessness
      3. Confusion

B. Accessory muscle use
C. Abnormal ABGs
   1. Elevated $PaCO_2$ (above acceptable limits)
   2. Decreased PaO_2 (below acceptable limits)
D. Decreasing pulse oximetry readings
2. Turn every 2 hours
3. Encourage incentive spirometer use every 1 to 2 hours
4. Maintain position of comfort, with head of bed elevated greater than 30 degrees (assist to tripod position, if desired)
5. Monitor effects of drug therapy (including oxygen therapy)
6. Encourage early ambulation
7. Assist patient to sit up in chair

Airway Clearance, Ineffective

Ineffective airway clearance is defined as "[i]nability to clear secretions or obstructions from the respiratory tract to maintain a clear airway" (Ulrich & Canale, 2001, p. 13).

Desired Patient Outcomes. Maintenance of effective airway clearance is evidenced by

1. Normal or improved lung sounds
2. No cyanosis
3. Normal respiratory rate and depth
4. No dyspnea

Independent Nursing Interventions
1. Assess for ineffective airway clearance
   A. Adventitious breath sounds
   B. Ineffective cough

C. Respirations greater than 24/min
D. Respiratory depth shallow
E. Presence of cyanosis
F. Complaint of dyspnea
2. Assist patient to cough and deep breathe every 1 to 2 hours
3. Encourage fluids to 2 to 2.5 L per 24 hours or 600 to 800 mL per 8-hour shift (if not contraindicated)
4. Perform tracheal suction as necessary
5. Monitor for effects of drug therapy (expectorants, mucolytics)
6. Monitor for and treat acute pain
7. Administer pain medications, as needed
8. Encourage self-care as tolerated
9. Encourage activity and early ambulation

In summary, there are three NANDA-approved respiratory-focused nursing diagnoses. In complex patients in whom all three problems are present, the alternative diagnosis *impaired respiratory function* may be used. Many of the desired patient outcomes and independent nursing interventions overlap among the three diagnoses. Regardless of the exact medical diagnosis attached to the patient, a plan of care can be developed if the nurse has an understanding of the underlying pathophysiologic problem.

SECTION SEVEN REVIEW

1. Evaluation of the effectiveness of interventions to resolve the nursing diagnosis ineffective breathing patterns is best measured by which of the following desired patient outcomes?
   A. usual mental status
   B. normal or improved lung sounds
   C. absent accessory muscle use
   D. normal respiratory rate, depth, and rhythm
2. The state in which a person experiences decreased passage of oxygen and/or carbon dioxide between the alveoli and the vascular system is the definition of
   A. impaired gas exchange
   B. ineffective breathing pattern
   C. ineffective airway clearance
   D. altered respiratory function
3. Assessments for impaired gas exchange in the early stage would include (choose all that apply)

   1. confusion
   2. increased lethargy
   3. decreased restlessness
   4. change in mental status
   A. 1, 2, and 3
   B. 2, 3, and 4
   C. 1, 2, and 4
   D. 2 and 4
4. Nursing interventions that would assist in maintaining effective airway clearance would include
   A. restrict fluids to 1 L/day
   B. cough and deep breathe every 1 to 2 hours
   C. minimize use of opioid analgesics
   D. restrict activities

Answers: 1. D, 2. A, 3. C, 4. B

POSTTEST

The following Posttest is constructed in a case study format. A patient is presented, and questions are asked based on available data. New data are presented as the case study progresses.

John Huang is a 68-year-old grocery store owner. He has a 45-year history of smoking one to two packs of cigarettes per day. He was diagnosed about 10 years ago with COPD. Mr. Huang is admitted to the hospital with severe dyspnea and a productive cough. He is diagnosed with right lower lobe pneumonia. He is currently receiving oxygen therapy per nasal prongs at 2 L/min.

1. Based only on available data, Mr. Huang's pneumonia condition would be considered an acute
   A. ventilatory failure
   B. obstructive disease
   C. respiratory failure
   D. restrictive disease

2. Mr. Huang's pneumonia affects expiratory airflow in which way?
   A. increases
   B. decreases
   C. no effect
   D. increases or decreases

3. His obstructive pulmonary disorder is associated with
   A. decreased tidal volumes
   B. increased inspiratory times
   C. decreased inspiratory airflow
   D. increased expiratory times

4. Assuming Mr. Huang is in a state of chronic respiratory insufficiency, he would most likely exhibit which clinical finding related to his chronic condition?
   A. increased blood pressure
   B. decreased respiratory rate
   C. increased temperature
   D. decreased pulse rate

5. If Mr. Huang develops acute ventilatory failure, you would anticipate which arterial blood gas finding?
   A. PaO_2 less than 60 mm Hg
   B. $PaCO_2$ greater than 50 mm Hg
   C. PaO_2 greater than 100 mm Hg
   D. $PaCO_2$ less than 35 mm Hg

6. According to the module, respiratory failure is clinically defined as
   A. $PaCO_2$ 50 mm Hg or greater with pH 7.30 and/or PaO_2 60 mm Hg or less
   B. $PaCO_2$ 60 mm Hg with a pH 7.30 and PaO_2 less than 60 mm Hg
   C. $PaCO_2$ 45 mm Hg with a pH 7.35 and/or PaO_2 80 mm Hg
   D. $PaCO_2$ 60 mm Hg with a pH 7.35 and PaO_2 80 mm Hg

7. ARDS is a pulmonary disorder that initially causes
   A. lung destruction
   B. ventilatory failure

   C. alveolar hypoventilation
   D. oxygenation failure

8. The nurse is developing a plan of care for the nursing diagnosis *impaired gas exchange*. Of the following, which desired patient outcome most accurately measures this diagnosis?
   A. ABG within normal limits for patient
   B. SaO_2 greater than 95 percent
   C. usual mental status
   D. no cyanosis

9. The nurse writes the nursing diagnosis *ineffective airway clearance* on Mr. Huang's care plan. All of the following are appropriate interventions to address this diagnosis EXCEPT
   A. administer pain medications as needed
   B. cough and deep breathe every 1 to 2 hours
   C. limit fluid intake to less than 1 L/24 hours
   D. tracheal suction as necessary

A 22-year-old female, Shelida W, was admitted to Trauma ICU after sustaining severe multiple trauma injuries in an automobile–tree collision. She has multiple abrasions on her head, arms, and legs; an open right femur fracture; right humeral fracture and pelvic fractures; and a ruptured spleen. She required multiple blood transfusions as a result of the development of hypovolemic shock. Since her admission, she has been on a mechanical ventilator. On day 5 postadmission, she developed sepsis.

10. Examine Shelida's presenting history. List three factors that place her at increased risk for development of ALI/ARDS.

   1. _____
   2. _____
   3. _____

It is now day 7 postadmission. Shelida has a pulmonary artery catheter and arterial line in place. The nurse is concerned with the deterioration in Shelida's SpO_2 regardless of supportive interventions. The nurse performs assessments and then contacts the physician who orders an immediate arterial blood gas and portable chest x-ray.

11. If Shelida is developing ALI/ARDS, the nurse would anticipate which values in her hemodynamic readings?
   A. deteriorating pulmonary artery pressures
   B. normal pulmonary artery wedge pressures
   C. elevated pulmonary artery pressures
   D. elevated pulmonary artery wedge pressures

The nurse calculates Shelida's PaO_2/FIO_2 ratio. It is 180 mm Hg.

12. True or False: Assuming that the medical team uses the ARDS consensus criteria, Shelida's PaO_2/FIO_2 ratio meets the criterion for ARDS.

13. Shelida's ABG result is pH 7.48; Pa_{CO_2} 32, Pa_{O_2} 64, and HCO_3 25. Which statement best explains the acid–base state reflected in her ABG result?
    A. she is triggering the ventilator at 28 to 32 breaths per minute
    B. her heart rate and blood pressure have been steadily increasing
    C. the oxygen concentration on her ventilator was increased 30 minutes ago
    D. she received pain medication 30 minutes ago

14. A bronchoalveolar lavage (BAL) fluid sample is taken from her lungs. If Shelida has ALI/ARDS, the fluid should contain
    A. no inflammatory cells
    B. low protein content
    C. high RBC content
    D. high protein content

Shelida is diagnosed with ARDS.

15. The nurse is explaining the concept of nonhydrostatic pulmonary edema to Shelida's family. Which statement, if made by the family, suggests that they understand the concept sufficiently?
    A. "Her disease has injured the membranes in her lung so that fluid is leaking into her lungs from the tiny blood vessels."
    B. "The high blood pressure in the left side of her heart is forcing fluid from her blood vessels into her lung tissue."
    C. "Infection in her lungs has harmed the small blood vessels there, causing blood to spill into the lung tissue."
    D. "The small air sacs have been destroyed, which has allowed air to enter into the blood vessels."

16. The nurse notes that Shelida's peak airway pressures are now above 50 cm H_2O. The reason for this development in the ALI/ARDS patient is
    A. onset of pneumonia
    B. development of microemboli
    C. development of $\dot{V}/\dot{Q}$ mismatch
    D. extensive atelectasis

17. Shelida's physician writes an order to maintain the peak airway pressure at less than 45 cm H_2O through permissive hypercapnia. The rationale for this intervention is based on which effect of carbon dioxide?
    A. anesthetic
    B. vasodilation
    C. analgesic
    D. vasoconstriction

18. Shelida is now receiving positive end expiratory pressure (PEEP). The medical team adheres to a "least PEEP" protocol. According to the module, least PEEP uses the minimum PEEP required to achieve a Sa_{O_2} of at least _____ percent with an F_{IO_2} (oxygen concentration) of _____ or less.

A. 75, 0.45 (45 percent)
B. 80, 0.50 (50 percent)
C. 85, 0.55 (55 percent)
D. 90, 0.60 (60 percent)

Brian J, 32 years old, is recovering from major surgery, in which he had left femur reconstruction performed. He has been immobilized for 7 days.

19. Based on Brian's available history, which factors of Virchow's triad are in place that make him at risk for development of deep-vein thrombosis? (check all that apply)
    _____ venous stasis
    _____ hypercoagulability
    _____ venous (endothelial) injury

Today, the nurse becomes concerned with an acute change in Brian's pulmonary status.

20. To assess Brian for a possible pulmonary embolus, for what common signs and symptoms would the nurse monitor him? (list all that apply)
    1. _____
    2. _____
    3. _____
    4. _____
    5. _____
    6. _____

21. The physician orders a D-dimer assay. The purpose of using this test initially is to
    A. confirm the presence of a pulmonary embolism
    B. rule out pulmonary embolism
    C. check for presence of hypercoagulability
    D. rule out pulmonary edema

22. Brian has an ABG drawn. Assuming that he has a pulmonary embolism, what ABG results would the nurse anticipate seeing?
    A. acute respiratory alkalosis with hypoxemia
    B. acute respiratory acidosis with hypoxemia
    C. acute metabolic alkalosis with hypoxemia
    D. acute metabolic acidosis with hypoxemia

23. The definitive diagnostic test for the presence of pulmonary embolism is
    A. $\dot{V}/\dot{Q}$ scan
    B. angiogram
    C. compression ultrasound
    D. D-dimer assay

24. True or False: Most diagnoses of pulmonary embolism are not made until postmortem.

25. True or False: Most pulmonary emboli are small and breakdown on their own.

26. What treatment options may be considered? (short answer)
    _____
    _____
    _____

Wen Wu, 43 years old, flew to Hong Kong to visit his family. Near the end of his visit, his sister (a nurse at a local hospital) became ill with what appeared to be a severe chest cold. Mr. Wu returned to his home in San Francisco the next day. Several days later, he became ill at work, complaining of sore muscles and feeling feverish. He was unable to work the next day and felt even worse than the day before. By day 7 of his illness, he developed a dry cough and was complaining of having difficulty breathing. His wife became alarmed and drove him to a local hospital emergency department.

27. In the emergency department, a portable chest x-ray was taken. If Mr. Wu has developed SARS, what will the chest x-ray show?
    A. presence of pneumonia
    B. enlarged right heart
    C. normal lungs
    D. pleural effusions

28. What should make the hospital emergency department staff suspicious of SARS rather than some other form of pneumonia?
    A. his Chinese heritage
    B. the fact that he flew (recirculating air)
    C. his recent trip to Hong Kong
    D. his chest x-ray results

29. The MOST COMMON presenting manifestations of SARS include (check all that apply)
    _____ fever greater than 100°F (37.8°C)
    _____ sore throat
    _____ severe myalgias
    _____ hemoptysis
    _____ mild headache
    _____ chest pain
    _____ extreme weakness
    _____ persistent dry cough
    _____ petechiae on trunk

30. The nurse is aware that about _____ percent of SARS patients progress to ALI/ARDS.
    A. 25
    B. 33
    C. 50
    D. 75

31. True or False: Mr. Wu's age (43) places him in the increased mortality category.

32. Mr. Wu has a battery of laboratory tests drawn, such as CBC with differential, blood cultures, and Gram stain and culture. For what primary reason are these tests performed in a patient who may have SARS? (short answer)

    _____

    _____

    _____

Based on Mr. Wu's history and presenting manifestations, he is tested for SARS-CoV.

33. What predictive value are the specialized tests for this virus, in the absence of confirmation of exposure to SARS-CoV?
    A. low predictive value
    B. high predictive value

34. You are the nurse assigned to Mr. Wu. As you prepare to enter his isolation room, the CDC recommends that you wear (check all that apply)
    _____ protective eyewear
    _____ booties
    _____ mask (N 96 or equivalent)
    _____ hair cover
    _____ one set of gloves
    _____ fluid resistant gown

35. Mr. Wu requires mechanical ventilation. Based on the reading, specify who should be in his room when intubation is being performed. (short answer)

    _____

    _____

36. What type of preintubation drug therapy is recommended for Mr. Wu as a patient with SARS?
    A. deep sedation
    B. nebulized local anesthesia
    C. small dose of IV diazepam
    D. neuromuscular blockade

37. Mr. Wu must be disconnected temporarily from the mechanical ventilator. Before detaching the connection, what ventilator setting should the ventilator be placed on and why?
    ■ Ventilator setting: _____
    ■ Rationale: _____

Clinical Update: Mr. Wu suddenly becomes more tachycardiac, his SpO$_2$ drops, and his peak inspiratory pressure increases. The nurse immediately auscultates his lungs and finds that he has no lung sounds in his right upper lung field. A chest x-ray confirms a right upper lobe pneumothorax. A chest tube is ordered.

38. The nurse is positioning Mr. Wu for the chest tube procedure. Which position would be most appropriate for insertion of a chest tube for a right pneumothorax?
    A. high-Fowler's position
    B. flat in the bed on his right side
    C. mild Trendelenburg position on left side
    D. right side with head of bed elevated 30 degrees

39. Mr. Wu has had his chest tube in place for 2 days. While assessing the chest drainage system, the nurse notes continuous vigorous bubbling in the water-seal chamber. The appropriate action to take would be
    A. decrease the amount of wall suction attached to the system
    B. check all connections for a leak
    C. check for subcutaneous emphysema
    D. place Mr. Wu on his left side

40. Mr. Wu is to have his chest tube removed today. Based on recent research regarding pain control during chest tube removal, which action is most effective (assuming that orders are present)?

A. place warm, dry heat over the dressing site directly following tube removal

B. give PO diazepam (Valium) 1 hour before the planned tube removal

C. provide Mr. Wu with a thorough explanation of the tube removal procedure

D. administer IV analgesia so that the drug's peak effect coincides with tube removal

POSTTEST ANSWERS

Question	Answer	Section
1	D	One
2	C	One
3	D	One
4	A	Two
5	B	Two
6	A	Two
7	D	Two
8	A	Seven
9	C	Seven
10	Multiple trauma, hypovolemic shock, blood transfusions	Three
11	B	Three
12	True; the criterion for P[a–A]O$_2$ ratio is set at 200 mm Hg. The Modified Lung Injury Scale, however, sets it at 175 mm Hg.	Three
13	A	Three
14	D	Three
15	A	Three
16	D	Three
17	B	Three
18	D	Three
19	Venous stasis and venous (endothelial) injury	Four
20	The most common signs and symptoms are dyspnea, tachypnea, pleural pain, crackles (rales), tachycardia, and cough.	Four
21	B	Four
22	A	Four
23	B	Four
24	True. PE is difficult to diagnose, particularly when the PE is severe enough to require emergency level interventions.	Four

Question	Answer	Section
25	True. It is believed that many PE go undetected, requiring no medical interventions.	Four
26	Anticoagulant therapy, thrombolytic therapy, surgical embolectomy, vena cava filter.	Four
27	A	Five
28	C	Five
29	Fever greater than 100°F (37.8°C), severe myalgias, mild headache, extreme weakness, persistent dry cough.	Five
30	A	Five
31	False. Sixty years old or older has increased risk.	Five
32	These tests rule out other, more common pathogens.	Five
33	A	Five
34	All except booties are required.	Five
35	Only the staff directly involved in the intubation procedure.	Five
36	A	Five
37	Stand-by; to prevent spraying of virus-contaminated fluid.	Five
38	A	Six
39	B	Six
40	D	Evidence-Based Practice Box

REFERENCES

Abcarian, P. W., Sweet, J. D., Watabe, J. T., & Yoon, H-C. (2003). Role of a quantitative D-dimer assay in determining the need for CT angiography of acute pulmonary embolism. *American Journal of Roentgenology, 182*(6),1377–1381.

ARDS Network (The Acute Respiratory Distress Syndrome Network). (n.d.). Available at: *http://www.ardsnet.org/index.php*. Accessed June 1, 2004.

ARDS Network (The Acute Respiratory Distress Syndrome Network).

(2000). Ventilation with lower tidal volumes as compared with traditional tidal volumes for acute lung injury and the acute respiratory distress syndrome. *New England Journal of Medicine, 342*(18), 1301–1308.

Ashbaugh, D. G., Bigelow, D. B., Petty, T. L., & Levine, B. E. (1967). Acute respiratory distress in adults. *Lancet, 2*(7511), 319–323.

Avendano, M., Derkach, P., & Swan, S. (2003). Clinical course and management of SARS in health care workers in Toronto: A case series. *Canadian Medical Association Journal, 168*(13), 1649–1659.

Awtry, E. H., & Loscalzo, J. (2001). Vascular diseases and hypertension. In C. C. J. Carpenter, R. C. Griggs, & J. Loscalzo (Eds.), *Cecil essentials of medicine* (5th ed., pp. 145–163). Philadelphia: W.B. Saunders.

Bigatello, L. M., & Hellman, J. (2003). Inhaled nitric oxide for ARDS: Searching for a more focused use. *Intensive Care Medicine, 29*(10), 1623–1626.

Breiburg, A. N., Aitken, L., Reaby, L., Clancy, R. L., & Pierce, J. D. (2000). Efficacy and safety of prone positioning for patients with acute respiratory distress syndrome. *Journal of Advanced Nursing, 32*(4), 922–929.

Carpenito-Moyet, L. J. (2004). *Nursing diagnosis: Application to clinical practice* (10th ed.). Philadelphia: Lippincott/Williams & Wilkins.

CDC [Centers for Disease Control]. (2004). Severe acute respiratory syndrome: In the absence of SARS-CoV transmission worldwide: Guidance for surveillance, clinical and laboratory evaluation, and reporting version 2. Available at: *www.cdc.gov/ncidod/sars/*. Accessed June 5, 2004.

Chunilal, S. D., Eikelboom, J. W., Attia, J., et al. (2003). Clinician's corner: Does this patient have a pulmonary embolism? *JAMA, 290*(21), 2849–2858.

Conrad, S. A. (2002). Venous air embolism? *E-medicine.* Available at: *www.emedicine.com/emerg/topic787.htm.* Accessed June 12, 2004.

Cooper, A., Joglekar, A., & Adhikari, N. (2003, October 14). A practical approach to airway management in patients with SARS. *Canadian Medical Association Journal, 169*(8).

Croce, M. A., Fabian, T. C., Davis, K. A., & Gavin, T. (1999). Early and late acute respiratory distress syndrome: Two distinct clinical entities. *Journal of Trauma-Injury Infection & Critical Care, 46*(3), 361–367.

Crouser, E. D., & Fahy, R. J. (2003). Acute lung injury, pulmonary edema, and multiple system organ failure. In R. L. Wilkins, J. K. Stoller, & C. L. Scanlan, *Egan's fundamentals of respiratory care* (8th ed., pp. 537–556). St. Louis: C. V. Mosby.

Curley, M. A. (1999). Prone positioning of patients with acute respiratory distress syndrome: A systematic review. *American Journal of Critical Care 8*(6), 397–405.

Davidson, T. A., Caldwell, E. S., Curtis, J. R., Hudson, L. D., & Steinberg, K. P. (1999). Reduced quality of life in survivors of acute respiratory distress syndrome compared with critically ill control patients. *Journal of American Medical Association, 281*(4), 354–360.

Davies, S. (2001). Amniotic fluid embolus: A review of the literature. *Canadian Journal of Anesthesia, 48,* 88–98.

Davis, K., Johannigman, J., Campbell, R., et al. (2001). The acute effects of body position strategies and respiratory therapy in paralyzed patients with acute lung injury. *Critical Care, 5,* 81–87.

Eisner, M. D., Thompson, T., Hudson, L. D., et al., & the Acute Respiratory Distress Syndrome Network. (2001). Efficacy of low tidal volume ventilation in patients with different clinical risk factors for acute lung injury and the acute respiratory distress syndrome. *American Journal of Respiratory and Critical Care Medicine, 164,* 231–236.

Gattinoni, L., Tognoni, G., Pesenti, A., et al. (2001). Effect of prone positioning on the survival of patients with acute respiratory failure. *New England Journal of Medicine, 345*(8), 568–573.

Gerlach, M., Keh, D., & Gerlach, H. (1999). Inhaled nitric oxide for acute respiratory distress syndrome. *Respiratory Care, 44*(2), 184–192.

Hite, R. D., & Morris, P. E. (2001). Acute respiratory distress syndrome. *Drugs 2001, 61*(7), 897–907.

Holmes, K. V. (2003). SARS-associated coronavirus. *New England Journal of Medicine, 348*(20), 1948–1951.

Houston, S., Hougland, P., Anderson, J., et al. (2002). Effectiveness of 0.12% chlorhexidine gluconate oral rinse in reducing prevalence of nosocomial pneumonia in patients undergoing heart surgery. *American Journal of Critical Care 11,*(6), 567–570.

Jassal, D., Sharma, S., & Maycher, B. (2004). Pulmonary hypertension. *E-medicine.* Available at: *www.emedicine.com/radio/topic583.htm.* Accessed June 12, 2004.

Lapinsky, S. E., & Hawryluck, L. (2003). ICU management of severe acute respiratory syndrome. *Intensive Care Medicine, 29*(6), 870–875.

Lew, T., Kwek, T-K., Tai, D., et al. (2003). Acute respiratory distress syndrome in critically ill patients with severe acute respiratory syndrome. *Journal of the American Medical Association, 290*(3), 374–380.

Lynn-McHale, D., & Carlson, K. (Eds.). (2001). *AACN procedure manual for critical care* (4th ed.). Philadelphia: W. B. Saunders.

Martin, A. (2001). Should continuous lateral rotation therapy replace manual turning? *Dimensions in Critical Care Nursing 2001, 20*(1), 42–49.

Matthay, M., Zimmerman, G., Esmon, C., et al. (2003). Future research directions in acute lung injury: Summary of a national heart, lung, and blood institute working group. *American Journal of Respiratory and Critical Care Medicine, 167,* 1027–1035.

Meduri, G. U., Headley, A. S., Golden, E., et al. (1998). Effect of prolonged methylprednisolone therapy in unresolving acute respiratory distress syndrome. *Journal of the American Medical Association, 280*(2), 159–165.

Mellor, A., & Soni, N. (2001). Fat embolism. *Anaesthesia, 56,* 145–154.

Miller, K., Lutz, A., & Durnisch, M. (2004). Case report: Use of prone positioning in late-phase ARDS. *RT: Journal for Respiratory Care Practitioners.*

MMWR. (2003). Update: Severe acute respiratory syndrome—United States. Available at: *www.cdc.gov/mmwr/preview/mmwrhtml/mm5220a2.htm.* Accessed May 4, 2004.

Moloney, E. D., & Griffiths, M. J. D. (2004). Protective ventilation of patients with acute respiratory distress syndrome. *British Journal of Anaesthesia, 92*(2), 261–270.

Murray, T. A., & Patterson, L. A. (2002). Prone positioning of trauma patients with acute respiratory distress syndrome and open abdominal incisions. *Critical Care Nurse, 22*(3), 52–56.

Newman, V., Gonzalez, R., Matthay, M., & Dobbs, L. (2000). A novel alveolar type 1 cell-specific biochemical marker of human acute lung injury. *American Journal of Respiratory and Critical Care Medicine, 161,* 990–995.

Porth, C. M. (2002). Alterations in respiration: Alterations in ventilation and gas exchange. In C. M. Porth (Ed.), *Pathophysiology: Concepts of altered health states* (6th ed., pp. 633–670). Philadelphia: J. B. Lippincott.

Puntillo, K., & Ley, S. J. (2004). Appropriately timed analgesics control chest pain due to chest tube removal. *American Journal of Critical Care, 13*(4), 292–303.

Quereshi, M., Shah, N., Hemmen, C., et al. (2003). Exposure of intensive care unit nurses to nitric oxide and nitrogen dioxide during therapeutic use of inhaled nitric oxide in adults with acute respiratory distress syndrome. *American Journal of Critical Care, 12*(2), 147–153.

Quinlan, D. J., McQuillan, A., & Eikelboom, J. W. (2004). Low-molecular-weight heparin compared with intravenous unfractionated heparin for treatment of pulmonary embolism. *Annals of Internal Medicine 140,*(3), 175–183.

Sakka, S. G., Klein, M., Reinhart, M. D., & Meier-Hellmann, A. (2002). Clinical investigations in critical care: Prognostic value of extravascular lung water in critically ill patients. *Chest, 122*(6), 2080–2086.

SARS Scientific Committee. (2003). Guidelines for the acute management of the patient with SARS in the hospital setting. British Columbia Center for Disease Control.

Stein, P. D., & Henry, J. W. (1997). Clinical characteristics of patients with acute pulmonary embolism stratified according to their presenting syndromes. *Chest, 112*(4), 974–979.

Uchiyama, K., Takano, H., Yanagisawa, R., Inoue, K., et al. (2004). A novel water-soluble vitamin E derivative prevents acute lung injury by bacterial endotoxin. *Clinical and Experimental Pharmacology and Physiology, 31,* 226–230.

Ulrich, S. P., & Canale, S. W. (2001). *Nursing care planning guides* (5th ed.). Philadelphia: W. B. Saunders.

Vollman, K. M., & Aulbach, R. K. (1998). Acute respiratory distress syndrome. In M. R. Kinney, S. B. Dunbar, J. A. Brooks-Brunn, N. Molter, & J. M. Vitello-Cicciu (Eds.), *AACN clinical reference for critical care nursing* (4th ed., pp. 529–564). St. Louis: C. V. Mosby.

WHO. (2003). Update 31—Coronavirus never before seen in humans is the cause of SARS. Available at: *www.who.int/csr/sarsarchive/2003_04_16?en/print.html.* Accessed June 6, 2004.

Mechanical Ventilation

Gail Priestley, Kathleen Dorman Wagner

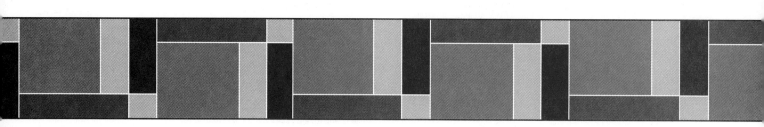

OBJECTIVES Following completion of this module, the learner will be able to

1. Correctly state why a mechanical ventilator is not a mechanical respirator.

2. Identify criteria used to determine the need for mechanical ventilator support.

3. Discuss the equipment necessary to initiate mechanical ventilation.

4. Describe the types of mechanical ventilators, based on mechanism of force and cycling mechanism.

5. Explain the commonly monitored ventilator settings.

6. Briefly explain two methods of providing noninvasive ventilatory support.

7. Discuss the major complications of mechanical ventilation.

8. Explain the cause and prevention of artificial airway complications.

9. Describe the care of the patient requiring mechanical ventilation.

10. Describe the weaning process.

This self-study module focuses on a variety of concepts related to initiation of mechanical ventilation and management of the patient on a mechanical ventilator. This module uses information covered in two other modules: Module 4 "Determinants and Assessment of Pulmonary Gas Exchange," and Module 5, "Alterations in Pulmonary Gas Exchange." It is suggested that the reader become familiar with the material in those two modules before reading this one.

This module is divided into 10 sections. Sections One through Six include such topics as criteria used for determination of the need for mechanical ventilation, required equipment to initiate mechanical ventilation, various types of mechanical ventilators, a brief discussion of the more commonly monitored ventilator settings, and noninvasive ventilatory support. In Sections Seven and Eight, the focus shifts to a discussion of how mechanical ventilation and artificial airways affect various parts of the body, including information about potential complications and methods to avoid them. Section Nine describes the nursing management of the mechanically ventilated patient. This section focuses on respiratory-related nursing diagnoses. The final section briefly describes the weaning process. Each section includes a set of review questions to help the learner evaluate his or her understanding of the section's content before moving on to the next section. All Section Reviews and the module Pretest and Posttest include answers. It is suggested that the learner review those concepts answered incorrectly in the review questions before proceeding to the next section.

 PRETEST

1. Mechanical ventilators are responsible for
   A. diffusion
   B. ventilation
   C. perfusion
   D. respiration

2. The most common indication for use of a mechanical ventilator is
   A. pneumonia
   B. chronic obstructive pulmonary disease (COPD)
   C. acute asthmatic attack
   D. acute ventilatory failure

3. Acute ventilatory failure is associated with
   A. alveolar hypoventilation
   B. severe hypoxemia
   C. alveolar hyperventilation
   D. severe hypocarbia

4. Acute respiratory acidosis can be defined clinically as
   A. pH greater than 7.50, PaO_2 less than 60 mm Hg
   B. pH less than 7.30, $PaCO_2$ greater than 50 mm Hg
   C. pH greater than 7.50, PaO_2 less than 35 mm Hg
   D. pH less than 7.30, $PaCO_2$ less than 30 mm Hg

5. The primary purpose of the endotracheal tube cuff is to seal off the
   A. lower airway from the upper airway
   B. lower airway from the esophagus
   C. oropharynx from the nasopharynx
   D. oropharynx from the esophagus

6. The most common type of airway access used during an emergency is
   A. tracheostomy
   B. nasal intubation
   C. pharyngeal airway
   D. oral intubation

7. A major advantage of volume-cycled ventilation is that it
   A. applies negative pressure to the thorax
   B. overcomes changes in lung compliance
   C. does not require an artificial airway
   D. automatically adjusts volume of gas delivered

8. A low tidal volume is associated most closely with
   A. hypoventilation
   B. hypocapnia
   C. hypoxia
   D. hypotension

9. The fraction of inspired oxygen (FIO_2) is correctly measured in
   A. decimals
   B. percentages
   C. centimeters of water pressure (cm H_2O)
   D. millimeters of mercury (mm Hg)

10. Synchronized intermittent mandatory ventilation (SIMV) is sensitive to
    A. rate of airflow
    B. respiratory rate
    C. concentration of oxygen
    D. the patient's ventilatory cycle

11. A common side effect of positive end-expiratory pressure (PEEP) is
    A. increased blood pressure
    B. decreased cardiac output
    C. decreased lung compliance
    D. increased venous return to the heart

12. During positive pressure ventilation, airflow will be greatest
    A. in areas that are diseased
    B. in areas that are nondependent
    C. in the peripheral lung areas
    D. in the lung apices

13. In what way does positive pressure ventilation affect intracranial pressure (ICP)?
    A. it has no effect
    B. it decreases ICP
    C. it increases ICP
    D. its effects are unknown

14. What effect does positive pressure ventilation have on renal function?
    A. urine output is unaffected
    B. urine output is decreased
    C. urine output is increased
    D. its effects are unknown

15. The term *barotrauma* refers to injury caused by
    A. oxygen
    B. friction
    C. temperature
    D. pressure

16. Oxygen toxity has what effect on lung tissue?
    A. it increases surfactant production
    B. it decreases mucous production
    C. it increases macrophage activity
    D. it increases lung compliance

17. Endotracheal cuff trauma can be avoided by maintaining cuff pressures in the range of
    A. 5 to 10 mm Hg
    B. 10 to 20 mm Hg
    C. 20 to 25 mm Hg
    D. 25 to 30 mm Hg

18. Noninvasive intermittent positive pressure ventilation (NIPPV) is most useful for the patient who
    A. requires only support of tidal volume
    B. cannot fully support his or her own expiratory effort
    C. requires only support for nocturnal hypercapnia and hypoxemia
    D. cannot fully support his or her own ventilatory effort over long periods of time

19. Common complications of noninvasive methods of ventilatory support include (choose all that apply)
    1. conjunctivitis
    2. nasal congestion
    3. hypoventilation
    4. otitis media
    A. 1, 2, and 4
    B. 2, 3, and 4
    C. 2 and 3
    D. 1, 2, and 3

20. The majority of difficult-to-wean patients have which problem?
    A. pneumonia
    B. congestive heart failure
    C. acute respiratory distress syndrome
    D. chronic pulmonary disease

21. The term _____ weaning is used to refer to weaning by intermittently removing the patient from the ventilator for increasing periods of time.
- **A.** manual
- **B.** ventilator

C. IMV/SIMV

D. pressure support ventilation

Pretest Answers: 1. B, 2. D, 3. A, 4. B, 5. A, 6. D, 7. B, 8. A, 9. A, 10. D, 11. B, 12. B, 13. C, 14. B, 15. D, 16. B, 17. C, 18. D, 19. D, 20. D, 21. A

GLOSSARY

acute ventilatory failure (AVF) A state of respiratory decompensation in which the lungs are unable to maintain adequate alveolar ventilation, losing the ability to eliminate carbon dioxide.

airway resistance (R_{aw}) The amount of opposition to airway flow through the conducting system.

alveolar ventilation ($\dot{V}A$) The air that fills the alveoli and is available for gas exchange.

assist-control mode (AC or ACMV) A mechanical ventilation mode that combines two single modes: assist, a patient-sensitive mode; and control, a time-triggered mode.

Auto-PEEP The unintentional buildup of positive end-expiratory pressure caused by airtrapping.

barotrauma Injury to pulmonary tissues as a result of excessive pressures.

compliance The amount of force required to expand the lungs; measured in mL/cm H_2O; normal is 50 to 100 mL/cm H_2O.

continuous positive airway pressure (CPAP) The application of positive pressure to the airway of a spontaneously breathing person (see positive end-expiratory pressure [PEEP]).

cycle The mechanisms by which the inspiratory phase is stopped and the expiratory phase is started.

deadspace ventilation ($\dot{V}D$) Air that fills the conducting airways and does not take part in gas exchange.

extubation Removal of an endotracheal or tracheostomy tube from the patient's airway.

fraction of inspired oxygen (F_{IO_2}) That portion of the total gas being inspired that is composed of oxygen; expressed in decimals from 0.21 to 1.0.

intermittent mandatory ventilation (IMV) A mechanical ventilator mode that allows the patient to breathe spontaneously through ventilator circuitry while interspersing mandatory mechanical breaths at even intervals via a preset rate.

negative inspiratory force (NIF) Also called maximum inspiratory force (MIF). The amount of negative pressure a person can exert during inspiration; normal is −50 to −100 cm H_2O.

noninvasive intermittent positive pressure ventilation (NIPPV) The application of positive pressure ventilation using a mechanical ventilator and a mask in place of an artificial airway.

P_{aCO_2} The partial pressure of carbon dioxide as it exists in the arterial blood; normal range is 35 to 45 mm Hg.

P_{aO_2} The partial pressure of oxygen as it exists in the arterial blood; normal range is 75 to 100 mm Hg.

peak airway pressure (PAP) Amount of pressure required to deliver a volume of gas.

positive end-expiratory pressure (PEEP) The application of positive pressure to the airway at the end of expiration such that the airway pressure never returns to ambient.

pressure support ventilation (PSV) A type of mechanical ventilatory support in which a preset level of positive pressure augments the inspiratory effort required to attain a tidal volume, thereby decreasing the work of breathing.

respiration The exchange of oxygen and carbon dioxide across a semipermeable membrane.

shunting The state in which pulmonary capillary perfusion is normal but alveolar ventilation is lacking.

sigh Intermittent hyperinflation of the lungs.

spontaneous breaths Breaths that use the patient's own respiratory effort and mechanics.

synchronous intermittent mandatory ventilation (SIMV) A form of intermittent mandatory ventilation (IMV) mode in which the mandatory breaths are synchronized to the patient's own breathing cycle.

tidal volume (TV or V_T) The volume of air moved in and out of the lungs during normal breathing.

ventilation The gross movement of air in and out of the lungs.

ventilation–perfusion ratio ($\dot{V}/\dot{Q}$) The relationship of pulmonary ventilation to pulmonary perfusion expressed as a ratio in L/min; normal is 4:5.

ventilator (mechanical) breath A breath, either patient or machine triggered, that delivers gas at prescribed ventilator settings.

vital capacity (VC) The volume of air that can be exhaled after maximum inhalation; an indication of respiratory muscle strength; normal is 65 to 75 mL/kg.

volutrauma Injury to pulmonary tissues as a result of excessive volumes

weaning Gradual withdrawal of mechanical ventilation.

ABBREVIATIONS

ABG	Arterial blood gases	**ARDS**	Acute respiratory distress syndrome
AC	Assist-control mode	**AVF**	Acute ventilatory failure

cm H$_2$O	Centimeters of water pressure		**NIPPV**	Noninvasive intermittent positive pressure ventilation
CNS	Central nervous system		**O$_2$**	Oxygen
CO$_2$	Carbon dioxide		**$\overline{PA}$**	Mean airway pressure
COPD	Chronic obstructive pulmonary disease		**Paco$_2$**	Partial pressure of arterial carbon dioxide
CPAP	Continuous positive airway pressure		**Pao$_2$**	Partial pressure of arterial oxygen
CPP	Cerebral perfusion pressure		**PAP**	Peak airway pressure; proximal airway pressure
CVP	Central venous pressure		**PEEP**	Positive end-expiratory pressure
EPAP	Expiratory positive airway pressure		**pH**	Hydrogen ion concentration
ET tube	Endotracheal tube		**PIP**	Peak inspiratory pressure
f	Rate of breathing (spontaneous or mechanical ventilator)		**PPV**	Positive pressure ventilation
FIO$_2$	Fraction of inspired oxygen		**PSV**	Pressure support ventilation
HCO$_3$	Bicarbonate		**Sao$_2$**	Saturation of arterial oxygen
HFJV	High-frequency jet ventilation		**SIMV**	Synchronous intermittent mandatory ventilation
ICP	Intracranial pressure		**SV**	Spontaneous ventilation
IMV	Intermittent mandatory ventilation		**SVR**	Systemic vascular resistance
IPAP	Inspiratory positive airway pressure		**TE**	Tracheoesophageal
IPPB	Intermittent positive pressure breathing		**$\dot{V}_A$**	Alveolar ventilation
MABP	Mean arterial blood pressure		**VAP**	Ventilator associated pneumonia
mm Hg	Millimeters of mercury		**VC**	Vital capacity
MMV	mandatory minute ventilation		**$\dot{V}_D$**	Deadspace ventilation
MPV	Microprocessor ventilator		**$\dot{V}_E$**	Minute ventilation
NIF	Negative inspiratory force		**$\dot{V}/\dot{Q}$**	Ventilation–perfusion ratio
			V$_T$	Tidal volume

SECTION ONE: Ventilator versus Respirator

At the completion of this section, the learner will be able to briefly explain why a mechanical ventilator is not a mechanical respirator.

To understand the concept of mechanical ventilation, one must first have a basic understanding of the difference between respiration and ventilation. **Ventilation** refers to the gross movement of air in and out of the lungs. It is composed of **deadspace ventilation ($\dot{V}_D$),** the air that fills the conducting airways and does not take part in gas exchange, and **alveolar ventilation ($\dot{V}_A$),** the air that fills the alveoli and is available for gas exchange (Fig. 6–1). Adequate alveolar ventilation is necessary to maintain normal arterial blood gas levels.

$\dot{V}_D$ is easily measured because it is equivalent to the ideal body weight of the person. For example, if the patient's ideal body weight is 150 pounds, the $\dot{V}_D$ would be 150 mL. $\dot{V}_A$ is easily calculated as the person's tidal volume (V$_T$) − $\dot{V}_D$.

$$\dot{V}_A = V_T - \dot{V}_D$$

Respiration is the exchange of oxygen and carbon dioxide across a semipermeable membrane. Respiration occurs both in the lungs (external respiration) and in the tissues (internal respiration).

Mechanical ventilators are sometimes referred to as respirators. This is a misnomer. Though the technology has become very sophisticated, the machines only cause gases to be moved in and out of the lungs, using negative or positive pressure. Although certain ventilator settings help maintain alveoli in an open state to facilitate respiration, the machines do not have the capability to diffuse gases. Respiration, then, remains dependent on adequate functioning of the lung tissues and pulmonary capillaries.

Figure 6–1 ■ Components of ventilation. Ventilation is composed of deadspace ventilation ($\dot{V}_D$) and alveolar ventilation ($\dot{V}_A$). $\dot{V}_D$ is the air located in the conducting airways. (The conducting airways begin at the mouth and nose and end at the terminal airways.) $\dot{V}_A$ is the air that is present in the alveoli.

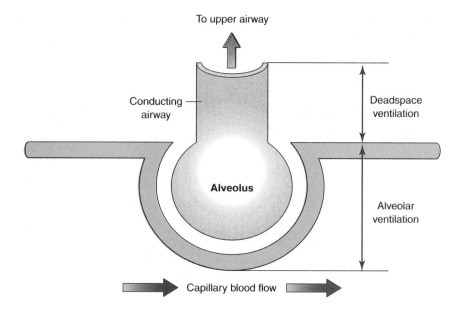

In summary, mechanical ventilation is a means by which the patient receives mechanical ventilatory support in maintaining adequate alveolar ventilation. Mechanical ventilators cannot cause diffusion of gases in the lungs. Rather, they facilitate the ventilatory process. Improved ventilatory status will enhance the ability of the gases to diffuse across the alveolar–capillary membrane.

SECTION ONE REVIEW

1. The primary purpose of mechanical ventilation is to
   A. support external respiration
   B. support alveolar ventilation
   C. prevent fatigue of the diaphragm
   D. prevent development of pneumonia
2. Deadspace ventilation refers to
   A. the amount of air left in the lungs after expiration
   B. the amount of carbon dioxide in venous blood
   C. the air in the lungs that does not take part in gas exchange
   D. the air in the lungs that leaks into the pulmonary interstitial space
3. Internal respiration refers to

A. gas exchange between the blood and tissues
B. gas exchange between the alveoli and blood
C. the movement of air into the alveoli
D. the movement of gases between alveoli

4. The term *alveolar ventilation* refers to
   A. gas exchange between the alveoli and the blood
   B. the intra-alveolar movement of air
   C. air in the alveoli that does not take part in gas exchange
   D. air that fills the alveoli and is available for gas exchange

Answers: 1. B, 2. C, 3. A, 4. D

SECTION TWO: Determining the Need for Ventilatory Support

At the completion of this section, the learner will be able to identify criteria used for determining the need for mechanical ventilatory support.

The decision to place a patient on a mechanical ventilator is a very serious one. The invasiveness of the artificial airway as well as the physiologic alterations associated with mechanical ventilation place the patient at substantial risk for development of serious complications. Therefore, the relative benefits and costs must be weighed.

Mechanical ventilation is a supportive intervention only. It is meant to support the patient's oxygenation and ventilation status while curative interventions are initiated to correct the underlying problem. Ventilatory support is probably best initiated as a "semielective" procedure before the patient's condition is severely compromised (i.e., cardiopulmonary arrest). Early support is thought to improve the patient's outcome.

How then is the decision made to place a patient on a mechanical ventilator? A variety of criteria have been established by pulmonary experts to aid the health care team in establishing rapidly which patients may require ventilatory support. These criteria generally are not based on specific medical diagnoses but rather on respiratory function status.

Acute Ventilatory Failure

Acute ventilatory failure (AVF) is probably the most common indication for ventilator support. Acute ventilatory failure is the inability of the lungs to maintain adequate alveolar ventilation. It is diagnosed on the basis of the acid–base imbalance it creates—acute respiratory acidosis, which is expressed as $PaCO_2$ greater than 50 mm Hg and pH less than 7.30. A variety of problems can cause AVF, such as head trauma, apnea of any etiology, neuromuscular dysfunction, and drug-induced central nervous system (CNS) depression. Essentially, any problem that decreases movement of air to and from the alveoli can precipitate AVF.

Generally speaking, AVF is a direct indication for rapid intubation and mechanical ventilatory support. A possible exception is the patient with chronic obstructive pulmonary disease (COPD, chronic airflow limitation). Patients with COPD live in a state of chronic (long-term) ventilatory insufficiency. They are at particularly high risk for development of complications if placed on a ventilator. For this reason, physicians often are reluctant to intubate and mechanically ventilate these patients unless it is absolutely necessary. Other criteria may be used, such as level of consciousness or a particular degree of respiratory acidosis, in making the decision to initiate mechanical support for this patient population.

Hypoxemia

The second major indication for mechanical ventilatory support is hypoxemia, which is frequently quantified as a PaO_2 of less than 50 mm Hg. A low **ventilation–perfusion ratio ($\dot{V}/\dot{Q}$)** is the most common cause of hypoxemia. A low $\dot{V}/\dot{Q}$ refers to a state in which there is an excess of perfusion in relation to ventilation. The cause of a low $\dot{V}/\dot{Q}$ often is an obstructing mucous plug in the distal airway, causing a reduction in alveolar ventilation. Examples of conditions that are associated with a low $\dot{V}/\dot{Q}$ include asthma, pneumonia, COPD, and atelectasis.

Low $\dot{V}/\dot{Q}$ is associated with a phenomenon called shunting. **Shunting** refers to the state in which pulmonary capillary perfusion is normal but alveolar ventilation is lacking. Pulmonary capillary blood that runs by a nonfunctioning alveolar unit cannot pick up oxygen from that alveolus. Although some shunting is normal, if many alveolar units become nonfunctioning, a significant decrease in oxygen saturation (SaO_2) will occur, causing hypoxemia. Severe shunting is associated with such conditions as respiratory distress syndromes of both the infant and adult and severe pneumonia.

Pulmonary Mechanics

Pulmonary function (pulmonary mechanics) testing may be used to decide if mechanical ventilatory support is needed. Such testing provides the clinician with crucial information about respiratory muscle strength and airflow. When evaluating the need for mechanical ventilation, pulmonary function tests can provide data regarding evidence of hypoventilation. Several of the more common tests used as criteria are **vital capacity (VC)**, **negative inspiratory force (NIF)**, and respiratory rate (f).

Special Considerations in the Elderly

Age-related changes in pulmonary physiology place the elderly at risk for respiratory failure. Phelan et al. (2002) suggest that these changes include decreased chest wall compliance, which increases the work of breathing; decreased oxygenation because of structural lung changes; and decreased lung volume and strength, which reduce cough effectiveness and increase the risk for infection. A reduced sensitivity to hypoxia and carbon dioxide plus changes in drug metabolism may increase the respiratory depressive effects of narcotics and sedatives. Many pulmonary diseases, such as COPD, become more evident with age. Age-related changes in other organs as well as comorbid conditions such as heart and renal disease impact respiratory function. Poor nutrition and decreased muscle strength can be additional risk factors. Thus, the elderly are at risk for respiratory failure due to pulmonary and non-pulmonary reasons.

The risks and benefits of critical care for the elderly, including the use of mechanical ventilation, has generated considerable controversy. Outcomes for this age group are related to disease severity and comorbid conditions; age alone is not predictive of survival or recovery (Sevransky & Haponik, 2003). Health care professionals may believe that the elderly do not benefit from critical care. Tullmann and Dracup (2000) caution against this "ageism" bias. The decision whether to institute mechanical ventilation should include a compassionate and realistic evaluation of the patient's status and wishes for care, and should not be based on age alone.

In summary, the decision as to whether to place a patient on a mechanical ventilator is a complex one, based on analysis of a variety of data. Actual criteria used to make this decision vary but generally include the patient's level of consciousness, arterial blood gas status, and pulmonary mechanics. A patient need not be in AVF or in severe hypoxemia to be placed on mechanical ventilation. If the clinician believes that the patient is in impending ventilatory failure, mechanical ventilation may be initiated as a semielective procedure. Table 6–1 summarizes some criteria that may be used to determine the need for mechanical ventilatory support.

TABLE 6–1   Criteria for Ventilatory Support

CRITERIA	CRITICAL VALUES
Acute ventilatory failure (AVF)	Pa_{CO_2} greater than 50 mm Hg, pH less than 7.30
Acute hypoxemia	Pa_{O_2} less than 50 mm Hg
Pulmonary mechanics	
Respiratory rate (f)	f greater than 35 breaths/min
Vital capacity (VC)	VC less than 15 mL/kg (normal: 65 to 75 mL/kg)
Negative inspiratory force (NIF)	NIF less than -20 cm H_2O (normal: -50 to -100 cm H_2O)
Minute ventilation ($\dot{V}E$)	$\dot{V}E$ greater than 10 L/min (normal: 5 to 10 L/min)

SECTION TWO REVIEW

1. The term *ventilatory failure* refers to the inability of the lungs to
   A. expand
   B. diffuse gases
   C. use oxygen and carbon dioxide
   D. maintain adequate alveolar ventilation
2. Acute respiratory acidosis is defined clinically as
   A. Pa_{CO_2} greater than 50 mm Hg and pH less than 7.30
   B. Pa_{O_2} less than 60 mm Hg
   C. Pa_{CO_2} greater than 45 mm Hg and pH less than 7.35
   D. Pa_{O_2} less than 80 mm Hg
3. Common causes of acute ventilatory failure include (choose all that apply)
   1. apnea
   2. head trauma
   3. myocardial infarction
   4. neuromuscular dysfunction
   A. 1, 2, and 3
   B. 2, 3, and 4

C. 1, 2, and 4
D. 1, 3, and 4
4. A low $\dot{V}/\dot{Q}$ exists when
   A. ventilation is in excess of perfusion
   B. perfusion is in excess of ventilation
   C. blood is shunted away from the alveoli
   D. there is an obstruction in the pulmonary capillaries
5. The term *pulmonary shunt* refers to
   A. movement of air directly from one alveolus to another
   B. normal pulmonary capillary perfusion, lacking alveolar ventilation
   C. an opening between the pulmonary artery and the heart
   D. normal alveolar ventilation, lacking pulmonary capillary perfusion

Answers: 1. D, 2. A, 3. C, 4. B, 5. B

SECTION THREE: Required Equipment for Mechanical Ventilation

At the completion of this section, the learner will be able to describe the equipment necessary for proper mechanical ventilation.

Mechanical ventilation is a complex intervention that requires a protocol of procedures and equipment. Adequate preparation before placement of the patient on the mechanical ventilator will facilitate smooth implementation.

Initial Equipment Necessary for Establishment of a Patent Airway

Mechanical ventilation requires the use of special artificial airways. Artificial airways can be divided into two groups: endotracheal tubes and tracheostomy tubes.

Endotracheal Tubes

The endotracheal (ET) tube is a specially designed semirigid radiopaque tube. Its slightly curved shaft is designed for ease of passage through the curved upper airway. In adults, the tubes require a cuff if positive pressure ventilation is to be initiated. The cuff is a balloon that is attached to the outside wall on the distal end of the ET tube. When it is inflated, the cuff seals off the lower airway from the upper airway and holds the tube in a stable position (Fig. 6–2). Neonatal and small pediatrics ET tubes do not have cuffs because in children younger than 5 years of age, the cricoid cartilage offers a sufficient seal once the tube is inserted.

Choice of Endotracheal Tube Size.   The size of the ET tube to be inserted will depend primarily on the age of the person to be intubated. ET tube sizes range from 2 mm to 11 mm, which reflects the diameter of the inside lumen. Table 6–2 lists recommended adult ET tube sizes by gender.

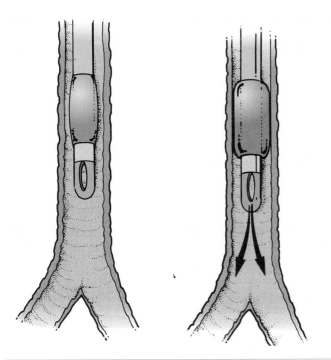

Figure 6–2 ▪ Endotracheal tube in the trachea. *A.* Balloon deflated. *B.* Balloon inflated. Air that is pushed through the tube enters the lungs because it cannot escape around the tube when the balloon is inflated. (From Martin, L. [1987]. *Pulmonary physiology in clinical practice: The essentials for patient care and evaluation [p. 198].* St. Louis: C.V. Mosby.)

TABLE 6–2   Recommended Sizes for Endotracheal Tubes in Adults

GENDER	INTERNAL DIAMETER (MM)	LENGTH (CM)
Female	7.5–8.0	19–24
Male	8.0–9.0	20–28

In the adult, the route of entry also determines ET tube size. A smaller-sized tube is required if it is to be inserted nasally because the nasal airway passage is significantly smaller than the oral airway passage. Many brands of ET tubes designate, on the tube, which route is appropriate for each size tube (i.e., nasal, nasal/oral, or oral).

Nasal intubation generally is performed blindly, that is, without viewing the vocal cords through a laryngoscope. It is most frequently performed when the procedure is a semielective (nonemergency) intubation. The nasal route is more comfortable for the patient once it is in place, and the tube is very stable. Oral intubation is most frequently used during an emergency because direct visualization of the vocal cords assures rapid proper placement in the lower airway. Figure 6–3 provides an illustration of a properly positioned ET tube.

Intubation Equipment.   The endotracheal tube is inserted by a specially trained member of the health care team. The following items must be gathered before intubation:

- Soft-cuffed ET tubes
- Stylet
- Topical anesthetic
- Laryngoscope handle with blade attached
- Magill forceps
- Suction catheters, Yankauers suction tip
- Syringe for cuff inflation
- Water-soluble lubricant
- Adhesive tape
- Personal protective equipment

Tracheostomy Tubes

Generally, when mechanical ventilation is initiated, a tracheostomy is not the entry of choice because it is more invasive and takes longer to perform. However, tracheostomy might be performed initially if the patient has received head or neck

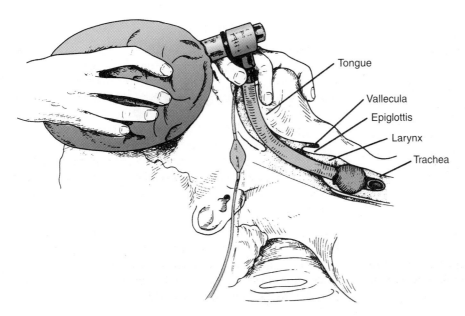

Tongue
Vallecula
Epiglottis
Larynx
Trachea

Figure 6–3 ▪ Orotracheal tube in place being used with a bag-valve resuscitator. *(From Marshak, A.B., & Scanlon, C.L. [1990]. Emergency life support. In C.L. Scanlon, R.L. Wilkins, & J.K. Stoller (eds.). Egans fundamentals of respiratory care, (5th ed.), [p. 533]. St. Louis: Mosby Year Book, with permission of Elsevier.)*

surgery or has an upper airway obstruction resulting from severe edema (such as burns) or a tumor obstruction. Tracheostomy is more commonly performed on the patient who requires prolonged intubation (over 2 to 3 weeks) because of failure to wean from the ventilator. Many hospitals have established guidelines for limiting the length of time a person is allowed to have an ET tube in place before receiving a tracheostomy.

Prolonged use of an ET tube is associated with many complications. Some of these complications can be avoided if a tracheostomy is performed in a timely manner. It should be noted that tracheostomy also is associated with a variety of complications. Currently, there is increasing controversy over when tracheostomy should be performed. (Artificial airway complications are discussed in Section Eight.)

Securing the Artificial Airway

Any type of artificial airway must be secured in place properly to prevent tube displacement and to minimize trauma to mucous membranes. Initially, in an emergency situation, the tube is se-

cured with adhesive tape. Figure 6–4 illustrates one method of securing an ET tube. This technique can be used with either nasal or oral ET tubes. Twill tape and a variety of commercially available stabilizers may be used in place of adhesive tape, particularly for prolonged use. Whatever method is used, stabilization of the tube is imperative. Tracheostomy tubes commonly are secured with twill tape or a commercially available tracheostomy band. The tracheostomy tube also may be sutured in place to prevent accidental dislodgment. Once the airway is secured, a chest x-ray should be performed to confirm correct placement.

Supportive Equipment

In addition to the artificial airway and mechanical ventilator, other supplies and equipment must be readily available.

- Two oxygen sources
  One for the ventilator
  One for the resuscitation bag, to provide 100 percent oxygen
- Suction equipment and at least one suction source

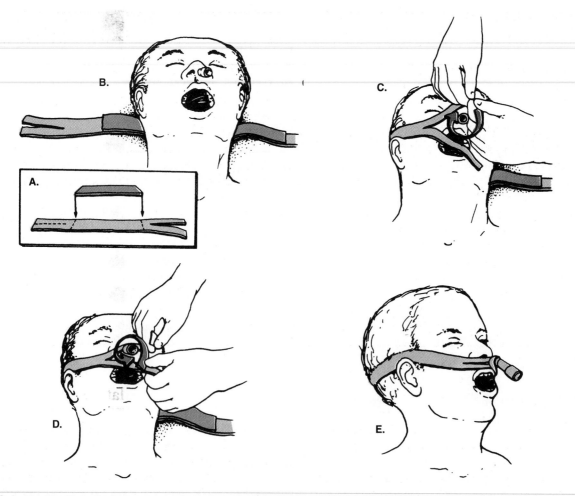

Figure 6–4 ■ The "head halter" technique for securing a nasotracheal tube. *A* demonstrates how the tape is cut on both ends with the middle section apposed by a tape section so that hair will not stick to the halter. *B* shows the tape under the patient's head. *C* demonstrates how one side is brought over the ear and the top leaf is wrapped around the tube in a clockwise fashion. *D* demonstrates the bottom leaf wrapped around the tube in a counterclockwise fashion. The procedure is repeated for the other side of the tape. (*From Shapiro, B. A. et al. [1991]. Clinical application of respiratory care, [4th ed., p. 164]. St. Louis: C.V. Mosby.*)

- Disposable sterile suction kits or sterile suction catheters, gloves, containers, sterile water
- Oral pharyngeal airway or a bite block if the oral route is used (to prevent closure of the airway if the patient should bite down on the tube)—also facilitates access to the oropharynx for suctioning
- Cuff manometer to check the cuff pressure on a regular basis
- A manual resuscitation bag to provide adequate backup in case of ventilator failure and for suctioning
- If positive end-expiratory pressure (PEEP) is to be used on the ventilator, a manual resuscitation bag with a PEEP attachment is recommended
- Secure intravenous access for medication administration
- Sedation and/or muscle relaxants

Postintubation Assessment

Immediately following intubation, the position of the endotracheal tube is assessed for proper placement in the trachea.

While the patient is receiving breaths via a manual resuscitation bag, both lung fields are auscultated for equal breath sounds. Air sounds or gurgling over the epigastric area indicates that the endotracheal tube is malpositioned in the esophagus. Additional methods of confirming proper tube placement are available, such as carbon dioxide monitors (capnography) or a disposable CO_2 detector. Chest radiograph is always used to confirm proper placement.

In summary, positive pressure mechanical ventilation requires the insertion of an artificial airway, either in the form of an ET tube, which can be inserted by the oral or nasal route, or by performing a tracheostomy. In an emergency, oral intubation using a laryngoscope most commonly is performed because of the speed and accuracy with which it can be placed. Adult artificial airways must have a cuff that is inflated for mechanical ventilation. Tracheostomy frequently is performed in those patients requiring prolonged mechanical ventilatory support or long-term assistance with airway clearance.

SECTION THREE REVIEW

1. In the adult, an inflated ET tube cuff is necessary for mechanical ventilation primarily because it
   A. prevents stomach contents from getting into the lungs
   B. seals off the nasopharynx from the oropharynx
   C. prevents air from getting into the stomach
   D. seals off the lower airway from the upper airway
2. The endotracheal tube size indicated on the tube reflects what measurement?
   A. the length of the tube
   B. the internal diameter of the tube
   C. the circumference size of the tube
   D. the length of the person's airway
3. In an emergency situation, the most common entry route for airway access is
   A. oral intubation
   B. nasal intubation

C. tracheostomy
D. oropharyngeal airway
4. Which of the following statements is true about securing the artificial airway?
   A. the inflated cuff provides sufficient securing
   B. the airway is generally sutured in place
   C. a nasotracheal tube does not require securing
   D. artificial airways must be secured directly to the patient.
5. When setting up a room for mechanical ventilator use, there must be
   A. one oxygen source
   B. two oxygen sources
   C. clean gloves for suctioning
   D. a backup ventilator in the room

Answers: 1. D, 2. B, 3. A, 4. D, 5. B

SECTION FOUR: Types of Mechanical Ventilators

At the completion of this section, the learner will be able to describe the types of mechanical ventilators, based on mechanism of force and cycling mechanism.

A common classification of ventilators uses mechanism of force, which is either negative or positive pressure. Figure 6–5 illustrates the mechanisms of force during spontaneous breathing as well as during negative and positive mechanical ventilation.

Negative Pressure Ventilators

According to Pilbeam (1998), negative pressure ventilators were the first ventilators to be experimented with, as early as the middle 1800s. The first model that achieved widespread success was developed in the United States in 1928 by Dr. Drinker and his associates. This model completely encased the body in an airtight tank, with only the patient's head being exposed to the outside. As an alternative design, first French physicians and then the inventor Alexander Graham Bell designed the cuirass (a French

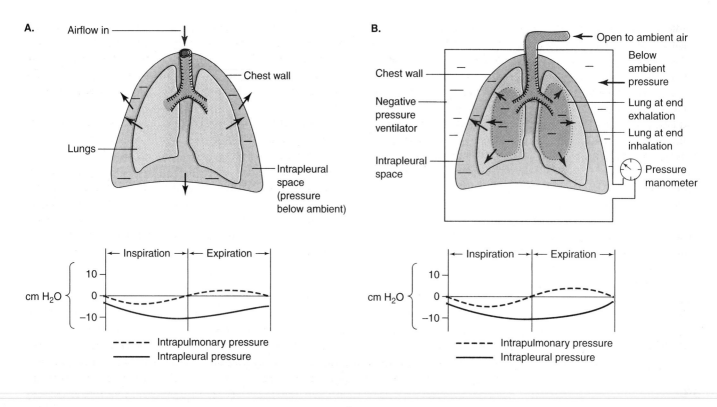

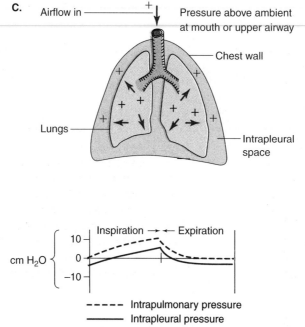

Figure 6–5 ■ The mechanics of breathing. *A.* The mechanics of spontaneous breathing and the resulting pressure waves. *B.* Negative pressure ventilation and the resulting lung mechanics and pressures. *C.* The mechanics and pressures associated with positive pressure ventilation. Intrapleural pressures are above ambient pressure during end-inspiration. *(From Pilbeam, S. P. [1998]. Mechanical ventilation: Physiological and clinical applications [3rd ed., pp. 31–35]. St. Louis: C.V. Mosby, permission of Elsevier.)*

word meaning "breastplate"). The cuirass negative pressure ventilator covers only the thoracic area (or the thorax and abdomen), somewhat like a turtle shell.

Negative pressure ventilation uses negatively applied pressure to the thorax by external means. To use a negative pressure

ventilator, the patient's entire body (e.g., in an iron lung) or thoracic region (e.g., in a cuirass) is encased in an airtight unit. At regular intervals, the air pressure in the sealed unit is reduced to below atmospheric pressure. The resulting negative pressure is transmitted through the thorax, which results in a pressure gradient that causes air to move into the lungs. The amount of negative pressure used is based on the desired tidal volume (VT)—the higher the desired VT), the higher the negative pressure required.

Negative pressure ventilation has several major advantages: (1) it does not require an artificial airway; (2) the patient can eat and talk normally; and (3) breathing mechanics are more normal, thereby decreasing the risk of physiologic complications. This type of ventilation also has a number of disadvantages, including (1) decreases venous return to the heart; (2) it may cause abdominal pooling of blood; and (3) the patient is relatively inaccessible for performance of activities of daily living (ADLs).

With the advent of positive pressure ventilators, negative pressure ventilators rapidly lost favor. Today, negative pressure ventilators are primarily used in the home, for long-term use in patients with relatively normal lung function. Examples of patients who might benefit from negative pressure ventilation include those with chronic hypoventilation and/or respiratory failure associated with neuromuscular diseases; those who require intermittent ventilatory support, such as during sleep; and, in certain cases, those with COPD.

Positive Pressure Ventilators

Positive pressure ventilators most commonly require an artificial airway to deliver ventilatory support. Gases are driven into the lungs through the ventilator's circuitry, which is attached to an artificial airway (ET or tracheostomy tube). Figure 6–6 shows an example of a positive pressure ventilator.

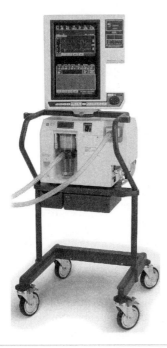

Figure 6–6 ■ Servo 300 series microprocessor-controlled positive pressure ventilator. *(Reprinted by permission of Nellcor Puritan Bennett Inc., Pleasanton, California)*

Positive pressure ventilators are commonly described on the basis of their cycling mechanism. The term **cycle** refers to the mechanism by which the inspiratory phase is stopped and the expiratory phase is started. There are four major cycling mechanisms: pressure-cycled, volume-cycled, time-cycled, and flow-cycled.

Because the cycling mechanisms actually limit the length of inspiration, the term *cycle* is often replaced by the term *limit* (i.e., pressure-limited). The newer ventilators provide more than one cycling device; however, only one cycling mechanism can be used at a time. With this increased flexibility, the health care team can alter the type of cycling based on the changing needs of the patient without switching ventilators. The remainder of this section briefly describes ventilators based on the cycling mechanism used.

Pressure-Cycled Ventilation

Pressure-cycled ventilation delivers a preset pressure of gas to the lungs. The pressure delivered (expressed in cm H_2O) is constant. The volume of air it delivers varies with the lung's compliance and airway resistance. This presents potentially serious support problems because stiffening lungs, a leak in the system, or a partially obstructed airway can significantly alter the volume of gas delivered. Maintaining an adequate VT is crucial for normal lung functioning. Pressure-cycled ventilation is increasingly used as a method to protect the injured lung from further damage from high pressures and is an option on most ventilators.

Volume-Cycled Ventilation

Volume-cycled ventilation delivers a preset volume of gas (measured in mL or L) to the lungs, making volume the constant and pressure the variable. Within a certain preset safety range (pressure limits), the ventilator will deliver the established volume of gas regardless of the amount of pressure it requires. This has the advantage of being able to overcome changes in lung compliance and airway resistance. For example, as lung compliance decreases or airway resistance increases, the pressure at which the gas is delivered to the lungs will increase sufficiently to deliver the desired volume of gas to the lungs.

Time-Cycled Ventilation

When time-cycled ventilation is used, the length of time allowed for inspiration is controlled. There are mechanical ventilators that solely use time-cycled ventilation, including the Servo 900c, Sechrist IV-100, and others. These ventilators hold time constant but volume and pressure may vary. Time-cycled ventilators frequently are referred to as time-cycled–pressure-limited ventilators because they also limit the amount of pressure that can be delivered. The microprocessor ventilators can use time cycling and also have the advantage of being able to limit volume and pressure.

Flow-Cycled Ventilation

Hess and Kacmarek (2002) describe pressure support as an example of flow-cycled ventilation. A preset pressure augments the patient's inspiratory effort and continues as long as the patient continues to inhale at a certain flow rate. As the patient reaches the end of inspiration, flow decreases. At a predetermined level of flow (e.g., 25 percent of peak inspiratory flow) inspiration ends. Tidal volume, rate, and time are variable.

In summary, negative pressure ventilators require sealing at least the chest of the patient in an airtight tank or shell. They do not require an artificial airway. Negative pressure ventilators are no longer seen commonly in acute care settings. Positive pressure ventilators directly force gases into the lungs using positive pressure. Various types of positive pressure cycling mechanisms are available. Pressure-cycled ventilation delivers a set amount of pressure to the lungs. Volume-cycled ventilation delivers a set amount of volume to the lungs. Volume cycling is commonly used because it is possible to adjust pressure to meet changes in airway resistance and compliance. Time-cycled ventilation uses inspiratory time as its major cycling parameter. Flow-cycled ventilation uses a decrease in inspiratory flow rate to determine when expiration will begin.

SECTION FOUR REVIEW

1. Negative pressure ventilators adjust the tidal volume by
   A. adjusting the amount of negative airflow
   B. adjusting the amount of positive airflow
   C. altering the amount of negative pressure applied
   D. altering the amount of positive pressure applied
2. The term *cycle* as it applies to mechanical ventilation refers to the mechanism by which
   A. the ventilator turns on and off
   B. inspiration ceases and expiration starts
   C. the concentration of oxygen is controlled
   D. the rate of airflow is maintained
3. Volume-cycled ventilation has an advantage over pressure-cycled ventilation because it
   A. adjusts volume as pulmonary pressure changes
   B. increases airflow as compliance increases
   C. decreases airflow as airway resistance decreases
   D. can adjust pressure to changes in lung compliance
4. Pressure-cycled ventilation uses which of the following as a constant?
   A. pressure
   B. time

C. volume
D. flow rate
5. Time-cycled ventilation is also referred to as time-cycled _____ limited ventilation.
   A. volume
   B. flow
   C. pressure
   D. time
6. When flow-cycled ventilation is used, _____ is preset.
   A. time
   B. pressure
   C. volume
   D. rate

Answers: 1. C, 2. B, 3. D, 4. A, 5. C, 6. B

SECTION FIVE: Commonly Monitored Ventilator Settings

At the completion of this section, the learner will be able to explain the commonly monitored ventilator settings.

Positive pressure ventilators offer many variables that can be manipulated to meet precisely the individual pulmonary needs of the patient. Certain settings and values related to each variable must be monitored by anyone taking care of a mechanically ventilated patient whether in a critical care unit, on a general floor, or in the home. The most commonly monitored settings include tidal volume (V_T), fraction of inspired oxygen (FIO_2), ventilation mode, respiratory rate (f), positive end-expiratory pressure (PEEP), continuous positive airway pressure (CPAP), pressure support (PS), peak inspiratory pressure (PIP), and alarms. Figure 6–7 shows the ventilator settings on a Servo 300 control panel.

Tidal Volume

Tidal volume (TV or V_T) is the amount of air that moves in and out of the lungs in one normal breath. Normal V_T ranges from 7 to 9 mL/kg (or 500 to 800 mL in an adult). If V_T is too low, hypoventilation will occur. If V_T is too high, the patient is at risk for pneumothorax and possible depression of the cardiovascular system.

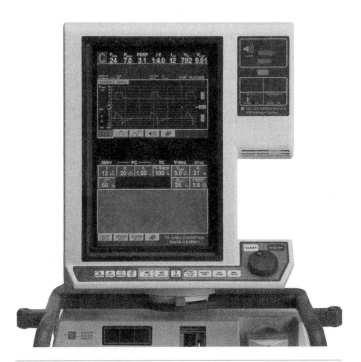

Figure 6–7 ▪ Mechanical ventilator control board. The control board of the Servo 300 microprocessor ventilator is divided into three sections. Patient Data—provides visual information regarding the patient's current ventilatory status. Ventilator Status—alerts the clinician to alarms and machine problems. Ventilator Settings—provide an active keyboard for manipulation of all the ventilator settings, such as mode, rate, volumes, and pressure limits. *(Reprinted by permission of Bennett Inc., Pleasanton, California)*

If volume-cycled ventilation is to be used, the desired VT must be set when mechanical ventilation is initiated. Opinions vary regarding how high to set the VT. Current trends in ventilator management are to use smaller tidal volumes and prevent high-peak pressures.

Adverse Effects of High Tidal Volumes

Traditionally, tidal volumes were set in the range of 10 to 15 mL/kg. According to Hess and Kacmarek (2002), a tidal volume of more than 12 mL/kg is no longer recommended because it overdistends the alveoli, causing lung damage. This damage may result in rupture of the alveolar membrane allowing air to enter the pleural space (pneumothorax) or tissue (subcutaneous emphysema). Such injury is termed *barotrauma*. Large tidal volumes can injure the basement membranes, epithelium, and endothelium of the lungs and stimulate an inflammatory response. This type of injury, *volutrauma*, increases the permeability of the lungs' microvasculature, which may result in pulmonary edema. The risk of lung injury increases as peak alveolar pressure increases. Though alveolar pressure is not measured directly, it can be approximated through measurement of the plateau pressure. Plateau pressure is easily measured at the end of inspiration by momentarily occluding the ventilatory circuit.

Normal-Volume Settings

Hess and Kacmarek (2002) suggest that the selection of tidal volume may range from 4 to 12 mL/kg of ideal body weight (adult) based on the patient's lung status. Patients with normal lungs can be ventilated in the higher range, whereas those with restrictive or obstructive disease should be managed with lower tidal volumes. The goal is to adequately ventilate the lungs while maintaining a plateau pressure of less than 30 cm H_2O. Some patients with pulmonary diseases cannot be adequately ventilated (i.e., normal $PaCO_2$) at these lower pressures and volumes. A technique called permissive hypercapnia may be considered for use in this patient population. The technique deliberately allows hypoventilation by using low tidal volumes. van Soeren and colleagues (2000) explain that the patient's $PaCO_2$ is allowed to slowly rise over a 24- to 48-hour period by slowly reducing minute ventilation. The health care team must determine how high the $PaCO_2$ and how low the pH will be permitted to drift.

Sigh

The term **sigh** refers to intermittent hyperinflation of the lungs. During normal spontaneous breathing, a person naturally takes an occasional deep breath (about one sigh every 6 minutes), which improves ventilation of the lungs. Use of manual and automatic sighs during mechanical ventilation was used widely in the 1960s to prevent development of atelectasis and to decrease shunt. When the practice of high tidal volume ventilation became common, use of the sigh controls was no longer considered necessary or desirable. Use of sighing remains controversial. When used, it is commonly set at a volume of 1.5 to 2 times the patient's VT and at a rate of 6 to 10 per hour.

Fraction of Inspired Oxygen

FIO_2 means the **fraction of inspired oxygen.** It is expressed as a decimal, although clinicians often discuss it in percentages, in terms of oxygen concentrations. At sea level, the room air that is inhaled into the alveoli is composed of oxygen that is 0.21 of the total concentration of gases in the alveoli. A mechanical ventilator is able to deliver a wide range of FIO_2, from 0.21 to 1.0 (an oxygen concentration of 21 percent to 100 percent).

Initially, in an emergency situation, FIO_2 is commonly set at 0.5 to 1.0 to deliver 50 percent to 100 percent oxygen to the patient. The setting is then increased or decreased based on the patient's PaO_2 and clinical picture. The goal is to maintain the PaO_2 within an acceptable range for the individual, using the lowest level of FIO_2. Prolonged use of FIO_2 greater than 0.60 may cause complications associated with oxygen toxicity (discussed in Section Seven).

In a semielective situation, the initial FIO_2 may be set at lower levels, based on more individualized oxygenation needs. The patient who retains carbon dioxide requires special consideration. When maintenance of some degree of patient-initiated breathing is desirable, care must be taken to set the FIO_2 at the lowest level that will deliver an acceptable PaO_2. The use of high concentrations of oxygen on such an individual may increase the PaO_2 excessively and obliterate the hypoxic drive to breathe.

Ventilation Mode

The ventilation mode refers to that which initiates the cycling of the ventilator to terminate expiration. The most common modes are **assist-control (AC or ACMV) mode** and **intermittent mandatory ventilation (IMV).**

Assist-Control Mode

Most ventilators have an assist mode, a control mode, and an assist-control mode. In assist mode, the ventilator is sensitive to the inspiratory effort of the patient. When the patient begins to inhale, the assist mode triggers the ventilator to deliver a breath at the prescribed settings (called a **ventilator** or **mechanical breath**). In the control mode, the ventilator delivers the breaths at a preset rate based on time. It is not sensitive to the patient's own ventilatory effort. Control mode generally is not used alone unless the patient is continuously apneic. A combination of assist and control modes generally is used. AC mode protects the patient in the following manner. The assist part of the mode is sensitive to spontaneous inspiratory effort of the patient, allowing the patient to maintain some control over breathing. At the same time, the control part of the mode acts as a backup should the patient decrease the breathing effort below the preset rate. When AC mode is used, every breath is a ventilator breath (V_T, and so on, as set by the clinician), which differentiates it from IMV. AC mode commonly is used initially, particularly in patients with acute respiratory failure or respiratory muscle fatigue because AC mode takes over the work of breathing.

Intermittent Mandatory Ventilation Mode

Using the IMV mode, the patient spontaneously breathes through the ventilator circuit, maintaining much of the work of breathing. Interspersed at regular intervals, the ventilator provides a preset ventilator breath. The intervals are based on the IMV rate set by the operator. For example, if the IMV is set at 12, the ventilator will deliver a breath approximately every 5 seconds. Between mandatory breaths, the patient's breathing will vary in V_T and rate because it is composed of **spontaneous breaths,** not ventilator breaths.

Synchronous intermittent mandatory ventilation (SIMV) is a type of IMV. The original IMV mode is not sensitive to the patient's own ventilatory cycle. Thus, an IMV breath can be stacked on top of the patient's own inhalation. SIMV synchronizes a mandatory breath to follow the patient's exhalation. The advantages of SIMV over IMV mode have not been proven because stacking of breaths has not been shown to be a physiologic hazard. SIMV, however, is more comfortable for the patient because it does not interfere with the normal breathing cycle.

IMV/SIMV have certain advantages over the other modes. They decrease the risk of hyperventilation and also provide a better ventilation–perfusion distribution. IMV/SIMV also facilitates the process of ventilator weaning.

Pressure Support Ventilation Mode

Pressure support ventilation (PSV) was introduced into the United States during the mid-1980s. Pressure support ventilation is defined as an adjunct weaning mode that enhances spontaneous inspiratory effort by application of positive pressure. In principle, PSV is similar to intermittent positive pressure breathing (IPPB). Both are triggered by the patient's spontaneous breathing effort and both decrease the effort (work) required to achieve a tidal volume. IPPB and PSV differ in what occurs upon achieving the preset level of pressure. IPPB ceases applying positive pressure as soon as the preset pressure is achieved. PSV, however, applies and maintains the preset pressure throughout the entire inspiration phase.

One use for PSV is to decrease the work of breathing by overcoming increased **airway resistance (R_{aw})** imposed by an artificial airway and ventilator circuitry. In this application, pressure support ventilation may be used as an aid to ventilator weaning. Patients on IMV/SIMV weaning mode are at increased risk for respiratory muscle fatigue and ventilatory failure because they must breathe harder than normal to maintain adequate tidal volumes due to increased airway resistance. In these patients, PSV decreases the work of breathing by supporting the tidal volume during spontaneous breaths.

Pressure support ventilation can also be used as a primary ventilatory mode to assist patients who are breathing spontaneously, including patients receiving continuous positive airway pressure. This application requires a stable lung condition as well as reliable respiratory control. Should the patient have an apneic spell while on PSV using only an assist mode, there is no timed backup present to take over ventilation.

Three major factors determine the patient's tidal volume: the preset pressure support level, the degree of patient effort, and the level of airway resistance and lung compliance. When using desired tidal volume as the basis for manipulating the level of PSV, the PSV level is increased until the desired tidal volume is reached. When the level of PSV is used to offset the resistance imposed by the artificial airway, the PSV level commonly is adjusted to provide just enough support to overcome an estimate of the resistance and increase patient comfort. Pressure support ventilation frequently is adjusted in increments of 5 cm H_2O, with levels commonly ranging from 5 to 15 cm H_2O.

Respiratory Rate

Properly setting the respiratory (breathing) rate (f) on the ventilator is important in establishing adequate minute ventilation ($\dot{V}_E$). Minute ventilation is the amount of air that moves in and out of the lungs in 1 minute. Normal $\dot{V}_E$ is 5 to 7 L/min. V_T (tidal volume) and f (rate) are the two variables that make up $\dot{V}_E$. It can be calculated using the following equation:

$$\dot{V}_E = V_T \times f$$

These variables are significant because if either one is manipulated, it will affect $\dot{V}_E$. If $\dot{V}_E$ becomes too low, hypoventilation will occur, possibly precipitating acute respiratory acidosis. In the carbon dioxide–retaining COPD patient, hyperventilation that results in decreased carbon dioxide levels can complicate weaning from the mechanical ventilator.

Hess and Kacmarek (2002) suggest that the most therapeutic ventilator rate depends on the characteristics of the patient's lungs. For example

- A patient with normal lungs
  V_T: 12 mL/kg; f: 8 to 12/min
- A patient with lung disease with increased C_L and R_{aw}
  V_T: 8 to 12 mL/kg; f: 6 to 10/min
- A patient with restrictive lung disease
  V_T: 8 to 10 mL/kg or less; f: 12 to 20/min

The SIMV rate is based on providing adequate ventilation for the patient. If the rate is set too slow, hypoventilation may develop, precipitating acute ventilatory failure (acute respiratory acidosis). If the rate is set too high, it may precipitate respiratory alkalosis by blowing off too much carbon dioxide.

PEEP and CPAP

For many years there has been an interest in perfecting a method to keep the alveoli open throughout the breathing cycle. Although this method (called **positive end-expiratory pressure, PEEP**) was first developed in the 1940s by the military, it was not used in medicine until 20 years later, in the late 1960s. In the early 1970s, it was introduced as a treatment for respiratory distress syndrome in newborns. Since that time, it has become the foundation for oxygenating the lungs in newborns and adults with respiratory distress syndrome (Pilbeam, 1998).

Positive end-expiratory pressure is applied to the lungs as either as **continuous positive airway pressure (CPAP)** or positive end-expiratory pressure (PEEP). PEEP is used with patients who are being mechanically ventilated and can be used in a variety of ventilator modes, including assist-control and SIMV. CPAP is used on patients who are spontaneously breathing. It does not require an artificial airway or a mechanical ventilator, although many ventilators have a CPAP setting. PEEP and CPAP provide the alveoli with a constant (preset) amount of positive pressure at the end of the expiratory phase of breathing, which prevents airway pressure from returning to zero. Normally, at the end of expiration, alveoli have a natural tendency to collapse. When positive pressure is provided during the expiration phase of the breathing cycle, it forces the alveoli to remain open, which (1) recruits previously collapsed alveoli, (2) prevents atelectasis, and (3) improves oxygenation (Fig. 6–8).

The primary indication for use of PEEP/CPAP is the presence of refractory hypoxemia (i.e., hypoxemia that is unresponsive to increasing concentrations of oxygen). PEEP is useful in treating acute diffuse lung disease processes (e.g., acute respiratory distress syndrome and cardiogenic pulmonary edema) and in treating postoperative atelectasis. Low levels of PEEP (e.g., 5 cm H_2O) are commonly used for intubated patients to prevent atelectasis (Hess & Kacmarek, 2002).

The level of PEEP can be monitored on most ventilators by observing the airway pressure manometer. When no PEEP is being applied, the manometer needle should fall back to zero at the end of each breath. When PEEP is present, the needle should fall back to the level of PEEP. For example, if PEEP is set at 10 cm H_2O, the needle should fall to 10 ± 2 cm H_2O rather than to zero.

The level of PEEP/CPAP is adjusted to meet the patient's oxygenation needs. Traditionally, this has been done by increasing the PEEP level in increments of 3 to 5 cm H_2O until adequate oxygenation is achieved at a safe F_{IO_2}. Hess and Kacmarek (2002) describe newer methods of selecting the optimal PEEP level using ventilator graphics that reflect levels of airway closure. They also caution that higher levels of PEEP require close cardiovascular monitoring and that PEEP should not be abruptly reduced.

The level of positive pressure required depends primarily on the severity of lung injury. Mild forms of lung injury usually require between 5 and 10 cm H_2O. In cases of more severe lung injury, the patient may require 10 to 20 cm H_2O. Levels of PEEP

		Example A			Example B		
Inspiration	Expiration	F_{IO_2}	Pa_{O_2}	Sa_{O_2}	F_{IO_2}	Pa_{O_2}	Sa_{O_2}
No PEEP O_2	No O_2	0.50	40	75	0.70	65	90
PEEP O_2	O_2	0.50	54	85	0.50	65	90

Figure 6–8 ■ Effect of PEEP on oxygenation. During expiration with PEEP, airways that would otherwise collapse are kept open, allowing continued oxygen transfer. In Example A, the Pa_{O_2} and Sa_{O_2} improve, and F_{IO_2} is unchanged. In Example B, the Pa_{O_2} is maintained at an acceptable level, whereas the F_{IO_2} is decreased from 0.70 to 0.50. (From Martin, L. [1987]. Pulmonary physiology in clinical practice: The essentials for patient care and evaluation [p. 212]. St. Louis: C.V. Mosby, with permission from Elsevier).

as high as 30 cm H_2O or more have been used; however, there is a trend away from using such high PEEP (sometimes referred to as "super PEEP") levels in favor of newer ventilator strategies that limit peak inspiratory pressures and use smaller tidal volumes.

PEEP can also be used to offset auto-PEEP. **Auto-PEEP** refers to an unintentional buildup of positive end-expiratory pressure caused by alveolar airtrapping. It is particularly associated with COPD. Airtrapping prevents the COPD patient from exhaling fully, which leaves a volume of air in the alveoli at the end of expiration. When a COPD patients' lungs become hyperinflated, they may not be able to inhale sufficiently to trigger the mechanical ventilator in an assist mode. Applying a small amount of PEEP externally, to match the level of auto-PEEP, can offset the effects of the auto-PEEP such that the patient can trigger the ventilator to cycle properly.

Although PEEP and CPAP are important in the treatment of severe hypoxemia, their use is associated with significant complications that can be as detrimental to patient outcomes as severe hypoxemia. The risk of complications increases as the amount of PEEP or CPAP is increased. The complications associated with PEEP can be categorized into two groups: barotrauma to the lungs and decreased cardiac output. Complications are discussed in Section Seven.

Peak Airway Pressure or Peak Inspiratory Pressure

When using volume-cycled ventilation, the tidal volume is preset to deliver a certain number of milliliters or liters. The pressure it takes to deliver that amount of volume varies depending primarily on airway resistance and lung compliance. The amount of pressure required to deliver the volume is called the **peak airway pressure (PAP)** or peak inspiratory pressure (PIP). PIP is measured in centimeters of water pressure (cm H_2O) and may be visualized on an airway pressure manometer or on a data screen. In the adult, PIPs of less than 40 cm H_2O are considered desirable. It is known that high PIPs greatly increase the risk of barotrauma and have negative effects on other body systems (see Section Seven). PIP should be recorded at regular intervals for trending—taking multiple measurements over an extended period of time to evaluate the parameter for a pattern of change.

Increasing Peak Inspiratory Pressure Trend

This signifies that increasing amounts of pressure are necessary to deliver the preset tidal volume. It is most commonly indicative of increased airway resistance or decreased lung **compliance.**

Decreasing Peak Inspiratory Pressure Trend

This signifies that less pressure is needed to deliver the tidal volume. It may indicate an improvement in airway resistance or lung compliance.

Alarms

The patient's life depends on correct functioning of the ventilator and maintenance of a patent airway. To protect the patient, ventilators are equipped with a system of alarms to alert the caregiver to problems. Two frequently triggered alarms are the low exhaled volume and high-pressure alarms.

The low exhaled volume alarm indicates that there is a loss of tidal volume or a leak in the system. When this alarm goes off, the nurse should focus rapidly on checking to see whether the ventilator tubing has become disconnected or whether the artificial airway cuff is inadequately filled with air or has a leak. The cuff can be checked by feeling for air leaking out of the nose and mouth. It may be noted that the patient can suddenly vocalize, which also indicates a leak or insufficiently inflated cuff. A leaking cuff may be checked by deflating and then reinflating the cuff to observe for its ability to attain and then maintain a tracheal seal. If the cuff is ruptured, the nurse must notify the medical team immediately and prepare for reintubation. If a cuff must be deflated for any reason, oral suctioning should precede deflation to prevent flooding the lower airway with contaminated secretions from the upper airway.

The high-pressure alarm is the most commonly heard alarm. Any patient problem that increases airway resistance can trigger it. Examples of clinical conditions that cause a high-pressure alarm include coughing, biting on the tube, secretions in the airway, or water in the tubing. Clearing the airway or tubing frequently will correct the problem.

Alarms should never be ignored or turned off. Some alarms can be muted temporarily, for example, during suctioning. Box 6-1 presents the rule regarding the proper response to an alarm.

Initial Ventilator Settings

When a patient is first placed on the mechanical ventilator, certain standard settings may be used as a guideline. Standard settings include

Tidal volume	5 to 12 mL/kg ideal body weight
Rate	8 to 12/minute
Mode	AC
FIO_2	0.5 to 1.0
Peak flow	40 to 60 L/min
Inspiratory sensitivity	-1 to -2 cm H_2O

Box 6-1   The Golden Rule of Ventilator Alarms

If the cause of an alarm is not immediately found or cannot be corrected immediately, the patient should be removed from the ventilator and manually ventilated using a resuscitation bag until the problem is corrected.

In most circumstances, the FIO_2 is initially set at 1.0 and can be titrated by pulse oximetry to maintain adequate oxygen saturation. Arterial blood gases are checked after the initiation of mechanical ventilation; adjustments in ventilator settings are made based on the patient's oxygenation, pH, and pCO_2.

In summary, positive pressure ventilators have many parameters that must be monitored by those persons who work directly with them. This section presents the most commonly monitored mechanical ventilator settings, including V_T, FIO_2, modes, rate, PEEP/CPAP, pressure support, PIP, and alarms. Special consideration is given to ventilator setting alterations for management of the patient with carbon dioxide–retaining COPD.

SECTION FIVE REVIEW

1. The normal tidal volume (V_T) in a spontaneously breathing adult is _____ mL/kg.
   A. 2 to 5
   B. 5 to 7
   C. 7 to 9
   D. 10 to 15

2. The common volume V_T setting range on a mechanical ventilator is _____ mL/kg.
   A. 2 to 5
   B. 5 to 12
   C. 7 to 9
   D. 10 to 15

3. If V_T is set too low on the ventilator, it will cause
   A. hypoventilation
   B. pneumothorax
   C. hypoxemia
   D. hypocapnia

4. A high PaO_2 is avoided in patients with COPD when possible because it could
   A. cause hyperventilation
   B. lead to hypocapnia
   C. obliterate the hypoxic drive
   D. precipitate metabolic acidosis

5. A major advantage of initial use of AC mode is that it allows
   A. the diaphragm to exercise
   B. the patient to rest
   C. increased work of breathing
   D. maintenance of some spontaneous breathing

6. SIMV is used primarily for
   A. weaning
   B. full support
   C. acute head injury
   D. acute pulmonary diseases

7. A low minute ventilation ($\dot{V}E$) can cause
   A. acute metabolic alkalosis
   B. acute respiratory alkalosis
   C. acute metabolic acidosis
   D. acute respiratory acidosis

8. PEEP affects the alveoli by
   A. increasing alveolar fluid
   B. decreasing their relative size
   C. sealing off nonfunctioning units
   D. maintaining them open at end expiration

9. PSV is used primarily for what purpose?
   A. to increase PIP
   B. to decrease oxygen need
   C. to decrease work of breathing
   D. to prevent atelectasis

10. An increasing PIP most commonly indicates
    A. increasing airway resistance and/or decreasing lung compliance
    B. decreasing airway resistance and/or decreasing lung compliance
    C. increasing airway resistance and increasing lung compliance
    D. decreasing airway resistance and decreasing lung compliance

11. The ventilator low exhaled volume alarm will trigger when
    A. the patient is coughing
    B. there is water in the tubing
    C. the patient is biting the ET tube
    D. there is a leak in the system

Answers: 1. C, 2. B, 3. A, 4. C, 5. B, 6. A, 7. D, 8. D, 9. C, 10. A, 11. D

SECTION SIX: Noninvasive Alternatives to Mechanical Ventilation

At the completion of this section, the learner will be able to explain briefly methods of providing noninvasive ventilatory support.

The combination of positive pressure ventilation and artificial airways places the patient at risk for multiple complications and significantly increases patient morbidity and mortality. In an effort to reduce some of the risks, several alternative noninvasive methods have been developed for delivery of positive airway pressure without requiring artificial airways. Noninvasive ventilatory methods have been shown to be effective alternatives to traditional invasive techniques in certain patient populations (Liesching et al., 2003). This section presents an overview of two major noninvasive alternatives to conventional mechanical ventilatory support: noninvasive intermittent positive pressure ventilation (NIPPV or NPPV) and continuous positive airway pressure (CPAP).

Noninvasive Intermittent Positive Pressure Ventilation (NIPPV or NPPV)

Noninvasive Intermittent Positive Pressure Ventilation (NIPPV) is a relatively new means of providing ventilatory support without requiring intubation. It is more comfortable, is easier to apply and remove, and has a lower incidence of nosocomial pneumonia than conventional mechanical ventilation (Mehta & Hill, 2001). It requires use of a positive pressure mechanical ventilator and an "interface," usually a mask.

Masks/Interfaces

NIPPV can be applied using a variety of masks, termed *interfaces,* in place of the invasive endotracheal or tracheostomy tube. In the acute care setting, the two most commonly used interfaces are oronasal and nasal masks. The oronasal mask covers both the mouth and the nose, and the nasal mask covers only the nose. Choice of mask primarily depends on patient comfort and effectiveness of ventilation. For example, a patient may find the oronasal mask to be claustrophobic and prefer the nasal mask. A distressed patient breathing through the mouth may get more benefit from the oronasal mask. Other interface options include nasal pillows (which fit into the nares), full-face masks, helmets, and a large, cannula-type device.

Unlike artificial airways, noninvasive interfaces commonly have air leaks. Leakage may occur at the edge of mask or through the patient's nose or mouth. Some air leakage is necessary when using a bilevel device (discussed later) because CO_2 accumulates in the single limb/hose. Air leakage is assured by special mask design with an exhalation port or by a special valve on the tubing/hose.

NIPPV Mechanical Ventilator

Any positive pressure mechanical ventilator can be used for NIPPV. Ventilators can be viewed as three basic types; standard ICU ventilators, smaller portable home ventilators, and bilevel devices.

Standard ICU Ventilators.   As described by Hess and Kacmarek (2002), standard ICU ventilators offer the advantages of increased monitoring and alarms and accurate titration of oxygen. Rebreathing CO_2 is not a problem using standard ventilators because the ventilator circuit consists of two tubes. Gas from the ventilator is delivered to the patient via the inspiratory limb or tubing. Exhaled air, including CO_2, is removed by a separate expiratory limb/tubing so the patient does not rebreathe

exhaled gas. ICU ventilators, however, may not be able to compensate for air leaks. Standard ventilators being used for NIPPV can be used in either volume or pressure modes (Mehta & Hill, 2001).

Portable Ventilators.   Smaller portable ventilators are primarily used in the home setting for patients with chronic respiratory failure. They can be used in either volume or pressure modes, depending on the ventilator model. The smaller size makes these ventilators a convenient option for long-term use. They have fewer alarms and monitoring capabilities than standard ventilators.

Bilevel Devices.   Bilevel devices were developed for noninvasive ventilation and were designed to compensate for the required NIPPV air leak. In addition, bilevel devices maintain a minimal PEEP level (usually about 4 cm H_2O) to continually flush CO_2 from the system. Smaller and less complex than standard ventilators, these devices provide positive pressure support to the patient throughout the breathing cycle. Bilevel devices have a single limb/hose that carries both inspired and exhaled gas. Gas from the bilevel device is delivered through the single limb/hose and the patient's exhaled air goes out through the same tube, making hypercapnia from rebreathing CO_2 a potential problem. To prevent hypercapnia, bilevel devices have continuous flow/PEEP to help expel exhaled CO_2 from the mask. In addition, either a special exhalation valve is used on the tubing, or the masks have an exhalation port. Bilevel devices are also designed to compensate for leaks. A backup breathing rate can be set for safety, but setting FIO_2 is usually less precise and they have fewer alarms and monitoring capabilities than a standard mechanical ventilator. Newer devices have more sophisticated monitoring and oxygen titration features.

Settings for bilevel devices use a different terminology than standard ventilators. The inspiratory positive airway pressure (IPAP) equates with the peak inspiratory pressure and the expiratory positive airway pressure (EPAP) equates with PEEP. The patient's level of support is the difference between the IPAP and EPAP. (Note: Clinicians often interchange the term *bilevel* with *BiPAP*™ which is a trade name for one of the first bilevel machines produced by Respironics).

Indications and Contraindications for Use

At home, NIPPV is used primarily for patients who cannot fully support their own ventilatory efforts for prolonged periods (e.g., with neuromuscular disease). In the ICU setting, NIPPV is used for patients in acute respiratory distress as a treatment option to avoid intubation. Liesching et al. (2003) explain that NIPPV has been used successfully for patients with hypercapnic failure, such as those with COPD or congestive heart failure, and with postoperative patients. It has also been used for immunocompromised patients who are at increased risk of bleeding and infection with intubation and for patients who do not wish to be intubated. NIPVPV has been used for patients with oxygenation respiratory failure (such as

ARDS and pneumonia), but the results have been mixed. Mehta and Hill (2001) caution that a critically ill patient using NIPPV requires intense monitoring so that intubation is not delayed if the patient's condition deteriorates further. Liesching et al. (2003) also suggest that NIPPV may be useful in supporting patients whose respiratory status has deteriorated after having been withdrawn from conventional mechanical ventilation to avoid reintubation.

There are a variety of contraindications for using NIPPV, including an unstable hemodynamic status, cardiac dysrhythmias or myocardial ischemia, apnea, the inability to clear one's own secretions or maintain airway patency, and the inability to attain a proper mask fit (Hess & Kacmarek, 2002).

Continuous Positive Airway Pressure (CPAP)

Continuous positive airway pressure (CPAP) is a mode of mechanical assistance that is closely related to NIPPV. CPAP provides a continuous level of positive airway pressure for a spontaneously breathing person. The level of pressure remains the same throughout the breathing cycle, hence, CPAP does not provide assisted ventilation on inspiration as does NIPPV. CPAP improves oxygenation by opening alveoli (similar to PEEP) and is used in pressures ranging from 5 to 12.5 cm H_2O (Mehta & Hill, 2001). CPAP does not require a mechanical ventilator; instead, it is delivered by a special flow generator (i.e., a blower) via a nasal or facial mask. The same type of masks/interfaces used with NIPPV can be used with CPAP.

CPAP is most commonly used to treat obstructive sleep apnea, a disorder in which the tissues of the oropharynx collapse, periodically obstructing the airway. The constant pressure of CPAP acts like a splint to hold the airway open (Malhotra et al., 2000). Flemons (2002) suggests that several methods are used to determine the desired level of CPAP. When employed as a treatment for obstructive sleep apnea, the desirable level of CPAP is determined through a sleep study in a laboratory setting. In establishing the correct level of CPAP, the goal is to set the CPAP level at the point at which the patient stops having the apnea episodes or when the frequency and duration of episodes is at an acceptable level. The CPAP level can also be determined at home rather than in a sleep laboratory setting. In the home setting, special equipment adjusts the level of positive pressure, and monitors apneic events, pressures, and oxygen saturation. Some of the newer CPAP units adjust airway pressure automatically, responding to snoring, apnea/hypopnea, or airflow limitation. CPAP is also used in the acute care setting to treat pulmonary edema.

Complications

Many of the potential complications associated with positive pressure ventilation, as described in Section Seven, also apply to noninvasive ventilation, although the severity and frequency of the complications are significantly reduced. Additional patient problems are associated with delivery of positive pressure through a mask, including conjunctivitis, gastric distention, nasal problems, skin irritation, and aspiration. In addition, hypoventilation is a common complication associated with mechanical problems.

Conjunctivitis is caused by air leaking out from the mask around the bridge of the nose and blowing on the eyes. This problem may be easily corrected by adjusting the mask to eliminate the leak or fitting of a new mask.

Gastric distention is caused by air swallowing. Inspiratory pressures used for NIPPV are usually less than 20 cm H_2O, which reduces air entry into the esophagus. Mehta and Hill (2001) suggest that simethicone may be helpful in reducing gastric distention. Fortunately, with long-term use, gastric distention often becomes less of a problem.

Nasal-related complaints include dryness, bleeding, and congestion. These problems may be relieved by use of heated humidification or nasal sprays.

Skin irritation and pressure sores may develop under the straps and mask. To minimize or prevent this problem, masks must be fitted carefully and not strapped tightly to the face. A protective skin covering can be used over the bridge of the nose. Alternating interfaces, for example, using nasal pillows, may also reduce skin irritation.

Aspiration is a rare, but serious, problem. It can be avoided by limiting NIPPV therapy to patients who can clear their own airways and who are not fed anything by mouth until stable (Mehta & Hill, 2001).

Hypoventilation is the major mechanical problem associated with NIPPV therapy. Hypoventilation can occur through two mechanisms: (1) when there is an inadequate seal to attain the preset pressure or (2) when there is inadequate airflow. Improving the seal or adjusting the flow (when possible) may relieve this problem.

Nursing Considerations

In the acute care setting, Mehta and Hill (2001) advise that NIPPV should be instituted before the patient is severely distressed and unable to cooperate. They stress the importance of explanations, patience, and coaching in the success of instituting NIPPV. The therapy should be explained and demonstrated at each step, giving the patient an opportunity to ask questions and adapt to the sensations of the masks and air pressures. Following is an example of steps that should be included in the initiation of NIPPV:

- Select the proper mask size
- Allow the patient to feel the airflow
- Hold the mask to the patient's face without straps, hose, and so forth
- Let the patient breathe through the mask briefly
- Connect the tubing to the mask (set IPAP low at 8 or less) to help the patient adjust to the feeling of positive airflow

- Continue to hold the mask in place
- As the patient becomes more comfortable, attach the head straps
- As the patient becomes more comfortable, gradually increase the pressure to the level desired

Patients are monitored for ventilator synchrony, air leaks, and patient status (e.g., comfort, relief of dyspnea). Positive patient outcomes include a decreasing respiratory rate, improved oxygenation, and decreased use of accessory muscles (Mehta & Hill, 2001).

Home ventilatory support therapy requires careful, thorough instructions to the patient or the primary caregiver. Teaching needs include

- Signs and symptoms of complications
- Circumstances under which to call the physician
- Proper use and maintenance of equipment
- Troubleshooting problems

Follow-up visits by a home health nurse or a respiratory therapist are usually ordered as a means of monitoring both the equipment and the patient.

In summary, noninvasive positive pressure ventilation (NIPPV) provides ventilatory support without requiring intubation. Positive pressure is usually applied using a mask that covers either the nose (nasal mask) or the nose and mouth (oronasal mask). There are three types of NIPPV mechanical ventilators: standard critical care ventilators, portable ventilators, and bilevel devices. In the home setting, NIPPV is used primarily for patients who cannot fully support their own ventilatory efforts for prolonged periods. In the hospital setting, NIPPV has been used as an alternative therapy for hypercapnic (ventilatory) failure, and for some immunocompromised patients when intubation is contraindicated. Use of NIPPV in the high acuity patient, however, requires intense monitoring for patient deterioration. Continuous positive airway pressure (CPAP) is closely related to NIPPV. It provides continuous positive airway pressure throughout the breathing cycle but does not provide breathing assistance on inspiration, as does NIPPV. CPAP is primarily used in the treatment of obstructive sleep apnea. Complications associated with noninvasive ventilation can be divided into types, mask-related complications (e.g., conjunctivitis and skin irritation), and mechanical problems (e.g., hypoventilation). Patients require explanations and support to adjust to this therapy. Patient and care provider teaching is crucial if home noninvasive ventilatory support is to be successful. Follow-up home visits by a home health nurse or respiratory therapist are also recommended, if not required.

SECTION SIX REVIEW

1. Which of the following statements describes NIPPV?
   A. it requires a flow generator (blower)
   B. it combines negative and positive pressure principles
   C. it uses a positive pressure mechanical ventilator
   D. it independently manipulates inspiratory and expiratory pressures
2. NIPPV is most useful for the patient who
   A. requires only support of tidal volume
   B. cannot fully support his or her own expiratory effort
   C. requires only support for nocturnal hypercapnia and hypoxemia
   D. cannot fully support his or her own ventilatory effort over long periods of time
3. Which statement best reflects nasal CPAP?
   A. it is used as a treatment of obstructive sleep apnea
   B. it requires a positive pressure mechanical ventilator
   C. the pressure level cannot be adjusted once it has been set
   D. it allows manipulation of inspiratory and expiratory pressures

4. Bilevel differs from CPAP because it
   A. requires an artificial airway
   B. can provide inspiratory positive pressure
   C. uses a standard positive pressure ventilator
   D. provides only nocturnal support
5. Common complications of noninvasive methods of ventilatory support include (choose all that apply)
   1. conjunctivitis
   2. nasal congestion
   3. hypoventilation
   4. otitis media
   A. 1, 2, and 4
   B. 2, 3, and 4
   C. 2 and 3
   D. 1, 2, and 3

Answers: 1. C, 2. D, 3. A, 4. B, 5. D

Major Complications of Mechanical Ventilation

At the completion of this section, the learner will be able to discuss the major complications of mechanical ventilation.

Positive pressure ventilation (PPV) affects virtually all body systems. These effects can lead to multiple system complications. Table 6–3 summarizes the multisystem effects of positive pressure ventilation.

Cardiovascular Complications

During normal spontaneous inhalation, air is drawn into the lungs because of a drop in intrathoracic pressure. At the same time, the decreased intrathoracic pressure increases venous return to the heart by drawing blood into the heart and the major thoracic vessels. As blood is moved into the right heart, the right heart chamber enlarges and stretches, enhancing right ventricular preload and stroke volume. During normal exhalation, there is an increase in the flow of blood from the pulmonary circulation to the left heart, increasing left ventricular preload and stroke volume. At the end of spontaneous exhalation, the output of blood decreases in both the right and left heart.

TABLE 6–3   Multisystem Effects of Positive Pressure Ventilation

SYSTEM	EFFECTS OF PPV
Cardiovascular	Decreased cardiac output
	Decreased right ventricular preload
	Decreased stroke volume
	Decreased left ventricular output
	Clinical manifestations: Decreased blood pressure (particularly in presence of hypovolemia); If compensation is present, normal blood pressure, increased heart rate, increased systemic vascular resistance
Pulmonary	Increased gas flow to nondependent lung and to central lung tissue
	Increased blood flow to peripheral lung tissues
	Clinical manifestations: Decreased Pa_{O_2}
Neurovascular	Decreased venous return from the head
	Decreased blood flow to head if cardiac output is decreased
	Clinical manifestations: Possible increased intracranial pressure; possible altered level of consciousness
Renal	Redistribution of blood flow through kidneys
	Decreased blood flow to the kidneys associated with decreased cardiac output
	Clinical manifestations: Decreased urine output; increased serum sodium and creatinine levels
Gastrointestinal	Decreased blood flow into the intestinal viscera
	Increased risk of gastric ulcer formation, gastrointestinal bleed, hepatic dysfunction (increased bilirubin)

When PPV is used, the positive pressure exerted on the lungs causes a relative increase in intrathoracic pressure, which is then transmitted to all structures in the thorax, including the heart, lungs, and major thoracic vessels. The major vessels become compressed, which creates an increase in central venous pressure (CVP). Blood return to the right heart is reduced because of a decreased pressure gradient. The resulting reduction in venous return to the heart causes right preload and stroke volume to decrease. Left ventricular output falls as a direct result of decreased right ventricular output.

PPV reduces cardiac output by decreasing venous return to the heart in three major ways. First, as described earlier, the presence of positive intrathoracic pressure prevents blood from being pulled into the major thoracic vessels and into the heart. Second, cardiac output is reduced through a squeezing of the heart by the lungs during the inspiratory phase of PPV. Third, the amount of pressure being exerted on the alveoli is the single most important factor influencing cardiac output when considering pulmonary influences. As the level of pressure is increased, venous return to the heart decreases. The more the heart and pulmonary capillaries are squeezed by the presence of positive pressure, the lower the cardiac output. This helps explain why high levels of PEEP can dramatically reduce cardiac output. Other factors that influence the effects of PPV on the cardiovascular system include lung and thoracic compliance, airway resistance, and the patient's volemic state.

Decreased cardiac output may be manifested as a reduction in arterial blood pressure, particularly if the patient is hypovolemic. However, a normal blood pressure frequently is maintained in PPV patients through the compensatory mechanisms of increased heart rate and increased systemic vascular resistance (SVR). Hemodynamic monitoring usually shows a decreased cardiac output, increased pulmonary artery wedge pressure, and increased right atrial pressure.

Pulmonary Complications

Normally, during spontaneous breathing, the relationship between ventilation and perfusion ($\dot{V}/\dot{Q}$) is relatively balanced, with most inhaled gases flowing toward the diaphragm. The distribution of gases to the alveoli normally favors the peripheral and dependent lung areas. Likewise, pulmonary perfusion normally is the greatest in dependent areas, thus matching the lung zones with the most ventilation with the lung zones with the most perfusion.

Altered Ventilation and Perfusion

PPV alters the relationship of ventilation to perfusion in the lungs. Gases flow through the path of least resistance, which during PPV increases ventilation to the nondependent lung areas and large airways. This is largely due to the decreased functioning and stiffening of the diaphragm associated with passive PPV. PPV gas flow increases ventilation to the healthy lung areas, whereas flow decreases to the diseased areas because it meets increased resistance in diseased lung tissue.

When PPV is being used, the positive pressure is transmitted to the pulmonary vessels, pushing the blood to the peripheral lung and to dependent areas. Because perfusion is now the greatest in the periphery and in the dependent lung areas and ventilation is greatest in the nondependent and larger airways, the relationship of ventilation to perfusion is altered to some degree. In areas with the most perfusion, there is decreased ventilation, and in areas with adequate ventilation, perfusion is reduced. This can create problems with oxygenation because of increased shunting, which can be reflected in deteriorating PaO_2 levels. Under certain circumstances, shunt and $\dot{V}/\dot{Q}$ matching can significantly improve during PPV. This is typically seen when PEEP is applied to treat refractory hypoxemia associated with increased shunt and decreased functional residual capacity (e.g., ARDS). In such a situation, shunt is often reduced, $\dot{V}/\dot{Q}$ matching is improved, and PaO_2 levels may significantly improve.

Barotrauma/Volutrauma

There is increasing evidence that the pulmonary injury associated with PPV results from alveolar distention created by a combination of excessive alveolar pressure (**barotrauma**) and volume (**volutrauma**). The higher the positive pressure or volume applied, the greater the risk of trauma. Patients who are at the highest risk for development of barotrauma/volutrauma are those requiring high levels of PEEP and high peak airway pressures (PAP, PIP) or high tidal volumes. Barotrauma/volutrauma can manifest itself as pneumothorax, subcutaneous emphysema, or pneumomediastinum. Clinically, it should be suspected if (1) the patient has a sudden onset of agitation and cough associated with a frequent high-pressure alarm, (2) the blood pressure and ABG rapidly deteriorate, (3) breath sounds suddenly are diminished or absent, or (4) subcutaneous emphysema can be palpated on the anterior neck or chest. If a pneumothorax or pneumomediastinum is diagnosed, insertion of a chest tube should be anticipated.

Oxygen Toxicity

Oxygen toxicity is associated with the use of an oxygen concentration of 60 percent or greater (FIO_2 of 0.6 or greater) for more than 48 hours. The use of 100 percent oxygen concentration (FIO_2 of 1.0) can cause pulmonary changes within 6 hours. Oxygen toxicity damages the endothelial lining of the lungs and decreases alveolar macrophage activity. It also decreases mucous and surfactant production. If it is allowed to continue for more than 72 hours, the patient may develop a pattern of symptoms similar to ARDS. The early signs and symptoms of oxygen toxicity are nonspecific (malaise, fatigue, and substernal discomfort). Because early symptoms are difficult to assess, the nurse should be aware of who is at risk for developing oxygen toxicity on the basis of the length of time that the patient has received an O_2 concentration of 60 percent or higher. Unfortunately, the signs and symptoms of oxygen toxicity are similar to changes that may be due to the underlying disease process or ventilator-induced lung injury. Hess and Kacmarek (2002) advise that although every effort should be made to decrease oxygen concentrations to nontoxic levels, maintaining adequate oxygenation and safe ventilatory pressures are paramount.

Nosocomial Pulmonary Infection: Ventilator-Associated Pneumonia (VAP)

Nosocomial pulmonary infection is a common major complication of mechanical ventilation. The passing of an ET tube from the upper airway into the lower airway introduces upper-airway contaminants into the lower airway. The presence of an artificial airway bypasses the normal upper airway defense mechanisms, reduces cough effectiveness, stimulates mucous production, and decreases the mucociliary motion that helps to remove bacteria. In addition, a biofilm rapidly forms on the endotracheal tube that provides an environment in which bacteria can multiply.

Because of the increased mortality and morbidity caused by ventilator-associated pneumonia, many studies have examined the factors that contribute to these infections. Chastre and Fagon (2002) found that gastric colonization with pathogenic bacteria that migrate to the lungs has been linked to stress ulcer prophylaxis that changes the normal acidity of the stomach. Placing the patient in a supine position increases the reflux of contaminated gastric fluid. Oral secretions pool between the endotracheal cuff and glottis, and can enter the lung by microaspiration around the endotracheal tube cuff. The presence of nasogastric tubes and feeding tubes has also been linked to increased risk of nosocomial pneumonia. Poor oral hygiene with the development of plaque makes the oropharynx a reservoir for pathogens (Munro & Grap, 2004).

Contamination also occurs as a result of failure to maintain strict aseptic technique during pulmonary suctioning or use of contaminated equipment. These factors, coupled with the physiologically compromised state of most mechanically ventilated patients and tearing of the mucous membranes with tracheal suctioning, places them at high risk for development of a pulmonary infection.

Signs and symptoms of a pulmonary infection include development of adventitious breath sounds and changes in sputum color or quantity. Systemically, infection may be evidenced by fever and increased white blood cell (WBC) count. Positive chest x-ray and sputum culture findings are important diagnostic tools.

Neurovascular Complications

PPV can cause a change in neurovascular status through two major mechanisms. First, intracranial pressure (ICP) can increase, and, second, cerebral perfusion pressure (CPP) can decrease. Patients who have existing intracranial or neurovascular problems are at particular risk when moderate to high ventilation pressures are required. The increased intrathoracic pressure associated with PPV decreases venous return from the head. The higher the pressure required to ventilate the patient, the greater the effects on the ICP.

Blood flow to the head (cerebral perfusion pressure) may be reduced. If cardiac output drops sufficiently to reduce systolic blood pressure, cerebral perfusion may become compromised. CPP is influenced by two factors: ICP and mean arterial blood pressure (MABP). This relationship is expressed as follows:

$$CPP = MABP - ICP$$

MABP is determined by the systolic and diastolic blood pressures. Therefore, as systolic blood pressure decreases, so will MABP, thus reducing CPP. If CPP drops too low, cerebral hypoxia can result.

Renal Complications

PPV is associated with decreased urinary output. The mechanisms for this decrease are multiple, and some are unclear. Pannu and Mehta (2002) describe three major mechanisms that may contribute to decreased renal function: decreased cardiac output, redistribution of renal blood flow, and hormonal alterations caused by positive pressure ventilation.

Decreased cardiac output is associated with reduced renal perfusion and reduced glomerular filtration rate, which can cause decreased urine output. In patients who are receiving PPV, arterial blood pressure generally is maintained through compensatory mechanisms.

It is suggested that when cardiac output has not been reduced significantly, the cause of low urine output may be associated with the redistribution of intrarenal blood flow that occurs with PPV. The redistribution of blood causes changes in kidney function. PPV seems to alter renal perfusion by decreasing blood flow to the outer renal cortex and increasing flow to the inner cortex and outer medullary tissue, where the juxtamedullary nephrons are located. This results in a 40 percent net decrease in urinary output, and less sodium and creatinine are excreted. When sodium is reabsorbed, water also is reabsorbed to maintain homeostasis, thus reducing urine output.

Finally, the cardiovascular changes induced by positive pressure may stimulate the release of antidiuretic hormone, renin, aldosterone, atrial natriuretic factor, and catecholamines. These hormones may affect renal blood flow and function but observed effects vary with a patient's clinical status, hydration, and underlying disease (Pannu & Mehta, 2002).

Gastrointestinal Complications

PPV can decrease blood flow into the intestinal viscera by increasing visceral vascular resistance. The increased resistance to flow can result in tissue ischemia, which causes increased permeability of the protective mucosal lining. This predisposes the ventilator patient to gastric ulcer formation and gastrointestinal bleeding. In addition, some patients develop hepatic dysfunction even if there is no history of liver disease.

Gastrointestinal bleeding occurs in approximately 25 percent of patients on mechanical ventilators through development of stress ulcers. Stress ulcers develop as a result of either gastric hyperacidity or, more commonly, from a transient visceral hypoxic episode. In the mechanically ventilated patient, the tissue hypoxia may have occurred related to acute respiratory failure or may be the result of increased resistance to blood flow in the viscera. Stress ulcers, which usually are shallow erosions in the mucosal lining, often cause slow bleeds and may, therefore, not be diagnosed early in their development. For this reason, it is important to check all stools for guaiac.

Clinically, the patient exhibits a decreasing hematocrit and guaiac positive stools. Stools may be black or dark red. If the ulcer is in the stomach, nasogastric aspirate will be guaiac positive, and the aspirate appears bright red to dark red. Because mechanical ventilation for greater than 48 hours has been identified as a risk factor for stress ulcers, preventive interventions are recommended. These include the use of antacids, histamine (H_2) antagonists, or proton pump inhibitors to maintain a gastric pH of greater than 3.5. Alternatively, sucralfate provides mucosal protection without pH alteration and may have advantages in reducing bacterial overgrowth in the stomach.

Mechanical ventilation, directly and indirectly, reduces gastrointestinal motility (Mutlu et al., 2001). Therapies often used in conjunction with mechanical ventilation such as sedatives and narcotics may further inhibit motility and complicate the provision of enteral nutrition.

In summary, there are many potential complications associated with mechanical ventilation. Cardiovascular complications are those associated with a significantly reduced cardiac output. PEEP is especially associated with cardiovascular compromise. Pulmonary complications include altered ventilation and perfusion and increased shunt, which can decrease oxygenation; barotrauma/volutrauma, associated mostly with higher levels of PEEP and high tidal volumes; oxygen toxicity, which occurs with higher levels of oxygen for a prolonged period of time (oxygen toxicity has been attributed to the development of ARDS); and nosocomial pulmonary infection. Neurovascular complications include increased intracranial pressure and decreased cerebral perfusion pressure. The primary renal complication is decreased urine output, which can be severely reduced. Gastrointestinal complications include development of stress ulcers, gastrointestinal bleeding, decreased gastric motility, and hepatic dysfunction.

SECTION SEVEN REVIEW

1. PPV affects the cardiovascular system by
   A. increasing cardiac output
   B. decreasing venous return to the heart
   C. increasing arterial blood pressure
   D. increasing venous return to the heart

2. Changes in cardiac output resulting from positive pressure ventilation are associated with which manifestation?
   A. increased arterial blood pressure
   B. increased urinary output
   C. arrhythmia development
   D. decreased pulse rate

3. PPV alters the relationship of ventilation to perfusion in what way?
   A. ventilation increases in nondependent lung areas
   B. ventilation increases in the small airways
   C. perfusion increases in the nondependent lung areas
   D. perfusion increases near the large airways

4. Which manifestation of pulmonary barotrauma/ volutrauma is secondary to mechanical ventilation?
   A. onset of increased lethargy
   B. increase in arterial blood pressure
   C. increase in breath sounds over a lung field
   D. increased cough with high-pressure alarm triggering

5. In which way does oxygen toxicity affect the pulmonary tissue?
   A. by decreasing macrophage activity
   B. by increasing mucous production
   C. by increasing surfactant production
   D. by decreasing peak inspiratory pressure (PIP)

6. Patients receiving mechanical ventilation are at increased risk of developing a nosocomial pulmonary infection because
   A. the lower airway is defenseless
   B. macrophage activity has been bypassed
   C. normal upper airway defenses are bypassed
   D. normal pulmonary mechanics have been interfered with

7. PPV influences ICP by
   A. decreasing intrathoracic pressure
   B. increasing cerebral perfusion pressure
   C. decreasing venous drainage from the head
   D. increasing MABP

8. The kidneys are affected by PPV in what way?
   A. decreased sodium retention
   B. redistribution of renal blood flow
   C. renal effects of increased cardiac output
   D. redistribution of urine flow through the kidneys

9. The gastrointestinal system may be adversely affected by PPV as a result of
   A. increased visceral vascular resistance
   B. increased blood supply to the viscera
   C. increased venous pooling in the viscera
   D. decreased visceral vascular resistance

10. Gastrointestinal bleeding secondary to mechanical ventilation most frequently manifests itself as
    A. grossly bloody stools
    B. guaiac-positive stools
    C. grossly bloody nasogastric drainage
    D. guaiac-negative nasogastric drainage

Answers: 1. B, 2. C, 3. A, 4. D, 5. A, 6. C, 7. C, 8. B, 9. A, 10. B

SECTION EIGHT: Artificial Airway Complications

At the completion of this section, the learner will be able to explain the cause and prevention of artificial airway complications. Artificial airways have their own set of complications that are primarily related to pressure damage.

Nasal Damage

Placing an artificial airway through the nasal passage is associated with trauma to nasal mucous membranes during the passing of the tube. In addition, ischemia and even necrosis of the nares may develop as a result of the pressure the tube exerts on the internal nasal wall. Anchoring the tube to the cheeks rather than to the top of the nose helps prevent pressure damage. Choice of the proper size tube also is important in minimizing the risk of damage. Nasotracheal tubes can cause inner ear problems related to their location. The nasotracheal tube can occlude the eustachian tubes, which increases the risk of development of ear pressure problems or inner ear infection.

Cuff Trauma

Although the use of tracheal cuffs is necessary to mechanically ventilate the patient properly, they are associated with potentially severe tracheal and laryngeal injuries. The use of excessive cuff pressures is the major contributing factor in these injuries. Arterial capillary blood flow pressure through the trachea is low

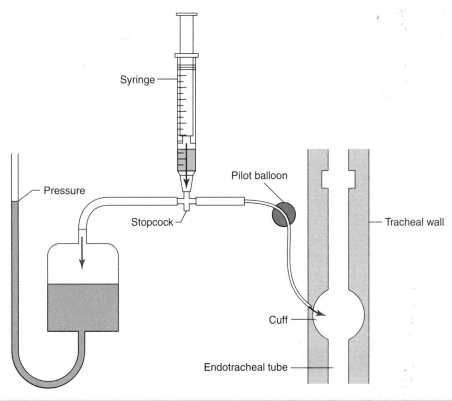

Figure 6–9 ■ The use of syringe, mercury manometer, and three-way stopcock for measuring cuff pressure. (*From Pilbeam, S. P. [1992]. Mechanical ventilation: Physiological and clinical applications, [3rd ed., p. 294]. St. Louis: C.V. Mosby, with permission from Elsevier*)

(less than 30 mm Hg). A high-pressure force, such as is delivered by an overinflated cuff, exerts a pressure that is higher than capillary pressure, causing circulation in the cuffed area to be compromised. Decreased or obliterated blood flow to an area of tissue causes ischemia, which, if allowed to continue for an extended period, can produce necrosis. Necrosis of the trachea, larynx, or both is associated with the development of fistulas, fibrosis, and ulceration.

Proper monitoring and control of cuff pressures decreases the risk of complications significantly. Cuff pressures must be monitored at least once every shift. Safe cuff pressure ranges from 20 to 25 mm Hg (27 to 34 cm H_2O). If a cuff manometer is not available, it is simple to make one using a three-way or four-way stopcock, a 10-mL syringe, and a sphygmomanometer (Fig. 6–9).

A minimum occluding pressure technique may also be used to reduce the risk of pressure-related cuff damage. Using this technique, the cuff is inflated only to the point at which it seals the airway during the mechanical ventilation. Cuff pressure should be regularly checked using this technique and should not exceed 20 to 25 mm Hg.

Artificial airways can damage one or both vocal cords as a result of the traumatic introduction of the tube or damage can be caused by the pressure of the tube against the cords. Fistula

formation is also a major concern. Should tracheal injury from a cuff cause a fistula to form between the trachea and esophagus, gastric secretions can be aspirated into the lungs. Tracheoesophageal (TE) fistulas should be suspected if tube feeding or food is aspirated during tracheal suctioning. This infrequent, but serious, complication is diagnosed with computed tomography (CT) scan and contrast studies. Proper cuff technique and use of correct tube size can minimize cuff-related complications.

In summary, the patient who requires an artificial airway is at risk for developing a complication related to its use. Artificial airway complications are primarily caused by the effects of pressure on delicate mucous membranes. Nasal damage may occur during passage of the tube or may be caused by the pressure of the tube against the nares or nasal passage. Cuff trauma is caused by excessive pressure being exerted against the trachea, compromising blood flow to the surrounding mucosa. Cuff pressures should be measured on a regular basis and should be maintained at 20 to 25 mm Hg (27 to 34 cm H_2O). The use of a minimum occluding pressure technique also can be used to reduce the chances of damage to the trachea. The presence of an artificial airway can damage one or both vocal cords. The formation of a TE fistula is a potentially serious complication that can cause aspiration of esophageal or stomach contents into the lower airways.

SECTION EIGHT REVIEW

1. The presence of a nasotracheal tube can affect the ears because it can
   A. occlude the eustachian tubes
   B. exert direct pressure on the inner ears
   C. cause inner ear ischemia
   D. directly damage the eustachian tubes
2. High endotracheal tube cuff pressures can damage the trachea when cuff pressure is
   A. increased during coughing
   B. reduced due to a leak
   C. lower than surrounding capillary pressure
   D. higher than surrounding capillary pressure
3. Normal tracheal capillary pressure is less than
   A. 10 mm Hg
   B. 20 mm Hg
   C. 30 mm Hg
   D. 40 mm Hg

4. Safe tracheal cuff pressure ranges are _____ mm Hg.
   A. 10 to 15
   B. 15 to 20
   C. 20 to 25
   D. 25 to 30
5. TE fistula formation secondary to tracheal cuff complications can cause
   A. sepsis
   B. aspiration pneumonia
   C. gastric ulcerations
   D. esophageal varices

Answers: 1. A, 2. D, 3. C, 4. C, 5. B

SECTION NINE: Care of the Patient Requiring Mechanical Ventilation

At the completion of this section, the learner will be able to describe care of the patient requiring mechanical ventilation.

Patient Care Goals

The general goals and outcome criteria appropriate to the management of a patient receiving mechanical ventilation may be divided into two major groupings: support of physiologic needs and support of psychosocial needs. Support of the patient's physiologic needs is accomplished through interventions that promote optimal oxygenation, treat impaired gas exchange, provide adequate ventilation, protect the airway, support tissue perfusion, and provide adequate nutrition. Support of the patient's psychosocial needs centers around interventions to reduce anxiety and pain, provide a balance of sleep and activity, promote communication, and support the family.

Nursing Management of Physiologic Needs

The patient's nursing management is planned around interventions to attain the patient care goals. The first three goals—promote optimal oxygenation, provide adequate ventilation, and protect the patient's airway—are all addressed through implementation of the three pulmonary-related nursing diagnoses, as follows.

Evidence-Based Practice

- *Daily interruption of infusions of sedative drugs in patients being mechanically ventilated decreased mechanical ventilation duration and ICU length of stay (Kress et al., 2000).*

- *Mechanically ventilated critically ill trauma patients who received ceftazidime by aerosol had a lower frequency of ventilator-associated pneumonia (VAP) than those who received placebo aerosol. Instillation of ceftazidime may also reduce lung proinflammatory response (Wood et al., 2002).*

- *In ALI/ARDS patients requiring mechanical ventilation, use of lower tidal volumes decreased mortality and number of days on mechanical ventilation (The Acute Respiratory Distress Syndrome Network, 2000).*

- *In a survey of critical care nurses at AACN's 2004 National Teaching Institute, 60 percent of nurses surveyed indicated that their ICU did not have an oral care protocol for prevention of ventilator-associated pneumonia (VAP) (Health & Medicine Week, 2004).*

Ineffective Airway Clearance

The patient who requires conventional positive pressure ventilation will have an endotracheal or tracheostomy tube inserted to access and seal off the lower airway. The length and relatively small internal diameter of artificial airways (particularly ET tubes) make it difficult, if not impossible, for the patient to clear his or her own airway. The problem of airway clearance is often compounded by general weakness and fatigue or diminished level of responsiveness, any of which also hinders airway clearance.

Airway clearance is a top-priority nursing goal in management of the patient with an artificial airway. If airway patency is not maintained, the patient's breathing and cardiovascular status eventually will fail as a result of hypoxia or hypercarbia.

> **Remember to apply the ABCs—Airway, Breathing, Circulation—in that order.**

The primary reason that airway patency becomes compromised is airway obstruction caused by excessive, thick, or pooled secretions. Each of these situations must be managed properly by the nurse.

Excessive Secretions.   Excessive secretions are removed by suctioning the artificial airway on an as-necessary basis, which may be every few minutes during initial intubation or several times a shift in chronic intubation. The patient's breath sounds should be assessed every 1 to 2 hours for the presence of secretions. If adventitious breath sounds are auscultated in the large airways, suctioning should be performed. Coughing, regardless of whether it sets off the ventilator's high-pressure alarm, may indicate a need for suctioning. The nurse often can hear the secretions without the use of a stethoscope, particularly during coughing. Coughing, however, can occur as a result of tracheal irritation or bronchospasm or because the tip of the airway is touching the carina. The last two situations can precipitate severe coughing spasms. Because coughing may occur without the presence of secretions in the large airways, the nurse should assess the situation first. Unnecessary suctioning causes needless trauma to the delicate mucous membranes in the trachea and also depletes oxygen levels. Good rules to apply are as follows:

- Always assess before suctioning.
- Do not suction unnecessarily.
- Follow approved protocols for suctioning.
- Monitor the patient closely for adverse effects of suctioning, such as arrhythmias and hypoxia.

In most circumstances, the nurse will maintain PaO_2 levels during suctioning if the following common protocol is maintained.

Step 1: **Hyperoxygenate/hyperventilate. Deliver 100 percent oxygen accompanied by manually ventilating the patient with a manual resuscitation (Ambu) bag for four to five breaths (two-handed ventilating will give significantly larger breaths than one-handed ventilating).**

Step 2: **Suction. Use moderate, not high, suction pressure. Apply suction only on withdrawal, rotating the catheter while using intermittent suction and withdrawing the catheter within 10 seconds. Repeat steps 1 and 2 until the airway is cleared.**

Step 3: **Return the patient to the ventilator.**

There are many variations to suctioning protocols. Some hospitals only hyperoxygenate by temporarily increasing the ventilator's oxygen concentration (FIO_2) to 100 percent (for 1 to 5 minutes). Hyperventilation may be part of such a policy. Hyperventilation can be accomplished through a sigh or other intermittent large inhaled volume mechanism on the ventilator that, when manually triggered, will deliver a breath that is 1.5 to 2 times the patient's set tidal volume. In patients with acute neurologic injury, protocol may call for initial hyperoxygenation/hyperventilation for 1 or more minutes before initiation of the suctioning protocol. The practice of instilling saline as part of the routine suctioning protocol remains controversial and may or may not be part of an institution's suctioning policy.

Suction catheters can be divided into two major groups: open and closed systems. Both systems are used for suctioning artificial airways, but only open systems are used without an artificial airway in place. Each type of system has its own suctioning protocol. Closed system catheters are self-contained within a sheath attached directly to the artificial airway. A closed-catheter system remains in the artificial airway system between suctionings, allowing it to be used multiple times. Open systems generally are single-use catheters and require introduction of the catheter into the artificial airway from outside the artificial airway system. Further discussion of suctioning systems is beyond the scope of this module.

If the patient is receiving PEEP, a different suctioning protocol may be required. Patients on PEEP often do not tolerate being detached from the ventilator for any reason. Loss of PEEP can precipitate oxygen desaturation and may make the patient hemodynamically unstable. Several approaches may be used: (1) the usual suctioning protocol; (2) the usual suctioning protocol using a manual resuscitation bag that has a special PEEP attachment, set at the prescribed PEEP level; or (3) suctioning without removing the patient from the ventilator by either an in-line closed-suction system or introducing a suction catheter into the closed system through a special port on top of the ventilator adaptor nozzle. Research is continuing on which type of suctioning system and protocol is best in specific situations. All types of suctioning have associated problems, including infection, hypoxia, trauma, arrhythmias, trauma to mucous membranes, and others.

Thick Secretions.   Thick secretions are a common challenge to maintaining effective airway clearance. Properly hydrating the patient is the most important means of thinning secretions because secretions are composed primarily of water. A fluid intake of 2 to 2.5 L/day is recommended unless it is contraindicated. Mechanically ventilated patients receive warmed, humidified gases that facilitate liquefying secretions. Intermittent nebulizer treatments of normal saline or mucolytics may be ordered to liquefy secretions.

Pooled Secretions.   Pooled secretions can cause obstruction of major airways or can plug the tip of the artificial airway. Proper suctioning, liquefying secretions, and turning the patient every 1 to 2 hours all help prevent obstruction by pooling. Percussion with postural drainage, prone positioning, and lateral rotation therapy beds are other therapies that have been used to enhance removal of secretions. Methods to improve cough effectiveness such as the assisted cough technique are used for specific populations (e.g., spinal cord injury patients).

Oral secretions also pool above the cuff of the endotracheal tube, presenting a risk of ventilator-associated pneumonia. Frequent oral care and oropharyngeal suctioning are important to reduce the volume of these secretions. Special endotracheal tubes that permit removal of subglottic secretions via an additional suction port are available. According to Collard et al. (2003), these tubes may be useful when prolonged intubation is anticipated.

Impaired Gas Exchange

Treatment of impaired gas exchange is the major reason for placing patients on a mechanical ventilator (i.e., impending ventilatory failure or acute respiratory failure). Ventilators can manipulate carbon dioxide levels directly by causing alveolar hyperventilation or hypoventilation.

Alveolar hyperventilation is associated with decreasing carbon dioxide levels and respiratory alkalosis. It can be patient induced if the patient is on the AC mode and is hyperventilating for any reason (e.g., anxiety, pain, head injury) because the patient can blow off too much carbon dioxide. It also can be induced mechanically by setting the rate or tidal volume too high on the ventilator. Sometimes, as in patients with increased intracranial pressure, mild respiratory alkalosis is induced intentionally to facilitate cerebral vasoconstriction through low carbon dioxide levels.

Alveolar hypoventilation is associated with increasing carbon dioxide levels and respiratory acidosis. Hypoventilation may be patient induced, for example, in the patient on SIMV mode (or other spontaneous breathing mode) whose breathing is very shallow. It also can be induced mechanically by setting the rate or tidal volume too low on the ventilator.

A changing ABG trend may indicate a change in the patient's respiratory or metabolic status, reflecting improvement or deterioration in his or her condition. The cause of the imbalance must be found and treated to correct the imbalance. It is the nurse's responsibility to monitor the ABG trends, observe the patient's condition, notify the physician of increasing abnormalities, follow up on orders received, and monitor the ventilator settings at established intervals. The nurse also can facilitate gas exchange by taking actions to maintain airway clearance and effective breathing patterns.

Ineffective Breathing Patterns

Patients may be placed on the mechanical ventilator because of ineffective breathing patterns, which consist of any significant changes in the breathing rate, rhythm, or depth from the patient's baseline normal values (e.g., tachypnea, bradypnea, apnea, hypoventilation, and hyperventilation). Changes in breathing patterns can affect oxygenation and acid–base status, as previously described.

Breathing patterns that remain too rapid must be controlled once the patient is placed on the ventilator to prevent hyperventilation problems. A variety of analgesics (e.g., IV morphine or fentanyl) or sedatives (e.g., benzodiazepines, such as midazolam/Versed and lorazepam/Ativan or propofol) may be ordered. In some patients, a neuromuscular blocking agent (e.g., cisatracurium or pancuronium) may be ordered if the breathing pattern is adversely affecting the patient's progress and cannot be controlled using analgesics or sedatives. The nurse should assess for possible causes of the rapid pattern and take steps to relieve the problem when possible. Rapid breathing patterns may stem from fear, anxiety, pain, or such physiologic problems as acid–base imbalance or head injury.

Protection of the Airway

Protecting the airway is a major goal in caring for the mechanically ventilated patient. Any artificial airway can be fairly easily dislodged, either partially or completely. Because of this, the nurse must always take steps to minimize the possibility of dislodgment, which could precipitate respiratory compromise. During bedside care, dislodgment is at the highest risk while moving the patient from side to side in bed or when transferring the patient into or out of bed. Certain nursing actions minimize this risk, such as (1) maintaining sufficient slack on the ventilator tubing to minimize tension on the airway during moving, (2) disconnecting the patient from the ventilator and manually ventilating during transfer into and out of bed, and (3) adequately securing the airway through correct taping or other stabilizing device. Tracheostomy tubes often are sutured in place as well as being tied around the neck. Securing an ET tube using twill tape may not stabilize the tube sufficiently to prevent accidental dislodgment.

If the patient is not fully oriented or is uncooperative, he or she may pull the airway out. Interventions to reorient and remind the patient are indicated as well as measures to relieve pain and anxiety. When less restrictive measures are not sufficient, soft wrist restraints may be necessary. When restraints are in use, neurovascular checks should be performed routinely distal to the restraints. The purpose of the restraints must be explained and intermittently reinforced to both the patient and family, emphasizing that the restraints are in place for protection of the airway. Patients and families frequently view restraints as a punishment or unnecessary restriction of freedom.

Alteration in Cardiac Output

The general goal, support tissue perfusion, can be addressed using the nursing diagnosis of *decreased cardiac output*. Positive pressure ventilation profoundly affects the normal hemodynamics of the body by increasing intrathoracic pressures and decreasing venous return to the heart, which decreases cardiac output. The use of PEEP further compromises cardiac output by further decreasing venous return. These effects are described in detail in Section Seven.

TABLE 6–4   Hemodynamic Effects of Mechanical Ventilation

MEASURED PULMONARY ARTERY	
CATHETER PARAMETER	TREND
Right atrial pressure	Increased
Pulmonary artery pressure	Increased
Pulmonary artery wedge pressure	Usually increased
Left atrial pressure	Usually increased
Peripheral arterial pressure	Unchanged or decreased
Cardiac output	Decreased

Hemodynamic Effects of Mechanical Ventilation.   While on the mechanical ventilator, the patient may have a pulmonary artery flow-directed catheter inserted to closely monitor hemodynamic status, particularly if there is a history of cardiovascular problems. Table 6–4 shows the hemodynamic trends associated with mechanical ventilation.

If the patient does not have a pulmonary artery catheter inserted, the nurse can assess for the clinical manifestations of decreased cardiac output, such as confusion, restlessness, decreased urine output, flattened neck veins, and clammy, cool skin. Management of the patient with decreased cardiac output is described in detail in the perfusion modules of the textbook.

Alteration in Nutrition

Many patients who require mechanical ventilation have preexisting malnutrition associated with chronic illness or inadequate nutritional support during hospitalization or a combination of both. This patient population is at high risk for altered nutrition (less than body requirements). During the acute phase of illness, the patient will receive nothing orally. The presence of an ET tube, even with a properly inflated cuff, places the patient at risk for aspiration of microparticles that can leak around the endotracheal cuff and contaminate the lower airway. This leakage can precipitate complications associated with aspiration. Food and fluids by the oral route are avoided while an endotracheal tube is in place. Elevating the head of the bed greater than 30 degrees is an inexpensive technique that reduces reflux and the incidence of nosocomial pneumonia (Collard et al., 2003).

Dental plaque and oropharyngeal secretions are emerging as important factors in ventilator-associated pneumonia. Effective oral hygiene should include brushing, rinsing, and frequent removal of oral secretions (Munro & Grap, 2004). Antimicrobial agents, such as chlorhexidine, may be effective.

Maintaining a malnourished state with its negative nitrogen balance will significantly decrease the patient's chances of successful weaning from the mechanical ventilator because of respiratory muscle atrophy and weakness. Regaining nutritional integrity is a crucial aspect of care management because it has a direct impact on the patient's ability to improve his or her condition.

While on mechanical ventilation, the patient has a small-bore feeding tube inserted, either nasogastric or nasoenteric. Feedings ideally are initiated within 3 days of artificial airway placement to prevent gastrointestinal complications and to initiate early nutritional support. Pulmonary patients may require special consideration of carbohydrate loading because of the high carbon dioxide by-product produced, which can further complicate acid–base balance. Constipation with abdominal distention can develop as a result of immobility, illness, and narcotics used for comfort. Patients should be assessed for the need for a bowel regimen to prevent abdominal distention that can restrict lung expansion and complicate ventilator weaning. Management of the patient with alterations in nutrition is detailed in Module 23, "Metabolic Responses to Stress."

Nursing Management of Psychosocial Needs

The psychosocial needs of the high-acuity patient are presented in depth in Module 1. The following is a brief discussion of psychosocial needs specific to the patient requiring mechanical ventilation.

Anxiety and Pain

The patient who is being mechanically ventilated is usually experiencing a high level of anxiety associated with the insertion of the ET tube, the mechanical ventilator, and the critical care environment. Anxiety is a common complaint of patients who have chronic respiratory problems. Many chronic pulmonary diseases are progressive in nature; thus, a pattern of increasing disability is experienced.

As many chronic pulmonary diseases progress, patients experience an increasing pattern of hospital admissions for complications of their diseases. Ultimately, at end-stage disease, these patients most commonly die of complications of their diseases, such as severe respiratory failure or cor pulmonale.

When patients are experiencing acute respiratory distress, they often are anxious. Severe dyspnea frequently is associated with fear of suffocation or dying. All energy is focused toward breathing when acute distress exists. Being placed on a mechanical ventilator may be received by the patient either with relief or with an increased state of anxiety. The nursing diagnosis to deal with this problem is *anxiety,* which is associated with the unfamiliar environment, unfamiliar invasive breathing assist device, loss of control, painful procedures, lack of understanding or procedures, and fear of dying.

Critically ill patients may also experience pain related to their underlying illness, procedures, immobility, and routine care, including the endotracheal tube and suctioning. Puntillo et al. (2004) recommend that patients be assessed for pain by their report, when possible and by nonverbal indicators when they cannot communicate. The nursing diagnosis of *pain* is used to address this aspect of care.

Management of the patient's anxiety and pain while on the mechanical ventilator combines collaborative and independent nursing interventions. Sedation commonly is ordered to decrease anxiety levels, which, in turn, helps the patient breathe with the ventilator. The sedation may be in the form of narcotics or sedatives. A high-anxiety state must be brought under control if the patient is to decrease the work of breathing and oxygen consumption. Narcotics are particularly useful if the breathing pattern must be subdued because they have a respiratory depressant side effect. This is sometimes the case in patients who have uncontrolled tachypnea. When oxygen consumption is very high, it may be decided to use a neuromuscular blocking agent to paralyze the respiratory muscles, producing rapid apnea and total skeletal muscle paralysis. Neuromuscular blocking agents do not alter the responsiveness level of the patient. Therefore, while in the paralyzed state, this group of patients should receive intermittent IV sedation and analgesia at regular intervals to reduce anxiety, relieve pain, and enhance mental rest. Nursing interventions regarding pain and anxiety include

- Monitoring for signs and symptoms of pain and anxiety
- Implementing measures to reduce anxiety and pain
- Maintaining a restful environment
- Explaining all procedures and diagnostic tests
- Assessing for therapeutic and nontherapeutic effects of sedation and analgesia

Sleep Pattern Disturbance

While on the ventilator, the patient experiences interruptions throughout the 24-hour day. Airway clearance and other maintenance nursing interventions frequently require disturbing a resting or sleeping high-acuity patient. The nursing diagnosis addressing this problem is *sleep pattern disturbance*. Tamburri et al. (2004) investigated sleep deprivation in patients in critical care units. They concluded that critically ill patients have "few uninterrupted periods for sleep" (p. 102). During the duration of the study, only 6 percent of patients were allowed to have 2 to 3 uninterrupted hours of rest and only one sleep intervention was charted by the nurse in 147 nights of care.

Management of this problem often is a matter of careful planning on the part of the nurse. Clustering activities to allow for prolonged periods of undisturbed rest, particularly during the night hours, is a nursing goal. Minimizing interruptions at night for suctioning and turning and other high-priority interventions requires coordination and good communication among the entire nursing team.

Communication and Sensation

The presence of an artificial airway prevents the patient from communicating verbally. This alteration is addressed using the nursing diagnosis, *impaired verbal communication*. The patient may require frequent reminders that he or she will be able to talk once the tube is removed, with a brief explanation of why speech is not possible at this time. The patient who is fully responsive may become very frustrated when he or she cannot be understood. Alternative communication methods are available. To evaluate appropriate types of communication alternatives, the nurse must evaluate the patient's visual status. If eyesight is poor or glasses are not available, communication alternatives are reduced significantly.

The nurse has a variety of communication alternatives from which to experiment for effectiveness; for example, an alphabet or picture board for the patient to point to. Alphabet boards are not very satisfactory for many patients because they cannot concentrate sufficiently or do not have the strength to point to multiple letters for writing a message. Some facilities have talking boards on which the patient touches the appropriate picture and the board verbally states the particular need. Use of any type of picture board depends on the patient's ability to see the pictures. Some patients are able to write on a board with paper and pencil or other type of writing board, such as a magic slate or small chalkboard.

Patience on the part of the nurse is a major component of successful communication with a mechanically ventilated patient. Simple needs often can be expressed through lip reading or hand signals. It is easier to lip read with a patient who has a nasotracheal tube rather than one with an orally placed tube.

Family Support

The psychosocial needs of the patient's family cannot be forgotten while the patient is being managed on the ventilator. Families vary on how they perceive the ventilator. The family may express relief that the patient's breathing status is now protected. This is particularly true of families of patients who have had several past intubations. The patient's family initially may find the presence of the artificial airway and mechanical ventilator a frightening experience. The frequent alarms and the patient's inability to communicate verbally are the basis of many of the questions asked of the nurse. Family members must be oriented to the equipment in direct simple terms. Frequent updates should be given on the patient's status in terms the family can understand. It also is appropriate to remind the family, as necessary, that the patient will be able to talk once the tube is removed if a temporary tracheostomy or ET tube is in place. The nurse may have to translate communications from the patient to his or her family members.

In summary, care of the patient requiring mechanical ventilation involves interdisciplinary support of physiologic and psychosocial needs. Pulmonary physiologic needs focus on promoting optimal oxygenation, treating impaired gas exchange providing adequate ventilation, and protecting the patient's airway. In addition, the physiologic needs of tissue perfusion and nutritional support require aggressive attention. Psychosocial problems include anxiety, pain, sleep pattern disturbance, and impaired verbal communication. The mechanically ventilated patient may require numerous additional nursing diagnoses based on specific functional needs associated with specific disease processes and multisystem dysfunction.

SECTION NINE REVIEW

1. The primary reason that airway patency becomes compromised in the mechanically ventilated patient is
   A. ineffective cough
   B. oversedation
   C. airway obstruction
   D. dehydration

2. Unless contraindicated, the patient should receive a fluid intake of _____ to _____ L/day to combat thick secretions.
   A. 1, 1.5
   B. 2, 2.5
   C. 3, 3.5
   D. 4, 4.5

3. The mechanically ventilated patient can develop respiratory alkalosis if the _____ and _____ settings on the mechanical ventilator are set too high.
   A. rate, tidal volume

B. peak airway pressure, rate
C. O_2 concentration, peak airway pressure
D. tidal volume, O_2 concentration

4. A mechanically ventilated patient who is malnourished is at high risk for failure to wean because of
   A. impaired gas exchange
   B. decreased cardiac output
   C. increased airway resistance
   D. respiratory muscle weakness

5. To treat the nursing diagnosis, *sleep pattern disturbance,* while managing the care of a mechanically ventilated patient, the best nursing action would be to
   A. cluster activities
   B. administer sedatives
   C. administer neuromuscular blocking agents
   D. space activities evenly throughout the 24-hour day

Answers: 1. C, 2. B, 3. A, 4. D, 5. A

SECTION TEN: Weaning the Patient from the Mechanical Ventilator

At the completion of this section, the learner will be able to describe the **weaning** process.

The term *mechanical ventilator weaning* refers to the activities involved in withdrawing a patient from mechanical ventilator support and attaining total independence from the ventilator. Withdrawing mechanical ventilator support is a multidisciplinary effort that requires coordination among the physician, respiratory therapist, nurse, and patient. Ventilator weaning may be a relatively simple and rapid withdrawal process or it may be complex and extremely slow. The majority of patients requiring mechanical ventilator support are weaned rapidly with little difficulty. The remaining few are those who require prolonged weaning or are unable to wean. This small but significant group primarily consists of patients who have a history of chronic pulmonary disease or who have required prolonged mechanical ventilation. This section presents a brief overview of the weaning process that will familiarize the learner with major assessments and interventions that are an integral part of the process.

Hess and Kacmarek (2002) divide patients who are being evaluated for ventilator weaning into three categories:

1. Patients whose removal is rapid when the reason for mechanical ventilation is resolved
2. Patients whose removal is slow and gradual and require more deliberate planning than the usual routine weaning activities

3. Patients who are considered unweanable (ventilator dependent) and may require long-term ventilatory support

The Weaning Process

Just as criteria are used in making the decision to place a patient on a mechanical ventilator, criteria are used when determining readiness for withdrawal from ventilator support. Successful weaning involves using a systematic approach, including determination of readiness to wean, weaning, and postextubation follow-up.

Determination of Readiness to Wean

Successful weaning depends largely on the physiologic and psychologic readiness of the patient. A variety of criteria are used to determine readiness; these criteria can be divided into initial and comprehensive patient screenings.

Initial Patient Screening. MacIntyre et al. (2001) suggest that consideration for readiness for weaning begins when the cause of respiratory failure is resolved or improving. Other necessary criteria include adequate oxygenation (while receiving FIO_2 less than 0.50 and PEEP less than 8), hemodynamic stability, and spontaneous ventilatory effort.

Comprehensive Patient Screening. The decision of when it is appropriate to begin the weaning process is not necessarily a clear one. Generally, prior to making a final decision, a multisystem assessment review is conducted, focusing on those physiologic systems that are particularly associated with ventilator dependence (respiratory, cardiovascular, CNS, renal, and metabolic).

TABLE 6–5   Mechanical Ventilator Weaning Criteria

CRITERIA	RESPONSES
I. Initial Criteria	
A. Is the patient clinically stable?	Yes/No
B. Is the patient's clinical condition improving?	Yes/No
C. Is the precipitating problem resolved?	Yes/No
D. Is $\dot{V}_E$ less than 10 L/min on AC or SIMV of 14 or less?	Yes/No
E. Is Spo_2 greater than 90 percent or greater at 0.40 Fio_2 or less?	Yes/No
F. Is A-a gradient less than 100 mm Hg?	Yes/No

If any "No" answers, quit here. Patient does not qualify for initiation of weaning. Reevaluate in 48 hours.

CRITERIA	RESPONSES
II. Comprehensive Criteria	
Is the patient:	
A. Hemodynamically stable?	
1. SBP 100–150, DBP 60–90 mm Hg at rest?	Yes/No
2. Heart rate 60–100 beats/min at rest?	Yes/No
3. Usual ECG pattern?	Yes/No
B. Systemically hydrated?	
1. Intake = Output	Yes/No
2. Urinary output greater than 620 mL/24 hr	Yes/No
3. BUN and creatinine: within normal limits	Yes/No
C. Without fever or new/unresolved pulmonary infection? (Chest x-ray within past 48 hr; temp. less than 100°F (37.8°c) orally)	Yes/No
D. Receiving support for nutritional status?	Yes/No
E. Have drugs been discontinued that	
1. Decrease respiratory drive?	Yes/No
2. Increase muscle weakness?	Yes/No
3. Increase anxiety?	Yes/No
III. Laboratory Values	
Are the following parameters in at least minimal acceptable ranges and current within the past 24 hours? Specify "Yes" if replacement therapy is occurring if value is below normal range.	
A. K (normal, 3.5–5.0 mEq/L)	Yes/No
B. Na (normal, 135–145 mEq/L)	Yes/No
C. PO_4 (normal, 3.0–4.5 mg/dL, acceptable greater than 2.0)	Yes/No
D. Ca (normal, 8.5–10.5 mg/dL)	Yes/No
E. Mg (normal, 1.5–4.5 mg/dL)	Yes/No
F. Prealbumin (normal, 24–30 mg/dL, acceptable 10 or higher)	Yes/No
G. CBC with differential, specifically:	
WBC (normal, 5,000–10,000/L)	Yes/No
Hgb (normal, greater than 10 g/dL)	Yes/No
Hct (normal, greater than 30 g/dL)	Yes/No
Calculated total lymphocyte count (normal, 1,500 or 2,000/mcL or greater)	Yes/No
H. Theophylline level (normal, less than 20 mcg/dL)	Yes/No
I. ABG while on ventilator within the past 12 hours:	
pH = 7.35–7.45	Yes/No
PO_2 = 60 mm Hg or greater on Fio_2 of 0.4 or less	Yes/No
PCO_2 = less than 50 mm Hg or within 10 mm Hg of baseline	Yes/No
Sao_2 = 90 percent or greater at 0.40 Fio_2 or less	Yes/No

If there are any "No" answers to the criteria in Sections II and III, the decision to initiate weaning will be closely evaluated. If the problem is easily correctable, appropriate interventions will be taken to correct the problem and the patient will be reevaluated after 24 hours.

Key: SBP: systolic blood pressure, DBP: diastolic blood pressure

Henneman (2001) and Burns et al. (2003) stress the importance of a comprehensive, multidisciplinary approach to weaning. Table 6–5 presents an example of a combined simple and comprehensive assessment form that might be used in helping to determine readiness for weaning. Note the number of criteria that focus on nutrition and metabolic function.

Assessment data provided by simple and comprehensive patient screenings identify potential barriers to successful weaning and actions that must be taken to resolve each problem. It is at this point in the weaning process that actions vary widely. Barriers to successful weaning are not necessarily considered equal and experts disagree regarding which criteria are absolute and which are relative contraindications. For this reason, weaning may be initiated on patients who do not meet all the simple or comprehensive criteria (e.g., presence of active but improving pneumonia; improving but not corrected malnutrition).

Alternative Indications of Readiness to Wean

The traditional criteria for readiness to wean are similar to the criteria used in deciding to place the patient on the mechanical ventilator. These criteria are useful primarily for assessing the readiness of short-term, relatively healthy individuals. They have not, however, been found to effectively predict weaning success in the elderly or those with chronic pulmonary disease (patients who make up a high proportion of the difficult-to-wean group). There is a strong interest in finding better indicators of weaning readiness and it is hoped that these new indicators will be more predictive of successful weaning in the difficult-to-wean population.

Weaning

Rapid Weaning (Short Term)

Frequently, a patient with no significant lung disease requires short-term mechanical ventilation (e.g., surgery, drug overdose). Once the underlying problem is corrected (e.g., reversal of anesthesia effects), the patient is evaluated for weaning. Hess and Kacmarek (2002) describe the use of a spontaneous breathing trial for patients who are likely to be weaned rapidly. If weaning criteria are met, the patient is placed on CPAP or removed from the ventilator and placed on a T-piece (or blow-by) for 30 to 120 minutes. During the trial period, the patient is monitored for comfort, cardiac rhythm status, and ABG status. If these criteria remain within acceptable limits (stable PaO_2, and pH above 7.30), the patient is extubated. Rapid weaning may also be accomplished using low levels of PSV or CPAP. The patient is given a brief trial period and then extubated. Figure 6–10 illustrates a typical T-piece (blow-by) configuration.

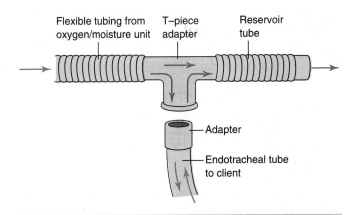

Figure 6–10 ■ T-piece (blow-by) configuration.

Slow Weaning (Long Term)

Patients who have underlying chronic lung disease (e.g., emphysema or pulmonary fibrosis) that is complicated by some acute problem (e.g., pneumonia) and patients who have had a prolonged illness frequently cannot be weaned as rapidly as patients with normal lungs. Slow weaning is performed on patients who are unable to wean for a variety of reasons. Problems associated with difficult weaning include excessive respiratory muscle work of breathing, respiratory muscle fatigue, anemia, malnutrition, excessive secretions, infection, unstable hemodynamic state, fear, and anxiety. Difficult-to-wean patients often are in a poorer state of general health than the fast-weaning group. Their ability to make the transition back to spontaneous negative pressure breathing from long-term positive pressure breathing is slow and requires retraining and strengthening of the respiratory muscles.

Slow weaning is a complex and difficult process for all involved. Over time, multiple weaning alternatives (IMV/SIMV, mandatory minute ventilation [MMV], PSV, manual weaning/spontaneous breathing trials) may need to be employed in response to changes in the patient's clinical status. Long-term weaning requires close monitoring of the patient's multisystem functions, as well as psychosocial status. Rapid, aggressive management of problems as they arise significantly improves the chances for successful weaning.

Methods of Weaning

Manual Weaning/Spontaneous Breathing Trials

Manual weaning was the original method of withdrawing a patient from a ventilator, and it is still used. Manual weaning is accomplished by following a schedule of removal from the mechanical ventilator for increasingly longer periods of time. When this method is used, the patient is taken off the ventilator and the artificial airway is attached to a humidified oxygen source using a T-piece. The nurse is responsible for closely monitoring the patient for signs of weaning intolerance. For example, respiratory rate greater than 30/min, a significant increase in blood pressure and pulse (often more than 10 mm Hg and 10/min, respectively), a minute ventilation of more than 10 L/min, cyanosis, or a decrease in oxygen saturation on pulse oximetry to below the patient's acceptable level. Other indicators of fatigue include diaphoresis, use of accessory muscles, and abdominal paradox.

Manual weaning requires close patient contact throughout the weaning period because the nurse plays a crucial part in patient monitoring and coaching correct breathing rate and depth for the trial period. The nurse's calm reassurance is instrumental in assisting the patient past the period of anxiety often associated with removal from the mechanical ventilator. Manual weaning is performed on an increasing schedule either throughout the 24-hour period or throughout the day and evening hours and maintaining the patient on mechanical ventilation throughout the night for rest. The amount of time the patient is kept off the ventilator may start at 5 minutes and increase to the entire day, except at night, before full independence. Manual weaning must be individually designed, based on the patient's changing status from day to day.

Manual weaning is a strengthening exercise for the respiratory muscles. Complete removal from the ventilator forces the respiratory muscles to take over complete work of breathing, without any assistance from the ventilator for increasing blocks of time. Muscle strength is increased through use of the weaning procedure and good nutrition and hydration. There are several disadvantages to manual weaning. First, it may be a frightening experience for the patient, who is more accustomed to positive pressure breathing. Abrupt removal from the ventilator may precipitate high anxiety, which can hinder the weaning process. Second, manual weaning is time consuming for the

nurse. During the period that the patient is off the ventilator, particularly in the early stages of weaning, the nurse is needed directly at the bedside to coach and monitor, and to give encouragement.

Spontaneous breathing trials can also be done using the ventilator. Rather than placing the patient on a T-piece, the patient is placed on CPAP with or without low levels of pressure support. The length of time of spontaneous breathing is increased as tolerated, similar to T-piece weaning (Hess & Kacmarek, 2002). Using the ventilator for spontaneous trials offers the advantages of maintaining CPAP, which may be important for some patients, and ventilator monitoring for safety.

Ventilator Weaning

Today, ventilator weaning (use of a ventilator mode) is more common than manual weaning. It is generally thought to be less traumatic for the patient because it does not involve intermittent removal from the ventilator. A variety of alternative modes are used for ventilator weaning, the most common ones being IMV/SIMV, PSV, and MMV. The choice of weaning mode is based on the clinician's preferences, the type of mode available based on equipment constraints, and the patient's needs and clinical status. Table 6–6 provides a summary of the common ventilator weaning modes.

IMV/SIMV Weaning.   Following is a brief description of one ventilator weaning protocol using IMV/SIMV. Using this ventilator mode, the patient is given mandatory mechanical (ventilator) breaths at preset intervals every minute. Between the mechanical breaths, the patient is able to exercise the respiratory muscles spontaneously. Initially, the IMV/SIMV rate may be set fairly high, near the patient's own respiratory rate. The rate of mandatory breaths is then decreased by 2-breath increments

TABLE 6–6   Common Ventilator Weaning Modes

WEANING MODE	DESCRIPTION	ADVANTAGES	DISADVANTAGES
IMV/SIMV	Frequency of mandatory ventilator breaths is slowly decreased, which requires the patient to gradually take over own work of breathing.	Maintains respiratory muscle strength and reduces atrophy Maintains more normal gas distribution Reduces cardiovascular side effects Maintains some of the work of breathing	May increase the work of breathing as a result of demand valve system Rate must be manually manipulated
PSV	Provides positive pressure during the inspiration phase to support tidal volumes and decrease work of breathing.	Decreased work of breathing Increased patient comfort Minimal cardiovascular side effects	All breaths are spontaneous Flow pattern may not be adequate Inspiratory flow rate may be too high or too low
MMV	Guarantees an ongoing stable level of minute ventilation ($\dot{V}_E$): As the patient increases or decreases ventilatory effort, the ventilator adjusts itself automatically to continue to provide the same level of $\dot{V}_E$.	Good control of $Paco_2$ Protection from hypoventilation during weaning Facilitates transition from ventilator to spontaneous breathing	May not respond quickly enough to an apneic episode Potential for development of hypercapnea in presence of a rapid shallow breathing pattern

Data from Pilbeam, S. P. (1998). Mechanical ventilation: Physiological and clinical applications, *(3rd ed.). St. Louis: C.V. Mosby.*

1 to 2 times per day (as tolerated) until the IMV/SIMV rate is down to 4 breaths per minute. Once the mandatory rate is at 4 breaths per minute, a spontaneous mode (such as PSV) or a T-piece trial is attempted for a minimum of 30 minutes. If the patient tolerates the weaning procedure and all parameters remain within acceptable boundaries, he or she can be extubated.

IMV/SIMV weaning is an endurance exercise for the respiratory muscles. The muscles work continuously over the entire day except when the IMV/SIMV breath triggers a positive pressure breath, which allows a single breath rest. Some patients do not tolerate decreasing IMV/SIMV rates. This tolerance may change on a day-to-day basis. Weaning often is not a smooth undertaking. In patients with underlying disease, changing status can require temporary cessation of weaning. This is particularly true if the patient should develop pneumonia. Such a status change may first manifest itself in a sudden intolerance to weaning.

Whatever the method used, evidence supports a comprehensive approach to weaning. Burns et al. (2003) and Henneman (2001) describe success in using structured, multidisciplinary protocols that guide the weaning process and ongoing patient assessments. Continuing efforts are made to optimize all aspects of care.

Special Considerations for the Elderly

Sevransky and Haponik (2003) explain that the elderly can have similar outcomes from mechanical ventilation as younger patients. They caution, however, that common complications of critical illness, such as delirium, side effects of sedative agents, and deconditioning, adversely prolong ventilation and length of stay. Higher mortality rates and poorer functional outcomes occur in patients with multiple organ failure or prolonged intubation. The best mode for weaning for elderly patients has not been identified.

Hart et al. (2002) identify the age-related reduction in reserve as a major factor in poor outcomes of hospitalized elderly. The elderly, without significant comorbid illness, become frail in this setting and vulnerable to complications. Although they are not limited to patients requiring mechanical ventilation, these researchers identify two major approaches to care of the older patient: avoiding fatigue and preventing complications.

To avoid fatigue, nursing care and procedures should be spaced at intervals allowing time for rest. Sleep can be enhanced by obtaining information on and trying to maintain the patient's usual schedule, promoting a day–night schedule, reducing noise, and following nonpharmacologic approaches.

Priorities for care include cautious use of sedative/hypnotic agents that can cause confusion because the elderly are at increased risk for developing delirium. All medications should be evaluated for potential adverse drug interactions. Efforts can be made to enhance quality stimulation and communication. Hearing aids and eyeglasses should be used if needed by the patient. Malnutrition may be present on admission or develop while the patient is in the hospital and can contribute to muscle weakness. Early aggressive reconditioning and physical therapy are needed to limit muscle atrophy from prolonged bedrest. Therapy may even include ambulation using a manual resuscitation bag (MacIntyre et al., 2001). These approaches are not limited to the care of the elderly, but represent important care for any critically ill patient. In the elderly, however, the approaches assume a greater imperative given the vulnerability of the aged and their reduced capacity to recover from severe insults.

Postextubation Follow-up

Extubation (removal of the artificial airway) is usually carried out as soon as it is determined that the patient can sustain spontaneous breathing. Removal of the artificial airway, however, requires that patients be able to maintain their own airways and cough adequately to mobilize secretions. Hess and Kacmarek (2002) suggest that an "air leak" test is helpful to evaluate the potential for airway obstruction postextubation. To conduct an air leak test, the oropharynx is suctioned, the ET cuff is deflated, and the patient is evaluated for the ability to breathe around the tube. When these criteria are met, rapid tube removal is recommended. Quick tube removal is important because the ET tube increases the work of breathing.

Following extubation, particular attention must be given to excellent pulmonary hygiene, including a routine of coughing, deep breathing, and incentive spirometry. Various aerosol therapies, percussion, and postural drainage may be ordered to prevent or treat complications, if necessary. Noninvasive ventilation may be helpful for patients at high risk for fatigue and reintubation (Hess & Kacmarek, 2002).

Jaber et al. (2003) suggest that postextubation stridor be closely watched for following extubation. It results from glottic edema and can be mild or severe. When severe, it can cause total obstruction of the airway requiring reintubation.

Postextubation, patients are also at risk for aspiration as a result of swallowing dysfunction. Ajemian et al. (2001) found a high incidence of aspiration (50 percent) in patients who had been intubated for more than 48 hours. Many of these patients (25 percent) had "silent aspiration," in that they did not cough. Aspiration may contribute to postextubation respiratory failure. Patients must be monitored carefully when oral intake is resumed and a formal swallow evaluation may be appropriate for high-risk patients.

In summary, withdrawal from mechanical ventilation (weaning) is a three-phase process, including (1) determination of readiness, an assessment phase; (2) weaning, an intervention phase; and (3) postextubation follow-up, an evaluation phase. Determination of readiness includes both simple and comprehensive weaning criteria that assess multiple body systems. There are two general types of weaning: rapid (short term) and slow (long term). Rapid weaning is performed on the majority of patients, usually those without significant lung disease. Slow weaning is required primarily in patients with significant lung disease and those with more serious health problems, and may involve the use of multiple weaning methodologies. The two general methods of weaning are manual and ventilator weaning. Manual weaning consists of intermittent removal of the patient from the ventilator for increasingly longer periods of time. Ventilator weaning uses manipulation of certain ventilator modes to wean the patient without disconnection from the ventilator.

Common ventilator weaning modes include IMV/SIMV, PSV, and MMV. Weaning considerations for the elderly include a focus on aspects of care to avoid fatigue and prevent complications. Postextubation follow-up includes close monitoring of the patient for development of postextubation respiratory distress, as well as interventions to facilitate adequate ventilation and oxygenation.

SECTION TEN REVIEW

1. The vast majority of patients requiring mechanical ventilation are weaned
   A. rapidly, with difficulty
   B. rapidly, without difficulty
   C. slowly, with difficulty
   D. slowly, without difficulty

2. The majority of difficult-to-wean patients have which condition?
   A. pneumonia
   B. congestive heart failure
   C. acute respiratory distress syndrome
   D. chronic pulmonary disease

3. Simple patient screening questions for weaning eligibility include
   A. Is the urinary output greater than 620 mL/24 hr?
   B. Is the prealbumin 10 mg/dL or greater?
   C. Is the patient's clinical condition improving?
   D. Have drugs been discontinued that decrease the respiratory drive?

4. Traditional weaning criteria most effectively predict readiness in patients who
   A. are elderly
   B. are relatively healthy
   C. have chronic pulmonary disease
   D. require prolonged mechanical ventilation

5. The term _____ weaning is used to refer to weaning by intermittently removing the patient from the ventilator for increasing periods of time.
   A. manual
   B. ventilator
   C. IMV/SIMV
   D. pressure support ventilation

6. IMV/SIMV weaning primarily is a(n) _____ exercise for the respiratory muscles.
   A. supportive
   B. resistance
   C. strengthening
   D. endurance

Answers: 1. B, 2. D, 3. C, 4. B, 5. A, 6. D

POSTTEST

The following Posttest is constructed in a case study format. A patient is presented. Questions are asked based on available data. New data are presented as the case study progresses.

Mary R, 55 years of age, has a 20-year history of smoking. She has been treated medically for emphysema for several years. Mary weighs 115 pounds. She is admitted to the hospital with a diagnosis of acute respiratory failure.

1. If Mary's tidal volume was 300 mL, her alveolar ventilation would be _____ mL.
   A. 8.4
   B. 50
   C. 185
   D. 300

2. To be clinically called acute ventilatory failure, which of the following arterial blood gas results must be present?
   A. pH less than 7.35
   B. Pa_{CO_2} greater than 50 mm Hg
   C. Pa_{O_2} less than 60 mm Hg
   D. HCO_3 less than 18 mm Hg

3. Mary has a low ventilation–perfusion ratio as a result of pulmonary shunting. Shunting refers to
   A. blood that does not go through the heart
   B. normal alveolar ventilation with poor perfusion
   C. diminished pulmonary ventilation and perfusion
   D. normal perfusion past unventilated alveoli

Mary is showing evidence of ventilatory fatigue. It is decided that she will require intubation and mechanical ventilation.

4. Mary's intubation is a semielective one. For increased comfort, she may have which type of artificial airway inserted?
   A. oral endotracheal tube
   B. nasotracheal tube
   C. tracheostomy tube
   D. oral pharyngeal airway

Mary is placed on volume-cycled ventilation.

5. The primary advantage of using volume-cycled ventilation is that it
   A. overcomes changes in airway resistance
   B. does not require a cuffed artificial airway
   C. automatically alters volume as pressure changes
   D. delivers higher levels of oxygen than other ventilators

6. Mary's tidal volume is set at 450 mL. A sufficiently large tidal volume is set on a mechanical ventilator to decrease
   A. peak airway pressure
   B. pneumothorax occurrence
   C. ventilator breaths
   D. atelectasis occurrence

Mary's minute ventilation is 5.6 L/min. Her ventilator settings are currently as follows: VT 700 mL, f 8/min. Her PaCO$_2$ has increased from 45 mm Hg in the past hour to the latest level of 55 mm Hg.

7. Assuming that the tidal volume cannot be manipulated further, how can the rate be manipulated to increase the minute ventilation to 7 L/min?
   A. decrease the rate to 6/min
   B. increase the rate to 10/min
   C. increase the rate to 12/min
   D. increase the rate to 14/min

8. If Mary was placed on 10 cm H$_2$O of PEEP, the level of PEEP could be monitored by the nurse in which manner?
   A. the PIP should increase by 10 cm H$_2$O during inspiration
   B. the PIP should decrease by 10 cm H$_2$O during inspiration
   C. the airway pressure manometer needle should fall only to 10 cm H$_2$O during expiration
   D. the airway pressure manometer needle should fall to negative 10 cm H$_2$O during expiration

Mary has improved and weaning from the ventilator has begun. The decision is made to place Mary on synchronous intermittent mandatory ventilation (SIMV) of 12/min with pressure support of 10 cm H$_2$O.

9. Pressure support ventilation is used for which of the following reasons?
   A. it makes inspiration easier
   B. it makes expiration easier
   C. it keeps alveoli open through the breathing cycle
   D. it increases PIP during inspiration

10. Mary's PIP has increased steadily for the past 3 hours. This trend may indicate
    A. increased lung compliance
    B. decreased airway resistance
    C. decreased lung compliance
    D. increased lung ventilatory capacity

11. Mary's low exhaled volume alarm keeps triggering. If the problem is not found immediately, the nurse should
    A. call the physician
    B. manually ventilate
    C. check connections again
    D. put more air in the tracheal cuff

12. When Mary was on PEEP, the nurse would expect which trend secondary to changes in cardiac output?
    A. decreased blood pressure, increased pulse
    B. increased blood pressure, increased pulse
    C. decreased blood pressure, decreased pulse
    D. increased blood pressure, decreased pulse

13. If Mary developed a right lower lobe (RLL) pneumonia while receiving mechanical ventilation, how would airflow be affected?
    A. ventilation would not be affected
    B. ventilation to RLL would increase
    C. ventilation to all right lung fields would decrease
    D. ventilation to RLL would decrease

14. Mary's urine output before mechanical ventilation was approximately 100 mL/hour over a 24-hour period. Once mechanical ventilation was initiated, the nurse should expect which trend for urine output?
    A. decrease
    B. increase slightly
    C. increase significantly
    D. remain approximately the same

15. While Mary is on the mechanical ventilator, the nurse will need to monitor her closely for development of a stress ulcer related to
    A. visceral tissue ischemia
    B. increased visceral blood flow
    C. increased visceral venous return
    D. decreased visceral vascular resistance

16. The nurse will need to monitor Mary for development of a nosocomial pulmonary infection. An assessment that would best support this problem is
    A. sputum is green
    B. lung sounds are clear
    C. a large quantity of sputum
    D. an increased serum white blood cell count

17. To prevent complications associated with endotracheal trauma, the nurse should maintain the cuff pressure within what range?
    A. 10 to 15 mm Hg
    B. 15 to 20 mm Hg
    C. 20 to 25 mm Hg
    D. 25 to 30 mm Hg

18. The nurse is having difficulty clearing Mary's airway of thick secretions. The most effective means of enhancing Mary's airway clearance is to
    A. increase frequency of suctioning
    B. increase fluid intake
    C. reposition her every 2 hours
    D. administer nebulizer treatments

Mary's ventilator settings were changed earlier today. The changes were as follows:

VT: increased from 500 mL to 700 mL

f: increased from 14 to 16 breaths/min

19. Mary has ABGs drawn. Based on the ventilator setting changes, which trend would be anticipated?
    A. increasing pH
    B. increasing Pa_{CO_2}
    C. decreasing pH
    D. decreasing Sa_{O_2}
20. The nurse is preparing to transfer Mary from her bed to a chair positioned next to the bed. Assuming Mary's respiratory status is stable, the safest method of transferring her is to
    A. closely observe the ventilator tubing during transfer
    B. have someone hold her head during transfer
    C. assure that the ET tube taping is secure prior to transfer
    D. disconnect her from the ventilator during transfer

The pulmonary team is considering initiating the weaning process. Mary's current status is as follows:

HR: 100/min, regular

RR: 28/min

Respiratory pattern: irregular

No palpable abdominal tensing on expiration

21. Which of Mary's assessments does not meet the simple criteria for weaning readiness?
    A. heart rate
    B. respiratory rate
    C. respiratory pattern
    D. abdominal tensing
22. Mary is weaned successfully using IMV/SIMV mode. This mode supports the weaning process by
    A. requiring Mary to gradually take over her own work of breathing
    B. supporting Mary's tidal volume during inspiration
    C. assuring that Mary maintains a stable minute ventilation
    D. supporting Mary by maintaining open alveoli at end expiration

POSTTEST ANSWERS

Question	Answer	Section	Question	Answer	Section
1	C	One	12	A	Five
2	B	Two	13	D	Seven
3	D	Two	14	A	Seven
4	B	Three	15	A	Seven
5	A	Four	16	A	Seven
6	D	Five	17	C	Eight
7	B	Five	18	B	Nine
8	C	Five	19	A	Nine
9	A	Five	20	D	Nine
10	C	Five	21	C	Ten
11	B	Five	22	A	Ten

REFERENCES

The Acute Respiratory Distress Syndrome Network. (2000). Ventilation with lower tidal volumes as compared to traditional tidal volumes for acute lung injury and the acute respiratory distress syndrome. *New England Journal of Medicine, 342*(18), 1301–1308.

Ajemian, M., Nirmul, G., Anderson M., et al. (2001). Routine fiberoptic endoscopic evaluation of swallowing following prolonged intubation. Implications for management. *Archives of Surgery, 136*, 434–437.

Burns, S., Earven, S., Fisher, C., et al. (2003). Implementation of an institutional program to improve clinical and financial outcomes of mechanically ventilated patients: One-year outcomes and lessons learned. *Critical Care Medicine, 31*, 2752–2763.

Chastre, J., & Fagon, J. (2002). Ventilator-associated pneumonia. *American Journal of Respiratory Critical Care Medicine, 165*, 867–903.

Collard, H., Saint, S., & Matthay, M. (2003). Prevention of ventilator-associated pneumonia: An evidence-based systematic review. *Annals of Internal Medicine, 138*, 494–501.

Flemons, W. (2002). Obstructive sleep apnea. *New England Journal of Medicine, 347*, 498–504.

Hart, B., Birkas, J., Lachmann, M., & Saunders, L. (2002). Promoting positive outcomes for elderly persons in the hospital: Prevention and risk factor modification. *AACN Clinical Issues, 13,* 22–33.

Health & Medicine Week Editors. (June 28, 2004). *Health & Medicine Week,* p. 997.

Henneman, E. (2001). Liberating patients from mechanical ventilation: A team approach. *Critical Care Nurse, 21*(3), 25, 27–33.

Hess, D., & Kacmarek, R. (2002). *Essentials of mechanical ventilation* (2nd ed.). New York: McGraw-Hill.

Jaber, S., Chanques, G., Matecki, S., et al. (2003). Post-extubation stridor in intensive care unit patients: Risk factors evaluation and importance of the cuff-leak test. *Intensive Care Medicine, 29,* 69–74.

Kress, J. P., Pohlman, A. S., O'Connor, M. F., et al. (2000). Daily interruption of sedative infusions in critically ill patients undergoing mechanical ventilation. *New England Journal of Medicine, 342* (20), 1471–1477.

Liesching, T., Kwok, H., & Hill, N. (2003). Acute applications of noninvasive positive pressure ventilation. *Chest, 124,* 699–713.

MacIntyre, N., Cook, D., Ely, E., et al. (2001). Evidence-based guidelines for weaning and discontinuing ventilatory support: A collective task force facilitated by the American College of Chest Physicians; the American Association for Respiratory Care; and the American College of Critical Care Medicine. *Chest, 120*(Suppl), 375S–395S.

Malhotra, A., Ayas, N., & Epstein, L. (2000). The art and science of continuous positive airway pressure therapy in obstructive sleep apnea. *Current Opinion in Pulmonary Medicine, 6,* 490–495.

Martin, L. (1987). *Pulmonary physiology in clinical practice: The essentials for patient care and evaluation.* St. Louis: C.V. Mosby.

Mehta, S., & Hill, N. (2001). Noninvasive ventilation. *American Journal of Respiratory and Critical Care Medicine, 163,* 540–577.

Munro, C., & Grap, M. (2004). Oral health and care in the intensive care unit: State of the science. *American Journal of Critical Care, 13,* 25–33.

Mutlu, G., Mutlu, E., & Factor, P. (2001). GI complications in patients receiving mechanical ventilation. *Chest, 119,* 1222–1241.

Pannu, N., & Mehta, R. (2002). Mechanical ventilation and renal function: An area for concern? *American Journal of Kidney Disease 39,* 616–24.

Phelan, B., Cooper, D., & Sangkachand, P. (2002). Prolonged mechanical ventilation and tracheostomy in the elderly. *AACN Clinical Issues, 13,* 84–93.

Pilbeam, S. P. (1998). *Mechanical ventilation: Physiological and clinical applications* (3rd ed.). St. Louis: C.V. Mosby.

Puntillo, K., Morris, A., Thompson, C., Stanik-Hutt, J., White, C., & Wild, L. (2004). Pain behaviors observed during six common procedures: Results from Thunder Project II. *Critical Care Medicine, 32,* 421–427.

Sevransky, J., & Haponik, E. (2003). Respiratory failure in elderly patients. *Clinical Geriatric Medicine, 19,* 205–224.

Tamburri, L. M., Di Brienza, R., Zozula, R., et al. (2004). Nocturnal care interactions with patients in critical care units. *American Journal of Critical Care, 13,* 102–113.

Tullmann, D., & Dracup, K. (2000). Creating a healing environment for elders. *AACN Clinical Issues, 11,* 34–50.

van Soeren, M., Diehl-Jones, W., Maykut, R., & Haddara W. (2000). Pathophysiology and implications for treatment of acute respiratory distress syndrome. *AACN Clinical Issues, 11,* 179–197.

Wood, G. C., Boucher, B.A., Croce, M. A., et al. (2002). Aerosolized ceftazidime for prevention of ventilator-associated pneumonia and drug effects on the proinflammatory response in critically ill trauma patients. *Pharmacotherapy, 22,* 972–982.

7 Nursing Care of the Patient with Altered Gas Exchange

Kathleen Dorman Wagner

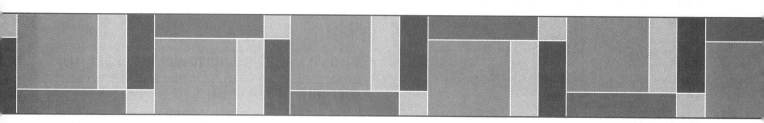

OBJECTIVES Following completion of this module, given a specific clinical situation, the learner will be able to

1. Interpret the significance of laboratory data.

2. Interpret the significance of assessment data.

3. Develop appropriate desired patient outcomes.

4. Apply knowledge of the patient with altered respiratory function to develop a plan of nursing interventions.

5. Describe the nursing management of the patient with restrictive and obstructive pulmonary diseases.

This module is designed to integrate the major points discussed in Modules 4 through 6, "Determinants and Assessment of Pulmonary Gas Exchange," "Alterations in Pulmonary Gas Exchange," and "Mechanical Ventilation." This module summarizes relationships between key concepts

and assists the learner in clustering information to facilitate clinical application. The module is divided into three sections. It applies content from Part 2: Pulmonary Gas Exchange in an interactive learning style. Using a case study format, the learner is encouraged to identify nursing actions based on the assessment of a patient with a restrictive pulmonary disease in Case Study 1, a patient with an obstructive pulmonary disease in Case Study 2, and a patient requiring mechanical ventilation in Case Study 3. Case Studies 1 and 2 include collaborative and independent nursing interventions typically used in planning the care of patients with restrictive and obstructive pulmonary disorders.

Case Study 1

MARY R, A PATIENT WITH RESTRICTIVE DISEASE

You are the nurse assigned to admit Mary R, 38 years old, who is a direct admission from a family practice clinic. No other information is available. You have just been informed that Mary has been brought to the floor and has been assisted into bed.

Initial Appraisal

On walking into her room for the first time, you quickly note the following.

GENERAL APPEARANCE. Mary is an African American female of small stature. She appears well nourished and is tidy in appearance. She is still fully clothed except for her shoes. She is wearing glasses.

SIGNS OF DISTRESS. Mary's respirations are rapid and appear shallow. She is moving restlessly in the bed. A frequent, harsh cough is heard, and secretions are audible during coughing. Perspiration is noted on Mary's face.

OTHER. You do not note any intravenous lines or oxygen in use. A man of approximately the same age is in the room with Mary, talking quietly to her. He identifies himself as James, her husband.

Focused Respiratory Assessment

Mary's clothing is exchanged quickly for a hospital gown to make assessment easier and make her more comfortable. Because Mary appears to be in acute respiratory distress, you immediately perform a rapid assessment focusing first on her pulmonary status. The results are as follows:

Mary is restless and oriented to person, place, and time. Her respiratory rate is 32/min, shallow, and regular. Her mucous membranes are dusky. Her respirations are labored. She is using accessory muscles in her neck during inspiration. Crackles and wheezes are auscultated in the right middle and right lower lobes of her lungs. A pleural friction rub is auscultated at the right anterior axillary line, fifth intercostal space. Her current blood pressure is 140/88 (baseline, according to her husband, is 130/76), pulse is 120/min, and temperature is 102°F (38.9°C) (orally). She is complaining of increased shortness of breath that does not improve when the head of the bed is raised. Though her cough is weak, she is expectorating a small amount of thick, green sputum.

After this initial assessment, you call her admitting physician. The physician gives the following stat phone orders:

- Arterial blood gas (ABG)
- Complete blood cell count (CBC)
- Electrolytes
- Portable chest x-ray
- Sputum for culture and Gram stain

QUESTION

Considering Mary's symptoms and assuming that the tests cannot all be performed at the same time, which test should you order to be done first?

A. electrolytes
B. portable chest x-ray
C. ABG
D. CBC

ANSWER

The correct answer is C. Because Mary appears to be in acute respiratory distress, priority tests would be, first, the ABG, which is a rapid, accurate method of measuring oxygenation and acid–base status. Discussion of incorrect options: The second priority is the chest x-ray, a rapidly performed diagnostic test that helps locate and differentiate the pulmonary problem. The CBC and electrolytes, although important, do not have a direct impact on Mary's respiratory status. The sputum specimen should be obtained as soon as possible. Results of the culture will not be available for several days.

Stat Test Results

Arterial blood gases (on room air): pH 7.45, $Paco_2$ 33 mm Hg, Pao_2 68 mm Hg, HCO_3 20 mEq/L, Sao_2 90 percent

CBC

WBC 15,000	(normal range 4,500–10,000/mcL)
RBC 4.8	(normal range $4.0–5.0 \times 10^{12}$/mcL in females)
Hgb 14	(normal range 12–15 g/dL in females)
Hct 42 percent	(normal range 36–46 percent in females)

Electrolytes (normal ranges are from Kee, 2002)

Sodium (Na) 142	(normal range 135–145 mEq/L)
Potassium (K) 4.5	(normal range 3.5–5.3 mEq/L)
Chloride (Cl) 104	(normal range 95–105 mEq/L)
Calcium (Ca) 9.2	(normal range 9–11 mg/dL)

Portable chest x-ray results: Right middle lobe (RML) and right lower lobe (RLL) infiltrates are consistent with pneumonia

Sputum for culture and Gram stain: Results pending on culture; Gram stain: gram-positive clustered cocci

QUESTION

Which statement is true regarding the laboratory or x-ray data?

A. the ABG shows evidence of acid–base balance with mild hypoxemia
B. the electrolytes show evidence of possible overhydration
C. the CBC does not show evidence of an infectious process
D. the Gram stain is consistent with a viral infection

ANSWER

The correct answer is A. The ABG shows acid–base balance with mild hypoxemia. Discussion of incorrect options: The electrolytes show evidence of possible dehydration in high–normal sodium and chloride levels. The increased white blood cell count on the CBC is consistent with the presence of an infectious process. The high–normal hematocrit may suggest dehydration when considered with the high–normal sodium and chloride levels. The presence of gram-positive clustered cocci in the sputum Gram stain is consistent with staphylococci. The Gram stain helps differentiate the causative agent before confirmation by the sputum culture results, which take several days.

Update

The results of the ABG are called to the physician immediately, and oxygen is initiated at 4 L/min per nasal cannula. The physician states that she will be at the hospital to see Mary shortly.

QUESTION

On closer examination of Mary's ABG results, the nurse would conclude that the acid–base values could best be explained by her

A. crackles and wheezes
B. pleural friction rub
C. respiratory rate
D. shallow breathing

ANSWER

The correct answer is C. Her rapid respiratory rate is blowing off CO_2, which has precipitated respiratory alkalosis (compensated). Though her breathing appears shallow, it is currently not causing her to hypoventilate. Respiratory alkalosis is a common early acid–base disturbance associated with conditions that cause a rapid respiratory rate (e.g., pneumonia, acute asthmatic episode). Crackles, wheezes, and pleural friction rub are adventitious breath sounds that do not directly affect acid–base balance.

QUESTION

You note that Mary is very restless in the bed. This assessment is most likely associated with her

A. decreased $Paco_2$
B. decreased Pao_2
C. increased pH
D. decreased HCO_3

ANSWER

The correct answer is B. Restlessness is a sign commonly associated with hypoxemia and general discomfort. You should assess Mary for possible etiologies of her restlessness before sedation or analgesia is considered because use of these drugs may or may not be the best treatment. For example, if Mary's shallow breathing is secondary to her pleural pain, analgesia therapy may well facilitate deeper breaths and improve oxygenation. If, however, sedation or analgesic therapy should depress her respiratory pattern further, it could worsen her hypoxemia.

Focused Nursing History

Because Mary is in too much distress to be interviewed directly, you decide to talk with her husband to obtain the most important critical historical data that may have an impact on Mary's present situation. The complete nursing database will be completed within the first 24 hours postadmission. Her husband gives the following history:

> Mary began exhibiting common cold symptoms approximately 10 days ago. About 4 days ago, Mary's fever began to increase, accompanied by severe chilling. Her cough became productive, with green sputum. The cough has prevented Mary from sleeping very much for the past several nights. She has been complaining of a pattern of increasingly severe shortness of breath. Mary is not currently taking any prescription drugs. She has been taking several over-the-counter medications to relieve her symptoms: a nonnarcotic cough preparation and acetaminophen. For the past several days, she has been complaining of a transient sharp pain in her lower right chest that increases with breathing. Mary is allergic to penicillin. She has a 20-year history of smoking 1/2 to 1 pack of cigarettes per day but has not been able to smoke for several days because of shortness of breath. She rarely drinks any alcoholic beverages.

QUESTION

Additional priority nursing history data that the nurse should obtain from Mary's husband is

A.   dietary preferences
B.   usual weight
C.   preexisting medical conditions
D.   date of last menstrual period

ANSWER

The correct answer is C. It is crucial to be aware of any preexisting medical conditions. Many high-acuity patients have preexisting conditions such as diabetes mellitus, chronic pulmonary diseases, or congestive heart failure that must be monitored and taken into consideration when developing the plan of care. The existence of preexisting chronic conditions may place the patient at increased risk for development of complications during the current acute illness. The other pieces of data, while adding to the overall database, can be obtained at a later time, as appropriate.

Systematic Bedside Assessment

Before the physician's arrival, you initiate a head-to-toe assessment.

HEAD AND NECK. Mary's overall skin coloring is difficult to assess because it is dark. Therefore, her mucous membranes are assessed, and they are dusky in color. Mary continues to be completely oriented but remains restless. Slight nasal flaring is noted. She has nasal cannula oxygen delivering 4 L/min. She does not have jugular vein distention. No other abnormalities of the head or neck are noted.

CHEST. Pulmonary status is as previously noted in the focused respiratory assessment. Cardiac status is as follows. Pulmonary adventitious sounds make it somewhat difficult to clearly discriminate sounds. S1 and S2 and no murmur are auscultated. Sounds are regular, with a rate of 122/min.

ABDOMEN. The abdomen is flat. Positive bowel sounds are auscultated in all quadrants. Mary denies any abdominal tenderness. It is soft to palpation.

PELVIS. Mary voided 125 mL of clear, dark amber urine, with a specific gravity of 1.030.

EXTREMITIES. There is poor skin turgor. The skin is hot and diaphoretic. No peripheral edema is noted. The nailbeds are difficult to assess because of her dark pigmentation. Peripheral pulses are palpable in all four distal extremities.

POSTERIOR. No skin breakdown is noted, and there is no sacral edema. Posterior breath sounds: crackles and wheezes present on the right side to midlung field.

QUESTION

Which statement best states the cause of Mary's right-sided crackles? Her crackles

A.   probably indicate exudate in the small airways
B.   are suggestive of bronchoconstriction
C.   are typical of secretions in the large airways
D.   result from inflammation of the parietal pleura

ANSWER

The correct answer is A. Crackles are heard in the small airways and indicate the presence of fluid, exudate, or atelectasis. Discussion of incorrect options: Wheezing is a musical sound commonly heard on expiration, indicating airway narrowing usually from bronchoconstriction or bronchospasm. Rhonchi are auscultated in the larger airways and indicate the presence of secretions or fluid. Inflammation of the parietal pleura is associated with pleural pain. A pleural friction rub is sometimes present over the inflamed area.

Development of Nursing Diagnoses

CLUSTERING DATA. You have just completed your head-to-toe assessment and are now ready to develop a problem list based on the subjective and objective data that you have collected thus far. To cluster your data, you look for abnormalities found during the assessment. During the initial appraisal you immediately noted Mary's labored, rapid, shallow respirations. These symptoms are sufficient to begin clustering similar data that can support or refute the presence of a pulmonary problem.

Cluster 1. (from previous history and physical assessment data):

Subjective data: Patient complaining of dyspnea unaffected by position changes. Cold symptoms for 10 days. Increasing pattern of shortness of breath that does not seem to be affected by changing height of head of the bed. Cough with green sputum is noted. Chills and fever that have worsened over several days. Complaining of a transient sharp pain in her lower right chest that increases with breathing. Has had difficulty sleeping because of frequent coughing.

Objective data: Labored, shallow respirations. Respiratory rate is 28/min. Accessory muscles are in use. Crackles and wheezes heard in RML and RLL in anterior fields and to midchest in posterior right field. Pleural friction rub is auscultated at right anterior axillary line, fifth intercostal space. ABG shows that mild hypoxemia is present. Chest x-ray indicates an RML/RLL infiltrate. Gram stain shows gram-positive clustered cocci. Her cough is weak. Secretions, which are very thick and green, are difficult for her to expectorate. Fever and chills are present.

QUESTION

Based on these data, which nursing diagnosis would you select as being appropriate in planning Mary's care?

- A. impaired gas exchange
- B. ineffective airway clearance
- C. ineffective breathing pattern
- D. all of the above

ANSWER

The correct answer is D. Mary's pulmonary problem is a complex one that requires a wide variety of medical and nursing interventions. NANDA has approved all of the three presented pulmonary-related nursing diagnoses as individual diagnoses. However, because all three apply to Mary, it is suggested that you choose *impaired respiratory function*.

- *Impaired gas exchange* related to alveolar consolidation and pooling of secretions
- *Ineffective airway clearance* related to thick secretions associated with pulmonary infection and dehydration, pleural pain, and ineffective cough
- *Ineffective breathing pattern:* hypoventilation related to weakness, pleural pain, and fatigue

QUESTION

List at least six desired patient outcomes (DPOs) that would be appropriate for Mary's nursing diagnosis, *impaired respiratory function:*

- impaired gas exchange
- ineffective airway clearance
- ineffective breathing pattern (Ulrich et al., 2001)

1.
2.
3.
4.
5.
6.

ANSWER

1. Normal respiratory rate, depth, and rhythm
2. Improved or clear breath sounds
3. Improving or no dyspnea
4. Usual mental status
5. Mucous membranes are pink
6. ABGs within acceptable limits for patient

For the purposes of Mary's case study, only the pulmonary-related nursing diagnoses are developed further. However, in a true clinical situation, as the nurse creating Mary's plan of care, you would continue to develop other clusters based on primary critical cues and supporting cues from the data already collected. If data are insufficient, you should follow through on collecting the necessary data to confirm or refute your hypotheses.

QUESTION

Based on the preliminary data collected on Mary, there is sufficient support to state some additional diagnoses. List at least three appropriate nursing diagnoses.

ANSWER

- Pain: pleural
- Risk for fluid volume deficit
- Self-care deficit
- Sleep pattern disturbance
- Altered nutrition: less than body requirements
- Potential complications:
    1. Exudative pleural effusion
    2. Atelectasis

Developing the Plan of Care

Mary's pneumonia is a restrictive pulmonary disease process. She has many signs and symptoms consistent with restrictive diseases.

Treatment goals based on the restrictive nature of her disease include (1) optimizing her oxygenation status, (2) promoting airway clearance, and (3) maintaining functional alveoli. These general goals are reflected in the nursing diagnoses and DPOs on the nursing care plan. For example, optimizing oxygenation status is addressed in the nursing diagnoses *impaired gas exchange* and *ineffective airway clearance*. Accomplishment of the goal is measured with such criteria as ABGs within normal limits for patient, usual skin color, usual mental status, and improved lung sounds.

Nursing interventions are based on activities to help Mary meet her DPOs. They consist of collaborative interventions, which are activities ordered by the physician but that require some actions by the nurse, and independent interventions, activities that are within the nursing scope of practice to write and carry out as nursing orders.

Collaborative Interventions Related to Pulmonary Status

The physician's orders may include the following:

1. **Pulmonary drug therapy.** Mary will be receiving several drugs while hospitalized. Oxygen therapy has been ordered to treat Mary's mild hypoxemia. In general, the minimal goal of oxygen therapy is to increase the Pao_2 to at least 60 mm Hg. Other types of drug therapy that probably will be ordered for Mary include antibiotics for treatment of pneumonia and analgesics for treatment of pleuritic pain. She may not receive a cough suppressant in this stage of her pneumonia because a productive cough is a protective reflex to help rid the lungs of unwanted secretions. If necessary, she also may receive drug therapy through a hand-held nebulizer or metered-dose inhaler.
2. **Laboratory and x-ray testing.** These may be ordered intermittently. Of particular interest will be the ABGs, CBC, and chest x-ray to follow progress of the therapeutic plan.
3. **Percussion (P) and postural drainage (PD).** P and PD may be ordered to facilitate airway clearance. In many hospitals, this is performed by a respiratory therapist. P and PD also can be done by the nurse if she or he is properly trained, as ordered by the physician, or it may be an independent nursing action, depending on hospital policy.
4. **Intravenous fluids.** These may be ordered to promote hydration, which is crucial in loosening secretions for improved airway clearance. An IV access site also is necessary for IV antibiotic therapy, if ordered.

Independent Nursing Interventions

Assess the patient for decreased respiratory function (report abnormals)

- Respirations less than 8/min or greater than 30/min
- Increasingly shallow, labored breathing
- Increasing dyspnea or central cyanosis
- Change in mental status
- Increased restlessness
- Increased lethargy
- Increasingly abnormal ABGs
- Increasingly abnormal breath sounds, adventitious sounds
- Change in sputum
- Accessory muscle use

QUESTION

Some of the remaining independent nursing interventions are incomplete. Fill in the spaces with the correct information as they apply to Mary's impaired respiratory function.

- **A.** Turn every _____ hours.
- **B.** Cough and deep breathe every _____ to _____ hours.
- **C.** Incentive spirometry every _____ to _____ hours.
- **D.** Encourage fluids: to _____ to _____ L/24 hours, or 600 to 800 mL/8-hour shift, unless contraindicated.
- **E.** Tracheal suction as needed.
- **F.** Position of comfort with head of bed _____.
- **G.** Monitor for effects of drug therapy (therapeutic and nontherapeutic).
- **H.** Monitor test results (report abnormals).
- **I.** Instruct patient and/or family regarding _____, _____, _____, and _____.
- **J.** Encourage self-care as tolerated.
- **K.** Assess for pleural pain every 4 hours and as needed. Administer analgesics as needed.

ANSWERS

- **A.** 2
- **B.** 1, 2
- **C.** 1, 2
- **D.** 2, 2.5
- **F.** elevated greater than 30 degrees
- **I.** condition, procedures, medications, treatment

Plan Evaluation and Revision

Mary's pulmonary plan of care is now developed and ready to execute. Her progress is monitored at regular intervals to evaluate the effects of the various therapeutic actions. If progress is not being noted toward the attainment of Mary's various desired patient outcomes, her plan may need revisions, examining alternative interventions that may be more effective.

Mary's plan of care is effective, and she responds rapidly to her antibiotic therapy and her pulmonary hygiene program. Because she does not have underlying pulmonary disease, her recovery is uncomplicated. Before discharge, she will need to receive teaching concerning continuing her antibiotic therapy as prescribed, increasing her activities slowly at home, smoking cessation, and pulmonary hygiene.

Case Study 2

PETER M, A PATIENT WITH OBSTRUCTIVE PULMONARY DISEASE

You are a registered nurse working on a general surgical floor in a 300-bed community hospital. You have, as part of your assignment, Mr. Peter M, a 68-year-old patient who had a transurethral resection (TUR) 3 days ago. You have just heard the shift report, in which you received the following information about Peter.

At 2:00 P.M., vital signs are blood pressure 150/90 (baseline is 130/84), pulse 100/min and slightly irregular, respiratory rate 38/min, temperature 98.6°F (37°C) (oral). He has 2 L of oxygen ordered per nasal cannula. Peter's lungs sound a little more congested, and breathing seems more labored. He has been on bedrest since surgery. Peter has a history of emphysema, his post-TUR status is stable and his urinary status has been uneventful since surgery. Urine is clear, and a three-way Foley catheter is in place. It will probably be discontinued today. His appetite has been poor. He has an IV of 5 percent dextrose in 0.45 percent normal saline in a right peripheral line. The nurse reporting off suggests that you watch Peter closely this evening, stating that he seems weaker today. He has been fully alert and awake throughout the day. The nurse also reports that Peter has gained 4 pounds (1.8 kg) over the past several days.

Significant History

Peter is a retired teacher. He was diagnosed with pulmonary emphysema approximately 10 years ago and congestive heart failure approximately 2 years ago. He states that he drinks an occasional glass of beer or wine but not on a regular basis. Over the past year, Peter has had increasing difficulty passing urine. Tests confirmed benign prostatic hyperplasia. His TUR was an elective procedure. He has no known allergies. His appetite has been poor for the past several days; he complains of nausea, though he has not been vomiting. Peter usually sleeps using two large pillows to help him breathe better.

QUESTION

In addition to what has already been obtained in the nursing history, the nurse should also obtain Peter's _____ history as a priority, at the time of admission.

- **A.** smoking
- **B.** complete medication
- **C.** diet
- **D.** usual activity level

ANSWER

The correct answer is B. Peter has a positive history of cardiopulmonary disease and is probably receiving long-term drug therapy to treat these medical conditions. It is important to know what medications he normally takes at home so that decisions can be made regarding continuation of these while he is hospitalized. In addition, certain drugs (e.g., digoxin, theophylline) may build up in the serum and precipitate adverse reactions. For this reason, the physician may order serum drug levels to be drawn to determine whether therapeutic levels are present. Discussion of incorrect options: Although information regarding his smoking, activity level, and diet history will be a useful part of the database, they are not as high a priority in helping to meet his immediate needs.

New Data Obtained During the Nursing History

Peter informs the nurse that he has been taking theophylline (Theo-Dur), digoxin, furosemide (Lasix), terbutaline inhalant, and prednisone. He has also been receiving home oxygen therapy for about 1 year. Peter has a history of smoking 2 to 2 1/2 packs per day for 40 years. This past year, he cut his intake to 1/2 pack per day. He has been on a low-sodium diet for at least 5 years. Peter states that he is "pretty good" at sticking with the diet. He indicates that he can usually perform his own activities of daily living. He complains that, over the past several months, he has become increasingly short of breath with climbing 15 steps to get to his bedroom, and he voices concern that he will not be able to do this much longer.

Initial Appraisal

It is now the beginning of your shift, and you are making your patient rounds with initial appraisals. On approaching Peter's bed, you note the following.

GENERAL APPEARANCE. Peter M is a Caucasian male. He is barrel-chested and poorly nourished in appearance, with little body fat noted. He is in bed sitting upright, leaning forward with his arms stretched out to his knees.

SIGNS OF DISTRESS. Respirations are rapid, with a prolonged expiratory phase. His breathing is noisy, with an expiratory wheeze heard while you are standing at the foot of the bed. His breathing appears labored and you note the use of accessory muscles during inspiration. His coloring appears dusky.

OTHER. There is approximately 50 mL of urine in his Foley bag. You note a three-way Foley catheter in place. Urine is clear and yellow. A bladder irrigant bag is hanging but is not running. The IV fluid is infusing at the correct rate. He has oxygen running at 2 L/min per nasal cannula. He is oriented to his name and the year but cannot tell you where he is. No one else is in the room with him.

QUESTION

Based only on Peter's history and initial appraisal, you would most appropriately perform a focused assessment of the _____ system as a priority.

- **A.** genitourinary
- **B.** integumentary
- **C.** gastrointestinal
- **D.** cardiopulmonary

ANSWER

D is correct. Because your initial appraisal of Peter included abnormal assessments that are overtly respiratory, you rapidly focus in on a more complete respiratory assessment followed by a cardiovascular assessment. You do this with the understanding that pulmonary signs and symptoms can be of pulmonary or cardiac origin.

Focused Assessment

His vital signs currently are respiratory rate 32/min and labored. Pulse 115/min; S1 and S2 are present though the sounds are hard to distinguish because of his loud adventitious breath sounds. Blood pressure is 156/92. You auscultate loud coarse rhonchi on both inspiration and expiration, and expiratory wheeze is heard bilaterally. Breath sounds can be heard distinctly in the apices but are progressively diminished from mid- to low lung fields bilaterally. He has a full rolling cough, but he is unable to clear the secretions from his lungs. His bedside chart shows an imbalance of 1,500 mL of intake over output during the past 24 hours.

Following respiratory data collection and based on Peter's history, you decide that his signs and symptoms may not be completely of pulmonary origin. You, therefore, quickly assess his cardiovascular status further.

CARDIOVASCULAR STATUS. You note positive jugular vein distention. Peter has +3 pitting edema of his lower legs. You cannot distinguish heart sounds sufficiently to assess for S3 and S4 reliably. His current urine output is 50 mL in a 2-hour period. Breath sounds are too diminished to clearly assess for presence of crackles in the bases.

Following your focused assessment, you call your report to the physician, who orders the following stat orders.

- Portable chest x-ray
- ABG
- Furosemide 40 mg IV now
- Aminophylline drip at 35 mg/hr
- Serum electrolytes
- Digoxin and theophylline levels
- Electrocardiogram (ECG)

QUESTION

Considering Peter's present condition and assuming that the orders cannot all be carried out at the same time, which stat physician order should you do first?

- **A.** IV furosemide
- **B.** ABG
- **C.** digoxin and theophylline levels
- **D.** chest x-ray

ANSWER

The correct answer is B. Obtaining the ABG first is a rapid and accurate method of measuring his oxygenation and acid–base status. Discussion of incorrect options: The IV furosemide would be next in priority to help relieve fluid volume excess problems. You should be aware, however, that Peter has been on long-standing digoxin therapy. It will be very important to check his electrolyte level at the earliest opportunity for possible hypokalemia, particularly because he is receiving furosemide, a potent loop diuretic that is very potassium depleting. Low-serum potassium associated with digoxin therapy can precipitate digoxin toxicity. The portable chest x-ray and ECG also can be ordered rapidly, but there often is a delay before these procedures are actually performed.

Stat Test Results

Portable chest x-ray: Right heart enlargement consistent with cor pulmonale. Hyperlucency is present, with flattening of the diaphragm. Increased antero-posterior (A/P) diameter is present. Bullous lesions are noted.

Arterial blood gases: pH 7.32, $Paco_2$ 75 mm Hg, Pao_2 70 mm Hg, HCO_3 36 mEq/L

Electrolytes: Na 138 mEq/L, K 4.0 mEq/L, Cl 102 mEq/L, Ca 9.2 mg/dL

Digoxin level: 2.2 ng/mL (therapeutic range 0.5–2 ng/mL)

Theophylline level: 15 mcg/mL (therapeutic range 5–20 mcg/mL)

ECG: Right ventricular leads show changes consistent with cor pulmonale. Changes also are noted consistent with digitalis effects. Unifocal premature ventricular contractions are present. (Therapeutic ranges are from Kee, 2002.)

QUESTION

Which statement is correct regarding the significance of laboratory and other test data?

- **A.** the ABG shows metabolic acidosis with mild hypoxemia
- **B.** the electrolytes are all within acceptable limits

- **C.** the chest x-ray finding of cor pulmonale is an uncommon finding in COPD
- **D.** the premature ventricular contractions are not of concern at this time

ANSWER

The correct answer is B. Peter's electrolyte levels are not significant at this time. However, they will need to be monitored carefully while he is receiving diuretics because of the potential for electrolyte depletion complications. Discussion of incorrect options: His portable chest x-ray showed evidence of cor pulmonale, right heart enlargement, and hypertrophy of pulmonary etiology. Cor pulmonale is frequently associated with some degree of right heart failure. The lung fields are consistent with emphysematous changes. His ABG showed acute respiratory acidosis with mild hypoxemia. Patients with chronic obstructive diseases frequently undergo progressive ABG alterations. Normal ABG values are relative numbers in patients with COPD.

If Peter has very severe emphysema, he may breathe normally on a hypoxic drive. He, like many COPD patients, may be tolerant of relatively low Pao_2 levels and high $Paco_2$ levels. His current pH is below the normal range, however, which tells you that at this time, he, for some reason, has moved from a state of chronic insufficiency to acute respiratory failure. (For review, see Modules 4 and 5.)

Peter's digoxin level is toxic. This is not uncommon in older patients receiving chronic digoxin therapy. Digoxin toxicity is potentially dangerous. As the nurse, you would hold the drug and inform the physician of the test results. Digoxin generally is held until levels return to therapeutic levels. His theophylline level is within the therapeutic range at this time. Patients on chronic theophylline therapy often become toxic, developing symptoms of nausea and vomiting, increased heart rate, dysrhythmias, insomnia, headache, and increased irritability.

Peter's ECG shows evidence of his chronic drug therapy and his cor pulmonale. The presence of premature ventricular contractions is significant because of his digoxin toxic state, which can precipitate many arrhythmias and conduction problems.

Systematic Bedside Assessment

Once you have completed the various stat activities on Peter, you begin your head-to-toe assessment.

HEAD AND NECK: Circumoral and earlobe duskiness is noted. Oxygen is in place at 2 L/min. Responsiveness level: He is oriented to name and month but not to place, although he has been reminded recently. His speech is breathless, and he is able to talk in one- to two-word phrases only. Purse-lip breathing is noted. Positive jugular vein distention is noted at 45 degrees.

CHEST: The chest is as previously assessed in the focused pulmonary and cardiac assessment.

ABDOMEN: His abdomen is distended and tight. He complains of tenderness in his right upper quadrant. Bowel sounds are auscultated in all four quadrants but are hypoactive.

PELVIS: A three-way Foley catheter is present. He denies pain at this time. Urine output in the bag is 50 mL for a 1-hour period. The urine color is clear and amber. No drainage is noted around the catheter at the meatus.

EXTREMITIES: Mild digital clubbing is noted. His nailbeds are dusky, and capillary refill is less than 3 seconds. His skin is warm and flaky dry. He has a peripheral IV in his right forearm. The site is negative for edema, redness, or heat; +1 edema is noted in both hands and +3 edema is noted in the lower legs. He has positive peripheral pulses. You are able to palpate his dorsalis pedis pulses but not his posterior tibial pulses.

POSTERIOR: No skin breakdown is noted at this time, but redness is noted in several areas along the spinous processes of the vertebrae and on the coccyx. Scattered rhonchi are auscultated throughout the posterior fields, and sounds are diminished.

Development of Nursing Diagnoses

CLUSTERING DATA: Following the systematic bedside assessment, there are sufficient data to develop nursing diagnoses. The first step is to cluster data based on major abnormal cues.

EXERCISE

You have hypothesized that Peter has an acute pulmonary problem. In the space provided, list the major abnormal data that have been obtained thus far to support this hypothesis.

Cluster 1

ANSWER

Subjective data: Peter has a long history of pulmonary emphysema. He continues to smoke, although he has decreased his intake to 1/2 pack per day. His at-home pulmonary medications include Theo-Dur, oxygen, prednisone, and terbutaline.

Objective data: Peter's respiratory rate is 32/min and labored. Pursed-lip breathing is noted. He is sitting upright in bed, leaning forward. His expiratory phase is noticeably longer than his inspiratory phase. He is using his accessory muscles to breathe. Loud rhonchi and wheezes are present. A full rolling cough is noted, but he is unable to cough up and expectorate the secretions. His pulse is 115/min and blood pressure is 156/92. His theophylline level is within normal limits. His latest ABG showed acute respiratory acidosis with mild hypoxia. He has oxygen per nasal cannula running at 2 L/min. Circumoral and earlobe duskiness are noted.

QUESTION

Based on these data, which nursing diagnosis would you select as being appropriate in planning Peter's care?
   A. impaired gas exchange
   B. ineffective airway clearance
   C. ineffective breathing pattern
   D. all of the above

ANSWER

The correct answer is D. Peter's critical cues show evidence of all three respiratory-related nursing diagnoses.
   - Impaired gas exchange related to ineffective airway clearance, ineffective breathing pattern, and decrease in functional lung surface area.
   - Ineffective airway clearance related to excessive secretions, ineffective cough, and pooling of secretions.
   - Ineffective breathing pattern related to anxiety and dysfunction of the muscles of respirations.

Desired patient outcomes (evaluative criteria) for Peter would include

1. Normal respiratory rate, depth, and rhythm
2. Decreased dyspnea
3. Usual or improved breath sounds
4. Usual mental status
5. ABGs within normal limits for patient

If Peter's emphysema is severe, his blood gases may never attain the usual normals. ABG normal values often are altered in patients with chronic obstructive diseases. His acceptable ranges might be

pH   7.35–7.45 (remains unchanged with disease)
$Paco_2$ less than 50 mm Hg (increases with obstructive disease)
Pao_2 greater than 50 mm Hg (decreases with obstructive disease)
Sao_2 85 percent or greater (decreases with obstructive disease)

QUESTION

In the space provided, state what additional effect Peter's age of 68 has on his Pao_2.

ANSWER

Peter's age of 68 influences his acceptable Pao_2 range. It is known that normal aging decreases the number of functioning alveoli. For this reason, Pao_2 has a normal tendency to decrease with age.

Peter's assessment had sufficient evidence to develop a picture consistent with a pulmonary problem and a possible cardiovascular problem. Because the pulmonary and cardiovascular systems actually exist as a single cardiopulmonary circuit, the possible cardiovascular problem is briefly explored.

EXERCISE

You have also hypothesized that Peter may have an acute cardiac problem. In the space provided, list the major abnormal data obtained thus far that would support this hypothesis, and state the major nursing diagnosis based on the cluster.

Cluster 2

Nursing Diagnosis:

ANSWER

Subjective data: Peter has a 2-year history of congestive heart failure. At-home cardiac-related medications include digoxin and furosemide. He usually sleeps with his head on two pillows.

Objective data: Jugular vein distention is present, and +3 edema is noted in his lower legs. His current urine output is 50 mL in a 2-hour period. Chest x-ray shows evidence of cor pulmonale. Digoxin level is greater than 2.0 (toxic). ECG results were consistent with cor pulmonale and showed premature ventricular contractions. He has experienced a 4-pound weight gain over the past several days.

Based on these data, a nursing diagnosis of *decreased cardiac output* related to ineffective right heart pumping associated with right heart hypertrophy is noted. Appropriate patient outcomes would need to be decided on and interventions performed to address this problem. This second cluster of data was included to exemplify the common cardiac complications associated with chronic respiratory disease. Nursing management of the patient with cardiovascular problems is addressed in Module 2: Alterations in Myocardial Tissue Perfusion.

Other nursing diagnoses supported by the existing data include

- Activity intolerance
- Nausea
- Altered nutrition: less than body requirements
- Anxiety
- Knowledge deficit
- Self-care deficit
- Risk for impaired skin integrity (Ulrich et al., 2001)

Developing the Plan of Care

Peter's emphysema is an obstructive pulmonary disease. He has many of the signs and symptoms that are typical of obstructive diseases.

Patients with COPD often are admitted to hospitals for reasons unrelated to their pulmonary disorder, such as was the case of Peter with his genitourinary problem. When a patient with COPD is admitted to the hospital for any reason, the health care team must incorporate management of the chronic problem with management of the acute problem if complications are to be avoided.

Many patients with COPD exist in a day-to-day state of chronic respiratory insufficiency; that is, they are able to maintain relatively normal (balanced supply-and-demand) acid–base and oxygenation states only at the expense of the other body systems. Normalcy is maintained through compensatory mechanisms.

QUESTION

What are the major clinical manifestations that indicate the presence of compensation activities by the following systems?

   A. cardiovascular system
   B. renal system
   C. pulmonary system
   D. hematopoietic system

ANSWER

   A. elevated blood pressure and pulse
   B. increased retention of bicarbonate
   C. increased respiratory rate and depth
   D. increased red blood cell production

Compensatory mechanisms, however, are finite in their abilities to compensate and vary in the length of time they take to respond to new demands. When a person, such as Peter, is placed under acute physiologic or psychologic stress (e.g., surgery, hospitalization, trauma, acute illness), the sudden increase in physiologic demand may go beyond the ability of the body to supply the necessary oxygen and eliminate the increased carbon dioxide. From the time of hospital admission, Peter has been under increased stress and, thus, is at increased risk for the development of multiple complications.

Overall goals in planning Peter's pulmonary care are consistent with his obstructive pulmonary disease needs and include (1) optimizing ventilation and (2) maintaining adequate oxygenation. A plan using both collaborative and independent interventions will be developed to accomplish these goals.

Collaborative Interventions Related to Peter's Pulmonary Status

The physician's orders may include the following:

1. **Pulmonary drug therapy.**   Peter, like many patients with COPD, is on long-term bronchodilator and steroid therapy. Bronchodilators dilate the smooth muscle of the bronchi, decreasing airway obstruction. There are two major groups of bronchodilators, the methylxanthines (e.g., aminophylline, theophylline) and the sympathomimetic bronchodilators (e.g., isoetharine, albuterol, terbutaline, metaproterenol). His bronchodilators may be administered orally, IV, by hand-held nebulizer, or by metered-dose inhaler. Corticosteroids sometimes are ordered for treatment of restrictive diseases but are used more commonly as treatment of obstructive diseases. This group of drugs reduces inflammation, promotes bronchodilation, and inhibits bronchoconstriction. In the presence of acute infection, corticosteroid therapy may be contraindicated because of its immunosuppressant activity. Prolonged use of corticosteroids is associated with many adverse effects, and thus their use is closely weighed in terms of benefits and risks before initiation of long-term therapy. Corticosteroids may be administered orally or by aerosol. Examples of commonly used drugs include prednisone, methylprednisone, and prednisolone.

    Oxygen therapy will be ordered carefully. If Peter is a carbon dioxide retainer, his respiratory center is driven by a hypoxic drive. Moderate to high oxygen concentrations may turn off his drive to breathe. Peter's oxygen concentration most likely will be maintained at 2 to 3 L/nasal cannula, or 28 percent Venti-mask. Analgesic therapy may be ordered to control Peter's postsurgical pain. His respiratory status must be monitored closely for signs and symptoms of respiratory depression, such as slowing respiratory rate or increasingly shallow respirations. Many analgesics are associated with respiratory depression, increasing the risk of acute ventilatory failure. This is of particular concern in patients with severe pulmonary problems.

2. **Laboratory and x-ray tests.**   Peter may have laboratory tests and x-rays ordered intermittently if significant clinical changes are noted in his status. They will, most likely, not be ordered on a regular basis. Of particular interest would be ABGs, electrolytes, and a CBC. A serum albumin may be ordered if the physician is concerned about possible malnutrition.

3. **Pulmonary function tests.**   Pulmonary function tests may be ordered if the physician wants to either (a) obtain baseline data concerning Peter's current pulmonary function status or (b) compare his current status with previously documented pulmonary function data.

4. **Diet.**   A special diet may be ordered that is low in carbohydrates, high in protein, and high in fat. Patients with chronic respiratory diseases frequently experience a loss of appetite from coughing, shortness of breath, general fatigue, excessive mucous production, and the side effects of drug therapy. Hypoxia, associated with advanced pulmonary disease, decreases the endurance of the respiratory muscles and increases energy consumption because of increased work of breathing. The combination of anorexia and hypoxia causes the chronic respiratory patient to lose weight. Ultimately, there is a decreased supply associated with an ever-increasing demand.

Chronic respiratory patients may need to control carbohydrate intake. Normally, carbohydrates comprise the majority of dietary intake. Carbohydrate metabolism causes CO_2 production that is higher than what is produced by fat or protein. A high carbohydrate diet may precipitate acute respiratory failure in the following way. The acutely ill respiratory patient is often in a malnourished state, which weakens the respiratory muscles, resulting in a decreased tidal volume. A decrease in tidal volume can result in alveolar hypoventilation. The combination of increased carbon dioxide in the alveoli and decreased alveolar ventilation causes increasing $Paco_2$ levels, which ultimately can cause acute respiratory acidosis.

The malnourished respiratory patient has a lower-than-normal protein level. Protein is vital to proper body function. Serum albumin (normal 3.5 to 5 g/dL) determination is a frequently used laboratory test to measure nonmuscle protein. Albumin is one of the best malnutrition predictors. Approximately 55 percent of plasma proteins in the blood is albumin. A serum-albumin level of less than 2.5 g/dL is considered critically low, decreasing the patient's chance of survival through an acute illness.

Independent Nursing Interventions

Nursing management of Peter, a patient with obstructive pulmonary disease, is essentially the same as management of the patient with restrictive pulmonary disease (refer to the independent nursing interventions in Case Study 1). Emphasis, however, is placed on airway clearance and pulmonary hygiene. Peter's nutritional status must be improved and monitored closely. His oxygenation status and therapy will require close assessment for therapeutic and nontherapeutic effects to prevent loss of his hypoxic drive to breathe if he is a CO_2 retainer. Encouraging him to maintain activities, such as getting up into a chair, or walking in the room or hall, will help maintain or strengthen activity tolerance and reduce the risk of immobility complications.

Plan Evaluation and Revision

Peter's plan of care should be evaluated at regular intervals. Evaluation will be based on the status of specific desired patient outcomes. If evaluation shows lack of forward progress toward attaining or maintaining goals, the plan must be revised, seeking alternatives to care that will be more successful.

Case Study 3

THE CONTINUING CASE OF PETER M, THE PATIENT REQUIRING MECHANICAL VENTILATION

In the first two case studies, Mary R and Peter M were successful in meeting their outcome criteria and were subsequently discharged home without further complications. In this case study, we are going to assume that Peter developed a complication of bedrest—pneumonia—and his condition has deteriorated.

Status Update

Today, Peter has demonstrated increasing respiratory distress and has been transferred to the critical care unit for close observation. Stat arterial blood gases are drawn (obtained while breathing room air) and the following results are called back to the nurse:

pH 7.28, $Paco_2$ 82 mm Hg, Pao_2 48 mm Hg, HCO_3 34 mEq/L, Sao_2 74 percent

EXERCISE

In the space provided, interpret the preceding ABG:

Acid–base status:

Oxygenation status:

ANSWER

Peter is in respiratory acidosis, either acute or partially compensated with moderate hypoxemia. If his elevated HCO_3 represents his baseline value, he is in an acute acidotic state.

Focused Respiratory Assessment

On transfer to the medical ICU, the nurse quickly performs a focused assessment of Peter's pulmonary and cardiovascular status, with the following results: Respiratory rate is 28/min, labored, and regular. Little air movement is heard on auscultation with distant breath sounds heard only in the central airway. Tongue and oral mucous membranes are dark and dusky, as are his lips and nail beds. He is sitting up on the side of the bed leaning on his bed stand. He is making heavy use of his accessory muscles. The respiratory therapist performs pulmonary mechanics, which result in a vital capacity (VC) of 952 mL [Peter weighs 150 lbs (68 kg)]; a minute ventilation ($\dot{V}_E$) of 12 L/min (normal is 5 to 10 L/min); and a negative inspiratory force (NIF) of 210 cm H_2O.

QUESTION

Based on the preceding assessment, which of Peter's data meet the criteria for ventilatory support? Circle "yes" or "no" beside each criterion.

1.	Respiratory rate	Yes	No
2.	pH and $Paco_2$	Yes	No
3.	Pao_2	Yes	No
4.	VC	Yes	No
5.	NIF	Yes	No
6.	$\dot{V}_E$	Yes	No

ANSWER

Some of the common critical values used for criteria for ventilatory support include $Paco_2$ of greater than 50 mm Hg with a pH of less than 7.30; Pao_2 of less than 50 mm Hg; respiratory rate of greater than 35 breaths/min; vital capacity of less than 15 mL/kg; NIF of less than 220 cm H_2O; and a $\dot{V}_E$ of greater than 10 L/min.

Based on these critical values, with the exception of respiratory rate, Peter currently meets all criteria. A person does not need to meet all of the criteria to be placed on a mechanical ventilator. Criteria are used to assist the clinician in decision making.

The decision is made to intubate Peter and place him on the mechanical ventilator to treat his acute respiratory failure. The nurse begins to assemble the necessary intubation equipment.

EXERCISE

List at least six pieces of equipment that must be assembled for an intubation:

1.
2.
3.
4.
5.
6.

ANSWER

Equipment needed for placement of an ET tube includes soft-cuffed ET tubes, stylet, topical anesthetic, laryngoscope handle with blade attached, Magill forceps, suction catheters, Yankauer suction tip, syringe for cuff inflation, water-soluble lubricant, and adhesive tape.

While Peter's ET tube is being placed, a mechanical ventilator is set up with initial settings. Depending on available support staff in a facility, a variety of people may be trained to set initial settings, including the respiratory therapist, the physician, or the nurse.

QUESTION

In the spaces provided, fill in the typical standard setting as described in Section Five of Module 6, "Mechanical Ventilation."

1. Tidal volume _____ to _____ mL/kg
2. Rate _____ to _____ breaths/min
3. Fio_2 _____ to _____
4. Mode AC or SIMV (circle one)

ANSWER

1.	Tidal volume:	5 to 7 mL/kg
2.	Rate:	8 to 12 breaths/min
3.	Fio_2	0.5 to 1.0 (50 to 100 percent oxygenation concentration)
4.	Mode	AC (Assist/Control)

Though mechanical ventilation was a necessary intervention to protect Peter's life, it has placed him at high risk for development of complications. The nurse will particularly need to monitor his cardiovascular status closely now that he is receiving positive pressure ventilation (PPV).

QUESTION

Based on what you know about Peter's history and assessments, why is the nurse particularly concerned about monitoring his cardiovascular status?

ANSWER

Positive pressure ventilation reduces cardiac output by decreasing venous return to the heart. Peter already has a history of congestive heart failure, and he was recently treated for an acute episode. He is extremely vulnerable for development of a recurrent congestive heart failure episode and he could potentially develop multiple system problems associated with reduced cardiac output.

A major general patient care goal used in guiding Peter's nursing interventions while he is receiving mechanical ventilation is support of physiologic needs. More specifically, Peter's pulmonary support will focus on protecting his airway and promoting ventilation and oxygenation. Endotracheal suctioning is a major intervention that helps meet his pulmonary needs.

QUESTION

Which open-system suctioning routines would best meet Peter's need for optimizing oxygenation? (Note: H/H = hyperoxygenate/hyperventilate)

A. Suction, H/H, return to ventilator
B. H/H, suction, suction, H/H, return to ventilator
C. Suction, H/H, suction, H/H, return to ventilator
D. H/H, suction, H/H, suction, H/H, return to ventilator

ANSWER

The correct answer is D. It is important to optimize oxygenation prior to initiating suctioning because the suction removes oxygenation as well as secretions. The hyperoxygenation/hyperventilation procedure should be repeated prior to each suctioning pass and prior to returning the patient to the ventilator to replace lost oxygen. Each suctioning pass should be limited to no longer than 10 seconds. As a reminder of the length of time for a single pass, some nurses hold their breath while suctioning. Breath holding becomes uncomfortable within 10 seconds for many people. If this easy procedure is used, the nurse can initially time her or his own breath holding to experience how it feels at 10 seconds. If the patient is attached to pulse oximetry, many nurses will also hyperoxygenate/hyperventilate the patient until the Spo_2 has returned to greater than 95 percent.

Scenario Update

Peter's pneumonia is now resolved and it is believed that he is ready for removal from the mechanical ventilator. It has been 7 days since he was first placed on mechanical ventilation. To initiate the weaning process, the clinicians will first need to determine his readiness to wean.

EXERCISE

List three simple questions that can be asked that can rapidly identify if Peter is NOT ready for weaning.

1.
2.
3.

ANSWER

Initially, it is simpler to decide if he is not ready for weaning because determination of actual readiness requires more thorough testing in patients with complex problems.

1. Has the problem that precipitated the need for mechanical ventilation resolved?
2. Is the patient's clinical condition stable?
3. Is the patient's clinical condition improving?

Peter's status does, in fact, meet the initial criteria. The clinicians decide to proceed with a more comprehensive patient screening. Because dysfunction of particular body systems increases the risk of Peter becoming ventilator dependent, the comprehensive screening focuses on function of those systems.

EXERCISE

List the five physiologic systems that are associated with failure-to-wean problems and list at least one test that might be performed to measure the function of each system.

Physiologic System	Test
1.	
2.	
3.	
4.	
5.	

ANSWER

Physiologic System	Test
1. Respiratory	ABG, $\dot{V}_E$, A–a gradient, Spo_2, chest x-ray
2. Cardiovascular	Blood pressure, heart rate, ECG pattern
3. CNS	Alert, cooperative, willing to be weaned
4. Renal	Intake = Output, adequate urine output, BUN, and creatinine
5. Nutritional/metabolic	Electrolytes, CBC with differential, albumin/prealbumin

It is determined that Peter meets the comprehensive patient-screening criteria sufficiently to warrant initiating weaning. Because of his history of chronic lung disease, it is anticipated that he will require a slow-ventilator weaning process, using SIMV mode with pressure support ventilation (PSV).

QUESTION

Which statement best describes SIMV weaning mode?

- A. guarantees an ongoing stable level of minute ventilation
- B. frequency of mandatory ventilator breaths is slowly decreased
- C. patient is removed from ventilator for increasing lengths of time
- D. provides positive pressure during the inspiration phase to support tidal volume

ANSWER

The correct answer is B. SIMV allows Peter to take over his own work of breathing gradually as he gains back his muscle strength. Discussion of incorrect options: A. Describes mandatory minute ventilation (MMV); C. Describes manual weaning; D. Describes pressure support ventilation (PSV).

Scenario Update

Peter has been successfully weaned from mechanical ventilation over a 5-day period. It is now time to extubate him.

QUESTION

Briefly explain the reason for rapid removal of the endotracheal tube once Peter no longer requires mechanical ventilation.

ANSWER

The presence of the endotracheal tube increases Peter's airway resistance and, thus, increases his work of breathing. It will be easier for him to breathe once the artificial therapy has been removed.

Following extubation, the nurse will monitor Peter closely for signs of acute respiratory distress. Such signs may occur immediately because of swelling of the airway associated with the trauma of tube removal; or it may occur later, usually as a result of respiratory muscle fatigue. He will immediately be placed on low-flow humidified (usually per mask) oxygen to maintain his oxygenation status.

REFERENCES

Kee, J. (2002). *Laboratory and diagnostic tests with nursing implications* (6th ed.). Upper Saddle River, NJ: Prentice Hall.

Ulrich, S. P., & Canale, S. W. (2001). *Medical–surgical nursing care planning guides* (5th ed.). Philadelphia: W.B. Saunders.

PART

3

Perfusion

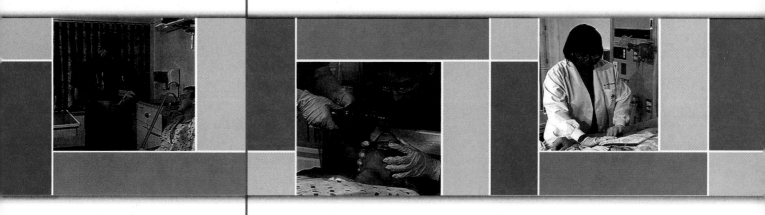

MODULE 8   Determinants and Assessment of Cardiac Output

MODULE 9   Hemodynamic Monitoring

MODULE 10   Electrocardiographic Monitoring and Conduction Abnormalities

MODULE 11   Alterations in Myocardial Tissue Perfusion

MODULE 12   Alterations in Cardiac Output

MODULE 13   Nursing Care of the Patient with Altered Myocardial Tissue Perfusion

Determinants and Assessment of Cardiac Output

Conrad Gordon, Karen L. Johnson

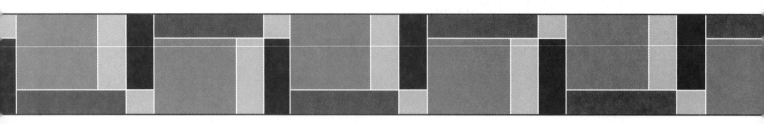

OBJECTIVES   Following completion of this module, the learner will be able to

1. Define and state adult normal values for cardiac output, cardiac index, heart rate, and stroke volume.

2. Discuss how preload, contractility, and afterload impact stroke volume.

3. Describe the relationship of stroke volume and preload in terms of the Frank–Starling law.

4. Describe the relationship among pressure, flow, and resistance and how these impact cardiac output.

5. Discuss factors that influence myocardial contractility.

6. State some of the conditions that affect heart rate, preload, contractility, and afterload.

7. Identify the common clinical assessments that evaluate heart rate, preload, contractility, and afterload.

8. Describe various cardiovascular diagnostic procedures used to evaluate the components of cardiac output.

9. Discuss nursing responsibilities in caring for a patient receiving cardiovascular diagnostic procedures.

This self-study module is intended for the novice nurse caring for the high acuity ill patient. This module focuses on the physiologic concepts that influence the function of the cardiovascular system, with particular focus on the heart. An understanding of these concepts will allow the nurse to apply them to a variety of clinical situations in order to understand assessment findings related to cardiovascular health and disease.

The module is composed of eight sections that define terms and normal values, describe key relationships among variables, identify common clinical conditions that influence these variables, and present the clinical assessments that can be made using these variables. Each section includes a set of review questions to help the learner evaluate his or her understanding of the section's content before moving on to the next section. All Section Reviews and the module Pretest and Posttest include answers. It is suggested that the learner review those concepts answered incorrectly in the review questions before proceeding to the next section.

 PRETEST

---

1. Stroke volume multiplied by heart rate equals the
   A. cardiac output
   B. cardiac index
   C. pulse pressure product
   D. left ventricular stroke work index

2. The normal cardiac output for an adult at rest is approximately
   A. 1.2 L/min
   B. 3.4 L/min
   C. 5.0 L/min
   D. 10.0 L/min

3. The resistance against which the heart must pump blood is known as
   A. preload
   B. afterload
   C. upload
   D. download

4. The most effective mechanism to increase cardiac output is to
   A. increase heart rate
   B. decrease contractility
   C. increase afterload
   D. decrease preload
5. The Frank–Starling law states that within physiologic limits, the heart will
   A. beat no faster than the body's demand for oxygen dictates
   B. pump the volume it receives
   C. completely empty of blood with each beat
   D. extract only the amount of oxygen needed from its blood supply
6. Too much preload results in a(n)
   A. decrease in heart rate
   B. increase in heart rate
   C. decrease in cardiac output
   D. increase in afterload
7. Blood pressure is the product of
   A. flow and volume
   B. cardiac output and afterload
   C. viscosity and resistance
   D. viscosity and volume
8. When afterload increases
   A. blood pressure decreases
   B. cardiac output decreases
   C. blood pressure increases
   D. both B and C are correct
9. Which of the following depresses myocardial contractility?
   A. epinephrine
   B. digitalis
   C. sympathetic nervous system activity
   D. hypoxemia

10. Which of the following increase(s) myocardial contractility?
    A. dopamine
    B. dobutamine
    C. digoxin
    D. all of the above
11. Profound hemorrhage initially results in
    A. decreased afterload
    B. decreased preload
    C. increased preload
    D. decreased heart rate
12. Which of the following conditions dilate arterioles?
    A. septic shock
    B. spinal cord injury
    C. anaphylactic shock
    D. all of the above
13. The number of heartbeats too weak to be transmitted to the periphery is measured by
    A. pulse pressure
    B. brachiopopliteal gradient
    C. electrocardiogram
    D. apical–radial pulse deficit
14. Which of the following is consistent with diminished preload to the right ventricle?
    A. ascites
    B. jugular venous distention
    C. hepatic engorgement
    D. poor skin turgor
15. Conscious sedation is required for which of the following cardiovascular diagnostic procedures?
    A. stress test
    B. transesophageal echocardiogram
    C. transthoracic echocardiogram
    D. electrocardiogram

Pretest Answers: 1. A, 2. C, 3. B, 4. A, 5. B, 6. C, 7. B, 8. D, 9. D, 10. D, 11. B, 12. D, 13. D, 14. D, 15. B

GLOSSARY

afterload   The resistance against which the ventricle pumps blood.

apical–radial pulse deficit   The difference between the apical and radial pulse rates, which reflects the number of heartbeats too weak to be transmitted to the periphery.

atrial gallop   S4 heart sound caused by atrial contraction.

body surface area (BSA)   A measure of overall body size using both height and weight in its calculation.

cardiac index (CI)   Cardiac output divided by body surface area.

cardiac output (CO)   The amount of blood pumped by the heart each minute.

contractility   The ability of a muscle to shorten when stimulated; in particular, the force of myocardial contraction.

C-reactive protein (CRP)   Peptide released by the liver in response to inflammation, infection, and tissue damage.

ejection fraction   The portion of ventricular end diastolic volume that is pumped from the ventricle in one beat.

hyperlipidemia   Elevated levels of lipids in the blood.

inotrope   Factors that influence myocardial contractility; a positive inotrope increases myocardial contractility; a negative inotrope decreased myocardial contractility.

palpitations   Subjective feeling of heart rhythm abnormalities; perceived as a "skipping" or "thumping"; related to premature cardiac beats.

preload   The degree of stretch in myocardial fibers at the end of diastole.

pulse pressure   Difference between diastolic and systolic pulse pressure.

pulsus alternans   Alternating weak and strong pulses.

stroke volume (SV)   The volume of blood pumped with each heartbeat.

summation gallop   S3 and S4 heart sounds are present; indicative of severe heart failure.

syncope   A temporary loss of consciousness, followed by a spontaneous and complete recovery.

troponin   A protein found in cardiac muscle; when present in the blood, it is used as a marker of myocardial cell death.

ventricular gallop   S3 heart sound caused by decreased ventricular compliance.

ABBREVIATIONS

ANP	A-type natriuretic peptide		**ICG**	Impedance cardiography
BNP	B-type natriuretic peptide		**JVD**	Jugular venous distention
Bpm	Beats per minute		**L/min**	Liters per minute
BSA	Body surface area		**LDL**	Low-density lipoprotein
CI	Cardiac index		**MRI**	Magnetic resonance imaging
CK-MB	Creatine kinase-myocardial bands		**MUGA**	Multigated angiographic scan
CO	Cardiac output		**PET**	Positron emission tomography
CRP	C-reactive protein		**PMI**	Point of maximal impulse
ECG	Electrocardiogram		**PTCA**	Percutaneous transluminal angioplasty
EPS	Electrophysiology studies		**SV**	Stroke volume
HDL	High-density lipoprotein		**TEE**	Transesophageal echocardiogram
HR	Heart rate			

SECTION ONE: Cardiac Output

At the completion of this section, the learner will be able to define and state adult normal values for cardiac output, cardiac index, heart rate, and stroke volume. These definitions and values will be applied to the content of later sections.

Cardiac output (CO) is the amount of blood pumped by the heart each minute. It is a critical aspect of cardiovascular function in both health and illness. Knowledge of how CO changes in response to various conditions permits an understanding of pertinent physical assessment findings when there is an alteration in cardiac output.

The normal CO is approximately 4.0 to 8.0 liters/minute (L/min). Normal CO for individuals can vary significantly depending on body size. Therefore, when CO is measured it is corrected to account for body size. The correction is calculated by dividing CO by **body surface area (BSA)** and is called the **cardiac index (CI)**. Normal CI is 2.4 to 4.0 L/min/m^2 . The BSA is calculated using the patient's height and weight. Extreme values of BSA in morbidly obese patients demonstrate the need for using CI rather than CO. For example, patient A is 70 inches tall and weighs 320 pounds and has a BSA of 2.5. Patient B is 70 inches tall and weighs 170 pounds and has a BSA of 2.0. Both patients have a "normal" CO of 5 L/min. However, when a CO of 5 L/min is indexed to BSA, patient A has a CI of 2.0 L/min/m^2 and patient B has a CI of 2.5 L/min/m^2. Both patients have a CI below normal.

The volume of blood pumped with each heartbeat is called the **stroke volume (SV).** CO is the product of SV and heart rate (HR). Given a normal heart rate of approximately 72 beats per minute (bpm) (range, 60 to 100) and CO of approximately 5 L/min, it is possible to determine that the usual stroke volume for an adult is 5,000 mL/min divided by 72 bpm = 69 mL/beat or approximately 70 mL per beat.

Changes in either the HR or SV will alter CO. Fortunately, the body uses the interrelationship between these two factors to maintain a normal CO. For example, if SV falls, HR increases to compensate and maintain CO. Conversely, if HR drops, SV increases to compensate and maintain CO. Of course, there is a limit to the capacity of the body to use these compensatory efforts to maintain CO.

In summary, CO is the product of SV and HR. Both SV and HR can be modified to ensure that CO is adequate to meet the body's needs.

SECTION TWO: Components of Stroke Volume

At the completion of this section, the learner will be able to define preload, contractility, and afterload and discuss how each of these components impact stroke volume.

There are four determinants of CO. Any condition or disease that affects one determinant causes a change in another determinant in an effort to maintain CO. The four determinants of CO are as follows:

- Heart rate (HR)
- Preload
- Contractility
- Afterload

Where is stroke volume? SV is determined by the interplay of preload, contractility, and afterload:

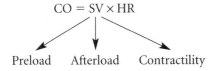

$$CO = SV \times HR$$

Preload   Afterload   Contractility

Heart Rate

If SV is held constant, any change in HR results in an immediate change in CO. For example, if the SV is 70 mL and the HR drops from 70 to 50 bpm, the CO drops from 4.9 L/min to 3.5 L/min. If HR increases from 70 bpm to 100 bpm and SV remains at 70 mL, CO increases from 4.9 L/min to 7.0 L/min.

The most effective mechanism to increase CO is to increase HR; however, this mechanism has limitations. A severe increase

in HR causes SV to decrease. A heart beating this fast spends too little time in diastole and the ventricles do not have time to fill with blood. Recall that the ventricles fill during diastole. Therefore, the faster the HR, the shorter the time spent in diastole, the less time available for ventricular filling, and less ventricular filling results in decreased preload and decreased SV.

Preload

Preload is the amount of stretch in the myocardial fibers at the end of diastole. Because blood volume affects the stretch of myocardial fibers, preload represents the volume of blood in the ventricle at end diastole. The greater the volume of blood in the ventricle, the greater the amount of stretch that the fibers experience. Preload is greatly affected by the volume of blood delivered to the heart from the venous system. If a large volume of blood returns from the venous system to the ventricle, the myocardial fibers will be very stretched. This represents a high preload. If a small volume of blood returns from the venous system to the ventricle, there will be less stretch and, therefore, less preload. High preload corresponds to high volume; low preload corresponds to low volume. Preload is discussed in greater detail later in Section Three.

Contractility

Contractility is defined as the force of myocardial contraction. Contractility reflects the ability of the heart muscle to work independently of preload and afterload; the ability to function as a pump. If the heart contracts forcefully, it pumps out most of the blood in the ventricle. If the heart pumps poorly, it pumps out less blood. Many variables affect the force with which the heart muscle contracts; however, anything that enhances or diminishes the ability of myocardial fibers to contract vigorously affects contractility. Contractility is discussed in further detail in Section Five of this module.

Even when working perfectly, the ventricle does not eject all the blood it contains. Usually, the ventricle ejects only 60 percent of the blood that it contains at the end of diastole. **Ejection fraction** is a measure of the percent of blood ejected with each stroke volume and is used as an index of myocardial function. The ejection fraction is the stroke volume divided by end diastolic volume. A normal ejection fraction is 60 percent.

Afterload

Afterload is the resistance against which the ventricle pumps blood. An optimal amount of resistance is necessary for the system to work properly. If afterload increases, stroke volume decreases because the ventricle is meeting increased resistance and cannot effectively pump out its volume. The major influence on afterload is the mechanical resistance to flow offered by the arterial system. If the arterial vessels are constricted, afterload to the left ventricle increases and stroke volume decreases. Other variables include the pulmonic and aortic valves, which may become stenotic and unable to fully open during systole. Afterload is discussed in greater detail in Section Four of this module.

In summary, cardiac output is the product of stroke volume and heart rate. There are three components of stroke volume: preload, contractility, and afterload. Preload is the volume of blood the heart has to pump, contractility is the ability of the heart to function as a pump, and afterload is the resistance the heart meets when it pumps out its volume. Therefore, the amount of CO depends on the volume of blood it receives, the ability of the heart to pump that volume, and the resistance the heart meets to pump out that volume times the number of times it does this each minute.

SECTION TWO REVIEW

1. The degree of stretch of myocardial fibers at the end of diastole is known as
   A. preload
   B. contractility
   C. compliance
   D. distensibility
2. A HR of 150 bpm would have what effect on CO?
   A. increase
   B. decrease
   C. no effect
   D. none of the above
3. The vigor of myocardial fibers' activities is known as
   A. automaticity
   B. conduction
   C. contractility
   D. afterload

4. The resistance against which the ventricle pumps blood is known as
   A. preload
   B. blood pressure
   C. compliance
   D. afterload
5. An increase in afterload has what effect on stroke volume?
   A. increase
   B. decrease
   C. no effect
   D. none of the above

Answers: 1. A, 2. B, 3. C, 4. D, 5. B

SECTION THREE: Preload

At the completion of this section, the learner will be able to describe the relationship of SV and preload in terms of the Frank–Starling Law.

Within limits, the heart pumps the amount of blood it receives with each beat. This is known as the Frank–Starling Law of the heart. In other words, as preload increases, so does SV, and as preload decreases, SV falls (Fig. 8–1A). Unfortunately, this law only applies within a certain range.

Note that until a critical point is reached, as preload increases, so does SV. An optimal preload results in optimal SV. Once past this point, an increase in preload results in a decrease in SV (Fig. 8–1B). If the heart receives too much preload, it cannot effectively pump out that volume and SV decreases. SV decreases because too much volume causes excessive stretching of the myocardial fibers and the ventricles cannot effectively contract.

A key assessment in high acuity patients is to determine how much preload provides an optimal SV. The nurse must be able to recognize assessment findings that indicate the patient has gone past that optimal point of preload and now has decreased SV. This will be discussed in greater detail in Section Seven.

In summary, the Frank–Starling Law of the heart demonstrates that an increase in preload results in an increase in SV to a certain point. Once that optimal preload is passed, more preload results in a decrease in SV because the myocardial fibers are too stretched. The heart cannot effectively pump out its volume.

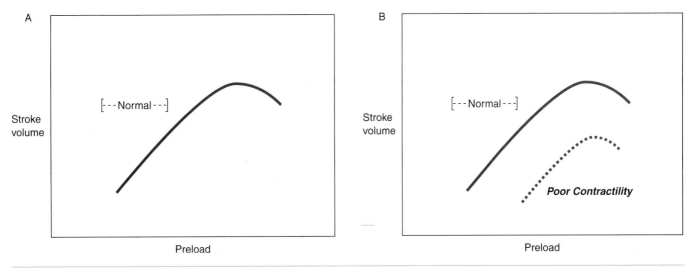

Figure 8–1 ■ Graphs demonstrating the Frank–Starling law of the heart.

SECTION THREE REVIEW

1. The Frank–Starling Law states that within physiologic limits the heart
   A. pumps as fast as it receives more blood
   B. pumps as much blood as it receives
   C. pumps less blood as it receives more blood
   D. pumps an unchanging amount of blood regardless of how much it receives

2. Disease may decrease the contractility of the myocardium. This means that if the preload decreases, SV
   A. increases
   B. decreases

C. stays the same
D. cannot be determined from this information

3. An increase in preload results in a(n)
   A. increase in SV
   B. decrease in contractility
   C. increase in HR
   D. decrease in afterload

Answers: 1. B, 2. B, 3. A

SECTION FOUR: Afterload

At the completion of this section, the learner will be able to describe the relationship among pressure, flow, and resistance. This relationship will help you understand the relationship between cardiac output, vascular resistance, and blood pressure. These relationships are often manipulated in acutely ill patients.

Recall from Section Two that afterload is the resistance the heart meets when it pumps out its SV. Most of the resistance the heart meets is related to the "size" of the arterial blood vessels—whether they are vasoconstricted or vasodilated. If they are vasoconstricted, afterload to the ventricle increases and SV decreases. If the vessels are vasodilated, afterload to the ventricle decreases and SV increases.

Imagine a system with a pump, a rigid tube, and a valve some distance from the pump, as shown in Figure 8–2. If the valve is half closed, the pressure in the tube increases as the rate of the liquid pumped increases. If the pump runs very fast and the valve is partially closed, the pressure in the pipe is high. If, however, the

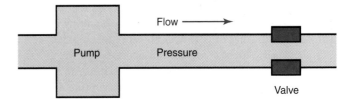

Figure 8–2 ■ Diagram demonstrating the hemodynamic concept of the relationship among flow, pressure, and resistance.

pump output remains constant and the valve is opened completely, there is little pressure in the tube. This relationship among flow, resistance, and pressure is expressed in Ohm's Law:

$$\text{Pressure} = \text{Flow} \times \text{Resistance}$$

Just as SV and HR compensate to maintain CO, flow and resistance compensate to maintain blood pressure (BP). Flow in the cardiovascular system is CO, resistance is afterload, and pressure is BP. Therefore, BP is the product of CO and afterload. When afterload increases (e.g., vasoconstriction), CO decreases and BP increases. This is what happens to patients with hypertension. When afterload decreases (e.g., vasodilation), CO increases and BP decreases. This is what happens to patients in septic shock. The relationship between BP, CO, and afterload have important clinical implications which are discussed in further detail in Modules 9 through 12.

In summary, blood pressure is the product of CO and vascular resistance. Blood pressure can be changed by adjustments in both CO and vascular resistance.

SECTION FOUR REVIEW

1. The mathematical relationship among flow, resistance, and pressure is
   A. flow = resistance/pressure
   B. resistance = flow/pressure
   C. pressure × flow = resistance
   D. flow × resistance = pressure
2. What is the flow in the cardiovascular system?
   A. cardiac output
   B. heart rate
   C. stroke volume
   D. blood pressure
3. What is the resistance in the cardiovascular system?
   A. preload
   B. afterload
   C. contractility
   D. compliance
4. If pressure drops and flow remains unchanged, resistance _____ to increase pressure.
   A. increases
   B. decreases
   C. remains unchanged
   D. cannot be determined
5. When afterload decreases
   A. BP increases
   B. CO increases
   C. BP decreases
   D. both B and C are correct

Answers: 1. D, 2. A, 3. B, 4. A, 5. D

SECTION FIVE: Contractility

At the completion of this section, the learner will be able to discuss factors that influence myocardial contractility.

Contractility refers to the ability of the heart to function as a pump. The contractile state is determined by biochemical and biophysical properties that govern the actin–myosin crossbridge formations and largely depends on the influx of calcium ions (Porth, 2005). Increased calcium release allows for greater interaction between actin and myosin filaments, resulting in greater contraction. Cardiac muscle does not store calcium like skeletal muscle; cardiac muscle contraction depends on this influx of calcium. Therefore, it is important for the nurse to recognize that when a patient's serum calcium is low, contractility of the heart may be decreased. Many drugs are given to increase calcium influx to produce greater myocardial contractility.

Factors that influence contractility are known as **inotropes.** Factors that increase myocardial contractility have a positive inotropic effect. Factors that decrease contractility have a negative inotropic effect. Positive inotropes include sympathetic nervous system stimulation, increased calcium release, and the administration of inotropic drugs, such as digoxin and dobutamine. Contractility decreases with hypoxemia; therefore, hypoxemia is considered to be a negative inotrope.

In acute care settings, inotropic drugs are often used to augment cardiac output. Digoxin, dopamine, and dobutamine are the most common medications used to increase CO by improving myocardial contractility.

In summary, contractility refers to the ability of the heart to function as a pump. Cardiac muscle contraction depends on calcium influx. Patients with a low serum calcium level may have decreased myocardial contractility. The nurse must recognize drugs and conditions that are positive and negative inotropes.

SECTION FIVE REVIEW

1. What electrolyte is important to cardiac contraction?
   A. calcium
   B. chloride
   C. sodium
   D. zinc
2. Sympathetic nervous system activation has what effect on myocardial contractility?
   A. increases myocardial contraction
   B. decreases myocardial contraction

C. has no effect on contractility
D. decreases heart rate, therefore, decreases cardiac output
3. Dobutamine is an example of a
   A. positive inotropic agent
   B. negative inotropic agent
   C. sympathomimetic
   D. B adrenergic blocking agent
4. Which of the following statements is true?
   A. cardiac muscle stores calcium
   B. skeletal muscle does not store calcium

C. cardiac muscle does not store calcium
D. both A and B are true
5. Which of the following is a negative inotrope?
   A. dopamine
   B. dobutamine
   C. digoxin
   D. hypoxemia

Answers: 1. A, 2. A, 3. A, 4. C, 5. D

SECTION SIX: Conditions That Affect Cardiac Output

At the end of this section, the learner will be able to state some of the conditions that affect heart rate, preload, contractility, and afterload. This information is important to apply in Modules 9 through 13.

Heart Rate

Heart rate is controlled by the heart's pacemaker sites, which are influenced by the interplay of the sympathetic and parasympathetic nervous systems. The sympathetic nervous system causes the fight-or-flight reaction, in which the body's resources are mobilized to counteract a real or perceived threat. The cardiovascular effects of sympathetic nervous system stimulation include increased HR, increased contractility, and vasoconstriction. The parasympathetic nervous system causes generally the opposite effects: decreased HR, decreased contractility, and vasodilation.

Any stressors that activate the sympathetic nervous system cause an increase in HR. Such stressors may include events or conditions perceived as threats, for example, speaking in front of large groups or fleeing a burning house. In the hospital environment, stimuli that activate the sympathetic nervous system include pain, anxiety, and sensory overstimulation, in addition to the physiologic causes. On a physiologic level, anything that causes a decrease in SV is likely to cause an increase in HR in an effort to compensate and hold CO constant. In addition, there are numerous other causes of increased HR, including cardiac conduction system dysfunction, drug effects, and hormone imbalances.

Heart rate is decreased by increased activity of the parasympathetic nervous system. There are numerous causes of low HR, ranging from drug effects and poisoning to straining hard to have a bowel movement. Other sources of a low HR include impaired impulse generation or conduction in the heart. Heart rate

may also be slowed by administration of drugs that either block sympathetic activity (beta blockers) or that inhibit calcium influx into myocardial fibers (calcium channel blockers). Conditions that affect HR are further discussed in Module 10.

Preload

Recall that preload is the amount of stretch of myocardial fibers at the end of diastole, and preload can be thought of as being the amount of blood in the ventricle at end diastole. Preload is altered by a change in the amount of blood delivered to the heart from the venous system.

A decrease in blood volume in the ventricle results in a decrease in preload. Loss of blood volume from hemorrhage, dehydration, diuretic use, or movement of fluid out of the vascular space into the extravascular compartment results in a decrease in preload. Diminished preload also can be caused by failure of an atrioventricular (AV) valve (either tricuspid or mitral) to allow free flow of blood into the ventricle. Vasodilation of the venous system causes the venous vessels to hold more blood, which results in less blood entering the ventricle and a decrease in preload. In addition, very fast HR shorten diastolic filling time. Therefore, there is insufficient time for the ventricle to fill adequately and the result is a decrease in preload.

An increase in blood volume results in an increase in preload. Conditions that cause an increase in blood volume include renal failure, fluid overload from IV therapy, increased aldosterone secretion (with retention of sodium and water), and excess sodium in the diet. Increased preload also occurs when the ventricle is unable to pump out its volume of blood. When this happens, there is still excess blood volume in the ventricle after ejection. When the ventricle fills during diastole, it already has a residual volume and now also has the blood volume recently pumped from the atria. At some point, the ventricle can no longer pump out all this volume and blood volume begins to "back up." This is precisely what happens in congestive heart failure: The heart pumps less blood than is delivered to it, and there is congestion in the venous system that drains into the affected ventricle. If the left ventricle fails, congestion occurs in the pulmonary vascular bed. If the right ventricle fails, the congestion occurs in the systemic venous system. These concepts are further discussed in Module 12.

Contractility

Contractility is much like HR in that it is strongly influenced by the autonomic nervous system. Sympathetic stimulation of the heart results in increased contractility, and, conversely, parasympathetic stimulation causes decreased contractility. Other major determinants of contractility include oxygenation (hypoxia or ischemia decrease contractility), myocardial disease (myocarditis, cardiomyopathy), and drug effects (many narcotics and anesthetic agents are direct myocardial depressants). Drugs that increase myocardial contractility include digitalis, epinephrine, and dobutamine.

Afterload

The major determinant of afterload is the resistance to flow caused by the arterial system. Most of the arterial resistance is caused by constriction of arterioles. Anything that changes arteriolar vascular tone changes afterload. For example, stimulation of the sympathetic nervous system causes constriction of the arterioles and an increase in afterload. Drugs that dilate or constrict the arterioles cause a prompt change in afterload. The arterioles are dilated during septic shock, spinal cord injury, or anaphylactic shock (Module 15). Further resistance to flow can be caused by failure of the pulmonic or aortic valve to allow free flow of blood from the ventricle to the artery. In this case, the stenosed valve causes an increase in afterload.

In summary, each determinant of CO can be affected by numerous clinical conditions. Thus, clinical conditions can have an impact on CO by their influence on preload, afterload, contractility, and HR.

SECTION SIX REVIEW

1. Decreased HR can be caused by
   A. decreased SV
   B. anxiety
   C. parasympathetic stimulation
   D. pain
2. Increased preload may occur with
   A. mitral stenosis
   B. vasodilation of venous vessels
   C. very fast HRs
   D. renal failure
3. Increased contractility can be caused by
   A. ischemia
   B. hypoxia
   C. cardiomyopathy
   D. sympathetic stimulation

4. Increased afterload can be caused by
   A. sympathetic stimulation
   B. septic shock
   C. anaphylaxis
   D. spinal cord injury
5. Decreased preload can be caused by
   A. too much IV fluid
   B. hemorrhage
   C. diuretics
   D. both B and C

Answers: 1. C, 2. D, 3. D, 4. A, 5. D

SECTION SEVEN: Assessment of Cardiac Output

At the completion of this section, the learner will be able to identify common clinical assessments that evaluate heart rate, preload, contractility, and afterload. Hemodynamic monitoring provides a means for invasive monitoring of CO which is discussed in Module 9. The first part of this section concentrates on the focused assessment of CO. The second part of this section focuses on diagnostic procedures that may be used to evaluate CO in acutely ill patients, and the nursing responsibilities associated with patients undergoing these diagnostic tests.

Focused Nursing Assessment

The key to accurately determining cardiac output lies in the assessment skills of the nurse. Assessment begins on admission. The nurse must obtain subjective data on admission, conduct a complete physical assessment, interpret lab results, use bedside monitoring equipment effectively, and apply knowledge gained via various diagnostic procedures. The nursing process, particularly in high acuity care, depends on a thorough assessment.

Nursing History

On admission, airway, breathing, and circulation are assessed prior to obtaining a nursing history to assure that the patient is sufficiently stable to be interviewed. This initial assessment is generally a rapid, limited one that may take no more than a minute. Appropriate priority interventions are then performed based on the assessed priority needs. Once the patient's safety and comfort has been attended to, the nurse obtains a nursing history including the patient's present illness and past medical history. It is important to assess perfusion regardless of whether the patient has a previous history of perfusion abnormalities.

Present Illness and Past Medical History

At the time of admission, the nurse may be interviewing the patient, a family member, or other person or persons. Eliciting a recent history of the present illness (i.e., the events leading up to this admission) provides the clinician with important data regarding the problem and possible etiologies, and the patient's ability to compensate for a cardiovascular stressor. Recent history information also helps identify areas where the patient may need external support in order to increase myocardial oxygen supply and decrease myocardial demand in order to regain or maintain a state of compensation.

A detailed patient history at the time of admission helps determine the plan of care. By using a variety of interviewing techniques and therapeutic communications, the nurse obtains demographic data, family history, diet, functional status, and prior medical history. Demographic data includes the patient's age, sex, race, and weight. Cardiovascular risk factors such as smoking history, exercise pattern, stress level, and obesity are assessed. Family history of cardiovascular disease and diet history are important data to elicit from the patient during the nursing history.

Knowledge about functional status prior to onset of illness allows for setting realistic goals of therapy and patient/family education. The patient's prior medical history provides information about comorbidities, medication and herbal use, and other interventions that have been used to maintain health. Certain medications impact physical assessment findings including changes in heart rate, blood pressure, and urine output.

Complaints of chest pain must be assessed as pain of cardiac origin or pain of pulmonary origin. The mnemonic PQRST is helpful in organizing assessment data related to pain. Eliciting information about precipitating factors (P), quality (Q), radiation and region (R), associated symptoms (S), and timing and treatment strategies (T) help the nurse determine the origin of the pain. Pain may not always be present in all patients with perfusion disorders. Diabetic patients and the elderly may not feel pain. Women may have "atypical" pain such as abdominal pain and fatigue. Chest pain is described in greater detail in Module 11.

A patient with a perfusion disorder may complain of **palpitations,** often described as a "skipping" or "thumping" of the heart. This symptom is related to the occurrence of premature cardiac beats. Palpation of the pulse will reveal premature beats. There will be irregular pulse amplitude because of the decreased blood volume associated with premature beats and the larger-than-normal volume of the beat immediately after the premature beat related to prolonged diastolic filling. The best way of detecting premature beats is by obtaining an electrocardiogram (ECG) and monitoring the patient's cardiac rhythm. These assessments are described in greater detail in Module 10.

A patient with a perfusion disorder may experience a change in level of consciousness related to a decreased CO or blockage of cerebral circulation. A diminished level of consciousness, confusion, or agitation may be signs of decreased perfusion to cerebral tissue. The patient may experience **syncope** (a temporary loss of consciousness, followed by complete, spontaneous recovery).

Nursing Physical Assessment

Techniques of physical assessment of cardiac output include inspection, palpation, and auscultation. Because of the rapid changes that can occur in the acute care setting, cardiac output is assessed frequently. By developing a systematic method of physical assessment, the nurse rapidly ascertains changes in hemodynamic status. Technology cannot substitute for physical assessment. Overreliance on the monitoring equipment alarms may lead to complacency, and subtle physical changes may be missed.

Inspection of the precordium may demonstrate rhythmic movement. Abnormal movement may be visualized in the aortic, pulmonic, or tricuspid areas (Jarvis, 2004). Normal movement is found in the area of the mitral valve. This is the apical impulse. It is usually seen in the area of the left 5th intercostal space along the midclavicular line.

Inspection and palpation of the periphery can also indicate variations in the patient's cardiac output. Changes in skin color are a late sign of hemodynamic compromise, as is clubbing of the fingers. A cooling of the skin is brought about by the vasoconstriction of the arterioles as blood is shunted to the internal organs. A decrease in cardiac output may be the cause. Cool distal extremities may be a useful marker of decreased

---

Evidence-Based Practice

- *In elderly patients, capillary refill does not correlate with objective measurements of hypovolemia (Gross et al., 1992).*

- *The sensitivity of capillary refill to blood loss is 6 percent; the specificity is 93 percent (Schringer & Baraff, 1991).*

- *Cool distal extremities correlate with other markers of hypoperfusion, such as base deficit, high lactate, and low mixed venous oxygen saturation (Kaplan et al., 2001).*

CO (Kaplan et al., 2001). Delayed capillary refill is often associated with decreased CO. However, capillary refill as an indicator of the adequacy of CO is controversial. It may be useful as a marker of hypovolemia and poor myocardial function in children, but in elderly patients it does not appear to be useful (Johnson, 2004).

The kidney is sensitive to changes in intravascular volume; therefore, the amount of urine output is frequently used to assess the adequacy of CO. Theoretically, a decrease in CO results in a decrease in urine output. However, there are conditions in which urine output does not reflect the adequacy of CO. These conditions may affect patients in compensatory shock states (see Module 15) and the elderly. The elderly may have chronic disease states and use medications that affect urine output.

The presence of peripheral edema may indicate too much preload to the right side of the heart. Edema is a palpable swelling produced by an accumulation of interstitial fluid volume. Pathophysiologic mechanisms that cause edema are listed below. Edema can be generalized or localized. Localized edema in the calf may indicate an obstruction of venous blood flow from a clot in a leg vein. Generalized edema is a physical assessment finding associated with congestive heart failure. See Module 3 for a more detailed discussion of edema.

Pathophysiologic mechanisms that cause edema

- Increase in capillary hydrostatic pressure
- Decrease in capillary colloid pressure
- Increase in capillary permeability that creates an increase in interstitial colloid pressure
- Obstruct lymphatic flow

The effects of edema are determined by its location: brain, larynx, lungs, hands, feet, face, or abdomen. Life-threatening situations occur with edema of the brain, larynx, or lungs. Edema of the extremities can interfere with mobility and can impair perfusion by compression on arterial vessels. Pitting edema occurs with an increase in capillary hydrostatic pressure, which pushes fluid from the vascular to the interstitial spaces. Nonpitting edema occurs with an increase in interstitial colloid pressure.

There are several methods to assess for edema including visual assessment by inspection, palpation, measurement of the affected part, and daily weight. Finger pressure can be used to assess the degree of pitting edema. Edema is measured on a 1-to-4 scale, with 4 being the most severe. Daily weights are helpful in monitoring trends in water gain or losses. One liter of water weighs 1 kilogram or 2.2 pounds. If a patient's weight increases in 24 hours by 1 kilogram, the interpretation is that the patient has gained 1 liter of fluid. If diuretics are given and the patient is weighed 24 hours later and has lost 1 kilogram, then the patient has diuresed 1 kilogram of water. Weights are particularly important for patients receiving renal dialysis because they provide an index of water balance before and after dialysis.

The presence of jugular venous distention may indicate too much preload to the right side of the heart. Jugular venous distention (JVD) may indicate a fluid distribution problem. The

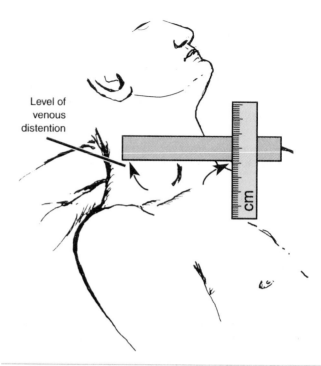

Figure 8–3 ■ Measurement of jugular venous distention.

venous system is a low-pressure system, and it is sensitive to right atrial pressure. Retention of blood in the right side of the heart (as in the case of heart failure or cor pulmonale) will increase right atrial pressure and subsequently produce jugular venous distention as a result of backflow through the vena cava. In assessing for venous distention, elevate the head of the bed to approximately 45 degrees. The patient's head is turned slightly away from the examiner. A penlight is used to shine a light tangentially across the neck (Fig. 8–3).

Palpation gives the nurse a tactile indication of cardiac output. Rolling the patient onto the left side moves the heart closer to the surface of the body. Precordial palpation may produce a vibration, also known as a thrill. This may correspond to a murmur, valvular stenosis, or increased afterload (Jarvis, 2004). The point of maximal impulse (PMI) corresponds to the location of the apical impulse. Heaves and lifts also indicate ventricular hypertrophy on either side. On the periphery, palpation of pulses is indicative of CO. Pulses should be of regular rate, strength, and rhythm. A hyperkinetic (bounding) pulse may indicate increased cardiac output because of thyrotoxicosis, fever, pain, or anxiety. A hypokinetic pulse may be the result of decreased cardiac output, with causes such as dysrhythmias, damaged myocardium, or cardiomyopathy. Severely depressed cardiac function may cause **pulsus alterans,** which is evidenced by alternating weak and strong pulses in a regular rhythm.

Auscultation is another technique to assess cardiac output. Knowledge of the auditory indicators of valvular dysfunction is essential. Recall, the function of heart valves is to provide unidirectional flow of blood through the heart. With valve dysfunction there is turbulent or decreased blood flow through the heart. This results in a decrease in CO. Heart valve disorders are discussed in greater detail in Module 12.

Auscultation of the precordium must be systematic and be performed using both the bell and the diaphragm of the stethoscope. The pattern of auscultation begins at the base of the heart using the diaphragm in the area of the aortic valve, and proceeds to the pulmonic, tricuspid, and mitral valves in order. Once completed, the bell is used in reverse sequence. Various extra heart sounds may be heard, such as high- and low-frequency murmurs, or extrasystolic sounds, such as clicks and rubs. Heart murmurs are evidence of turbulent blood flow, and can be due to stenotic or incompetent valves. They can be heard during systole or diastole. Table 8–1 outlines the grading system used to classify murmurs.

Diastolic filling sounds may help determine why cardiac output is reduced. The S3 sound, heard early in diastole, is a ventricular filling sound caused by decreased ventricular compliance and is a sign of early heart failure. It is also known as **ventricular gallop.** S4 is also a ventricular filling sound but occurs late in diastole. It is heard during atrial contraction, and it, therefore, is known as **atrial gallop.** It is a result of myocardial infarction, ventricular hypertrophy, and increased afterload. A **summation gallop,** when both S3 and S4 sounds are heard, is often indicative of severe heart failure (Jarvis, 2004).

Shortness of breath results from fluid movement out of the pulmonary capillaries and into the lung interstitial space, thereby decreasing oxygen diffusion from the alveoli into the pulmonary capillaries. The presence of wet-sounding crackles (rales) on auscultation of the lungs indicates pulmonary edema. Severe pulmonary edema is associated with frothy, pink sputum production.

Auscultatory techniques can also be used on the peripheral vasculature system. Bruits along the carotid arteries may indicate areas of occlusion. These partial blockages represent potential compromise to the cerebral vasculature and account for some signs and symptoms also attributable to decreased cardiac output. Renal artery bruits may indicate renal artery stenosis, which leads to systemic hypertension. The resulting increase in afterload may compromise cardiac output. A dialysis graft should be auscultated. The bruit heard indicates patency of the graft and corresponds to the thrill described earlier.

TABLE 8–1   Grading System Used to Classify Murmurs

I/VI	Very faint
II/VI	Faint
III/VI	Loud; moderate in intensity
IV/VI	Loud; palpable thrill
V/VI	Loud enough to be heard with head of stethoscope partially off chest wall; palpable thrill
VI/VI	Loud enough to be heard with head of stethoscope completely off chest wall; palpable thrill

Diagnostic Laboratory Tests

There are numerous diagnostic lab parameters used to assess CO, which is adversely affected by myocardial damage. When the myocardium is damaged as a result of ischemia, myocardial cells die and release their intracellular contents, including enzymes, into the general circulation. Since the enzymes are not normally present in the blood, elevated serum levels are indicative of myocardial cell death. These enzymes will be briefly described in this module and are described in greater detail in Module 11.

Creatine kinase-myocardial band (CK-MB) is a myocardial enzyme that is released 4 to 12 hours after the onset of myocardial necrosis and is very specific for myocardial damage (Newby, 2004). Because of these varying times of release, CK-MB and other cardiac enzymes are often obtained on a serial basis, meaning they are assessed every couple of hours over the course of 24 hours after the patient complains of chest pain. Serial CK-MB measurement resulting in an elevation or upward trend is a cardiac marker for acute myocardial infarction or "heart attack." The major limitation of CK-MB is that levels do not start to rise until 4 hours after the onset of myocardial damage. This can delay diagnosis and treatment of myocardial infarction.

Troponin is a protein found in cardiac muscle. It is part of a protein complex for the binding of myosin and actin, the myofilaments that regulate contraction. Troponin can appear in the blood as early as 3 to 4 hours after myocardial damage. Troponin has a higher sensitivity and specificity for identifying even minor myocyte necrosis than CK-MB (Casey, 2004).

C-reactive Protein (CRP) is a peptide released by the liver in response to systemic inflammation, infection, and tissue damage. Atherosclerosis is considered to be a chronic inflammatory process and studies have shown CRP levels increase with the atherosclerotic disease process. Several large studies have shown CRP to be predictive of coronary disease in postmenopausal women (Ridker et al., 2000), the elderly (Kop et al., 2002), and in individuals with average levels of cholesterol (Ridker et al., 2001). The American Heart Association suggests that in patients with stable coronary disease, CRP measurement may be useful as a marker of prognosis for myocardial injury and death (Pearson et al., 2003). CRP results of less than 1.0 mg/L are considered low risk, 1 to 3 mg/L as average risk, and CRP results greater than 3 mg/L are considered high risk (Casey, 2004).

B-type natriuretic peptide (BNP) is a hormone released from the ventricles. This peptide, which is released in response to increased preload, causes urinary excretion of sodium and diuresis, and counteracts the effects of the renin–angiotensin–aldosterone system (Gordon & Rempher, 2003). This results in a reduction of preload. When BNP is present in the blood, it is indicative of heart failure (Module 12). BNP can also be used as a therapeutic agent (Nesiritide, a recombinant form of BNP) in patients with heart failure (Prahash & Lunch, 2004).

Hyperlipidemia, high levels of lipids in the blood, is associated with high risk for coronary heart disease. High risk lipids include elevated total cholesterol, increased low-density lipoprotein (LDL) cholesterol, decreased high-density lipoprotein (HDL), and elevated triglycerides. HDLs are the "good" cholesterol (remember H stands for "happy" or "healthy"). LDLs are the "bad" cholesterols. Higher levels of HDLs than LDLs are desirable. The ratio should be at least 1:5 with 1:3 being ideal. These lab values are discussed in greater detail in Module 11.

There are several electrolytes that affect cardiac output and are important to monitor. These include potassium, calcium, magnesium, and sodium. Imbalances of potassium, calcium, and magnesium often produce changes in heart rate and rhythm and are often detected by an ECG (Module 10).

Assessment of Specific Components of Cardiac Output

Preload, like contractility and afterload, are difficult to assess at the bedside because the cardiovascular structures where these exist are embedded deeply in the chest and are unavailable for examination. Direct measures of these determinants of CO require invasive monitoring devices (such as a pulmonary artery catheter) and are discussed in Module 9. Without invasive monitoring devices, the nurse must use indirect measures that permit an estimation of preload, contractility, or afterload.

Heart Rate

Evaluating HR is relatively easy. A simple count of the radial pulse is useful for determining the number of heartbeats that are strong enough to reach the periphery. A count of the apical HR is useful to determine the total HR. Usually, these two rates are equal, but there may be a deficit between the apical rate and the radial rate caused by irregular heart rhythms that result in SV varying from beat to beat, which results in some beats being too weak to be felt at the radial artery (this is called the **apical–radial pulse deficit**). For example, a radial pulse would give a better indication of the adequacy of peripheral perfusion in a person complaining of dizziness than an apical pulse. It is recommended that the clinician use a 60-second counting interval when assessing a patient for the first time, if the patient is unstable, if the cardiac rhythm is irregular, or treatment decisions are based on HR (Jarvis, 2004).

Preload

Preload for the right ventricle is assessed by evaluating the systemic venous system. The assessment findings of increased and decreased right ventricular preload are summarized in Table 8–2. Increased preload to right heart typically manifests as signs of too much fluid in the peripheral tissues and organs as fluid backs up from the right side of the heart. Preload for the left heart is assessed by evaluating the pulmonary venous system. Assessment findings are summarized in Table 8–3. Increased

TABLE 8–2   Assessment of Right Heart Preload

INCREASED RIGHT HEART PRELOAD	DECREASED RIGHT HEART PRELOAD
Jugular venous distention (JVD) (immediate sign)	Poor skin turgor
Ascites	Dry mucous membranes
Hepatic engorgement	Orthostatic hypotension
Peripheral edema	Flat jugular veins

preload to the left heart typically manifests as signs of too much fluid in the pulmonary circulation as fluid backs up from the left side of the heart.

Unfortunately, there are no noninvasive assessments currently available that specifically indicate diminished left ventricular preload. Usually, if the left heart has insufficient preload, the right heart has the same situation, and signs of diminished right ventricular preload are present. In some situations S1 and S2 may be muffled.

Contractility

Assessing the force of myocardial contraction is done by assessing the quality of the heartbeat when isolated from HR. The character of the pulse is noted at the radial artery. Increased contractility will demonstrate a bounding, vigorous pulse, whereas diminished contractility will demonstrate a weak, thready pulse. A splitting of S2 indicates that one ventricle is emptying earlier or later than the other, usually because of a structural (e.g., valve defect), mechanical (e.g., heart failure), or electrical (e.g., alternate pacemaker) problem. Contractility may be diminished. It is important to note that contractility is difficult to measure indirectly by physical signs because so many other factors may alter the character of the pulse. Decreased contractility usually is determined by exclusion of other causes of poor cardiac output.

The **pulse pressure** is the difference between diastolic and systolic blood pressures. It reflects how much the heart is able to raise the pressure in the arterial system with each beat. Pulse pressure increases when SV increases or in arteriole vasoconstriction. Pulse pressure drops with decreased SV or vasodilation (e.g., some shock states). The normal pulse pressure is approximately 30 to 40 mm Hg. Within the restrictions noted,

TABLE 8–3   Assessment of Increased Left Heart Preload

INCREASED LEFT HEART PRELOAD
Dyspnea
Cough
Third heart sound (S3)
Fourth heart sound (S4)

the pulse pressure can be a useful, objective, and noninvasive indicator of myocardial contractility.

Afterload

Recall that indirect assessment of right ventricle afterload is difficult because of the location of the pulmonary arterial system deep in the chest. However, it is possible to assess the systemic arterial system for signs of increased or decreased afterload. Even though signs of altered afterload may be present in some patients, they are not present in all patients with altered afterload. It is necessary to remember once again that all of these determinants of CO are interrelated, and it can be difficult to isolate individual factors at the bedside without invasive diagnostic tests.

Signs of increased systemic afterload include cool, clammy extremities. These signs may indicate that peripheral arterioles are constricted. Nonhealing wounds and thick brittle nails are indicators of chronic poor perfusion of the extremities. Signs of decreased systemic afterload include warm, flushed extremities, which may indicate peripheral vasodilation.

In summary, the key to accurately assessing CO lies in the assessment skills of the acute care nurse. A focused nursing assessment begins with the nursing history to identify cardiovascular risk factors, chest pain, abnormal heart rhythms, or changes in mentation. Physical assessment of CO should be done frequently in acutely ill patients and include techniques of inspection, palpation, and auscultation. A focused assessment may reveal signs of impaired CO, including skin color and temperature, edema, changes in weight and urine output, and auscultation of murmurs. Certain lab values are important as indicators of CO, including CK-MB, troponin, CRP, BNP and ANP, lipoproteins, and electrolytes.

SECTION SEVEN REVIEW

1. Pitting edema is associated with
   A. an increase in capillary hydrostatic pressure
   B. an increase in interstitial colloid pressure
   C. obstruction of lymph flow
   D. B and C are correct
2. Mr. Z gains 2 kg over the past 24 hours. Estimate the amount of fluid he has retained.
   A. one-half liter
   B. 1 liter
   C. 2 liters
   D. unable to determine with data provided
3. JVD may be a sign of
   A. elevated left ventricular preload
   B. decreased left ventricular preload
   C. hypertension
   D. elevated right ventricular preload
4. Which of the following cardiac enzymes appear in the blood within three hours of myocardial cell death?
   A. ANP
   B. BNP
   C. CK-MB
   D. troponin
5. Signs of decreased contractility include
   A. bounding pulse
   B. diminished pulse pressure
   C. ascites
   D. poor skin turgor
6. Signs of increased afterload for the left ventricle include
   A. cool, clammy extremities
   B. thin, flexible toenails
   C. liver engorgement
   D. peripheral edema

Answers: 1. A, 2. C, 3. D, 4. D, 5. B, 6. A

SECTION EIGHT: Cardiovascular Diagnostic Procedures

At the end of this section, the learner will be able to describe various cardiovascular diagnostic procedures used to evaluate the components of cardiac output and discuss nursing responsibilities in caring for a patient receiving these diagnostic procedures.

Imaging Techniques

A chest x-ray is used to view the size and position of the heart. Pulmonary edema caused by decompensated heart failure may be visualized. An enlarged cardiac silhouette may be evidence of cardiac tamponade or dilated cardiomyopathy. Chest x-rays may be taken daily for patients with acute cardiovascular problems. Patients who require continuous ECG monitoring but are stable do not typically require a daily chest x-ray unless there is a change in status. It is important for the nurse to help the patient with proper positioning when the x-ray is obtained to ensure a high-quality film.

Magnetic resonance imaging (MRI) technology has improved to where coronary mapping, blood flow, and cardiac structures can be visualized. The patient cannot wear any metal, and patients with cardiac pacemakers are prohibited from having the procedure performed.

Radionuclide testing can be used to evaluate myocardial perfusion and left ventricular function. A small amount of a radioisotope is injected intravenously and the heart is scanned with a radiation detector. Ischemic or infarcted cells in the myocardium do not take up the radioisotope.

Exercise Electrocardiogram

Exercise ECG, commonly known as a "stress test," evaluates heart muscle and its blood supply during physical stress (exercise). This can identify myocardial ischemia that may not be present at rest. If for some reason the patient cannot tolerate exercise, a simulated stress is given to the heart muscle by the administration of dobutamine, a positive inotropic drug.

Prior to the procedure, the patient may be anxious and may fear having a heart attack during the test. The patient should be assured of close monitoring during the procedure.

The stress test consists of the patient exercising on either a stationary bicycle or a treadmill. The patient's blood pressure and ECG are closely monitored as the exercise workload is increased. The patient is reminded to let the health care team know if chest pain, palpitations, or dyspnea occur. The test is discontinued when a predetermined heart rate is reached and maintained, signs of insufficient cardiac output appear, or ECG changes occur. The nurse conducting the exam must be familiar with cardiac dysrhythmias and emergency procedures. Emergency medications and a defibrillator should be present. Once the patient has returned to baseline hemodynamic status, the patient either returns to the hospital room or is allowed to go home. Some outpatients are admitted to the hospital for further diagnostic testing if they have unfavorable results from the exercise ECG. ECG and telemetry monitoring are discussed in detail in Module 10.

Echocardiogram

Another common cardiovascular diagnostic test is the echocardiogram. There are two forms of this test: transthoracic echocardiogram and transesophageal echocardiogram (TEE). Echocardiograms are particularly useful for visualizing blood, cardiac valves, the myocardium, and the pericardium. Ultrasound technology can be used to assess and diagnose cardiomyopathies, valvular function, cardiac tumors, and left ventricular function. An estimate of ejection fraction is also obtained.

Transthoracic echocardiograms are noninvasive tests that can be performed at the bedside or in the outpatient setting by a technologist. The patient is usually placed in a semifowler, left lateral, or supine position. The position is determined by the patient's overall condition, the patient's ability to tolerate the position, and the position that will give the best view of the structures to be visualized. Lubricant is placed on the skin and a transducer is placed on the skin. The transducer emits ultrasound waves and receives a signal back from the reflected waves. Nursing responsibilities may include dimming of the lights in the room and ensuring patient privacy and warmth.

The TEE is much more invasive. An ultrasound probe is inserted orally into the patient's esophagus and advanced until it is close to the heart. The TEE provides a more definitive representation of the heart. TEE produces images of intracardiac structures and the entire thoracic aorta. It produces high-quality images of both atrial chambers and is the procedure of choice to detect clots in the left atrium, atrial septal defects, infections on valve leaflets, and valve dysfunction.

Conscious sedation is used with the TEE, so nursing care is much more involved. Prior to the procedure, the nurse reviews the patient's chart, obtains a detailed history, and inserts a peripheral intravenous catheter. Suction equipment should be available in case the patient vomits. During the procedure, the nurse administers sedation, monitors vital signs and pulse oximetry saturations every 3 to 5 minutes, adjusts fluid and oxygen, and documents patient condition. During and immediately after the procedure, the nurse monitors for complications, which include respiratory depression and aspiration. Movement of the probe in the esophagus may stimulate the vagus nerve resulting in bradycardia or hypotension. Vital signs are monitored as the patient awakens from the procedure. The patient recovers in 1 to 2 hours. If the transesophageal echocardiogram was performed in an outpatient setting, the patient must be released to a responsible adult, in case there are residual effects of the sedation.

Cardiac Catheterization

Cardiac catheterization can be performed on either the left or right side of the heart. Catheterization of the left side of the heart is primarily performed to determine the patency of the coronary vessels, but it can also be used to observe blood flow through the chambers and valves of the heart or to deliver a thrombolytic agent directly into the coronary vessels. Chamber pressures may also be measured.

The nurse in the prep area is responsible for initial assessment and history, vital signs, initiating intravenous access, and placing electrocardiogram leads. A thorough review of the patient's medications and allergies is required. The prep nurse must ensure that metformin (Glucophage) and warfarin (Coumadin) have been held to prevent potential complications. Metformin has been shown to interfere with renal clearance of the dye used, resulting in acute renal failure in some cases. The anticoagulation properties of warfarin can result in additional bleeding complications. The dye used during this fluoroscopic procedure is iodine based, so inquiries as to a patient's allergies to iodine or seafood are imperative. Because this is an invasive procedure, informed consent must be obtained.

An interventional cardiologist, who is assisted by a nurse and a cardiovascular technician, performs the procedure. The nurse prepares the insertion site, monitors vital signs, and gives medications for conscious sedation. It is important to monitor the patient's airway during conscious sedation. The nurse also monitors the patient for any abnormalities in heart rate or rhythm during the procedure.

The procedure is conducted via the arterial system. The most common insertion route is the femoral artery, although recent reports indicate that the radial artery is a safe and effective route (Nickolaus et al., 2001). After local anesthesia is given, a catheter is passed up through the aortic arch, and dye is injected to visualize the coronary vessels. The patient remains sedated but awake enough to follow commands, such as requests to reposition and to hold the breath. The diagnostic portion of the procedure lasts 30 to 60 minutes.

If a lesion is discovered, then an intervention is performed. This intervention is called an "angioplasty" or percutaneous transluminal angioplasty (PCTA). For this intervention, a balloon is inserted and inflated, then a stent (wire basket) is placed to hold the vessel lumen open (Fig. 8–4). If this type of intervention is performed, the patient stays overnight for observation of potential complications, such as bleeding, dysrhythmias, or signs of vessel reocclusion.

After the cardiac catheterization procedure the patient remains in the cardiovascular lab for frequent nursing assessments until the patient is discharged to home or to the telemetry unit. The patient is monitored postprocedure for complications. Vascular complications occur in 0.1 to 2 percent of patients, with an increased risk caused by the presence of peripheral vascular disease or obesity (Nickolaus et al., 2001). Complications include hematoma, bleeding, and pseudoaneurysm (McCabe et al., 2001). The nurse monitoring the patient postprocedure assesses the access site for bleeding or hematoma formation. Pedal pulses are assessed bilaterally. One important assessment is to check the patient's flanks for signs of retroperitoneal bleeding. This complication is difficult to diagnose and can be life threatening (Nickolaus et al., 2001). The patient is required to remain supine for the first hour postprocedure. The patient must be reminded to keep the procedural leg straight to reduce stress on the procedure site. For example, the patient should be instructed to compress the insertion with her or his hand when coughing.

There are several means of closing the access site: pressure, collagen plug, or suturing. If a collagen plug or sutures were used to close the procedure site, the patient is usually discharged within a few hours after closure of the access site. If pressure was used to close the site, the patient typically remains for several more hours.

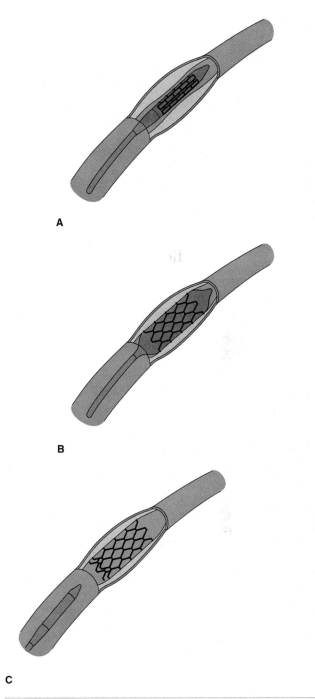

A

B

C

Figure 8–4 ■ Placement of balloon expandable intracoronary stent.

If the patient is going home, patient education must include information about activity restrictions. Driving, bathing, and climbing stairs should be avoided for 72 hours. The patient is prohibited from driving postprocedure because in the event of a need to brake the car suddenly, the increased pressure at the catheterization site can cause rupture of the weakened femoral vessel. The resulting hemorrhage could be fatal. A similar risk is present when walking up and down stairs. The puncture site should not be submerged for 7 days to reduce the chances of infection. The vasodilatory effect of the warm water can also cause vessel rupture.

If the patient is an inpatient, he or she will return to the telemetry unit. It is important for the nurse in the receiving unit to know of the events during the procedure. Pre- and postprocedure checklists are one way to optimize communication, thereby improving patient care between the telemetry unit and the cardiac catheterization lab (Coloff, 2003). These checklists help ensure continuity of care.

Electrophysiology Study

The electrophysiology study (EPS) is another invasive procedure that evaluates the cardiac conduction system and helps classify cardiac arrhythmias. Electrode catheters are placed in the right atrium and an intracardiac ECG is obtained. Arrhythmias can be induced and classified. Various therapies can be used to treat the induced arrhythmias. The nurse's role is similar to that during a catheterization, except that the bleeding risk is reduced because access is gained via the low-pressure venous system.

Other diagnostic tests used to diagnose cardiac dysfunction include the multigated angiographic (MUGA) scan, myocardial nuclear perfusion imaging (Persantine-thallium test), positron emission tomography (PET) scans, and impedance cardiography (ICG). Nursing care is focused on the patient and is dependent on the invasiveness of the procedure. The more risk of complications, the greater the involvement of the nurse in monitoring the patient. The nursing roles have been detailed previously.

In summary, there are several cardiovascular diagnostic procedures used to assess the components of CO. The nurse has specific responsibilities while caring for patients before, during, and after these cardiovascular diagnostic procedures. Imaging techniques include x-rays and MRIs. Exercise ECG evalutes heart muscle and coronary perfusion during exercise to identify myocardial ischemia. The nurse conducting the exam must be familiar with ECG interpretations and emergency procedures. Echocardiogram is an ultrasound technique used to assess cardiac and valve function and to estimate ejection fraction. The TEE is an invasive echocardiogram that produces high-quality images of intracardiac structures; however, conscious sedation must be used and this requires vigilance from the nurse to assess for complications during and after the procedure. Cardiac catheterization is used to evaluate coronary tissue perfusion. Postcatheterization nursing care includes monitoring for complications, particularly bleeding and patient education. EPS focuses on diagnosing problems in the cardiac conduction system.

SECTION EIGHT REVIEW

1. Which of the following patients is prohibited from having an MRI scan performed?
   A. the 77-year-old patient 4 days postcardiac catheterization
   B. the 24-year-old woman with dilated cardiomyopathy
   C. the 17-year-old patient with a titanium plate in his skull
   D. the 55-year-old man with type II diabetes currently on Meformin (Glucophage)
2. The nurse preparing a patient for cardiac catheterization must notify the cardiologist when
   A. the diabetic patient's fasting blood glucose is 244 mg/dL
   B. the patient states he has an allergy to shellfish
   C. the patient's Warfarin has been held for 5 days
   D. the patient complains of nervousness
3. The primary complication the nurse must monitor for after a cardiac catheterization is
   A. bleeding
   B. parasthesia

C. increased urine output
D. pain at the site of vascular access
4. The transthoracic echocardiogram is
   A. an invasive procedure requiring an overnight stay in the hospital postprocedure
   B. used to directly measure ejection fraction
   C. used to evaluate structures within the heart, such as the septum and valves
   D. the primary means of evaluating pulmonary artery pressures
5. The EPS is used to
   A. determine cardiac output
   B. determine cause of arrhythmias
   C. measure intracardiac pressures
   D. evaluate blockages with the coronary artery system

Answers: 1. C, 2. B, 3. A, 4. C, 5. B

POSTTEST

1. What is the relationship among stroke volume, cardiac output, and heart rate?
   A. $SV \times CO = HR$
   B. $SV \times HR = CO$
   C. $CO \times HR = SV$
   D. $CO = HR/SV$

2. Mr. P has morbid obesity. Which of the following parameters best reflects the amount of blood pumped by the heart each minute for this patient?
   A. CO
   B. CI
   C. SV
   D. ejection fraction

3. The degree of stretch in the myocardial fibers at the end of diastole is called
   A. preload
   B. contractility
   C. afterload
   D. compliance

4. Which of the following variables does not affect stroke volume?
   A. preload
   B. afterload
   C. contractility
   D. ejection fraction

5. In the healthy heart, an increase in preload will have what effect on SV?
   A. increase
   B. decrease
   C. stay the same
   D. cannot be determined from the available data

6. Which of the following statements is true?
   A. a decrease in preload results in an increase in SV
   B. an increase in preload results in a decrease in contractility
   C. preload does not have an effect on stroke volume
   D. an increase in preload results in an increase in SV up to a certain point

7. If afterload increases and CO remains the same, blood pressure will
   A. increase
   B. decrease
   C. stay the same
   D. cannot be determined from the available data

8. As afterload increases, what effect does this have on CO?
   A. increase
   B. decrease
   C. stay the same
   D. cannot be determined from the available data

9. Decreased oxygen delivery to myocardial cells (hypoxemia) will affect
   A. preload
   B. afterload

   C. contractility
   D. vascular tone

10. The actin–myosin crossbridge formations in the heart muscle largely depend on
    A. potassium
    B. sodium
    C. magnesium
    D. calcium

11. Sudden physiologic stress, such as escaping a burning building, will result in
    A. increased heart rate and increased afterload
    B. increased heart rate and decreased afterload
    C. decreased heart rate and increased afterload
    D. decreased heart rate and decreased afterload

12. Increased preload can occur with
    A. renal failure
    B. congestive heart failure
    C. hypovolemic shock
    D. A and B

13. Following hemorrhage, the presence of cool and clammy skin suggests
    A. increased contractility
    B. decreased contractility
    C. increased afterload
    D. decreased afterload

14. Mr. P complains of dyspnea. On auscultation of his heart sounds, you note the presence of S3 and S4. Mr. P has signs of
    A. increased right heart preload
    B. decreased right heart preload
    C. increased left heart preload
    D. decreased left heart preload

15. Which of the following is a complication of PTCA?
    A. bleeding
    B. dysrhythmias
    C. vessel reocclusion
    D. all of the above

16. Conscious sedation is required for which of the following cardiovascular diagnostic procedures?
    A. transthoracic echocardiogram
    B. transesophageal echocardiogram
    C. dobutamine stress test
    D. cardiac catheterization

17. The most common insertion site for cardiac catheterization is the
    A. femoral artery
    B. femoral vein
    C. carotid artery
    D. A and C

POSTTEST ANSWERS

Question	Answer	Section	Question	Answer	Section
1	B	One	10	D	Five
2	B	One	11	A	Six
3	A	Two	12	D	Six
4	D	Two	13	C	Seven
5	A	Three	14	C	Seven
6	D	Three	15	D	Eight
7	A	Four	16	B	Eight
8	B	Four	17	A	Eight
9	C	Five			

REFERENCES

Casey, P. (2004). Markers of myocardial injury and dysfunction. *AACN Clinical Issues, 15,* 547–557.

Coloff, K. (2003). Pre-procedures: Make a list and check it twice. *Nursing Management, 34*(11), 45–47.

Gordon, C., & Rempher, K. J. (2003). Brain (B-type) natriuretic peptide: Implications for heart failure management. *AACN Clinical Issues, 14,* 532–542.

Gross, C. R., Linquist, R. D., Woolley, A. C., et al. (1992). Clinical indicators of dehydration severity in elderly patients. *Journal of Emergency Medicine, 10,* 267–274.

Jarvis, C. (2004). *Physical examination and health assessment* (4th ed.). St. Louis: C. V. Mosby.

Johnson, K. L. (2004). Diagnostic measures to evaluate oxygenation in critically ill adult patients: Implications and limitations. *AACN Clinical Issues, 15,* 506–524.

Kaplan, L. J., Partland, K., Santora, T. A., & Trooskin, S. Z. (2001). Start with a subjective assessment of skin temp to identify hypoperfusion in intensive care unit patients. *Journal of Trauma: Injury, Infection and Critical Care, 50,* 620–628.

Kop, W. J., Gottdiener, J. S., Tangen, C., et al. (2002). Inflammation and coagulation factors in persons over 65 years of age with symptoms of depression but without evidence of myocardial ischemia. *American Journal of Cardiology, 89,* 419–424.

McCabe, P. M., McPherson, L. A., Lohse, C. M., & Weaver, A. L. (2001). Evaluation of nursing care after diagnostic coronary angiography. *American Journal of Critical Care, 10,* 330–340.

Newby, L. K. (2004). Markers of cardiac ischemia, injury, and inflammation. *Progress in Cardiovascular Disease, 46,* 404–416.

Nickolaus, M. J., Gilchrist, I. C., & Ettinger, S. M. (2001). The way to the heart is all through the wrist: Transradial catheterization and interventions. *AACN Clinical Issues, 12,* 62–71.

Pearson, T. A., Mensah, G. A., Alexander, R. W., et al. (2003). Markers of inflammation and cardiovascular disease. Application to clinical and public health practice: A statement for health care professionals from the Centers for Disease Control and the American Heart Association. *Circulation, 107,* 499–511.

Porth, C. (2005). Control of cardiovascular function. In C. Porth, (Ed.), *Pathophysiology: Concepts of altered health states* (7th ed.). Philadelphia: Lippincott Williams & Wilkins.

Prahash, A., & Lunch, T. (2004). B-type natriuretic peptide: A diagnostic, prognostic, and therapeutic tool in heart failure. *American Journal of Critical Care, 13,* 47–55.

Ridker, P. M., Hennekens, C. H., Buring, J. E., & Rifai, N. (2000). C-reactive protein and other markers of inflammation in the prediction of cardiovascular disease in women. *New England Journal of Medicine, 342,* 836–843.

Ridker, P. M., Rifai, N., Clearfield, M., et al. (2001). Air Force/Texas coronary atherosclerosis prevention study investigators: Measurement of c-reactive protein for the targeting of statin therapy in the primary prevention of acute coronary events. *New England Journal of Medicine, 344,* 1959–1965.

Schringer, D. L., & Baraff, L. J. (1991). Capillary refill: Is it a useful predictor of hypovolemic states? *Annals of Emergency Medicine, 20,* 601–605.

Hemodynamic Monitoring

Kara Adams

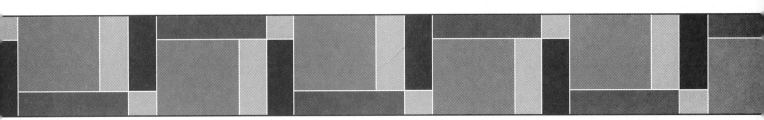

OBJECTIVES Following completion of this module, the learner will be able to

1. Describe the purpose and functional components of a basic pulmonary artery catheter.

2. Explain how cardiac output is measured in the clinical setting.

3. Recognize a normal right atrial waveform pattern.

4. Relate right ventricular preload to right atrial pressure.

5. Identify common physical findings and nursing interventions related to abnormal right atrial pressures.

6. Recognize a normal right ventricular waveform.

7. Identify appropriate nursing interventions related to right ventricular waveforms.

8. Recognize a normal pulmonary artery waveform pattern.

9. Identify common physical findings and nursing interventions related to abnormal pulmonary artery pressures.

10. Recognize a normal pulmonary artery wedge waveform.

11. Relate left ventricular preload to pulmonary artery wedge pressure.

12. Identify common physical findings and appropriate nursing interventions related to abnormal pulmonary artery wedge pressures.

13. Understand the physiology underlying the systemic arterial waveform.

14. Identify the components of a normal arterial waveform.

15. Understand the implications of selected derived hemodynamic parameters.

16. Calculate cardiac index, stroke volume index, mean arterial pressure, systemic vascular resistance, pulmonary vascular resistance, left ventricular stroke work index, and right ventricular stroke work index.

The high-acuity patient has complex nursing needs. This self-study module focuses on the integration of hemodynamic concepts and physical findings in the nursing assessment of the high-acuity patient. The nurse requires a working knowledge of the determinants of cardiac output: preload, afterload, and contractility (Module 8). These determinants of cardiac output are linked to the data available through hemodynamic monitoring with a pulmonary artery catheter. This knowledge, coupled with astute observation and sharp assessment skills, guides critical thinking at the bedside and provides a high level of nursing care for the high-acuity patient. The module is composed of eight sections. Each section includes a set of review questions to help the learner evaluate his or her understanding of the section's content before moving on to the next section. All Section Reviews and the module Pretest and Posttest include answers. It is suggested that the learner review those concepts answered incorrectly in the review questions before proceeding to the next section.

PRETEST

1. Filling pressure of the right ventricle (right ventricular preload) is measured through the pulmonary artery catheter port opening into the
   A. superior vena cava
   B. right atrium
   C. right ventricle
   D. pulmonary artery

2. Potential risks associated with insertion of a PA catheter include
   A. acute respiratory failure
   B. pneumothorax
   C. arrhythmias
   D. B and C

3. Bolus thermodilution cardiac output measurements should be taken
   A. during inspiration
   B. at end expiration
   C. randomly throughout the respiratory cycle
   D. every 2 minutes

4. Continuous cardiac output measurements would be MOST beneficial for a patient with
   A. fluid volume excess
   B. fluid volume deficit
   C. fever
   D. septic shock

5. All of the following conditions lead to an elevated right atrial pressure EXCEPT
   A. sepsis
   B. pulmonic valve stenosis
   C. pulmonary hypertension
   D. cardiac tamponade

6. The right ventricular end-diastolic pressure is marked in the RAP tracing by the
   A. "a" wave
   B. "v" wave
   C. "x" deflection
   D. "y" deflection

7. The greatest potential for dysrhythmias occurs when the pulmonary artery catheter passes through the
   A. superior vena cava
   B. right atrium
   C. right ventricle
   D. pulmonary artery

8. RV diastolic pressure remains essentially the same as
   A. RV systolic pressure
   B. RAP
   C. PAWP
   D. B and C

9. Which of the following pressures fall within the normal range?
   A. PAP = 40/22, PAWP = 18
   B. PAP = 26/12, PAWP = 10
   C. PAP = 18/7, PAWP = 3
   D. PAP = 34/26, PAWP = 23

10. The dicrotic notch on the pulmonary artery waveform represents
    A. atrial contraction
    B. closure of the pulmonic valve
    C. closure of the aortic valve
    D. the beginning of ventricular systole

11. The right atrial waveform and the _____ waveform are similar in appearance.
    A. pulmonary artery wedge
    B. right ventricular
    C. pulmonary artery
    D. systemic arterial

12. Preload of the left ventricle is measured indirectly by
    A. cardiac output
    B. pulmonary artery systolic pressure
    C. pulmonary artery diastolic pressure
    D. pulmonary artery wedge pressure (PAWP)

13. Normal MAP is
    A. 60 to 70 mm Hg
    B. 140/80 mm Hg
    C. 70 to 90 mm Hg
    D. 100 to 120 mm Hg

14. The dicrotic notch on the systemic arterial pressure waveform represents
    A. closure of the aortic valve
    B. closure of the pulmonic valve
    C. opening of the aortic valve
    D. mean arterial pressure

15. The left ventricle stroke work index is compared with which of the following when assessing left ventricle function?
    A. right atrial pressure
    B. cardiac output
    C. cardiac index
    D. pulmonary artery wedge pressure

16. Afterload to the left ventricle is estimated by determining the
    A. PAWP
    B. right atrial pressure
    C. cardiac index
    D. systemic vascular resistance

Pretest Answers: 1. B, 2. D, 3. B, 4. A, 5. A, 6. A, 7. C, 8. B, 9. B, 10. B, 11. A, 12. D, 13. C, 14. A, 15. D, 16. D

GLOSSARY

afterload   The resistance to ventricular contraction; pressure the ventricles have to overcome to eject blood into the circulation.

cardiac index (CI)   Cardiac output divided by body surface area.

cardiac output (CO)   The amount of blood pumped by the heart each minute.

mean arterial pressure (MAP)   Average pressure within the arterial system throughout the cardiac cycle.

phlebostatic axis   An imaginary point determined by the intersection of two lines; 4th intercostal space midpoint between the anterior and posterior diameter; this is the correct level for positioning transducers used for hemodynamic monitoring.

preload   Pressure or stretch exerted on the walls of the ventricle by the volume of blood filling the ventricles at the end of diastole; used as an indication of volume status.

pulmonary artery diastolic (PAD) pressure   Reflects diastolic filling pressure in the left ventricle.

pulmonary artery systolic (PAS) pressure   Pressure generated by the right ventricle during systole.

pulmonary artery wedge pressure (PAWP)   Pressure obtained when the inflated balloon wedges in a small branch of the pulmonary artery, reflecting pressures from the left heart.

pulmonary vascular resistance (PVR)   Afterload of the right ventricle; the resistance the right ventricle must overcome to open the pulmonic valve and eject the stroke volume into the pulmonary artery.

right atrial pressure (RAP)   A measure of the pressure in the right ventricle at end diastole; represents right ventricular preload.

stroke volume   The volume of blood pumped with each heart beat.

stroke volume index   The volume of blood pumped with each beat, indexed to body size.

systemic vascular resistance (SVR)   Afterload of left ventricle; the resistance the left ventricle must overcome to open the aortic valve and eject the stroke volume into the aorta.

thermodilution   Method used to obtain cardiac output with a pulmonary artery catheter; uses theory of a known amount of volume infused at a known temperature and change in blood temperature over time as a result of that infusion.

ventricular stroke work index   The work involved in moving blood in the ventricle with each heartbeat against afterload.

HEMODYNAMIC PARAMETERS AND NORMAL VALUES

HEMODYNAMIC PARAMETERS	NORMAL VALUES
$CI = CO/BSA$	2.4 to 4.0 L/min/m^2
$CO = HR \times SV$	4 to 8 L/min
$LVSWI = [(MAP - PAWP) \times (SVI) \times (0.0136)]$	50 to 62 g/m^2/beat
$MAP = [(SBP) + 2 (DBP)]/3$	70 to 90 mm Hg
Mean PAP $= [(systolic) + 2 (diastolic)]/3$	12 to 20 mm Hg
PAD	20 to 30 mm Hg
PAS	8 to 15 mm Hg (2 to 5 mm Hg higher than PAWP)
PAWP	4 to 12 mm Hg
$PVR = [(Mean\ PAP) - (PAWP) \times 80]/CO$	50 to 250 dynes $\cdot$ sec $\cdot$ cm^{-5}
$PVRI = [(Mean\ PAP) - (PAWP) \times 80]/CI$	255 to 315 dynes $\cdot$ sec $\cdot$ cm^{-5}/m^2
RAP	2 to 6 mm Hg
RV pressures (RV systolic/RV diastolic)	20 to 30 mm Hg/2 to 8 mm Hg
$RVSWI = [(Mean\ PAP - RAP) \times (SVI) \times (0.0136)]$	7.9 to 9.7 g/m^2/beat
$SVI = CI/HR$	25 to 45 mL/beat/m^2
$SV = CO/HR$	50 to 100 mL/beat
$SVR = [(MAP) - (RAP) \times 80]/CO$	800 to 1,200 dynes $\cdot$ sec $\cdot$ cm^{-5}
$SVRI = [(MAP) - (RAP) \times 80]/CI$	1,970 to 2,390 dynes $\cdot$ sec $\cdot$ cm^{-5}/m^2

ABBREVIATIONS

ABG	Arterial blood gas	**CO**	Cardiac output
ACE	Angiotensin converting enzyme	**ECG**	Electrocardiogram
BPM	Beats per minute	**HR**	Heart rate
BSA	Body surface area	**IV**	Intravenous
CI	Cardiac index	**LA**	Left atrium

L/min	Liters per minute		**PVRI**	Pulmonary vascular resistance index
LV	Left ventricle		**RA**	Right atrium
LVEDP	Left ventricular end-diastolic pressure		**RAP**	Right atrial pressure
LVSWI	Left ventricular stroke work index		**RV**	Right ventricle
MAP	Mean arterial pressure		**RVEDP**	Right ventricular end-diastolic pressure
PA	Pulmonary artery		**RVSWI**	Right ventricular stroke work index
PAD	Pulmonary artery diastolic		**SV**	Stroke volume
PAP	Pulmonary artery pressure		**SVI**	Stroke volume index
PAS	Pulmonary artery systolic		**Svo$_2$**	Mixed venous oxygen saturation
PAWP	Pulmonary artery wedge pressure		**SVR**	Systemic vascular resistance
PVR	Pulmonary vascular resistance		**SVRI**	Systemic vascular resistance index

SECTION ONE: The Pulmonary Artery Catheter

At the completion of this section, the learner will be able to describe the purpose and functional components of a basic pulmonary artery catheter. Various terms are used by health care professionals to refer to a pulmonary artery catheter, including right heart catheter, Swan or Swan–Ganz catheter, flow-directed thermodilution catheter, and pulmonary artery catheter. This module uses the term *pulmonary artery catheter*.

Purpose

The pulmonary artery (PA) catheter is an invasive diagnostic tool that can be used at the bedside for the following purposes:

1. To determine the pressures within the right heart and PA, and for indirect measurement of left heart pressures
2. To determine cardiac output (CO)
3. To sample mixed venous blood (Svo$_2$) from the PA
4. To infuse fluids

Hemodynamic data are used to make clinical management decisions in high-acuity patients. There are three steps of hemodynamic assessment with the PA catheter that the nurse must follow (Adams, 2004).

1. Obtain accurate data. It is a nursing responsibility to ensure the proper calibration of the equipment used for hemodynamic monitoring.
2. Correctly perform waveform analysis.
3. Integrate the data with other assessment parameters.

These three steps will be discussed in further detail throughout this module.

Basic Construction

The PA catheter is constructed of a radiopaque polyvinylchloride. Several sizes and various options are available. Most have a heparin coating to reduce the risk of thrombus formation. All PA catheters have color-coded extrusions or "ports" on the proximal end that provide access to the various catheter lumens. The catheter is marked at 10-cm intervals to facilitate correct placement. A typical PA catheter has five lumens, as shown in Figure 9–1.

Special Pulmonary Artery Catheters

Special PA catheters are also available. These catheters are almost identical to the one pictured in Figure 9–1. However, additional options are present. One special catheter has an integrated port for pacing wires that allows for synchronized atrial and ventricular pacing. Another catheter uses special technology to provide continuous monitoring of the cardiac output, as opposed to the individual "spot check" measurements traditionally obtained by the clinician. This technology is discussed in Section Two. Another special PA catheter allows for continuous measurement of the mixed venous oxygen saturation (Module 14). Keep in mind that these special catheters provide all the functions of the basic catheter described in this section but include special features that permit additional functions.

Components and Pertinent Points

Following are discussions of each section of the basic PA catheter. When indicated, special nursing considerations are included with the descriptive information.

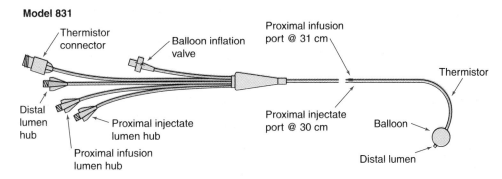

Figure 9–1 ■ A five-lumen pulmonary artery catheter.   *(Reprinted with permission. Copyright © 2000 Edwards Lifesciences. Swan-Ganz® is a trademark of Edwards Lifesciences Corporation, registered in the U.S. Patent and Trademark Office)*

Proximal Injectate Lumen/Hub

- This lumen terminates in the most proximal chamber of the heart, the right atrium.
- Most catheter manufacturers imprint the word *proximal* on either the hub or the tubing close to the hub. Look for it.
- On most catheters, the tubing of this port is blue for rapid visual identification. One way to remember this is to link the blue tubing of this port to the "blue" desaturated blood found in the right atrium.
- This port allows for monitoring or sampling of the right atrial pressure (RAP) when it is connected to a transducer.
- The injectate used to determine cardiac output is pushed through this lumen.
- IV fluids can also be infused through this port. To avoid inadvertent bolus of potent medications, do not infuse vasoactive medications through this lumen when it is used for thermodilution cardiac output measurements.

Proximal Infusion Lumen/Hub (Optional)

- When present, this extra lumen terminates in the right atrium and is labeled *infusion* on the hub or the tubing near the hub.
- On most catheters, the tubing of this port is white or clear for rapid visual identification.
- This port is primarily used as the "central line" for intravenous (IV) fluid infusions such as total parenteral nutrition. This is especially helpful in patients with poor peripheral venous access.
- This port can be used for obtaining cardiac output determinations if the proximal injectate lumen occludes. However, the individual values obtained from this port may not be as reproducible as those obtained from the proximal injectate port. To avoid inadvertent bolus of potent medications, do not infuse vasoactive medications through the lumen selected for bolus thermodilution cardiac output determinations.

Distal Lumen/Hub

- This lumen terminates in the PA.
- Most catheter manufacturers imprint the word *distal* on either the hub or the tubing close to the hub. Look for it.
- On most catheters, the tubing of this port is yellow for rapid visual identification.
- This port is always connected to a transducer for continuous monitoring of the PA pressure (PAP) and waveform (see the following discussion).
- Pulmonary artery wedge pressure (PAWP) is obtained through this port by careful balloon inflation (discussed later).
- Mixed venous blood oxygen saturation (SvO_2) is obtained or "sampled" from this port. Remember that this port terminates in the PA. The venous blood returning from all parts of the body has been "well mixed" in the right atrium and ventricle before it is pumped into the PA.
- Medications and IV solutions are not infused through this port, except under certain conditions by a physician.

Thermistor Wire/Connector

- The thermistor wire terminates near the tip of the catheter and is exposed to the blood flowing through the PA.
- This wire detects changes in the temperature of the blood, which is an essential part of cardiac output determination.
- It allows for continuous monitoring of core body temperature.
- The proximal end attaches to a cable linking it with the device used for measuring cardiac output. This will either be a cardiac output module compatible with the bedside monitoring system or a freestanding cardiac output computer.

Balloon Inflation Lumen/Valve

- This lumen is contiguous with the small balloon at the distal end of the catheter.
- A "gate valve" mechanism on the hub locks this port in an open or closed position.

Figure 9–2 ■ Hemodynamic monitoring equipment.

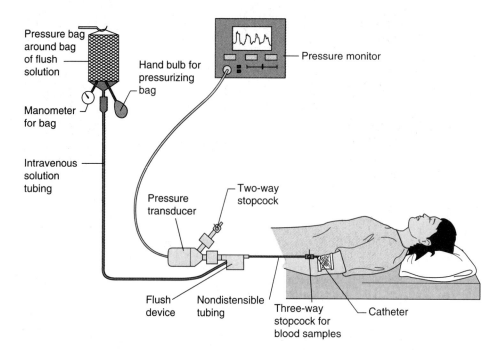

- The balloon is slowly inflated using a syringe provided with the catheter while the PA waveform is continuously monitored. Inflation is stopped as soon as the waveform changes to a PA wedge waveform.
- The maximum recommended inflation volume provided with catheter instructions should not be exceeded.
- Deflation is always passive. Manual deflation may damage balloon integrity.
- Never leave the balloon in the inflated position.

Hemodynamic Monitoring Equipment

A typical hemodynamic monitoring set is shown in Figure 9–2. The system components, except for the catheter, are the same as for pulmonary arterial pressure monitoring or systemic arterial pressure monitoring (Section Seven).

Transducer

Measurement of pressures within the heart and PA is accomplished using a transducer. A transducer is a "translator." It translates mechanical energy sensed by the catheter and converts it to electrical energy displayed on the monitor screen as a waveform. It is a nursing responsibility to ensure the transducer is translating correctly. To ensure the transducer is translating correctly, the nurse must level and zero the catheter according to unit or hospital policies and procedures. Leveling the transducer corrects for hydrostatic pressure changes in vessels above and below the heart. Zeroing the transducer corrects for any drift or deviation from baseline that may occur in the transducer. The **phlebostatic axis** approximates the level of the right atrium and is considered to represent the level of the catheter tip. The transducer is leveled and zeroed at the phlebostatic axis. In the supine

position, the external landmark for the left atrium is the 4th intercostal space at the midpoint of the anterior and posterior diameter (Darvic, 2002). Improper positioning of the transducer leads to very different readings. Once the correct location for the phlebostatic axis is identified, a mark should be placed on the chest wall (Keckeisen et al., 1998).

Pressure Bag

To overcome the arterial pressure and prevent blood from backing up into the pressure tubing, a pressure bag is placed around the flush solution bag and inflated to 300 mm Hg. Depending on hospital policy, the flush solution may or may not contain heparin.

Insertion

Insertion of a PA catheter is performed in critical care units, cardiac catheterization laboratories, and operating rooms. The complication rate related to this procedure is low; however, the insertion of a PA catheter is not without risks. Potential risks include pneumothorax, damage to the blood vessels or heart, arrhythmias, infection or bleeding, or bleeding at the insertion site and death. Except in emergency situations, informed consent should be obtained prior to catheter insertion.

Patients may be awake when the catheter is inserted, and it can be a frightening experience if the patient does not know what to expect. The patient should know that the purpose of the catheter is to assess heart function and fluid status, allowing more precise management of his or her condition. Explain to the patient that the site will be scrubbed with an antiseptic solution, and that a pinch, sting, or burning sensation may be felt when the local anesthetic is injected. A temporary sensation of pressure should be expected when a large IV catheter (the sheath) is inserted into the subclavian, jugular, or femoral vein. Once positioned, the sheath is typically sutured in place. The patient should know that the long, thin, balloon-tipped catheter will not be felt as it is threaded through the sheath, floated through the right heart, and positioned in the PA. Most patients find it helpful during the procedure to receive general information on how things are going and an estimated time to completion. After the procedure, the patient should expect to be attached to multiple IV lines that will restrict some freedom of movement. The family should be prepared to see additional equipment prior to the first visit postprocedure.

The insertion of a PA catheter is always a sterile procedure. Along with the physician, the nurse is responsible for careful observation and monitoring of the patient during the insertion process. Once the catheter has been inserted, the nurse assumes responsibility for patient safety, comfort, and system maintenance. The nurse is responsible for catheter site maintenance, documentation of pressures in the heart and PA, and obtaining valid cardiac output measurements. Postprocedure, a chest x-ray is obtained to confirm catheter position and assess for pneumothorax. The catheter is not used for infusion of medications or fluids until proper placement of the catheter has been confirmed by chest x-ray. It is the nurse's responsibility to recognize abnormal waveforms and trends, and intervene appropriately, including notification of the physician when indicated. The nurse must know unit-specific policies and procedures related to hemodynamic monitoring.

Provider Competency

Hemodynamic monitoring in the high-acuity patient population requires competency in both technical and physiological aspects. As is true for all diagnostic tests, the information obtained is only as good as the data collected. Assessment of the hemodynamic profile is taken in three steps:

1. **Obtain accurate data.** Obtaining accurate data includes appropriate leveling and zeroing, use of minimal transducer tubing, maintenance of system patency, square wave testing, and patient position (Ahrens, 1999).
2. **Assess the waveform.** Studies suggest that assessment of waveforms is best performed when printed graphically and correlated with the electrocardiogram (ECG) and respiratory cycles (Ahrens & Shallom, 2001). Certain modes of mechanical ventilation and rapid and spontaneous respirations make locating end-expiration difficult. There is some literature to support the use of capnography to identify physiological end expiration (Ahrens & Sona, 2003).
3. **Integrate data with the patient assessment.** Integration is accomplished by looking at all the data in the hemodynamic profile collectively. Data in the hemodynamic profile will be discussed in detail in this module; however, recognize that this data must be correlated with findings in the physical assessment of CO (Module 8).

> **Box 9–1 Hemodynamic Monitoring: Educational Resources**
>
> - *Pulmonary artery catheter education project: http://www.pacep.org*
> - *Darvic, G. O. (2002). Hemodynamic monitoring: Invasive and non-invasive clinical application. (3rd ed.). Philadelphia: W. B. Saunders*
> - *American Association of Critical Care Nurses: Essentials of critical care education (ECCO)*
> - *American Association of Critical Care Nurses: Protocols for practice: hemodynamic monitoring series*

This module will focus on each of these steps. However, it is important to recognize that ongoing education is needed to ensure patient safety and positive clinical outcomes. Resources for ongoing education are outlined in Box 9–1.

Interpretation of Data

Data collection is not the end point of hemodynamic monitoring. Abnormal pressures and changes in trends must be recognized, correlated with the patient's condition, and acted on. Careful clinical assessment, integrated with the data collected from a PA catheter, provides a basis for nursing interventions and manipulation of potent vasoactive medications or fluids.

Several complications may occur from invasive hemodynamic monitoring. Infection may result. Air emboli or thromboembolism can occur from loose connections or improper flushing, respectively. Fluid overload may result from fluid infusion through multiple lumens or lack of surveillance of IV pumps. Exsanguination may occur if a stopcock remains open or tubing becomes disconnected.

The following guidelines are used when interpreting readings.

1. Always look at patient trends and not an isolated reading.
2. Question abnormal readings. Recheck the reading after zeroing and calibrating the equipment. Assess the patient for additional data to support the reading.
3. Compare the patient's readings with his or her normal values and not with the normal values listed in a textbook.
4. Do not be fooled by normal readings. The patient may have normal readings temporarily because of compensatory mechanisms. Continue to assess the patient.
5. Assess the interrelationships among the readings. The goal is to obtain a picture of the patient's hemodynamic status and not simply a number.

Patient Positioning

Studies in a variety of patient populations have found that PAP and RAP measurements are accurate when the head of the bed is elevated to any angle between 0 and 60 degrees, as long as the patient is in the supine position (Quaal, 2001).

Reading at End Expiration

Changes in intrathoracic pressure during respiration significantly alter hemodynamic pressures. Obtaining accurate measurements requires reading pressure waveforms at end expiration. Digital readouts on the bedside monitor reflect pressures obtained throughout the respiratory cycle. These pressures are significantly different from end-expiratory pressures (Ahrens & Shallom, 2001). Therefore, pressure should be read at end expiration.

In summary, the PA catheter is a tool used in the care of critically ill patients. Changes in therapy can be guided by the information obtained from a PA catheter with the goal of producing improved patient outcomes. An understanding of the functional components of a PA catheter and the clinical interpretation of the data obtained from a PA is important and will be expanded on in each of the remaining sections of this module.

SECTION ONE REVIEW

1. Which port of the PA catheter is used to obtain RAP?
   A. proximal port
   B. distal port
   C. thermistor wire port
   D. balloon inflation port
2. Which lumen is used for obtaining CO determinations?
   A. proximal port lumen
   B. distal port lumen
   C. thermistor wire lumen
   D. balloon inflation port lumen
3. The pressure reading from which lumen is always continuously monitored?
   A. proximal
   B. distal
   C. thermistor wire
   D. balloon port

4. Why should vasoactive drugs never be infused through the port used for thermodilution CO determinations?
   A. the size of the lumen is too small
   B. a bolus injection of a potent drug will occur every time CO is obtained
   C. CO readings will be less accurate
   D. some vasoactive drugs are not compatible with the catheter material
5. What is the best way to deflate the balloon on the PA catheter?
   A. slowly pull back on the syringe plunger
   B. quickly pull back on the plunger to limit inflation time
   C. allow the balloon to deflate passively
   D. remove the syringe from the hub directly after inflation

Answers: 1. A, 2. A, 3. B, 4. B, 5. C

SECTION TWO: Hemodynamic Monitoring and Determination of Cardiac Output

At the completion of this section, the learner will explain how cardiac output is measured in the clinical setting. Recall from Module 8 that **cardiac output (CO)** is the amount of blood ejected from the heart into the circulation each minute. It is expressed in liters per minute.

The formula used to derive the CO is simple. CO is the product of the heart rate (HR) multiplied by the **stroke volume** (SV) (i.e., the amount of blood ejected by each heartbeat). The formula for CO is CO = HR × SV. Changes in heart rate will affect CO; in fact, acceleration of heart rate is one of the first compensatory mechanisms when CO decreases. Stroke volume is also variable and is altered by the effects of preload, afterload, and contractility. These terms were introduced in Module 8 but will be briefly reviewed again because an understanding of the concepts of preload, afterload, and contractility is key to understanding hemodynamic monitoring.

Preload

Preload is the pressure or stretch exerted on the walls of the ventricle by the volume of blood filling the ventricle at the end of diastole. Preload is typically used as an indication of the volume status of the patient. Too little preload (volume) will not adequately stretch the ventricular muscle to get the best contraction (i.e., the best stroke volume). Too much preload (volume) acts to overstretch the ventricular muscle, resulting in poor contractility, a reduced stroke volume, and a drop in CO. Preload, then, has to be "just right" to maximize Frank–Starling's Law to get the best ventricular contraction and the most optimal CO. Although emphasis is often placed on left ventricular preload, keep in mind that both ventricles have the property of preload.

An estimate of preload is obtained from a PA catheter. For the left heart, the **pulmonary artery wedge pressure** (PAWP) is used as an indirect measure of pressure in the left ventricle at the end of diastole. Left ventricular end-diastolic pressure provides an estimate of the "volume status" of the patient. It is obtained from the distal port after the catheter balloon has been inflated and allowed to float into "wedge" position. The normal range of the PAWP is 4 to 12 mm Hg. However, every patient must be considered in the context of his or her health history. Patients with impaired myocardial function (myocardial infarction) may need more volume to stretch an impaired ventricle to get the best contraction. Consequently, a higher PAWP of 15 mm Hg may be necessary to get the best possible contraction of the ventricle. Right heart preload is obtained by using a transducer to measure the RAP from the proximal port of the PA catheter. The normal range of the RAP is 2 to 6 mm Hg. RAP and PAWP are the topics of Sections Three and Six, respectively.

Afterload

Afterload is the resistance to ventricular contraction. Simply stated, afterload is the pressure the ventricle has to overcome to open the aortic or pulmonic valve and push blood out of the ventricle into the systemic or pulmonary circulation. An estimate of afterload to the left heart is obtained by using a formula to calculate the **systemic vascular resistance** (SVR). An estimate of afterload to the right heart is obtained by using a formula to calculate the **pulmonary vascular resistance (PVR)**. These measures are discussed further in Section Eight.

Afterload can be viewed as the pressure in the aorta pushing against the valve to hold it in the closed position. However, fixed lesions, such as aortic stenosis, and anomalies, such as coarctation of the aorta, also represent afterload the ventricle must overcome before it can eject the stroke volume. As afterload increases, the heart works harder, which requires more oxygen. When afterload is high, the ventricle does not fully empty, which translates into a reduced stroke volume and low CO.

Afterload can also be too low. When the pressure or resistance in the aorta is low, the left ventricle needs to generate very little pressure to open the aortic valve and eject blood into the circulation. It will not contract vigorously. The net effect is a weak contraction, resulting in a reduced CO and a low systolic blood pressure. Similar to preload, afterload needs to be "just right" for the best CO.

Contractility

Contractility is the property of the heart that allows it to shorten muscle fibers and contract. A vigorous contraction will improve CO by increasing the SV. When contractility is compromised, as in heart failure or hypovolemia, the amount of blood volume that is ejected with each beat is reduced and reflected in the SV. A normal stroke volume is 50 to 100 mL/beat. This value may be indexed to body size, known as the **stroke volume index (SVI)** (25 to 45 mL/beat/m^2). Stoke volume or stroke volume index must be assessed in the context of both the cardiac output and the preload values.

Contractility is optimized when preload and afterload are optimized. If the CO remains low after both preload and after-

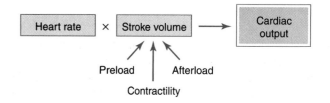

Figure 9–3 ■ The determinants of cardiac output.

load have been optimized, inotropic agents to improve CO may be considered. Increasing the contractile force of a weak ventricle improves SV and CO. Contractility is assessed by calculating a parameter called the **ventricular stroke work index**. The ventricular stroke work index is the work involved in moving blood in the ventricle with each heartbeat against afterload. This will be further discussed in Section Eight.

It becomes clear that preload, afterload, and contractility interact to determine the CO by their effects on stroke volume (Fig. 9–3). Traditionally, primary emphasis has been placed on the left ventricle because it is the capacity of the left ventricle to function as a pump that determines patient outcome. It is important to keep in mind that these properties are important to the function of both ventricles.

Cardiac Output

The normal range for CO is 4 to 8 L/min. Recall from Module 8, that this important parameter does not address the effect of body size on CO requirements. Consider the CO required by a large and muscular professional football player versus the CO needed by a petite female. If each has a CO of 4 L/min, technically, both COs fall within the normal range of 4 to 8 L/min. A quick bedside physical assessment would tell us that more information is needed. Although 4 L/min may well serve the needs of the petite female, it would likely be inadequate for the needs of a large, muscular professional football player.

The **cardiac index** (CI) references the CO to body size. This information is more useful because the CO is now individualized to a specific patient. The CI is obtained by dividing the CO by the patient's body surface area (BSA) to individualize the CO to the patient. A normal CI is 2.4 to 4.0 L/min/m^2. Most monitors calculate the CI if the patient's height and weight are entered. The CI is far more meaningful than the CO during bedside clinical decision making. As a derived parameter, the CI will be discussed further in Section Eight.

How Is Cardiac Output Obtained?

Various methods exist for determining CO. The focus of this section will be the traditional "bolus" **thermodilution** method of CO measurement. With this method, intermittent "spot" checks of CO are obtained at the discretion of the clinician or by a schedule dictated by policy or procedure. Other methods of obtaining CO will be briefly discussed at the end of this section.

The thermodilution method uses temperature change over time to calculate CO. The distal end of the thermistor wire terminates in an exposed bead 1.6 in. (4 cm) below the tip of the catheter (refer to Fig. 9–1). This thermistor bead is exposed to the blood flowing past it in the PA. It senses the temperature of the blood and allows for constant monitoring of core body temperature. It also monitors changes in the temperature of the blood and the duration of the temperature change. This information is relayed to the computer through a special cable attached to the thermistor connector at the proximal end of the PA catheter.

In the traditional method of thermodilution CO, a 10-mL bolus of fluid is injected through the proximal injectate port of the PA catheter into the right atrium. The temperature of this fluid is cooler than blood temperature. The injectate fluid temperature is sensed by an in-line temperature probe and then relayed to the CO computer. The CO computer now has two temperatures stored in it: the temperature of the blood and the temperature of the fluid bolus. The injection of the fluid bolus must be smooth, rapid, and completed within a 4-second interval. This fluid "bolus" mixes with blood as it is pumped through the right ventricle and into the PA. The mixture of the cooler fluid bolus with the blood results in a transient drop in the temperature of the blood flowing through the PA. As blood continues to be pumped into the PA, the blood temperature will warm to prebolus level. The blood temperature change and the duration of the blood temperature change are sensed by the exposed thermistor bead positioned in the PA. This information is relayed to the CO computer where it is analyzed and a time–temperature CO "curve" is formed (Fig. 9–4). The area under the curve represents the CO.

This area is calculated by the computer and displayed digitally in liters per minute (L/min). There is an inverse relationship between the size of the curve and the CO. A small curve indicates a rapid return of the blood to its baseline temperature and, therefore, a high CO. A large curve indicates a slow return to baseline temperature and, therefore, a low CO. A notched or uneven curve indicates poor injection technique, and the value obtained should not be accepted.

Equipment Preparation

Obtaining valid CO determinations is an important nursing responsibility. To calculate CO accurately, the computer must know the catheter model, fluid bolus volume, and fluid temperature selected for use. A number or "constant" that represents this information is entered into the computer before starting. This constant is obtained from a chart on a package insert provided with the catheter. It is important that the correct constant is entered prior to obtaining COs. If the volume or temperature of the injectate is changed during the course of hemodynamic monitoring, a new constant is entered or the CO determinations will be inaccurate.

Fluid Bolus

Normal saline is used as the injectate fluid (Keckeisen et al., 1998). The volume of the bolus injectate used varies according to hospital policy and patient condition. The most common volume is 10 mL; however, if volume overload is a problem, 5 mL can be used. The literature reports that a 10-mL bolus provides the most reproducibility (Gould et al., 2001). An important nursing consideration is to be consistent and not vary the volume of the bolus. A common practice is to obtain three sequential CO measurements, using 10 mL of saline for each determination. If one of the CO results varies more than 10 percent from the others, it is rejected. An average of at least two "similar" values (within 10 percent of each other) is accepted for the CO.

Bolus Temperature

Selection of either room temperature or iced injectate is generally considered acceptable (according to unit policy) as long as the proper constant is entered into the CO computer. Although there remains some controversy, research suggests that there is no significant difference between iced injectate and room temperature injectate (O'Malley et al., 2000). In hypothermia the temperature difference between the injectate and the patient's temperature may not be wide enough to ensure accuracy. Once the choice is made to use either iced or room temperature injectate, that decision should be followed through the course of that patient's hemodynamic monitoring. If the injectate temperature is changed, a new constant must be entered into the CO computer.

Timing of Bolus Injection

The timing of the bolus injection must coincide with the end-expiratory phase of the patient's breathing cycle. This is thought to provide more consistency in the results.

Conditions Affecting Pulmonary Artery Temperature

Many conditions produce a change in venous return that can alter the PA temperature. These include coughing, restlessness, shivering, and the administration of peripheral IV fluids of a different temperature through the venous infusion port of the PA catheter.

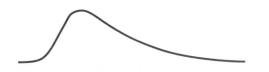

Figure 9–4 ■ A normal cardiac output curve. *(Reprinted with permission. Copyright © 2000 Edwards Lifesciences. Swan-Ganz ® is a trademark of Edwards Lifesciences Corporation, registered in the U.S. Patent and Trademark Office)*

Method of Bolus Injection

The bolus injection should be rapid and smooth. The entire bolus should be injected within a 4-second interval at end expiration. Improper injection technique affects accuracy.

Continuous Cardiac Output Measurement

There are several limitations with traditional bolus thermodilution CO measurements. They are a "snapshot" in time; time consuming to obtain; subject to operator error; and require administration of additional fluid, which may be contraindicated in some patients. Because of these limitations, a PA catheter for the determination of CO on a continuous basis was developed. This type of catheter uses a modified thermodilution method. Similar to a traditional catheter, there is a balloon tip, a proximal injectate port, an infusion port, a thermistor wire, and a distal port. The primary difference is a thermal filament on the exterior of the catheter between the infusion port and the balloon tip. When the catheter is properly positioned, this heating filament lies in the right ventricle. Random pulses of energy from the monitor raise the temperature of the filament to 111°F (44°C). The thermistor located downstream near the catheter tip detects the blood temperature change and relays it to the computer, which uses a formula to develop the familiar CO curve. The small amount of heat emitted is safe for the patient and does not have an adverse effect on blood cells.

The CO is continuously displayed on the bedside monitor and values are updated every 3 minutes. The displayed values represent an average of the CO of the previous 3 minutes. By entering the patient's height and weight, a continuous CI is displayed. The accuracy of this modified technique, using heat "pulses" to replace the traditional fluid bolus, is not dependent on user technique. The patient is spared multiple fluid boluses. Several research studies compared this method to the traditional intermittent bolus thermodilution method. Data support the fact that these two methods to obtain CO agree (Ott et al., 2001).

In summary, cardiac output is the amount of blood ejected from the heart per minute. Preload, afterload, and contractility determine cardiac output. Cardiac index references cardiac output to body size. Cardiac output can be measured through a thermistor wire in a pulmonary arterial catheter. In the traditional thermodilution method of measurement, a 10-mL fluid bolus is injected through the proximal injectate port of the pulmonary arterial catheter. In the continuous measurement method, heat pulses replace the fluid bolus. There is support for both methods.

SECTION TWO REVIEW

1. The thermodilution method of CO determination is based on
   A. a change in blood temperature over time
   B. the length of time it takes for dye to be circulated
   C. the temperature of the injectate
   D. the volume of the injectate
2. To increase the accuracy of CO determinations, which of the following techniques is used?
   A. inject slowly and smoothly over 1 minute
   B. inject smoothly within a 4-second interval
   C. inject rapidly over 8 seconds
   D. intermittently inject the volume over 30 seconds
3. Which of the following are disadvantages associated with bolus thermodilution CO measurements?
   A. they are time consuming
   B. multiple measurements may subject patients to fluid overload

   C. accuracy is affected by user technique
   D. all of the above
4. Continuous CO measurements
   A. are less accurate than bolus thermodilution CO measurements
   B. provide two updates on CO readings every hour
   C. depend on user technique for accuracy
   D. agree with bolus thermodilution measurements
5. Mr. S has fluid volume overload and pulmonary edema. A PA catheter is inserted to monitor his CO. Which method would you recommend to obtain CO measurement in this patient?
   A. bolus thermodilution with 10 mL of normal saline
   B. continuous cardiac output monitoring
   C. bolus thermodilution with 10 mL of dextrose
   D. A and C

Answers: 1. A, 2. B, 3. D, 4. D, 5. B

SECTION THREE: Right Atrial Pressure

At the completion of this section, the learner will be able to relate right ventricular preload to right atrial pressure, recognize a normal right atrial waveform, and identify common physical findings and nursing interventions related to abnormal right atrial pressures.

Right atrial pressure (RAP) is obtained from the proximal port of the PA catheter, which opens into the right atrium. The RAP is always read as a mean pressure, and the normal range is 2 to 6 mm Hg (Fig. 9–5).

Figure 9–5 ■ A right atrial waveform with the *a* and *v* wave components identified. (*Reprinted with permission. Copyright © 2000 Edwards Lifesciences. Swan-Ganz ® is a trademark of Edwards Lifesciences Corporation, registered in the U.S. Patent and Trademark Office*)

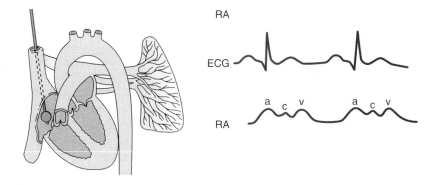

RAP is an estimate of right ventricular preload (i.e., the volume status of the right heart). Recall from Section Two that preload is the stretch exerted on the walls of the ventricle by the volume of blood filling the ventricle at the end of diastole. RAP is also known as right ventricular end-diastolic pressure (RVEDP). Measurement of RVEDP is possible because the tricuspid valve remains open until the end of right ventricular diastole, allowing right ventricular pressure to be transmitted to the right atrium. This is why RAP can be used as a measure of RVEDP.

Obtaining RAP Measurements

The RAP waveform is monitored by attaching a transducer to the proximal (blue) port of the PA catheter. The right atrial waveform has a characteristic undulating pattern, consisting of three positive and two negative excursions. These undulations are a result of mechanical events in the cardiac cycle. The positive excursions consist of *a*, *c*, and *v* waves. The rise in atrial pressure during atrial systole forms the *a* wave. Closure of the tricuspid valve early in systole produces the *c* wave (not always well visualized). The *v* wave is produced by an increase in pressure from passive atrial filling during ventricular systole. The negative excursions consist of the *x* and *y* deflections. The *x* descent follows the *a* and *c* waves and is a result of the drop in atrial pressure after atrial systole. The *y* descent is a result of passive right atrial emptying into the right ventricle when the tricuspid valve opens just prior to atrial systole. Refer to Figure 9–6 for a labeled atrial waveform.

Assessment of the waveform begins with obtaining a graphic readout from the bedside or central monitoring system (Ahrens & Shallom, 2001). This printout should include both the ECG and RAP tracings in order to correlate the mechanical events of the heart (RAP tracing) with the electrical events (ECG tracing) (Daily, 2001). The RVEDP is marked in the RAP tracing by the *a* wave. The *a* wave represents atrial systole and, therefore, follows the *P* wave on the ECG tracing. Find the correlation between the *a* wave and the *P* wave in Figure 9–5.

Any pressure in the thoracic cavity is transmitted to the great vessels and the cardiac chambers. Thus, measurement of the right atrial pressure is obtained at end-expiration to eliminate intrathoracic pressures. Spontaneously breathing patients generate a negative pressure breath on inspiration. This is reflected in the RAP waveform as a downward deflection. Patients on a ventilator with mandatory positive pressure breaths show a rise in their RAP waveform on inspiration. Addition of positive end-expiratory pressure greater than 10 cm H_2O may result in elevation of the entire waveform above the baseline pressure. Interpretation of the RAP is based on trends in data and not the absolute number. Find the end-expiration phase of the RAP waveform in the mechanically ventilated patient in Figure 9–7.

Conditions Leading to an Elevated RAP

Pressure and volume are proportional: An increase in volume can generate an increase in pressure. This is the basis for using pressures as proxies for volume status. There are circumstances, however, where an increase in pressure may occur without an increase in volume. Consider a balloon that is inflated with a given volume of water. Imagine squeezing the balloon: The pressure inside the balloon increases, but the volume does not change. Clinically, this is seen in circumstances such as cardiac tamponade or tension pneumothorax.

Figure 9–6 ■ A labeled right atrial waveform.

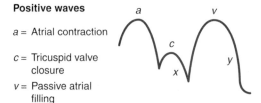

Positive waves

a = Atrial contraction

c = Tricuspid valve closure

v = Passive atrial filling

Negative waves

x = Decrease in atrial pressure after atrial systole

y = The passive emptying of atrium into right ventricle

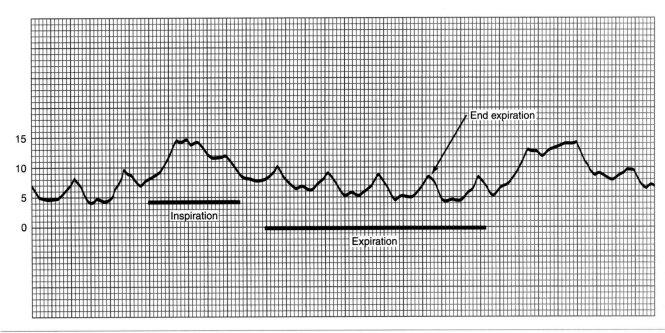

Figure 9–7 ■ End-expiration phase on RAP waveform in a patient receiving mechanical ventilation.

Pulmonic Valve Stenosis

The right ventricle has to overcome the fixed resistance (fixed afterload) of a stenotic or "tight" pulmonary valve to eject the stroke volume into the PA. As a result, there is reduced emptying of the right ventricle and an increase in the resistance to further ventricular filling. This is reflected by an elevated RAP.

Pulmonary Hypertension

Pulmonary hypertension increases the afterload to the right ventricle. As a result of higher afterload in the pulmonary circuit, there is reduced emptying of the right ventricle, and this is reflected by an elevated RAP.

Chronic or Severe Left Heart Failure

Inadequate cardiac output from the left ventricle results in "backward failure." The increased volume in the pulmonary circulation results in inadequate emptying of the right ventricle and increased resistance to ventricular filling. An elevated RAP will be seen.

Cardiac Tamponade

The right heart is a low-pressure system. As a result of this, any rapid fluid buildup in the pericardial space results in resistance to right ventricular filling. The RAP will be elevated.

Clinical Findings Associated with Elevated RAP

Clinical findings associated with an increased RAP vary according to the cause and duration. Signs and symptoms may include all or some of the following: distended neck veins, tachycardia, a right ventricular gallop (S3, S4, or both), right upper quadrant tenderness from liver engorgement, dependent or generalized edema, and ascites.

When elevated RAP is a result of left heart failure, signs and symptoms of left ventricular failure also will be found. These are discussed later in this module.

Collaborative and Independent Interventions for Elevated RAP

Interventions for elevated RAP are determined by the cause. In general, care is directed toward optimizing preload by reducing volume. Overall goals are to decrease venous return to the right heart, increase contractility, and decrease the workload of the heart. Preload is reduced by fluid and sodium restrictions, and administration of diuretics or vasodilating medications.

Nursing care includes careful and frequent assessment of the patient's response to interventions. This includes meticulous keeping of intake and output records, and obtaining daily weights. A plan of care to decrease patient energy requirements is implemented. A dietary consult is obtained to provide patient and family education on sodium and fluid restrictions. Patient education includes information on the purpose and importance of all medications.

Conditions Leading to a Low RAP

A low right atrial pressure indicates low preload of the right heart. This is the result of either an actual or relative hypovolemia. Poor venous return to the heart for any reason is demonstrated in a low RAP.

Fluid Deficit

There are two types of fluid deficit. First, an actual hypovolemia results from loss of volume from the vascular system. Causes include hemorrhage, diuresis, dehydration from vomiting or diarrhea, and loss of body fluids from extensive burns.

Second, a relative hypovolemia results from vasodilation. Certain medications cause vasodilation, including IV and oral nitrates, some calcium channel blockers, angiotensin converting enzyme (ACE) inhibitors, hydralazine, and analgesics (morphine). Although intravenous nitroprusside is primarily used for its action on the arterioles, it is included here because it also dilates the venous bed. Use of these medications may cause a relative hypovolemia; fluid volume is not lost but only temporarily displaced in the venous system. This reduces venous return to the right heart and produces a low RAP, reflecting low preload.

Severe systemic infections are associated with a relative hypovolemia. Mediators released from bacterial cell walls produce dilation of the vascular smooth muscle that lines the arterioles and increase intravascular permeability that allows third spacing. Fevers, often associated with these infections, may also be present. These conditions produce a relative hypovolemia as more fluid stays in the peripheral vascular system and less returns to the right atrium (Module 15).

Clinical Findings Associated with Decreased RAP

Clinical findings accompanying decreased RAP depend on the severity of the condition. Typical findings include tachycardia, hypotension, diminished pulse amplitude, flat neck veins in a supine position, reduced CO, thirst, poor skin turgor, dry mucous membranes, and decreased urine output. If right heart preload (volume) is severely reduced, the signs and symptoms of shock also will be present (Module 15).

Interventions for Decreased RAP

Interventions for a low RAP are determined by the cause. Interventions are directed toward optimizing preload by restoring volume. Dehydration from overly vigorous diuresis, burns, vomiting, or diarrhea is corrected by oral replacement when possible or by careful intravenous hydration. Hemorrhage may need surgical correction. Crystalloid IV fluids replace volume lost by hemorrhage; however, when hemorrhage is significant, blood replacement is necessary to increase oxygen carrying capacity. The hypovolemia or low-preload state related to sepsis is treated with replacement fluids; the administration of appropriate antibiotics to treat the sepsis; and careful adjustment of vasoconstricting medications, such as dopamine and norepinephrine. Vasodilating medications are also a potential cause of low preload because pooling of blood in a dilated vascular system reduces venous return to the heart. Intravenous nitrates and nitroprusside are typically titrated by the nurse, based on physician orders. Oral medications with vasodilating properties should be identified and administration of these agents should be discussed with the physician prior to administration. The nurse provides careful and frequent assessment of the patient's response to the interventions previously described. Intake and output are monitored and evaluated. Patient weight changes provide important information.

In summary, the RAP is an indicator of right heart preload. It is obtained from the proximal port of the PA catheter, and the normal range is 2 to 6 mm Hg. Treatment of either low or high RAP is guided by an ongoing evaluation of the hemodynamic response to interventions. Nursing care consists of both collaborative and independent interventions.

SECTION THREE REVIEW

1. RAP is measured through which port of the catheter?
   A. proximal port
   B. distal port
   C. thermistor wire port
   D. balloon inflation port
2. RAP is a reflection of
   A. PAWP
   B. preload of the right heart
   C. afterload of the right heart
   D. left heart function
3. Normal mean RAP is
   A. less than 4 mm Hg
   B. 2 to 6 mm Hg
   C. 6 to 12 mm Hg
   D. 14 to 20 mm Hg
4. Right heart failure results in a RAP that is
   A. lower than normal
   B. above normal
   C. within normal range
   D. unchanged
5. Hypovolemia results in a RAP that is
   A. lower than normal
   B. above normal
   C. within normal range
   D. unchanged

Answers: 1. A, 2. B, 3. B, 4. B, 5. A

SECTION FOUR: Right Ventricular Pressure

At the completion of this section, the learner will be able to recognize the normal right ventricular (RV) waveform, and identify appropriate nursing interventions related to RV waveforms.

RV pressure is not continuously monitored with a traditional PA catheter but is observed and documented during insertion of the catheter. It is the responsibility of the nurse to recognize a RV waveform.

The normal RV systolic pressure is 20 to 30 mm Hg. This represents the pressure necessary to exceed the pressure in the PA (RV afterload), open the pulmonary valve, and eject blood into the pulmonary circulation. RV diastolic pressure range is low (2 to 8 mm Hg). This right end-diastolic pressure directly reflects the preload status of the right ventricle and should approximate the RAP.

The RV waveform has a characteristic pattern. It consists of a steep upstroke and a sharp downstroke (Fig. 9–8). Compare this waveform to the right atrial waveform in Figure 9–5. Although there is a marked increase in systolic pressure, the RV diastolic pressure remains essentially the same as the RAP. That is important information in identifying the waveform of a catheter that has slipped back into the right ventricle.

The RV waveform is typically seen on only two occasions:

1. During insertion, as the catheter is floated through the RV
2. If the catheter tip retreats from its proper position in the PA into the RV

Observation of this waveform at any time other than insertion indicates that the catheter tip has retreated from its proper position in the PA. This has important implications from both a technical and a patient safety standpoint. All parameters obtained from the catheter, including the CO, are incorrect. Most importantly, the patient is at risk for cardiac arrhythmias. Irritation of the right ventricular endothelium by the catheter tip causes abnormal cardiac rhythms (premature ventricular con-

tractions, ventricular tachycardia; refer to Module 10). In addition, the right bundle branch portion of the cardiac conduction system lies close to the surface of the right ventricular septum. Therefore, irritation can cause cardiac conduction disturbances (heart block, bundle branch blocks; refer to Module 10). For these reasons, it is important to recognize the RV waveform and its corresponding pressures.

The cardiac rhythm and waveforms are monitored by the nurse as the catheter is floated into the PA. Once the catheter has been properly positioned in the PA, a change to an RV waveform should be reported immediately to the physician to expedite repositioning of the catheter. Some hospitals or units have specific nursing protocols to follow when a PA catheter retreats into the RV. It is the responsibility of the nurse to be aware of unit policy and state licensure guidelines related to manipulating the catheter to a different location. In addition to observing for arrhythmias and notifying the physician for repositioning, some facilities have specific protocols that instruct the nurse to pull the catheter back into the right atrium or inflate the balloon to foster flotation of the catheter tip back into the PA.

Once the catheter has been inserted, the exposed portion of the catheter is considered contaminated and should not be advanced unless a sterile sleeve was placed over the catheter before insertion. Use of these optional sleeves allows repositioning of the catheter without increasing the risk of infection.

In summary, RV waveforms should be seen only during insertion and removal of the catheter. The presence of the RV waveform at any other time indicates improper positioning and puts the patient at an increased risk for the development of dysrhythmias. Careful observation of the patient and the cardiac rhythm is indicated when the catheter is in the RV. Once the catheter has been inserted, the exposed portion of the catheter is considered contaminated and should not be advanced unless a sterile sleeve was placed over the catheter prior to insertion. Use of these optional sleeves allows repositioning of the catheter without increasing the risk of infection.

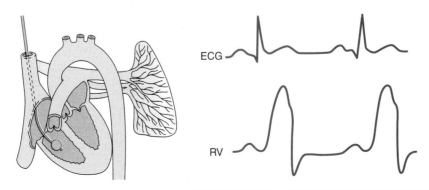

Figure 9–8 ■ Right ventricular (RV) waveform. *(Reprinted with permission. Copyright © 2000 Edwards Lifesciences. Swan-Ganz ® © is a trademark of Edwards Lifesciences Corporation, registered in the U.S. Patent and Trademark Office)*

SECTION FOUR REVIEW

1. The normal range for RV systolic pressure is
   A. 10 to 20 mm Hg
   B. 20 to 30 mm Hg
   C. 30 to 40 mm Hg
   D. 40 to 50 mm Hg
2. The normal range for RV diastolic pressure is
   A. 2 to 8 mm Hg
   B. 4 to 10 mm Hg
   C. 6 to 12 mm Hg
   D. 8 to 14 mm Hg
3. The BEST description of an RV waveform is
   A. a soft undulating pattern
   B. a steep upstroke followed by a sharp downstroke
   C. sharply notched with a slow downstroke
   D. almost flat

4. The greatest potential for abnormal cardiac rhythms occurs when the PA catheter is in the
   A. superior vena cava
   B. right atrium
   C. right ventricle
   D. PA
5. The RV waveform is typically seen by the nurse
   A. during insertion of the PA catheter
   B. if the catheter retreats from its original position in the PA
   C. on a continuous basis
   D. A and B

Answers: 1. B, 2. A, 3. B, 4. C, 5. D

SECTION FIVE: Pulmonary Artery Pressure

At the completion of this section, the learner will be able to recognize a normal PA waveform and identify common physical findings and nursing interventions related to abnormal PA pressures.

Pulmonary artery pressure (PAP) is read as a systolic and diastolic pressure. It is obtained from the distal port of the PA catheter. Under normal conditions, the PAP is considered to reflect both right and left heart pressures.

The **pulmonary artery systolic (PAS) pressure** reflects the highest pressure generated by the RV during systole. The normal range is 20 to 30 mm Hg. The **pulmonary artery diastolic (PAD) pressure** is normally 2 to 5 mm Hg higher than the pulmonary artery wedge pressure (PAWP). In the absence of chronic obstructive pulmonary disease, pulmonary embolism, mitral stenosis, and heart rates greater than 125 beats per minute (BPM), the PAD pressure is used to estimate the left ventricular preload status. This is possible because there are no valves to impede the transmission of left atrial pressure to the PA. The normal range for PAD pressure is 8 to 15 mm Hg. Once

the PAD pressure has been demonstrated to correlate with the PAWP, it is used to monitor left ventricular preload status.

Taking Measurements

The PA waveform is monitored continuously by a transducer attached to the distal port of the catheter. The PA waveform has a characteristic pattern (Fig. 9–9). It consists of a steep upstroke and a downstroke that is distinguished by a dicrotic notch formed by the closure of the pulmonic valve.

On entering the PA from the right ventricle, the top of the waveform stays essentially the same height, but the bottom or diastolic portion of the waveform elevates. Another identifying feature of the PA waveform is the dicrotic notch on the downstroke. The dicrotic notch is formed by the closure of the pulmonic valve. If the catheter tip retreats into the right ventricle, the diastolic pressure drops, and the dicrotic notch is lost. Knowledge of these waveform properties allows the nurse to identify catheter position correctly. This is important because catheter retreat into the right ventricle could result in dysrhythmias (see Section Four).

Figure 9–9 ■ PA waveform. (*Reprinted with permission. Copyright © 2000 Edwards Lifesciences. Swan-Ganz ® is a trademark of Edwards Lifesciences Corporation, registered in the U.S. Patent and Trademark Office*)

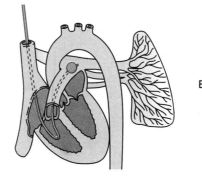

The PA pressure waveform represents arterial pressure on the right side of the heart. The systolic upstroke of the PA pressure tracing represents right ventricular ejection and is preceeded by ventricular electrical depolarization. The PA pressure may be obtained clinically by printing out both the ECG and PA pressure tracings. The PA systolic pressure will follow the *QRS* wave of the ECG. Correlate the ECG with the PA pressure tracing in Figure 9–9.

Elevated Pulmonary Artery Systolic Pressure

The PA pressure is generated by the right ventricle. Anything that increases the afterload of the right ventricle (i.e., increases the pulmonary vascular resistance) results in an elevated PAS pressure. Examples include pulmonary hypertension from any cause, including chronic lung disease, pulmonary embolism, and hypoxemia.

Clinical Findings

Symptoms vary according to the cause, severity, and duration of the elevated pressure. Assessment of the patient with pulmonary hypertension may reveal signs of right heart failure, including distended neck veins, peripheral edema, a tender liver, and ascites. Palpation may reveal a right ventricular lift. Auscultation may reveal S3 and S4 heart sounds. Patients with chronic lung disease have a chronically elevated PAS pressure. A pulmonary embolus increases PAS pressure. The patient with a pulmonary embolus may present as a medical emergency with dyspnea, chest pain, hemoptysis, and hemodynamic instability.

Elevated Pulmonary Artery Diastolic Pressure

Conditions that affect the left heart, such as angina or myocardial infarction, fluid overload, mitral stenosis, and left-to-right intracardiac shunts, are associated with a high PAD pressure.

Clinical Findings

Clinical findings associated with left heart failure may result in some or all of the following signs and symptoms: dyspnea, tachycardia, S3 or S4, and bilateral crackles in the lungs. CO is reduced and PAWP is elevated.

Interventions

Interventions for an elevated PAS or PAD pressure are determined by the cause. In general, care is directed toward reducing preload by administering diuretics and restricting fluid and sodium intake. Cardiac contractility is improved by the use of inotropic medications, such as digoxin, dobutamine, dopamine, and amrinone. When indicated, the use of an intra-aortic balloon pump reduces the afterload of a failing heart as well as increases the blood supply to the heart by augmenting the patient's diastolic pressure. Nursing care includes careful administration of potent medications, intake and output measurements, and daily weights. Care is directed also toward reducing the workload of the heart by planning activities to allow rest periods.

Low Pulmonary Artery Diastolic Pressure

Low PAD pressure typically indicates a low preload state related to inadequate venous return to the left heart.

Clinical Findings

Clinical findings associated with low preload states include tachycardia, flat neck veins, clear lungs, dry oral mucosa, poor skin turgor, hypotension, and decreased urine output. If severe, the signs and symptoms of advanced shock, such as cool and clammy skin, also may be seen.

Interventions

Interventions are directed toward improving left ventricle (LV) preload through volume replacement. Nursing care includes managing fluid replacement through an ongoing assessment of the patient's hydration status and hemodynamic parameters. Changes in patient weight and intake and output data are important to assess.

In summary, under normal conditions, the PAS and PAD pressures provide a means for assessing both right and left heart function. Knowledge of the typical PA waveform helps the nurse recognize incorrect catheter placement. Integrating hemodynamic parameters with careful physical assessment findings allows the nurse to plan interventions to improve patient outcome.

SECTION FIVE REVIEW

1. The normal range for PAS pressure is
   A. 10 to 20 mm Hg
   B. 20 to 30 mm Hg
   C. 30 to 40 mm Hg
   D. 40 to 50 mm Hg

2. The normal range for PAD pressure is
   A. 2 to 8 mm Hg
   B. 4 to 10 mm Hg
   C. 6 to 12 mm Hg
   D. 8 to 15 mm Hg

3. The BEST description of a PA waveform is a
   A. soft undulating pattern
   B. steep upstroke followed by a sharp downstroke
   C. sharply notched upstroke with a steep downstroke
   D. steep upstroke and a downstroke distinguished by a dicrotic notch

4. Under normal conditions, a high PAD pressure suggests
   A. hypovolemia (low preload)
   B. hypervolemia (high preload)
   C. good left heart function
   D. right heart failure

5. A PAD is 2 mm Hg. The nurse should anticipate which of the following interventions?
   A. administer diuretics and implement fluid restrictions
   B. volume replacement
   C. administer a positive inotropic agent
   D. no intervention because 2 mm Hg is acceptable

Answers: 1. B, 2. D, 3. D, 4. B, 5. B

SECTION SIX: Pulmonary Artery Wedge Pressure

At the completion of this section, the learner will be able to recognize a normal pulmonary artery wedge pressure waveform (PAWP), relate left ventricular preload to PAWP, and identify common physical findings and appropriate nursing interventions related to abnormal PAWP pressures.

Preload is defined as the pressure or stretch exerted on the wall of the ventricle by the volume of blood filling it at end diastole. The Frank–Starling Law of the heart states that the greater the myocardial fibers are stretched during diastole, the more they will shorten (contract) during systole, and the greater the force of contraction will be until a physiologic limit has been reached (refer to Module 8). The way myocardial fibers are stretched is through preload or volume.

This concept of preload applies to both the right and left ventricles, but emphasis is placed on the left ventricle because it is the capacity of the left ventricle to function as a pump that determines patient outcome. Left ventricular preload is measured directly only during a cardiac catheterization or following open heart surgery when a left atrial line is placed. Left ventricular preload is indirectly measured with a PA catheter through measurement of PAWP. It is obtained through the distal port of the PA catheter. The normal range is 4 to 12 mm Hg. Similar to the RAP, the PAWP is always read as the mean of the *a* wave. The PAWP waveform (Figure 9–10) is similiar in appearance to the right atrial waveform (Figure 9–5).

To obtain a PAWP, the catheter balloon is inflated slowly, allowing the catheter to float and "wedge" in a small branch of the PA. Inflation of the balloon is stopped as soon as the characteristic PAWP pattern is observed (Fig. 9–11). The inflated balloon stops the forward flow of blood through that vessel. Because

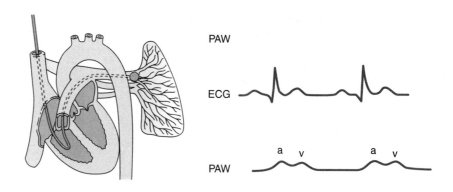

Figure 9–10 ■ Pulmonary artery wedge waveform. *(Reprinted with permission. Copyright © 2000 Edwards Lifesciences. Swan-Ganz ® is a trademark of Edwards Lifesciences Corporation, registered in the U.S. Patent and Trademark office)*

Figure 9–11 ■ A labeled PAW waveform.

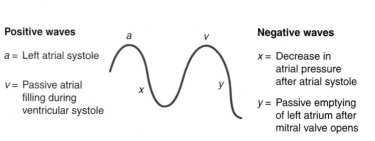

Positive waves

a = Left atrial systole

v = Passive atrial filling during ventricular systole

Negative waves

x = Decrease in atrial pressure after atrial systole

y = Passive emptying of left atrium after mitral valve opens

there are no valves in the pulmonary circulation, the catheter sitting in the PA "sees" through the pulmonary capillaries, pulmonary vein, left atrium, and into the left ventricle. Because the mitral valve remains open until the end of ventricular diastole, the left atrium and ventricle essentially function as one open chamber until the mitral valve closes. This is why the PAWP reflects the pressure in the left ventricle at end diastole. In the absence of mitral valve disease, the PAWP is considered an accurate estimate of left ventricular preload. It provides information about the volume status of the left ventricle and aids in the evaluation of left ventricular compliance. An elevated PAWP suggests a stiff, noncompliant left ventricle that contracts poorly. A low PAWP indicates that preload is low.

PAWP Waveform Analysis

The first positive wave is the *a* wave, produced by the rise in atrial pressure caused by left atrial contraction. The second positive wave is the *v* wave, formed as the left atrium fills during ventricular systole. The *c* wave, not typically seen on the PAWP waveform, is produced by closure of the mitral valve at the initiation of ventricular systole.

The two negative PAWP waveforms are the *x* and *y* descents. The first negative descent is the *x* wave, which reflects decreased volume in the left atrium after atrial systole. The *y* descent results from the pressure drop in the left atrium when the mitral valve opens just prior to atrial contraction, permitting passive emptying of the left atrium (see Fig. 9–11).

Obtaining the PAWP is done in the same manner as that for the RAP. The tracing is printed out simultaneously with the ECG. Similar to the RAP, the *a* wave is found following the *P* wave of the ECG. Because the left side of the heart is more muscular, depolarization takes slightly more time (approximately 0.20 seconds) so the *a* wave may be located by drawing a line from the *P* wave and measuring 0.20 seconds further or as a "buried" wave in the *QRS* wave (Quaal, 2001). The mean of the *a* wave is documented. Find the correlation between the *a* wave of the PAWP tracing and the ECG in Figure 9–10.

There are two primary differences in the RAP and PAWP waveforms. First, the *c* wave sometimes present on the RAP waveform is rarely seen on a PAWP waveform. Second, normal PAWPs are higher than normal RAPs.

Key Points to Follow When Obtaining Pulmonary Artery Wedge Pressure

There are several technical points the nurse must consider when obtaining a PAWP measurement.

- Observe the waveform constantly during inflation, and stop inflation as soon as the PAWP is identified.
- Use the smallest inflation volume possible, and do not exceed the maximum recommended volume (typically less than 1.25 mL). This reduces the risk of balloon rupture.

- Maintain inflation only long enough to obtain a stable reading.
- Obtain the PAWP at end expiration, when intrathoracic pressure is most stable and less affected by respiratory variation.
- If resistance is felt during balloon inflation, stop! Do not continue! Allow the balloon to passively deflate. Call the physician.
- Allow the balloon to deflate passively to avoid damaging the balloon.

Pulmonary infarction can result from leaving the PA balloon inflated for too long or when a deflated balloon becomes lodged in the pulmonary capillary bed. A PAWP waveform will appear on the monitor. The patient should be turned or made to cough to relieve a lodged balloon. Open the stopcock on the port and remove the syringe to allow passive deflation of the balloon. The balloon may rupture from repeated overfilling. If you are unable to obtain a PAWP waveform after instilling the proper amount of air through the PA catheter balloon port, turn the balloon lumen off to the patient. Label the lumen "Do not use." Notify the physician.

Elevated Pulmonary Artery Wedge Pressure

Any condition that increases the left ventricular end-diastolic blood volume results in an elevated PAWP. The following conditions are associated with elevated PAWP

- **Fluid overload.** Occurs with overly aggressive fluid replacement, although normal kidneys usually compensate. Patients with acute and chronic renal failure often have fluid overload.
- **Left ventricular failure.** Poor contractility results in inadequate emptying of the ventricle.
- **Ischemia.** An ischemic myocardium becomes "stiff" and resistant to ventricular filling.
- **Mitral stenosis.** Mitral stenosis creates a high left atrial pressure, which is transmitted back into the pulmonary vasculature.
- **Cardiac tamponade.** Accumulation of fluid between the pericardium and the heart results in resistance to ventricular filling. The RAP, PAD, and PAWP elevate, and all three values are similar. This is known as diastolic equalization and is a hallmark of cardiac tamponade.

Clinical Findings

Clinical findings related to an elevated PAWP vary according to the degree of elevation but typically include tachycardia, exertional dyspnea, orthopnea, paroxysmal nocturnal dyspnea, crackles in the lung fields, and an S3 or S4 gallop at the apex. Neck veins are distended.

Interventions

Interventions are directed toward optimizing preload by administration of diuretics and vasodilators along with sodium and fluid restrictions. Intravenous and oral nitrates dilate the venous bed and displace fluid, which lower preload by reducing the venous return to the heart. Control of dysrhythmias helps the heart to pump more effectively. Afterload is reduced by administration of arteriole vasodilators, such as nitroprusside (Nipride), and ACE inhibitors, such as captopril (Capoten). By dilating the peripheral arterioles, these drugs reduce afterload, promote emptying of the ventricle, and effectively reduce cardiac work and myocardial oxygen requirements. Contractility is enhanced by careful titration of inotropic medications, such as digoxin, dobutamine (Dobutrex), and amrinone (Inocor). If these interventions fail to improve PAWP and CO, an intra-aortic balloon pump may be required (Module 15).

The nurse is responsible for careful titration of potent vasoactive medications to improve hemodynamics. Manipulation of medications and treatments is based on astute physical assessments correlated with current hemodynamic parameters obtained from the PA catheter. Critical thinking at the bedside is crucial to improved patient outcomes. Frequent nursing assessments, meticulous intake and output records, and daily weights are crucial to follow the response to treatment.

Low Pulmonary Artery Wedge Pressure

A low PAWP typically is related to inadequate circulating blood volume.

Clinical Findings

Clinical findings include flat neck veins, clear lungs, low pulse pressure, decreased urine output, hypotension, tachycardia, and likely complaints of thirst.

Interventions

Interventions include careful replacement of fluid or blood products by correlating the PAWP with an ongoing assessment of the patient's response to treatment. Hourly urine output, careful intake and output records, and daily weights are indicated.

SECTION SIX REVIEW

1. What is the normal range of the PAWP?
   A. 2 to 10 mm Hg
   B. 4 to 12 mm Hg
   C. 8 to 16 mm Hg
   D. 10 to 18 mm Hg
2. The BEST description of a PAWP waveform is a
   A. soft undulating pattern
   B. steep upstroke followed by a sharp downstroke
   C. sharply notched with a slow downstroke
   D. sawtooth pattern
3. In a hypovolemic patient, the PAWP is
   A. well within the normal range
   B. low-normal or below normal range
   C. high-normal or above normal range
   D. high or low

4. In congestive heart failure, the expected PAWP is
   A. well within the normal range
   B. low-normal or below normal range
   C. high-normal or above normal range
   D. high or low
5. Which waveform most closely resembles the PAWP waveform?
   A. right atrial waveform
   B. right ventricular waveform
   C. PA waveform
   D. systemic arterial waveform

Answers: 1. B, 2. A, 3. B, 4. C, 5. A

SECTION SEVEN: Systemic Arterial Pressure

At the completion of this section, the learner will be able to discuss the physiology underlying the systemic arterial waveform and identify the components of a normal systemic arterial waveform.

Blood pressure is a function of blood flow (CO) and the elasticity of the blood vessels. Systolic blood pressure normally ranges between 100 and 140 mm Hg. Systolic pressure reflects the highest pressure exerted by the left ventricle as it ejects the stroke volume into the aorta. Diastolic blood pressure normally ranges between 60 and 80 mm Hg. The **mean arterial pressure (MAP)** is the average arterial pressure throughout the cardiac cycle. It normally ranges between 70 and 90 mm Hg (Section Eight). Advantages of direct (invasive) blood pressure monitoring in the high-acuity patient include the following:

■ Knowledge of minute-to-minute changes in blood pressure
■ Increased accuracy of measurement in the hypotensive patient
■ More precise titration of medications and fluids
■ The capacity to obtain arterial blood gases (ABGs) and blood samples without pain and discomfort to the patient

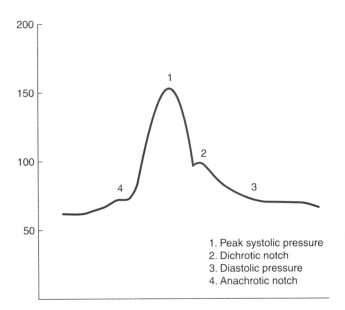

Figure 9–12 ■ Components of the systemic arterial pressure waveform. *(Reprinted with permission. Copyright © 2000 Edwards Lifesciences. Swan-Ganz ® is a trademark of Edwards Lifesciences Corporation, registered in the U.S. Patent and Trademark Office)*

1. Peak systolic pressure
2. Dichrotic notch
3. Diastolic pressure
4. Anachrotic notch

represents the diastolic pressure and is reflected digitally on the monitor.

Arterial pressure monitoring is common in high-acuity settings. The nurse typically is responsible for setting up the equipment for catheter insertion, calibrating the equipment to ensure accurate readings, and assisting the physician with the procedure. The two most common insertion sites for arterial monitoring include the radial and femoral arteries.

Once the arterial catheter is in place, the nurse is responsible for patient safety and comfort, and maintenance of the system as discussed in Section One. Securing the pressure tubing to prevent dislodgement and possible exsanguination is an important nursing responsibility.

Monitoring circulation distal to the insertion site is another important nursing function. The skin color and temperature and all pulses distal to the insertion site are regularly assessed and documented. Any alteration in circulation is promptly brought to the attention of the physician. The site is observed frequently for signs of infection: redness, warmth, edema, and drainage. Unit-specific protocols and responsibilities related to arterial monitoring are typically described in hospital policy and procedure manuals.

Arterial monitoring provides the capacity to monitor the patient's blood pressure on a continuous basis. Depending on specific monitor characteristics, digital blood pressure readings are usually updated at 4- to 6-second intervals. This allows the nurse to monitor the patient's response to interventions without having to disturb the patient to take a manual blood pressure reading.

The common practice of comparing systemic arterial pressure measured with the arterial line against a noninvasive blood pressure is not supported by the literature (Bridges & Middleton, 1997). Each patient should be assessed to determine which system is appropriate for monitoring blood pressure and then the system is optimized. The two pressures do not always agree.

In summary, there are several advantages of invasive blood pressure monitoring in the high-acuity patient. The equipment is the same as the equipment used to monitor pulmonary artery pressures. The catheter is inserted into a peripheral artery. The arterial waveform is a classic morphology related to the cardiac cycle. There are specific nursing responsibilities related to care of the patient with arterial blood pressure monitoring.

The equipment needed to monitor systemic arterial blood pressures is the same as the equipment used to monitor PA pressures, except a small catheter is used and inserted into a peripheral artery (Fig. 9–2).

The arterial waveform has a characteristic morphology that is related to the cardiac cycle (Fig. 9–12). When the aortic valve opens, blood is ejected into the aorta. This forms a steep upstroke on the arterial waveform, called the anacrotic limb. The top of this limb represents the peak, or highest systolic pressure, which appears digitally on the monitor as the systolic pressure. After this peak pressure, the waveform descends. This descent forms the dicrotic limb and represents systolic ejection of blood that is continuing at a reduced force. The descending, or dicrotic, limb is disrupted by the dicrotic notch, which is an important point on the waveform. The dicrotic notch represents closure of the aortic valve and the beginning of ventricular diastole. The lowest portion of the waveform (baseline)

SECTION SEVEN REVIEW

1. The dicrotic notch on the descending limb of the arterial waveform represents
   A. opening of the aortic valve
   B. closure of the aortic valve
   C. the beginning of ventricular systole
   D. the diastolic pressure

2. The highest point on the arterial waveform denotes the
   A. anacrotic limb
   B. peak systolic pressure
   C. mean arterial pressure
   D. diastolic pressure

SECTION EIGHT: Derived Parameters

At the completion of this section, the learner will be able to discuss the implications of selected derived hemodynamic parameters and calculate the following derived hemodynamic parameters: cardiac index, stroke volume index, mean arterial pressure, systemic vascular resistance, and pulmonary vascular resistance, left ventricular stroke work index, and right ventricular stroke work index.

Cardiac Index

As discussed in Section Two, CO is the amount of blood ejected from the heart in 1 minute. The normal range is 4 to 8 L/min. As a generic or raw value, the CO does not take the size of the patient into account. The cardiac index (CI) individualizes the CO to the patient by taking body size into consideration. Knowledge of the CO and body surface area (BSA) are all that is necessary to determine the CI. The formula is

$$CI = CO/BSA$$

The normal CI is 2.4 to 4.0 L/min/m^2. The BSA is simply a function of height and weight. Most monitors will calculate the BSA when the patient's height and weight are entered. The following example demonstrates the importance of calculating the CI.

	Patient A	Patient B
Height	6'0"	5'0"
Weight	216 lb	118 lb
BSA	2.22 m^2	1.50 m^2
CO	4.0 L/min	4.0 L/min
CI	1.89 L/min/m^2	2.4 L/min/m^2

Both patients have a CO of 4.0 L/min, which falls within the normal range, but the CI of patient A is well below normal and suggests a shock state. Using the CO alone does not indicate the gravity of the patient's hemodynamic status. The CI provides meaning to the CO and is the more important parameter to consider when making clinical decisions.

Stroke Volume and Stroke Volume Index

As discussed in Section Two, the stroke volume (SV) and stroke volume index (SVI) are used to assess cardiac function and cardiac contractility. With the traditional PA catheter, the SV is not directly measured. Stroke volume is a helpful parameter in interpreting the hemodynamic profile. A decreased stroke volume is seen in hypovolemia, cardiac failure, increased afterload, or in patients with cardiac valve problems. An increase in the stroke volume is seen with a reduction in afterload values. The cardiac output and cardiac index are assessed in the context of the preload values as well as the SV and SVI.

SV = Cardiac output/HR (normal SV = 50 to 100 mL/beat)

SI = Cardiac index/HR (normal SI = 25 to 45 mL/beat/m^2)

Mean Arterial Pressure

The MAP is an approximation of the average pressure in the systemic circulation throughout the cardiac cycle. Normal range is 70 to 90 mm Hg. The MAP is provided as a digital readout when an arterial line or automatic blood pressure equipment is in use. The MAP obtained from an arterial line is the most accurate because the mean actually is measured rather than calculated.

When direct arterial monitoring is not available, the MAP must be calculated. Keep in mind that MAPs calculated from cuff pressures (automatic or manual) have a potential for error because of extraneous factors, such as wrong size cuff, differences in hearing, sensitivity of the instrument, and patient movement.

The formula for MAP reflects the components of the cardiac cycle. In normal heart rates, systole accounts for one third of the cycle and diastole for two thirds of the cycle.

$$MAP = SBP + 2 (DBP)/3$$

Use the MAP formula to calculate the MAP for a patient with a blood pressure of 90/40 mm Hg. The correct answer is 57 mm Hg.

Systemic Vascular Resistance and Systemic Vascular Resistance Index

Systemic vascular resistance (SVR) is an estimate of left ventricular afterload. It represents an average of the resistance of all the vascular beds. Recall from Section Two that afterload is the resistance the left ventricle must overcome to open the aortic valve and eject the stroke volume into the systemic circulation. Afterload is one of the primary determinants of myocardial oxygen demand. The harder the heart works to pump blood out of the ventricle, the higher the myocardial oxygen requirements. A high SVR can reduce SV and CO. This is an important aspect to consider during regulation of potent vasoactive medications. These medications may improve MAP and afterload, but may also decrease SV.

Most monitors will calculate the SVR. However, it is helpful to understand the components that make up the formula. Recall from Module 8, that Ohm's Law describes afterload. Left ventricular afterload is the product of a change in pressure (MAP − RAP) divided by flow (CO):

$$SVR = \frac{(MAP - RAP) \times 80}{CO}$$

(80 is a conversion factor). The SVR is expressed in dynes·sec·cm^{-5}, and the normal range is 800 to 1,200 dynes·sec·cm^{-5}. To individualize SVR to the patient, the CI is substituted for the CO in the formula. The formula for the SVR index (SVRI) is

$$SVRI = \frac{(MAP - RAP) \times 80}{CI}$$

The normal range for the SVRI is 1,970 to 2,390 dynes·sec·cm^{-5}/m^2. The indices of CI and SVRI are far better indicators of the patient's hemodynamic status than the CO and SVR alone because the indices are referenced to body size.

Elevated Systemic Vascular Resistance

A high SVR may be the result of multiple causes. In hypothermia, peripheral vasoconstriction occurs as a compensatory mechanism to keep core body temperature warm. In this circumstance, warming the patient may be the only intervention necessary to dilate the constricted peripheral vasculature, normalize SVR, and improve CO.

Hypovolemia can produce an elevated SVR. Inadequate circulating blood volume induces vasoconstriction. This mechanism results in the shunting of as much peripheral blood volume as possible back to the vital organs (heart, lungs, and brain). Careful fluid replacement normalizes the SVR.

In cardiac failure, hypotension initiates similar compensatory mechanisms. The peripheral vascular beds constrict in an attempt to increase the blood return to the heart, thereby increasing the blood pressure. However, in this situation, returning more blood (more preload) to an already failing heart does not help. The vasoconstriction itself results in an increased afterload, which means the already-struggling heart must now overcome more pressure to open the aortic valve and eject the stroke volume. This patient needs help on both preload and afterload reduction. Diuretics and nitrates reduce preload. Afterload reduction is done cautiously in a patient with low blood pressure. Vasodilators, such as nitroprusside (Nipride), or an ACE inhibitor, such as captopril (Capoten), may be administered. Amrinone (Inocor) is an inotrope that improves myocardial contractility and causes vasodilation to reduce both afterload and preload. Reducing afterload makes it easier for the heart to eject SV, lessens cardiac work and myocardial oxygen demand, and improves CO.

Low Systemic Vascular Resistance

Physiologic responses to shock states, such as sepsis, neurogenic shock, and anaphylactic shock, initiate vasodilation. This results in low SVR. Low SVR results in low blood pressure. (Treatment of specific shock states is discussed in Module 15.) SVR is improved with careful titration of vasoconstricting medications, such as dopamine, neosynephrine, or norepinephrine (Levophed).

Pulmonary Vascular Resistance

Pulmonary vascular resistance (PVR) is an estimate of right ventricular afterload. It represents an average of the resistance of pulmonary vascular beds. A high PVR reduces right ventricular SV and CO. Most monitors calculate PVR. However, it is helpful to understand the components that make up the formula. Recall from Module 8, Ohm's Law describes afterload. Right ventricular afterload is the product of change in pressure (mean PAP − PAWP) divided by flow (CO):

$$PVR = \frac{(Mean\ PAP - PAWP) \times 80}{CO}$$

(80 is a conversion factor). The normal range is 50 to 250 dynes·sec·cm^{-5} (much less than SVR). To individualize PVR to the patient, CI is substituted for CO in the formula. The formula for the PVR index (PVRI) is

$$PVRI = \frac{(Mean\ PAP - PAWP) \times 80}{CI}$$

The normal range for the PVRI is 255 to 315 dynes·sec·cm^{-5}/m^2.

PVR or PVRI is elevated with acute lung injury, acute respiratory distress syndrome, pulmonary hypertension, and pulmonary congestion. Like SVR, vasodilators decrease PVR.

Left Ventricular Stroke Work Index

Left ventricular stroke work index (LVSWI) is the amount of work involved in moving blood in the left ventricle with each heartbeat. A lot of information goes into calculating the LVSWI because it represents work performed that is influenced by both pressure the heart beats against and the volume the heart must pump. Variables in the calculation of LVSWI are first collected. These include SVI, MAP, and PAWP. Once all the information is obtained, it is placed in the following equation:

$$LVSWI = [(MAP - PAWP) \times (SVI) \times (0.0136)]$$

MAP − PAWP = a measure of the pressure the left ventricle is ejecting against

SVI = the volume the left ventricle must eject

0.0136 = a constant that converts work to pressure

Normal values for LVSWI range from 50 to 62 $g/m^2/beat$. There are situations in which it helps to compare the LVSWI with the PAWP. PAWP reflects volume. LVSWI represents pressure. When the left ventricle becomes stiffer (decreased compliance), the PAWP does not accurately reflect the workload of the left ventricle because the relationship between volume and pressure is not direct. It is best to calculate LVSWI.

Once the LVSWI is obtained, it is plotted on the y axis of a ventricular function curve (Fig. 9–13). PAWP is plotted on the x axis. This provides a picture of how the left ventricle is performing in light of the pressure and volume conditions. As noted in the diagram, an LVSWI between 40 and 60 $g/m^2/beat$, and a PAWP between 8 and 20 mm Hg, is best for left ventricular ejection.

Low LVSWI may be an indication that the patient is hypovolemic or has cardiac failure. In situations in which both the LVSWI and the PAWP are low, more volume may be needed to improve contractility. High LVSWI may be an indication of hypervolemia. In situations in which both the LVSWI and the PAWP are high, diuretics and vasodilators may be needed.

Right Ventricular Stroke Work Index

Right ventricular stroke work index (RVSWI) is the amount of work involved in moving blood in the right ventricle with each beat. The formula represents the pressure generated (mean PAP) multiplied by the volume pumped (SVI). Similar to LVSWI, the RVSWI increases or decreases because of changes in either pressure (mean PAP) or volume pumped (SVI). Normal values are 7.9 to 9.7 $g/m^2/beat$. Increased and decreased values are treated much the same as for LVSWI.

$$RVSWI = [(mean\ PAP) - (RAP) \times (SVI) \times (0.00136)]$$

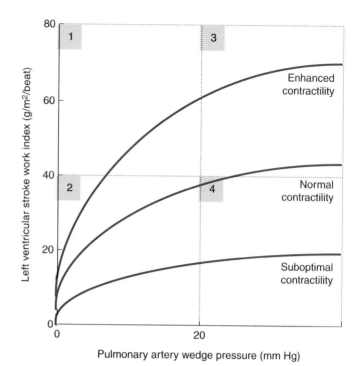

Quadrant 1: Optimal fuction; Quadrant 2: Hypovolemia; Quadrant 3: Hypervolemia; Quadrant 4: Cardiac failure

Figure 9–13 ■ Ventricular function curve.

In summary, the derived parameters of CI, SVI, MAP, SVR, SVRI, PVR, PVRI, LVSWI, and RVSWI provide important information about CO (see the following chart). Correlating hemodynamic parameters with physical assessment can assist the nurse in clinical decision making at the bedside. Integration of this knowledge can enable the nurse to provide both independent and collaborative interventions.

SV Component	Right Heart	Left Heart
Preload	RAP	PAWP
Afterload	PVR, PVRI	SVR, SVRI
Contractility	RVSWI	LVSWI

SECTION EIGHT REVIEW

1. Normal range for MAP is
   A. 60 to 80 mm Hg
   B. 70 to 90 mm Hg
   C. 80 to 100 mm Hg
   D. 90 to 110 mm Hg

2. Using the following hemodynamic parameters:
   MAP = 90 mm Hg, RAP = 6 mm Hg, CO = 6.2 L/min, BSA = 1.8 m^2, calculate the CI.
   A. 2.00   C. 4.50
   B. 3.44   D. 2.96

3. Using the hemodynamic parameters in question 2, calculate the SVR.
   A. 1,832 dynes·sec/cm^{-5}
   B. 622 dynes·sec/cm^{-5}
   C. 1,083 dynes·sec/cm^{-5}
   D. 1,274 dynes·sec/cm^{-5}
4. Calculate the SVRI.
   A. 3,200 dynes·sec/cm^{-5}/m^2
   B. 1,020 dynes·sec/cm^{-5}/m^2
   C. 2,195 dynes·sec/cm^{-5}/m^2
   D. 1,953 dynes·sec/cm^{-5}/m^2
5. What is the normal range for the SVRI?

   A. 800 to 1,200 dynes·sec/cm^{-5}/m^2
   B. 250 to 680 dynes·sec/cm^{-5}/m^2
   C. 1,970 to 2,390 dynes·sec/cm^{-5}/m^2
   D. 1,200 to 1,500 dynes·sec/cm^{-5}/m^2
6. The LVSWI should be used instead of the PAWP in assessing left ventricular function in cases of
   A. hypovolemia
   B. congestive heart failure
   C. decreased compliance
   D. hypervolemia

Answers: 1. B, 2. B, 3. C, 4. D, 5. C, 6. C

 POSTTEST

1. IV fluids can be infused through which port on the PA catheter?
   A. proximal port
   B. distal port
   C. yellow port
   D. balloon port
2. A PA catheter is an invasive diagnostic tool used to
   A. determine right and left heart pressures
   B. determine CO
   C. sample Svo$_2$
   D. all of the above
3. In viewing a CO curve, a large curve indicates
   A. a normal CO
   B. a high CO
   C. a low CO
   D. an error in technique
4. CI is more specific than CO because
   A. CI is a direct measurement instead of an estimate
   B. CI takes the size of the patient into consideration
   C. CO can be affected by afterload
   D. CO depends on patient position
5. The hemodynamic measurement for right heart preload is
   A. PAWP
   B. PAS pressure
   C. RAP
   D. CO
6. Which of the following conditions cause a decreased RAP?
   A. sepsis
   B. cardiac tamponade
   C. pulmonary hypertension
   D. pulmonic valve stenosis

7. It is important to recognize a right ventricular waveform because
   A. a catheter in the right ventricle can induce dysrhythmias
   B. this pattern is the one that should be monitored constantly
   C. this is the best indicator of hemodynamic status
   D. this is the patient's pulmonary end diastolic pressure
8. The nurse notes an RV waveform on the bedside monitor during routine hemodynamic monitoring. Which of the following actions should the nurse institute?
   A. nothing; this is normal
   B. assess for altered CO
   C. auscultate lungs for crackles
   D. notify the physician immediately
9. A normal PA pressure waveform demonstrates which of the following characteristics?
   A. a soft undulating pattern
   B. a steep upstroke followed by a sharp downstroke
   C. a sharply notched upstroke with a steep downstroke
   D. a steep upstroke and a downstroke distinguished by a dicrotic notch
10. All of the following clinical findings are associated with elevated PAD pressures EXCEPT
    A. dyspnea
    B. S3 or S4
    C. crackles
    D. flat neck veins
11. PAWP is the hemodynamic measurement for
    A. right ventricular preload
    B. right ventricular contractility
    C. left ventricular preload
    D. left ventricular afterload

12. The nurse would expect the primary intervention for a symptomatic patient with a PAWP of 3 mm Hg to be
    A. fluid restriction
    B. decreasing preload
    C. volume replacement
    D. decreasing afterload
13. The dicrotic notch on the systemic arterial pressure waveform represents
    A. left ventricular end-diastolic volume
    B. right ventricular end-diastolic volume
    C. beginning of ventricular diastole
    D. beginning of ventricular systole
14. To overcome the arterial pressure and prevent blood from backing up into the pressure tubing, the pressure bag is inflated to
    A. 90 mm Hg
    B. 100 mm Hg
    C. 200 mm Hg
    D. 300 mm Hg
15. To assess the afterload status of the left ventricle, one should
    A. calculate the pulmonary vascular resistance
    B. calculate the systemic vascular resistance
    C. determine the mean arterial pressure
    D. determine the CI
16. Which is the most important parameter to follow when titrating inotropic drugs on a patient with poor left ventricular function?
    A. CO
    B. CI
    C. MAP
    D. RAP

POSTTEST ANSWERS

Question	Answer	Section	Question	Answer	Section
1	A	One	9	D	Five
2	D	One	10	D	Five
3	C	Two	11	C	Six
4	B	Two	12	C	Six
5	C	Three	13	C	Seven
6	A	Three	14	D	Seven
7	A	Four	15	B	Eight
8	D	Four	16	B	Eight

REFERENCES

Adams, K. L. (2004). Hemodynamic assessment: The physiologic basis for turning data into clinical information. *AACN Clinical Issues, 15,* 534–546.

Ahrens, T. (1999). Hemodynamic monitoring. *Critical Care Nursing Clinics of North America, 11*(1), 19–31.

Ahrens, T., & Shallom, L. (2001). Comparison of pulmonary artery and central venous pressure waveform measurements via digital and graphic measurement methods. *Heart and Lung, 30,* 26–38.

Ahrens, T., & Sona, C. (2003). Capnography application in *acute* and critical care. *AACN Clinical Issues, 14,* 123–132.

Bridges, E. J., & Middleton, R. (1997). Direct arterial versus oscillometric monitoring of blood pressure: Stop comparing and pick one. *Critical Care Nurse, 17*(3), 58–72.

Daily, E. K. (2001). Hemodynamic waveform analysis. *Journal of Cardiovascular Nursing, 15*(2), 6–12.

Darvic, G. O. (2002). *Hemodynamic monitoring: Invasive and non-invasive clinical application* (3rd ed.). Philadelphia: W. B. Saunders.

Gould, K., Hartigan, C., & Keane, S. (2001). Cardiac output measurement techniques. In D. Lynn-McHale & K. Carlson (Eds.), *AACN procedure manual for critical care* (4th ed., pp. 389–401). Philadelphia: W. B. Saunders.

Keckeisen, M., Chulay, M., & Gawlinski, A. (1998). Pulmonary artery pressure monitoring. In *AACN's protocols for practice: Hemodynamic monitoring series.* Aliso Viejo, CA: AACN.

O'Malley, P., Smith, B., Hamlin, R., et al. (2000). A comparison of bolus versus continuous cardiac output in an experimental model of heart failure. *Critical Care Medicine, 28,* 1985–1990.

Ott, K., Johnson, K. L., & Ahrens, T. S. (2001). New technologies in the assessment of hemodynamic parameters. *Journal of Cardiovascular Nursing, 15*(2), 41–55.

Quaal, S. J. (2001). Improving the accuracy of pulmonary artery catheter measurements. *Journal of Cardiovascular Nursing, 15*(2), 71–82.

Electrocardiographic Monitoring and Conduction Abnormalities

Ted Rigney

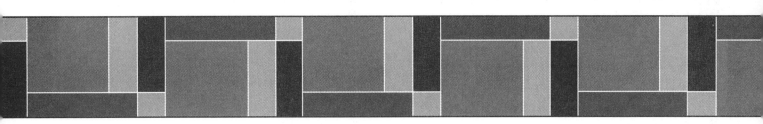

OBJECTIVES Following completion of this module, the learner will be able to

1. Describe the membrane permeability changes of cardiac cells.

2. Discuss the relationship between membrane permeability and serum electrolyte levels.

3. Describe the cardiac conduction system and a normal ECG complex and state nursing responsibilities for a patient requiring cardiac monitoring.

4. Identify a system for interpreting ECG patterns.

5. Identify factors that place a person at risk for developing dysrhythmias.

6. Identify common dysrhythmias arising from the sinoatrial (SA) node and describe the treatment of these dysrhythmias.

7. Identify basic atrial dysrhythmias and describe the treatment of these dysrhythmias.

8. Identify common junctional dysrhythmias and describe the treatment of these dysrhythmias.

9. Identify common ventricular dysrhythmias and describe the treatment of these dysrhythmias.

10. Compare and contrast atrial and ventricular premature beats, identify their origins, and describe the treatment of these premature beats.

11. Differentiate three conduction abnormalities and describe treatment for cure.

12. Identify common drug classifications used in treating cardiac dysrhythmias and state the nursing responsibilities associated with administration of these agents.

13. Discuss nursing responsibilities associated with cardioversion and defibrillation.

14. Discuss indications for pacemaker and implantable cardioverter/defibrillation therapy, types of devices, and nursing implications for the patient receiving these therapies.

This self-study module is written at the core knowledge level for individuals who provide nursing care for acutely ill patients. The module translates the cardiac cycle in order to promote understanding of the implications of dysrhythmias. Guidelines for electrocardiogram (ECG) interpretations are included. The module does not attempt to discuss every potential dysrhythmia a nurse may encounter in the clinical setting. Instead, it provides a systematic approach to understanding automaticity and conduction that can then be applied to practical situations. The learner must go to outside sources for additional experience in ECG interpretation. Section One discusses automaticity. Sections Two and Three include guidelines for interpreting ECG patterns and normal sinus rhythm. Section Four addresses conditions that produce dysrhythmias. Sections Five through Ten cover basic dysrhythmias. Sections Eleven and Twelve discuss basic pharmacology and electrical treatment of common dysrhythmias. Each section includes a set of review questions to help the learner evaluate his or her understanding of the section's content before moving on to the next section. All Section Reviews and the module Pretest and Posttest include answers. It is suggested that the learner review those concepts answered incorrectly in the review questions before proceeding to the next section.

PRETEST

1. The isoelectric line on the ECG pattern represents
   A. depolarization of cardiac cells
   B. an ectopic pacemaker
   C. the resting membrane potential
   D. cellular influx of potassium

2. Which of the following statements reflects events during the relative refractory period?
   A. there is a temporary decrease in excitability
   B. the cell can respond to a stimulus of greater intensity than normal
   C. depolarization occurs
   D. a flux of negatively charged ions out of the cell occurs

3. Which of the following patients may need the skin prepared in order to obtain a good connection for the monitoring electrode?
   A. dyspneic patient
   B. diaphoretic patient
   C. obese patient
   D. elderly patient

4. *P* waves in sinus rhythms
   A. are always positively deflected
   B. should precede the *QRS* complex
   C. are 0.08 second in length
   D. are followed immediately by a *T* wave

5. You measure the *PR* interval. It is 0.24 seconds. This represents
   A. a normal *PR* interval
   B. atrial fibrillation
   C. a conduction delay
   D. delayed conduction in the ventricles

6. Hyperkalemia produces
   A. tall, peaked *T* waves
   B. absent *T* waves
   C. flat *T* waves
   D. inverted *T* waves

7. A decrease in stroke volume produces
   A. bradycardia
   B. tachycardia
   C. atrial fibrillation
   D. ventricular fibrillation

8. In a fast-paced rhythm (greater than 100 beats per minute), which of the following is the most plausible?
   A. the parasympathetic nervous system is stimulated
   B. the atrioventicular (AV) node is pacing the heart
   C. ventricular conduction is slowed
   D. decreased cardiac output occurs

9. Sinus dysrhythmia is usually
   A. a warning sign of impending heart failure
   B. life threatening
   C. harmless
   D. related to chronic coronary problems

10. Supraventricular tachycardia is
    A. produced by a ventricular pacemaker
    B. the result of delayed atrioventricular conduction
    C. produced by a cell functioning as a pacemaker above the ventricles
    D. associated with sympathetic response to pain

11. The ventricular rate in atrial flutter is
    A. greater than 250 beats per minute
    B. dependent on the number of impulses that pass through the AV node
    C. regular
    D. greater than the atrial rate

12. Junctional rhythms commonly occur
    A. as a protective mechanism in sinoatrial (SA) node abnormalities
    B. in response to ventricular escape beats
    C. as an indication of reperfusion in thrombolytic therapy
    D. when a pacing device fails to capture

13. All of the following circumstances warrant close observation of premature ventricular contractions (PVCs) EXCEPT
    A. 2 to 5 PVCs per minute
    B. PVCs occurring in couplets
    C. multifocal PVCs
    D. four PVCs in a row

14. The treatment of choice for premature ventricular contractions (PVCs) is
    A. defibrillation
    B. cardioversion
    C. lidocaine
    D. amiodarone

15. In ventricular tachycardia, the
    A. *P* waves are inverted
    B. *QRS* complexes are less than 0.12 second
    C. R–R interval is irregular
    D. *P* waves are usually buried in the *QRS* complexes

16. Which of the following dysrhythmias is the most common cause of sudden death?
    A. ventricular defibrillation
    B. ventricular tachycardia
    C. atrial fibrillation
    D. atrial flutter

17. The difference between type I and type II second-degree AV block is
    A. dropping of a *QRS* complex
    B. rate of the rhythm
    C. progressive lengthening of the *PR* interval
    D. widening of the *QRS* complex

18. A patient with first-degree AV block who becomes hypotensive may be treated with
    A. dopamine
    B. cardioversion
    C. atropine
    D. isoproterenol

19. Which of the following anti-arrhythmic categories are contraindicated in patients with asthma?
   A. class I
   B. class II
   C. class III
   D. class IV

20. The typical first voltage used in cardioversion is
   A. 50 joules
   B. 200 joules
   C. 300 joules
   D. 400 joules

21. Failure to sense means that an artificial pacing device is
   A. not producing depolarization
   B. competing with the patient's own rhythm

   C. allowing ectopic beats to occur
   D. producing conduction delays

22. A pacemaker is inserted to pace the ventricles. In the ECG you would note a spike
   A. before the *QRS*
   B. during the *QRS*
   C. after the *QRS*
   D. before the *P* wave

Pretest Answers: 1. C, 2. B, 3. B, 4. B, 5. C, 6. A, 7. B, 8. D, 9. C, 10. C, 11. B, 12. A, 13. A, 14. C, 15. D, 16. A, 17. C, 18. C, 19. B, 20. A, 21. B, 22. A

GLOSSARY

absolute refractory period   The period after an action potential when a stimulus cannot produce a second action potential no matter how strong the stimulus is.

action potential   Signal produced from rapid change in membrane permeability that is transmitted from one part of the nerve or muscle cell to another.

automaticity   Ability to initiate an impulse.

bigeminy   A cardiac rhythm of one SA node–generated beat followed by one premature ventricular contraction.

cardioversion   A synchronized direct current electrical countershock that depolarizes all the cells simultaneously, allowing the SA node to resume the pacemaker role.

contractility   The ability of a muscle to shorten when stimulated; in particular, the force of myocardial contraction.

defibrillation   An unsynchronized direct current electrical countershock that depolarizes all the cells simultaneously, allowing the SA node to resume the pacemaker role.

ejection fraction (EF)   Ratio of stroke volume to volume of blood remaining in the ventricle at the end of diastole.

excitability   Ability to respond to an impulse.

isoelectric   Occurs when the muscle is completely polarized or depolarized; no potential is recorded on the ECG.

plateau phase   Part of the repolarization when the calcium channels open to allow movement of calcium into the cell to help maintain the cell in a depolarized state.

relative refractory period   The period after an action potential when a stimulus can produce a second action potential if the stimulus is greater than the threshold level.

repolarization   Return of the cellular membrane to its resting membrane potential.

resting membrane potential   Point at the end of repolarization when the membrane is relatively permeable to potassium but is almost impermeable to sodium; thus, intracellular concentration of potassium is greater than extracellular concentration.

sarcolemma   Cell membrane of a muscle fiber.

slow response action potential   Action potential of a pacemaker cell characterized by the slow movement of sodium into the cell because the sarcolemma is permeable to sodium ions.

stroke volume   Amount of blood ejected with each beat.

supranormal period   The period after an action potential during which a stimulus that is slightly less than normal can precipitate another action potential.

trigeminy   A cardiac rhythm of two SA node–generated beats followed by one premature ventricular contraction.

ABBREVIATIONS

AV node	Atrioventricular node	**ICD**	Implantable cardioverter/defibrillator
BBB	Bundle branch block	**PAC**	Premature atrial contraction
Bpm	Beats per minute	**PVC**	Premature ventricular contraction
CO	Cardiac output	**SA node**	Sinoatrial node
ECG	Electrocardiogram	**SV**	Stroke volume
EF	Ejection fraction	**SVT**	Supraventricular tachycardia
J	Joules	**VT**	Ventricular tachycardia

SECTION ONE: Membrane Permeability

At the completion of this section, the learner will be able to explain briefly membrane permeability changes in cardiac cells and discuss the relationship between membrane permeability and serum electrolyte levels.

The resting membrane potential of cardiac cells is represented by an **isoelectric** line on the ECG pattern. There is no deflection because there is no movement of ions across the **sarcolemma.** Normally, the intracellular concentration of potassium is greater than the extracellular concentration. The concentration of sodium ions is greater extracellularly. Calcium also has a much higher concentration outside of the cell. The intracellular potential becomes increasingly negative because potassium diffuses out of the cell. In addition, proteins and phosphates remain inside the cell, and they are negatively charged.

There are five phases of an **action potential** as shown in Figure 10–1: depolarization (phase 0), early repolarization (phase 1), plateau phase (phase 2), repolarization (phase 3), and resting membrane potential (phase 4). During depolarization, the cell is almost impermeable to sodium unless a stimulus oc-

curs. This stimulus may be electrical in origin, such as the firing of the sinoatrial (SA) node or defibrillation. Chemical changes also may precipitate depolarization. Hypoxia and its accompanying respiratory acidosis as well as pharmaceutical agents (e.g., sodium bicarbonate) may serve as chemical stimuli. In depolarization, more sodium moves into the cell through the fast sodium channels and creates a fast response action potential. The inside of the cell becomes positively charged.

The process of **repolarization** takes place over phases 1, 2, and 3 (Fig. 10–1). In early repolarization, sodium channels close. During the **plateau phase,** calcium channels open. These channels are slow in relation to the preceding sodium channels. The influx of calcium maintains the positive charge (depolarization) a little longer. Chemical blockage of the channels is used to treat cardiac abnormalities. In phase 3, repolarization, potassium moves back into the cell to create the original electrochemical gradient.

During the **resting membrane potential** phase (phase 4), repolarization is completed, and the original electrochemical gradient is in place. The cell is ready to be depolarized again. The **absolute refractory period** begins in phase 0 and lasts until the midpoint of phase 3. During this period, the cell cannot

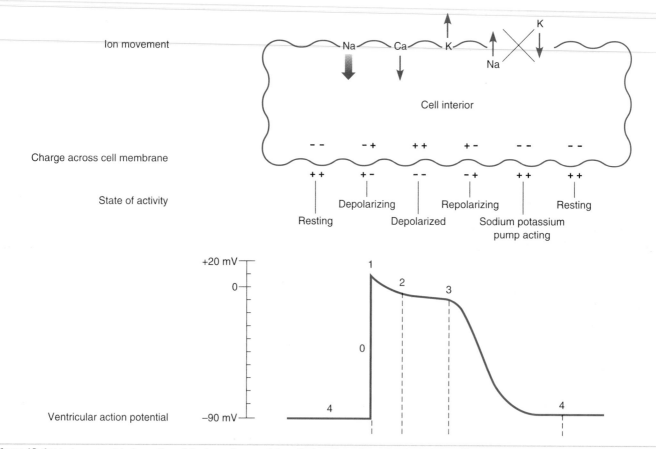

Figure 10–1 ■ Action potential of a cardiac cell. In the resting state (phase 4), the cell membrane is polarized: the cell's interior has a negative charge compared to that of extracellular fluid. On depolarization (phase 0), sodium ions diffuse rapidly across the cell membrane into the cell, and calcium channels open. In the fully depolarized state (phase 1), the cell's interior has a net positive charge compared to its exterior. During the plateau period (phase 2), calcium moves into the cell and potassium diffusion slows, prolonging the action potential. In phase 3, calcium channels close, the sodium-potassium pump removes sodium from the cell, and the cell membrane again becomes polarized with a net negative charge.

respond to another stimulus regardless of the strength of the stimulus. The **relative refractory period** begins at the midpoint of phase 3 and lasts until the beginning of phase 4. A stronger than normal stimulus can produce depolarization. During the **supranormal period** (phase 4), a weaker than normal stimulus can produce depolarization. A common example of a stimulus producing depolarization during the supranormal or relative refractory period is premature atrial and ventricular beats. These are discussed later in the module. Table 10–1 summarizes the phases of the action potential. The pacemaker cells in the sinoatrial node have a constant sodium influx; thus, they slowly depolarize at a steady rate until threshold is reached and an action potential created, referred to as **automaticity.** This impulse is then transmitted to the surrounding myocardium (Bond, 2000).

In summary, it is helpful to remember that sodium, calcium, and potassium always are intracellular and extracellular

TABLE 10–1 Phases of an Action Potential

Phase 0	Depolarization	Movement of sodium into cell (fast channels open)
Phase 1	Early repolarization	Closure of fast sodium channels
Phase 2	Plateau	Calcium moves into cell (slow channels open)
Phase 3	Repolarization	Potassium moves into cell
Phase 4	Resting membrane potential	Electrochemical gradient returned to potential normal Sarcolemma almost impermeable to sodium

electrolytes. The total of these electrolytes remains the same. The action potential changes where the total is distributed, at the location of the ions. Figure 10–2 depicts the ion changes throughout the action potential.

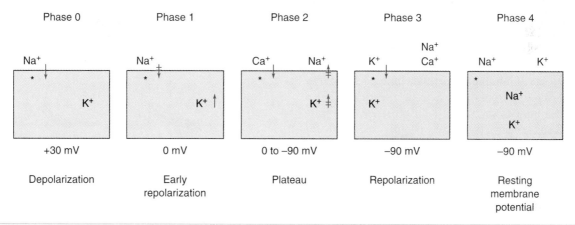

Figure 10–2 ■ Membrane permeability changes in nonpacemaker myocardial cells. Cell permeability changes throughout depolarization and repolarization. * = protein⁻, phosphate⁻; ↑↓ = rapid; ≠ = slow.

SECTION ONE REVIEW

1. Depolarization may occur in direct response to all of the following EXCEPT
   A. chemical stimuli
   B. acidosis
   C. defibrillation
   D. hyperglycemia
2. Potassium is located primarily
   A. intracellularly
   B. in skeletal muscle
   C. extracellularly
   D. in cardiac muscle
3. During the relative refractory period
   A. a larger-than-normal stimulus occurs
   B. the SA node fires

   C. depolarization may occur
   D. the cardiac cell is not able to be stimulated
4. The three major electrolytes associated with automaticity are
   A. sodium, potassium, and calcium
   B. potassium, glucose, and sodium
   C. calcium, phosphate, and proteins
   D. potassium, calcium, and phosphate
5. The movement of calcium into the cell promotes
   A. depolarization
   B. repolarization
   C. the refractory period
   D. closure of the slow channels

Answers: 1. D, 2. A, 3. C, 4. A, 5. A

SECTION TWO: Cardiac Conduction

At the completion of this section, the learner will be able to describe the cardiac conduction system, the normal ECG complex, and nursing responsibilities for a patient requiring cardiac monitoring.

There are two types of myocardial cells: working cells and pacemaker cells. Pacemaker cells have a **slow response action potential.** The resting membrane potential of pacemaker cells is unstable, and the cell membrane is somewhat permeable to sodium. The slow diffusion of sodium into the cell precipitates depolarization without a preceding impulse. Only pacemaker cells possess automaticity, or the ability to initiate an impulse. Conversely, the working cells have a stable resting membrane potential. In order for depolarization to occur, a stimulus must be present. Working cells are responsible for **contractility.** Both working and pacemaker cells have the ability to respond to stimuli (**excitability**) and regularity (rhythmicity) and to conduct impulses.

The SA node is the pacemaker of the heart because it controls the heart rate normally between 60 and 100 beats per minute (bpm). When abnormalities occur with the firing of the SA node, another cardiac cell will discharge. An ectopic pacemaker is a new site of impulse formation within the heart. The impulse is transmitted from the atria to the ventricles along a cardiac conduction pathway (Fig. 10–3). Myocardial contraction occurs when the ventricular muscle is stimulated. The combined events of depolarization and repolarization comprise the electrical phases of the cardiac cycle.

The normal ECG complex consists of several components (Fig. 10–4). The *P* wave indicates atrial depolarization, stimulated by the firing of the SA node. The *PR* interval depicts atrial conduction of the impulse, through the atrioventricular (AV) node to the ventricles. The normal length of the *PR* interval is 0.12 to 0.20 second. A longer *PR* interval suggests a conduction delay, usually in the area of the AV node.

The *QRS* complex reflects ventricular depolarization and atrial repolarization. Atrial repolarization is overpowered by ventricular depolarization because the ventricular muscle mass is larger than that of the atria. Therefore, atrial repolarization is not seen on the ECG. *QRS* complexes may be of various sizes and configurations. Figure 10–5 illustrates common *QRS* configurations. The *QRS* segment is 0.10 second or less in length. A prolonged *QRS* complex indicates abnormal impulse conduction through the ventricles.

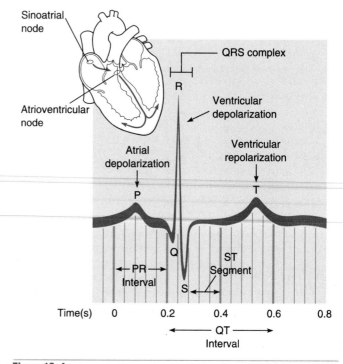

Figure 10–4 ■ Normal ECG waveform and intervals.

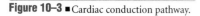

Figure 10–3 ■ Cardiac conduction pathway.

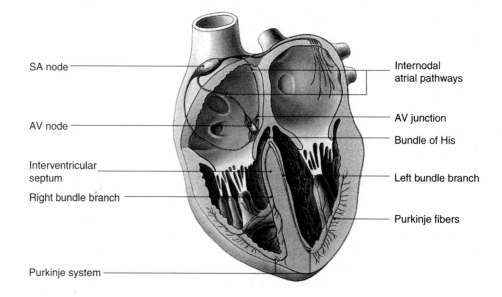

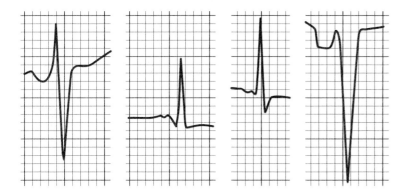

Figure 10–5 ■ Examples of different types of *QRS* complexes. *(From Hutchisson, B., Cossey, S., & Wheeler, R. M. [2003]. Basic electrocardiogram interpretation for perioperative nurses. AORN Journal 78(4):585. Copyright 2000–2004 by the AORN Journal. Reprinted with permission of the author.)*

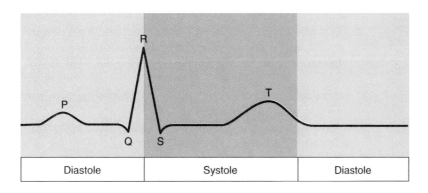

Figure 10–6 ■ Relationship between ECG and cardiac cycle (diastole and systole). *(From Dracup, K. [1995]. Meltzer's intensive coronary care: A manual for nurses [5th ed., p. 127]. East Norwalk, CT: Appleton & Lange)*

The *ST* segment demonstrates ventricular conduction. It represents the completion of ventricular depolarization and the beginning of ventricular repolarization. The segment should be isoelectric, with no deflections present because positive and negative charges are balanced. Deflections in the *ST* segment usually indicate ventricular muscle injury. The *T* wave depicts ventricular repolarization (Fig. 10–4). *T* waves also are affected by ventricular muscle injury because of interference with repolarization. An example of a clinical condition with potential ventricular muscle injury is acute myocardial infarction.

The *QT* interval represents ventricular depolarization and repolarization (Fig. 10–4). It is measured from the beginning of the *QRS* complex to the end of the *T* wave. The *QT* interval is usually less than 0.40 second in length, depending on heart rate. The *QT* interval is less than half the R–R interval. As heart rate increases, the *QT* interval shortens. If the heart rate decreases, the *QT* interval lengthens.

Electrical transmission is usually connected with mechanical events of the heart, although certain conditions (prolonged hypoxia, acidosis) can cause depolarization without mechanical contraction. Diastole occurs during atrial depolarization and at the end of ventricular repolarization. This is depicted by the end of the *T* wave to the *R* wave on the ECG. During diastole the aortic and pulmonic valves close and the mitral and tricuspid valves open, allowing ventricle filling. Systole begins at the peak of the *QRS* complex (ventricular depolarization) and continues to the end of the *T* wave (ventricular repolarization). During systole, the ventricles contract. The increased intraventricular pressure causes the mitral and tricuspid valves to close. The intraventricular pressure exceeds the pressure within the aorta and pulmonary arteries, causing the pulmonic and aortic valves to open. The ventricles eject blood (known as the stroke volume) into the aorta and pulmonary arteries. **Stroke volume** is the amount of blood ejected from the ventricle with each beat. The **ejection fraction (EF)** is the ratio of the stroke volume to the volume of blood remaining in the ventricle at the end of diastole. Normal left ventricular EF should be greater than 55 percent and the normal is 65 percent (Bond, 2000).

Abnormalities in ventricle depolarization decrease stroke volume and EF. This relationship helps explain why cardiac output is affected when a dysrhythmia occurs. Figure 10–6 illustrates the relationship between the ECG and the cardiac cycle.

Nursing Care of a Patient Requiring Cardiac Monitoring

Cardiac monitoring is used whenever it is necessary to continuously monitor a patient's heart rate and rhythm. Although there are many types of monitors, all systems use three basic components: an oscilloscope display system, a monitoring cable, and electrodes. Electrodes are placed on the patient's chest to record electrical activity generated by the heart (Fig. 10–7). The electrical signal is then carried by the monitoring cable to an oscilloscope where it is displayed. In telemetry monitoring, no direct wire connection is used between the patient and the cardiac monitor. Electrodes are connected by a short monitoring cable to a small transmitter that is kept with the patient.

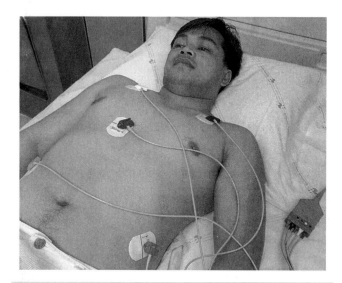

Figure 10–7 ■ Placement of electrodes.

All cardiac monitors use lead systems to record cardiac electrical activity. A lead system is composed of three electrodes: one positive, one negative, and one ground. Each lead system looks at cardiac depolarization from a different location and thus produces *P* waves and *QRS* complexes of varying configuration.

Although a minimum of three electrodes is required, often five electrodes are used, either to monitor two leads simultaneously or to allow selection of different leads. Typical placement of five electrodes in a multilead system is shown in Figure 10–7. Accurate lead placement is essential for accurate cardiac monitoring. Lead placement is verified at the beginning of each shift.

There are several nursing actions for a patient requiring cardiac monitoring. The chest wall is shaved and treated with an adhesive (i.e., tincture of benzoin, skin preparation) before placement of the electrodes, especially for individuals who are diaphoretic. This will help ensure a good connection. Sites are rotated every 24 to 48 hours to prevent skin breakdown. Clean gel residue from previous sites and document skin condition under the pads. The sensitivity knob of the cardiac monitor may need to be adjusted to view complexes. Alarms on the monitor are set typically at 20 bpm higher and lower than the patient's baseline rates. The alarms are left on and audible to the nurse. An ECG strip is recorded and placed in the nursing record on a regular basis per unit protocol, when the cardiac rhythm changes, or with any change in patient condition. Each strip is analyzed using the six step process outlined in Section Three.

Patients need to know why they require cardiac monitoring. They need reassurance that they are protected from electric shocks from the equipment. They need to know that the alarms can sound as a result of patient movement and other factors, in addition to cardiac abnormalities.

In summary, the ECG reflects the cardiac conduction pathway. Abnormalities in conduction appear on the ECG. The cardiac cycle depends on proper electrical transmission and conduction in order to maintain an adequate cardiac output. The normal ECG (normal sinus rhythm [NSR]) has a rate between 60 and 100 bpm. The SA node paces the rhythm (*P* wave), and the impulse is transmitted to the ventricles within 0.20 second (*PR* interval). The ventricles depolarize, representing contraction or systole, within 0.10 second. The complete sequence of ventricular events occurs within 0.40 second (*QT* interval). The nursing care of a patient who requires cardiac monitoring includes decreasing the patient's fear and increasing his or her knowledge regarding the procedure.

SECTION TWO REVIEW

1. Abnormalities in the firing of the SA node usually
   A. result in cardiac arrest
   B. result in the discharging of another pacemaker cell
   C. produce tachydysrhythmias
   D. result in heart blocks
2. A *PR* interval greater than 0.20 second
   A. is normal
   B. indicates a pacemaker other than the SA node is firing
   C. indicates a delay in conduction
   D. is too fast to maintain adequate cardiac output
3. Atrial repolarization is reflected in the
   A. *P* wave
   B. *PR* interval
   C. *T* wave
   D. *QRS* complex
4. All cardiac monitors use lead systems to record
   A. cardiac electrical activity
   B. cardiac output
   C. stroke volume
   D. the cardiac cycle
5. The chest wall is shaved and treated with an adhesive for individuals who are
   A. elderly
   B. diabetic
   C. hairy
   D. diaphoretic

Answers: 1. B, 2. C, 3. D, 4. A, 5. D

SECTION THREE: Interpretation Guidelines

At the completion of this section, the learner will be able to identify a system for interpreting ECG patterns.

The ECG is printed on graph paper (Fig. 10–8). Each small block of the graph paper is equal to 1 mm, or 0.04 second, on the horizontal axis. The horizontal axis of the graph paper represents time. The vertical axis of the graph paper represents voltage. Each small block is equivalent to 1 mm (0.1 mV) on the vertical axis. Each large box is 5 mm (0.5 mV). For the purposes of basic ECG interpretation, time is the most important factor to consider. Because each small block equals 0.04 second, a large block, composed of five small blocks, equals 0.20 second. Five large blocks represent 1 second. There are six steps to follow when interpreting an ECG:

1. Measure the heart rate.
2. Examine the R–R interval.
3. Examine the *P* wave.
4. Measure the *PR* interval.
5. Determine if each *P* wave is followed by a *QRS* complex.
6. Examine the *QRS* complex.

Measure rate. There are two methods commonly used to determine heart rate by visual examination of an ECG strip. These methods are used only when the rate is regular. Using the first method, the number of 0.20-second boxes are counted between two *R* waves and divided into 300. The second method is based on a 6-second cardiac strip. ECG paper is marked at the top margin in 3-second intervals. *QRS* complexes in a 6-second strip (30 large blocks) are multiplied by 10 to get the heart rate by minute (6 × 10 = 60 seconds). Figure 10–9 demonstrates these methods of rate calculation.

Examine the R–R interval. Next, the *R* waves are examined. If the *R* waves appear in regular intervals (are constant), the rhythm is a regular rhythm. If the *R* waves do not occur in a regular pattern, a dysrhythmia is present.

Examine the *P* wave. Normally, *P* waves precede each *QRS* complex. If the SA node is not serving as pacemaker and a cell other than the SA node is serving as the pacemaker, *P* waves

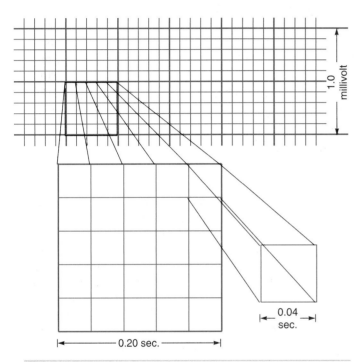

Figure 10–8 ■ ECG paper is a graph divided into millimeter squares. Time is measured on the horizontal axis. With a paper speed of 25 mm/sec, each small (millimeter) box equals 0.04 second and each larger (5-mm) box equals 0.2 second. The amplitude of any wave is measured on the vertical axis in millimeters.

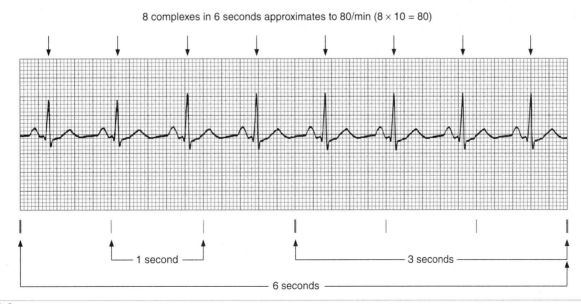

8 complexes in 6 seconds approximates to 80/min (8 × 10 = 80)

Figure 10–9 ■ Calculation of heart rate.

have an altered shape or are absent. Cardiac cells in the area of the AV node pace the heart at a rate of 40 to 60 bpm. Pacemaker cells in the Purkinje fibers and ventricles pace at a rate less than 40 bpm. Generally, if the atria are discharging chaotically, the rate is greater than 60 bpm. If the atria are not discharging and the pacer is outside the SA node, the rate is usually less than 60 bpm.

Measure the *PR* interval. The next step in ECG interpretation is to measure the *PR* interval. If it is greater than 0.20 second in length, a delay in conduction is present.

P waves precede each *QRS*. Next, determine if each *P* wave is followed by a *QRS* complex. If a prolonged *PR* interval (greater than 0.20 second) is followed by a *QRS* complex, a first-degree heart block is present (Section Ten). If *P* waves are present but they are not followed consistently by a *QRS* complex, a second- or third-degree heart block (Section Ten) is present.

Examine the *QRS* complex. The final step involves examination of the *QRS* complexes. The complex should be 0.10 second or less in length unless there is a delay in the impulse reaching the ventricles. A widened *QRS* complex means delayed conduction through the bundle branches, abnormal conduction within the ventricles, or early activation of the ventricles through a bypass route.

Figure 10–10 illustrates the application of the principles discussed in this section. The system outlined in this section should provide a consistent and comprehensive approach to ECG interpretation.

In summary, there are six steps to follow when interpreting an ECG: (1) Measure the heart rate; (2) Examine the R–R interval—they should be regular; (3) Examine the *P* waves—they should look alike; (4) Measure the *PR* interval—it should be less than 0.20 seconds; (5) Determine if each *P* wave is followed by a *QRS*; (6) Examine the *QRS* complexes—they should be less than 0.10 seconds.

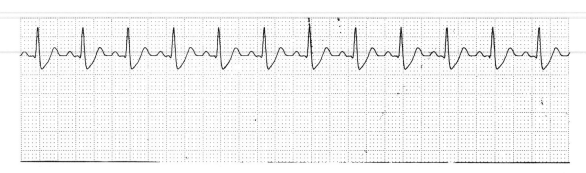

Figure 10–10 ■ Interpretation of ECG using six-step process.
1. Measure the rate.
2. Examine the R-R interval. The interval is regular; therefore, the rhythm is regular.
3. Examine the *P* wave. The *P* waves are the same configuration.
4. Measure the *PR* interval. The interval is constant and measures 4 small boxes (0.4) or 0.16 seconds.
5. Check to see whether the *P* waves are followed by a *QRS* complex. *P* waves are followed by *QRS* complex.
6. Examine the *QRS* complex. The complexes are the same configuration and measure 2 small boxes (0.04) or 0.08 seconds.

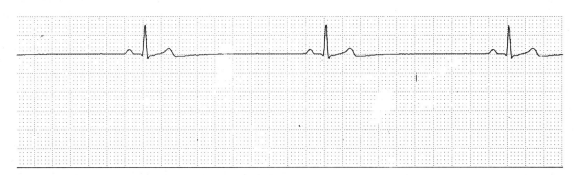

Figure 10–11 ■ Section Three Review: Review questions 1 & 2.

SECTION THREE REVIEW

1. Using the large-block method (0.20 second), the heart rate in the ECG in Figure 10–11 is
   A. 35 bpm
   B. 30 bpm
   C. 40 bpm
   D. 45 bpm
2. Measure the *PR* interval in Figure 10–11.
   A. 0.04 second
   B. 0.12 second
   C. 0.20 second
   D. 0.28 second
3. Using the number of *QRS* complexes in the 6-second strip method, the heart rate in the ECG in Figure 10–12 is
   A. 120 bpm
   B. 140 bpm

C. 130 bpm
D. 70 bpm
4. Measure the *QRS* complex in Figure 10–12.
   A. 0.08 second
   B. 0.12 second
   C. 0.20 second
   D. 0.28 second
5. The *QRS* complex should
   A. be greater than 0.12 second
   B. precede the *P* wave
   C. differ in configuration
   D. precede the *T* wave

Answers: 1. B, 2. C, 3. A, 4. A, 5. D

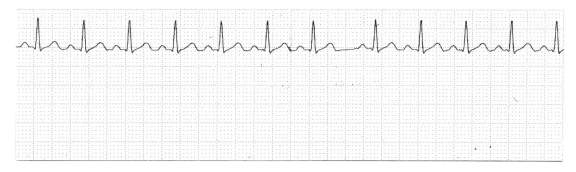

Figure 10–12 ■ Section Three Review: Questions 3 & 4.

SECTION FOUR: Risk Factors for Development of Dysrhythmias

At the completion of this section, the learner will be able to identify factors that place a person at risk for developing dysrhythmias.

An alteration in myocardial tissue perfusion as a result of coronary artery disease predisposes the development of dysrhythmias (abnormal rhythms) because of potential myocardial ischemia. The ventricles are not able to depolarize as effectively (*QRS* complex), and repolarization is inefficient (*T* wave). Thus, abnormal ventricular beats or blocks in conduction occur.

Tachydysrhythmias, rapid abnormal rhythms, are noted in patients with a fluid volume deficit. The heart rate increases in response to a diminished stroke volume. Fluid volume overload can result in ventricular enlargement and decreased contractility. Premature beats, cardiac conduction blocks, and abnormalities in heart rate can appear in response to excess fluid volume.

Electrolyte abnormalities increase the risk of developing dysrhythmias. Hypokalemia decreases the amount of positive ions available to produce depolarization. Depolarization becomes more difficult and repolarization is extended. Therefore, the *PR* interval is longer, and the *T* wave is flat. The *QT* interval lengthens. An extra wave follows the *T* wave (*U* wave). Bradydysrhythmias and conduction blocks are common. Premature ventricular contractions (PVCs) can occur. Hyperkalemia produces easier depolarization and short repolarization. Tall, peaked *T* waves are present. The *QT* interval shortens. Eventually the cell becomes too positive to respond and depolarize, and asystole (no heartbeat) occurs. Before asystole, the *PR* interval lengthens, and the *QRS* complex widens.

Other electrolyte imbalances can potentiate the development of dysrhythmias. Increased levels of calcium strengthen contractility and shorten ventricular repolarization, shortening the QT interval. Hypocalcemia prolongs the QT interval (Jacobson, 2000). Decreased levels of magnesium increase the irritability of the nervous system and can produce dysrhythmias. Prominent U waves and a flattening of the T wave can occur, as well as prolongation of the QT interval (Jacobson, 2000). Increased levels of magnesium can produce a prolonged PR interval; wide QRS complexes; bradycardia; and tall, peaked T waves.

Hypothermia decreases the electrical activity of the heart. Thus, bradycardia (rate of less than 60 bpm), prolongation of the PR and QT intervals, and wide QRS complexes may occur.

In summary, a person may be at risk for developing cardiac dysrhythmias if an alteration in tissue perfusion, fluid volume, electrolyte values, or temperature is present.

SECTION FOUR REVIEW

1. An alteration in myocardial tissue perfusion predisposes the development of dysrhythmias because
   A. the ventricles are not able to depolarize effectively
   B. of a diminished stroke volume
   C. calcium leaks from cells
   D. the heart muscle is hypothermic
2. Excess fluid volume increases the risk for dysrhythmias because it
   A. increases automaticity
   B. decreases contractility
   C. increases cardiac conduction
   D. produces an influx of sodium ions
3. Hypokalemia results in
   A. delayed conduction
   B. increased automaticity

C. tall, peaked T waves
D. inverted P waves

4. Hypocalcemia results in
   A. decreased sodium influx into the cell
   B. delayed repolarization
   C. prolonged QT interval
   D. spontaneous conduction
5. Hypothermia can result in all of the following EXCEPT
   A. bradycardia
   B. prolonged PR intervals
   C. prolonged QT intervals
   D. tall, peaked T waves

Answers: 1. A, 2. B, 3. A, 4. C, 5. D

SECTION FIVE: Sinus Dysrhythmias

At the completion of this section, the learner will be able to identify common dysrhythmias arising from the SA node and describe the treatment of these dysrhythmias.

Sinus node dysfunction, typically associated with heart disease, results from blockages to the right coronary artery or the circumflex artery (Mangrum & DiMarco, 2000). These arteries provide blood flow to the SA node. Sinus node dysfunction produces bradycardia.

Sinus bradycardia is described as a heart rate less than 60 bpm and originates from the SA node, as evidenced by a regular P wave preceding each QRS complex. The only abnormality noted in this rhythm is the rate. This rhythm can be present in athletes because they have strong cardiac muscle contractions (Maron, 2003); therefore, a slower heart rate can still maintain an efficient CO. Sinus bradycardia is not treated unless the person experiences symptoms of decreased CO, such as syncope, hypotension, and angina. If the rate drops too low, the chance of ectopic (abnormal) pacemakers firing increases. Lethal ventricular dysrhythmias can result. Sinus bradycardia is treated by administering atropine because it blocks the parasympathetic innervation to the SA node, allowing normal sympathetic innervation to gain control and increase SA node firing. Figure 10–13 illustrates sinus bradycardia.

Sinus tachycardia has a rapid rate, from 100 to 150 bpm. There are no other abnormal characteristics associated with this rhythm. The rapid rate results from sympathetic nervous stimulation. This stimulation can be in response to fear, increased activity, hypermetabolic states (such as fever), pain, and decreased CO as a result of hypovolemia or ventricular failure. Sinus tachycardia can produce angina if the CO decreases to the point of reducing coronary circulation or if myocardial oxygen demand is increased without an increase in coronary circulation. Treatment is aimed at relieving the cause of increased sympathetic stimulation. Nursing measures, such as imagery, distraction, and promoting a calm environment, as well as drug

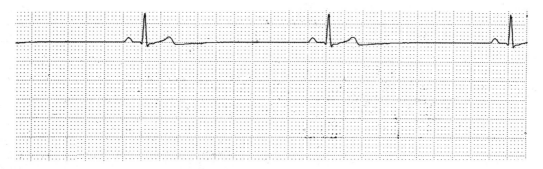

Figure 10–13 ■ Sinus bradycardia
1. Rate = 30
2. R–R interval: regular
3. *P* wave has same configuration
4. *PR* interval = 0.20
5. *P* wave precedes *QRS*: yes
6. *QRS* complex = 0.08

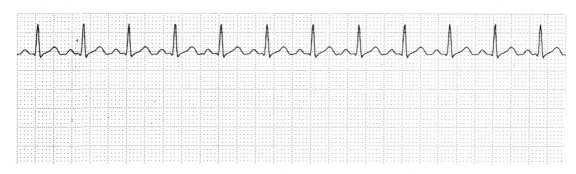

Figure 10–14 ■ Sinus tachycardia
1. Rate = 120
2. R–R interval: regular
3. *P* wave has same configuration
4. *PR* interval = 0.12 − 0.14
5. *P* wave precedes *QRS*: yes
6. QRS complex = 0.06 − 0.08

therapy, are necessary. Sedatives, tranquilizers, antianxiety agents, analgesics, and antipyretics are used. Figure 10–14 is an ECG tracing of sinus tachycardia.

In cases of sinus node dysfunction, atrial conduction becomes less effective, and "rescue" rhythms originating elsewhere in the atria occur to maintain cardiac output (e.g., atrial flutter and atrial fibrillation; see Section Six). Ultimately, a pacemaker may be required (see Section Twelve).

In summary, sinus dysrhythmias are characterized by regular rates. They usually are harmless unless CO becomes compromised. The nurse assesses the patient for signs of decreasing level of consciousness, hypotension, and angina. When these symptoms occur, the dysrhythmia is treated. Table 10–2 compares sinus dysrhythmias.

TABLE 10–2 Summary of Differences in Sinus Dysrhythmias

RHYTHM	CHARACTERISTIC	TREATMENT STRATEGY
Sinus bradycardia	Rate less than 60 bpm	Atropine
Sinus tachycardia	Rate greater than 100 bpm and less than 150 bpm	Antianxiety measures
		Pain relief measures
		Antipyretics
		Oxygen
		Calcium channel blockers
		Beta-blocking agents

SECTION FIVE REVIEW

1. Sinus bradycardia originates from
   A. delayed AV conduction
   B. the AV nodal area
   C. Purkinje fibers
   D. the SA node
2. Atropine is used to treat sinus bradycardia because it
   A. inhibits the AV node
   B. stimulates the sympathetic nervous system
   C. blocks the parasympathetic nervous system
   D. enhances ventricular conduction
3. Sinus tachycardia results from all of the following EXCEPT
   A. parasympathetic stimulation
   B. anxiety

C. pain
D. fever

4. What interventions are used to treat sinus tachycardia?
   A. imagery
   B. promoting a calm environment
   C. defibrillation
   D. A and B
5. Decreasing levels of consciousness associated with sinus dysrhythmias indicates
   A. decreased ventricular contractility
   B. decreased cardiac output
   C. increased atrial filling
   D. decreased AV conduction

Answers: 1. D, 2. C, 3. A, 4. D, 5. B

SECTION SIX: Atrial Dysrhythmias

At the completion of this section, the learner will be able to identify basic atrial dysrhythmias and describe the treatment of these dysrhythmias.

Common atrial dysrhythmias are supraventricular tachycardia, atrial flutter, and atrial fibrillation. Each of these dysrhythmias is characterized by a rapid rate. Most patients when experiencing these dysrhythmias describe a fluttering sensation in the chest, dyspnea, lightheadedness, or angina. The rapid heart rate decreases ventricular filling time and stroke volume.

Supraventricular tachycardia (SVT) has a rate between 150 and 250 bpm. The rhythm is regular, but *P* waves are not distinguishable because they are buried in the preceding *T* wave. The *QRS* complex appears normal because ventricular conduction is not affected. Normal *QRS* complexes indicate that the ectopic pacemaker is located above the ventricles. The exact location is not distinguishable without a 12-lead ECG. At times SVT is mistaken for ventricular tachycardia (VT) (see Section Nine). However, in VT, the *QRS* complex is greater than 0.14 second, and the rate is usually between 130 and 170 bpm. Treatment remains the same regardless of pacemaker origin (Gilbert, 2001). If the patient is not experiencing symptoms, drug therapy is initiated to slow the rate. SVT can be treated with Valsalva's maneuver or adenosine, an endogenous nucleoside. Because it is a naturally occurring body substance, it is rapidly removed from the circulation. Adenosine (6 to 12 mg IV) temporarily inhibits AV node conduction and blocks reentry of impulses from the ventricles. Consequently, heart rate decreases and conduction of impulses through the AV node slows. Adenosine clarifies whether the

ECG pattern is SVT or VT (Gilbert, 2001). Only dysrhythmias involving the AV node convert while VT remains unchanged. Adenosine has a very short half-life (approximately 10 seconds). A brief period of asystole (up to 15 seconds) is common after rapid administration. Side effects include facial flushing, dyspnea, and chest pressure. Calcium channel blocking agents are used to prevent the influx of calcium into the cell and to prevent depolarization. Verapamil, digitalis preparations, propranolol, or quinidine can also be used. In cases in which the patient is experiencing distress or is unresponsive to drug therapy, electric cardioversion is used to rapidly correct the dysrhythmia. Figure 10–15 is an example of SVT.

Atrial flutter has a faster rate than SVT. The atrial rate is greater than 250 bpm. The ventricular rate depends on the number of impulses that pass through the AV node. The ventricular rate can be irregular if some of the impulses are blocked. The atrial oscillations appear as sawtooth waves. A fast ventricular rate decreases SV in the absence of digitalis toxicity. Cardioversion is the preferred method of treating this dysrhythmia. Calcium channel blockers, beta-blocking agents, and digitalis preparations may be used (Section Eleven). Atrial flutter is described by the number of atrial oscillations (*f waves*) between each *QRS* complex (Fig. 10–16).

Atrial fibrillation is one of the most common heart disturbances in clinical practice, and the incidence is expected to increase as the population ages (Navas, 2003). Atrial fibrillation is a condition in which the atria are contracting so fast that they are unable to refill before contraction. Therefore, the ventricles are inadequately filled and SV is diminished. The atria are not able to empty completely because of the fast rate of depolarization. Blood that remains in the atria is prone to forming clots, which increases the risk of thrombotic stroke.

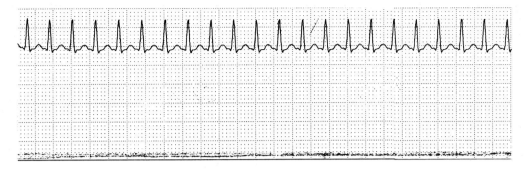

Figure 10–15 ■ Supraventricular tachycardia (*Note:* This is not a 6-second strip.)
1. Rate = 250
2. R–R interval: regular
3. *P* wave: difficult to distinguish
4. *PR* interval: cannot calculate
5. *P* wave precedes each *QRS*: cannot identify
6. *QRS* complex = 0.06

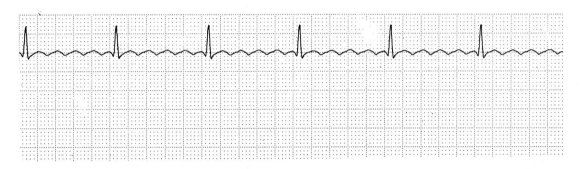

Figure 10–16 ■ Atrial flutter.
1. Rate: atrial = 250,
   ventricular = 60
2. R–R interval: regular
3. *P* wave: cannot distinguish, flutter wave present
4. *PR* interval: cannot calculate
5. *P* wave precedes each *QRS*: cannot identify
6. *QRS* complex = 0.06

Atrial fibrillation has an irregular ventricular response. The *QRS* complexes are normal in appearance but occur at irregular intervals. This is manifested clinically as a difference between the apical heart rate and the peripheral pulse rate because the SV is inadequate with some beats to produce a peripheral pulse. The atria can be discharging at a rate greater than 400 bpm. Absent *P* waves and irregular *QRS* intervals are characteristic of this dysrhythmia. Control of the ventricular rate is important in atrial fibrillation. Drugs that are particularly effective in controlling ventricular rate are digoxin, beta-adrenergic blocking agents, and calcium channel blocking agents. Conversion of the atrial fibrillation to a normal sinus rhythm improves hemodynamics. Conversion is achieved by direct current cardioversion and/or class IA, IC, and III antiarrhythmics (Section Eleven). In some cases, atrial fibrillation is resistant to conversion by either method. Atrial fibrillation is not treated if it is of long-standing duration and does not produce symptoms. Figure 10–17 is an example of atrial fibrillation.

In summary, atrial dysrhythmias have a rapid atrial response and are characterized by absent *P* waves. A complication of these dysrhythmias is decreased CO if the ventricular response is rapid, resulting in inadequate ventricular filling. Table 10–3 compares atrial dysrhythmias.

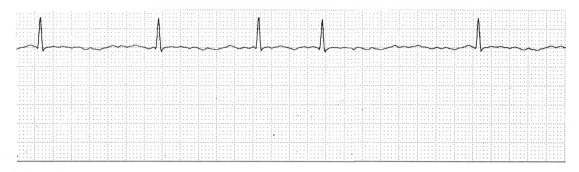

Figure 10–17 ■ Atrial fibrillation.
1. Rate: atrial: unable to calculate, ventricular = 50
2. R–R interval: irregular
3. *P* wave: undistinguishable
4. *PR* interval: cannot calculate
5. *P* wave precedes each *QRS*: cannot identify
6. *QRS* complex = 0.06

TABLE 10–3 Summary of Differences in Atrial Dysrhythmias

RHYTHM	CHARACTERISTIC	TREATMENT STRATEGY
Superventricular tachycardia	R–R interval regular Atrial rate 150 to 250 bpm	Adenosine Beta-blocking agents (propranolol) Calcium channel blocking agents Digitalis Cardioversion Overdrive pacing
Atrial flutter	R–R interval may be regular or irregular Atrial rate may be up to 350 bpm Sawtoothed waves	Cardioversion Digitalis
Atrial fibrillation	R–R interval irregular Atrial rate greater than 350 bpm	Digitalis Cardioversion Calcium channel blocking agents Class IA, IC, and III agents

SECTION SIX REVIEW

1. Atrial dysrhythmias produce symptoms of lightheadedness or angina because
   A. cardiac output is decreased
   B. ventricular conduction is delayed
   C. the SA node is competing for pacemaker status
   D. coronary vasodilation occurs
2. Adenosine may be used to treat supraventricular tachycardia because it
   A. increases AV conduction
   B. prevents reentry of impulses from the ventricles
   C. prolongs repolarization
   D. blocks potassium movement extracellularly
3. Atrial fibrillation predisposes a person to a stroke because it produces
   A. cardiac fatigue
   B. inadequate emptying of the atria
   C. ventricular exhaustion
   D. decreased cerebral circulation
4. Which of the following distinguishes SVT from VT?
   A. prolonged *PR* interval
   B. appearance of sawtooth waves
   C. irregular *QRS* pattern
   D. *QRS* complex greater than 0.14 seconds
5. Atrial flutter typically has an atrial rate
   A. between 150 and 250 bpm
   B. less than 60 bpm
   C. greater than 250 bpm
   D. greater than 400 bpm

Answers: 1. A, 2. B, 3. B, 4. D, 5. C

SECTION SEVEN: Junctional Dysrhythmias

At the completion of this section, the learner will be able to identify common junctional dysrhythmias and describe the treatment of these dysrhythmias.

Junctional dysrhythmias occur because the SA node fails to fire. They have a protective function. The junctional area is located around the AV node. Pacemaker cells in this area have an intrinsic rate of 40 to 60 bpm. Once the pacemaker cell discharges, it spreads upward to depolarize the atria and downward to depolarize the ventricles. Because the ventricles usually are depolarized in a downward fashion, the *QRS* complex appears normal. The atria are depolarized in an abnormal manner so the *P* wave can be inverted. The timing of the *P* wave is abnormal. It may precede the *QRS* complex, but the *PR* interval is shorter than 0.12 seconds. The *P* wave can be buried in the *QRS* complex and be indistinguishable or it can follow the *QRS* complex.

The term *junctional tachycardia* refers to a junctional rhythm with a rate greater than 100 bpm. If the rate of the rhythm is between 60 and 100 bpm, it is called an *accelerated junctional rhythm.* Figure 10–18 shows an accelerated junctional rhythm pattern.

Digitalis increases the automaticity of the AV node; therefore, digitalis toxicity can precipitate junctional rhythms (Ma et al., 2001). The dysrhythmia is treated by withholding the

TABLE 10–4 Summary of Differences in Junctional Dysrhythmias

RHYTHM	CHARACTERISTIC	TREATMENT STRATEGY
Junctional rhythm	Rate 40 to 60 bpm Inverted or absent *P* waves	May not be treated if patient is asymptomatic Atropine Pacemaker insertion
Junctional tachycardia	Rate greater than 100 bpm Inverted or absent *P* waves	May not be treated if patient is asymptomatic Pacemaker insertion Withhold digitalis if associated with digitalis toxicity

medication. Usually, the patient can tolerate junctional rhythms; however, if the patient experiences symptoms of decreased CO because the rate is too slow, atropine is administered. A pacemaker may be inserted as a protective measure in case the junction fails or if the patient is symptomatic. Table 10–4 compares junctional rhythms.

In summary, junctional rhythms are a protective mechanism when the SA node fails to discharge appropriately. Depolarization of the atria is abnormal; therefore, the *P* wave may fall before, during, or after the *QRS* complex.

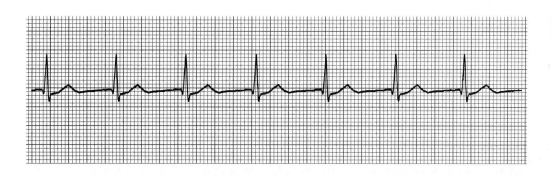

Figure 10–18 ■ Accelerated junctional rhythm.

SECTION SEVEN REVIEW

1. Junctional rhythms are
   A. precursors to ventricular dysrhythmias
   B. protective mechanisms
   C. generated by the SA node
   D. considered atrial dysrhythmias
2. Junctional tachycardia is classified as a junctional rhythm with a rate
   A. greater than 40 bpm
   B. greater than 60 bpm
   C. greater than 100 bpm
   D. between 60 and 100 bpm
3. The *P* wave in a junctional rhythm
   A. is bizarre in configuration
   B. is always absent

C. can appear anywhere in relation to the *QRS* complex
   D. is flat
4. An accelerated junctional rhythm has a rate of
   A. less than 60 bpm
   B. 60 to 100 bpm
   C. 100 to 120 bpm
   D. greater than 150 bpm
5. Interventions for junctional rhythms may include
   A. administration of digitalis
   B. atropine
   C. a pacemaker
   D. B and C

Answers: 1. B, 2. C, 3. C, 4. B, 5. D

SECTION EIGHT: Premature Contractions

At the completion of this section, the learner will be able to compare and contrast atrial and ventricular premature beats, identify their origin, and describe the treatment of these premature beats.

Premature heart beats originate from an excitable focus outside of the normal SA node pacemaker (an ectopic pacemaker). Premature heart beats are a relatively common phenomenon and in healthy people they are benign. In the presence of cardiovascular disease, however, ectopic pacemakers can trigger potentially life-threatening cardiac dysrhythmias. Premature heart beats are usually caused by enhanced automaticity of cardiac cells resulting from a stimulus such as caffeine, nicotine, alcohol, or stress. In patients with cardiovascular disease, the most dangerous cause is cardiac ischemia.

Premature atrial contractions (PACs) originate from one (unifocal) or more (multifocal) ectopic pacemakers located in the atria. A *P* wave is visible, unless it is hidden in the preceding *T* wave. The premature *P* wave may look different from the normal *P* wave, depending on the location of the originating impulse.

The underlying rhythm is usually regular with the PAC causing a brief irregularity. There is a characteristic short pause following a PAC called a *noncompensatory pause* (i.e., the R-R interval from the *R* wave preceding the PAC to the *R* wave following the PAC is less than two regular R-R intervals measured on the underlying regular rhythm). Figure 10–19 shows an example of a PAC.

Premature ventricular contractions (PVCs) originate from one or more ectopic pacemakers in the ventricles. Since the electrical stimulus is originating outside of the atria, there is no *P* wave preceding the PVC. The wave form of a PVC is usually large (higher voltage on ECG monitor and wider than 0.12 seconds). The wave form is also bizarre appearing and is generally in the opposite direction of the person's usual QRS complex. There is a characteristic full *compensatory pause* (i.e., the R-R interval from the *R* wave preceding the PVC to the *R* wave following the PVC is equal to two regular R-R intervals of the underlying rhythm). Unifocal PVCs (Fig. 10–20) originate from same location so their configuration is the same. Multifocal PVCs (Fig. 10–21), however, originate from two or more locations and therefore have different configurations. Ventricular diastole following a PVC is ineffective and does not contribute significantly to cardiac output.

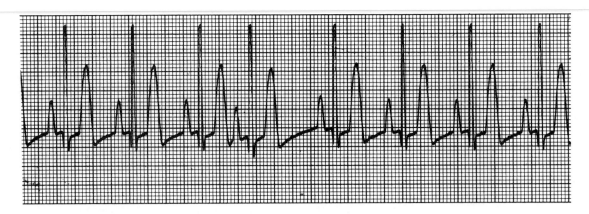

Figure 10–19 ■ Premature atrial contractions. Note the PAC that occurs following the third *QRS* complex. This is followed by a normal appearing *QRS* and a short (noncompensatory) pause.

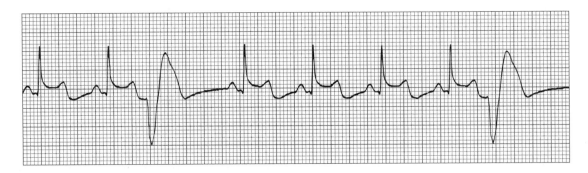

Figure 10–20 ■ Unifocal PVCs. Note that the two PVCs are bizarre in appearance and the wave forms are in opposite directions of the underlying *QRS* complexes.

Certain circumstances warrant close observation of PVCs because they are associated with development of ventricular tachycardia (VT) and ventricular fibrillation (VF). These circumstances include:

1. More than six PVCs per minute
2. PVCs occurring together (couplet)
3. Multifocal PVCs (from more than one ectopic focus)
4. A run of ventricular tachycardia (more than three PVCs in a row)
5. R-on-T phenomenon (PVC that occurs on the down-stroke of the *T* wave preceding the PVC. The down-stroke of the

T wave is a relative refractory or vulnerable period whereby a strong enough stimulus can excite the heart and trigger VT or VF).

A major responsibility of the nurse is to determine factors that contribute to the development of PVCs. The nurse assesses and describes the patient's underlying cardiac rhythm and the type of PVC (uniformed versus multiformed). The timing of the PVCs is described if they occur in a repeatable pattern. For example, **bigeminy** is a pattern of one normal SA node–initiated beat followed by one PVC (Fig. 10–22). **Trigeminy** is a pattern of two normal beats followed by one PVC (Fig. 10–23).

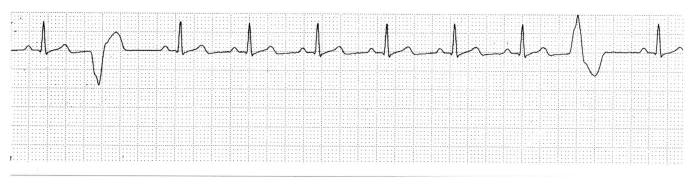

Figure 10–21 ■ Multifocal PVC's. [*Note:* Strip is longer than 6 seconds = 37 (0.20) boxes.] Note the differences in PVC configurations.

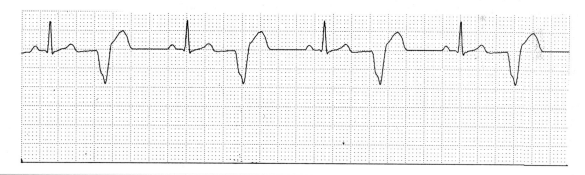

Figure 10–22 ■ Ventricular bigeminy. Note that the heart rate is actually 40 bpm since PVCs do not contribute to the cardiac output.

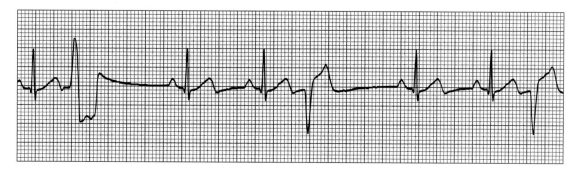

Figure 10–23 ■ Ventricular trigeminy.

Lidocaine is administered if PVCs occur in the setting of myocardial ischemia or infarction. Prophylactic use of lidocaine is not recommended (Trappe et al., 2003). Amiodarone or procainamide is administered if the PVCs are refractory to lidocaine.

In summary, PACs are harmless and are not treated unless they are present at a rate of six or greater a minute. PVCs can be life threatening because they indicate ventricular irritability. Multiple PVCs, multifocal PVCs, a couplet of PVCs, and a run of VT are treated with lidocaine if the patient has underlying cardiac disease because they can potentiate life-threatening dysrhythmias. Table 10–5 compares premature contractions.

TABLE 10–5 Summary of Differences in Premature Contractions

CONTRACTION	CHARACTERISTIC	TREATMENT STRATEGY
Premature atrial contraction	*PR* interval may be normal or prolonged *QRS* normal	May not be treated if patient is asymptomatic Reduce caffeine, alcohol intake Beta-blocking agents (propranolol)
Premature ventricular contraction	*PR* interval absent in premature beat *QRS* greater than 0.12	May not be treated if patient is asymptomatic Reduce caffeine intake Decrease stress Lidocaine

SECTION EIGHT REVIEW

1. Which of the following statements best describes premature beats?
   A. they originate anywhere along the cardiac conduction pathway
   B. they originate in the atria
   C. they originate in the ventricles
   D. they originate in the junctional (AV nodal) area
2. PACs are treated when they
   A. occur as pairs
   B. originate from different sites
   C. occur greater than six per minute
   D. occur in a repeatable pattern
3. PVCs are associated with
   A. hyponatremia
   B. hypocalcemia
   C. hypoglycemia
   D. hypokalemia
4. In PVCs, the *QRS* complex is
   A. greater than 0.12 second
   B. negatively deflected
   C. isoelectric
   D. preceded by a *T* wave
5. PVCs that are refractory to lidocaine are treated with
   A. defibrillation
   B. amiodarone
   C. digitalis
   D. cardioversion

Answers: 1. A, 2. C, 3. D, 4. A, 5. B

SECTION NINE: Ventricular Dysrhythmias

At the completion of this section, the learner will be able to identify common ventricular dysrhythmias and describe treatment of these dysrhythmias.

Ventricular dysrhythmias can be lethal. Inadequate ventricular ejection produces inadequate SV. If prolonged, coronary and peripheral ischemia results, producing ischemia and cell death. Two common ventricular dysrhythmias are ventricular tachycardia and ventricular fibrillation.

Ventricular tachycardia (VT) is classified as three or more consecutive PVCs occurring at a rapid rate, usually greater than 100 bpm. Although the SA node continues to fire, ectopic pacemakers in the ventricles fire spontaneously and bear no relationship to the SA node–initiated impulse. *P* waves are not identifiable because they are buried in the *QRS* complexes. The R–R interval is often regular, and the *QRS* complex is greater than 0.12 second. Short runs of VT (less than 30 seconds) generally can be tolerated. A danger of VT is that it may deteriorate into ventricular fibrillation. Patients can be alert while experiencing VT, and a carotid pulse can be present; however, as CO diminishes, loss of consciousness ensues. Witnessed VT is treated with a precordial thump over the sternum. Cardioversion may be used. Pharmacological treatment of VT includes amiodarone, lidocaine, and magnesium (Asselin & Cullen, 2001). Figure 10–24 is an example of VT.

Ventricular fibrillation is the most common cause of sudden death. The ECG pattern is chaotic. It is impossible to identify any *PQRST* waves, and the rhythm is grossly irregular (Fig. 10–25). The patient will be unresponsive, without a pulse, and requires emergency treatment and cardiopulmonary resuscitations. **Defibrillation** is the treatment of choice and is used beginning with 200 J and progressing up to 360 J for a total of three times

(AHA-ILCR, 2000). A bolus of vasopressin (preferred) or epinephrine is administered. If the patient remains pulseless, attempts at defibrillation continue. For persistent or recurrent pulseless ventricular tachycardia or fibrillation, amiodarone, lidocaine, magnesium, and procainamide are used. Once the patient has converted from ventricular fibrillation and has a pulse, a continuous infusion of the last drug used to convert the rhythm is initiated. Myocardial infarction and premature ventricular beats can precede the development of ventricular fibrillation.

In summary, ventricular dysrhythmias are more life threatening than other dysrhythmias and require immediate treatment. They are recognizable by absent *P* waves and regular, wide *QRS* complexes or, if *P* waves are present, they are not associated with the *QRS* complex. In the case of ventricular fibrillation, chaotic waveforms are seen. Table 10–6 compares ventricular dysrhythmias.

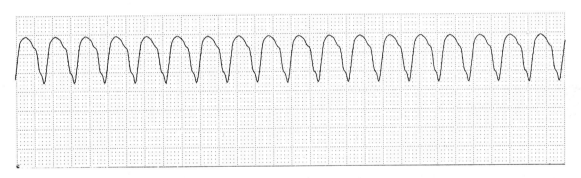

Figure 10–24 ■ Ventricular tachycardia.

1. Rate: atrial: unable to calculate
   ventricular = 180
2. R–R interval: regular
3. *P* wave: undistinguishable
4. *PR* interval: none
5. *P* wave precedes each *QRS*: no
6. *QRS* complex = 0.28

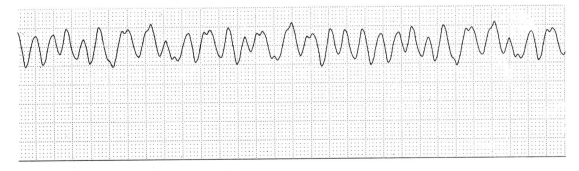

Figure 10–25 ■ Ventricular fibrillation.

1. Rate: atrial: none
   ventricular: none
2. R–R interval: undeterminable
3. *P* wave: none
4. *PR* interval: none
5. *P* wave precedes each *QRS*: no
6. *QRS* complex: none

TABLE 10–6　Summary of Differences in Ventricular Dysrhythmias

RHYTHM	CHARACTERISTIC	TREATMENT STRATEGY
Ventricular tachycardia	R–R interval usually regular, but can be irregular	Lidocaine
	Absent *P* waves or *P* waves not associated with *QRS* complex	Magnesium
	Wide *QRS* but somewhat uniform	Amiodarone
	Rate greater than 100 bpm	Cardioversion
Ventricular fibrillation	R–R interval undeterminable	Cardiopulmonary
	Absent *P* wave	Defibrillation
	Absent *QRS*	Epinephrine
	Rate undeterminable	Lidocaine
	Chaotic waveform	Vasopressin
		Amiodarone

SECTION NINE REVIEW

1. Ventricular tachycardia
   A. may be harmless
   B. is defined as three or more consecutive PVCs
   C. results from SA node fatigue
   D. produces ventricular rates less than 100 bpm
2. Which of the following is considered a "short run" of VT?
   A. 1 minute
   B. 45 seconds
   C. 30 seconds
   D. two PVCs
3. In ventricular fibrillation, the ECG pattern
   A. is chaotic
   B. has recognizable *QRS* complexes
   C. has inverted *T* waves
   D. has a regular atrial rate

4. The treatment of choice in ventricular fibrillation is
   A. lidocaine
   B. epinephrine
   C. cardioversion
   D. defibrillation
5. Once the patient has converted from ventricular fibrillation and has a pulse, which of the following interventions should be initiated?
   A. defibrillation at 360 J
   B. a bolus of vasopressin
   C. a bolus of epinephrine
   D. a continuous infusion of the last drug used to convert the rhythm

Answers: 1. B, 2. C, 3. A, 4. D, 5. D

SECTION TEN: Conduction Abnormalities

At the completion of this section, the learner will be able to distinguish the three conduction abnormalities and describe the treatment for each.

Cardiac impulse conduction can become inhibited anywhere along the conduction pathway. A variety of factors can slow conduction, such as cardiac ischemia, digitalis, antiarrhythmic agents, and increased parasympathetic activity. When the delay occurs at the atrioventricular (AV) node area, it is called an AV block (Fig. 10–3). Acute AV blocks are associated with myocardial infarction while chronic AV blocks develop from coronary artery disease. AV blocks are classified as first-degree, second-degree, or third-degree, based on the relationship of the *P* wave to the *QRS* complex.

A *first-degree AV block* is denoted by a prolonged *PR* interval (greater than 0.20 second). There is a delay in conduction

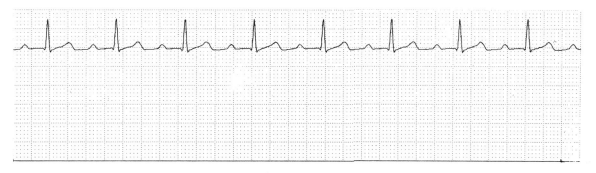

Figure 10–26 ▪ First degree AV block. Note the prolonged *PR* interval and the 1:1 relationship between the *P* waves and *QRS* complexes.

through the AV node; however, the P wave and *QRS* complex maintain a 1:1 relationship. The rest of the ECG is normal. The patient is usually asymptomatic, and no treatment is necessary. While first-degree AV block is usually benign, in the presence of acute MI or coronary artery disease, the conduction delay can increase, leading to second-or third-degree AV block, requiring treatment. Figure 10–26 is an example of first-degree AV block.

In *second-degree AV block,* a SA node impulse is conducted with a delay or it is completely blocked in the AV nodal area. Therefore, a *P* wave is present, but the *PR* interval is irregular or unmeasureable because of the missing *QRS* complexes. In some cases, the *PR* interval lengthens progressively before the dropping *QRS* complex (Wenckebach or Mobitz type I second-degree heart block). In Mobitz type II second-degree AV block, the *PR* intervals are of constant duration before dropping the *QRS* complex. *QRS* complexes are wide because the block is usually lower in the conduction system (bundles). This type of AV block is less common but is considered more serious because it is associated with third-degree AV block and asystole (Hand, 2002). The nurse determines the ventricular rate (number of *QRS* complexes) of the rhythm and the frequency of dropped beats. Angina, light-headedness, and dyspnea can occur because of decreased cardiac output. In the case of type I second-degree AV block, if the rate is below 60 bpm and the patient is asymptomatic, no treatment is initiated. The patient is observed. A patient with type II second-degree AV block, whether symptomatic or asymptomatic, will receive a transvenous pacemaker. The point at which the pacemaker is inserted may vary because symptoms are initially managed with medications. Regardless of the type of second-degree block, if the patient experiences symptoms, atropine is administered. If isoproterenol is used, it is used with extreme caution, particularly

in the setting of ischemic heart disease (Kaushik et al., 2000). Dopamine or epinephrine are used in severe symptomatic bradycardia. A transvenous pacemaker may be inserted for symptomatic patients with type I second-degree AV block. Transcutaneous pacing is extremely effective. If bradycardia is severe and the patient is unstable, transcutaneous pacing is performed immediately (Kaushik et al., 2000). Figure 10–27 is an example of type I second-degree AV block, and Figure 10–28 is an example of type II second-degree AV block. If two *QRS*s are dropped in a row, the AV block is called advanced heart block (Fig. 10–29).

Third-degree (complete) AV block requires emergency treatment because the atria and ventricles are contracting independently. Thus, CO is greatly diminished because of inadequate filling of the ventricles. Impulses are not conducted through the AV node. The atria and ventricles fire at a regular rate, but they do not function as a single unit. The P–P wave interval is regular, as is the R–R wave interval, but the *PR* interval varies. There is no relationship between the *P* wave and the *QRS* complex because the atria and the ventricles are paced by a separate pacemaker. The *QRS* complex is usually wide because of the ventricular origin of the stimulus. Complete heart block is usually associated with myocardial infarction. In rare cases, the ventricular rate is fast enough to maintain CO, and symptoms are less severe. Usually, the patient experiences an alteration in mental status and syncope. Complete heart block can progress to ventricular fibrillation. Treatment of complete heart block is the same as that for type II second-degree heart block. If symptomatic, the patient is administered atropine, dopamine, or epinephrine, and if isoproterenol is used, it is used with extreme caution. External pacing, and transvenous pacing may also be used. Figure 10–30 is an example of complete heart block.

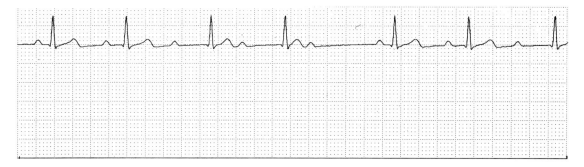

Figure 10–27 ■ Type I second degree block. Note the regularity of the *P-P* intervals and increasing *P-R* intervals that end in a nonconducted (dropped) *QRS*.

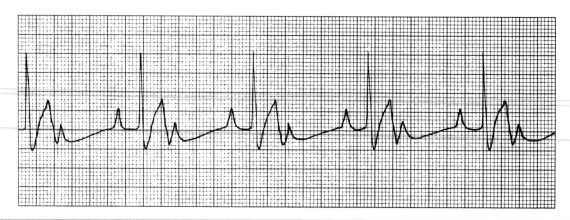

Figure 10–28 ■ Type II second degree block. Note the *P-P* interval regularity and that every other *P* wave is nonconducted (a 2:1 block). The conducted *P* waves have a stable *P-R* interval.

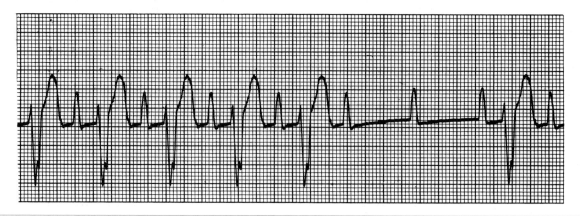

Figure 10–29 ■ Advanced AV heart block. Note the 3:1 block after the fifth *QRS* complex.

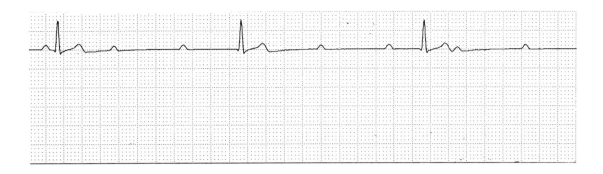

Figure 10–30 ■ Third-degree (complete) heart block. Note that the P-P and R-R intervals are regular but have no relationship to each other.

Once the impulse enters the ventricles, its conduction through the right and left bundle branches can be impaired. This is called a bundle branch block (BBB). The bundle branches are divided into right and left. The impulse travels slowly through the blocked side; thus, one ventricle depolarizes faster than the other. On the ECG, the *QRS* complex is prolonged and its appearance varies, depending on the affected side (right or left). Treatment is not necessary except in the case of a new onset left BBB in which the patient may be experiencing a myocardial infarction (Cunningham et al., 2000).

In summary, abnormalities can occur along the cardiac conduction pathway that interfere with transmission of the impulse from the atria to the ventricles. The least severe of these abnormalities is first-degree AV block. The impulse is transmitted to the ventricles, but there is a delay at the AV nodal area. Impulses from the atria to the ventricles are periodically blocked in second-degree AV block. In type I, the *PR* interval progressively lengthens before the blocked impulse. In type II, the *PR* interval remains constant. Third-degree AV block is a medical emergency. Cardiac output is decreased because the atria and ventricles are contracting independently. It is treated with transcutaneous pacing followed by placement of a temporary transvenous pacing catheter. Table 10–7 compares atrioventricular blocks.

TABLE 10–7 Summary of Differences in Atrioventricular (AV) Blocks

BLOCK	CHARACTERISTICS	TREATMENT STRATEGIES
First degree	*PR* interval > 0.20 R–R interval is regular	Usually not treated unless patient is symptomatic Atropine
Second degree, Mobitz type I	Atrial rate is greater than ventricular rate R–R interval is irregular *PR* interval gradually lengthens until a *P* wave is blocked (no *QRS* follows the *P* wave)	Withhold digitalis associated with digitalis toxicity Atropine Transcutaneous pacemaker Permanent pacemaker insertion
Second degree, Mobitz type II	Atrial rate is greater than ventricular rate No consistent pattern to the blocking of the *P* wave R–R interval usually irregular	Atropine Transcutaneous pacemaker Permanent pacemaker insertion
Advanced AV block	Atrial rate is greater than ventricular rate Two *QRS* complexes in a row are blocked R–R interval is irregular	Atropine Transcutaneous pacemaker Permanent pacemaker insertion
Third degree, complete	*PR* interval varies R–R interval regular *QRS* may be widened	Transcutaneous pacemaker Permanent pacemaker insertion

SECTION TEN REVIEW

1. Which of the following may produce blocks in impulse conduction?
   A. ischemia
   B. sympathetic stimulation
   C. fever
   D. antipyretic agents
2. The difference between type I and type II second-degree AV block is
   A. dropping of the *QRS* complex
   B. regularity of the rhythm
   C. length of the *PR* interval
   D. *P* wave configuration
3. Complete heart block is characterized by
   A. a constant *PR* interval
   B. a heart rate less than 50 bpm
   C. *QRS* complexes less than 0.12 second
   D. regular *P–P* and *R–R* intervals

4. First-degree AV block should be treated if the
   A. *PR* interval is irregular
   B. patient is symptomatic
   C. *PR* interval is isoelectric
   D. *PR* interval is negatively deflected
5. Advanced AV heart block is characterized by
   A. two blocked *QRS* complexes in a row
   B. a heart rate less than 60 bpm
   C. dropping of *P* waves
   D. shortening of the *PR* interval

Answers: 1. A, 2. C, 3. D, 4. B, 5. A

SECTION ELEVEN: Pharmacologic Interventions and Nursing Implications

At the completion of this section, the learner will be able to identify common drug classifications used in treating cardiac dysrhythmias, state nursing implications associated with administration of these agents, and discuss nursing responsibilities associated with cardioversion and defibrillation. The learner is referred to a pharmacology text for specific information on dosages and administration. Cardioversion and defibrillation are discussed because of the relationship between drug therapy and electric shock with some agents.

Antiarrhythmic Agents

Antiarrhythmic agents are used in treating cardiac conduction disturbances. The antiarrhythmics have several subcategories, class I through class IV. Each of these drugs is capable of producing new dysrhythmias or worsening current dysrhythmias (proarrhythmics). Therefore, constant ECG monitoring is required as these medications are initiated (Table 10–8).

Class I drugs are fast sodium channel blockers. By blocking these channels, these drugs slow impulse conduction through the atria and ventricles. There are three categories of Class I drugs: IA, IB, and IC. Class IA drugs reduce automaticity and prolong the refractory period of the heart. They are indicated in the treatment of atrial dysrhythmias and PVCs. Class IB drugs decrease refractory periods but do not affect automaticity to a great extent. These drugs are used chiefly in the treatment of ventricular dysrhythmias. Class IC agents decrease spontaneous

depolarization. They are also used in treating ventricular dysrhythmias. These drugs are used with caution because they can induce dysrhythmias (Sanguinetti & Bennett, 2003).

Class II agents block the effects of catecholamines (e.g., epinephrine). They decrease SA node automaticity and slow AV conduction velocity and myocardial contractility. Their exact effects depend on which catecholamine receptor they block. Catecholamines can affect four different receptors: alpha$_1$, alpha$_2$, beta$_1$, and beta$_2$. For example, phentolamine (Regitine) is an alpha-blocking agent, therefore, it produces peripheral vasodilation. However, most of the agents used to treat dysrhythmias in this category are beta-blocking agents. Thus, they decrease cardiac stimulation and may produce vasoconstriction and bronchoconstriction. Drugs in this category are used in treating tachydysrhythmias. These drugs are not be used in patients with congestive heart failure, severe bradycardia, and second-degree or higher heart block because of decreased cardiac stimulation. They are contraindicated in asthma because of bronchoconstriction. Because class II drugs decrease the heart rate, the heart rate may be unable to increase to maintain CO in some situations, such as exercise. In cases of cardiac arrest, the heart may be less sensitive to sympathomimetic drugs (i.e., epinephrine) because of the beta-blocking effect.

Class III agents block potassium channels, thereby delaying repolarization and prolonging the refractory period. They increase the fibrillation threshold (making the cell more resistant). They are indicated in the treatment of ventricular dysrhythmias. Sotalol is an agent in this category. Amiodarone, another class III agent, is a first-line medication for VT and VF resistant to defibrillation (Asselin & Cullen, 2001).

Class IV agents are calcium channel blockers. These drugs block the entry of calcium through the cell membranes,

TABLE 10–8 Comparison of Antiarrhythmic Agents

CATEGORY	EXAMPLES	EFFECTS	INDICATIONS
Class IA	Quinidine (Cardioquin) Procainamide (Pronestyl) Disopyramide (Norpace)	Reduced automaticity Prolonged refractory period	PVCs Atrial fibrillation and flutter
Class IB	Lidocaine (Xylocaine) Mexiletine (Mexitil) Tocainide (Tonocard)	Decreased refractory period	PVCs Ventricular tachycardia or fibrillation
Class IC	Encainide (Enkaid) Flecainide (Tambocor) Propafenone Moricizine (Ethmozine)	Decreased spontaneous depolarization	PVCs Ventricular tachycardia
Class II	Propanolol (Inderal) (Beta blockers) Esmolol (Brevibloc) Acebutolol (Sectral)	Decreased automaticity Decreased conduction	Atrial/supraventricular dysrhythmias
Class III	Amiodarone (Cordarone) Bretylium (Bretylol) Sotalol (Butilide)	Prolonged refractory period	Ventricular tachycardia or fibrillation Atrial fibrillation/flutter
Class IV	Verapamil (Calan) Diltiazem (Cardiazem) Nifedipine (Procardia)	Decreased conduction	Supraventricular dysrhythmias and hypertension
Digitalis glycosides	Digoxin (Lanoxin)	Decreased conduction through AV node	Tachydysrhythmias
Endogenous nucleoside	Adenosine (Adenocard)	Blocks reentry of ventricular impulses through the AV node into the atria	Supraventricular dysrhythmias

thereby decreasing depolarization. Verapamil and Diltiazem are commonly used calcium channel blockers for tachydysrhythmias.

Adenosine and digoxin do not fit within the major classes. Both of these drugs reduce AV node automaticity and slow AV conduction.

Prior to administration of antiarrhythmic agents, the nurse assesses the following baseline data: vital signs; ECG interpretation using the six-step process; and a physical assessment of the cardiac, respiratory, and neurologic systems. These data are monitored during drug administration. An infusion pump is used when these drugs are administered by the IV route. The patient is be instructed to report dizziness, palpitations, skin rashes, or wheezing. It must be noted that although the goal of these drugs is to suppress dysrhythmias, virtually all antiarrhythmic drugs also have prodysrhythmic effects, meaning they can worsen existing dysrhythmias and precipitate new ones.

Cardioversion and Defibrillation

Cardioversion delivers electrical current that is synchronized with the patient's heart rhythm. It is used to treat SVT that is resistant to medication, atrial fibrillation or atrial flutter, and ventricular tachycardia in an unstable patient. The unstable patient may be hypotensive; dyspneic; experiencing chest pain; or have evidence of congestive heart failure, myocardial infarction, or ischemia. Analgesia is provided before the electric shock. A synchronizer button is pushed on the defibrillator machine, which allows the machine to discharge after the *R* wave and before the downstroke of the *T* wave. Initially, low voltages are delivered (50 to 100 joules, depending on the size of the patient). Cardioversion is repeated using higher voltages if it is unsuccessful at lower voltages.

The nurse assists with cardioversion by obtaining an ECG strip prior to, during, and after the procedure. Informed consent is obtained and IV access is confirmed before the procedure. The patient is given a sedative prior to treatment to minimize discomfort. Any serum electrolyte abnormalities are reported to the physician (especially calcium, magnesium, and potassium). Oxygen and all metallic objects are removed from the patient. Conductive pads are placed on the chest below the right clavicle to the right of the sternum, and in the midaxillary line on the left. After the procedure, the nurse assesses for complications, including emboli (especially cerebral), respiratory depression, skin burns, and dysrhythmias.

Defibrillation is an emergency procedure used to treat ventricular tachycardia in an unresponsive patient and ventricular fibrillation. Defibrillation is an unsynchronized electric shock that usually administers a larger number of joules (J) than cardioversion (200 J up to 360 J). With defibrillation, conductive paste or gel pads are applied on the chest wall at the apex and base of the heart (Fig. 10–31). A continuous ECG recording is obtained during the procedure. Only those health care providers with advanced cardiac life support certification can deliver defibrillation therapy. Initial defibrillation is performed at 200 J. The person delivering the current announces "All clear!" prior to dispensing the electrical current to ensure that no one is touching the patient or the bed. After each attempt, the cardiac rhythm and pulse are assessed. If the first attempt is unsuccessful, the energy level is increased and second and third attempts are made. If the treatment is unsuccessful after three defibrillation attempts, additional pharmacologic agents are administered.

In summary, antiarrhythmic agents are classified in four large categories. They usually act by decreasing automaticity or by affecting the refractory period. Impulse conduction can be delayed. Antiarrhythmic agents can help correct or worsen a dysrhythmia. Cardioversion and defibrillation are procedures that deliver electrical currents to the heart in attempts to restore normal sinus rhythm. Nursing responsibilities for both administration of these drugs and electrical therapies include careful monitoring of the patient's ECG pattern and clinical response to treatment.

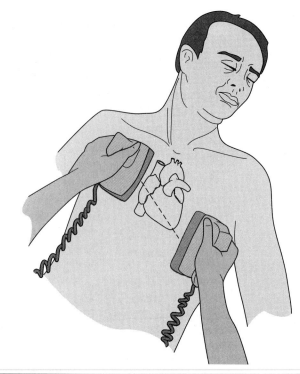

Figure 10–31 ■ Placement of paddles for defibrillation.

SECTION ELEVEN REVIEW

1. Beta blockers (class II agents) may produce which of the following side effects?
   A. weight gain
   B. hypokalemia
   C. wheezing
   D. hives
2. The difference between cardioversion and defibrillation is
   A. defibrillation uses a lower amount of joules
   B. cardioversion is synchronized
   C. defibrillation cannot be repeated
   D. cardioversion is used only to treat atrial dysrhythmias
3. Nursing responsibilities in administering antiarrhythmic agents include
   A. administering all IV drugs with an infusion pump
   B. obtaining an ECG strip before, during, and after administration
   C. obtaining vital signs before, during, and after administration
   D. all of the above

4. Which of the following classes of antiarrhythmics is a fast sodium channel blocker?
   A. class I
   B. class II
   C. class III
   D. class IV
5. Which of the following is a complication of cardioversion?
   A. nausea
   B. chest pain
   C. cerebral emboli
   D. ventricular fibrillation

Answers: 1. C, 2. B, 3. D, 4. A, 5. C

SECTION TWELVE: Long-Term Electrical Therapy

At the completion of this section, the learner will be able to identify indications for pacemaker and implantable cardioversion/defibrillation therapy, types of devices, and nursing implications for the patient receiving these therapies.

Pacemakers

A pacemaker is a pulse generator used to provide an electrical stimulus to the heart when the heart fails to conduct or generate impulses on its own at a rate that maintains CO. The pulse generator is connected to leads (wires) that provide an electrical stimulus to the heart when necessary. Pacemakers are used in addition to drug therapy when one of three conditions exists: failure of the conduction system, failure to initiate an impulse spontaneously, or failure to maintain primary pacing control (spontaneous impulses may occur, but they are not synchronized). There are three commonly used pacing mechanisms: external, epicardial, and endocardial.

External pacing is a temporary measure. It delivers electric impulses to the myocardium transthoracically through two electrode pads placed anteriorly and posteriorly on the chest. However, during periods of hypoxia and acidosis, the myocardium is less responsive to external pacing (Felver, 2000). When caring for a patient receiving external pacing, the nurse notes the date and time external pacing is initiated, as well as pacing rate, mode, and the amount of current needed for capture. An ECG strip is obtained and analyzed before, during, and after the procedure. The presence of an adequate pulse and blood pressure demonstrates mechanical capture (the ability of the heart to respond to the electrical impulse).

Permanent pacemakers use an internal pulse generator. This generator is located in a subcutaneous tissue pocket in the chest or abdominal wall. The leads are sewn directly into the heart (epicardial pacing; Fig. 10–32) or passed transvenously into the heart (endocardial pacing; Fig.10–33). Epicardial pacers are inserted during open heart surgery; electrodes are placed directly on the surface of the heart. Endocardial pacers are usually inserted through the subclavian, jugular, or femoral veins into the right ventricle, where they are lodged.

Pacemakers are programmed to pace different areas of the heart at specific time intervals and in response to a level of stimulation. Most pacemakers are designed to pace the ventricles. In this case, a spike will occur before the *QRS* complex (Fig. 10–34). This method of pacing is used when transmission of impulses from the atria is blocked (i.e., complete heart block; see Section Ten). The atria can also be paced. A spike will appear before the *P* wave (Fig. 10–35). This method of pacing is used with sinus node disease. AV sequential pacing is used to synchronize heart depolarization in order to maintain CO. In this type of pacing, both the atria and the ventricles are

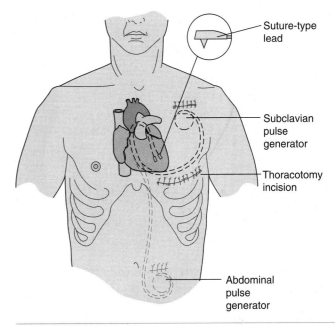

Figure 10–32 ■ Epicardial pacing.

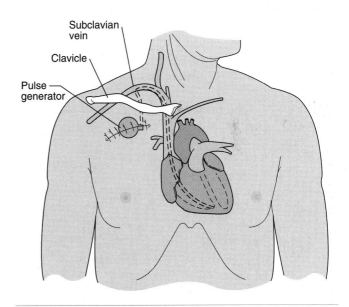

Figure 10–33 ■ Endocardial pacing.

paced (dual chamber). Spikes appear before the *P* wave and the *QRS* complex (Fig. 10–36).

A pacemaker can be programmed to function in the inhibited mode, where a pacing impulse is initiated only when an intrinsic beat is not sensed. If it is programmed in a triggered mode, it fires an impulse in response to sensing electrical activity (e.g., ventricular fibrillation). A double function pacemaker reacts to both inhibition and triggering.

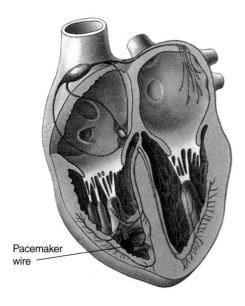

Pacemaker
wire

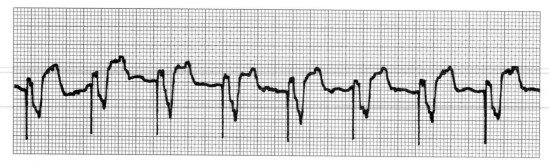

Figure 10–34 ■ Ventricular pacemaker spikes occur before the *QRS*.

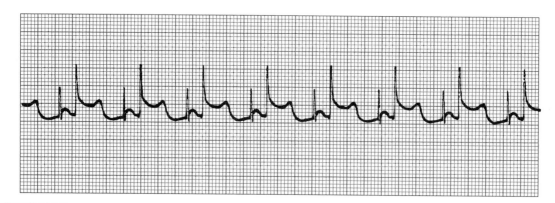

Figure 10–35 ■ Atrial pacemaker spikes occur before the *P* wave.

The number of times the pacemaker fires is determined by the sensitivity setting of the pacemaker. If the sensitivity is low, the pacemaker does not sense the patient's cardiac electrical activity and will pace more frequently. If the sensitivity is high, the pacemaker is better able to sense the patient's cardiac electrical activity and is inhibited from firing. Most are set on demand, with a high-sensitivity setting. A paced beat occurs only when the patient's atria or ventricles fail to discharge. Fixed-rate pacing is used only with individuals whose inherent rhythm is exceedingly slow. If the pacemaker competes with the patient's own impulse generation, the term *failure to sense* is used (Fig. 10–37). This is a potentially dan-

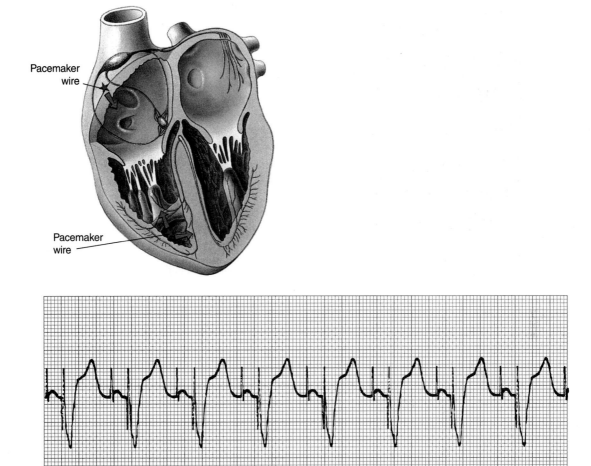

Figure 10-36 ■ AV sequential pacing: both atria and ventricles are paced.

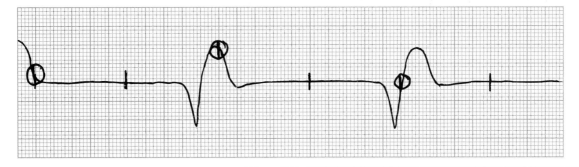

Figure 10-37 ■ Failure to sense.

gerous situation because the pacemaker can discharge an impulse during the relative refractory or supranormal periods of ventricular repolarization, precipitating ventricular fibrillation. The term *failure to capture* is used to describe the situation in which the pacemaker initiates an impulse but the stimulus is not strong enough to produce depolarization. A

pacing spike is present, but *P* waves or *QRS* complexes or both are absent (Fig. 10–38). For sensing and capturing to occur, the pulse generator must have adequate battery function, the leads must be firmly attached to the pacemaker and the myocardium, and the lead wires must be intact (Reynolds & Apple, 2001).

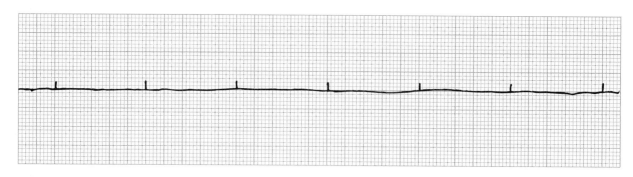

Figure 10–38 ■ Failure to capture.

TABLE 10–9 Generic Pacemaker Code

FIRST LETTER CHAMBER PACED	SECOND LETTER CHAMBER SENSED	THIRD LETTER PACEMAKER RESPONSE	FOURTH LETTER PROGRAMMABLE FUNCTIONS	FIFTH LETTER ANTITACHYCARDIA FUNCTIONS
Atrium	Atrium	Triggered	Programmable	Pacing
Ventricle	Ventricle	Inhibited	Multiprogrammable	Shock
Dual	Dual	Double	Communication	Dual
0×5	0	0	Rate modulated	0
			0	

Key: O = None

Pacemakers are classified according to a uniform system that is universally used to describe how the device functions according to where the pacing leads are and the mode of pacing (Jackson & Gerity, 2000). Pacemaker code is written using a five-letter format and using no more letters than necessary (Bernstein et al., 2000) (Table 10–9). A DDD pacemaker is a dual-chamber pacemaker that is able to pace and sense. A DDDR pacemaker is rate responsive, which means that it can detect the metabolic need for rate adjustment (e.g., during exercise) and adjust accordingly if the native pacemaker fails to achieve this rate.

Implantable Cardioverter/Defibrillator

An implantable cardioverter/defibrillator (ICD) is placed in patients who have had prior aborted sudden cardiac death or proven sustained ventricular tachycardia (Gregoratos et al., 2002). It also may be placed prophylactically in high-risk groups, such as those with various forms of cardiomyopathy (Saksena & Madan, 2002). The device is a fully implantable, battery-operated system designed to recognize and terminate ventricular tachyarrhythmias that can cause sudden death. The device discharges to override the ectopic ventricular pacemaker. The most recent ICDs are capable of distinguishing ventricular tachycardia (VT) from ventricular fibrillation (VF) (thus delivering defibrillation shocks only when absolutely necessary); antitachycardia pacing (to treat VT without resorting to cardioversion shocks unless necessary); providing backup bradycardia pacing (eliminating the need for a standard pacemaker);

and storing cardiac events so that they can be retrieved for analyzing the patient's response to treatment. Generator longevity depends on how often the device's features are used but generally is at least 4 years (Saksena & Madan, 2002).

Implantation of the ICD is accomplished percutaneously through the subclavian or cephalic vein. The lead is positioned in the heart transvenously and the generator is implanted subcutaneously in the upper chest. Once in place the device is programmed and tested using electrophysiologic studies. In essence, VF is intentionally induced in a controlled environment. The ICD is set to deliver shocks at the rate necessary to convert the VF to a sinus rhythm.

If the ICD malfunctions, it may be necessary to deactivate the device by applying a special magnet over the ICD. The nurse must be familiar with the correct procedure for deactivating the device. If the ICD malfunctions, or if the heart does not respond to shocks delivered, life-support measures are initiated. During cardiopulmonary resuscitation (CPR), the rescuer can feel a mild shock (similar to a static electricity shock) if the device fires. External defibrillation is performed using anterior–posterior paddle placement. If temporary external pacing is required, the ICD is deactivated.

Patients who need an ICD require extensive teaching. Patients must understand the difference between heart attack and cardiac arrest. The ICD does not prevent a myocardial infarction, but it does prevent cardiac arrest. The patient is taught that the ICD can "reorganize" his or her heart rhythm as well as stimulate the heart (pacemaker action is available on most recent models). Patients are encouraged to keep a diary of shocks received, activities before and after treatment, symptoms, and response after shock. They should contact their cardiologist when they receive a shock.

Patients with ICDs may be restricted from driving in some states (Edelman et al., 2003). They must avoid high magnetic fields because these can deactivate the device. These patients should not receive diathermy treatment, magnetic resonance imaging, or lithotripsy. Arc welders and large industrial motors should be avoided. Cellular phones can interfere with the operation of all defibrillators if held closer than 6 inches from the pulse generator.

An automatic external defibrillator may be used by some medical and nursing service personnel and lay persons to treat ventricular tachycardia and ventricular fibrillation. The ECG pattern is detected through paddles placed on the patient's chest. If a lethal dysrhythmia is detected, the paddles discharge to defibrillate the patient.

Caring for a patient with a pacemaker or ICD requires specialized nursing care, including preparing the patient for insertion of an endocardial pacemaker or applying an external pacing device correctly. The ECG pattern is monitored to determine if the pacemaker is pacing at the correct rate (demand versus fixed), capturing with each impulse, and sensing the patient's own rhythm. Additionally, the nurse assesses the threshold (minimal amount of output required to initiate depolarization) of the pacemaker. The learner is referred to the literature associated with each pacing and defibrillation device to determine the correct method of checking the threshold for that device. It is helpful if patients with histories of dysrhythmias carry copies of their most recent ECGs. Patients are encouraged to obtain MedicAlert bracelets to identify themselves as having pace-

Evidence-Based Practice

- *Patients with ICDs perceive the devices as "life extenders" but are anxious about the batteries running out and technical failure of their devices (Duru et al., 2001).*

- *Women are more concerned than men about how the pacemaker site and scar make them feel about their bodies, clothes, and wearing swimsuits (Davis et al., 2004).*

- *Participation in a support group for patients with ICDs augments patients' knowledge, dispels misconceptions, facilitates social exchange, normalizes fears and concerns, and provides emotional support (Dickerson et al., 2000).*

- *Older ICD recipients appear to need psychosocial interventions to help retain their physical functioning after ICD insertion and improve their health status (Hamilton & Carroll, 2004).*

makers or ICDs. The type of device, manufacturer, and model number should be readily available.

In summary, there are three routes of electrical therapy: external, epicardial, and endocardial. The atria or the ventricles may be paced. The rate is set on a demand or continuous setting. The pacing device may fail to sense and compete with the patient's own rhythm. The device may fail to capture by initiating an impulse that is not sufficient to depolarize myocardial cells. ICD devices are capable of pacing, cardioverting, and defibrillating (unless they are older models). In cases in which the device malfunctions or the heart does not respond mechanically to treatment, CPR is initiated without hesitation. Nursing care focuses on assisting with insertion or application; and monitoring the threshold, capture, and sensitivity of the device.

SECTION TWELVE REVIEW

1. An external pacing device
   A. is used only to treat supraventricular dysrhythmias
   B. is a temporary measure
   C. requires the patient to be alert in order to function
   D. can be set only in continuous mode

2. An epicardial pacing device is
   A. placed through the subclavian vein
   B. applied to the chest wall
   C. inserted in open heart surgery
   D. used exclusively for AV sequential pacing

3. Failure to sense means
   A. the pacing device is turned off
   B. depolarization is not occurring
   C. the patient is tachycardic
   D. the pacing device is competing with the patient's own rhythm

4. Failure to capture means
   A. depolarization does not occur after a pacer-generated impulse

   B. atria and ventricles are not contracting in a synchronous manner
   C. the pacing device needs to be replaced
   D. the patient will require cardioversion

5. When a pacemaker is functioning in an inhibited mode
   A. a pacing impulse is generated when an intrinsic beat is not sensed
   B. it fires an impulse in response to sensing electrical activity
   C. the SA node is overriding the pacing rate
   D. the device is malfunctioning

6. A patient with an ICD complains of multiple repeated shocks. He is in sinus tachycardia on the heart monitor. The nurse should
   A. hold a magnet over the ICD
   B. cardiovert the patient
   C. notify the physician to obtain a deactivation order
   D. roll the patient to his left side

Answers: 1. B, 2. C, 3. D, 4. A, 5. A, 6. C

POSTTEST

1. Depolarization is precipitated by
   A. potassium moving into the cell
   B. calcium moving out of the cell
   C. sodium moving into the cell
   D. sodium moving out of the cell

2. When the SA node is pacing the heart, the heart rate will be
   A. irregular
   B. less than 50 bpm
   C. 60 to 100 bpm
   D. regular

3. The *ST* segment should be
   A. less than 0.20 second
   B. isoelectric
   C. positively deflected
   D. peaked

4. *QRS* complexes should be
   A. preceded by a *T* wave
   B. isoelectric
   C. positively deflected
   D. less than 0.10 second

5. Time is represented by the
   A. vertical axis of the ECG paper
   B. color of ink on the ECG paper
   C. horizontal axis on the ECG paper
   D. asterisk at the bottom of the ECG paper

6. Which of the following are normal values?
   A. *PR* interval less than 0.20 second; *QRS* complex less than 0.10 second
   B. *PR* interval less than 0.04 second; *QRS* complex less than 0.10 second
   C. *PR* interval less than 0.20 second; *QRS* complex less than 0.20 second
   D. *PR* interval less than 0.10 second; *QRS* complex less than 0.20 second

7. Fluid volume deficit primarily produces
   A. tachydysrhythmias
   B. cardiac conduction blocks
   C. bradydysrhythmias
   D. wide *QRS* complexes

8. Hypercalcemia results in
   A. increased automaticity
   B. PACs
   C. shortened *QT* interval
   D. tall, peaked *T* waves

9. Sinus bradycardia may be normal in
   A. athletes
   B. persons experiencing stressful situations
   C. elderly patients
   D. persons with hypertension

10. Sinus dysrhythmias are usually harmless. They should be treated when the patient develops
    A. a decreased level of consciousness
    B. hypotension
    C. angina
    D. all of the above

11. Atrial flutter is characterized by
    A. sawtoothed *P* waves
    B. regular *QRS* intervals
    C. absent *P* waves
    D. atrial rate less than 250 bpm

12. Which of the following drugs temporarily inhibits AV node conduction?
    A. Propanolol
    B. Digoxin
    C. Adenosine
    D. Verapamil

13. Junctional tachycardia is differentiated from an accelerated junctional rhythm by
    A. presence of *P* wave
    B. length of *PR* interval
    C. rate of the rhythm
    D. *QRS* configuration

14. Which of the following is true about *P* waves in a junctional dysrhythmia?
    A. *P* wave may be inverted
    B. *P* wave may precede *QRS*
    C. *P* wave may follow *QRS*
    D. all of the above

15. PACs are usually
    A. preceded by a hypoxic episode
    B. a signal of ventricular irritability
    C. harmless
    D. associated with digitalis toxicity

16. Which of the following statements is FALSE?
    A. hypoxia can cause PVCs
    B. acidosis can cause PVCs
    C. digitalis toxicity can cause PVCs
    D. hyperkalemia can cause PVCs

17. Pharmacologic treatment of VT includes
    A. amiodarone
    B. lidocaine
    C. magnesium
    D. all of the above

18. Defibrillation is the treatment of choice for
    A. ventricular tachycardia
    B. ventricular defibrillation
    C. atrial fibrillation
    D. atrial flutter

19. Type II second-degree AV block
   A. is associated with ventricular irritability
   B. is more ominous than type I second-degree AV block
   C. is less than 50 bpm
   D. requires treatment with Verapamil

20. Which of the following requires emergency treatment because the atria and ventricles are contracting independently?
   A. complete heart block
   B. atrial fibrillation
   C. ventricular fibrillation
   D. Mobitz type II heart block

21. The major difference between cardioversion and defibrillation is
   A. the number of times each can be repeated
   B. one method is synchronized to discharge directly following the *R* wave
   C. one method is used to treat delays in cardiac conduction
   D. one method requires the patient to be alert

22. Which of the following classes of antiarrhythmics block potassium channels?
   A. class I
   B. class II
   C. class III
   D. class IV

23. Failure to capture means the artificial pacing device
   A. is competing with the patient's own rhythm
   B. is not producing depolarization
   C. needs new batteries
   D. is causing PVCs

24. Which of the following therapies may be used for a patient who has had prior aborted sudden cardiac death?
   A. DDD pacemaker
   B. epicardial pacemaker
   C. external pacing
   D. ICD

POSTTEST ANSWERS

Question	Answer	Section	Question	Answer	Section
1	C	One	13	C	Seven
2	C	Two	14	D	Seven
3	B	Two	15	C	Eight
4	D	Two	16	D	Eight
5	C	Three	17	D	Nine
6	A	Three	18	B	Nine
7	A	Four	19	B	Ten
8	C	Four	20	A	Ten
9	A	Five	21	B	Eleven
10	D	Five	22	C	Eleven
11	A	Six	23	B	Twelve
12	C	Six	24	D	Twelve

REFERENCES

AHA-ILCR (American Heart Association in association with The International Liaison Committee on Resuscitation). (2000). Guidelines 2000 for cardiopulmonary resuscitation and emergency cardiovascular care. An international consensus on science. *Circulation, 102*(8), I1–I384.

Asselin, M. E., & Cullen, A. (2001). New ACLS guidelines. *Nursing, 31*(4), 48.

Bernstein, A. D., Daubert, J. C., Fletcher, R. D., et al. (2000). The revised NASPE/BPEG generic code for antibradycardia, adaptive-rate, and multisite pacing. *PACE, 25,* 260–264.

Bond, E. F. (2000). Cardiac anatomy and physiology. In S. L. Woods, E. S Froelicher, & S. A. Motzer (Eds.), *Cardiac nursing* (4th ed., pp. 3–50). Philadelphia: Lippincott Williams & Wilkins.

Cunningham, S., DelBene, S., & Vaughan, A. F. (2000). Myocardial ischemia pathogenesis of atherosclerosis. In S. L. Woods, E. S Froelicher, & S. A. Motzer (Eds.), *Cardiac nursing* (4th ed., pp. 479–540). Philadelphia: Lippincott Williams & Wilkins.

Davis, L. L., Vitale, K. A., Irmiere, C. A., et al. (2004). Body image changes associated with dual chamber pacemaker insertion in women. *Heart and Lung: The Journal of Acute and Critical Care, 33,* 273–280.

Dickerson, S. S., Posluszny, M., & Kennedy, M. (2000). Help seeking in a support group for recipients of implantable cardioverter defibrillators and their support persons. *Heart and Lung: The Journal of Acute and Critical Care, 29,* 87–96.

Duru, F., Buchi, S., Klaghofer, R., et al. (2001). How different from pacemaker patients are recipients of implantable cardioverter defibrillators with respect to psychosocial adaptation, affective disorders, and quality of life? *British Heart Journal, 85,* 375–379.

Edelman, S., Lemon, J., & Kidman, A. (2003). Psychological therapies for recipients of implantable cardioverter defibrillators [Issues in cardiovascular nursing]. *Heart and Lung: The Journal of Acute and Critical Care, 32*(4), 234–240.

Felver, L. (2000). Acid–base balance and imbalances. In S. L. Woods, E. S. Froelicher, & S. A. Motzer (Eds.), *Cardiac nursing* (4th ed., pp. 153–161). Philadelphia: Lippincott Williams & Wilkins.

Gilbert, C. J. (2001). Common supraventricular tachycardias: Mechanisms and management. *AACN Clinical Issues: Advanced Practice in Acute Critical Care, 12*(1), 100–133, 167–169.

Gregoratos, G., Abrams, J., Epstein, A. E., et al. (2002). ACC/AHA/NASPE 2002 guideline update for implantation of cardiac pacemakers and antiarrhythmia devices: A report of the American College of Cardiology/American Heart Association Task Force on Practice Guidelines. *Circulation, 106,* 2145–2161.

Hamilton, G. A., & Carroll, D. L. (2004). The effects of age on quality of life in implantable cardioverter defibrillator recipients. *Journal of Clinical Nursing, 13,* 194–200.

Hand, H. (2002). Common cardiac arrhythmias. *Nursing Standard, 16*(28), 43–53, 58.

Jackson, C., & Gerity, D. (2000). Pacemaker and implantable defibrillators. In S. L. Woods, E. S. Froelicher, & S. A. Motzer (Eds.), *Cardiac nursing* (4th ed., pp. 661–698). Philadelphia: Lippincott Williams & Wilkins.

Jacobson, C. (2000). Arrhythmias and conduction disturbances. In S. L. Woods, E. S. Froelicher, & S. A. Motzer (Eds.), *Cardiac nursing* (4th ed., pp. 297–362). Philadelphia: Lippincott Williams & Wilkins.

Kaushik, V., Leon, A. R., Forrester, J. S., & Trohman, R. G. (2000). Bradyarrhythmias, temporary and permanent pacing. *Critical Care Medicine, 28*(10 Suppl), N121–128.

Ma, G., Brady, W. J., Pollack, M., & Chan, T. C. (2001). Electrocardiographic manifestations: Digitalis toxicity. *Journal of Emergency Medicine, 20*(2), 145–152.

Mangrum, J., & DiMarco, J. P. (2000). Primary care: The evaluation and management of bradycardia. *New England Journal of Medicine, 342*(10), 703–709.

Maron, B. J. (2003). Medical progress: Sudden death in young athletes. *New England Journal of Medicine, 349*(11), 1064–1075.

Navas, S. (2003). Atrial fibrillation: Part 2. *Nursing Standard, 17*(38), 47–54.

Reynolds, J., & Apple, S. (2001). A systematic approach to pacemaker assessment [Cardiovascular nursing]. *AACN Clinical Issues: Advanced Practice in Acute Critical Care, 12*(1), 114–126.

Saksena, S., & Madan, N. (2002). Management of the patient with an implantable cardioverter-defibrillator in the third millennium [Clinician update]. *Circulation, 106*(21), 2642–2646.

Sanguinetti, M. C., & Bennett, P. B. (2003). Antiarrhythmic drug target choices and screening. *Circulation Research, 93*(6), 491–499.

Trappe, H. J., Brandts, B., & Weismueller, P. (2003). Arrhythmias in the intensive care patient. *Current Opinion in Critical Care, 9*(5), 345–355.

Alterations in Myocardial Tissue Perfusion

Clifford C. Pyne,* Karen L. Johnson

11

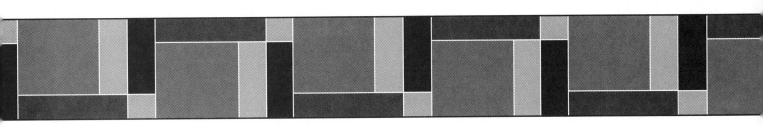

OBJECTIVES Following completion of this module, the learner will be able to

1. Describe the pathophysiology of atherosclerosis.
2. Identify modifiable and nonmodifiable risk factors for atherosclerosis.
   - List nursing diagnoses appropriate for the patient with risk factors for atherosclerosis.
   - Discuss collaborative interventions to reduce and manage risk factors for atherosclerosis.
3. Describe normal coronary artery anatomy and regulation of coronary perfusion.
4. Identify subjective data associated with coronary artery disease.
   - Differentiate types of angina including stable angina, unstable angina, and variant angina.
   - Discuss the focused physical assessment for a patient who complains of chest pain.
5. Identify electrocardiogram changes associated with myocardial ischemia and myocardial infarction.

- Identify cardiac markers that, when present in the serum, indicate myocardial muscle damage.
- Discuss the purpose of three commonly used diagnostic tests available for assessment of myocardial tissue perfusion.

6. Define acute coronary syndromes, unstable angina, and myocardial infarction.
   - List nursing diagnoses appropriate for a patient with an acute coronary syndrome.
7. Discuss initial collaborative management of a patient presenting with chest pain.
   - State the collaborative interventions commonly used to restore myocardial tissue perfusion.
   - Discuss nursing management priorities for patients requiring thrombolytic therapy, percutaneous coronary intervention, and coronary artery bypass surgery.

This self-study module focuses on disease processes that alter myocardial perfusion, signs and symptoms of altered myocardial perfusion, collaborative interventions used in the high-acuity setting to restore myocardial tissue perfusion, and nursing care of patients who require these myocardial tissue reperfusion interventions. The module is composed of seven sections. Section One reviews the pathophysiology of atherosclerosis. Section Two discusses the assessment and management of risk factors for atherosclerosis. Section Three reviews

normal coronary tissue perfusion. Section Four presents the signs and symptoms associated with decreased myocardial tissue perfusion. Section Five considers the diagnostic studies used in the evaluation of myocardial tissue perfusion. Section Six presents the acute coronary syndromes, and Section Seven reviews collaborative interventions to restore myocardial tissue perfusion, and discusses nursing management priorities for patients who receive myocardial reperfusion therapies. Each section includes a set of review questions to help the learner evaluate his or her understanding of the section's content before moving on to the next section. All Section Reviews and the module Pretest and Posttest include answers. It is suggested that the learner review those concepts answered incorrectly in the review questions before proceeding to the next section.

*The views expressed in this article are those of the author and do not necessarily reflect the official policy or position of the Department of the Navy, Department of Defense, or the U.S. Government.

PRETEST

1. Fatty streaks are
   A. a group of foam cells
   B. flat, thick, yellow lesions that get progressively bigger
   C. found in children
   D. all of the above

2. The basic lesion associated with atherosclerosis is a(n)
   A. fibrous atheromatous plaque
   B. atheroma
   C. type I lesion
   D. foam cell

3. Which of the following is NOT a modifiable risk factor for atherosclerosis?
   A. hypercholesterolemia
   B. type 2 diabetes
   C. age
   D. hypertension

4. High-density lipoprotein (HDL)
   A. is the major cause of atherosclerosis
   B. contains high-density protein and low amounts of cholesterol
   C. deposits in the intimal lining of arteries
   D. should be less than 100 mg/dL

5. Blood supply to the lateral walls of the left ventricle is from the
   A. left anterior descending artery
   B. left main coronary artery
   C. left circumflex artery
   D. right coronary artery

6. Currents of injury result in
   A. hyperacute *T* waves
   B. *ST* elevation
   C. *T* wave inversion
   D. all of the above

7. A troponin I level is 1.0 mcg/L. This level indicates
   A. significant damage to the left ventricle
   B. a normal level
   C. less than 25 percent cardiac muscle damage
   D. a myocardial infarction has occurred

8. Patients with ischemic *ST* changes and presence of serum cardiac markers are diagnosed as having
   A. unstable angina
   B. stable angina
   C. non-*ST* elevation myocardial infarction (MI)
   D. *ST* elevation

9. Morphine is given for patients with chest pain for all of the following reasons EXCEPT
   A. to increase cardiac output
   B. to cause vasodilation
   C. to decrease myocardial workload
   D. because it has a direct action on pain receptors

10. Postpercutaneous coronary intervention procedures require the patient to remain supine for _____.
    A. 24 hours
    B. 12 hours
    C. 6 hours
    D. 1 hour

11. Which of the following is NOT a sign associated with Beck's triad?
    A. elevated right atrial pressure
    B. hypotension
    C. muffled heart sounds
    D. pulsus paradoxus

12. Blood flow through the coronary arteries is regulated by
    A. the sympathetic nervous system
    B. the parasympathetic nervous system
    C. aortic pressure
    D. calcium

13. Which of the following is the easiest and most cost effective diagnostic test to assist in evaluating the adequacy of myocardial tissue perfusion?
    A. ECG
    B. cardiac markers
    C. exercise stress test
    D. myocardial perfusion imaging

14. Changes in the _____ is the most sensitive electrographic indicator of ischemia and injury to the myocardium.
    A. *PR* interval
    B. *QRS* complex
    C. *ST* segment
    D. *T* wave

Pretest Answers:
1. D, 2. A, 3. C, 4. B, 5. A, 6. D, 7. B, 8. C, 9. A, 10. C,
11. D, 12. C, 13. A, 14. C

GLOSSARY

akinesis   Lack of myocardial wall movement.

angina pectoris   Chest pain that is usually precipitated by exercise and relieved by rest.

anginal equivalents   Symptoms suggestive of coronary artery disease but that do not include angina (examples include dyspnea, fatigue, dizziness).

atheroma   Complicated atherosclerotic lesion that is calcified and contains hemorrhage, ulceration, and scar tissue deposits.

atherosclerosis   Immune-inflammatory disorder characterized by formation of plaque in the intimal lining of medium and large arteries.

Beck's triad Classic signs of cardiac tamponade that include elevated right atrial pressure, hypotension, and muffled heart sounds.

cardiac markers Proteins that necrotic myocytes release into the blood; when present in the serum, they signal myocardial damage.

cardiac tamponade A life-threatening postoperative complication of coronary artery bypass surgery caused by bleeding into the pericardial sac.

dyskinesis Myocardial wall movement in the opposite direction.

echocardiography Imaging technique used to assess functional structures of the heart using ultrasound waves.

ejection fraction (EF) The amount of blood ejected from the left ventricle per each heartbeat; normal is above 50 percent.

endothelium Thin inner layer of blood vessels composed of endothelial cells.

fatty streaks Type II atherosclerotic skin lesions characterized by macrophage migration across the endothelium and smooth muscle cells that contain lipid droplets.

fibrous atheromatous plaque Basic lesion associated with atherosclerosis; lesion filled with lipids, collagen, scar tissue, and vascular smooth muscle cells.

high-density lipoprotein (HDL) Lipoprotein molecule that has a high density (amount) of protein and a small amount of cholesterol; commonly known as the "good" cholesterol.

hypercholesterolemia High levels of serum cholesterol.

hypokinesis Decreased myocardial wall movement.

lipoproteins Cholesterol bound to protein and carried in the blood.

low-density lipoprotein (LDL) Lipoprotein molecule that has a low density (amount) of protein and a large amount of cholesterol; commonly known as the "bad" cholesterol.

modifiable risk factors Risk factors that can be altered through either lifestyle modification or medications (examples include obesity and smoking).

nonmodifiable risk factors Risk factors that, regardless of therapy, cannot be altered (examples include genetics and age).

percutaneous coronary intervention (PCI) The use of angioplasty balloons and coronary stents to alleviate stenoses of arteries and reestablish blood flow to ischemic myocardium.

perfusionist A specially trained technician who controls the cardiopulmonary bypass machine during coronary artery bypass surgery.

precursor lesions Types II and III atherosclerotic lesions that form during the teenage years.

prinzmetal's angina See variant angina.

pulsus paradoxus Exaggerated decrease (greater than 10 mm Hg) in systolic blood pressure during inspiration.

stable angina Chest pain that is predictable and relieved with rest or nitrates.

unstable angina Chest pain that is not predictable, and that occurs with rest or with minimal activity.

variant angina Chest pain that is not predictable, may occur at night, and is caused by coronary artery spasm; also known as Prinzmetal's angina.

xanthoma A cholesterol-filled skin lesion.

ABBREVIATIONS

ACC	American College of Cardiology
ACS	Acute coronary syndromes
AHA	American Heart Association
aPTT	Activated partial thromboplastin time
ASA	Acetylsalicylic acid (aspirin)
CABG	Coronary artery bypass graft
CAD	Coronary artery disease
CCSC	Canadian Cardiology Society Classification
CI	Cardiac index
CK	Creatine phosphokinase
CK-MB	Creatine phosphokinase–myocardial bands
CO	Cardiac output
CPB	Cardiopulmonary bypass
CPP	Coronary perfusion pressure
cTn	Troponin
cTnI	Troponin-I
cTnT	Troponin-T
DBP	Diastolic blood pressure
EBL	Estimated blood loss
ECG	Electrocardiogram
EF	Ejection fraction
EST	Exercise stress test
GP	Glycoprotein
HDL	High-density lipoprotein
IV	Intravenous
LAD	Left anterior descending artery
LCX	Left circumflex artery
LDL	Low-density lipoprotein
LIMA	Left internal mammary artery
LMCA	Left main coronary artery

LMWH	Low molecular weight heparin	PVD	Peripheral vascular disease
MI	Myocardial infarction	RCA	Right coronary artery
MPI	Myocardial perfusion imaging	RIMA	Right internal mammary artery
NSTEMI	Non-*ST* elevation myocardial infarction	STEMI	*ST* elevation myocardial infarction
PAWP	Pulmonary artery wedge pressure	SVG	Saphenous vein graft
PCI	Percutaneous coronary intervention	UA	Unstable angina
PDA	Posterior descending artery	UH	Unfractionated heparin

SECTION ONE: Pathophysiology of Atherosclerosis

At the completion of this section, the learner will be able to describe the pathophysiology of atherosclerosis.

Atherosclerosis, commonly referred to as "hardening of the arteries," accounts for almost 75 percent of deaths as a result of cardiovascular disease (CVD) in the United States and is the primary underlying cause of peripheral artery disease (PAD), coronary artery disease (CAD), and cerebrovascular disease (AHA, 2003). Atherosclerosis and its associated disorders are pervasive and affect both men and women.

A normal artery consists of three concentric layers: the innermost layer is the tunica intima, the middle layer is the tunica media, and the outermost layer is the tunica adventitia (Fig. 11–1A). **Atherosclerosis** is an immune–inflammatory disorder associated with injury to the intimal lining. It is a progressive disease characterized by formation of plaque in the intimal lining of medium and large arteries, including those in the aorta and its branches, the coronary arteries, and large vessels that supply the brain.

Although the precise mechanisms are unknown, atherosclerosis appears to begin with chronic injury or inflammation to the endothelial cells that line blood vessels. Collectively, all these endothelial cells are called the **endothelium.**

Sources of chronic injury and inflammation may include such things as hypertension, smoking, viruses, high cholesterol, and high glucose. These factors damage the endothelium causing endothelial cells to separate. This allows monocytes from the bloodstream to enter into the intimal lining and become macrophages. Macrophages release substances that oxidize low-density lipoproteins (LDL) which are toxic to endothelial cells. This causes further endothelial cell dysfunction. Macrophages engulf LDL and become "foam cells." A group of foam cells becomes a "fatty streak" along the vessel wall (Fig. 11–1A). **Fatty streaks** are flat, thick, yellow lesions that progressively get thicker and bigger, and protrude into the lumen of the artery. Fatty streaks have been found in the arteries of children (Gotto & Pownall, 2003).

Some fatty streaks develop into another type of atherosclerotic lesion called a **fibrous atheromatous plaque.** This is the basic lesion associated with atherosclerosis. Inside this lesion is an accumulation of lipids, collagen, scar tissue, and vascular smooth muscle cells (Matfin & Porth, 2005) (Fig. 11–1B). As these lesions grow, they become more complex and thick. Eventually, they narrow the vessel lumen and reduce blood flow.

Some of these lesions advance to a more complicated lesion called an **atheroma.** Atheromas are calcified lesions that contain hemorrhage, ulceration, and scar tissue deposits (Porth, 2005). Decreased or sluggish blood flow past the lesion can result in the formation of a thrombus on the lesion. The formation of this thrombus is dangerous because not only does it further reduce blood flow but it can also break off to become an embolus.

American Heart Association Classification

The American Heart Association (AHA) uses a classification system to distinguish among lesion progressions. Type I lesions are small lesions that are not visible to the unaided eye and can be present in children. As atherosclerosis development continues with advancing age, other types of lesions form. Types II and III lesions (**precursor lesions**) begin to form as early as the teenage years. Type II lesions are the fatty streaks. A significant amount of research is currently underway to identify the causative factors that result in the formation of these lesions at such a young age. Type III lesions are intermediate lesions and form a bridge between type II lesions and atheromas (Braunwald et al., 2002).

Advanced atherosclerotic lesions (types IV through VII) are responsible for the majority of the symptoms commonly attributed to atherosclerotic disease. These are the lesions that cause significant narrowing of the arterial lumen and ischemia to the organs distal to the lesion.

In summary, atherosclerosis is an immune–inflammatory disease that is associated with injury to the intimal lining as a result of chronic injury to the endothelium. Chronic injury causes endothelial cells to separate, allowing monocytes to enter the intimal lining of arteries. Macrophages engulf LDL and become foam cells. A group of foam cells becomes a fatty streak. Fatty streaks, present in children, may be the precursor to fibrous atheromatous plaque, the basic lesion of atherosclerosis and the more advanced lesion called an atheroma. These lesions obstruct blood flow distal to the lesion.

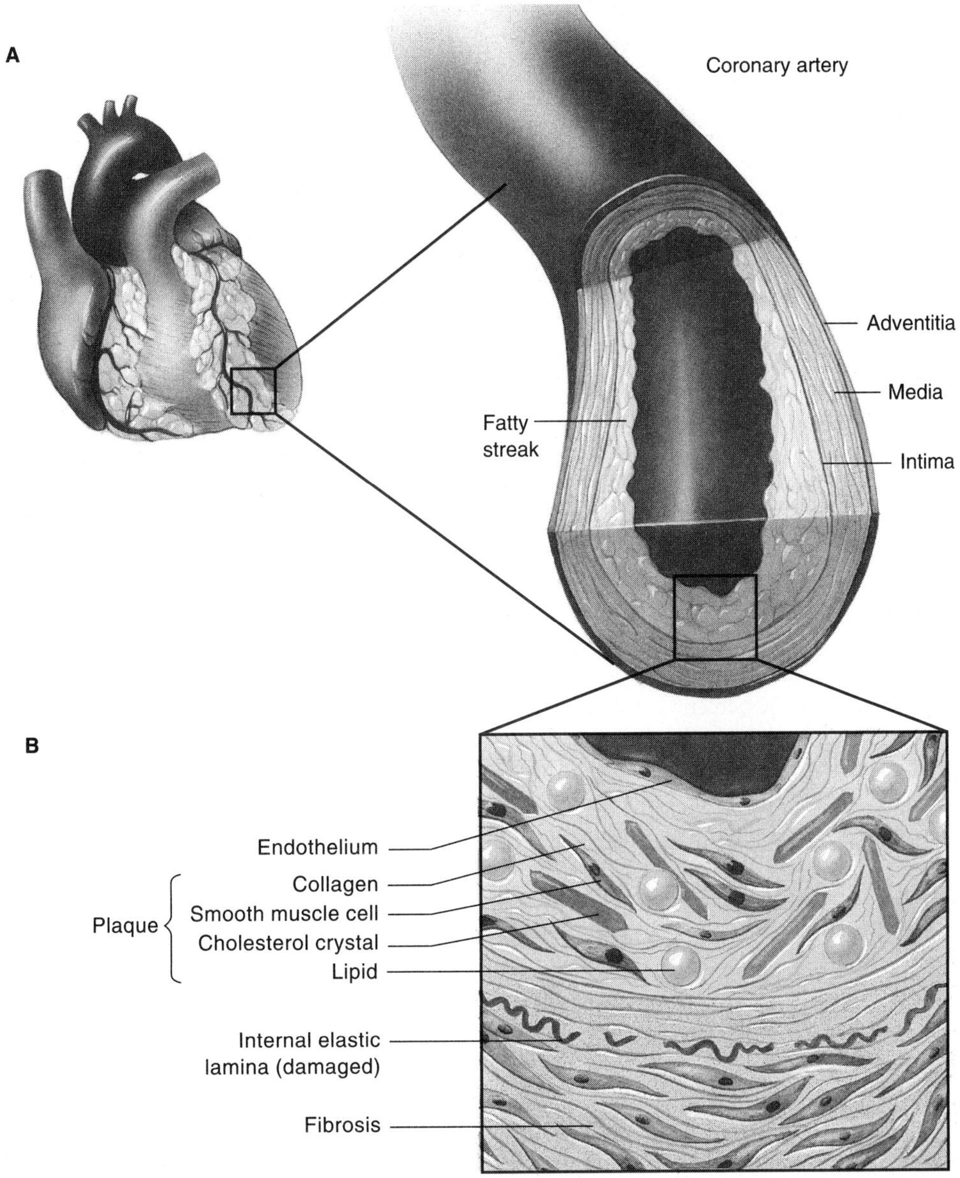

Figure 11–1 ■ The normal artery layers: intima, media, and adventitia.

A

Coronary artery

Adventitia

Media

Intima

Fatty streak

B

Endothelium

Collagen

Plaque { Smooth muscle cell

Cholesterol crystal

Lipid

Internal elastic lamina (damaged)

Fibrosis

SECTION ONE REVIEW

1. Atherosclerosis is a disease associated with injury to
   - A. intimal lining of arteries
   - B. medial lining of arteries
   - C. fibrous atheromatous plaque
   - D. macrophages
2. Sources of chronic endothelial cell injury include
   - A. hypertension
   - B. smoking
   - C. high cholesterol
   - D. all of the above
3. Foam cells are
   - A. cells that secrete peroxidase
   - B. cells that secrete hydrogen peroxide
   - C. macrophages that have engulfed LDL
   - D. endothelial cells with LDL
4. Type I lesions may be present in
   - A. children
   - B. 20 year olds
   - C. 30 year olds
   - D. people with advanced atherosclerosis
5. Types IV through VII lesions are
   - A. precursor lesions
   - B. responsible for symptoms of atherosclerotic disease
   - C. present in children
   - D. filled with HDL

Answers: 1. A, 2. D, 3. C, 4. A, 5. B

SECTION TWO: Assessment and Management of Risk Factors for Atherosclerosis

At the completion of this section, the learner will be able to identify modifiable and nonmodifiable risk factors for atherosclerosis, list nursing diagnoses appropriate for the patient with risk factors for atherosclerosis, and discuss collaborative interventions to reduce and manage risk factors for atherosclerosis.

Although the exact cause of atherosclerosis is not known, epidemiologic studies have found certain risk factors that, when present, seem to predispose the development of atherosclerosis. Risk factors are categorized as either modifiable or nonmodifiable. **Modifiable risk factors** include those risk factors that can be altered through either lifestyle modification or medication. **Nonmodifiable risk factors** include those risk factors that, regardless of therapy, cannot be altered.

Nonmodifiable Risk Factors

Nonmodifiable risk factors are summarized in Table 11–1. Increasing age is a nonmodifiable risk factor. More than 50 percent of heart attack victims are 65 or older (Lemone & Burke, 2004). Men are at a greater risk for developing atherosclerosis than premenopausal women. Estrogen may have some type of protective effect on endothelial cells. After menopause, the risk of atherosclerosis-related diseases increases in women. African Americans have a higher incidence of hypertension. Hypertension is believed to be one of the forces that causes chronic injury to endothelial cells and promotes the development of atherosclerotic lesions. Atherosclerosis appears to run in families because persons from families with strong histories of atherosclerotic-associated diseases (stroke, heart disease) are at greater risk for developing atherosclerosis than those with negative family histories (Matfin & Porth, 2005).

Unfortunately people with nonmodifiable risk factors cannot do anything about them. However, people with these risk factors must take special precautions to reduce further risks by decreasing their modifiable risk factors.

Modifiable Risk Factors

Modifiable risk factors are summarized in Table 11–2.

Hypercholesterolemia, or elevated serum cholesterol levels, is a major risk factor for the development of atherosclerosis. Cholesterol is carried in the bloodstream bound to proteins.

TABLE 11–1   Nonmodifiable Risk Factors for Atherosclerosis

Age	African American
Male sex	Genetics

TABLE 11–2   Modifiable Risk Factors for Atherosclerosis

Hypercholesterolemia	Obesity
Elevated LDL levels	Physical inactivity
Type 2 diabetes	Smoking
Metabolic syndrome	Diet
Hypertension	

When cholesterol is bound to proteins, this combination forms a molecule called a **lipoprotein.** There are different amounts, or densities, of proteins and cholesterol that form lipoprotein molecules. Recall from Module 8, when a lipoprotein molecule contains a high amount of cholesterol and low-density protein, it is called a **low-density lipoprotein (LDL),** commonly referred to as "bad" cholesterol. When a lipoprotein molecule contains a small amount of cholesterol and high-density protein, it is called **high-density lipoprotein (HDL),** commonly referred to as "good" cholesterol. The LDLs accumulate in the intimal lining of arteries and promote formation of atherosclerotic lesions. Recommended levels for serum cholesterol and LDL are listed in Table 11–3.

Other diseases, including type 2 diabetes, metabolic syndrome, hypertension, and obesity, are risk factors for the development of atherosclerosis. Although the exact mechanisms are not known, these diseases participate in the chronic injury to endothelial cells. Control of the risk factor diseases with medications and changes in health care behaviors can reduce the risk of developing atherosclerosis and may reduce disease progression.

There are several modifiable risk factors that can be altered with lifestyle changes. These include physical inactivity, obesity, smoking, and diet. Components of cigarettes cause endothelial damage and vasoconstriction. Obese individuals (body weight greater than 30 percent more than ideal body weight) have higher rates of hypertension, hyperlipidemia, and diabetes. The cardiovascular benefits of exercise are well established. Individuals who engage in regular exercise programs have lower risk of development of cardiovascular diseases related to atherosclerosis.

TABLE 11–3   Classification of Serum Cholesterol and LDL Values[a]

	TOTAL CHOLESTEROL (mg/dL)	LDL CHOLESTEROL (mg/dL)
Very high		Greater than 190
High	Greater than 240	Greater than 160
Borderline high	200 to 239	130 to 159
Desirable	Under 200	100 to 129
Optimal		Less than 100

[a] As defined by National Cholesterol Education Program (2001).

Collaborative Management of Risk Factor Reduction

Nursing diagnoses may include imbalanced nutrition: more than body requirements, and ineffective health maintenance. Aggressive reduction and management of risk factors is crucial to reducing the incidence and progression of atherosclerosis. Identification of risk factors begins with a thorough history. Laboratory testing to assess risk factors may include serum cholesterol and lipid profiles (triglycerides, LDL, HDL levels).

When people stop smoking, the risk of atherosclerotic heart disease is greatly reduced. All people who smoke are advised to quit. Dietary recommendations to reduce cholesterol and LDL levels are listed in Table 11–4. People who are overweight or obese are encouraged to lose weight through a program that includes diet and exercise. Unless contraindicated, most individuals should participate in at least 30 minutes of moderate-intensity physical activity 5 to 6 days a week.

Control of hypertension is vital to reducing atherosclerosis. Management strategies include a low sodium diet, regular exercise, stress management, and compliance with medication regimens. (Refer to Module 12 for additional information on hypertension.)

An integral part of reducing atherosclerotic disease progression is drug therapy to reduce serum cholesterol and LDL levels. Drug therapy must be used in combination with a diet that is low in fats and cholesterol. The first-line drugs used are the "statins": Lovastatin (Mevacor), Provastatin (Pravachol), Simvastatin (Zocor), Fluvastatin (Lescol), and Atorvastatin (Lipitor). These drugs lower LDL by creating more LDL re-ceptors on liver cells. LDL receptors bring in LDL from the blood into liver cells where LDL is further broken down. Other classes of cholesterol reducing drugs include bile acid sequestrants (Cholestyramine [Questran], Colestipol [Colestid], and Colesevelam [Welchol]) and fibric acid derivatives (Gemfibrozil [Lopid], Fenofibrate [Tricor], and Clofibrate [Atromid-S]).

In summary, there are modifiable and nonmodifiable risk factors in the development of atherosclerosis. Modifiable risk factors can be modified with lifestyle or medication changes. Aggressive reduction and management of risk factors is crucial to preventing/controlling the development of atherosclerosis.

TABLE 11–4 Dietary Recommendations to Reduce Total Cholesterol and LDL[a]

NUTRIENT	RECOMMENDATION
Total Fat	25 to 35 percent of total calories
▪ Saturated fat	▪ Less than 7 percent of total calories
▪ Polysaturated fat	▪ Up to 10 percent of total calories
▪ Monosaturated fat	▪ Up to 20 percent of total calories
▪ Cholesterol	▪ Less than 200 mg per day
Carbohydrates	50 to 60 percent of total calories
Dietary fiber	20 to 30 grams per day
Protein	About 15 percent of total calories

[a] According to the National Cholesterol Education Program (2001).

SECTION TWO REVIEW

1. Which of the following is a nonmodifiable risk factor for atherosclerotic disease?
   A. age
   B. smoking
   C. obesity
   D. hypercholesterol

2. A lipoprotein that contains a high amount of cholesterol and a low-density protein is called a
   A. high-density lipoprotein
   B. low-density lipoprotein
   C. hypercholesterolemia
   D. lipoprotein A

3. When people stop smoking, the risk of atherosclerotic heart disease
   A. does not change
   B. decreases after 15 years
   C. is greatly reduced
   D. actually is greater

4. Desirable levels of cholesterol are _____ mg/dL and LDL is _____ mg/dL.
   A. greater than 240; greater than 160
   B. 200 to 300; 130 to 159
   C. less than 100; greater than 190
   D. less than 200; 100 to 129

5. Statins work to reduce atherosclerotic disease progression by
   A. increasing LDL receptors on liver cells
   B. increasing HDL concentration
   C. decreasing total body cholesterol
   D. sequestering cholesterol in bile

Answers: 1. A, 2. B, 3. C, 4. D, 5. A

SECTION THREE: Myocardial Tissue Perfusion

At the completion of this section, the learner will be able to describe normal coronary artery anatomy and regulation of coronary perfusion.

Coronary Artery Anatomy

The main coronary arteries lay along the epicardial surface of the heart. There are four primary coronary arteries consisting of the left main coronary artery (LMCA), left anterior descending artery (LAD), left circumflex artery (LCX), and right coronary artery (RCA) (Fig. 11–2). The LAD and the LCX are branches of the LMCA after its bifurcation. The RCA pre-

dominantly supplies the right ventricle and atrium and gives rise to the posterior descending artery (PDA). The LAD supplies the anterior aspect of the left ventricle and septum, and the LCX supplies the lateral walls of the left ventricle. As the arteries cross the epicardial surface, small feeder arterioles penetrate the chamber walls giving rise to a dense network of thousands of capillaries per square millimeter called arteriosinusoidal channels. This dense network of capillaries ensures that each myocyte is in contact with a bordering capillary (Califf, 2003).

There are no connections between the large coronary arteries, but there are collateral channels between the smaller arteries. These channels become important when the large arteries occlude. The collateral channels enlarge to provide an alternate route for myocardial tissue perfusion.

Regulation of Coronary Perfusion

Blood flow through the coronary arteries is regulated primarily by aortic pressure. The coronary arteries fill with blood after closure of the aortic valve during diastole. Coronary blood flow is greatest just after closure of the valve and gradually slows during diastole. One way to evaluate the effectiveness of coronary perfusion is to calculate the coronary perfusion pressure (CPP). The CPP is derived by subtracting the pulmonary artery wedge pressure (PAWP) from the diastolic blood pressure (DBP): (DBP − PAWP). CPP should be maintained above 50 mm Hg to provide adequate blood flow to the myocardium (Berne & Levy, 2001).

In summary, there are four main arteries that supply the myocardium. Collateral channels provide an alternate route for myocardial tissue perfusion if one or more of these arteries becomes obstructed. Blood flow through the coronary arteries is determined by aortic pressure and can be calculated by subtracting pulmonary artery wedge pressure from diastolic blood pressure.

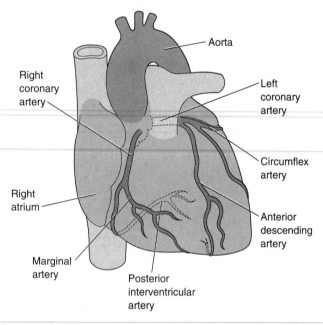

Figure 11–2 ■ Coronary arterial circulation.

SECTION THREE REVIEW

1. There are _____ primary coronary arteries.
   A. two
   B. three
   C. four
   D. five
2. The artery that supplies the right ventricle and right atrium is the
   A. right coronary artery
   B. right descending artery
   C. right circumflex artery
   D. posterior descending artery
3. Coronary perfusion pressure is calculated as
   A. mean arterial pressure minus right atrial pressure
   B. diastolic blood pressure minus pulmonary artery wedge pressure
   C. mean arterial pressure minus cerebral perfusion pressure
   D. systolic blood pressure minus right atrial pressure
4. Coronary collateral channels
   A. occur between smaller arteries
   B. provide an alternate route for myocardial tissue perfusion

C. become important when large arteries occlude
D. all of the above
5. Mr. T has a blood pressure of 90/50 and a PAWP of 12 mm Hg. What is your interpretation of his CPP?
  A. it is 38 mm Hg and this is an inadequate CPP
  B. it is 38 mm Hg and this is a normal CPP

C. it is 78 mm Hg and this is an inadequate CPP
D. it is 50 mm Hg and this is a normal CPP

Answers: 1. C, 2. A, 3. B, 4. D, 5. A

SECTION FOUR: Signs and Symptoms of Impaired Myocardial Tissue Perfusion

At the completion of this section, the reader will be able to identify subjective data associated with coronary artery disease; differentiate types of angina, including stable angina, variant angina, and unstable angina; and discuss the focused physical assessment for a patient who complains of chest pain.

Subjective Data

The classic presenting symptom of CAD is **angina pectoris.** Angina is chest pain that is usually precipitated by exercise and relieved by rest. It is caused by a decrease in myocardial oxygen supply as a result of occluded coronary arteries and an increase in myocardial oxygen demand. When myocardial cells do not have an adequate oxygen supply for aerobic metabolism, they switch to anaerobic metabolism. The by-product of anaerobic metabolism is lactate. Lactate, an acid, irritates nerve endings and causes pain.

Patients may describe their angina as tightness, heaviness, or a vise-like sensation in the chest. It may be accompanied by diaphoresis, shortness of breath, and lightheadedness. Patients will often report that the pain radiates to the left arm and hand, jaw, and shoulder. They also may report symptoms of nausea, shortness of breath, or fatigue.

Time is an important variable to consider when assessing a patient complaining of angina symptoms. Temporal questions to consider include the time of onset of the pain, the activity in which the patient was participating when the pain began, and the length of the anginal episodes. Typically, angina begins gradually and peaks over a period of minutes as the precipitating activity continues. Chest pain that lasts several seconds or constant pain over a period of hours is not typical pain associated with altered myocardial tissue perfusion.

Quantifying the level of pain is important because treatment decisions may be based on the initial intensity and the response of the patient to the pain therapy. Patients are asked to describe the pain using a numerical scale of 0 to 10, with 0 indicating no pain and 10 representing pain of maximum intensity.

Symptoms that are suggestive of CAD but do not include angina are called "**anginal equivalents.**" These symptoms include dyspnea, fatigue, and lightheadedness (dizziness). Patients reporting a history of exertional or resting dyspnea require close scrutiny because these symptoms strongly correlate with CAD.

When assessing a patient presenting with angina symptoms it is helpful to employ the mnemonic PQRST as an assessment tool. The *P* stands for the precipitating conditions at the onset of the pain. These may include activities such as mowing the lawn, exercising, or engaging in sexual activity, or low-level activities such as watching TV or sleeping. *Q* stands for the quality or quantity of the pain. This includes a rating of the pain on a scale of 0 to 10 and a description of the pain quality. *R* stands for the regional location of the pain (substernal or precordial) and radiation of pain (neck, jaw, arms, shoulders), as well as for relieving factors, such as rest, nitroglycerine, or position change. The *S* stands for accompanying symptoms. This may include dyspnea, pallor, tachycardia, anxiety, or fear. And *T* is the temporal nature of the pain—when does the pain occur?

Anginal severity is classified using the Canadian Cardiovascular Society Classification which describes anginal symptoms based on the level of activity that precipitates the angina symptoms (Braunwald et al., 2002) (Table 11–5).

There are three types of angina: stable angina, Prinzmetal's angina, and unstable angina. **Stable angina** is chest pain that is predictable. It occurs with a predictable level of activity. Often patients know they will get chest pain if they participate in a certain amount of activity. For example, a patient will state "I get chest pain when I walk three blocks. I know I'm okay at two

---

TABLE 11–5   Grading of Angina Pectoris by the Canadian Cardiovascular Society Classification System

Class I	Ordinary physical activity, such as walking or climbing stairs, does not cause angina. Angina occurs with strenuous, rapid, or prolonged exertion at work or recreation.
Class II	Slight limitation of ordinary activity. Angina occurs with walking or climbing stairs rapidly; walking uphill; walking or stair climbing after meals, in the cold, or in the wind; emotional stress; or only during the few hours after wakening. Walking more than two blocks on the level and climbing more than one flight of ordinary stairs at a normal pace and in normal condition.
Class III	Marked limitations of ordinary physical activity. Angina occurs with walking one to two blocks on the level and climbing one flight of stairs in normal conditions and at a normal pace.
Class IV	Inability to carry on any physical activity without discomfort—anginal symptoms may be present at rest.

From Campeau, L. (1976). Grading of angina pectoris. Circulation, 54, *S22–S23. Copyright 1976, American Heart Association, Inc. Used with permission.*

blocks, but three blocks does it." Stable angina is relieved by rest or nitroglycerin tablets. The typical sequence is activity–chest pain, rest–relief.

Prinzmetal's angina, or **variant angina,** is chest pain that is not related to physical activity. It often occurs at night and may be related to coronary artery spasms. The exact cause of these spasms is not known.

Unstable angina is chest pain that is not predictable. It occurs with rest or minimal activity and it occurs with increased frequency and severity.

Not all patients with altered myocardial tissue perfusion have chest pain symptoms. Silent ischemia can occur. Women are more likely to have silent ischemia. They more often complain of fatigue or upper arm weakness. Some women with chest pain attribute the pain to heartburn. Older people have a greater incidence of silent ischemia. They often have vague complaints of shortness of breath, dizziness, or confusion.

Objective Data: Physical Assessment

After obtaining the patient's history, a focused physical assessment on the cardiovascular and pulmonary systems is completed. Patients with CAD may or may not exhibit any outward signs of the disease. They may be of normal weight and have normal vital signs. An attempt should be made to correlate subjective data with physical signs.

The vital signs are reviewed for evidence of hypertension and alterations in the heart and respiratory rates. The overall appearance of the patient is noted, taking into account the patient's weight, skin color and tone, posture, and level of functional ability. The skin is examined for evidence of cyanosis and **xanthomas** (cholesterol-filled lesions). The color and temperature of the extremities are evaluated along with the intensity of the peripheral pulses. Peripheral edema is evaluated and graded according to the severity of pitting identified. Alterations in these findings may indicate peripheral vascular disease (PVD) or left ventricular dysfunction. PVD and left ventricular dysfunction are common correlates of CAD.

The chest and abdomen are inspected. Heart sounds are auscultated. Any abnormalities in rhythm and rate, any murmurs, rubs, or gallops are reported. Abnormal or additional heart sounds can be associated with left ventricular failure and fluid volume overload caused by an ischemic left ventricle (refer to Module 12). Respirations are assessed for depth and adventitious sounds. The abdomen is auscultated for bowel sounds and the presence of abdominal bruits. The presence of abdominal bruits can be an indication of renal artery stenosis or abdominal aortic aneurysm.

In summary, the classic symptom of CAD is angina pectoris. It is important to use the PQRST mnemonic when assessing chest pain. Angina is classified in four classes based on level of activity that precipitated the symptoms. There are three types of angina. Subjective data should correlate with physical signs.

Evidence-Based Practice

- *Women who experience chest discomfort may not use the word pain; instead, they may use descriptors, such as aching, tightness, or pressure (McSweeney et al., 2003).*

- *Despite initiatives to raise awareness that heart disease is important for women, women underestimate the significance of chest pain (Richards et al., 2002).*

- *Critical factors that can improve the rapid identification of coronary artery disease in women include cardiac screening of women who present with cardiac risk factors and careful attention to less anticipated symptoms (fatigue, shortness of breath, edema, and transient nonspecific chest discomfort) (Miller, 2002).*

SECTION FOUR REVIEW

1. The classic presenting symptom(s) of CAD is (are)
   A. angina pectoris
   B. chest pain with nausea
   C. elevated lactate with chest pain
   D. nausea, vomiting, heartburn
2. Mr. G is now unable to walk a block or climb one flight of stairs without getting chest pain. What classification of angina pectoris would he have?
   A. I
   B. II
   C. III
   D. IV
3. Chest pain that is not related to physical activity and often occurs at night is called
   A. unstable angina
   B. Prinzmetal's or variant angina
   C. stable angina
   D. silent myocardial ischemia
4. Xanthomas are
   A. atherosclerotic lesions in the intimal lining of arteries
   B. pockets of cyanosis in nail beds
   C. symptoms of upper arm numbness and weakness
   D. cholesterol filled skin lesions
5. Renal artery stenosis may be evidenced by
   A. abdominal bruits
   B. abdominal distention
   C. decreased urine output
   D. absent bowel sounds

Answers: 1. A, 2. C, 3. B, 4. D, 5. A

SECTION FIVE: Collaborative Assessment of Myocardial Tissue Perfusion

At the completion of this section, the reader will be able to identify electrocardiogram changes associated with myocardial ischemia and myocardial infarction; identify cardiac markers that, when present in the serum, indicate myocardial muscle damage; and discuss the purpose of three commonly used diagnostic tests available for assessment of myocardial tissue perfusion.

Electrocardiogram

Several diagnostic tests are available to assist in evaluating the adequacy of myocardial tissue perfusion. The easiest and most cost effective to perform is the 12-lead electrocardiogram (ECG). Thousands of ECGs are performed each year. All patients being evaluated for chest pain have a 12-lead ECG performed to document baseline cardiac rhythm. The ECG aids in the identification of QRS or ST segment abnormalities indicating ischemia or injury to the myocardium.

The standard ECG includes 12 leads. ECG leads are categorized as limb leads (leads I, II, III), augmented limb leads (aVR, aVL, aVF), and the precordial leads (V1 through V6). Each lead overlies a specific area of the myocardium and provides an electrographic snapshot of electrochemical activity taking place at the level of the cell membrane (Pyne, 2004). The basic components of the ECG, as discussed in-depth in Module 10, are depicted in Figure 11–3.

The ST segment represents the early stage of ventricular recovery, and corresponds with the plateau phase of the ventricular action potential. It begins as the S wave of the QRS complex returns to the isoelectric line (baseline) and ends when the T wave becomes isoelectric as shown in Figure 11–3. As can also be seen on Figure 11–3, the point where the S wave returns to the isoelectric line is described as the J point. It is important to note that in the normal ECG, the S wave may dip below the baseline briefly or return directly to the baseline.

The T wave is a graphical representation of ventricular repolarization and should be isoelectric at its conclusion. Changes in the ST segment are the most sensitive electrographic indicators of ischemia and injury to the myocardium (Channer, 2002). When blood flow is reduced or occluded to an area of the myocardium, depolarization changes take place. These changes result in a decrease in the resting membrane potential (from a more negative to a less negative value) and a reduction in the action potential. These changes, called "currents of injury," result in ST depression, hyperacute T waves, ST elevation, and T wave inversion (Conover, 2003) (Fig. 11–4).

Continuous ST segment monitoring provides valuable information for the management of patients at risk for a myocardial infarction (MI), and for those who have experienced an MI, undergone revascularization procedures, or require ECG monitoring after noncardiac surgery (Pyne, 2004). Current monitoring technology includes the ability to monitor ST segments continuously and by doing so, ST segment changes can be identified early and appropriate therapy implemented.

Myocardial regions and their corresponding leads are listed in Table 11–6. The nurse must be familiar with the leads to ensure rapid identification of which area of the myocardium may be ischemic or damaged. This is crucial because treatment options and potential conduction abnormalities differ depending on the myocardial region affected (Zimetbaum & Josephson, 2003).

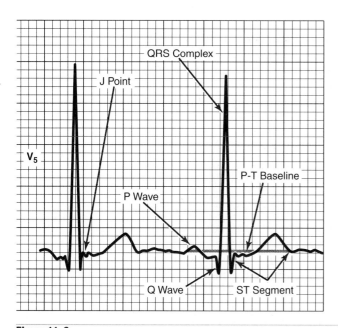

Figure 11–3 ■ Components of a normal ECG.

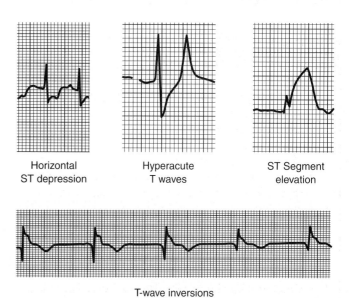

Horizontal ST depression   Hyperacute T waves   ST Segment elevation

T-wave inversions

Figure 11–4 ■ ECG ischemia and injury patterns: Horizontal ST depression, hyperacute T waves, ST segment elevation, and T wave inversions.

TABLE 11–6   Anatomical Regions of the Myocardium and Their Corresponding Leads

ANATOMICAL REGION	CORONARY ARTERY	ECG LEADS	CLINICAL IMPLICATIONS
Anteroseptal wall	LAD	V1, V2, V3, V4	Potential for significant muscle damage leading to pump failure and shock. Septal necrosis can lead to prolonged *PR* interval and heart block.
Left lateral wall	LCX	I, aVL, V5, V6	Some muscle damage and possible arrhythmias secondary to sinoatrial nodal dysfunction.
Inferior wall	RCA, LCX	II, III, aVF	Inferior wall infarctions result from occlusion of the RCA in about 80 percent of the cases and LCX in 20 percent of the cases. *ST* elevation greater in lead III than II suggests RCA, whereas *ST* elevation greater in lead II than III suggests LCX occlusion.
Right ventricular infarction	RCA	V4$_R$, *ST* elevation in V1, II, III, aVF	Requires increased preload. Use of nitrates may be contraindicated.
Posterior wall	RCA	Tall *R* wave and *ST* depression in right precordial leads V1 and V2. V7 to V9 *ST* elevation.	

Adapted from Morton, P. G. (1996). Using the 12-lead ECG to detect ischemia, injury, and infarction. Critical Care Nurse, 16(2), 85–95.

Cardiac Markers

Proteins released by necrotic myocytes into the bloodstream are referred to as serum **cardiac markers.** When present in the blood, these markers signify myocardial muscle damage. These markers include the troponins (cTn), creatine phosphokinase (CK), and creatine phosphokinase–myocardial bands (CK-MB). These different markers appear in the blood at different times, and often the higher the marker, the worse the amount of necrotic cardiac muscle damage. Cardiac markers, discussed in greater detail in Module 8, are summarized in Table 11–7.

CK is an enzyme found in the brain, skeletal muscle, and cardiac muscle. Therefore, it is not specific to heart muscle damage when it is present in the blood. The CK-MB is a subset of CK that is specific to cardiac muscle. A level greater than 5 percent is usually considered a positive indicator of cardiac muscle damage. The cardiac muscle troponins, troponin-I (cTnI) and troponin-T (cTnT), are the most specific indicators of cardiac muscle damage. Troponins are proteins that are part of the actin–myocin unit. They are not normally in the blood, unless there is damage to the actin–myocin units of cardiac muscle.

Even if there is a small amount of cardiac muscle damage, they appear in the blood.

For most patients who complain of chest pain, cardiac markers are obtained on admission (or when the patient complains of chest pain if already admitted to the hospital). They are repeated daily for 3 successive days. Serial levels determine the extent of myocardial damage.

Exercise Stress Test

The exercise stress test (EST) is one of the most commonly used diagnostic tests available for the assessment of a patient suspected of having CAD. ESTs combine the use of exercise (on a treadmill or bicycle) and continuous ECG monitoring to evaluate the patient's likelihood of having altered myocardial tissue perfusion. Patients with CAD may have a normal ECG at rest when myocardial oxygen supply meets myocardial oxygen demand. However, in some patients when myocardial oxygen demand increases (as with exercise), myocardial oxygen supply is not sufficient to meet this increased demand. This imbalance of myocardial oxygen demand and supply produces altered myocardial tissue perfusion and the resultant ECG changes.

TABLE 11–7   Cardiac Markers

MARKER	NORMAL LEVEL	ONSET	PEAKS	DURATION
CK	Male: 12 to 80 U/L Female: 10 to 70 U/L	3 to 6 hours	12 to 24 hours	24 to 48 hours
CK-MB	0 to 3 percent	4 to 8 hours	18 to 24 hours	72 hours
cTnT	Less than 0.2 mcg/L	2 to 4 hours	24 to 36 hours	10 to 14 days
cTnI	Less than 3.1 mcg/L	2 to 4 hours	24 to 36 hours	7 to 10 days

CK = creatine phosphokinase; CK-MB = creatine phosphokinase-myocardial bands; cTnT = Troponin-T; cTnI = Troponin-I.

Not all patients can exercise. Patients who cannot exercise may include those with arthritis, amputation, severe peripheral vascular disease, or chronic obstructive pulmonary disease. These patients undergo a pharmacologic stress test. An inotropic drug is given, such as dobutamine, to increase myocardial contractility and workload similar to that which would occur with exercise.

Indications of myocardial ischemia during an EST include the development of angina, *ST* segment depression of 1 mm or more, failure to increase systolic blood pressure to 120 mm Hg or more, or a sustained decrease of 10 mm Hg or more with progressive increase in exercise. EST is less specific in young or middle-aged women than in men.

In preparation for the EST, the patient is instructed not to eat, smoke, or drink beverages containing caffeine for several hours prior to the test. Certain drugs, such as beta-blockers, may be held for 24 hours prior to the procedure. Patients are instructed to wear comfortable shoes.

Echocardiography

Echocardiography is an imaging technique used to assess the functional structures of the heart using ultrasound waves. Ultrasound waves are applied to the chest wall through a transducer and transect the heart at different planes providing pictures of various cardiac structures. The echocardiogram identifies structural abnormalities of valves, the chamber size of the atria and ventricles, great vessels, and heart wall motion. Echocardiography can be done in conjunction with EST.

An echocardiogram is performed at the patient's bedside in the high-acuity unit. During the test the patient's ECG is monitored for abnormalities and the myocardial walls are evaluated for ischemia-induced motion abnormalities. Myocardial wall motion abnormalities noted may include **hypokinesis** (decrease in movement), **akinesis** (lack of movement), **dyskinesis** (movement in the opposite direction).

Myocardial Perfusion Imaging

Radionuclide myocardial perfusion imaging (MPI) is performed by injecting an intravenous nucleotide during peak exercise. Pictures are taken of the myocardial walls with a special type of camera. This procedure is very helpful in identifying specific areas of myocardial ischemia and damage. The perfusion images help differentiate between exertional and resting myocardial perfusion abnormalities. Perfusion is reported as being without defect (normal), a fixed defect, or a reversible defect.

In summary, there are several diagnostic tests available to evaluate the adequacy of myocardial tissue perfusion. The ECG is an easy, cost-effective method to identify myocardial ischemia and injury by evaluation of the *ST* segment and *T* wave changes. Cardiac markers, when present in the blood, signify myocardial muscle damage. These markers include CK-MB, troponin-I, and troponin-T. Other diagnostic tests include the exercise stress test, echocardiography, and myocardial perfusion imaging.

SECTION FIVE REVIEW

1. Changes in the _____ are the most sensitive electrographic indicators of ischemia and injury to the myocardium.
   A. *ST* segment
   B. *U* wave
   C. *QRS* complex
   D. *P* wave
2. *T* wave inversion and *ST* segment depression in two or more contiguous leads are hallmarks of
   A. myocardial infarction
   B. myocardial ischemia
   C. conduction defect
   D. good myocardial tissue perfusion
3. A CK-MB level greater than _____ is indicative of cardiac muscle damage.
   A. 2 percent
   B. 5 percent
   C. 10 percent
   D. 15 percent

4. Mr. B. has an echocardiogram that revealed evidence of hypokinesis in the left ventricle. What is your understanding of how his left ventricle is working?
   A. it is working just fine; these are normal findings
   B. his left ventricle is not moving at all
   C. his left ventricle is moving in the opposite direction
   D. there is a decrease in movement in his left ventricle
5. An exercise stress test may be ordered to
   A. assess the functional structures of the heart
   B. induce the release of cardiac markers in the blood
   C. evaluate the patient's likelihood of having altered myocardial tissue perfusion
   D. identify specific areas of myocardial ischemia and damage

Answers: 1. A, 2. B, 3. B, 4. D, 5. C

SECTION SIX: Impaired Myocardial Tissue Perfusion: Acute Coronary

Syndromes

At the completion of this section, the learner will be able to define acute coronary syndromes, unstable angina, and myocardial infarction; list nursing diagnoses appropriate for a patient with an acute coronary syndrome; and discuss initial collaborative management of a patient presenting with chest pain.

Diagnosis of Acute Coronary Syndromes

Coronary heart disease is commonly divided into two types of disorders: chronic ischemic heart disease and the acute coronary syndromes (ACS). Chronic ischemic heart disease includes stable angina and variant angina (Section Four). ACS represents a continuum of the atherosclerotic disease processes described in Section One and include unstable angina and myocardial infarction.

The ACS are characterized by an imbalance between myocardial oxygen supply and demand. As blood flow is reduced, the affected myocardium becomes ischemic, leading to symptoms of angina. Thrombi that partially occlude arteries produce symptoms of unstable angina (UA). Total occlusion of the artery results in cell necrosis, release of cardiac markers, and MI distal to the occlusion.

Classification of ACS has changed based on a clearer understanding of plaque disruption and thrombus development. Not all patients with symptoms of chest pain are experiencing an acute MI, but many have a nonocclusive thrombus on pre-existing plaque (Braunwald et al., 2002).

The Joint European Society of Cardiology/American College of Cardiology Committee (2000) established the following diagnostic criteria:

1. Patients with ECG changes suggestive of ischemia, but without the presence of serum biomarkers, are diagnosed as UA.
2. Patients with ischemic *ST* segment changes and the presence of serum cardiac markers are diagnosed as having non-*ST* elevation myocardial infarction (NSTEMI).
3. Patients with *ST* segment elevation and the presence of serum cardiac markers are diagnosed as having *ST* elevation MI (STEMI) (Alpert, Thygesen, et al., 2000).

T wave inversion and *ST* segment depression in two or more contiguous leads are hallmarks of myocardial ischemia. In patients suspected of having ACS, symmetrical *T* wave inversion 2 mm (0.2 mv) or greater strongly suggests acute ischemia. *ST* segments that are depressed from the baseline by 0.5 mm (0.05 mV) or greater and are horizontal or down slop-

ing in two contiguous leads are also suggestive of ischemia. Nonspecific *ST* segment changes can complicate the picture of a patient presenting with symptoms suggestive of ACS. Nonspecific changes are usually defined as *T* wave inversion less than 2 mm or *ST* segment variations of less than 0.05 mV (0.5 mm).

ECG criteria indicative of acute MI include hyperacute *T* waves (early), *ST* segment elevation of 1 mm (0.1 mV) or greater in two contiguous leads, and the presence of new or presumably new left bundle branch block.

Patients presenting with symptoms suggestive of ACS require a rapid assessment and ECG. Chest pain that is suggestive of acute MI typically lasts longer than 20 minutes, but less than 12 hours. Patients may describe the pain as crushing or gripping or they may report chest heaviness and a sense of impending doom. UA is defined as having three possible presentations: symptoms of angina at rest (usually prolonged, greater than 20 minutes), new-onset angina of ordinary physical activity (such as walking one or two blocks), and increasing angina that has become more frequent and longer in duration. Some patients (for example, women, the elderly, and diabetics) may not have chest pain but may present with exertional symptoms of jaw, neck, arm, or epigastric pain; fatigue; nausea; or unexplained worsening of exertional dyspnea.

Initial Collaboratative Management

Nursing diagnoses that may be pertinent for the patient with ACS are listed in Table 11–8. Nursing care priorities include relieving chest pain and reducing myocardial oxygen demand. Psychosocial support for the patient and family is important at this time because they are faced with potential mortality.

Medical management of ACS varies depending on the initial 12-lead ECG findings, risk stratification, and evidence of serum cardiac markers. In 2002, American Heart Association (AHA) and American College of Cardiology established guidelines for the management of patients with UA, STEMI, and NSTEMI (Braunwald et al., 2002). The guidelines recommend that an initial ECG be obtained within 10 minutes of presen-

---

TABLE 11–8   Nursing Diagnoses for the Patient with ACS

Ineffective tissue perfusion: Cardiopulmonary

Decreased cardiac output

Acute pain

Activity intolerance

Ineffective individual coping

Ineffective health maintenance

Anxiety

tation to the emergency department (or in the high-acuity unit, an ECG is obtained within 10 minutes of the patient complaining of chest pain). This ECG is used to differentiate patients with *ST* elevation (potential candidates for reperfusion) from UA and NSTEMI. Evidence supports that mortality is decreased and myocardium preserved when this critical treatment decision is made within 30 minutes of the patient's presentation.

Initial management of all patients with chest pain includes rapid triage to immediate care and placement in a treatment area established to manage such emergencies. After a 12-lead ECG is obtained, acetylsalicylic acid (ASA [aspirin]) is administered. Oxygen by nasal cannula is applied and intravenous (IV) access is obtained. Administration of ASA has been shown to significantly reduce mortality in patients with ACS and begins to decrease platelet aggregation and clot formation by blocking thromboxane A_2 as soon as 10 minutes after oral administration (Kleinschmidt, 2001). Supplemental oxygen raises the partial pressure of oxygen in the blood supplying more oxygen to the ischemic myocardium. At the time that IV access is obtained, blood is drawn for serum cardiac markers. Nitroglycerin may be administered sublingually for ongoing chest pain. Intravenous nitroglycerin may be given for the first 24 to 48 hours. Nitroglycerin, a direct vasodilator, decreases ischemic pain by decreasing afterload and, subsequently, myocardial oxygen demand. If chest pain is not relieved with nitroglycerin, morphine IV is given. Morphine decreases pain through direct action on pain receptors, decreases anxiety, and causes vasodilation to further decrease myocardial workload (Opie & Gersh, 2001; Braunwald et al., 2002). Morphine is administered intravenously in small doses (2 to 4 mg) and repeated every 5 minutes until chest pain is relieved. Repeated doses of morphine requires the nurse to monitor the patient for respiratory depression. Use of a pulse oximeter aids in detection of impaired ventilation.

If the preliminary ECG is normal or nondiagnostic (meaning there are no specific changes), the patient may be monitored in a chest pain unit. Here, serial serum cardiac markers and ECGs are obtained every 6 hours. The patient is "ruled out" for an MI if subsequent ECGs and serum cardiac markers remain unchanged for 12 to 24 hours. Most patients will undergo some form of noninvasive testing (stress test or noninvasive cardiac imaging) prior to discharge.

In addition to the therapies just described, patients with UA and NSTEMI are admitted to cardiac high-acuity units where they receive continuous ECG monitoring. ECG monitoring with continuous *ST* segment monitoring technology is particularly helpful in monitoring these patients.

Pharmaceutical management may include beta blockers. Beta blockers are administered to block catecholamine stimulation, decrease myocardial oxygen demand (by slowing heart rate), and decrease the likelihood of dysrhythmias. Commonly used beta blockers include metoprolol and atenolol.

Pharmaceutical management may include an antithrombin regimen including unfractionated heparin (UH) or low molecular weight heparin (LMWH), glycoprotein (GP) IIb/IIIa inhibitors, and, in many cases, thienopyridines (clopidogrel). Heparin exerts its effect by increasing the effect of antithrombin. This results in inactivation of factors IIa, IXa, and Xa of the coagulation cascade. Heparin is given as an initial bolus dose followed by a continuous infusion. Serum activated partial thromboplastin time (aPTT) is monitored at 6, 12, and 24 hours until the aPTT is maintained at 2 to 2.5 times the normal reference value. Patients are monitored for evidence of bleeding. Incidence of cerebral bleeding increases with an aPTT greater than 2.5 times normal; therefore, elevated aPTTs are reported to the physician and the heparin dose is appropriately adjusted (Jneid et al., 2003).

LMWH (enoxaparin) has also demonstrated excellent efficacy when used in conjunction with ASA in patients with UA and NSTEMI. Advantages to the use of LMWH include its subcutaneous administration, safety, and its ability to be administered without aPTT monitoring. Enoxaparin is dosed at 1 mg/kg every 12 hours.

In addition to ASA, thienopyridines may be administered to patients with ACS. Clopidogrel blocks platelet aggregation and is recommended for patients with UA and NSTEMI.

GP IIb/IIIa inhibitors are selective antagonists of the IIb/IIIa receptor expressed on the surface of activated platelets. Once activated, this receptor binds with fibrinogen resulting in platelet aggregation. GP IIb/IIIa inhibitors are indicated in patients with UA and NSTEMI. Currently available GP IIb/IIIa inhibitors include abciximab (Reopro), tirofiban (Aggrastat), and eptifibatide (Integrelin). GP IIb/IIIa inhibitors are typically administered as a bolus dose followed by an infusion for 18 to 24 hours. Adverse side effects include bleeding and thrombocytopenia. Complete blood counts are monitored at regular intervals and the patients are monitored for signs of bleeding.

In summary, patients with ECG changes suggestive of ischemia, but without the presence of serum biomarkers, are diagnosed as having unstable angina. Patients with ischemic *ST* segment changes and the presence of serum cardiac markers are diagnosed as having non-*ST* elevation myocardial infarction. Patients with *ST* segment elevation and the presence of serum cardiac markers are diagnosed as having *ST* elevation MI. Patients with symptoms suggestive of ACS require rapid assessment and a 12-lead ECG within 10 minutes. After the ECG, ASA is administered, IV access is obtained and blood for serum markers are sent, and nitroglycerin is given. Morphine may be required if pain is not relieved. Patients are ruled out for an MI if ECG and serum cardiac markers remain unchanged for 12 to 24 hours. Pharmaceutical management includes beta blockers, and an antithrombin regimen including UH, LMWH, GP inhibitors, and, in many cases, thienophridines.

SECTION SIX REVIEW

1. Patients with ECG changes suggestive of ischemia, but without the presence of serum biomarkers, are diagnosed as having
   A. unstable angina
   B. non-*ST* elevation myocardial infarction
   C. *ST* elevation myocardial infarction
   D. stable angina
2. ECGs indicative of an acute MI include all of the following EXCEPT
   A. hyperacute *T* waves
   B. *ST* segment elevation
   C. presence of new left bundle branch block
   D. chest pain
3. Current guidelines recommend that an ECG is obtained within _____ of the complaint of chest pain in the high-acuity unit.
   A. 1 minute
   B. 10 minutes

   C. 30 minutes
   D. 1 hour
4. After an initial ECG is obtained, what is the first drug that is usually administered?
   A. oxygen
   B. nitroglycerin
   C. aspirin
   D. morphine
5. A patient is ruled out for an MI if
   A. ECG and cardiac markers remain unchanged for 12 to 24 hours
   B. chest pain subsides within 30 minutes
   C. there are no *ST* changes on the ECG
   D. serum cardiac markers return to normal after 6 hours

Answers: 1. A, 2. D, 3. B, 4. C, 5. A

SECTION SEVEN: Collaborative Interventions to Restore Myocardial Tissue

Perfusion

At the completion of this section, the learner will be able to state the collaborative interventions commonly used to restore myocardial tissue perfusion; and discuss nursing management priorities for patients requiring thrombolytic therapy, percutaneous coronary intervention, and coronary artery bypass surgery.

As noted in Section Six, patients with chest pain, *ST* elevation greater than or equal to 1 mm (1 mv) in two contiguous leads, or new bundle branch blocks in the absence of ECG cofounders are diagnosed with STEMI. Patients with STEMI have a high likelihood that a thrombus is the cause of the infarct. As discussed in Section Six, the initial collaborative management of patients presenting with STEMI includes rapid triage, administration of oxygen, ASA, nitroglycerin, analgesics, beta blockers, and antithrombins (e.g., UH). The goal of these interventions is to promote reperfusion of the affected artery within 30 minutes (Maynard et al., 2000).

Rapid reperfusion of the affected artery reduces the amount of damage to the myocardium and preserves ventricular function. Maximum damage occurs approximately 6 hours after the initial occlusion. The amount of damage depends on the artery occluded and the location of the thrombus. Survival and quality of life are significantly improved if the function of the left ventricle is preserved. Left ventricular (LV) function is typically gauged by measuring the LV **ejection**

fraction (EF). EF is the ratio of blood ejected from the left ventricle with each beat. Normal is greater than 50 percent. EFs between 40 and 50 percent are considered mildly depressed, and LV dysfunction is defined by an EF of less than 40 percent (Berne & Levy, 2001).

Interventions to restore myocardial tissue perfusion include administration of thrombolytic therapy, percutaneous coronary intervention, and coronary artery bypass surgery.

Thrombolytic Therapy

Thrombolytic therapy includes the use of drugs that break up blood clots. These drugs activate the fibrinolytic system to dissolve the blood clot and restore blood flow to the obstructed artery. This actually changes the course of an MI by reducing the area of infarction, decreasing mortality, decreasing the likelihood that the patient will develop *Q* waves on an ECG, and increasing the likelihood that LV function will be preserved (Braunwald et al., 2002).

Candidates for thrombolytic therapy include those whose time of onset of symptoms was less than 12 hours and those who are less than 75 years of age. Contraindications are typically categorized as absolute or relative based on the degree of bleeding risk. Table 11–9 summarizes contraindications to thrombolytic therapy. The learner should be aware that the literature is not conclusive regarding contraindications or their classification as absolute or relative. Risks and benefits must be carefully weighed. Where the risks outweigh the benefit of thrombolytic therapy, other reperfusion therapies are considered.

Nursing responsibilities for the patient receiving thrombolytics include monitoring for evidence of bleeding, hemody-

TABLE 11–9 Contraindications to Thrombolytic Therapy*

Absolute

Active internal bleeding

Cardiovascular: Acute myocardial infarction resulting from dissected aortic aneurysm, severe uncontrolled hypertension

CNS: Aneurysm, AV malformation, neoplasm, or previous hemorrhagic stroke within the past year or CNS surgery or trauma within 2 months

Known predisposition for bleeding

Previous hypersensitivity response

Relative

Age: Older than 75

Cardiovascular:

High risk for cardiac thrombosis, hypertension, subacute bacterial endocarditis, current oral anticoagulant therapy

Conditions that have been associated with increased risk for bleeding

End-stage diseases

History of stroke (brain attack)

Pregnancy

Recent major surgery, trauma (to include CPR), GI bleed or active ulcer disease

Terminal cancer

CNS: Central nervous system, INR: International normalized ratio, PT: Prothrombin time

*Each thrombolytic agent provides product-specific contraindications information and consensus on absolute and relative contraindications has not been established for thrombolytic agents.

Data from: Gahart, B. L., & Nazareno, A. R. (2005). Intravenous medications, (21st ed.) St. Louis: Elsevier/Mosby; and Genentech (2005). Tenecteplase. Accessed April 1, 2005. Available online at: http://www.gene.com/gene/products/information/cardiovascular/tnkase/index.jsp.

namic instability, reperfusion, and reocclusion. The risk for intracranial hemorrhage is relatively low but increases in patients older than 65 years of age, those with low body weight, those with hypertension, and females. The first 24 hours after fibrinolytic administration holds the highest risk for intracranial hemorrhage. Routine neurologic checks are performed to detect evidence of a change in the level of consciousness. Change in level of consciousness is a very sensitive indicator of increased intracranial pressure secondary to intracranial hemorrhage (refer to Module 20). IV sites and wounds are monitored closely for evidence of bleeding, and pressure dressings may be required at IV removal sites. Hemodynamic instability may be an indication of hemorrhage or allergic reaction.

Thrombolysis and reperfusion of the affected myocardium is indicated by resolution of *ST* segment elevation, pain resolution, and the occurrence of reperfusion arrhythmias, such as premature ventricular complexes or ventricular tachycardia. Antiarrhythmics, such as lidocaine or amiodarone, are necessary for sustained ventricular arrhythmias that influence hemodynamic stability. Continuous *ST* segment monitoring is useful in this setting to identify evidence of reperfusion. Reocclusion

remains a problem with thrombolytics and occurs in 5 to 20 percent of patients. Reocclusion is indicated by reoccurrence of chest pain and *ST* segment elevation. Reocclusion most commonly occurs within the first 24 hours. Intravenous heparin is administered for 24 to 48 hours after thrombolytics to minimize the incidence of reocclusion (Opie & Gersh, 2001).

Patients not eligible for revascularization will typically be admitted to a high-acuity cardiac unit for observation and continued medical management. Patients who are not eligible for revascularization include those who are advanced age and are accompanied by significant comorbidities (e.g., renal failure, chronic obstructive pulmonary disease, advanced cancer, and significant LV dysfunction). In these patients, the risks of the procedure outweigh the potential benefit. Patients admitted to the high-acuity unit may require short-term support with an intra-aortic balloon counter pulsation device or inotropic support for cardiogenic shock (Module 15). Vital signs and fluid balance are closely monitored. Continuous ECG monitoring allows for prompt treatment of dysrhythmias.

Percutaneous Coronary Intervention

Primary **percutaneous coronary intervention (PCI)** is the procedure of choice for patients with STEMI. PCI is especially useful for patients who are elderly, not candidates for thrombolytics, or those who have experienced reocclusion after receiving thrombolytic therapy. The 1999 AHA/ACC guidelines recommend that hospitals performing PCI as a primary therapy in STEMI use experienced interventional cardiologists and operate within a "corridor of outcomes" that include balloon dilation within 90 minutes of diagnosis, documented clinical success rates, an emergency bypass surgery rate less than 5 percent, and a mortality rate less than 10 percent (Ryan et al., 1999).

Patients considered for PCI receive all the appropriate therapies used in the management of STEMI with the exception of thrombolytics, LMWH, and clopidogrel. Thrombolytics are not necessary in the setting of acute PCI because their intended purpose is to lyse the thrombus. LMWH is not recommended in the setting of STEMI and can increase the incidence of bleeding. Clopidogrel may be administered in the catheterization lab once the need for emergent coronary artery bypass surgery is ruled out. PCI is performed in an angiography lab (Fig. 11–5) under the direction of an interventional cardiologist and a catheterization team.

Preparing the Patient for PCI

Prior to the procedure, nursing responsibilities include continued monitoring of the patient's vital signs, timely medication administration, and patient and family education. Some institutional protocols may include a shave prep of the patient's groin area. Bilateral groin shave preps are recommended in the event that the cardiologist is unable to access the femoral artery from either side. The time of the patient's last meal is assessed

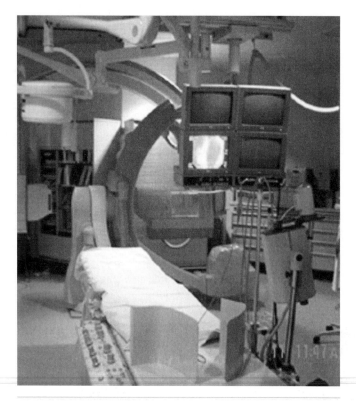

Figure 11–5 ■ Angiography lab.

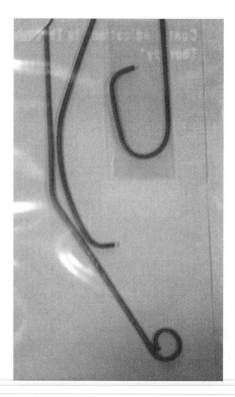

Figure 11–6 ■ Guiding catheters used in coronary angiography.

and documented. Renal function is assessed (blood urea nitrogen and serum creatinine). Renal function can be altered by contrast dye used during the procedure. Patients with renal insufficiency may receive N-acetylcysteine (mucomyst) prior to the procedure to decrease the renal toxic effects of contrast dye. Patients with IV contrast allergy or allergies to shellfish are premedicated with benadryl and corticosteroids to help prevent allergic reactions to the contrast dye. Diabetic patients who have taken their oral medications may require finger stick glucose checks during the procedure. Patients should void prior to being transported to the catheterization lab and women may require a Foley catheter.

PCI Procedure

The procedure typically involves the insertion of an introducer catheter into the femoral or radial artery. Guiding catheters, similar to those shown in Figure 11–6, are inserted through the introducer and the target vessel is engaged. The coronary anatomy is assessed using fluoroscopy, and the offending thrombus is located. Figure 11–7 shows how a thrombus looks using fluoroscopy.

A key decision at this point is whether the occlusion can be removed and a balloon angioplasty performed safely or whether the patient needs to be transported to the operating room for emergent bypass surgery. Indications for surgery include severe LMCA disease, LMCA equivalent disease, and three or more proximal coronary artery obstructions.

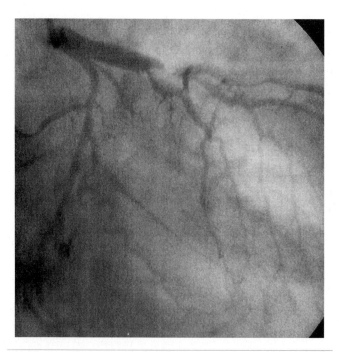

Figure 11–7 ■ Thrombus identified by fluoroscopy during PCI.

Once the decision has been made to procede with the intervention, the cardiologist crosses the occlusion with a guidewire and removes the thrombus. A thrombectomy device, an Angio-jet™ (Possis Corporation, 2004), may be used to remove the

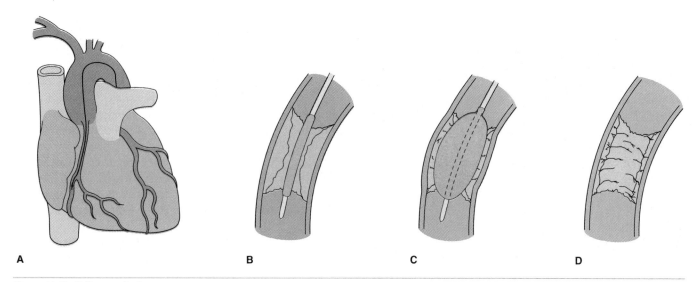

Figure 11–8 ■ Balloon angioplasty

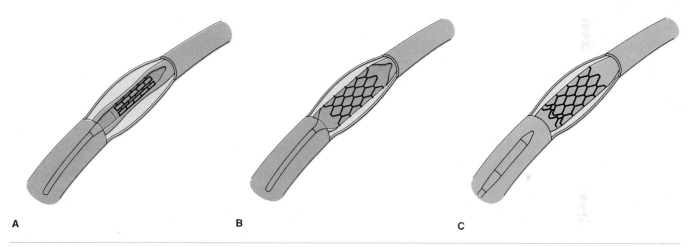

Figure 11–9 ■ Placement of the balloon expandable intracoronary stent

thrombus. The Angiojet uses a catheter and high-pressure saline jets to create a vacuum effect that removes the thrombus. The lesion is then predilated with an angioplasty balloon (Fig. 11–8).

Once the lesion is satisfactorily predilated, another balloon catheter is inserted over the balloon metal stent. The balloon is inflated in the artery and the stent is seated across the lesion (Fig. 11–9).

Metal stents are commonly used for PCI procedures and have significantly reduced the potential for acute closure and restenosis of the dilated coronary artery. Restenosis rates average 30 to 50 percent with plain balloon angioplasty. Additionally, stents have decreased the need for emergent bypass surgery resulting from failed angioplasty attempts (Braunwald et al., 2002; Ryan et al., 1999). New metal stents are available with special coatings (drug-eluting) that help decrease the likelihood of restenosis.

The catheters, guidewires, and introducer are removed and the patient is prepared for transport to a recovery area.

Depending on the location of the insertion site, either direct pressure or a closure device are used to achieve homeostasis at the insertion site. Examples of currently available closure devices include the Angio-seal and Perclose devices. The Angio-seal device uses an anchoring device and a collagen plug to achieve arterial homeostasis and the Perclose device uses sutures. Homeostasis of radial artery insertion sites is achieved using direct pressure with a hemoband. The advantage of closure devices is the ability to allow the patient to ambulate within 3 hours after the procedure (Abbott Laboratories, 2002; St. Jude Medical, 2002).

Care of the Patient Post-PCI

Postprocedure management of the PCI patient includes monitoring vital signs and the ECG, and assessing the access site. Routine blood work typically includes complete blood count, chemistry panel, and coagulation studies. IV infusions may include a GP IIb/IIIa inhibitor and crystalloid solutions. GP IIb/IIIa inhibitors are continued for a minimum of 18 hours post-PCI unless contraindicated. Clopidogrel and ASA may be ordered. IV hydration continues until just prior to discharge if the patient is to go home the same day. If the patient is admitted to a high-acuity unit, IV hydration may continue for another 10 to 12 hours.

Patients whose access site was sealed using a closure device must remain flat for approximately 30 minutes. After this time, the head of the bed may be elevated to 30 degrees. Access sites closed with direct pressure require that the patient remain supine for approximately 6 hours with the affected leg straight. Palpation of pedal pulses and observation of the access site are important nursing assessments that are made frequently after the procedure.

The most common postprocedure complications include chest pain, hypotension, and bleeding at the access site. Chest pain shortly after PCI can indicate acute closure. If the patient complains of chest pain, the nurse obtains vital signs, an ECG, and notifies the cardiologist. Acute closure requires the patient to return to the catheterization lab. Hypotension can be caused by bleeding at the access site, retroperitoneal bleeding, or delayed IV contrast reaction. Patients are instructed to notify the nurse if they feel wetness or warmth around the affected leg, are dizzy or lightheaded, or experience backache. If the patient becomes hypotensive, tachycardic, or experiences an unexplained vagal episode, bleeding may be present and the cardiologist is notified immediately. A computed tomography (CT) scan is required if a retroperitoneal bleed is suspected.

Coronary Artery Bypass Surgery

Coronary artery bypass graft (CABG) has been performed in the United States since the late 1960s. Advances in surgical technique, cardiopulmonary bypass (CPB), conduit selection, and cardioplegic solutions have improved their outcomes and made the procedure available to a broader selection of patients. In elective CABG surgery, operative mortality ranges between 1 and 4 percent, depending on patient selection, surgeon experience, and comorbidities. Operative mortality increases with advanced age, an EF less than 30 percent, female sex, diminished renal function, and when done as a result of failed PCI. Emergent CABG mortality rates are very high if cardiogenic shock is present or cardiac arrest occurs.

In the setting of ACS, CABG is performed after angiography has determined that the lesion or lesions associated with the ACS are not amenable to PCI. Indications for CABG include severe LMCA disease, LMCA equivalent disease, and three or more proximal artery obstructions. Additionally, CABG may be performed as a rescue procedure for acute restenosis or rupture of a coronary artery. Additional factors that influence the suitability of a patient for bypass include the size of the native coronary artery, muscle viability, left ventric-ular function, and extent of disease distal to the stenotic lesion. The primary goal of CABG surgery performed under emergency conditions is prompt restoration of blood flow to the ischemic portion of the myocardium.

CPB is a technique used during surgery whereby blood is directed from the vascular system and circulated through a system of reservoirs and pumps (Fig. 11–10). The system that performs this function is referred to as extracorporeal circulation.

Blood that filters through the bypass system undergoes oxygenation, filtration, and cooling, and is returned to the systemic circulation. Moderate hypothermia is achieved by cooling the patient's temperature to approximately 28 to 32°C. This cooling process helps protect target organs and the myocardium from damage.

Monitoring of the bypass machine is under the control of specially trained technicians called **perfusionists.** During the procedure, the perfusionist monitors the CPB machine, and administers heparin and other medications to maintain anticoagulation and hemodynamic stability. CPB is exclusively used for heart surgery. Factors associated with bypass that influence the patient's postoperative course include hypothermia, hemodilution, catecholamine release, hormone release, and platelet damage (Finkelmeier, 2000).

Bypass of the coronary artery lesion is performed under general anesthesia using blood vessels from the right or left internal mammary artery (RIMA, LIMA), saphenous vein grafts (SVG), or a combination of both (Fig. 11–11).

The grafts are harvested from either the anterior chest wall (in the case of IMA grafts) or the saphenous veins of the legs. Many surgeons prefer the use of IMA grafts (depending on lesion location) over the SVG because of the higher patency rates and increased longevity (10 to 15 years) of the IMA grafts. Alternate (but not commonly used) graft conduits include the gastroepiploic artery, inferior gastric artery, and radial artery. Great care is taken during the harvesting of the grafts to prevent injury to the vessel.

CABG surgery is classically performed through a median sternotomy incision. In order to reduce the risk of myocardial ischemia the heart is infused with cold cardioplegia solution, which inhibits membrane depolarization and action potential propagation. This produces a temporary diastolic arrest (stopping the heart) that allows the surgeon to perform the delicate grafting procedure. The distal anastomoses are performed first so that cardioplegia solution may be infused into the vein graft. The proximal aortic anastomoses are performed as rewarming of the patient begins. The aortic cross clamps are removed and the rewarming process is completed. Once rewarming has taken place and the heart begins beating, the anastomoses sites are checked for leaks and final preparations are made for completion of the procedure. Epicardial pacing wires and mediastinal chest tubes are inserted. The sternotomy incision is closed using stainless steel wires after homeostasis is achieved. Usually five or six wire sutures secure the sternum prior to skin closure.

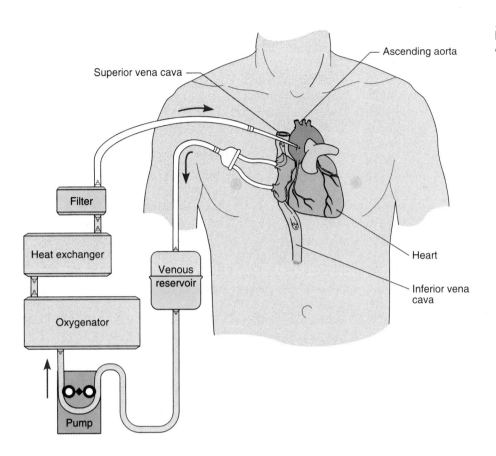

Figure 11–10 ■ A diagrammatic representation of cardiopulmonary bypass.

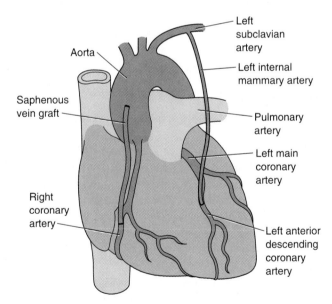

Figure 11–11 ■ Coronary artery bypass grafting using the internal mammary artery and a saphenous vein graft.

TABLE 11–10 Nursing Diagnoses for Patients Who Have Had CABG Surgery

Decreased cardiac output

Fluid volume deficit

Hypothermia

Acute pain

Ineffective airway clearance

Risk for infection

Disturbed thought processes

Dedicated surgery teams that include surgeons, anesthesiologists, perfusionists, nurses, and operating room and Intensive Care Unit (ICU) staffs are available at most hospitals that provide bypass surgery. This team approach provides the best outcomes for patients undergoing this procedure. Clinical pathways, patient care guidelines, and protocols are typically used to manage patients in the postoperative period. These patients are cared for by nurses who have received specialized education and training.

Care of the Patient Post-CABG Surgery

Nursing diagnoses that may be pertinent for patients after CABG surgery are listed in Table 11–10. After the surgical procedure is completed, the patient is transported by the operating room team to the ICU. On arrival in the ICU, the first nursing priority is to confirm a patent airway by assessing endotracheal tube placement and auscultating breath sounds. Ventilator settings are verified.

The patient is connected to continuous ECG monitoring. Because the mediastinum was opened during surgery, negative intrathoracic pressure is restored through the use of mediastinal tubes (or chest tubes) connected to wall suction. Depending on unit protocol, patients will return to the ICU with either a central venous line or a pulmonary artery catheter. Continuous blood pressure is monitored through the use of an arterial catheter. The nurse must ensure hemodynamic monitoring equipment is reproducing accurate data (Module 9). A nasogastric tube for gastric decompression may be present. Atrial and ventricular pacing wires are insulated with gauze and secured to the patient's chest with tape.

After this initial assessment, the nurse receives a report from a member of the operating room team. Key information that is communicated includes the length of time the patient was on CPB, estimated blood loss (EBL), number of bypass grafts that were performed and where these were harvested from, current medications, and blood transfusions received. All medications infusing by IV route are assessed for accuracy.

Management during the initial postoperative period is frequently guided by unit protocols and guidelines. Nursing responsibilities during the early postoperative period include frequent and ongoing physical assessments, and monitoring of vital signs, hemodynamics, and ECG rhythms.

Ongoing physical assessments include not only the cardiopulmonary systems but also the neurologic, gastrointestinal, and renal systems. An ECG and chest x-ray are obtained shortly after arrival at the ICU. Initial postoperative laboratory tests are obtained. Vital signs are taken frequently initially to ensure that hemodynamic instability is detected early and treated promptly. Temperature is monitored to ensure the patient's temperature returns to normal.

If a pulmonary artery catheter is in place, hemodynamic parameters, including mean arterial pressure, right atrial pressure, pulmonary artery wedge pressure, cardiac output (CO), and cardiac index (CI), are obtained to assess adequacy of cardiac output and tissue perfusion (Module 9).

During the initial postoperative period, betadine (used as a skin prep during surgery) is removed from the skin. Early removal of betadine minimizes irritation to the skin and allows the nurse to visualize wounds and dressings for drainage.

The nurse must be vigilant in detecting problems in the postoperative period, including hypovolemia associated with postoperative bleeding, diuresis, and vasodilation. Additional problems that can occur include low CO, hypotension or hypertension, electrolyte imbalances, and postoperative arrhythmias (Inwood, 2002).

Low CO resulting from hypovolemia and inadequate preload is a common problem during the initial postoperative period. Low CO exists when the CI is less than 2.0 L/min/m². Clinical manifestations of low CO include cool, clammy extremities, tachycardia, decreased urine output, and diminished pulses. Hypovolemia is the most common cause of diminished preload and low CO. Hypovolemia associated with bleeding may result from disruption of an anastomosis site or coagulopathies. Chest tube drainage is monitored frequently for evidence of excessive bleeding that may require reexploration. Chest tube drainage greater than 300 to 500 mL/h for the first hour or greater than 200 to 300 mL/h during the second hour is reported to the physician (Marolda & Finkelmeier, 2000). If coagulation abnormalities are present, they are promptly corrected.

Diuresis (greater than 2 to 3 L/h) is significant during the initial postoperative period. Patients undergoing bypass surgery typically gain several kilograms of body weight as a result of fluid shifts (third spacing) and neurohormonal activation. Prior to being taken off the bypass pump, the perfusionist may administer a diuretic. This counteracts some of the fluid retention associated with CPB. Volume repletion may be necessary to maintain hemodynamic parameters and is usually guided by institution protocols.

Decreased CO in spite of increased preload may indicate impaired cardiac function. Impaired cardiac function can result from preexisting heart failure, perioperative MI, reperfusion injuries, or cardiac tamponade. Inotropic medications are used to treat impaired ventricular function. Commonly used medications include dopamine, dobutamine, epinephrine, norepinephrine, and milrinone.

Cardiac tamponade is a life-threatening postoperative complication. Cardiac tamponade is caused by bleeding into a nonflexible sac. The accumulating pressure around the heart increases intracardiac pressures, impairs ventricular filling, and decreases CO. **Pulsus paradoxus** is one of the classic signs of cardiac tamponade. This is an exaggerated decrease (greater than 10 mm Hg) of the systolic blood pressure during inspiration. Other clinical manifestations include distant heart sounds (muffled by the increased pericardial fluid) and a pericardial friction rub. Right atrial pressures are usually elevated. **Beck's triad,** which includes elevated right atrial pressure, hypotension, and muffled heart sounds, may be present.

Treatment of cardiac tamponade requires the physician to open the chest incision to drain the blood by a procedure called pericardiocentesis (Module 8). Many ICUs require that wire cutters, chest trays, and staple removers are readily available for this purpose.

Elevated systemic vascular resistance and cardiac dysrhythmias can also exacerbate low CO states. If systemic vascular resistance is elevated, this represents increase afterload for the heart. Vasodilators, such as sodium nitroprusside and nitroglycerin, are used to decrease afterload. Caution must be taken to ensure that adequate preload exists prior to administration of vasodilators to avoid unexpected hypotension. Antiarrhythmics, such as lidocaine, are required for ventricular dysrhythmias that precipitate low cardiac output states.

Electrolyte imbalances are frequently associated with diuretic use, fluid volume shifts, and volume repletion. Common electrolytes that require replacement include potassium, magnesium, and calcium.

During the initial postoperative period, the patient is typically rewarmed to a temperature of 37°C using a warming blanket. Care must be taken to avoid excessive peripheral rewarming, which can lead to vasodilation and cardiac decomposition. Vital signs and central temperature are closely monitored during the rewarming phase to avoid potential complications.

Ventilation management includes pulmonary hygiene, turning the patient every 2 hours, and suctioning. If there are no pulmonary complications postoperatively, the patient is extubated within a few hours of surgery. Postoperative analgesia is usually accomplished with IV morphine. Benzodiazepines may be administered to control anxiety.

Within 24 hours of surgery, most patients are extubated. The pulmonary artery catheter, nasogastric tube, and Foley catheter are removed. Patient-controlled analgesia is initiated. The patient receives aggressive pulmonary hygiene, including coughing and deep breathing exercises with incentive spirometry. Patients begin preparation for getting out of bed by dangling their feet over the edge of the bed. Patients may get out of bed to sit in a chair.

Diet is advanced as tolerated. At this time, if they are stable, patients are transferred from the ICU to a cardiac high-acuity unit.

Discharge planning is multidisciplinary and includes health care team members from physical therapy, occupational therapy, and nutritional support. Patient recovery, discharge planning, and patient and family education continues until the patient is discharged, usually 5 to 7 days after surgery.

Nursing responsibilities include continued physical assessment, medication administration and education, evaluation of vital signs, psychological support, and patient and family education. Nurses use their experience to develop individualized patient goals, based on established protocols, which assist the patient to smoothly transition through the various stages of the postoperative period.

In summary, interventions to restore myocardial tissue perfusion include administration of thrombolytic therapy, percutaneous coronary intervention, and coronary bypass surgery. Thrombolytic therapy uses drugs to break up blood clots. But this therapy is not for everyone. PCI is the procedure of choice for patients with STEMI. Indications for CABG include severe LMCA and three or more proximal artery obstructions. Nursing care before, during, and after these procedures to restore myocardial tissue perfusion is highly specialized.

SECTION SEVEN REVIEW

1. The goals of thrombolytic therapy include all of the following EXCEPT
   A. reducing the area of infarction
   B. decreasing the likelihood of developing Q waves on ECG
   C. increasing the likelihood that LV function will be preserved
   D. containing the clot in a localized area

2. Which of the following signs may indicate that reocclusion has occurred after thrombolytic therapy?
   A. hypotension
   B. chest pain
   C. ST segment depression
   D. change in level of consciousness

3. The advantage of using closure devices post-PCI is that
   A. patients can ambulate within 3 hours
   B. they are associated with less bleeding
   C. they require less nursing time
   D. they are associated with lower rates of occlusion

4. Which of the following assessments is made frequently after PCI?
   A. PTT levels
   B. ST segment measurements

   C. palpation of pedal pulses
   D. Glascow Coma Scale

5. All of the following blood vessels can be used for CABG surgery EXCEPT
   A. left internal mammary artery
   B. right internal mammary artery
   C. saphenous vein
   D. jugular vein

6. Patients who have CABG surgery will require a chest tube
   A. only if the lungs are injured during the operative procedure
   B. to drain blood from the mediastinum
   C. to keep pressure off the heart
   D. for at least a week

7. Which of the following is NOT a sign of cardiac tamponade?
   A. high peak pressures on the ventilator
   B. elevated right atrial pressures
   C. muffled heart sounds
   D. pulsus paradoxus

Answers: 1. D, 2. B, 3. A, 4. C, 5. D, 6. B, 7. A

POSTTEST

1. An atheroma is
   A. a foam cell
   B. a group of foam cells
   C. a calcified lesion containing hemorrhage and scar tissue
   D. a type I lesion that is not visible to the unaided eye
2. Macrophages release substances that oxidize
   A. low-density lipoproteins
   B. high-density lipoproteins
   C. endothelial cells
   D. foam cells
3. Current recommendations to reduce cholesterol and LDL state that total fat should be _____ of total calories.
   A. less than 7 percent
   B. up to 10 percent
   C. up to 20 percent
   D. 25 to 35 percent
4. Which of the following is a TRUE statement about the use of statins as part of reducing atherosclerotic disease progression?
   A. statins must be used in conjunction with a low fat/cholesterol diet
   B. a major side effect of these drugs is bleeding and hemorrhage
   C. statins reduce HDL and increase LDL levels
   D. statins reduce hypertension and total cholesterol
5. Coronary perfusion pressure should be maintained above
   A. 25 mm Hg
   B. 50 mm Hg
   C. 75 mm Hg
   D. 100 mm Hg
6. Mr. P states his chest pain starts after he walks three blocks. When he sits and rests for 5 minutes, it goes away. You would define his angina as
   A. unstable angina
   B. variant angina
   C. stable angina
   D. Prinzmetal's angina
7. Women who complain of chest pain often have
   A. silent ischemia
   B. complaints of fatigue

C. complaints of heart burn
D. all of the above
8. Which of the following ECG findings is indicative of myocardial ischemia?
   A. *ST* segment depression in two or more contiguous leads
   B. *ST* segment elevation
   C. elevated *T* wave
   D. irregular *QRS* complex
9. Which of the following is the MOST specific indicator of cardiac muscle damage?
   A. CK
   B. lactate
   C. LDH
   D. troponin
10. Unstable angina is defined as having all of the following presentations EXCEPT
    A. symptoms of angina at rest
    B. new onset of angina with ordinary activity
    C. angina that lasts greater than 20 minutes
    D. angina that is more frequent
11. The first drug given in the initial management of all patients with chest pain is
    A. oxygen
    B. aspirin
    C. nitroglycerine
    D. morphine
12. Thrombolytic therapy would be appropriate for which of the following situations?
    A. a patient with chest pain for less than 24 hours
    B. a patient with chest pain for less than 12 hours
    C. a patient with chest pain for less than 30 minutes
    D. a patient older than 75 years of age
13. Chest tube drainage greater than _____ mL/hr for the first hour after CABG surgery should be reported to the physician immediately.
    A. 100
    B. 1,000
    C. 500 to 800
    D. 300 to 500

POSTTEST ANSWERS

Question	Answer	Section
1	C	One
2	A	One
3	D	Two
4	A	Two
5	B	Three
6	C	Four
7	D	Four

Question	Answer	Section
8	A	Five
9	D	Five
10	C	Six
11	B	Six
12	B	Seven
13	D	Seven

REFERENCES

Abbott Laboratories. (2002). Perclose: What you need to know about closure of your femoral artery access site [Brochure]. Abbott Park, IL.: MediMark, Author.

AHA (American Heart Association). (2003). *Heart disease and stroke statistics* (2004 update). Dallas, TX: Author.

Alpert, J. S., Thygesen, K., Antman, E., & Bassand, J. P. (2000). Myocardial infarction redefined—a consensus document of The Joint European Society of Cardiology/American College of Cardiology Committee for the redefinition of myocardial infarction. *Journal of American College of Cardiology, 36*(3), 959–969.

Berne, R. M., & Levy, M. N. (2001). *Cardiovascular physiology* (8th ed.). Philadelphia: C. V. Mosby.

Braunwald, E., Antman, E. M., Beasley, J. W., et al. (2002). ACC/AHA 2002 guideline update for the management of patients with unstable angina and non-*ST*-segment elevation myocardial infarction: A report of the American College of Cardiology/American Heart Association task force on practice guidelines. Available at: *http://www.acc.org/clinical/guidelines/unstable/unstable.pdf*. Accessed December 20, 2003.

Califf, R. M. (2003). *ACS essentials.* Royal Oak, MI: Physician's Press.

Campeau, L. (1976). Grading of angina pectoris. *Circulation, 54,* S22–S23.

Channer, F. M. (2002). ABC of clinical electrocardiography in myocardial ischemia. *British Medical Journal, 324,* 1023–1026.

Conover, M. B. (2003). *Electrocardiography.* Baltimore, MD: C. V. Mosby.

Finkelmeier, B. A. (2000). *Cardiothoracic surgical nursing* (2nd ed.). Philadelphia: Lippincott Williams & Wilkins.

Gotto, A. M., & Pownall, H. J. (2003). Atherosclerosis: Overview and histologic classification of lesions. In A. M. Gotto & H. J. Pownall (Eds.), *Manual of lipid disorders* (pp. 68–79). Philadelphia: Lippincott Williams & Wilkins.

Inwood, H. (2002). *Adult cardiac surgery: Nursing care and management.* London: Whurr.

Jneid, H., Bhatt, D. J., Corti, R., Badimon, J. J., Foster, V., & Francis, G. S. (2003). Aspirin and clopidogrel in acute coronary syndromes. *Archives of Internal Medicine, 63,* 1145–1153.

Kleinschmidt, K. (2001). *Acute coronary syndromes (ACS): Pharmacotherapeutic interventions—Treatment guidelines for patients with and without procedural coronary intervention (PCI). Cardiology Consensus Reports.* Atlanta, GA: American Health Consultants.

Lemone, P., & Burke, K. (2004). Nursing care of clients with coronary heart disease. In P. Lemone & K. Burke (Eds.), *Medical surgical nursing: Critical thinking in client care* (pp. 804–831). Upper Saddle River, NJ: Prentice Hall.

Marolda, D., & Finkelmeier, B. (2000). Postoperative patient management. In B. Finkelmeier (Ed.), *Cardiothoracic surgical nursing.* Philadelphia: Lippincott Williams & Wilkins.

Matfin, G., & Porth, C. M. (2005). Disorders of blood flow in the systemic circulation. In C. M. Porth (Ed.), *Pathophysiology: Concepts of altered health states* (7th ed., pp. 474–503). Philadelphia: Lippincott Williams & Wilkins.

Maynard, S. J., Scott, G. O., Riddell, J. W., & Adgey, A. A. (2000). Management of acute coronary syndromes. *British Medical Journal, 321*(7255), 220–223.

McSweeney, J. C., Cody, M., O'Sullivan, P., et al. (2003). Women's early warning symptoms of acute MI. *Circulation, 108,* 2619–2623.

Miller, C. L. (2002). A review of symptoms of coronary artery disease in women. *Journal of Advanced Nursing, 39*(1), 17–23.

National Cholesterol Education Program. (2001). *Adult treatment panel III report.* National Cholesterol Expert Panel on Detection, Evaluation, and Treatment of High Blood Cholesterol in Adults.

Opie, L. H., & Gersh, B. J. (2001). *Drugs for the heart* (5th ed.). Philadelphia: W. B. Saunders.

Porth, C. M. (Ed.). (2005). *Pathophysiology: Concepts of altered health states* (7th ed.). Philadelphia: Lippincott Williams & Wilkins.

Possis Cooperation. (2004). Technical manual pertaining to the Angiojet thrombectomy device [Brochure]. Available at: *http://www.possis.com*. Accessed January 20, 2004.

Pyne, C. C. (2004). Classification of acute coronary syndromes using the 12-lead electrocardiogram as a guide. *AACN Clinical Issues, 15,* 558–567.

Richards, H. M., Reid, M. E., & Watt, G. C. M. (2002). Why do men and women respond differently to chest pain? A qualitative study. *Journal of the American Medical Women's Association, 57*(2), 79–81.

Ryan, T. T., Antman, E. M., Brooks, N. H., Califf, R. M., Hillis, L. D., Hiratzka, L. F., et al. (1999). ACC/AHA guidelines for the management of patients with acute myocardial infarction: 1999 update: A report of the American College of Cardiology/American Heart Association task force on practice guidelines. Available at: *http://www.acc.org/clinical/guidelines*. Accessed November 18, 2003.

St. Jude Medical. (2002). The Angio-seal device patients' information guide [Brochure]. St. Jude Medical: Author.

The Joint European Society of Cardiology/American College of Cardiology Committee. (2000). Myocardial infarction redefined: A consensus document of the Joint European Society of Cardiology/American College of Cardiology committee for the redefinition of myocardial infarction. *Journal of the American College of Cardiology, 36*(3), 959–969.

Zimetbaum, P. J., & Josephson, M. E. (2003). Use of the electrocardiogram in acute myocardial infarction. *New England Journal of Medicine, 348*(10), 933–939.

MODULE
12
Alterations in Cardiac Output

Nancy Munro

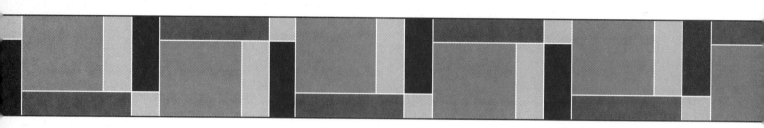

OBJECTIVES   Following completion of this module, the learner will be able to

1. Describe the pathophysiologic mechanisms of cardiac valve dysfunction, including valvular stenosis, valvular regurgitation, and infective endocarditis.

- Identify cardiac murmurs that occur with valve dysfunction.

- List two nursing interventions for patients with valvular dysfunction.

2. Define heart failure.

- Describe the pathophysiologic and compensatory mechanisms that occur during heart failure.

- Discuss the pharmacologic therapies used in the collaborative management of heart failure.

3. Define the ranges of systolic and diastolic blood pressure for prehypertension, stage 1 hypertension, and stage 2 hypertension.

- Explain the pathophysiologic mechanisms that contribute to hypertension.

- Discuss collaborative and nursing interventions for the patient with hypertension.

The cardiac system plays a pivotal role in pumping and transporting oxygen to tissues. As with any other organ, the heart is composed of various components that must work congruently in order to function optimally. Conceptually, the cardiac system is a sophisticated "plumbing system" where the heart is the pump that has valves to direct blood flow into the "pipes" (the vascular system). Pump, valve, or pipe dysfunction can lead to alterations in cardiac output. This module addresses these alterations in cardiac output, which include pump dysfunction (heart failure and cardiomyopathy), valve dysfunction (stenosis and regurgitation), and "pipe" dysfunction (hypertension).

This self-study module is divided into three sections. Section One discusses valvular heart disease and infective endocarditis. Section Two reviews heart failure and cardiomyopathy and Section Three discusses hypertension. For each section the clinical manifestations, pathophysiologic mechanisms, collaborative management, and nursing interventions are presented. Each includes a set of review questions to help the learner evaluate his or her understanding of the section's content before moving on to the next section. All Section Reviews and the module Pretest and Posttest include answers. It is recommended that the learner review those concepts answered incorrectly before proceeding to the next section.

PRETEST

1. With mitral stenosis, the following hemodynamic changes occur
   - A. left atrial pressure increases and left ventricular diastolic pressure decreases
   - B. left atrial pressure increases and pulmonary artery pressures increase
   - C. left atrial pressure decreases and left ventricular diastolic pressure decreases
   - D. Left atrial pressure and left ventricular diastolic pressures do not change

2. Aortic regurgitation is caused primarily by
   A. rheumatic heart disease
   B. myocardial infarction
   C. ventricular hypertrophy
   D. chronic renal disease

3. Subacute infective endocarditis is commonly caused by
   A. *Staphylococcus aureus*
   B. *Pseudomonas aeruginosa*
   C. *Candida albicans*
   D. *Streptococcus viridans*

4. A compensatory mechanism that plays a major role in sodium and water retention in heart failure is
   A. the parasympathetic nervous system
   B. the sympathetic nervous system
   C. the renin–angiotension–aldosterone system
   D. reflex tachycardia

5. Mr. P has been diagnosed with heart failure. He is asymptomatic. Which of the following drugs would most likely be used to manage his condition?
   A. ACE inhibitor
   B. beta blocker
   C. digitalis
   D. A and B

6. Patients in heart failure present with the following signs and symptoms

A. fatigue
B. orthopnea
C. dyspnea
D. all of the above

7. Prehypertension is defined as
   A. SBP less than 120 mm Hg or DBP less than 80 mm Hg
   B. SBP greater than 160 mm Hg or DBP greater than 100 mm Hg
   C. SBP between 140 and 159 mm Hg or DBP between 90 and 99 mm Hg
   D. SBP of 120 to 139 mm Hg and DBP of 80 to 89 mm Hg

8. Nursing interventions for the hypertensive patient include
   A. lifestyle modifications
   B. education about medications
   C. education about monitoring blood pressure
   D. all of the above

9. Target organ damage from hypertension occurs to which of the following organs?
   A. eyes
   B. kidneys
   C. peripheral vasculature
   D. all of the above

Pretest Answers: 1. B, 2. A, 3. D, 4. C, 5. D, 6. D, 7. D, 8. D, 9. D

GLOSSARY

aortic regurgitation (AR)   Aortic valve insufficiency that allows blood to flow back into the left ventricle from the aorta during diastole.

aortic stenosis (AS)   A narrowing of the aortic valve orifice so that blood flow is obstructed from the left ventricle into the aorta during systole.

cardiomyopathy   End-stage heart failure (class IV); the patient has symptoms of HF at rest and cannot perform activities of daily living.

constrictive cardiomyopathy   Condition associated with normal left ventricular size and a slightly depressed ejection fraction with a marked decrease in cardiac muscle compliance.

diastolic dysfunction   Heart failure characterized by impairment of ventricular relaxation.

dilated cardiomyopathy   Condition associated with left ventricular dilation and decreased ejection fraction.

drug allergy   Refers to an immune-based hypersensitivity reaction (for example, rash, or hypotension).

drug side effect   Refers to a predictable or expected undesirable effect of a drug.

echocardiogram   Noninvasive technology that allows visualization of the valves; their movement; as well as the size, thickness, and function of the aorta and ventricles.

heart failure (HF)   Clinical syndrome that can result from structural or functional cardiac disorders that decrease the ability of the ventricle to fill or eject.

hypertrophic cardiomyopathy   Condition associated with left ventricular hypertrophy that decreases the ability of the chamber to relax (diastolic dysfunction).

infective endocarditis (IE)   A disease caused by microbial infection of the endothelial lining of the heart, usually presenting with vegetations on a heart valve.

mitral regurgitation (MR)   Incompetent mitral valve allows blood to flow back into the left atrium during systole because the mitral valve does not fully close.

mitral stenosis (MS)   A narrowing of the mitral valve orifice so that blood flow is obstructed from the left atrium into the left ventricle during diastole.

mitral valve prolapse   A type of mitral valve insufficiency that occurs when one or both of the mitral valve cusps flow into the atria during ventricular systole.

orthopnea   Sensation of shortness of breath in the supine position.

prehypertension   Defined as systolic blood pressure of 120 to 139 mm Hg and diastolic blood pressure of 80 to 89 mm Hg.

regurgitation   Backward blood flow through the chambers of the heart.

stenosis   Valve leaflets fuse together and cannot fully open or close.

systolic dysfunction.   Heart failure characterized by ejection fraction less than 40 percent.

target organ damage   Dysfunction that occurs in organs affected by high blood pressure.

ABBREVIATIONS

ACE	Angiotensin-converting enzyme	**IE**	Infective endocarditis
AICD	Automatic implantable cardioverter/defibrillator	**INR**	International normalized ratio
ANP	Atrial natriuretic peptide	**LA**	Left atrium
AR	Aortic regurgitation	**LV**	Left ventricle
ARB	Angiotensin receptor blocker	**MR**	Mitral regurgitation
AS	Aortic stenosis	**MS**	Mitral stenosis
AV	Atrioventricular	**NYHA**	New York Heart Association
BB	Beta blocker	**PA**	Pulmonary artery
BNP	Brain natriuretic peptide	**PND**	Paroxysmal nocturnal dyspnea
BPM	Beats per minute	**PT**	Prothrombin time
CCB	Calcium channel blocker	**PTT**	Partial prothromboplastin time
CO	Cardiac output	**PVR**	Pulmonary vascular resistance
DASH	Dietary approaches to stop hypertension	**RA**	Right atrium
DBP	Diastolic blood pressure	**RV**	Right ventricle
ECG	Electrocardiogram	**SBP**	Systolic blood pressure
EF	Ejection fraction	**SV**	Stroke volume
HF	Heart failure	**VAD**	Ventricular assistive device
HR	Heart rate		

SECTION ONE: Valvular Heart Disease

At the completion of this section, the learner will be able to describe the pathophysiologic mechanisms of disorders of cardiac valve dysfunction, including valvular stenosis, valvular regurgitation, and infective endocarditis; identify cardiac murmurs that occur with valve dysfunction; and list two nursing interventions for patients with valvular dysfunction.

Structure and Function of Cardiac Valves

There are four heart valves, which are thin, paperlike structures that allow forward blood flow, prevent **regurgitation** (or backward flow of blood), and open and close in response to changes in pressure gradients (Fig. 12–1). When the pressure is higher in the preceding chamber, the valve opens. When the gradient reverses, the valve closes. The flimsy structure of the valves enables them to perform these functions easily. The tricuspid and mitral valves are referred to as the atrioventricular (AV) valves. They direct blood flow from the atria to ventricles. The pulmonic and

aortic valves are referred to as the semilunar valves. They direct blood flow from the ventricle into the circulation.

During diastole when the ventricles are filling, the AV valves are open (Fig. 12–2A) and the semilunar valves are closed (Fig. 12–2B). During systole when the ventricles are contracting, the semilunar valves are open (Fig. 12–2C) and the AV valves are closed (Fig. 12–2D). The opening and closing of the valves during the cardiac cycle allows for forward unidirectional movement of blood through the four chambers of the heart. When valve dysfunction occurs, this forward unidirectional movement of blood flow through the heart is affected. The two major categories for valvular dysfunction are stenosis and regurgitation.

Valve Stenosis

Stenosis of a valve occurs when valve leaflets fuse together and the valve cannot fully open or close. With stenosis, valve components become thickened and the valve orifice narrows. This causes resistance of blood flow across the valve (Fig. 12–3). The chamber before the valve is exposed to an increased afterload

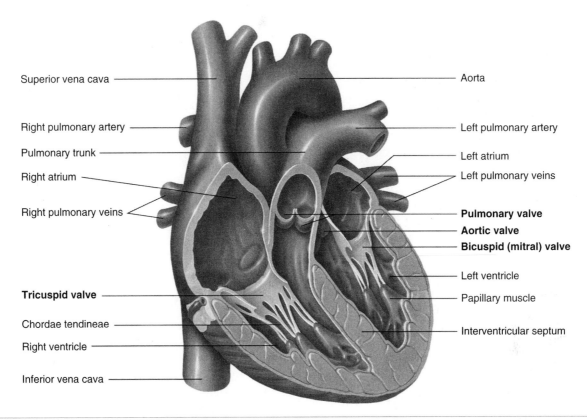

Figure 12–1 ■ The four chambers and four valves in the heart.

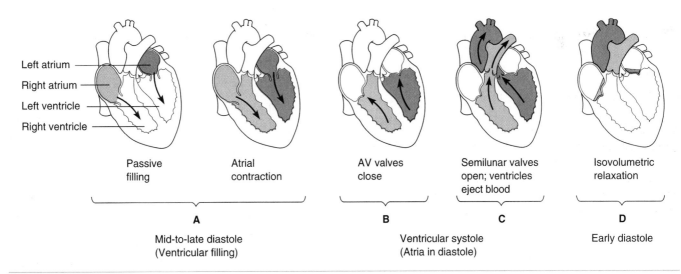

Figure 12–2 ■ Opening and closing of the heart valves during the cardiac cycle.

because flow through the valve is more difficult. The blood from that chamber "backs up" to the preceeding chamber. Stenosis of a valve may be caused by calcification, congenital factors, or rheumatic fever (Braunwald, 2000). Risk factors for the development of stenosis are listed in Table 12–1.

Mitral Valve Stenosis

Mitral stenosis (MS) is a narrowing of the mitral valve orifice that obstructs blood flow from the left atrium into the left ventricle during diastole. It is predominantly caused by rheumatic fever and occurs more frequently in women (Braunwald, 2000).

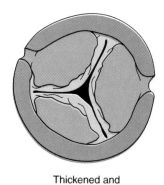

Thickened and
stenotic valve leaflets

Figure 12–3 ■ Stenosis of a heart valve.

TABLE 12–1 Risk Factors for the Development of Valve Disorders

Stenosis

MITRAL	AORTIC
Rheumatic heart disease	Congenital
Female gender	Acquired
	Age-related

Regurgitation

MITRAL	AORTIC
Abnormalities of the leaflets	Rheumatic heart disease
Rheumatic heart disease	Calcification
Infective endocarditis	Infective endocarditis
Collagen–vascular disease	Trauma
Abnormalities of the annulus	Congenital (less common)
Cardiomyopathy	
Abnormalities of the chordae tendineae or papillary muscle	
Ischemic heart disease	
Mitral valve prolapse	

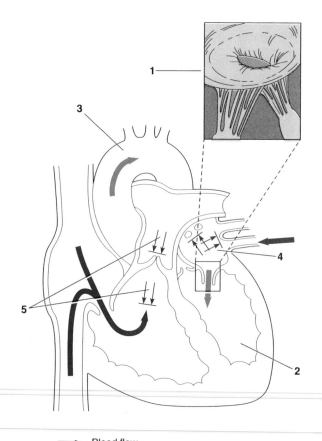

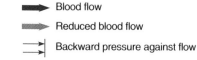

➡ Blood flow

➡ Reduced blood flow

⇥ Backward pressure against flow

Figure 12–4 ■ Mitral stenosis.

evated LA pressures lead to LA dilatation and changes in the LA electrical refractory period, which may precipitate atrial fibrillation (Braunwald, 2000). A vicious cycle occurs if the HR is not controlled.

Aortic Valve Stenosis

Aortic stenosis (AS) is a condition in which the aortic valve is narrowed and blood flow is obstructed from the LV into the aorta during systole. AS can be caused by congenital or acquired conditions. Acquired causes include rheumatic heart disease and aging. Through the aging process, degenerative calcifications occur.

In aortic stenosis, the valvular orifice narrows, increases the pressure gradient between the LV and aorta, and causes a "backup phenomen." The LV end-diastolic pressure increases and the LV hypertrophies (Fig. 12–5). LA contractility increases to eject volume against higher LV pressures. However, in the event of a loss of an effective atrial contraction, such as that which occurs with atrial fibrillation (Module 10), immediate decompensation can occur (Braunwald, 2000).

Left atrial (LA) pressure increases with MS and eventually causes an increase in pulmonary artery (PA) pressure and pulmonary vascular resistance (PVR) (Fig. 12–4). Cardiac output (CO) can be normal with mild MS, but as the MS becomes more severe, CO decreases. With severe MS, an increase in PVR causes the right ventricle (RV) and right atrium (RA) to fail. Left ventricular (LV) diastolic pressure also increases because the pressure gradient across the valve is higher.

An important factor to consider with MS is heart rate (HR). Recall from Module 8 that during ventricular diastole the ventricle relaxes and fills. If a patient with MS experiences a sudden increase in HR, diastolic filling time is shortened. This results in a substantial decrease in CO and an increase in LA pressure. El-

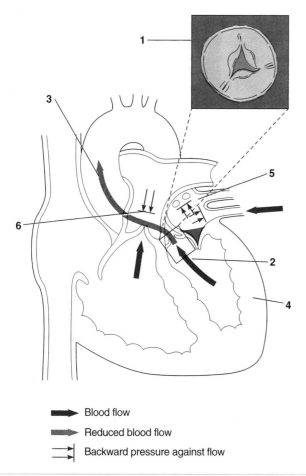

Figure 12–5 ■ Aortic stenosis.

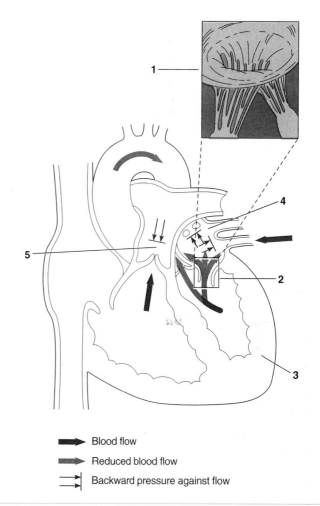

Figure 12–7 ■ Mitral regurgitation.

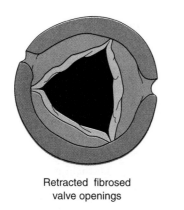

Retracted fibrosed
valve openings

Figure 12–6 ■ An incompetent or regurgitant valve.

Valvular Regurgitation

Insufficient or incompetent valves that do not close completely are called regurgitant valves (Fig. 12–6). This allows regurgitation of blood through the valve and back into the chamber that the blood just left. Risk factors for the development of regurgitant valves are summarized in Table 12–1.

Mitral Valve Regurgitation

Mitral regurgitation (MR) occurs when the mitral valve does not completely close and allows blood to flow back into the LA during systole. This causes regurgitation of a portion of the ventricular stroke volume (SV) into the LA (Fig. 12–7).

Causes of MR are categorized into (1) abnormalities of the leaflets, (2) abnormalities of the annulus, or (3) abnormalities of the chordae tendineae or papillary muscle. When the leaflets are abnormal (especially with chronic rheumatic heart disease), they shorten, become more rigid and deformed, and retract. This causes the leaflets not to close properly during ventricular systole. The annulus or ring around the valve can either be dilated, calcified, or both. The annulus does not constrict properly during systole and regurgitation occurs. Finally, the supporting structures, the chordae tendineae, and papillary muscles can be damaged.

Mitral valve prolapse is a type of mitral valve insufficiency that occurs when one or both of the mitral valve cusps flow into the LA during ventricular systole. Excess tissue in the valve leaflets and elongated chordae tendineae impair mitral valve

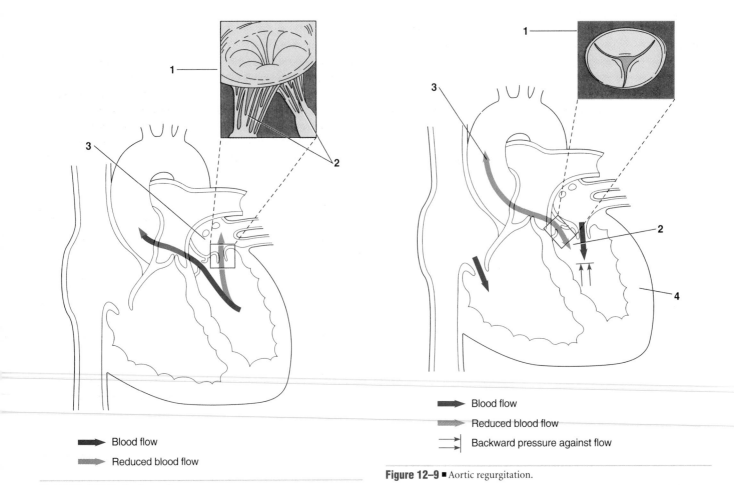

Figure 12–8 ■ Mitral valve prolapse.

Figure 12–9 ■ Aortic regurgitation.

closure during systole and some ventricular blood regurgitates (Fig. 12–8). The large volume of blood ejected backward into the LA over time causes the LV to dilate and hypertrophy in response to the increased preload of the LA. In an acute situation, such as a myocardial infarction and rupture of the papillary muscle, the LA and LV cannot acutely compensate. Elevated left heart pressures "back up" to the pulmonary vasculature and acute pulmonary edema occurs.

Aortic Valve Regurgitation

Aortic regurgitation (AR) is caused by an incompetent aortic valve that allows blood to flow back into the LV from the aorta during diastole. It occurs primarily as a result of rheumatic heart disease. The leaflets' structures are altered because of infiltration of fibrous tissue. The fibrous tissue causes the leaflets to retract and, therefore, they do not completely close during systole.

With AR, regurgitation of part of the ventricular SV back into the LV leads to ventricular hypertrophy (Fig. 12–9). This is structurally different than the hypertrophy that develops with AS. The hypertrophy associated with AR is more severe and significantly decreases SV (Braunwald, 2000).

Infective Endocarditis

When valves have structural abnormalities, it increases their susceptibility to infection. **Infective endocarditis (IE)** is a disease caused by a microbial infection of the endothelial lining of the heart. The process starts with damage to the endothelium of a valve. Damage may be the result of congenital diseases (e.g., rheumatic heart disease) or iatrogenic (with the introduction of intracardiac catheters or other devices). The disrupted surface of the endothelium attracts platelets that adhere to the surface and starts the development of nonbacterial thrombi. The next phase of IE is the introduction of bacteria in the blood through portals of entry, such as wounds, biopsy sites, pacemakers, intravenous and arterial catheters, urinary catheters, or through other invasive mechanisms, such as dental or gastrointestinal (colonoscopy) procedures. Once bacteria enter the blood, they settle on the thrombi on the heart valve. The infected thrombi enlarge with time and increases valve dysfunction (Sande et al., 2001).

There are groups of patients that are more susceptible to this possible infection, including patients with preexisting heart disease, children, the elderly, intravenous drug abusers, patients infected with human immunodeficiency virus, patients postcardiac surgery, and patients who require hemodialysis. These patients have weakened local and systemic defense mechanisms that are unable to destroy the bacteria and stop the infectious process. The course of the disease can develop over months (subacute), or it can be very rapid, developing within a few days (acute). There are several bacteria that can cause IE but the more common species are *streptococci* (*alpha-hemolytic* or *viridans*) and *staphylococcus aureus*. The *streptococci viridans* is found in the oropharyngeal and gastrointestinal flora and is a low-grade pathogen that is usually responsible for subacute endocarditis. *Staphylococcus aureus* is a more virulent organism and is the leading cause of acute bacterial endocarditis (Sande et al., 2001). Although all heart valves can be affected by this disease, aortic stenosis and mitral regurgitation most commonly occur as a result of IE.

The treatment goal for IE is appropriate and aggressive administration of antibiotics over the course of several weeks. Timely administration of antibiotics is imperative so that adequate levels can be maintained and resistance of bacteria to antibiotics can be reduced. If valvular dysfunction is severe, valve replacement may be required. In high-risk patient populations, antibiotic prophylaxis is suggested prior to procedures that may introduce bacteria. This practice is still followed although there is little evidence to support this intervention (Sande et al., 2001).

Assessment and Diagnosis

The assessment process starts with a thorough physical assessment. Because turbulent blood flow is the result of valvular dysfunction, auscultation of the heart can reveal a murmur. The key to understanding the timing of murmurs in the cardiac cycle is to think about the valve position in relation to ventricular systole or diastole. Table 12–2 includes a summary of heart murmurs, their timing in the cardiac cycle, and characteristics.

The mitral valve is open during ventricular diastole, so the murmur of MS occurs during diastole. The aortic valve is open during ventricular systole, so the murmur of AS occurs during systole.

The opposite timing for murmurs applies for regurgitation. The mitral valve is closed during systole, so the murmur of MR occurs during systole. The aortic valve is closed during diastole, so the murmur of AR occurs during diastole.

With AS, angina can occur because of possible disturbance of blood flow through the coronary arteries because the opening of these arteries is located close to the aortic valve. Symptoms specific to AS include syncope on exertion as a result of decreased cerebral perfusion. If valvular dysfunction is critical, the patient can experience heart failure or pulmonary edema. Dyspnea, tachypnea, crackles in the lungs, tachycardia, and chest pain can be present. A chest x-ray may reveal pulmonary edema or an enlarged LA.

TABLE 12–2 Heart Murmurs Timing and Characteristics

MURMUR	CARDIAC CYCLE TIMING	AUSCULTATION SITE	CONFIGURATION OF SOUND	CONTINUITY
Mitral stenosis	Diastole	Apical	S_1 — S_2	Rumble that increases in sound toward the end, continuous
Mitral regurgitation	Systole	Apex	S_1 — S_2	Holosystolic (occurs throughout systole), continuous
Aortic stenosis	Midsystolic	Right sternal border (RSB) 2nd intercostal space (ICS)	S_1 — S_2	Crescendo-decrescendo, continuous
Aortic regurgitation	Diastole (early)	3rd ICS, LSB	S_2 — S_1	Decrescendo, continuous
Tricuspid stenosis	Diastole	Lower LSB	S_2 — S_1	Rumble that increases sound toward the end, continuous
Tricuspid regurgitation	Systole	4th ICS, LSB	S_2 — S_1	Holosystolic, continuous

From Lemone, P. & Burke, K. (2004). Medical surgical nursing: Critical thinking in client care. (3rd ed.) Upper Saddle River, NJ: Prentice Hall, Inc. Copyright 2004 Pearson Education.

Another assessment tool that is helpful in the diagnosis of valvular disease is an echocardiogram. The **echocardiogram** is noninvasive technology that allows visualization of the valves as well as the size, thickness, and function of the atria and ventricles. Abnormal findings in the echocardiogram can be confirmed by cardiac catheterization (Module 11). During this procedure, the valves can be thoroughly examined, and intracardiac pressures and pressure gradients across the chambers can be measured.

Collaborative Management

Patients who are asymptomatic with a valvular dysfunction usually do not require medical intervention. As the dysfunction becomes more severe, HR is controlled with drugs such as beta blockers (BB), calcium channel blockers (CCB), and digoxin. Examples of these drugs are listed in Table 12–3. The major therapeutic goal is to maintain normal sinus rhythm and avoid atrial fibrillation. If atrial fibrillation does occur, immediate treatment with cardioversion may be required (Module 10). If heart failure (HF) occurs, diuretics and sodium and fluid restriction may be required. With regurgitation, afterload reduction is very important. Reducing afterload lessens the degree of regurgitation and significantly improves symptoms. Angiotensin-converting enzyme (ACE) inhibitors are particularly effective for afterload reduction and controlling hypertension.

Surgical intervention is required if valvular dysfunction is severe. The valve is replaced with either a tissue or mechanical, artificial valve. Mechanical valves last longer, but anticoagulation is required because the foreign material causes clot formation. The type of valve used depends on patient age and tolerance of anticoagulation. Anticoagulation is also required if chronic atrial fibrillation is present. Advancement in medical management has decreased mortality and improved quality of life in patients with valvular disease.

Nursing Management

Nursing diagnoses for a patient with a valve disorder may include decreased cardiac output, activity intolerance, fatigue, risk for infection, ineffective protection, and ineffective health maintenance. Nursing priorities include assessing and maintaining CO, assessing for side effects of the disorder, preventing complications, administering pharmacologic therapies, and providing patient education.

All valve disorders affect ventricular filling or emptying and result in decreased CO. Vital signs are carefully monitored. Hypotension and tachycardia indicate decreased CO. If a PA catheter is present, hemodynamic findings may include decreased CO and elevated pulmonary artery wedge pressure and right atrial pressure. These findings are associated with pulmonary congestion. Auscultation of heart sounds is performed regularly. Atrial fibrillation may be averted by aggressive repletion of potassium and magnesium as needed and administration of antiarrhythmics as prescribed.

Failure of the heart to function as a pump results in decreased oxygen delivery to tissues and impaired tissue perfusion. An early sign of valve disease is dyspnea with exertion. The nurse monitors the patient's vital signs before and during activities. A change of heart rate of more than 20 beats per minute (bpm) or change in blood pressure of more than 20 mm Hg indicates activity intolerance. Other signs of activity intolerance include shortness of breath, chest pain, fatigue, diaphoresis, dizziness, or syncope. Activities and self-care activities are gradually increased. Rest periods between activities is helpful and decreases oxygen demand of the heart. A shower chair during bathing saves valuable energy. A physical therapy consult is initiated to help the patient regain and maintain physical strength. Asymptomatic patients are counseled about exercise tolerance, the importance of compliance with medications, and the need for periodic exams with their health care provider to monitor valve function.

Discharge planning includes education about the importance of monitoring blood pressure and HR. Because a therapeutic goal is to maintain a regular HR, the nurse educates the patient and family about monitoring pulse rate. They are observed for proper technique. Patient education includes information about medications, their action, and possible side effects.

Ineffective protection can occur as a result of anticoagulation therapy. The patient is at risk for bleeding. Therefore, vigilant assessment is necessary of serum coagulation studies, such as prothromboplastin time (PT), international normalized ratio (INR), and partial prothromboplastin time (PTT) as well as hemoglobin and hematocrit. If the patient is on coumadin (Warfarin), an INR goal is set. The nurse must be cognizant of this INR goal. Aspirin may also be prescribed. Patients receiving anticoagulant therapy are monitored for signs of bleeding, such as

TABLE 12–3 Brief Listing of Common Drugs by Classes

THIAZIDE DIURETICS	LOOP DIURETICS	ACE INHIBITORS	ANGIOTENSIN RECEPTOR BLOCKERS	BETA BLOCKERS	CALCIUM CHANNEL BLOCKERS
Chlorothiazide (Diuril)	Bumetanide (Bumex)	Captopril (Capoten)	Losartan (Cozaar)	Atenolol (Tenormin)	Diltiazem (Cardizem)
Metolazone (Zaroxolyn)	Furosemide (Lasix)	Enalapril (Vasotec)	Valsartan (Diovan)	Metoprolol (Lopressor)	Verapamil (Calan)
		Lisinopril (Zestril, Prinivil)	Irbesartan (Avapro)	Nadolol (Corgard)	
		Ramipril (Altace)		Propanolol (Inderal)	

unexplained bruises, bleeding gums, and blood in stools. Patients who go home on anticoagulant therapy must receive patient education about monitoring for signs of bleeding, the need for drawing blood samples, taking the medication in the evening, and avoiding foods that have a high vitamin K content.

Although this intervention is controversial, patients with artificial or abnormal valves may require antibiotic prophylaxis when undergoing certain procedures, such as dental work or endoscopies. They are encouraged to wear emergency identification tags about this condition.

In summary, the patient with valvular disease can have a single disease process or can be in a very complex later stage of the disease. The heart and compensatory mechanisms can adapt to some degree but the patient will then become symptomatic. Medical management maintains the patient's lifestyle but surgical intervention may be required. Anticoagulation is a major component of care for most patients with valve disease. Astute assessment and comprehensive patient education are the main components of nursing care.

SECTION ONE REVIEW

1. If a patient is on Coumadin, which lab value guides the therapeutic goal?
   A. activated clotting time
   B. thrombin time
   C. partial prothromboplastin time
   D. INR
2. When a patient has MS, the abnormal heart sound would be
   A. diastolic murmur
   B. systolic murmur
   C. S_3
   D. S_4
3. A condition in which the orifice of the mitral valve has narrowed and blood flow is obstructed during diastole is called
   A. mitral stenosis
   B. mitral regurgitation

   C. aortic stenosis
   D. infective endocarditis
4. Which of the following patients are susceptible to infective endocarditis?
   A. patients with preexisting heart disease
   B. patients with human immunodeficiency virus
   C. patients that require hemodialysis
   D. all of the above
5. When a patient has MR, the abnormal heart sound is
   A. diastolic murmur
   B. systolic murmur
   C. S_3
   D. S_4

Answers: 1. D, 2. A, 3. A, 4. D, 5. B

SECTION TWO: Heart Failure

At the completion of this section, the learner will be able to define heart failure, describe the pathophysiologic and compensatory mechanisms that occur during heart failure, and discuss the pharmacologic therapies used in the collaborative management of heart failure.

Heart failure (HF), a major health problem in our society today, is a clinical syndrome that results from any structural or functional cardiac disorder that decreases the ability of the ventricle to fill or eject.

Clinical manifestations of heart failure include dyspnea and fatigue that limit exercise tolerance, and fluid retention that leads to pulmonary congestion and peripheral edema. Because not all patients have fluid volume excess at the time of evaluation, the term *heart failure* is considered a better description of this condition than the older term *congestive heart failure* (Hunt et al., 2001). Symptoms of patients with HF are a result of impairment of LV function.

The New York Heart Association (NYHA) developed a classification of HF based on functional limitations. There are four classes (Francis et al., 2001):

■ Class I includes patients with cardiac disease but without resulting limitations of physical activity

■ Class II includes patients with cardiac disease resulting in slight limitations of physical activity

■ Class III includes patients with cardiac disease resulting in marked limitations of physical activity

■ Class IV includes patients with cardiac disease resulting in inability to carry on any physical activity without discomfort

There are two categories of HF: (1) **systolic dysfunction,** characterized by an ejection fraction (EF) less than 40 percent and (2) **diastolic dysfunction,** characterized by an impairment of ventricular relaxation (Hunt et al., 2001). In two thirds of patients with HF, the cause of the syndrome is coronary artery disease, whereas the final one third of the HF patients have a cardiomyopathy.

TABLE 12–4 Conditions That Trigger Heart Failure

Hypertension	Rheumatic fever
Diabetes	Exposure to cardiotoxic agents (some chemotherapies)
Hypercholestolemia	
Coronary artery disease	Illicit drug use
Valvular heart disease	Alcohol abuse
Peripheral vascular disease	

HF is a progressive disease and causes cardiac remodeling. The LV dilates, hypertrophies, and becomes more spherical. The mechanism that causes HF is not clearly understood. Current theories support its development as the result of a sequence of events. Heart failure begins with a primary event that results in a loss of myocardium or excessive overload on the muscle. Many conditions can trigger heart failure. Table 12–4 summarizes these conditions.

Whatever the cause, some cardiomyocytes are destroyed, whereas other cells try to adapt by increasing their size and elongating. The cardiac muscle hypertrophies in order to sustain the increased workload. When the muscle can no longer maintain that workload, the LV dilates in order to maintain SV even though the EF has decreased. Compensatory neurohormonal mechanisms help achieve this adaptive response.

Sodium and water retention occurs in an effort to increase preload and cardiac output. The renin–angiotensin system stimulates aldosterone release and increases sodium retention. As CO decreases, the sympathetic nervous system releases norepinephrine and vasopressin to increase blood pressure, HR, and contractility. All these mechanisms help with short-term adaptation but have untoward long-term effects. A chronic increase in afterload eventually causes a decrease in cardiac output. A lower cardiac output leads to pulmonary congestion and peripheral edema. Prolonged increases in adrenergic activity lead to dysrhythmias, increased cardiac cellular activity, increased energy utilization, and cell death (Francis et al., 2001).

Recall from Module 8 the counterregulatory hormones atrial natriuretic peptide (ANP) and brain natriuretic peptide (BNP) are released in response to distention of heart chambers. ANP is released in response to atrial distention and BNP is released in response to ventricular distention. Both hormones cause vasodilation and induce natriuresis (loss of sodium).

Assessment and Diagnosis

A careful history and physical examination provide important information. HF has multisystem effects (Fig. 12–10). Dyspnea, orthopnea, and paroxysmal nocturnal dyspnea (PND) are classic respiratory symptoms of patients with HF. **Orthopnea** is the sensation of shortness of breath in the supine position, whereas PND is sudden dyspnea at night that may awaken patients. Fatigue is another hallmark symptom. Jugular vein distention is a sign of fluid volume excess. Peripheral edema may also be present as a sign of fluid volume excess, although it can result from noncardiac causes. Crackles is an unreliable sign of heart failure. Most patients with chronic HF do not have crackles. A third heart sound (S_3) is an important assessment finding.

The single most useful diagnostic test for HF is the two-dimensional echocardiogram with doppler flow studies. With these studies, an EF is obtained and pericardial, valvular, or myocardial dysfunction is visualized (Hunt et al., 2001). A chest x-ray gives an estimate of heart size and pulmonary congestion. A 12-lead electrocardiogram (ECG) can demonstrate myocardial infarction, ventricular hypertrophy, or dysrhythmia. However, the chest x-ray and electrocardiogram do not provide specific information to make the diagnosis of HF. Cardiac catheterization may also be needed to provide further information about coronary artery or valvular disease (refer to Module 8).

It is important to remember that HF is a syndrome with many presentations, including decreased exercise tolerance, fluid retention, or symptoms of another cardiac or noncardiac disorder (Hunt et al., 2001).

Collaborative Management

The American College of Cardiologists and the American Heart Association established evidence-based guidelines for the management of HF (Hunt et al., 2001). Therapy is divided into four categories:

- Stage A includes patients at high risk for developing LV dysfunction
- Stage B includes patients with LV dysfunction who have not developed symptoms
- Stage C includes patients with LV dysfunction with current or prior symptoms
- Stage D includes patients with refractory end-stage HF

The focus of treatment for patients at high risk for HF is to control risk factors. Management of hypertension, diabetes, and hyperlipidemia reduces the risk of developing HF. Counseling patients on the hazards of recreational substances, such as tobacco, alcohol, and illicit drugs, provides a strong impetus for patients to reduce the use of these agents. There is no evidence that controlling dietary sodium intake and exercise helps prevent HF, but these habits can promote general health.

First-line drug management for HF usually includes an ACE inhibitor and a BB. This regimen controls the neurohormonal and sympathetic compensatory responses and decreases the occurrence of HF. Once patients display symptoms of HF, a combination of four types of drugs are used: diuretics, ACE inhibitors, BBs, and digitalis (Hunt et al., 2001).

Furosemide (Lasix) is the most common diuretic used. If two diuretics are needed to obtain the desired response, the two drugs used typically act on different sections of the nephron. For example, furosemide, a loop diuretic, acts on the loop of Henle, and metolazone (Zaroxolyn), a thiazide diuretic, works on blocking sodium reabsorption at the proximal tubule (Hardman & Limbird, 2000).

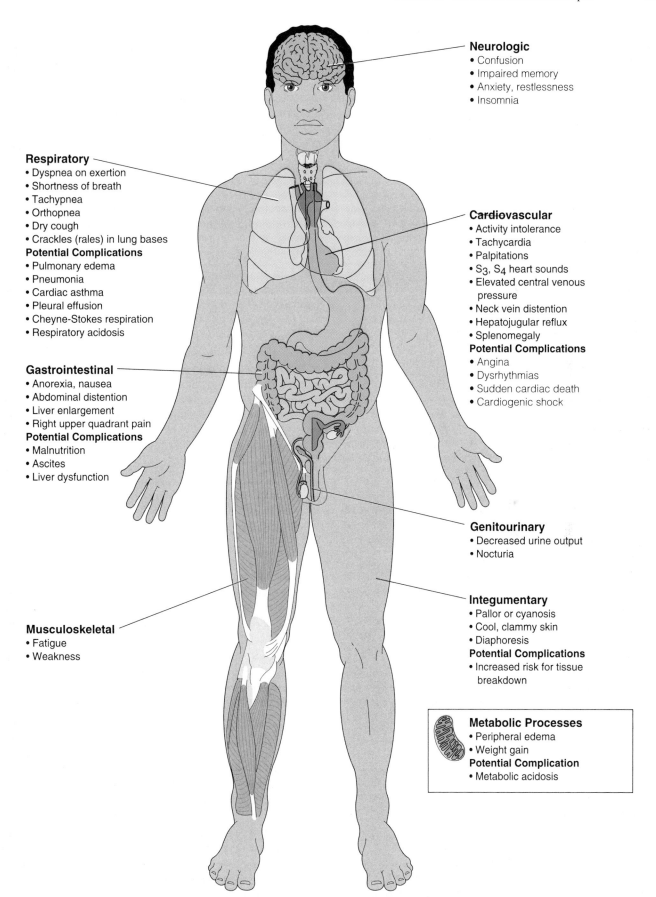

Neurologic
• Confusion
• Impaired memory
• Anxiety, restlessness
• Insomnia

Respiratory
• Dyspnea on exertion
• Shortness of breath
• Tachypnea
• Orthopnea
• Dry cough
• Crackles (rales) in lung bases
Potential Complications
• Pulmonary edema
• Pneumonia
• Cardiac asthma
• Pleural effusion
• Cheyne-Stokes respiration
• Respiratory acidosis

Cardiovascular
• Activity intolerance
• Tachycardia
• Palpitations
• S_3, S_4 heart sounds
• Elevated central venous
  pressure
• Neck vein distention
• Hepatojugular reflux
• Splenomegaly
Potential Complications
• Angina
• Dysrhythmias
• Sudden cardiac death
• Cardiogenic shock

Gastrointestinal
• Anorexia, nausea
• Abdominal distention
• Liver enlargement
• Right upper quadrant pain
Potential Complications
• Malnutrition
• Ascites
• Liver dysfunction

Genitourinary
• Decreased urine output
• Nocturia

Integumentary
• Pallor or cyanosis
• Cool, clammy skin
• Diaphoresis
Potential Complications
• Increased risk for tissue
  breakdown

Musculoskeletal
• Fatigue
• Weakness

Metabolic Processes
• Peripheral edema
• Weight gain
Potential Complication
• Metabolic acidosis

Figure 12–10 ■ Multisystem effects of heart failure.

ACE inhibitors are commonly administered. However, there are important contraindications to the use of ACE inhibitors of which nurses must be aware. Contraindications include previous severe adverse reactions to ACE inhibitors, serum creatinine greater than 3 mg/dL, systolic blood pressure less than 80 mm Hg, and serum potassium levels greater than 5.5 mEq/L (Hunt et al., 2001). Beta blockers may be administered to patients who do not have fluid retention. Spironolactone (Aldactone) may be used if the patient with HF has adequate renal function and a normal potassium level.

Angiotensin receptor blockade (ARB) may be used for patients who cannot tolerate an ACE inhibitor because of a side effect or allergic reaction (Hunt et al., 2001). The ARB drugs can have similar clinical results as the ACE inhibitors. Figure 12–11 depicts how ARB and ACE inhibitors work to block the renin–angiotensin–aldosterone system. ARBs do not have some of the adverse effects that are associated with ACE inhibitors, such as cough.

Nursing Management

Nursing diagnoses that may apply to the patient with HF include decreased cardiac output, activity intolerance, excess fluid volume, knowledge deficit: low-sodium diet, and ineffective health maintenance.

Failure of the heart to function as a pump results in heart failure and decreased CO. A major nursing goal is to decrease the patient's oxygen demands because oxygen supply is severely decreased. This goal is accomplished by ensuring adequate rest, administering medications as prescribed to decrease preload and improve contractility, assessing patient response to medications, and helping the patient manage the symptoms of this disease.

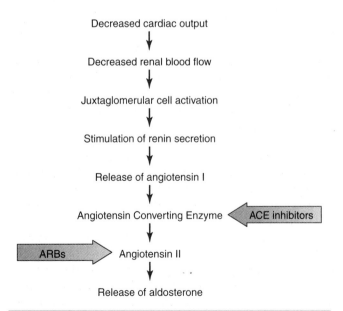

Figure 12–11 ■ACE inhibitors and ARBs block the renin–angiotensin–aldosterone system.

As the heart fails to function as a pump, less oxygen is delivered to tissues and ineffective tissue perfusion results. Many of the nursing interventions listed for the patient with valve disease are pertinent for the patient with heart failure. Nursing assessments focus on astute observation of the patient for signs of decompensation. Vital signs are monitored for signs of decreased CO. Palpation of the apical pulse can be located to the left of the midclavicular line because of LV enlargement. Heart sounds are auscultated regularly. An early sign of heart failure is an S_3 heart sound. Lung sounds are monitored for the development of crackles. Cardiac rhythm, exercise tolerance, and renal function are assessed for early signs of deterioration.

Continuous telemetry monitoring is recommended for patients in the high-acuity setting because BBs, digitalis, and other medications affect HR. Because digitalis and BBs slow the heart rate, patients are instructed on how to correctly take their pulse and when to call the health care provider if pulse parameters are violated.

The patient with HF may have activity intolerance and fatigue from a couple of sources. First, the disease process itself causes fatigue because of decreased oxygen delivery to peripheral tissues. Fluid volume excess in the lungs interferes with pulmonary gas exchange. BBs cause fatigue, a significant side effect that often causes patients to discontinue taking the drug. It is important for patients to know that the fatigue may disappear after the first several weeks of therapy. The patient is encouraged to rest between activities and to gradually increase activities. The nurse monitors the patient's activity tolerance. This includes taking vital signs before, during, and after an activity.

Because fatigue is one of the major symptoms of HF, proper sleep and sleeping habits are very important to maintain quality of life. The nurse recognizes that these patients have sleep disturbances and obtains a brief sleep history, ensuring that other causes of sleep disturbances, such as depression or sleep apnea, are ruled out. The hospital environment is optimized to promote sleep using relaxation techniques, sleep protocols, and a quiet environment. Sleep disturbances are treated by (1) reviewing good sleep habits; (2) considering alternative practices, such as relaxation, or cognitive or behavioral therapy; or (3) suggesting structured changes in sleep habits (Erickson et al., 2003). Family focused care is another helpful intervention that is explored and implemented to maintain compliance with the health care regimen (Clark & Dunbar, 2003).

Careful monitoring of fluid status is important for patients with HF. Diuretics can deplete circulating volume and cause hypovolemia, as well as potassium and magnesium deficits. These electrolytes are replaced either by oral/IV supplements or food source supplementation. Potassium depletion is further exacerbated if digitalis is used with a diuretic. A decreased urine output can indicate a significant decrease in CO and renal perfusion. Monitoring weight trends is also very important in controlling fluid retention. Obtaining and recording daily weights is vital. Typically, a weight gain of 2.2 pounds (1 kg) equates to fluid retention of a liter. For discharge planning, the patient is given tools for recording daily weights and advised to call a

Evidence-Based Practice

- *Health care professionals must assess the level of control perceived by spouses of patients with advanced heart failure and provide information and counseling directed toward increasing their sense of control (Dracup et al., 2004).*

- *Exercise training in adults with heart failure increases exercise tolerance and perceived physical function (Collins et al., 2004).*

- *Spouses of patients with heart failure need information about the disease, medications, diet restrictions, fluid limitations, importance of daily weights, diuretic regime for weight gain, and warning signs of decompensation (Martensson et al., 2001).*

health care provider if he or she gains 3 or more pounds (1.4 kg) in 24 hours (MacKlin, 2001).

Nursing interventions focus on patient education in an effort to improve patient compliance with the prescribed drug regimen. Drug therapy is a major component of management of this condition. One of the most important concepts for patients to understand is the difference between a drug side effect and a drug allergy. A **drug allergy** refers to some display of anaphylactic shock, such as a rash, airway compromise (edema of the tongue or larynx), or hypotension. A **drug side effect** is a reaction to some action of the drug other than anaphylaxis. A patient may say that he or she has an allergy to a drug but it is really a side effect. For example, a patient thinks that he or she has an allergy to ACE inhibitors because they cause a cough. Cough is really a side effect of ACE inhibitors, not an allergy. Coughing is the result of the release of kinins that cause coughing with prolonged therapy (Hunt et al., 2001). It would be unfortunate for this patient to not reap the benefits of ACE inhibitors because of wrong information.

It is also important to understand any financial constraints that the patient has in order to make sure that he or she is able to obtain needed drugs.

Cardiomyopathy

End-stage HF is referred to as **cardiomyopathy** and is classified class IV HF. At this stage, symptoms of HF occur at rest and the patient cannot perform activities of daily living.

The disease progression is diffuse and affects all heart chambers, although it may be more extensive in one chamber than others. Cardiomyopathies are classified into three categories according to clinical and structural findings: dilated cardiomyopathy, hypertrophic cardiomyopathy, and constrictive cardiomyopathy. The causes, pathophysiology, manifestations, and management of each of these cardiomyopathies are summarized in Table 12–5.

Dilated cardiomyopathy is associated with LV dilation and decreased EF. **Hypertrophic cardiomyopathy** is associated with LV hypertrophy that decreases the ability of the chamber to relax (diastolic dysfunction). **Constrictive cardiomyopathy** is associated with normal LV size, slightly depressed EF, and a marked decrease in cardiac muscle compliance. Depending on the type of cardiomyopathy, collaborative management may differ, but the same general principles of HF treatment continue.

Control of volume overload is aggressive. A loop diuretic and a second diuretic are usually needed. ACE inhibitors or BBs are used cautiously. Typically, these patients are very unstable. Patients with refractory HF may also require intermittent hospitalization for infusion of positive ionotropic medications (such as dobutamine or milrinone) and vasodilators (such as nitroprusside or nitroglycerin) (Hunt et al., 2001). These drugs improve contractility and decrease afterload. Another newer drug that may be used is nesiritide (Natrecor). This drug, given as an IV infusion, mimics brain natriuretic peptide and is given to enhance diuresis (Gordon & Rempher, 2003).

Other interventions have demonstrated some improvement in symptoms and are being used more frequently. Fast cardiac rhythms that quickly cause decompensation are controlled with an automatic implantable cardioverter/defibrillator (AICD) (Branum, 2003). Biventricular pacing is another intervention that improves both right and left ventricular electrical activity and enhances ventricular mechanical performance (Mardell, 2004).

Surgical intervention may include mitral valve replacement to decrease LV dilatation (Hunt et al., 2001). Removal of a hypertrophied LV, known as the Batista procedure, is another surgical option. Cardiomyoplasty is a procedure that uses muscle or other material to "wrap" the heart, thereby mechanically increasing the contractility of the heart muscle. Final surgical interventions that may be considered are placement of ventricular assist devices (VAD) and cardiac transplantation. These interventions are reserved for when heart failure has become unresponsive to conventional medical treatment (Hunt et al., 2001).

Patient and family education is ongoing. Continuity of care with the same health care team is very important. All the nursing interventions previously described for the patient with HF are applicable to this patient population. However, monitoring is more intense because these patients are more unstable. Blood pressure monitoring is pivotal. Subtle changes in mental status indicate a change in cerebral perfusion and the physician is notified immediately. Renal function is monitored because of diuresis and decreased renal perfusion as a result of decreased CO. Patient education about pacing or AICD is very important if these interventions are used. Consideration is given to end-of-life care in this patient population. The nurse plays a vital role in assisting these patients in developing and implementing advance directives and the use of hospice care (Hunt et al., 2001).

In summary, the patient with heart failure is very complex and requires careful and vigilant collaborative care and nursing management. The compensatory mechanisms of the body are attempting to maintain reasonable cardiac performance. Monitoring heart rhythms, blood pressure, and exercise tolerance for subtle changes may prevent or anticipate clinical deterioration of the patient's condition.

TABLE 12–5 Classifications of Cardiomyopathy

	DILATED	HYPERTROPHIC	RESTRICTIVE
Causes	Usually idiopathic; may be secondary to chronic alcoholism or myocarditis	Hereditary; may be secondary to chronic hypertension	Usually secondary to amyloidosis, radiation, or myocardial fibrosis
Pathophysiology	Scarring and atrophy of myocardial cells	Hypertrophy of ventricular muscle mass	Excess rigidity of ventricular walls restricts filling
	Thickening of ventricular wall	Small left ventricular volume	Myocardial contractility remains relatively normal
	Dilation of heart chambers	Septal hypertrophy may obstruct left ventricular outflow	
	Impaired ventricular pumping	Left atrial dilation	
	Increased end-diastolic and end-systolic volumes		
	Mural thrombi common		
Manifestations	Heart failure	Dyspnea, anginal pain, syncope	Dyspnea, fatigue
	Cardiomegaly	Left ventricular hypertrophy	Right-sided heart failure
	Dysrhythmias	Dysrhythmias	Mild to moderate cardiomegaly
	S_3 and S_4 gallop; murmur of mitral regurgitation	Loud S_4	S_3 and S_4
		Sudden death	Mitral regurgitation murmur
Management	Management of heart failure	Beta blockers	Management of heart failure
	Implantable cardioverter-defibrillator (ICD) as needed	Calcium channel blockers	Exercise restriction
	Cardiac transplantation	Antidysrhythmic agents	
		ICD, dual-chamber pacing	
		Surgical excision of part of the ventricular septum	

From Lemone, P. & Burke, K. (2004). Medical surgical nursing: Critical thinking in client care. (3rd ed., p. 912). Upper Saddle River, NJ: Prentice Hall, Inc. Copyright 2004 Pearson Education.

SECTION TWO REVIEW

1. Weight gain of greater than 3 pounds might dictate which drug category would be increased
   A. ACE inhibitor
   B. diuretic
   C. beta blocker
   D. digitalis
2. Mr. M has a blood pressure of 75/45 mm Hg. You are the nurse and it is time to administer his ACE inhibitor. Which nursing action is MOST appropriate?
   A. give the drug immediately; it will improve his blood pressure
   B. wait 1 hour and recheck the blood pressure

   C. notify the physician and ask if the dose should be held
   D. discuss the issue with your colleague
3. ANP and BNP cause
   A. myocardial infarction
   B. hypertension
   C. vasoconstriction and fluid retention
   D. vasodilation and diuresis
4. Which of the following are classic respiratory symptoms of patients with HF?
   A. dyspnea
   B. orthopnea

C. paroxysmal nocturnal dyspnea
D. all of the above
5. Normal LV size, slightly depressed EF, and a marked decrease in compliance of cardiac muscle describes
A. constrictive cardiomyopathy

B. dilated cardiomyopathy
C. hypertrophic cardiomyopathy
D. stage II heart failure

Answers: 1. B, 2. C, 3. D, 4. D, 5. A

SECTION THREE: Hypertension

At the completion of this section, the learner will be able to define the ranges of systolic and diastolic blood pressure for prehypertension, stage 1 hypertension, and stage 2 hypertension; explain the pathophysiologic mechanisms that contribute to hypertension; and discuss collaborative and nursing interventions for the patient with hypertension.

The focus on hypertension and its early detection, prevention, and treatment is a top priority in health care because hypertension contributes to an increased risk of heart attack, heart failure, stroke, and kidney disease. Hypertension can be found in the young as well as the elderly, and frequently patients do not have symptoms. Risk factors for the development of hypertension have been identified (Table 12–6).

Parameters for hypertension are defined in the *Seventh report of the Joint National Committee on Prevention, Detection, Evaluation and Treatment of High Blood Pressure* (Chobanian, 2003) for adults over 18 years. In this report, normal blood pressure is defined as a systolic blood pressure (SBP) less than 120 mm Hg and a diastolic blood pressure (DBP) less than 80 mm Hg. A new category for blood pressure classification, **prehypertension** assists with earlier identification of those at risk for developing hypertension. Prehypertension is defined as a SBP of 120 to 139 mm Hg and DBP of 80 to 89 mm Hg. Definitions of the classifications of blood pressure, as summarized by Chobanian (2003), are listed in Table 12–7.

Although a lot of research has focused on identifying the cause of hypertension, the exact cause has not been identified (Kaplan, 2000). Neurohormonal mechanisms appear to be key to the development of hypertension. The sympathetic nervous system plays a major role by releasing catecholamines that result in increased heart rate and vasoconstriction. The renin–angiotensin system also influences the development of hypertension by secreting aldosterone to promote sodium and water retention. Hyperinsulinemia and insulin resistance may contribute to the development of hypertension. Although the mechanism is not clear, peripheral tissues do not use insulin. Insulin may act as a vasopressor. Nitric oxide, produced by endothelial cells, normally causes vasodilation; however, with hypertension, it appears that nitric oxide release is inhibited (Kaplan, 2000). Endothelin-1, a factor produced by endothelial cells, has significant vasoconstrictor properties and appears to contribute to the development of hypertension (Kaplan, 2000).

TABLE 12–6 Risk Factors for the Development of Hypertension

Hypertension
Cigarette smoking
Obesity
Physical inactivity
Hyperlidemia
Diabetes mellitus
Estimated glomerular filtration rate less than 60 mL/min
Age (older than 55 for men; 65 for women)
Family history of premature cardiovascular disease

TABLE 12–7 Classification of Blood Pressure

BLOOD PRESSURE CLASSIFICATION	SYSTOLIC BLOOD PRESSURE (mm Hg)	DIASTOLIC BLOOD PRESSURE (mm Hg)
Normal	Less than 120	Less than 80
Prehypertension	120 to 139	80 to 89
Stage 1 hypertension	140 to 159	90 to 99
Stage 2 hypertension	160 or greater	100 or greater

Adapted from Chobanian, A. V. (2003). Seventh report of the Joint National Committee on prevention, detection, evaluation and treatment of high blood pressure. *Washington, DC: National Institutes of Health, National Heart, Lung and Blood Institute.*

Assessment and Diagnosis

The diagnosis of hypertension is based on measurement of blood pressure. Measurements are done on both arms and obtained on at least two different occasions before the diagnosis is made. Once hypertension has been identified, the patient is assessed for identifiable causes, possible lifestyle changes, and for the presence of target organ damage (Chobanian, 2003). **Target organ damage** refers to dysfunction that occurs in organs affected by high blood pressure. Cardiovascular consequences of hypertension can include LV hypertrophy, angina or myocardial infarction, heart failure, stroke, and peripheral arterial disease. Target organ damage may also include renal dysfunction and retinopathy.

Patient assessment is focused on detection or limitation of target organ involvement. An initial physical examination includes opthalmoscopic visualization of the optic fundi; auscultation of the carotid, abdominal, and femoral arteries; assessment of lower extremities for pulses and edema; a thorough exam of the heart, lungs, and abdomen (for enlarged kidneys); and a neurologic assessment (Chobanian, 2003).

Before initiating therapy, routine laboratory assessment includes an electrocardiogram; urinalysis; and serum evaluations of glucose, hematocrit, potassium, creatinine, calcium, and lipid profiles (Chobanian, 2003). Once hypertension has been diagnosed, further testing may be indicated.

Collaborative Management

The ultimate goal of therapy is to lower the SBP. DBP usually decreases before SBP. Management centers on pharmacologic agents and lifestyle changes. For patients who are overweight or obese, the dietary approaches to stop hypertension (DASH) eating plan is implemented. This plan consists of a diet rich in calcium and potassium, sodium reduction, physical activity, and moderation of alcohol consumption (Chobanian, 2003). If these interventions do not achieve the target blood pressure, pharmacologic treatment is initated.

Pharmacologic treatment is evidence based and includes the use of several classes of drugs previously described in this module, including ACE inhibitors, ARBs, BBs, CCBs, and thiazide-type diuretics (Chobanian, 2003). Thiazide diuretics are the basis of antihypertensive therapy. These diuretics are used either alone or in combination with another drug for initial therapy. For stage 1 hypertension, thiazide diuretics are most commonly prescribed. For stage 2 hypertension, a two-drug combination is usually needed (a thiazide diuretic and an ACE inhibitor, ARB, BB, or CCB).

Hypertension along with certain comorbidities requires special consideration. In patients with ischemic heart disease, BBs and ACE inhibitors are the first drugs of choice. Patients with heart failure also attain good blood pressure control with BB and ACE inhibitors unless they become symptomatic, in which case aldosterone blockers and loop diuretics are recommended. Diabetic hypertension responds better to ACE inhibitors or ARBs. Chronic kidney disease is treated aggressively and may require three or more types of drugs (Chobanian, 2003).

Nursing Management

Nursing diagnoses that may be appropriate for the patient with hypertension include altered peripheral tissue perfusion, excess fluid volume, ineffective health maintenance, and risk for noncompliance.

Nursing management of patients with hypertension starts with accurate blood pressure measurement. The patient should be in a sitting or supine position for 5 minutes with the arm supported at heart level. An appropriately sized cuff is one that has at least 80 percent of the cuff bladder encircling the arm. Measurements are taken in both arms in an initial screening. In the acute care setting, noninvasive blood pressure machines are commonly used. All the same techniques in obtaining accurate blood pressure measurement are applied when using these machines. All blood pressure equipment is properly calibrated and checked at regular intervals. Patients and family are also instructed on how blood pressure is measured at home.

Patient education is a major component in nursing management in this patient population. Patients and families need significant teaching to manage this chronic condition. Patients and family members should understand the medications, their actions, and side effects. The nurse assists the patient to develop a medication administration schedule. Drugs that block the sympathetic nervous system (ARB, BBs) cause orthostatic hypotension. The nurse instructs the patient to slowly rise from a supine position.

Diuretics cause potassium and magnesium depletion. Patients receiving diuretics have these serum electrolytes monitored on a regular basis. Patients must know how to correctly take their pulse. Dietary restrictions of fluid and salt are part of routine patient education. Exercise programs are introduced using the expertise of other disciplines, such as physical therapy.

SECTION THREE REVIEW

Mr. G is an 85-year-old man with a past medical history of diabetes mellitus, hypertension, and coronary artery disease. He had coronary artery bypass surgery 10 years ago. He is now admitted for increasing fatigue and shortness of breath with minimal exertion. His blood pressure is 160/120 mm Hg. His serum creatinine is 2.3 mg/dL.

1. Which of the following risk factors does Mr. G have for the development of hypertension?
   A. diabetes mellitus
   B. poor renal function
   C. advancing age
   D. all of the above
2. What may be the cause of Mr. G's high serum creatinine?
   A. target organ damage
   B. chronic aldosterone secretion
   C. release of endothelin-1
   D. release of nitric oxide
3. Mr. G needs education about his diet. Which of the following plans would be most beneficial for him?
   A. a diet rich in calcium and potassium
   B. a restricted-sodium-intake diet
   C. a diet rich in vitimin K
   D. A and B
4. To accurately measure Mr. G's blood pressure, what cuff size would be appropriate?
   A. any cuff as long as it is an adult cuff
   B. a cuff that has at least 80 percent of the cuff encircling the arm
   C. it would be best to use a noninvasive machine cuff
   D. one that is two thirds the diameter of his arm
5. Patient education for those receiving antihypertensive agents should include information about
   A. orthostatic hypotension
   B. potassium intake
   C. magnesium intake
   D. weight changes

Answers: 1. D, 2. A, 3. D, 4. B, 5. A

POSTTEST

1. The cardiac dysrhythmia that can cause immediate decompensation in a patient with significant aortic valve stenosis is
   A. premature ventricular contractions
   B. premature atrial contractions
   C. atrial fibrillation
   D. sinus bradycardia
2. A patient with infective endocarditis may require antibiotics for
   A. 24 hours
   B. 72 hours
   C. 7 to 10 days
   D. several weeks
3. Which of the following heart murmurs would be heard between S_1 and S_2?
   A. mitral regurgitation
   B. aortic stenosis
   C. tricuspid regurgitation
   D. all of the above
4. Why are two diuretics (such as furosemide and zaroxolyn) used in the management of patients with heart failure?
   A. the two drugs act on different sections of the nephron
   B. it is a common mistake and should not be done
   C. they have different time releases
   D. they act synergistically
5. Cardiomyopathy can be categorized into what categories?
   A. dilated
   B. hypertrophic
   C. constrictive
   D. all of the above
6. Which of the following are important nursing interventions for patients with HF?
   A. monitor weight trends
   B. promote sleep
   C. provide family-focused care
   D. all of the above
7. Orthostatic hypotension can be minimized by
   A. skipping medications
   B. getting up more slowly from supine position
   C. decreasing ACE inhibitors
   D. increasing ARBs
8. Normal blood pressure is _____ mm Hg (systolic) and _____ mm Hg (diastolic).
   A. less than 120; less than 80
   B. 130; 85
   C. 140; 90
   D. 160; 100
9. The ultimate therapeutic goal for the treatment of hypertension is
   A. the ability to exercise without shortness of breath
   B. to lower SBP
   C. to lower DBP
   D. all of the above

POSTTEST ANSWERS

Question	Answer	Section	Question	Answer	Section
1	C	One	6	D	Two
2	D	One	7	B	Three
3	D	One	8	A	Three
4	A	Two	9	B	Three
5	D	Two			

REFERENCES

Branum, K. (2003). Management of decompensated heart failure. *AACN Clinical Issues, 14*, 498–511.

Braunwald, E. (2000). Valvular heart disease. In E. Braunwald, D. P. Zipes, & P. Libby (Eds.), *Heart disease: A textbook of cardiovascular medicine* (6th ed.). Philadelphia: W. B. Saunders.

Chobanian, A. V. (2003). *Seventh report of the Joint National Committee on prevention, detection, evaluation and treatment of high blood pressure.* Washington, DC: National Institutes of Health; National Heart, Lung and Blood Institute.

Clark, P. C., & Dunbar, S. B. (2003). Family partnership intervention: A guide for family approach to care of patients with heart failure. *AACN Clinical Issues, 14*, 467–477.

Collins, E., Langbein, W. E., Dilan-Koetje, J., et al. (2004). Effects of exercise on aerobic capacity and quality of life in individuals with heart failure. *Heart and Lung: The Journal of Acute and Critical Care, 33*, 154–161.

Dracup, K., Evangelista, L., Doering, L., et al. (2004). Emotional well being in spouses of patients with advanced heart failure. *Heart and Lung: The Journal of Acute and Critical Care, 33*, 354–361.

Erickson, V. S., Westlake, C. A., Dracup, K. A., Woo, M. A., & Hage A. (2003). Sleep disturbances in patients with heart failure. *AACN Clinical Issues, 14*, 477–487.

Francis, G. S., Gassler, J. P., & Sonnenblick, E. H. (2001). Pathophysiology and diagnosis of heart failure. In V. Fuster, R. A. Alexander, & R. A. O'Rourke (Eds.), *Hurst's the heart* (10th ed.). New York: McGraw-Hill Medical Publishing Division.

Gordon, C., & Rempher, K. J. (2003). Brain (b-type) natriuretic peptide: Implications for heart failure management. *AACN Clinical Issues, 14*, 532–542.

Hardman, J., & Limbird, L. (2000). *Goodman and Gillman's the pharmacological basis of therapeutics* (10th ed.). New York: McGraw-Hill Medical Publishing Division.

Hunt, S. A., Baker, D. W., Chin, M. H., et al. (2001). ACC/AHA guidelines for the evaluation and management of chronic heart failure in the adult. Available at: *http://www.acc.org/clinical/guidelines/failure/hf_index.htm*. Accessed February 22, 2005.

Kaplan, N. M. (2000). Hypertensive and atherosclerotic disease. In E. Braunwald, D. P. Zipes, & P. Libby (Eds.), *Heart disease: A textbook of cardiovascular medicine* (6th ed.). Philadelphia: W. B. Saunders.

MacKlin, M. (2001). Managing heart failure: A case study approach. *Critical Care Nurse, 21*(2), 36–51.

Mardell, P. (2004). Biventricular pacing and cardiac resynchronization therapy: A fresh approach to heart failure and intraventricular conduction delay. *Canadian Journal of Cardiovascular Nursing, 14*(1), 29–38.

Martensson, J., Dracup, K., & Fridlund, B. (2001). Decisive situations influencing spouses' support of patients with heart failure: A critical incident technique analysis. *Heart and Lung: The Journal of Acute and Critical Care, 30*, 341–350.

Sande, M. A., Kartalija, M., & Anderson, J. (2001). Infective endocarditis. In V. Fuster, R. A. Alexander, & R. A. O'Rourke (Eds.), *Hurst's the heart* (10th ed.). New York: McGraw-Hill Medical Publishing Division.

Nursing Care of the Patient with Altered Tissue Perfusion

Karen L. Johnson

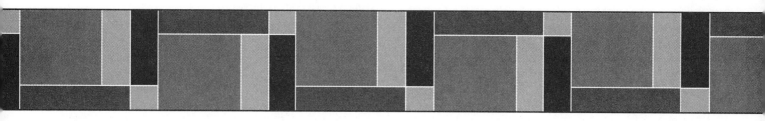

OBJECTIVES Following completion of this module, the learner will be able to

1. Cluster assessment data to formulate perfusion patterns.
2. Appraise a patient's perfusion status based on a nursing assessment.
3. Identify priorities in nursing care for a patient experiencing an alteration in perfusion.
4. Explain rationale for nursing actions that support perfusion.

This self-study module is designed to integrate the major points discussed in Modules 8, 9, 10, 11, and 12 and to summarize relationships between key concepts while assisting the learner in clustering information to facilitate clinical application. The module is divided into two case studies. Both case studies apply the content in an interactive learning style. The learner is encouraged to identify nursing actions based on patient assessment in a case study format. Nursing care of a patient with a fluid volume deficit is addressed in Case Study 1. Nursing care of a patient with a fluid volume excess is addressed in Case Study 2. Consequences of selecting particular actions are discussed, and the rationale for correct actions is presented. The module ends with a summary of nursing priorities in caring for patients with altered tissue perfusion.

ABBREVIATIONS

ABG	Arterial blood gas	**IV**	Intravenous
ACE	Angiotensin converting enzyme	**LDH**	Lactic dehydrogenase
AST	Aspartate aminotransferase	**LVSWI**	Left ventricular stroke work index
bpm	Beats per minute	**MAST**	Military antishock trousers, also known as pneumatic antishock garment
CBC	Complete blood cell count		
CI	Cardiac index	**PAP**	Pulmonary arterial pressure
CK-MB	Creatinine phosphokinase–myocardial bands	**PAWP**	Pulmonary artery wedge pressure
CO	Cardiac output	**RAP**	Right atrial pressure
CT	Computerized tomography	**SVR**	Systemic vascular resistance
IABP	Intra-aortic balloon pump		

Case Study 1

SUE S, A PATIENT WITH A FLUID VOLUME DEFICIT

Sue S is a 24-year-old, gravida 1 female who is 12 weeks pregnant. Her husband brought her to the emergency department when she passed out at home. Sue began vomiting en route and complaining of severe, continuous right lower quadrant abdominal pain that extended to her suprapubic area. She also complained of pain in the right shoulder area. Sue is admitted into your zone by the triage nurse.

Initial Appraisal

On walking into Sue's room, you note the following.

GENERAL APPEARANCE. Sue is diaphoretic. She is of moderate stature. Weight is appropriate for height. She is fully clothed.

SIGNS OF DISTRESS. Sue is moaning. She is lying on her left side with her knees drawn to her chest. She is clutching a man's hands.

OTHER. You do not note any intravenous (IV) lines or oxygen in use. The man identifies himself as her husband.

Focused Circulatory Assessment

You quickly place Sue in a hospital gown, noting her profuse diaphoresis and cool, clammy skin. Because Sue appears to be in acute distress, you immediately perform a rapid assessment, focusing on her perfusion status. The results are as follows.

Sue is restless but alert and oriented to person, place, time, and reason for being at the hospital. Her blood pressure is 90/70 mm Hg (baseline according to her husband is 128/70 mm Hg), pulse is 126 beats per minute (bpm), respiratory rate is 28/min. Her respirations are shallow. Sue's radial pulse is regular. S1 and S2 are present without murmur. No extra heart sounds are auscultated. Breath sounds are clear bilaterally. Her capillary refill is 3 seconds. Her nailbeds are dusky. No bowel sounds are auscultated after 1 minute. Her abdomen is firm. Sue's pain increases dramatically on palpation of any part of her abdomen. She complains of increased pain unrelieved by change in position. Her oral temperature is 99°F (37.2°C).

After this initial assessment, you alert the emergency physician, Dr. P, who is busy examining a patient experiencing an acute myocardial infarction. Until she is able to examine Sue, Dr. P orders the following:

- 1,000 mL lactated Ringer's solution to be infused at 200 mL/hr through a large-bore IV line
- Stat complete blood cell count (CBC)
- Type and crossmatch for 4 units of blood
- Cardiac monitor
- Place urinary catheter
- Urinalysis and urine for pregnancy test
- Serum HCG
- Electrolyte panel
- Computed tomography (CT) scan of the abdomen
- Oxygen 2 L per nasal cannula

QUESTION

Considering Sue's presenting symptoms, prioritize the following orders. Which order should be implemented first?

A. CT scan of the abdomen
B. serum HCG
C. cardiac monitor
D. IV access

ANSWER

The correct answer is D. Because Sue's blood pressure is low compared with her normal value and she has had an episode of syncope at home, the IV line is initiated first. IV access provides a means of administering fluid boluses or volume expanders if necessary. Blood is obtained at the same time for the laboratory tests. Oxygen is administered next because tachycardia increases myocardial demands for oxygenation. Next, Sue is connected to the cardiac monitor because of her fast heart rate. The CT scan is ordered to determine the source of Sue's hypotension. Finally, the urinalysis is obtained. The status of Sue's pregnancy is determined by the serum HCG. The urine pregnancy test and urinalysis provide supplemental data.

STAT TEST RESULTS

CBC

WBC = 15,000/mL	(normal range 5,000 to 10,000/mL)
RBC = 5.0×10^6/mL	(normal range 4.2 to 5.4×10^6/mL)
Hgb = 12 g/dL	(normal range 12 to 16 g/dL in females)
Hct = 37 percent	(normal range 28 to 47 percent in females)

Electrolytes

Sodium (Na) = 146 mEq/L	(normal range 136 to 146 mEq/L)
Potassium (K) = 3.5 mEq/L	(normal range 3.5 to 5.5 mEq/L)
Chloride (Cl) = 95 mEq/L	(normal range 96 to 106 mEq/L)
Calcium (Ca) = 8.8 mg/dL	(normal range 8.5 to 10.5 mg/dL)
Glucose = 140 mg/dL	(normal range 80 to 120 mg/dL)
Serum HCG (pending)	
CT abdomen (scan positive for diffuse abdominal bleeding)	

QUESTION

What is the significance of the laboratory and radiographic data?

ANSWER

The WBC count is elevated, perhaps in response to an infectious or inflammatory process. The CBC, Hgb, and Hct are on the low side of normal because of abdominal bleeding. It generally takes several hours after hemorrhage begins to detect a noticeable decrease in the Hct. The high-normal sodium is related to an increase in aldosterone secretion to maintain blood volume. Thus, renal excretion of sodium decreases. Renal excretion of potassium increases because of this same response as evidenced by Sue's low-normal level. Her glucose is elevated because of sympathetic stimulation. The CT scan suggests a ruptured ectopic pregnancy originating in the right fallopian tube. This finding is consistent with Sue's history of being

3 months pregnant. Ectopic pregnancy is a life-threatening event because of associated internal bleeding. The results of the CT scan confirm that Sue requires surgical intervention.

Focused Nursing History

While Sue is in the radiology department with the emergency medicine resident, you speak with her husband to obtain critical historical data that may have an impact on Sue's present situation. Her husband gives the following history.

Sue diagnosed her pregnancy using an over-the-counter pregnancy detection kit. Both she and her husband are excited about the pregnancy; they had been trying to conceive for more than 2 years. Sue has not had any problems during the pregnancy. Before trying to conceive, Sue was using birth control pills. Her last menstrual period was 86 days ago. She has not had a previous pregnancy. For the past 2 days, she has complained of abdominal pain that has gradually increased in intensity. She has had nausea but did not begin vomiting until in the car on the way to the emergency department. Sue fainted when she got up to answer the phone after lying on the couch to try to relieve her abdominal pain. She has never fainted before. Sue does not have any medical conditions. She is not allergic to any medication. Her last meal was 6 hours ago. She has had two glasses of water since her last meal.

The Systematic Bedside Assessment

Sue returns from having a CT scan. You complete a head-to-toe assessment because you will be caring for Sue until the operating suite is ready. Sue signs a consent for an exploratory laparotomy.

HEAD AND NECK. Sue remains oriented, but she is restless. She is receiving 2 liters of oxygen through a nasal cannula. Her neck veins are slightly filled at an angle of 30 degrees. No other abnormalities of the head and neck are noted.

CHEST. Cardiac status. As previously noted, apical heart rate is 138 bpm. The pattern on the cardiac monitor is shown in Figure 13–1. Blood pressure is 88/70 mm Hg. Lactated Ringer's solution is infusing at 200 mL/hr via a 16-gauge IV catheter in the right forearm. The IV site is without edema or redness.

QUESTION

The pattern in Figure 13–1 is
A. normal sinus rhythm
B. sinus tachycardia
C. supraventricular tachycardia
D. atrial fibrillation

ANSWER

The correct answer is B. Sinus tachycardia; the rate is regular and greater than 100 bpm and *P* waves precede the *QRS* complex.

PULMONARY STATUS. As previously noted, the respiratory rate has increased to 32/min. Respirations remain shallow.

ABDOMEN. The abdomen is firm and tight. No bowel sounds are auscultated. Sue complains of increased pain in all quadrants and in her right shoulder on light palpation.

PELVIS. A urinary catheter is in place draining light yellow urine, 40 mL in the last hour.

EXTREMITIES. The skin is diaphoretic, cool, and clammy. The nailbeds are dusky. Capillary refill is sluggish. Peripheral pulses are palpable but faint in all extremities.

POSTERIOR. Posterior breath sounds are diminished in bilateral lower lung fields. No sacral edema is noted.

Development of Nursing Diagnoses

CLUSTERING DATA You have just completed your head-to-toe assessment and are ready to list appropriate nursing diagnoses for Sue. To cluster the data, look for abnormal results found during the assessment. Sue's major symptoms at this time are her intense pain and hypotension. These primary symptoms can initiate your first cluster of critical cues.

CLUSTER 1

Subjective data. Sue complains of continuous abdominal pain unrelieved with change in position. Pain has increased over the past 2 days. The pain increases with abdominal palpation and radiates to all four quadrants

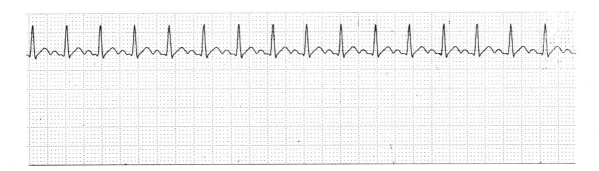

Figure 13–1 ■ Sue's current cardiac rhythm strip.

and the right shoulder (Kehr's sign). Nausea and vomiting are present, and the patient fainted once at home.

Objective data. Blood pressure is 88 to 90/70 mm Hg. The heart rate is 126 to 138 bpm. Respirations are 28 per minute. Hgb and Hct are borderline low. Potassium is borderline low, and sodium is borderline high. Urine output is 40 mL/hr. The last menstrual period was 86 days ago, and she had a positive over-the-counter pregnancy test. The CT scan was positive for abdominal bleeding.

QUESTION

Based on these data, which of the following nursing diagnoses would you select as being appropriate in planning Sue's care?

   A. fluid volume deficit
   B. decreased cardiac output (CO)
   C. altered tissue perfusion: renal, peripheral
   D. all of the above

ANSWER

The correct answer is D. All three are present in Sue's case. However, the decreased cardiac output and tissue perfusion are directly related to an actual fluid volume deficit. Therefore, focusing your nursing interventions on addressing the fluid volume status will improve her cardiac output and tissue perfusion. The most appropriate of the three diagnoses is *fluid volume deficit* related to abdominal bleeding.

Desired patient outcomes for Sue include

1. Systolic blood pressure greater than 90 mm Hg
2. Heart rate between 60 and 100 beats per minute
3. Respirations 12 to 16/min
4. Absence of abdominal pain
5. Urine output of at least 30 mL/hr
6. Absence of dizziness and syncope

For the purposes of Sue's case study, only the perfusion-related nursing diagnosis will be developed further. In a true clinical situation, however, other clusters would be developed based on primary critical cues from the collected data. If data are insufficient, you should collect additional data to confirm or refute your hypotheses.

Based on Sue's available data, these additional nursing diagnoses also pertain to her case:

- *Infection:* related to abdominal irritation as evidenced by elevated white blood cell (WBC) count
- *High risk for altered tissue perfusion:* Renal, related to decreased circulating blood volume
- *Alterated nutrition:* Less than body requirements related to increased metabolic rate
- *Acute pain:* related to abdominal irritation
- *High risk for disturbance in self-concept, role performance, and body image:* related to surgical incision, loss of pregnancy, and potential loss of reproductive abilities

Sue's fluid volume deficit is related to hemorrhage. Severe dehydration also may produce a fluid volume deficit. Sue's treatment goals will focus on stopping the source of her bleeding, restoring vascular volume, and optimizing perfusion. These general goals are reflected in the nursing diagnoses and ex-

pected patient outcomes. For example, restoring vascular volume is addressed in the nursing diagnosis *fluid volume deficit*. Accomplishment of this goal is measured in such criteria as systolic blood pressure greater than 90 mm Hg, heart rate between 60 and 100 bpm, and urine output of at least 30 mL/hr.

Development of the Plan of Care

Nursing interventions are based on activities that will achieve expected patient outcomes. They consist of collaborative interventions that are both multidisciplinary and interdisciplinary. Independent interventions are activities that are within the scope of nursing practice and do not require a physician's order.

COLLABORATIVE INTERVENTIONS RELATED TO CIRCULATORY STATUS. The physician's orders include the following:

1. **Volume replacement.** Crystalloids or colloids may be used to expand the vascular volume. Usually, lactated Ringer's solution is used initially because it contains potassium and calcium as well as lactate. Lactate is converted to bicarbonate to provide additional compensation for acidosis, which is encountered commonly in shock states. Packed red blood cells will be administered once the typing and crossmatching are performed. Whole blood is rarely given because the aim of the transfusion is to increase oxygen delivery to the tissue and not merely to increase circulating blood volume. Albumin and plasma may be administered in situations in which the fluid volume deficit is related to fluid shifting from the vascular space into the interstitial space.

2. **Vasopressor therapy.** Vasopressors may be ordered to increase venous return and, ultimately, CO. Vasopressors are administered after adequate fluid volume has been restored. The most commonly used vasopressor in hypovolemic shock states is norepinephrine. The major problem associated with the use of vasoconstrictors is decreased renal perfusion because the renal arterioles are already vasoconstricted as a result of sympathetic stimulation.

3. **Oxygen.** Oxygen is administered to ensure oxygen delivery to tissues. High-flow oxygen is preferred in hypovolemic states. A nonrebreather mask connected to 10 liters of oxygen promotes hemoglobin saturation and prevents respiratory acidosis. Because Sue's condition has not improved, the physician probably will change the route and amount of oxygen she is receiving.

4. **Hemodynamic monitoring.** A pulmonary arterial catheter (PAC) is inserted to evaluate and monitor CO and preload. This will also provide another access route for IV fluid replacement and blood specimen removal as well as pressure monitoring.

5. **Laboratory and x-ray testing.** Serial Hgb and Hct levels are obtained to monitor the degree of hemorrhage. A chest x-ray is obtained to evaluate Sue's baseline pulmonary status and to confirm proper PAC placement. A lactate level is obtained to monitor cellular oxygenation.

INDEPENDENT NURSING INTERVENTIONS

1. Elevate Sue's legs to promote venous drainage from the legs.
2. Facilitate and maintain a position of comfort to decrease Sue's pain and anxiety and thus oxygen requirements.
3. Maintain accurate intake and output records.
4. Keep Sue NPO in anticipation of surgery.

5. Monitor vital signs continuously.
6. Monitor the effects of drug therapy and fluid replacement.
7. Monitor test results (report abnormal results).
8. Keep the patient and husband informed about the plan of care.
9. Assess for decreased perfusion (report abnormal results):
   - Systolic blood pressure less than 90 mm Hg
   - Narrowing of pulse pressure
   - Respirations less than 8 or greater than 30/min
   - Presence of bradycardia, tachycardia, or premature beats
   - Change in responsiveness
   - Urine output less than 30 mL/hr
   - Flat neck veins

Plan Evaluation and Revision

Sue's perfusion plan of care is now developed and ready to be executed. Her progress is monitored at regular intervals to evaluate the effects of the various therapeutic actions. If Sue's desired patient outcomes are not met, her plan will be revised to include alternative interventions that may be more effective.

Sue's condition worsens. Her systolic blood pressure is 66 mm Hg. She is unresponsive. You call for the physician and adjust her IV fluids to a wide open rate. The blood from the blood bank arrives. Dr. P decides to insert a peripheral artery catheter. You assist her while another nurse hangs the blood through the peripheral IV line.

Nursing Care of a Patient Requiring Hemodynamic Monitoring

The goals and outcome criteria that are appropriate to the management of Sue while she is being hemodynamically monitored can be divided into two major groupings: support of her physiologic needs and support of her psychosocial needs.

SUPPORT OF PHYSIOLOGIC NEEDS. Sue's physiologic needs are met through nursing interventions that promote adequate fluid volume and distribution, and prevent infection and other hemodynamic monitoring complications. Sue's nursing management is planned around interventions to attain these goals. These goals are addressed through the nursing diagnoses of *decreased cardiac output, fluid volume deficit, altered tissue perfusion: peripheral, risk for infection,* and *risk for injury.*

A pulmonary arterial catheter is inserted. Initial readings are RAP 2 mm Hg, pulmonary artery pressure (PAP) 17/6 mm Hg, and pulmonary artery wedge pressure (PAWP) 3 mm Hg. These readings are low, indicating a fluid volume deficit. Her CO is 3.2 L/min. The mean arterial pressure is 65 mm Hg. Her systemic vascular resistance (SVR) is 1,575 dynes · sec · cm^{-5}, indicating vasoconstriction as the sympathetic nervous system compensates for the low venous return. Sue's cardiac index (CI) is 1.7 L/m^2. Her left ventricular stroke work index (LVSWI) is 11.3 g/m^2. The low PAWP and low LVSWI indicate hypovolemia.

Decreased Cardiac Output

Sue's CO, CI, and SVR measurements provide information about the response to fluid and medication administration. Sue's SVR reading indicates the degree to which her sympathetic nervous system is trying to compen-

sate for the low stroke volume. Her heart rate and pattern are assessed to determine her hemodynamic response to changes in fluid volume. Dysrhythmias and tachycardia further diminish CO. Improvement in Sue's level of responsiveness indicates improvement in her CO. Her urine output provides another parameter for monitoring CO because 20 percent of the CO goes to the kidneys.

Fluid Volume Deficit

Sue's preload is monitored to determine her response to volume replacement. The impact of inotropes and vasopressors on preload are examined by comparing RAP and PAWP measurements before and after these interventions. Hemoglobin and hematocrit values provide information regarding how much volume has been lost. She is at risk for exsanguination if the hemodynamic monitoring tubing becomes disconnected or a stopcock is left open. To prevent this from occurring, keep all catheter connecting sites visible and reassess their security frequently. Keep monitor alarms on to detect changes in blood pressure.

Altered Tissue Perfusion: Peripheral

Sue has a fluid volume deficit; therefore, her tissue perfusion is compromised. Assess capillary refill, distal pulses, and skin temperature frequently. She also has a peripheral artery catheter in place and she is at risk for further compromise in her peripheral perfusion if a thrombus or thrombophlebitis develops. The insertion site is examined at least every 8 hours for tenderness, redness, and skin temperature. A loss in arterial pulsation distal to the placement of the catheter indicates arterial insufficiency related to thrombus formation.

Risk for Infection

The catheter dressing, tubing, stopcocks, and transducer are changed according to institution protocol. Aseptic technique is used when obtaining blood specimens and flushing the catheter. Ports are cleansed of all blood after obtaining samples. Sue's WBC count is monitored for further increases. Her temperature is evaluated. If an infection is suspected related to the PAC, cultures will be obtained from Sue's blood and the catheter.

Risk for Injury

If the pulmonary artery catheter tip falls into the right ventricle, Sue may experience life-threatening dysrhythmias. If you notice a right ventricular waveform pattern, the physician is notified. The PAC balloon is inflated either by the physician or nurse (depending on hospital policy). This allows the catheter to float back into the pulmonary artery. If Sue has hemoptysis and abnormal arterial blood gases (ABGs) and respirations, she may be experiencing a pulmonary infarction from permanent wedging of the balloon or lodging of the deflated balloon in the pulmonary capillary bed. Open the stopcock on the pulmonary artery balloon port and remove the syringe to allow for passive deflation of the balloon.

SUPPORT OF PSYCHOSOCIAL NEEDS. Support of Sue's psychosocial needs center around interventions that reduce anxiety and promote a balance between sleep and activity.

Anxiety Related to Equipment

Sue went from having one pattern monitored, her cardiac rhythm, to having three patterns monitored: cardiac rhythm, PAP, and arterial pressure. Family members may become alarmed when they notice the oscilloscope at the patient's bedside. Most individuals are accustomed to peripheral IV lines, but insertion of a catheter into the neck may be a foreign concept. Sue was unresponsive at the time the catheter was inserted. When she becomes responsive, the nurse needs to explain the purpose of the catheters and warn Sue not to touch any of the tubing or connections.

The operating suite is ready for Sue. Her hemodynamic lines are secured. Blood and lactated Ringer's are infusing through her PAC. She is still receiving 10 liters of oxygen through a nonrebreather mask. Sue remains in sinus tachycardia. The report is given to the operating room nurse. Sue's husband is escorted to the surgical waiting area.

Case Study 2

MRS. G., A PATIENT EXPERIENCING FLUID VOLUME EXCESS

You are the nurse assigned to care for Mrs. G. Mrs. G. was admitted to the telemetry floor with a diagnosis of angina: Rule out myocardial infarction. She was admitted through the emergency department 16 hours ago.

Initial Appraisal

On walking into the room, you note the following.

GENERAL APPEARANCE. Mrs. G. is a Hispanic female of moderate stature. She is overweight and tidy in appearance.

SIGNS OF DISTRESS. Mrs. G. is diaphoretic. Her respirations are fast and shallow. She is sitting upright in bed.

OTHER. You note that she is receiving oxygen by nasal cannula. An IV solution of D5W is infusing.

Focused Respiratory and Circulatory Assessment

Because Mrs. G. appears to be in acute distress, you immediately perform a rapid assessment, focusing on her cardiopulmonary status. The results are as follows.

Mrs. G. is restless but oriented to person, place, time, and reason for hospitalization. Her respiratory rate is 28/min, shallow and regular. On auscultation of her chest, you note bilateral crackles in the lower lung fields, left greater than right. S1 and S2 are present. No murmurs are noted, but an S3 is auscultated. Her blood pressure is 156/106 mm Hg, and her pulse is 104 bpm. She is complaining of chest pain, sharp in nature, that is radiating down her left arm. She is in the cardiac rhythm shown in Figure 13–2.

QUESTION

The pattern in Figure 13–2 is

- **A.** atrial flutter
- **B.** complete heart block
- **C.** atrial fibrillation
- **D.** artifact

ANSWER

The correct answer is C. *P* waves are not distinguishable. The R–R interval is irregular.

Following this initial assessment, you check her admission orders. Mrs. G has the following medications ordered.

- Nitroglycerin grain 1/150 SL PRN chest pain
- Morphine sulfate 4 mg IVP PRN q 2 to 3 hrs for chest pain

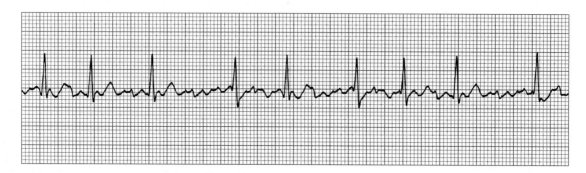

Figure 13–2 ■ Mrs. G.'s current cardiac monitor rhythm strip.

QUESTION

What effect will these medications have on Mrs. G.'s perfusion status?

ANSWER

All the medications will help improve Mrs. G.'s CO. Nitroglycerin is a fast-acting drug that produces peripheral vasodilation, thus redistributing blood away from the congested pulmonary bed. Nitroglycerin also increases collateral circulation to the myocardium. The vasodilation should decrease her pain. Morphine decreases preload by producing peripheral vasodilation. It decreases anxiety, which increases myocardial oxygen consumption. Morphine also relaxes airway smooth muscle, so it may decrease Mrs. G.'s respiratory rate by improving gas exchange.

You administer both of the medications and place a call to her cardiologist. In the interim, Mrs. G.'s morning laboratory results come back.

Electrolytes

Sodium (Na) = 142 mEq/L	(normal range 136 to 146 mEq/L)
Potassium (K) = 3.5 mEq/L	(normal range 3.5 to 5.5 mEq/L)
Chloride (Cl) = 104 mEq/L	(normal range 96 to 106 mEq/L)
Calcium (Ca) = 9.0 mg/dL	(normal range 8.5 to 10.5 mg/dL)

Cardiac Enzymes

Creatinine phosphokinase–myocardial bands (CK-MB) = 3 percent
   (normal range 0 to 3 percent)
Troponin I = 1.0   (normal range less than 3.1)

QUESTION

What is the significance of these laboratory results?

ANSWER

Mrs. G.'s electrolyte values are within normal limits. Thus, she is not predisposed to cardiac dysrhythmias resulting from electrolyte disturbances. However, her potassium level is borderline low. You need to check her chart to see if she has been taking diuretics at home. If digitalis is prescribed because of her beginning pulmonary edema (as suspected based on the presence of crackles on pulmonary auscultation), Mrs. G. may be predisposed to digitalis toxicity. However, angiotensin-converting enzyme (ACE) inhibitors will be prescribed in most cases before digitalis.

The normal cardiac enzyme and marker levels indicate that Mrs. G. has not had a myocardial infarction. When the heart muscle is damaged, enzymes are released. CK-MB is the isoenzyme associated with damage to cardiac muscle. CK-MB levels begin to rise 4 to 8 hours postinfarction. It does not rise during angina. Troponin I levels begin to increase 2 to 4 hours after myocardial ischemia occurs, peak at 24 to 36 hours, and remain elevated for 7 to 10 days. Detection of cardiac troponin I in serum is very specific for myocardial injury because this protein is found only in myocardial cells.

Mrs. G.'s pain has not decreased. She is complaining of shortness of breath. Her blood pressure has decreased to 114/72 mm Hg. Her heart rate is 92 bpm. Respirations remain at 28/min. Her daughter arrives in the room to see you administering a second nitroglycerin tablet to her mother.

Focused Nursing History

Because Mrs. G. is still experiencing pain, you decide to speak with her daughter to obtain important critical historical data that may have an impact on Mrs. G.'s present situation. Her daughter gives the following history.

Mrs. G. started to experience chest pain the morning of her admission after she moved a piece of bedroom furniture. She has complained of "heartburn" after eating heavy meals for the past 6 months. The pain yesterday would not go away after Mrs. G. rested. She called her daughter, who drove over to Mrs. G.'s house and convinced Mrs. G. to go to the hospital. Mrs. G. is not allergic to any medicine. She has a history of smoking one pack of cigarettes a day for 40 years. She is 60 years old and has a history of hypertension. She takes Lasix 10 mg orally daily for her hypertension. She does not take potassium supplements, but her daughter states that Mrs. G. eats many bananas.

Even though most of this information should already be recorded in Mrs. G.'s chart, you have not had time to read her chart. This information was important to obtain and will help you as you perform your systematic assessment.

The Systematic Bedside Assessment

HEAD AND NECK. Mrs. G. has an olive complexion. Perspiration is noted on her forehead. She remains oriented and alert. Oxygen is infusing through her nasal cannula at 2 L/min. She is in a semi-Fowler's position at 30 degrees. Her jugular veins are full but not distended.

CHEST

Pulmonary status. Her crackles have increased since your initial assessment. Crackles in her right and left lung fields are equal in intensity. Respirations are 26/min.

Cardiac status. It is more difficult to hear her heart sounds because of the crackles. However, S1, S2, and S3 are still audible. Her apical heart rate is irregular without a distinctive pattern. Her blood pressure is 92/70 mm Hg.

ABDOMEN. Her abdomen is soft and obese. Hypoactive bowel sounds are auscultated. No pain is elicited on palpation. Liver borders are nonpalpable.

PELVIS. Mrs. G. voided 100 mL in the past hour. Her urine is yellow and clear.

EXTREMITIES. She has bilateral nonpitting pedal edema. Pedal pulses are faint (+1) but palpable. Capillary refill is 2 seconds in all extremities. Her skin is damp from perspiration.

POSTERIOR. No sacral edema is noted. Posterior breath sounds reveal bilateral coarse crackles in the lower to midlung fields.

Development of Nursing Diagnoses

Clustering Data

You are now ready to develop nursing diagnoses based on the available subjective and objective data. To cluster your data, look for abnormal values discovered during the assessment. Mrs. G.'s major symptoms at this time are chest pain, decreasing blood pressure, and increasing pulmonary crackles. Thus, these primary symptoms can initiate your first cluster of critical cues.

Cluster 1

Subjective data. The patient is complaining of increasing chest pain not relieved with nitroglycerin SL × two or morphine sulfate 4 mg IVP. She also is complaining of shortness of breath despite oxygen administration at 2 liters per nasal cannula. She has a previous history of hypertension and heartburn.

Objective data. Mrs. G. is diaphoretic with full neck veins, bilateral pedal edema. Crackles are auscultated in the bilateral posterior lung fields. S3 is auscultated. Atrial fibrillation with rapid ventricular response is noted. On admission, cardiac enzymes were normal.

QUESTION

Based on the preceding data, which of the following nursing diagnoses is the priority diagnosis at this time for Mrs. G.?

- **A.** decreased cardiac output
- **B.** impaired gas exchange
- **C.** altered tissue perfusion: peripheral
- **D.** fluid volume excess

ANSWER

The correct answer is D. Although you might expect a decreased CO to be present, you lack data to confirm this diagnosis because Mrs. G. is still voiding an appropriate amount and she remains alert. It is true that her blood pressure has decreased, but it may be decreased as a normal response to the vasodilating medications. Arterial blood gases (ABGs) have not been obtained, so *impaired gas exchange* cannot be supported. However, if Mrs. G.'s tachypnea continues and her crackles continue to increase, impaired gas exchange probably will occur. *Altered peripheral tissue perfusion* cannot be supported adequately because even though her pedal pulses are faint (+1), they are present, and capillary refill is normal. *Fluid volume excess* is the most plausible diagnosis because of her increasing crackles and shortness of breath. She is also in atrial fibrillation, a pattern commonly associated with heart failure. Mrs. G.'s admission diagnosis of angina and her history of hypertension suggests that she is susceptible to heart failure. Several factors contribute to fluid overload: increased fluid intake, decreased fluid elimination, or altered fluid distribution. Mrs. G.'s fluid volume overload is related to altered distribution. The volume has remained unchanged. Her left ventricle has decreased contractility as a result of distention probably related to chronic hypertension.

The physician calls, and you inform him of Mrs. G.'s present status. He orders a stat electrocardiogram (ECG), portable chest x-ray, cardiac enzymes, ABGs, and a nitroglycerin IV drip at 5 mg/min. He is coming to see Mrs. G. She will be transferred to the coronary care unit as soon as a bed is available.

When you return to Mrs. G.'s room, you notice that she is less responsive and responds to touch instead of verbal stimuli. Her daughter is crying and saying, "Momma don't die!" Mrs. G.'s cardiac rhythm in lead II has changed to that shown in Figure 13–3.

QUESTION

The pattern in Figure 13–3 indicates which of the following?

- **A.** ectopic pacemaker
- **B.** infarction
- **C.** conduction abnormality
- **D.** ischemia

ANSWER

The correct answer is D. You recognize this pattern as indicating myocardial ischemia. The *ST* segment should be isoelectric. An alteration from isoelectric occurs from delayed repolarization.

You rush to start the IV nitroglycerin. Fortunately, Mrs. G.'s vital signs have not changed. The stat ECG and portable chest x-ray are completed. A blood specimen for enzyme analysis is obtained. A respiratory therapist obtains the ABG.

The physician arrives and reads the ECG and portable chest film. Based on her history and the ECG, he determines she has had an acute anterolateral infarction. The chest x-ray reveals cardiomegaly with bilateral infiltrates, consistent with acute pulmonary edema. She is transferred immediately to the coronary care unit.

Quick Review

Mrs. G's initial symptoms demonstrated compensatory efforts to maintain CO. The changes in the ECG indicate that myocardial oxygen supply is diminished, probably because of a blockage in the coronary arteries. Mrs. G.'s pain is secondary to a decreased myocardial oxygen supply. Injured myocardial tissue cannot contract adequately, and blood remains in the left ventricle. As the left ventricle becomes stretched, contractility further decreases once the point of maximum elasticity is reached. The Frank–Starling Law addresses the limits of cardiac compensation. The heart rate initially increases

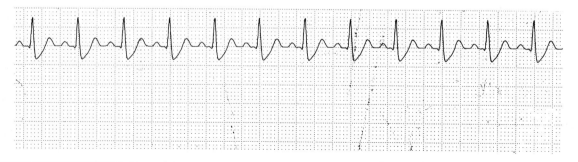

Figure 13–3 ▪ Mrs G.'s cardiac rhythm strip associated with acute changes in her clinical status.

in an effort to maintain CO. The sympathetic nervous system is stimulated, and peripheral vasoconstriction produces the symptoms of nausea and diaphoresis. Mrs. G.'s CO has now decreased, as evidenced by her decreased responsiveness.

More data are now available. Therefore, it is time to reassess nursing diagnoses appropriate for Mrs. G. Mrs. G.'s perfusion problem is complex. The perfusion problem involves a fluid volume excess related to altered fluid distribution and decreased CO related to decreased myocardial contractility.

Desired patient outcomes for Mrs. G. include

1. Absence of crackles on auscultation
2. Absence of dyspnea
3. Stable vital signs: Systolic blood pressure greater than 90 mm Hg and less than 140 mm Hg
4. Absence of S3
5. Absence of jugular venous distention
6. Absence of ascites and abdominal tenderness
7. Alert and oriented
8. Urine output greater than 30 mL/hr
9. ABGs within normal limits
10. Cardiac enzymes negative
11. Absence of chest pain

For the purposes of this case study, only the perfusion-related nursing diagnoses are further developed. However, in a true clinical situation, as the nurse creating Mrs. G.'s plan of care, you would continue to develop other clusters based on assessment data. If data are insufficient, you follow through on collecting the necessary data to confirm or refute your hypotheses.

Based on the preliminary data collected, there is sufficient support to state the following nursing diagnoses:

- *Chest pain:* related to myocardial ischemia
- *Altered tissue perfusion:* Cerebral related to decreased myocardial contractility
- *High risk for impaired gas exchange:* related to pulmonary interstitial fluid
- *High risk for anxiety:* related to impending transfer to coronary care unit
- *High risk for fear:* related to severity of illness

Treatment goals for Mrs. G. focus on increasing the blood supply to the heart, decreasing the demands placed on the heart, and improving the blood flow distribution. These general goals are reflected in the nursing diagnoses and desired patient outcomes on the nursing care plan. For example, decreasing the demands placed on the heart is addressed in the nursing diagnosis of fluid volume overload. Accomplishment of the goal is measured in such criteria as patient will be pain free.

Development of the Plan of Care

Nursing interventions are based on activities that will help meet the desired patient outcomes. They consist of collaborative interventions ordered by the physician but require nursing actions and independent interventions that the nurse implements without a physician's order.

COLLABORATIVE INTERVENTIONS RELATED TO PERFUSION STATUS. The physician's orders may include the following:

1. **Cardiovascular drug therapy.** Mrs. G. will receive several drugs while hospitalized. Thrombolytics may be ordered to dissolve a thrombus

and improve coronary artery perfusion, limit the extent of the myocardial ischemia, and improve left ventricular function. The major nursing concern associated with administering thrombolytic agents is to monitor for complications. The most frequent complications include bleeding and an allergic reaction. Reperfusion dysrhythmias may occur with lysis of the thrombus and restoration of blood flow in the coronary arteries but these are self-limiting and usually do not require treatment.

Inotropic agents, such as dobutamine and digitalis, may be administered. These agents increase myocardial contractility and improve ventricular function. A negative effect of these agents is that they increase myocardial oxygen consumption.

Vasodilators may be ordered. Frequently used IV vasodilators are nitroprusside and nitroglycerin. These drugs improve stroke volume and CO by decreasing afterload. The heart is able to eject against less resistance. Vasodilators are used cautiously in right ventricular infarctions because a decrease in preload can worsen myocardial ischemia.

QUESTION

Which of the following may be an undesirable side effect of vasodilators?
- **A.** decreased SVR
- **B.** decreased CO
- **C.** increased PAWP
- **D.** increased CVP

ANSWER

The correct answer is B. Hypotension and a further decrease in CO may occur if preload is diminished as a result of venous vasodilation.

QUESTION

A diuretic is ordered for Mrs. G to
- **A.** prevent renal failure
- **B.** increase the PAWP
- **C.** decrease vasoconstriction
- **D.** reduce preload

ANSWER

The correct answer is D. Diuretics are given to reduce preload and pulmonary venous congestion.

Loop diuretics are the preferred drug of choice in cases of heart failure. Furosemide has vasodilating and diuretic properties and, thus, has a greater potential of decreasing preload. The nurse must monitor for electrolyte abnormalities and fluid volume deficit that may occur with diuresis.

Oxygen therapy is ordered to meet cellular energy requirements.

2. **Mechanical support.** If Mrs. G.'s heart failure worsens, she may need an intra-aortic balloon pump (IABP). This device improves coronary artery perfusion by inflating during diastole and increasing the coronary artery perfusion pressure. It deflates during systole, rapidly decreasing the coronary artery pressure and ventricular ejection resistance. The nurse caring for a patient with an IABP requires special training in order to adjust balloon inflation and deflation correctly.

3. **Dietary restrictions.** Mrs. G. is placed on a sodium-restricted diet. Use of table salt and salt in food preparation is eliminated. She is placed

on fluid restriction until her fluid distribution problem is corrected. The nurse monitors Mrs. G.'s sodium level and intake and output record. Family members need to know the dietary restrictions so they do not bring food that would be detrimental to Mrs. G.'s fluid volume status.

4. **Hemodynamic monitoring.**   Mrs. G. may have a PAC placed once she is in the coronary care unit. Nursing responsibilities associated with hemodynamic monitoring are discussed Module 9. You expect Mrs. G.'s hemodynamic readings to be abnormal because of her fluid volume overload. Before initiation of drug therapy, Mrs. G.'s RAP, PAP, and PAWP measurements would be elevated because of increased volume. Her CO and CI would be decreased. Mrs. G.'s LVSWI would be decreased due to diminished contractility. Mrs. G.'s SVR would be elevated initially to try to compensate for her decreased stroke volume. However, her blood pressure has been decreasing, and a nitroglycerin IV drip was initiated. Her SVR should now be decreased. Medications will be administered and titrated to decrease her CVP, PAP, and PAWP while increasing her CO. The combination of inotropes and vasodilators can be confusing to a novice nurse because they appear to have opposite actions. However, the goal of using both of these agents is the same—improvement of CO.

5. **Laboratory and x-ray testing.**   Cardiac enzymes or markers probably are ordered every 6 to 8 hours to determine the severity of Mrs. G.'s myocardial infarction. ABGs are ordered intermittently to monitor gas exchange. Pulse oximetry is used to monitor arterial oxygen saturation. Periodic chest x-rays assist in evaluating the effects of interventions. The cardiomegaly and pulmonary infiltrates should resolve.

Independent Nursing Interventions Related to Perfusion Status

1. Assess for decreased perfusion
   - Systolic blood pressure less than 90 mm Hg
   - Heart rate less than 60 or greater than 100 beats per minute
   - Urine output less than 30 mL/hr
   - Decreased responsiveness
   - Diminished peripheral pulses
   - Capillary refill greater than 4 seconds
   - Pedal edema
   - Dysrhythmias
2. Assess for fluid overload
   - Metabolic or respiratory acidosis
   - Dyspnea

- Abnormal breath sounds
- Extra heart sounds
- Jugular venous distention
- Ascites
- Weight gain
- Abnormal electrolyte levels

3. Implement measures to reduce cardiac workload
   - Place Mrs. G. in semi-Fowler's position
   - Allow for frequent rest periods
   - Monitor intake and output
   - Monitor for side effects of drug therapy
   - Maintain oxygen therapy
   - Administer pain medication as ordered and use imagery and other diversional activities
   - Decrease patient anxiety
     A. Refer to support services as necessary (e.g., chaplain, social services)
     B. Assist patient with identifying coping behaviors
     C. Explain procedures, environment, and equipment to degree of patient satisfaction

Plan Evaluation and Revision

Mrs. G.'s plan of care is now ready to be executed. Her progress is monitored at regular intervals to evaluate the effects of various therapeutic actions. If desired patient outcomes are not achieved, Mrs. G.'s plan of care is revised.

Summary

This module addressed the nursing care of patients who are experiencing alterations in perfusion. Concepts from the perfusion-related modules (Modules 8 to 12) have been applied in a case study approach. It is impossible to address specifically each perfusion problem a nurse may encounter in the clinical setting. However, these problems can be managed by applying basic principles. These principles can be classified into conditions of fluid volume excess and fluid volume deficit. Two case studies were used to illustrate nursing care responsibilities with these conditions. Review questions were integrated throughout the case study to encourage application of material in other modules and assimilation of content within this module. Nursing interventions for a patient being hemodynamically monitored were addressed specifically because this intervention is used for patients experiencing both fluid overload and fluid deficit.

PART

4

Oxygenation

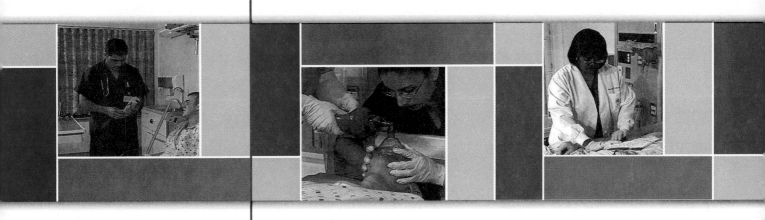

MODULE 14	Oxygenation
MODULE 15	Shock States
MODULE 16	Multiple Organ Dysfunction Syndrome
MODULE 17	Nursing Care of the Patient with Impaired Oxygenation

Determinants and Assessment of Oxygenation

Karen L. Johnson

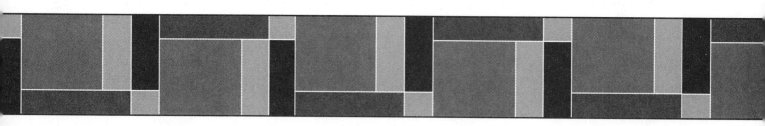

OBJECTIVES Following completion of this module, the learner will be able to

1. Explain the concept of oxygenation.
2. Discuss pulmonary gas exchange.
3. Describe the physiologic components of oxygen delivery.
4. Describe oxygen consumption in terms of aerobic and anaerobic metabolism.
5. Define pathophysiologic conditions that result in impaired oxygenation.
6. Identify techniques to assess oxygenation status in relation to pulmonary gas exchange, oxygen delivery, and oxygen consumption.

This self-study module focuses on the physiologic as well as the pathophysiologic processes involved in oxygenation. The module is composed of six sections. Section One considers the underlying general principles involved in the oxygenation process. Sections Two through Four review the processes of pulmonary gas exchange, oxygen delivery, and oxygen consumption. In Section Five, definitions of clinical conditions that occur as a result of impaired oxygenation are given. Section Six reviews oxygenation assessment techniques. Each section includes a set of review questions to help the learner evaluate his or her understanding of the section's content before moving on to the next section. All Section Reviews and the module Pretest and Posttest include answers. It is suggested that the learner review those concepts answered incorrectly in the review questions before proceeding to the next section.

 PRETEST

1. Oxygenation is
   A. a concept that involves multisystem coordination of the intake, delivery, and use of oxygen for energy
   B. a process that occurs in the lungs
   C. a process that involves the transportation of oxygen to cells
   D. a process that depends on ventilation, diffusion, and perfusion

2. Gas exchange depends on
   A. ventilation and diffusion
   B. ventilation, diffusion, and perfusion
   C. oxygen content in the alveoli
   D. oxygen diffusion across alveolar–capillary membranes

3. Oxygen delivery is affected by
   A. hemoglobin and the oxygen content of arterial blood
   B. cardiac output, autoregulation, and the oxygen content of arterial blood
   C. cardiac output, autoregulation, and autonomic nervous system input
   D. cardiac output, autoregulation, autonomic nervous system input, and oxygen content of arterial blood

4. Ninety-seven percent of oxygen carried to tissues is
   A. dissolved in the plasma
   B. carried as oxyhemoglobin
   C. unavailable for cellular use
   D. delivered to cells by the heart

5. The most effective mechanism of oxygen consumption occurs by
   A. aerobic metabolism
   B. anaerobic metabolism
   C. producing two ATP molecules, lactate and pyruvate
   D. oxygen extraction
6. Completion of a nursing assessment would have what impact on oxygen consumption?
   A. none
   B. increase consumption by 10 percent
   C. increase consumption by 20 percent
   D. increase consumption by 30 percent
7. Impaired oxygenation can result in
   A. hypoxemia and hypoxia
   B. hypoxemia, hypoxia, and dysoxia
   C. hypoxemia, hypoxia, dysoxia, and shock states
   D. hypoxemia, hypoxia, dysoxia, shock states, and multiple organ dysfunction
8. Hypoxemia is defined as
   A. PaO_2 <50 mm Hg
   B. $PaCO_2$ >50 mm Hg

C. inadequate amount of oxygen in arterial blood
   D. hemoglobin < 10 mg/dL
9. Clinical assessment of oxygenation includes assessment of
   A. arterial blood gases
   B. the cardiovascular and pulmonary systems
   C. pulmonary gas exchange and oxygen delivery
   D. pulmonary gas exchange, oxygen delivery, and oxygen consumption
10. An indirect assessment of oxygen consumption is made using
   A. mixed venous oxygen saturation
   B. arterial blood gases
   C. serum hemoglobin levels
   D. serum adenosine triphosphate levels

Pretest Answers: 1. A, 2. B, 3. D, 4. B, 5. A, 6. B, 7. D, 8. C, 9. D, 10. A

GLOSSARY

aerobic metabolism   The mechanism used by the body for energy generation in the presence of oxygen.

affinity   The degree to which hemoglobin releases oxygen.

anaerobic metabolism   The mechanism used by the body for energy generation in the absence of oxygen.

autoregulation   Mechanism used by tissues to regulate their own blood supply by dilating or constricting local blood vessels.

cardiac output (CO)   The amount of blood pumped by the ventricles each minute.

diffusion   Movement of gases across a pressure gradient from an area of high concentration to one of low concentration.

dysoxia   Condition characterized by an inability of the cells to use oxygen properly despite adequate levels of oxygen delivery.

hypoxemia   Condition characterized by an inadequate amount of oxygen in the blood as a result of impaired gas exchange, frequently quantified as a PaO_2 of < 50 mm Hg.

hypoxia   An inadequate amount of oxygen available at the cellular level.

oxygen consumption (VO_2)   The amount of oxygen used by cells.

oxygen delivery (DO_2)   The process of transportation of oxygen to cells, dependent on cardiac output, hemoglobin saturation with oxygen, and the partial pressure of oxygen in arterial blood.

oxygen extraction   The process by which cells take oxygen from the blood.

pulmonary gas exchange   The process that involves the intake of oxygen from the external environment into the internal environment and is carried out by ventilation, diffusion, and perfusion.

ventilation   The mechanical movement of air to and from the atmosphere and the alveoli.

ABBREVIATIONS

ABG	Arterial blood gas	**CaO₂**	Oxygen content of arterial blood
ARDS	Acute respiratory distress syndrome	**CvO₂**	Oxygen content of venous blood
ATP	Adenosine triphosphate	**2, 3 DPG**	Diphosphoglycerate
AV̇	Alveolar ventilation	**DO₂**	Oxygen delivery
CO	Cardiac output	**FIO₂**	Fraction of inspired oxygen
CO₂	Carbon dioxide	**H₂O**	Water

Hb	Hemoglobin		Qs/Qt	Intrapulmonary shunt
HbO_2	Oxyhemoglobin		RR	Respiratory rate
MODS	Multiple organ dysfunction syndrome		Sao_2	Oxygen saturation of arterial blood
$M\dot{V}$	Minute ventilation		$S\dot{v}o_2$	Oxygen saturation of mixed venous blood
O_2	Oxygen		V_T	Tidal volume
Pao_2	The amount of oxygen physically dissolved in arterial blood, unattached to hemoglobin		VC	Vital capacity
Pao_2	The partial pressure of alveolar oxygen		VO_2	Oxygen consumption
Pvo_2	The amount of oxygen physically dissolved in venous blood			

SECTION ONE: Oxygenation

At the completion of this section, the learner will be able to explain the concept of oxygenation.

Oxygenation is a concept of multisystem integration and coordination in the intake, delivery, and use of oxygen for energy metabolism. Oxygenation cannot be understood solely by understanding the pulmonary system or the cardiovascular system. Oxygenation involves the integration and coordination of pulmonary, cardiovascular, neurologic, hematologic, and metabolic processes.

Unlike the heart, which has intrinsic rhythmic properties to work independently, the respiratory system requires continuous input from the nervous system. Depending on various internal and external stimuli, the nervous system regulates the respiratory system to meet identified body needs for oxygen. Oxygen is brought into the internal environment via the respiratory system during the process of ventilation. Oxygen crosses alveolar–capillary membranes by diffusion, combines with hemoglobin, and is transported via the pulmonary vein to the left side of the heart. The heart pumps oxygenated blood into the vascular system where it is transported to cells. Oxygenated blood then leaves the capillaries by diffusion and enters cells. Depending on cellular energy requirements, each cell extracts the amount of oxygen it needs to fulfill its metabolic requirements. Cells use oxygen to convert food substrates into energy. Carbon dioxide and "unused" oxygen are carried to the right side of the heart and back to the lungs for elimination and reuse.

The concept of oxygenation involves three physiologic components for the intake, delivery, and use of oxygen for energy: pulmonary gas exchange, oxygen delivery, and oxygen consumption, as summarized in Figure 14–1. Adequacy of oxygenation depends on the integration of these physiologic

Figure 14–1 ■ Johnson's conceptual model of oxygenation depicts oxygenation as a process involving the intake, delivery, and use of oxygen for energy metabolism. (*Adapted, with permission, from Taylor, C.R., & Weibel, E.R. [1981]. Design of the mammalion respiratory system, Respiration Physiology, 41 [p. 2]. Copyright © 1981 by Elsevier Science.*)

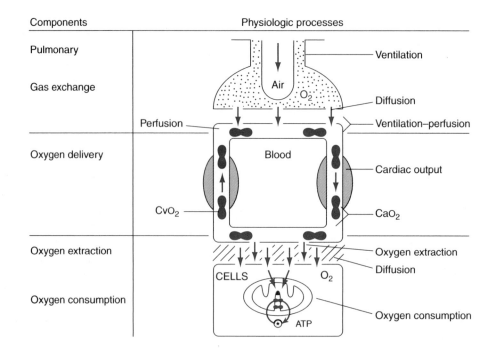

components. **Pulmonary gas exchange** involves the intake of oxygen from the external environment into the internal environment and is carried out by the processes of ventilation, diffusion, and perfusion. Oxygen delivery (DO_2) is the process of transportation of oxygen to cells and is dependent on cardiac output (CO), hemoglobin saturation with oxygen, and the partial pressure of oxygen in arterial blood (PaO_2). Oxygen consumption (VO_2) involves the use of oxygen at the cellular level to generate energy for cells to use to perform their specific functions. Impaired oxygenation can result from impaired pulmonary gas exchange, decreased oxygen delivery, or impaired oxygen consumption.

In summary, the concept of oxygenation requires an understanding that the intake, delivery, and use of oxygen for energy involves multisystem integration and coordination involving three physiologic components: pulmonary gas exchange, oxygen delivery, and oxygen consumption. Adequacy of oxygenation depends on these three components. Any disease or condition that affects these processes will affect oxygenation.

SECTION ONE REVIEW

1. Oxygenation is
   A. a process that occurs in the pulmonary system
   B. a process that involves ventilation, diffusion, and perfusion
   C. a process that involves the transportation of oxygen to cells
   D. a concept that specifies that the intake, delivery, and use of oxygen requires multisystem integration and coordination

2. Which of the following are the physiologic processes involved with oxygenation?
   A. pulmonary gas exchange, oxygen delivery, and oxygen consumption
   B. diffusion, ventilation, and perfusion
   C. cardiac output and hemoglobin saturation with oxygen
   D. the pulmonary and cardiovascular systems

3. Pulmonary gas exchange is carried out by which of the following?
   A. inspiration of oxygen by the process of ventilation
   B. expiration of carbon dioxide by the process of diffusion
   C. ventilation, diffusion, and perfusion
   D. ventilation, oxygen consumption, and perfusion

4. Oxygen consumption
   A. depends on cardiac output and hemoglobin saturation with oxygen
   B. involves the use of oxygen to generate energy
   C. involves the intake of oxygen from the external environment
   D. is the process of transporting oxygen to cells

Answers: 1. D, 2. A, 3. C, 4. B

SECTION TWO: Pulmonary Gas Exchange

At the completion of this section, the learner will be able to discuss pulmonary gas exchange. For more detailed information, please refer to Module 4, "Determinants and Assessment of Pulmonary Gas Exchange." An understanding of FIO_2, PAO_2, PaO_2, and PvO_2 is necessary to understand this section.

The initial component of oxygenation involves pulmonary gas exchange. Pulmonary gas exchange involves the inspiration and delivery of oxygen from the external environment to the alveoli and diffusion across the alveolar–capillary membrane, where oxygen combines with hemoglobin in the pulmonary capillaries. Adequate blood flow must exist to "carry away" the oxygenated blood to the left side of the heart and the systemic circulation. These functions are carried out by physiologic processes involving ventilation, diffusion, and perfusion (Fig. 14–2).

Ventilation is the movement of air to and from the atmosphere and the alveoli. It involves the actual work of breathing and requires adequate functioning of the ventilatory muscles, thorax, lungs, conducting airways, and nervous system. Decreased functioning of any one of these systems can affect ventilation and impair oxygenation.

Diffusion is the movement of gas across a pressure gradient from an area of high concentration to one of low concentration. Diffusion is the mechanism by which oxygen moves across the alveoli and into the pulmonary capillary. There are three factors that affect diffusion across the alveolar–capillary membrane: pressure gradient, surface area, and thickness. The greater the difference between alveolar oxygen and pulmonary capillary oxygen pressures, the greater the diffusion of oxygen from the alveoli to the pulmonary capillaries. The greater the available alveolar–capillary membrane surface area, the greater the amount of oxygen that can diffuse across it. Many conditions can cause a significant reduction in functional surface area. The thickness of the alveolar–capillary membrane affects diffusion of oxygen from the alveoli to the pulmonary capillary. Conditions that increase the thickness of the alveolar–capillary membrane can decrease diffusion.

Figure 14–2 ■ Initial process of oxygenation: pulmonary gas exchange.

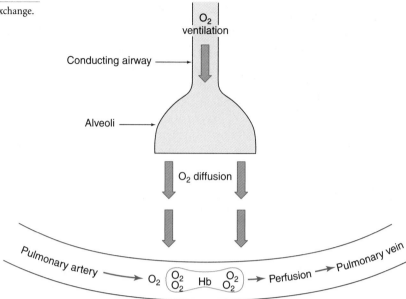

The third component of gas exchange involves perfusion. Three factors affect perfusion: hemoglobin (Hb) concentration, affinity of oxygen to Hb, and blood flow. When oxygen diffuses across the alveolar–capillary membrane, it combines with hemoglobin in the pulmonary capillary and is carried to the left side of the heart. Certain factors affect the affinity of oxygen to hemoglobin, including body temperature, acid–base balance, 2, 3 diphosphoglycerate (2, 3 DPG), and CO_2. Refer to Module 5 for factors that affect the oxyhemoglobin dissociation curve. Perfusion of alveoli has an effect on oxygenation. A decrease in blood flow through the pulmonary vasculature results in an imbalance between ventilation and perfusion. Any disease or condition that impairs pulmonary perfusion impairs pulmonary gas exchange. Some conditions and diseases that affect oxygenation as a result of impaired gas exchange are summarized in Table 14–1.

In summary, the initial component of oxygenation is pulmonary gas exchange. Gas exchange depends on three processes: ventilation, diffusion, and perfusion. Any disease or condition that affects gas exchange can impair oxygenation.

TABLE 14–1 Conditions That Impair Pulmonary Gas Exchange

Ventilation Impairment

Inspiratory muscle weakness or trauma (Guillian-Barré, spinal cord injury)

Decreased level of consciousness

Obstruction or trauma to airways, lung, thorax (flail chest, mucous plug)

Restrictive pulmonary disorders

Diffusion Impairment

Decrease in alveolar–capillary membrane surface area (atelectasis, lung tumors, pneumonia)

Increase in alveolar–capillary membrane thickness (acute respiratory distress syndrome, pulmonary edema, pneumonia)

Decreased pressure gradient for oxygen ($\downarrow$ Fio_2)

Perfusion Impairment

Decreased Hb (anemia, carbon monoxide poisoning)

Decreased perfusion ($\downarrow$ cardiac output, hemorrhage, pulmonary embolism)

Pulmonary vasoconstriction (pulmonary hypertension, hypoxemia)

SECTION TWO REVIEW

1. Which of the following conditions has an effect on ventilation?
   A. low hemoglobin levels
   B. upper airway obstruction
   C. pulmonary embolism
   D. hypovolemic shock

2. A Pao_2 of 100 mm Hg and a pulmonary Pao_2 of 40 mm Hg would
   A. facilitate diffusion
   B. decrease diffusion
   C. decrease ventilation
   D. facilitate perfusion

3. Atelectasis results in a decrease in functional alveolar–capillary membrane surface area. This results in a(n)
   A. increased alveolar–capillary pressure gradient
   B. decreased alveolar–capillary pressure gradient
   C. decrease in oxygen diffusion across alveolar–capillary membranes
   D. increase in oxygen diffusion across alveolar–capillary membranes
4. Anemia affects which component of the gas exchange process?
   A. ventilation
   B. diffusion

C. $P_{A}O_{2}$
D. perfusion
5. Impaired gas exchange results in
   A. oxygenation impairment
   B. ventilation impairment
   C. diffusion impairment
   D. perfusion impairment

Answers: 1. B, 2. A, 3. C, 4. D, 5. A

SECTION THREE: Oxygen Delivery

At the completion of this section, the learner will be able to describe the physiologic components of oxygen delivery.

The second component of oxygenation is oxygen delivery. **Oxygen delivery** involves the process of transporting oxygen to cells. The amount of oxygen delivered to tissues is approximately 1,000 mL/min. (When indexed to consider body surface area, oxygen delivery is approximately 600 mL/min/m^2.) Factors that affect oxygen delivery include cardiac output (CO), autoregulation, oxygen content of arterial blood (CaO_2), and autonomic nervous system innervation.

Cardiac output (CO) is the amount of blood pumped by the heart each minute (see Module 8). The greater the cardiac output, the greater the amount of oxygen delivered to the tissues per minute. Conversely, conditions that cause a decrease in cardiac output result in a decrease in the amount of oxygen delivered to tissues per minute.

Under normal circumstances, the volume of oxygenated blood pumped by the heart is proportional to the body's demands. When tissues require more oxygen, heart rate will increase in an attempt to augment cardiac output in the delivery of more oxygenated blood. Tissues have the ability to regulate their own blood supply by dilating or constricting local blood vessels through the mechanism of **autoregulation.** Tissues have varying energy requirements and use autoregulation to meet their metabolic demands. When the body is at rest, not all tissue capillaries are open at the same time. Increased metabolic rate (e.g., during exercise) and arterial hypoxemia (decreased PaO_2) open more tissue capillaries, thereby allowing more oxygen to be extracted by tissue beds. Autoregulation serves to protect tissues by controlling blood flow and oxygen delivery in response to individual tissue needs.

Oxygen is carried in arterial blood in two forms: It can be combined with hemoglobin or it can be dissolved in the plasma. The content of oxygen in arterial blood (CaO_2) depends on the amount of Hb available to carry oxygen, the amount of oxygen

carried in the blood in the "nondissolved" form (PaO_2), and the saturation of hemoglobin with oxygen (SaO_2). Normal CaO_2 is 20 mL/100 mL of blood. Almost 97 percent of all oxygen delivered to cells is in the form of oxyhemoglobin (HbO_2), and the remaining 3 percent is delivered partially dissolved in plasma.

Each molecule of hemoglobin has the ability to carry four oxygen molecules. When hemoglobin is fully saturated with oxygen, oxyhemoglobin is formed. Each hemoglobin molecule can be thought of as a bus that carries four oxygen passengers to tissues. The measurement of SaO_2 by arterial blood gas (ABG) analysis is a measurement of the ratio of oxygenated hemoglobin to total hemoglobin (see Module 5). For example, if the SaO_2 is 95 percent, it can be interpreted that 95 percent of all the available seats on the "hemoglobin bus" are occupied by oxygen. Because the majority of oxygen is carried to tissues by hemoglobin, any condition or disease that decreases hemoglobin content will severely decrease the amount of oxygen carried to tissues.

Many conditions impair oxygen delivery. High-acuity patients are particularly at risk for impaired oxygen delivery as a result of decrease in heart function, such as that occurring with arrythmias or heart failure (Schallom & Ahrens, 1999). An uncompensated decrease in cardiac output, hemoglobin, or SaO_2 can significantly reduce oxygen delivery. Patients who have what may appear to be clinically insignificant decreases in all three factors can have a significant decrease in oxygen delivery when they are considered together.

The autonomic nervous system exerts partial control of oxygen delivery through excitatory or inhibitory effects on the heart, lungs, and blood vessels. Specific cell receptors present in the cardiovascular and respiratory systems, when stimulated, result in a target cell response. The types of cell receptors and their physiologic responses are summarized in Table 14–2.

In summary, oxygen delivery is the process of transporting oxygen to cells. Four factors affect oxygen delivery: cardiac output, autoregulation, oxygen content of arterial blood, and autonomic nervous system innervation. An uncompensated decrease in cardiac output, hemoglobin, or SaO_2 can cause a significant reduction in the amount of oxygen delivered to cells.

TABLE 14–2 Alpha, Beta, and Dopaminergic Receptor Stimulation and Physiologic Response

RECEPTOR	LOCATION	RESPONSE
Alpha	Vessels of intestines, kidneys, muscles, skin	Vasoconstriction of arterioles
Beta 1	Heart	Increase in heart rate, conduction, and contraction
Beta 2	Bronchial and vascular smooth muscles	Bronchodilation Vasoconstriction of arterioles
Dopaminergic	Renal vasculature Mesenteric vasculature	Increased renal blood flow Increased mesenteric blood flow

SECTION THREE REVIEW

1. Oxygen delivery is the
   A. amount of oxygen in arterial blood
   B. process of transporting oxygen to cells
   C. process of utilizing oxygen for energy
   D. amount of blood pumped by the heart per minute
2. Factors that affect oxygen delivery include
   A. ventilation, diffusion, and perfusion
   B. cardiac output, hemoglobin concentration, and ventilation
   C. cardiac output, autoregulation, and oxygen content of arterial blood
   D. cardiac output, autoregulation, oxygen content of arterial blood, and autonomic nervous system innervation
3. A patient who has suffered a myocardial infarction is at risk for impaired oxygenation primarily related to
   A. overactive autoregulation
   B. impaired autonomic nervous system innervation
   C. decreased cardiac output
   D. decreased oxygen content of arterial blood
4. Ninety-seven percent of all oxygen delivered to cells
   A. is in the form of oxyhemoglobin
   B. is dissolved in plasma
   C. is carried as PaO_2
   D. is carried as HCO_3
5. Administration of a drug that stimulates beta 1 receptors
   A. decreases blood pressure
   B. increases heart rate
   C. increases renal blood flow
   D. decreases afterload

Answers: 1. B, 2. D, 3. C, 4. A, 5. B

SECTION FOUR: Oxygen Consumption

At the completion of this section, the learner will be able to describe oxygen consumption in terms of aerobic and anaerobic metabolism.

The third component of oxygenation is oxygen consumption. **Oxygen consumption (VO_2)** (Fig. 14–3) is the process by which cells use oxygen to generate energy. Oxygen enables the energy contained in food to be converted into a usable form of energy. Ingested carbohydrates, fats, and proteins are broken down into substrates that are converted in the Krebs cycle into energy in the form of adenosine triphosphate (ATP). This process is called **aerobic metabolism** (Fig. 14–4). The purpose of forming ATP is to create intracellular energy stores. When energy is needed, ATP is broken down and energy is released. Aer-

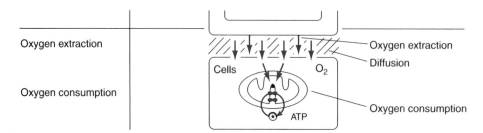

Figure 14–3 ■ Oxygen consumption: Cells extract and use oxygen to generate energy. *(Adapted, with permission, from Taylor, C. R., & Weibel, E. R. [1981], Design of the mammalian respiratory system,* Respiration Physiology, *41 [p. 2]. Copyright © 1981 by Elsevier Science.)*

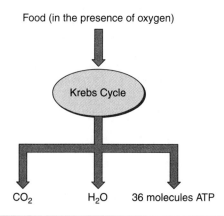

Figure 14–4 ■ Aerobic metabolism.

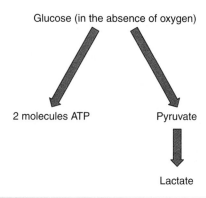

Figure 14–5 ■ Anaerobic metabolism.

TABLE 14–3　Aerobic Versus Anaerobic Metabolism

AEROBIC METABOLISM	ANAEROBIC METABOLISM
Generation of energy through the use of oxygen	Generation of energy in the absence of oxygen
Carbohydrates, fats, proteins broken down into substrates	Carboyhydrates broken down into substrates
Produces 36 ATP molecules	Produces 2 ATP molecules, lactate, and pyruvate
Generates large amount of energy	Generates small amount of energy

obic metabolism results in the creation of 36 molecules of ATP. Cells use ATP molecules as their energy source to perform all their necessary functions. Without the ATP energy stores, cellular processes break down and cells cannot function. The primary value of oxygen is its ability to develop ATP.

As a "backup" mechanism, cells have the ability to generate energy in the absence of oxygen by the process of **anaerobic metabolism** (Fig. 14–5). When anaerobic metabolism is used, carbohydrates are broken down to generate ATP. Carbohydrates are the only food substrates that can be broken down to generate ATP without the use of oxygen. Anaerobic metabolism produces only two ATP molecules and produces the by-products pyruvate and lactate. When cells use anaerobic metabolism, lactate (an acid) accumulates in the body and results in lactic acidosis. The acidic environment alters cellular structure and greatly impairs cellular function. Anaerobic metabolism is less efficient than aerobic metabolism and results in some potentially harmful by-products. Table 14–3 compares aerobic and anaerobic metabolism.

The process by which cells take oxygen from the blood is called **oxygen extraction.** Normal DO_2 is approximately 1,000 mL/min, and approximately 250 mL of this oxygen is required by tissue metabolic processes (VO_2); therefore, the usual oxygen

extraction is 25 percent (Hameed, Aird, & Cohn, 2003). Under normal circumstances, oxygen is loosely attached to hemoglobin so that oxygen is readily released from the hemoglobin. The degree to which hemoglobin releases oxygen is called **affinity.** The affinity of oxygen to hemoglobin is determined by the oxyhemoglobin dissociation curve (see Module 4). Release of oxygen from hemoglobin at the cellular level depends on the relationship demonstrated in the oxyhemoglobin dissociation curve. A shift of the curve to the right results in decreased affinity of hemoglobin for oxygen. This decreased affinity increases the release of oxygen and is beneficial for tissue oxygenation. For example, a shift to the right occurs when there is an increase in body temperature. Increased body temperature increases metabolic rate and a greater need for oxygen. A shift to the left increases the capacity of hemoglobin to carry oxygen but decreases unloading of oxygen to tissues. Oxygen dissociates from hemoglobin in response to local tissue oxygen demands. When cells have increased energy demands, they extract more oxygen from the blood. For example, during exercise, muscle cells extract more oxygen than they do when at rest.

The amount of oxygen actually used (or "consumed") by cells is normally 250 mL/min. When indexed to body surface area, oxygen consumption is 110 to 130 mL/min/m^2.

Numerous conditions alter the oxygen consumption of high-acuity patients (Table 14–4). Coexisting conditions can have an additive effect on oxygen consumption. For example, a patient with a fever, infection, and increased work of breathing can have an oxygen consumption two times the resting oxygen consumption.

TABLE 14–4　Conditions That Alter Oxygen Consumption

Increase O$_2$ consumption	Hyperventilation, hyperthermia, trauma, sepsis, anxiety, stress, hyperthyroidism, increased muscle activity
Decrease O$_2$ consumption	Hypoventilation, hypothermia, sedation, neuromuscular blocking agents, anesthesia, hypothyroidism, inactivity

TABLE 14–5 Activities That Increase Oxygen Consumption

ACTIVITY	APPROXIMATE INCREASE ABOVE RESTING OXYGEN CONSUMPTION (%)
Nursing assessment	10
Repositioning patient	30
Dressing change	10
Bed bath	20
Weighing patient on sling bed scale	40
Visitors	18
Restlessness/agitation	18

Routine nursing care increases oxygen consumption in critically ill patients (Swinamer et al., 1987). Table 14–5 lists some routine activities that increase oxygen consumption.

In summary, oxygen consumption is the process by which cells use oxygen to generate energy in the form of ATP. Under normal circumstances, this is done by aerobic metabolism. When insufficient oxygen is available, cells use anaerobic metabolism. Anaerobic metabolism is inefficient and results in lactic acidosis. When cellular energy demands increase, oxygen extraction and oxygen consumption increase. Research has demonstrated that various clinical conditions and activities increase oxygen consumption.

SECTION FOUR REVIEW

1. A continuous supply of oxygen is
   A. not necessary because oxygen is stored in cells
   B. required for adequate ATP synthesis
   C. dependent on the amount of blood ejected from the left ventricle
   D. dependent on adequate supplies of hemoglobin
2. A blood sample for a newly admitted trauma patient reveals a high level of lactate. This is indicative of
   A. adequate oxygen delivery
   B. anaerobic metabolism
   C. adequate oxygen consumption
   D. aerobic metabolism
3. Which of the following conditions increases oxygen consumption?
   A. hypoventilation
   B. sedation
   C. bedrest
   D. temperature of 102°F
4. All of the following statements are true EXCEPT
   A. aerobic metabolism produces 36 molecules of ATP
   B. aerobic metabolism generates a small amount of energy
   C. anaerobic metabolism produces 2 ATP molecules
   D. anaerobic metabolism generates energy in the absence of oxygen

Answers: 1. B, 2. B, 3. D, 4. B

SECTION FIVE: Impaired Oxygenation

At the completion of this section, the learner will be able to define pathophysiologic conditions that result in impaired oxygenation.

Sections Two through Four of this module reviewed the three physiologic components of oxygenation: pulmonary gas exchange, oxygen delivery, and oxygen consumption. Any condition or disease that affects one or more of these components will result in impaired oxygenation (e.g., acute respiratory distress syndrome, anemia, hyperventilation). These conditions represent a "continuum" of oxygen disturbances. Life-threatening oxygenation impairments usually involve deficiencies of all three components of oxygenation.

Matching of ventilation to perfusion is essential for gas exchange; otherwise, impaired oxygenation occurs. Conditions such as pulmonary embolus or pneumothorax can produce ventilation–perfusion mismatching. The mismatching of ventilation to perfusion is a common cause of hypoxemia. **Hypoxemia** is a condition characterized by an inadequate amount of oxygen in the blood as a result of impaired gas exchange. Hypoxemia is frequently quantified as a PaO_2 of less than 50 mm Hg (see Module 4). If allowed to progress, hypoxemia can result in hypoxia. **Hypoxia** is defined as an inadequate amount of oxygen available at the cellular level such that cells experience anaerobic metabolism. **Dysoxia** is a condition characterized by an inability of the cells to use oxygen properly despite adequate levels of oxygen delivery.

If left untreated, hypoxemia, hypoxia, or dysoxia can lead to more life-threatening oxygenation impairments, including shock states and multiple organ dysfunction syndrome (MODS). Shock states are characterized by an imbalance of oxygen supply and demand (see Module 15). MODS is characterized by a continuing impairment of oxygenation, mediated by the inflammatory process (refer to Module 16 for more information).

In summary, any disease or condition that affects one or more of the three components will result in impaired oxygenation. Impaired oxygenation can result in ventilation–perfusion disturbances, including hypoxemia, hypoxia, dysoxia, and shock states.

SECTION FIVE REVIEW

1. Hypoxemia is defined as
   A. an inadequate amount of oxygen in the blood
   B. an inadequate amount of oxygen available at the cellular level
   C. $Paco_2$ of less than 50 mm Hg
   D. an imbalance of oxygen supply and demand
2. Hypoxia is defined as
   A. an inadequate amount of oxygen in the blood
   B. an inadequate amount of oxygen available at the cellular level
   C. $Paco_2$ of less than 50 mm Hg
   D. the inability of cells to use oxygen properly
3. Dysoxia is defined as
   A. an inadequate amount of oxygen in the blood
   B. an inadequate amount of oxygen available at the cellular level

C. $Paco_2$ of less than 50 mm Hg
D. the inability of cells to use oxygen properly
4. Shock states are characterized by
   A. an inadequate amount of oxygen in the blood
   B. an inadequate amount of oxygen available at the cellular level
   C. $Paco_2$ of less than 50 mm Hg
   D. an imbalance of oxygen supply and demand
5. MODS is characterized by
   A. continuing hypoxemia
   B. continuing hypoxia
   C. continuing impairment of oxygenation mediated by the inflammatory response
   D. continuing dysoxia mediated by the inflammatory response

Answers: 1. A, 2. B, 3. D, 4. D, 5. C

SECTION SIX: Assessment of Oxygenation

At the completion of this section, the learner will be able to identify techniques to assess oxygenation status in relation to pulmonary gas exchange, oxygen delivery, and oxygen consumption.

Monitoring oxygenation is an important component of a nursing assessment. Accurate assessment and treatment of oxygenation disturbances may determine whether patients survive. Identification of impaired oxygenation requires an understanding of the three components of oxygenation: pulmonary gas exchange, oxygen delivery, and oxygen consumption. Each of these three components of oxygenation may vary independently in response to pathophysiologic conditions and therapeutic interventions. Therefore, it is necessary to accurately assess all three components of oxygenation.

There are two goals in the assessment of oxygenation: (1) to determine overall adequacy of oxygenation and (2) to determine which component of oxygenation dysfunction should be manipulated. Oxygenation can be assessed using direct and indirect assessment techniques.

Pulmonary Gas Exchange

Assessment of gas exchange must include techniques to assess ventilation, diffusion, and perfusion. Techniques to assess for pulmonary gas exchange are summarized in Box 14–1.

Box 14–1   Assessment of Pulmonary Gas Exchange
ABG (Pao_2, $Paco_2$)
Auscultation
End-tidal CO_2
Assessment of respiratory muscle efficiency
(VT, MV̇, AV̇, RR, VC, pulmonary function tests)
Calculation of intrapulmonary shunt (Qs/Qt)
Pao_2/Fio_2 ratio

Auscultation of the lungs is a common and easy assessment technique to assess ventilation. The key physiologic disturbance that auscultation detects is a change in airflow. It is important for the nurse to convey the assessment accurately, using correct terminology. Crackles should be used to describe a discontinuous sound and wheeze should be used to describe a continuous sound. Ventilation is the only mechanism of eliminating carbon dioxide. Therefore, assessment of $PaCO_2$ provides valuable information about this physiologic process. Ventilatory failure is commonly defined as a $PaCO_2$ greater than 50 mm Hg. Carbon dioxide can also be assessed using end-tidal CO_2 measurements whereby a sensor is placed at the end of the endotracheal tube to measure the amount of exhaled CO_2.

Assessment of respiratory muscle efficiency is accomplished by pulmonary function tests (see Module 4) and includes measurements of tidal volume (V_T), minute ventilation ($\dot{M}V$), alveolar ventilation ($\dot{A}V$), respiratory rate (RR), and vital capacity (VC).

Calculation of intrapulmonary shunt can be made for patients who have peripheral arterial and pulmonary artery catheters in place. Intrapulmonary shunt (Qs/Qt) is the proportion of blood that flows past alveoli without participating in gas exchange. An elevated intrapulmonary shunt indicates a large proportion of blood is flowing past alveoli without participating in gas exchange. Elevated intrapulmonary shunt can be attributed to a diffusion impairment or abnormalities in the ventilation to perfusion ratio. Data needed to calculate Qs/Qt are obtained by drawing simultaneous mixed venous and arterial blood gases. It is a complex formula to calculate, although most bedside monitoring systems in the ICU have the capability to calculate Qs/Qt once mixed venous and arterial blood gas data are available. Normal intrapulmonary shunt is less than 5 percent. A Qs/Qt of 30 percent would mean that 30 percent of blood is flowing past alveoli without participating in gas exchange.

Because Qs/Qt requires simultaneous mixed venous and arterial blood gases, simpler, less cumbersome formulas for the determination of intrapulmonary shunt are often used. The simplest formula to estimate intrapulmonary shunt is the PaO_2/FIO_2 ratio. A normal value is more than 286, with a value less than 200 suggesting a large intrapulmonary shunt (Schallom & Ahrens, 1999). For example, a patient with a PaO_2 of 80 mm Hg on 40 percent FIO_2 (80/0.40) = 200.

Oxygen Delivery

Assessment of oxygen delivery must include the components of oxygen delivery, including cardiac output, Hb, SaO_2, and PaO_2.

Physical assessment of oxygen delivery is difficult because oxygen is a colorless, odorless gas. Physical assessments of oxygen delivery can be made using skin color and temperature assessments and capillary refill. *Cyanosis,* a term used to describe bluish skin discoloration, is difficult to use because of subjectivity. Cool extremities indicate poor perfusion (Kaplan et al.,

2001). Capillary refill may be a useful assessment parameter in children, but is not as useful in elderly patients (Johnson, 2004).

Direct measurement of PaO_2, SaO_2, and hemoglobin can be made with an ABG. Although PaO_2 minimally contributes to oxygen delivery (less than 3 percent of all oxygen delivered to tissues), it is still used in the evaluation of oxygen delivery. Arterial oxygen saturation, the ratio of oxygenated hemoglobin to total hemoglobin, can be measured by ABG (SaO_2) or by pulse oximetry (SpO_2). Pulse oximetry is used for continous noninvasive measurement of arterial oxygenation saturation. Pulse oximetry is recommended for any patient at risk for hypoxemia because desaturation is detected earlier by pulse oximetry than by clinical observation (Grap, 2002).

Cardiac output can be assessed directly or indirectly. An indirect assessment of cardiac output would include an evaluation of heart rate and stroke volume, including the components of preload and afterload (see Module 8). Direct measurement of cardiac output can be made using a pulmonary artery catheter. Cardiac output measurements can be made using thermodilution techniques or by the use of a special pulmonary artery catheter that measures cardiac output continuously (see Modules 8 and 9). Oxygen delivery (DO_2) can also be calculated for these patients. Calculation of oxygen delivery requires a cardiac output measurement, serum hemoglobin analysis, and ABG analysis for SaO_2 and PaO_2. Oxygen delivery can be calculated as the product of cardiac output and oxygen content of arterial blood as follows:

$$DO_2 = (CO \times [Hb \times 1.34 \times SaO_2] + [PaO_2 \times 0.003]) \times 10^*$$

*10 is a conversion factor

Oxygen Consumption

Assessment of oxygen consumption must include techniques that assess the availability and use of oxygen at the cellular level. Direct assessment of oxygen consumption in the clinical setting is currently not possible. There are no physical assessment parameters that can be used to evaluate oxygen consumption. Traditional means of assessing oxygenation (ABGs, cardiac output, etc.) do not reflect oxygen availability at the cellular level. Future technologies will focus on measuring oxygenation at the cellular level.

Current methods of assessing oxygen consumption are limited to indirect measurement techniques including measurement of serum lactate levels, base deficit, and mixed venous oxygen saturation monitoring.

Under conditions of inadequate oxygen delivery, cells convert from aerobic metabolism to anaerobic metabolism. The byproduct of anaerobic metabolism is lactate. Normal serum lactate levels are less than 2 mMol/L. The underlying cause of high serum lactate levels may be inadequate oxygen delivery to meet cellular oxygen needs. Serum lactate levels, evaluated using serial measurements (for example, every 4 to 8 hours), can be used as an indicator of improving or worsening oxygen delivery in relation to oxygen consumption. Serum lactate levels must be interpreted with caution in patients with liver or renal disease and alcohol intoxication (Johnson, 2004).

Base deficit is defined as the amount of base (mMol) required to titrate 1 L of arterial blood to a normal pH. It is calculated from an ABG. Normal base deficit is +3 mMol to −3 mMol. It is used as an approximation of acidosis. A base deficit results from an imbalance between oxygen delivery and oxygen consumption, which results in a lactic acidosis secondary to anaerobic metabolism. Positive values reflect metabolic alkalosis and negative reflect metabolic acidosis. Base deficit can be classified as mild (−2 to −5 mMol), moderate (−6 to −14 mMol), and severe (greater than −15 mMol). Administration of sodiumbicarbonate, hypothermia, and hypocapnea can affect base deficit (Johnson, 2004).

Mixed venous oxygen saturation (SvO_2) reflects the balance between oxygen supply and oxygen demand. Measuring SpO_2 provides information about the oxygen saturation of arterial blood. Measuring SvO_2 provides information about the oxygen saturation of venous blood. Monitoring both of these parameters allows clinicians to make an assessment about the amount of oxygen delivered to tissues and the amount of oxygen returned from tissues.

When the supply of oxygen to the tissues is sufficient, tissues extract the amount of oxygen needed for their metabolic processes. Each organ system requires a different amount of oxygen. The kidneys actually have a relatively low demand for oxygen because much of their function uses passive transport. The oxygen saturation of the venous blood leaving the kidney averages 74 percent. Conversely, the heart requires a large amount of oxygen for its work. The oxygen saturation of blood leaving the coronary circulation averages only 30 percent. Each body part extracts a certain percentage of the oxygen depending on the metabolic rate of that organ system. The venous blood from all organ systems is transported to the right heart. The venous blood from all body systems is considered "mixed" when it has reached the pulmonary artery. The saturation of this mixed venous blood (SvO_2) represents an average of the venous saturation of blood from all parts of the body. Normal mixed venous oxygen saturation is 60 to 80 percent.

Evidence-Based Practice

- *Elderly trauma patients have lower mean levels of oxygenation parameters (lower CO, DO_2, and VO_2) (Epstein et al., 2002).*

- *The presence of cool extremities should trigger consideration that the patient may be hypoperfused and, in such case, markers of inadequate oxygenation should be assessed (base deficit, lactate) (Kaplan et al., 2001).*

- *PaO_2/FiO_2 remains the most important clinical physiologic variable used in the diagnosis and assessment of ARDS (Offner & Moore, 2003).*

- *Critically ill surgical patients whose lactate levels return to normal within 24 hours have a lower mortality than those who take 96 hours to return to normal levels (McNelis et al., 2001).*

- *An SpO_2 greater than 94 percent appears necessary to ensure an SaO_2 greater than 90 percent (Van de Louw et al., 2001).*

If the oxygen delivery to tissues is adequate for tissue demands, oxygen saturation of the blood in the pulmonary artery will be 60 to 80 percent. The SvO_2 provides information about the adequacy of CO. The patient's blood gases and CO may be within normal limits, but if the SvO_2 is below 60 percent, oxygen delivery is inadequate for tissue oxygen demands. A low SvO_2 means that less oxygen is returning to the right heart; the cells are not getting enough oxygen to meet their needs. Conversely, a low CO of 3.0 L/min in a post operative patient may not be of concern if the patient's SvO_2 is between 60 and 80 percent. These patients are hypothermic, sedated, intubated, and mechanically ventilated so their tissue oxygen demands are very low. A normal SvO_2 indicates that oxygen delivery is adequate for tissue oxygen demands. Causes of decreased and increased SvO_2 are summarized in Table 14–6.

To illustrate how SvO_2 monitoring can be used to assess oxygen consumption, consider the following patient example. Mr. X has an SaO_2 of 100 percent and an SvO_2 of 75 percent. Mr. Z has an SaO_2 of 98 percent and an SvO_2 of 40 percent. Mr. X's SaO_2 indicates that the oxygen content of arterial blood is fully saturated and that the oxygen saturation of the blood returning to the right side of the heart is 75 percent. If 100 percent was delivered and 75 percent was returned, it appears that the cells extracted 25 percent of the oxygen they received. This is a normal oxygen extraction. Mr. X appears to have a normal oxygen supply-and-demand balance. Now consider Mr. Z's values. The SvO_2 value is below normal. This is interpreted as a decrease in oxygen delivery compared with oxygen demand. Thus, more oxygen is extracted at the cellular level. The alteration in this SvO_2 value does not indicate which of the determinants of oxygen delivery has changed but implies an oxygenation impairment. The nurse should then assess for changes in cardiac output, SaO_2, and hemoglobin, or for conditions that cause an increase in oxygen consumption (e.g., fever). (Conditions that increase oxygen consumption were discussed in Section Four of this module.)

SvO_2 can be measured intermittently by blood gas analysis of a mixed venous blood sample drawn from the distal port of a pulmonary artery catheter. SvO_2 can be measured continuously through the use of a special fiber-optic pulmonary artery catheter. A fiber-optic filament in the catheter emits a constant beam of light on the red blood cells flowing past it in the pulmonary artery. The amount of emitted light reflected back to the computer through a receiving fiber-optic depends on the oxygen saturation of the red blood cells flowing past it. The computer uses this information to determine the oxygen saturation of mixed venous blood. A digital readout of the SvO_2 is updated several times each minute. Trends in SvO_2 can be used to assess patient tolerance to interventions (Fig. 14–6).

In summary, monitoring oxygenation is one of the most important components of a nursing assessment. Clinical assessment of oxygenation should include techniques that assess the three components of oxygenation: pulmonary gas exchange, oxygen delivery, and oxygen consumption. Assessment of gas exchange must include techniques to assess ventilation, diffusion, and perfusion.

TABLE 14–6 Causes of Decreased and Increased Svo_2

Decreased Svo_2

1. Decreased oxygen supply
   - Decreased cardiac output
     - Heart failure
     - Hypovolemia
     - Dysrhythmias
     - Cardiac depressants (i.e., beta blockers)
   - Decreased oxygen saturation
     - Respiratory failure
     - Pulmonary infiltrates
     - Suctioning
     - Ventilator disconnection
   - Decreased hemoglobin
     - Anemia
     - Hemorrhage
2. Increased oxygen consumption
   - Hyperthermia
   - Seizures
   - Shivering
   - Pain
   - Increased work of breathing
   - Increased metabolic rate
   - Exercise
   - Agitation

Increased Svo_2[a]

1. Increased oxygen supply
   - Increased cardiac output
     - Inotropic drugs
     - Intra-aortic balloon pump
     - Afterload reduction
     - Early septic shock
   - Increased oxygen saturation
     - Increased Fio_2 (inspired oxygen)
     - Improvement in lung problem
   - Increased hemoglobin
     - Blood transfusion
2. Decreased oxygen demand
   - Hypothermia
   - Fever reduction
   - Sepsis (late stages)
   - Paralysis
   - Pain relief
   - Anesthesia

[a]A wedged pulmonary artery catheter may result in a falsely elevated Svo_2.

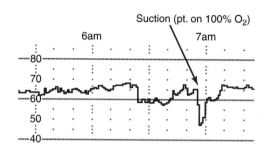

A. Endotracheal suctioning

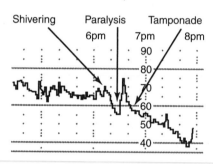

B. Cardiac tamponade

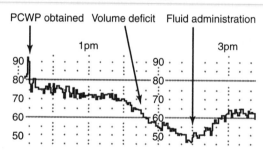

C. Fluid volume deficit

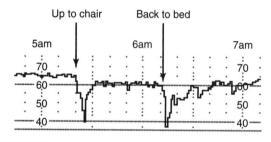

D. Increased O_2 consumption

Figure 14–6 ■ Comparison of Svo_2 patterns. *(Used with permission from Cathe-lyn, J. L., & Samples, D. A. (1998). Svo_2 monitoring: Tool for evaluating patient outcomes. Dimensions of Critical Care in Nursing, 17(2), 58–66. Copyright © Springhouse Corporation/www.springnet.com.)*

Assessment of oxygen delivery includes cardiac output, hemoglobin, SaO_2, and PaO_2. Current methods of assessing oxygen consumption are limited to indirect measurement techniques, including serial measurements of lactate, base deficit, and SvO_2.

SECTION SIX REVIEW

1. The "gold standard" for the assessment of oxygen delivery is
   A. PaO_2
   B. cardiac output
   C. SvO_2
   D. auscultation
2. Direct measurement of oxygen consumption
   A. is made using SvO_2 monitoring
   B. is made using transcutaneous oxygen measurements
   C. is not clinically possible
   D. can be calculated as the product of cardiac output and oxygen content of arterial blood
3. A patient has the following values: SaO_2 100 percent and SvO_2 55 percent. Which one of the following assessments would be helpful in determining the source of the oxygenation imbalance?
   A. auscultating lung fields
   B. taking temperature
   C. drawing an arterial blood gas
   D. measuring preload
4. Calculation of oxygen delivery requires all of the following EXCEPT
   A. cardiac output measurement
   B. serum hemoglobin analysis
   C. ABG analysis
   D. measurement of blood pressure

Answers: 1. B, 2. C, 3. B, 4. D

POSTTEST

1. The concept of oxygenation involves
   A. pulmonary gas exchange, oxygen delivery, and oxygen consumption
   B. integration of the pulmonary and cardiovascular systems
   C. ventilation, diffusion, and perfusion
   D. oxygen extraction and oxygen consumption
2. Your patient's postoperative hemoglobin is 6 mg/dL. What impact would this have on the initial component of oxygenation?
   A. none
   B. ventilation impairment
   C. diffusion impairment
   D. perfusion impairment
3. A pulmonary embolism would result in impaired gas exchange as a result of
   A. ventilation impairment
   B. diffusion impairment
   C. perfusion impairment
   D. decreased oxygen content of arterial blood
4. Which of the following contributes minimally to oxygen delivery?
   A. PaO_2—50 mm Hg
   B. SaO_2—70 percent
   C. CO—3 L/min
   D. Hb—6 mg/dL

Mr. B is admitted with a diagnosis of pneumonia. His data on admission are as follows:

ABG: PaO_2 45, $PaCO_2$ 50, SaO_2 70 percent, pH 7.30, HCO_3 28
Lactate: 8 mMol/L
Hb: 10 mg/dL
CO: 3 L/min
SvO_2:   60 percent

Questions 5, 6, and 7 pertain to Mr. B.

5. Based on the preceding data, Mr. B has impaired oxygen consumption as evidenced by
   A. PaO_2 of 45, $PaCO_2$ of 50
   B. $PaCO_2$ of 50, SaO_2 of 70 percent
   C. lactate 8 mMol/L and SvO_2 of 60 percent
   D. Hb 10 mg/dL and CO of 3 L/min
6. Based on the data on Mr. B, you determine that Mr. B has
   A. multiple organ dysfunction syndrome
   B. shock
   C. hypoxemia and hypoxia
   D. dysoxia
7. Based on the data on Mr. B, calculate the oxygen delivery.
   A. 282 mL/min
   B. 28,142 mL/min
   C. 125 mL/min
   D. 243 mL/min

8. Which of the following would decrease oxygen consumption?

A. administration of an antibiotic

B. preoperative anxiety

C. nursing assessment

D. administration of a sedative

9. The clinical condition characterized by inadequate oxygen in arterial blood is

A. hypoxia

B. hypoxemia

C. dysoxia

D. shock

10. Which of the following represents the most complete oxygenation assessment?

A. arterial blood gas, auscultation, and calculation of intrapulmonary shunt

B. auscultation of lung fields, measurement of cardiac output, and SvO_2

C. cardiac output, serum measurement of hemoglobin, SaO_2, and PaO_2

D. serum lactate level, SvO_2, and arterial blood gas

POSTTEST ANSWERS

Question	Answer	Section	Question	Answer	Section
1	A	One	6	C	Five
2	D	Two	7	A	Six
3	C	Two	8	D	Four
4	A	Three	9	B	Five
5	C	Four	10	B	Six

REFERENCES

Epstein, C. D., Peerless J., Mart J., et al. (2002). Oxygen transport and organ dysfunction in older trauma patients. *Heart and Lung, 31,* 315–326.

Grap, M. J. (2002). Protocols for practice: Pulse oximetry. *Critical Care Nurse, 22,* 69–76.

Hameed, S. M., Aird, W. C., & Cohn, S. M. (2003). Oxygen delivery. *Critical Care Medicine, 31* (12 suppl), S658–S667.

Johnson, K. L. (2004). Diagnostic measures to evaluate oxygenation in critically ill adults. Implications and limitations. *AACN Clinical ISS, 15,* 506–524.

Kaplan, L. J., McPartland, K., Santora T. A., et al. (2001). Start with a subjective assessment of skin temperatures to identify hypoperfusion in intensive care unit patients. *Journal of Trauma, 50,* 620–628.

McNelis, J., Marini, C. P., Jurkiewicz, A., Szom Stein, S., Simms, H. H., Ritter, G., et al. (2001). Prolonged lactate clearance is associated with increased mortality in the surgical intensive care unit. *American Journal of Surgery, 182,* 481–485.

Offner, P. J., & Moore E. E. (2003). Lung injury severity scoring in the era of lung protective mechanical ventilation: The PaO_2/FIO_2 ratio. *Journal of Trauma, 55,* 285–289.

Schallom, L., & Ahrens, T. (1999). Using oxygenation profiles to manage patients. *Critical Care Nurse Clinics of North America, 11,* 437–446.

Swinamer, D. L., Phang, P. T., Jones, R. L., Grace, M., & King, E. G. (1987). Twenty-four hour energy expenditure in critically ill patients. *Critical Care Medicine, 15,* 637–643.

Van De Louw A., Cracco C., & Cerf C. (2001). Accuracy of pulse oximetry in the ICU. *Intensive Care Medicine, 27,* 1606–1613.

Shock States

Adam DaDeppo, Karen L. Johnson

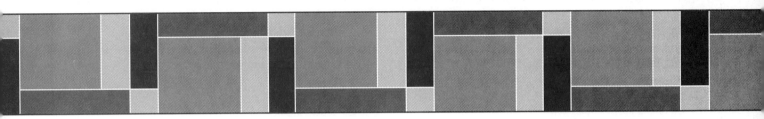

OBJECTIVES Following completion of this module, the learner will be able to

1. Describe the mechanism of impaired oxygenation for each of the four functional classifications of shock states.

2. Describe the compensatory mechanisms that occur in response to shock states.

3. List the clinical manifestations of each of the four functional shock states.

4. State the medical and nursing interventions used in the treatment of shock states that optimize oxygen delivery and decrease oxygen consumption.

The major function of the cardiovascular system is to deliver blood, oxygen, and nutrients to the cells, tissues, and organs of the body and to remove metabolic wastes. When this fails to occur, a state of shock develops.

Defining *shock* is more difficult than defining other disease entities. No one seems to agree on one concise definition because shock is a syndrome, a complex of signs and symptoms that describe a sequence of changes that occur when tissue oxygen supply does not meet oxygen demand. The relationship between oxygen supply (delivery) and oxygen demand (consumption) serves as the conceptual framework for shock in this module.

This self-study module is composed of four sections. Section One describes the mechanisms of impaired oxygenation for each of four functional classifications of shock. Section Two reviews the compensatory mechanisms that occur in response to shock states. In Section Three, clinical manifestations for each of the four functional shock states are given. The final section describes medical and nursing interventions that optimize oxygen delivery and decrease oxygen consumption. Each section includes a set of review questions to help the learner evaluate his or her understanding of the section's content before moving on to the next section. All Section Reviews and the module Pretest and Posttest include answers. It is suggested that the learner review those concepts answered incorrectly in the review questions before proceeding to the next section.

PRETEST

1. Common to all shock states is
   A. blood pressure of 90 mm Hg, heart rate greater than 100 beats per minute
   B. loss of blood volume
   C. decreased oxygen delivery with decreased oxygen consumption
   D. inadequate oxygen delivery to meet cellular oxygen demands

2. Which of the following shock states have similar pathologic mechanisms?
   A. neurogenic and septic shocks
   B. anaphylactic and cardiogenic shocks
   C. left ventricular myocardial infarction and cardiac tamponade
   D. carbon monoxide poisoning and cardiac tamponade

3. Which of the following is NOT one of the sympathetic nervous system's fight-or-flight responses?
   A. increased heart rate
   B. dilation of pupils
   C. increased respiratory rate
   D. increased intestinal peristalsis
4. Which of the following is a potent vasoconstrictor?
   A. renin
   B. aldosterone
   C. angiotensin II
   D. antidiuretic hormone (ADH)
5. In neurogenic shock, signs and symptoms are related to
   A. loss of spinal fluid
   B. damaged parasympathetic cells
   C. loss of hypothalamic control
   D. loss of sympathetic innervation
6. Shock states result from
   A. an imbalance of oxygen delivery and oxygen consumption
   B. an increase in oxygen delivery and oxygen consumption
   C. a decrease in oxygen delivery and oxygen consumption
   D. inadequate blood pressure, heart rate, and urine output
7. Transport shock states are the result of
   A. an increase in vessel diameter

B. a dysfunctional or inadequate amount of hemoglobin
   C. a barrier to flow of oxygenated blood
   D. failure of the heart to adequately pump blood
8. All of the following are stages of shock EXCEPT
   A. initial
   B. compensatory
   C. noncompensatory
   D. progressive
9. A systemic response to infection that includes a temperature greater than 38°C and a heart rate greater than 90 beats per minute characterizes
   A. sepsis
   B. severe sepsis
   C. septic shock
   D. septic syndrome
10. All of the following may be used in the treatment of cardiogenic shock EXCEPT
   A. a ventricular assist device
   B. an intra-aortic balloon pump
   C. a cardiac transplantation
   D. isoproterenol

Pretest Answers: 1. D, 2. A, 3. D, 4. C, 5. D, 6. A, 7. B, 8. C, 9. A, 10. D

GLOSSARY

oxygen consumption   The amount of oxygen used by the body; described as a product of cardiac output and the difference between arterial oxygen content and venous oxygen content.

pulsus paradoxus   Exaggerated decrease (greater than 10 mm Hg) of systolic blood pressure during inspiration.

ABBREVIATIONS

ACTH	Adrenocorticotropic hormone
ADH	Antidiuretic hormone
APC	Activated protein C
CO	Cardiac output
GI	Gastrointestinal
Hb	Hemoglobin
Hct	Hematocrit
HR	Heart rate
IABP	Intra-aortic balloon pump
LVAD	Left ventricular assist device
MAP	Mean arterial pressure
MDF	Myocardial depressant factor

MI	Myocardial infarction
MODS	Multiple organ dysfunction syndrome
O$_2$	Oxygen
Pa$_{CO_2}$	Partial pressure of dissolved carbon dioxide in the plasma of arterial blood
PAP	Pulmonary artery pressure
PAWP	Pulmonary artery wedge pressure
PTCA	Percutaneous transluminal coronary angioplasty
RAP	Right atrial pressure
SVR	Systemic vascular resistance
VAD	Ventricular assist device
WBC	White blood cell

TABLE 15–1 Functional States of Shock, Causes, and Pathologic Mechanisms

FUNCTIONAL STATE	ETIOLOGY	MECHANISM OF IMPAIRED O₂ DELIVERY
Hypovolemic	Fluid volume loss (dehydration, burn injuries, third spacing)	Loss of intravascular volume

	Vasodilation (neurogenic shock, anaphylactic shock, septic shock)	Increase in vessel diameter due to
		    Loss of sympathetic tone
		    Histamine release
		    Endotoxin release

Transport	Diminished supply of Hb to carry O₂ (anemia, hemorrhage, carbon monoxide poisoning)	Dysfunction or inadequate amount of Hb to bind with O₂

Obstructive	Mechanical barriers to blood flow (pulmonary embolism, tension pneumothorax, cardiac tamponade)	Barrier to flow of oxygenated blood due to
		    Pulmonary artery blocked
		    Great vessels kinked
		    Ventricles unable to fill or eject blood volume

Cardiogenic	Heart fails to function as a pump (myocardial infarction, dysrhythmias)	Ischemic muscles fail to contract Irregular rate/rhythm causes heart to fail its function as a pump

Compiled from Clochesy, J. M. (Ed.), (1988). Essentials of critical care nursing *(p. 127). Rockville, MD: Aspen Publishing.*

SECTION ONE: Functional Classifications of Shock States

At the completion of this section, the learner will be able to describe the mechanism of impaired oxygenation for each of the four functional classifications of shock states.

Common to all shock states is inadequate oxygen delivery to meet cellular oxygen demand. Traditionally, shock states have been classified according to their etiology (e.g., septic shock, hemorrhagic shock, neurogenic shock). More recently, shock states have been categorized into functional shock states. Several functional classifications have been used. For this module, shock is classified into four categories: hypovolemic, transport, obstructive, and cardiogenic (Clochesy, 1988). This classification system groups shock states not according to the cause of the shock state but according to similar mechanisms responsible for impaired oxygenation.

Hypovolemic shock states have impaired oxygenation because of inadequate cardiac output (CO) as a result of decreased intravascular volume. Transport shock states have impaired oxygenation because of a diminished supply of hemoglobin (Hb) in which to carry oxygen to tissues. Obstructive shock states have impaired oxygenation because of a mechanical barrier to blood flow. Cardiogenic shock states have impaired oxygenation because the heart fails to function as a pump to deliver oxygenated blood. The functional states, causes, and mechanisms of impaired oxygen delivery are summarized in Table 15–1.

Hypovolemic Shock States

Hypovolemia can result from two conditions: The fluid volume in the circulation has decreased or the size of the intravascular compartment has increased in proportion to fluid volume. When either or both of these conditions exist, venous return to the right atrium decreases. This reduces ventricular filling pressure, stroke volume, cardiac output, and blood pressure.

Loss of intravascular volume can be caused by loss of blood volume (hemorrhage), loss of intravascular fluid from the skin (as with dehydration or burns), loss of fluid from persistent vomiting or diarrhea, or loss of fluid from the intravascular compartment to interstitial spaces (third spacing). A diminished fluid volume leads to a decreased cardiac output (CO), resulting in impaired oxygen delivery.

When the size of the intravascular compartment has increased in proportion to the amount of fluid in the intravascular compartment, the body interprets this as a state of hypovolemia. Blood volume may be normal, but the intravascular space has increased without a proportional increase in blood volume. Vasodilation causes the intravascular compartment to increase without a corresponding increase in volume. Vasodilation can occur with neurogenic shock, anaphylactic shock, and septic shock.

Neurogenic shock may occur with a spinal cord injury. When there is injury to the spinal cord above the midthoracic region, impulses from the sympathetic nervous system cannot reach the arterioles. The loss of sympathetic innervation prohibits vasoconstriction of blood vessels, but blood vessels continue to receive parasympathetic innervation, allowing vasodilation. Blood then pools in the dilated peripheral venous system. The right heart receives an inadequate venous return, and cardiac output decreases. As CO decreases, delivery of oxygen-carrying blood decreases.

Anaphylactic shock occurs in response to a severe allergic reaction to such things as foods (peanuts, fish, eggs, milk), drugs (nonsteroidal anti-inflammatory drugs, aspirin, antibiotics, blood products), insect venoms, and latex (Kemp & Lockey, 2002). Massive amounts of vasoactive substances (e.g., histamine and kinins) are released from mast cells. This causes vasodilation and increases capillary permeability. Vasodilation increases the size of the intravascular compartment. Increased capillary permeability allows fluid to move from intravascular to interstitial spaces. As fluid is lost from the vascular compartment, a relative hypovolemia develops. The net consequences of combined massive vasodilation and increased capillary permeability are a decrease in venous return, decrease in CO, and a decrease in oxygen delivery.

Septic shock is a systemic response to invading microorganisms of all types: gram-positive and gram-negative bacteria, fungi, or viruses. The systemic response to infection triggers a complex series of cellular and humoral events (Fig. 15–1). These organisms release endotoxins that invade the bloodstream and stimulate the release of cytokines (tumor necrosis factor and interleukins). These substances produce vasodilation and increased capillary permeability. This reduces venous return, and cardiac output decreases. A second fluid alteration that occurs with septic shock is a maldistribution of circulating blood volume. Some organs receive more blood than needed as a result of vasodilation, whereas others (skin, lungs, kidneys) do not receive the blood needed. Altered fluid volume related to vasodilation, increased capillary permeability, and maldistribution of circulating volume characterize septic shock.

Transport Shock States

The common pathologic mechanism in transport shock states is a diminished supply of Hb to carry O_2 to tissues. Recall that Hb is the bus that carries O_2 molecules to tissues (Module 14). Anemia and hemorrhage are characterized by a decrease in red blood cells and Hb for O_2 to bind to.

Carbon monoxide toxicity represents another form of transport shock state. Carbon monoxide is a colorless, odorless gas that, when inhaled, rapidly binds to Hb to form carboxyhemoglobin. The Hb bus seats are occupied by carbon monoxide, leaving no room for O_2. Oxygen cannot be transported to tissues. The presence of carbon monoxide interferes with the release of O_2 from Hb and also interferes with the cell's ability to use O_2 properly (Hampson et al., 2001). A state of shock occurs as the transport of O_2 to tissues is severely limited.

Obstructive Shock States

Obstructive shock states occur as a result of a mechanical barrier to blood flow that blocks O_2 delivery to tissues. Causes include pulmonary embolism, tension pneumothorax, or cardiac tamponade.

Pulmonary embolism can range from clinically unimportant thromboembolism to massive embolism with sudden death. Hypercoagulability leads to formation of thrombi in the deep veins of the legs, pelvis, or arms. The thrombi dislodge and embolize to the pulmonary arteries. Pulmonary arteries become partially obstructed, which results in an increase in alveolar dead space and a ventilation–perfusion mismatch, which impairs gas exchange. Obstruction of the pulmonary arteries by emboli also results in increased pulmonary vascular resistance (Torbicki et al., 2000). As right ventricular afterload increases, right ventricular dysfunction can occur. Shock states in response to a pulmonary embolism can result from inadequate systemic O_2 delivery because of impaired gas exchange and cardiac dysfunction.

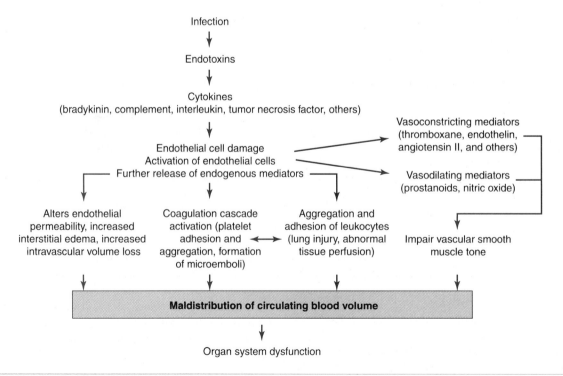

Figure 15–1 ■ Pathophysiology of septic shock.

A tension pneumothorax occurs when air enters the pleural space during inspiration but cannot leave during expiration. The progressive accumulation of air within the thoracic cavity leads to a shift of the mediastinal structures and compression of the opposite lung. The increased pleural pressure impedes venous return and serves as a barrier to O_2 delivery.

Cardiac tamponade is caused by bleeding into a nonflexible pericardial sac. The accumulating pressure around the heart impairs ventricular filling and decreases CO.

Cardiogenic Shock States

Cardiogenic shock states occur as a result of impaired O_2 delivery due to cardiac dysfunction. Dysfunction of either the right or left ventricle can lead to cardiogenic shock. Failure can occur when the right ventricle fails to pump the volume of blood it receives or when the left ventricle fails to pump oxygenated blood into the systemic circulation. Causes of cardiogenic shock include extensive acute myocardial infarction, mechanical complications (papillary muscle rupture), or other conditions (cardiomyopathy). Among patients with myocardial infarction, shock is more likely to develop in those who are elderly, diabetic, have an anterior infarction, or a history of previous infarction (Hollenberg, 2001).

An infarction in the left ventricle produces a necrotic area that impairs contractility and CO. The ventricle cannot propel oxygenated blood forward into the systemic circulation for delivery to tissues. As stroke volume decreases, so do CO and blood pressure. Because the damaged left ventricle cannot propel all of its contents forward, blood begins to "back up" into the pulmonary system, causing pulmonary congestion. Increased pulmonary congestion leads to increased afterload for the right ventricle. These changes can occur rapidly or can progress over several days.

In cardiogenic shock due to dysfunction of the right ventricle, the right ventricle ejects too little blood and, therefore, less blood enters the left ventricle. As left ventricular stroke volume decreases, CO and blood pressure decrease. Because the right ventricle cannot effectively pump all the blood it receives, blood begins to "back up" into the systemic circulation.

In summary, shock states can be classified according to the common pathologic mechanisms that produce impaired oxygenation: hypovolemic, transport, obstructive, and cardiogenic shock states. Independent of etiology or pathologic mechanisms, altered tissue perfusion with impaired oxygen delivery in relation to oxygen consumption is common to all forms of shock.

SECTION ONE REVIEW

1. Which of the following conditions produces a hypovolemic shock state?
   A. carbon monoxide poisoning
   B. tension pneumothorax
   C. pulmonary emboli
   D. third spacing (movement of fluid from the vascular to the interstitial space)
2. Which of the following conditions can produce a transport shock state?
   A. carbon monoxide poisoning
   B. dehydration
   C. cardiac tamponade
   D. anaphylactic shock
3. Which of the following conditions can produce an obstructive shock state?
   A. myocardial infarction
   B. anemia
   C. pulmonary emboli
   D. sepsis

4. Which of the following characterizes septic shock?
   A. occurs as a result of fluid shifts and vasoconstriction
   B. inadequate oxygen delivery and impaired oxygen consumption
   C. loss of sympathetic nerve innervation prohibits vasoconstriction
   D. occurs in response to an allergic reaction
5. Which of the following characterizes cardiogenic shock?
   A. increasing stroke volume in the face of decreasing cardiac output
   B. the heart fails to function as a pump
   C. increasing stroke volume in the face of increasing cardiac output
   D. cardiogenic shock as the result of a massive myocardial infarction

Answers: 1. D, 2. A, 3. C, 4. B, 5. B

SECTION TWO: Physiologic Response to Shock

At the completion of this section, the learner will be able to describe the compensatory mechanisms that occur in response to shock states.

Shock occurs when O_2 delivery does not support tissue O_2 demands. In an attempt to stabilize this life-threatening situation, a pattern of responses, or compensatory mechanisms, occurs.

Compensation in Shock

Complex neuroendocrine responses are triggered to overcome ineffective circulating blood volume. Low-pressure stretch receptors in the right atrium sense a decrease in circulating blood volume when there is a decrease in venous return to the right atrium. Baroreceptors in the aorta and carotid arteries sense a decrease in blood volume and CO. Carotid body chemoreceptors sense alterations in pH and partial pressure of arterial carbon dioxide ($PaCO_2$). The baroreceptors and chemoreceptors alert the hypothalamus to activate the sympathetic nervous system's fight-or-flight response. This system releases a massive amount of norepinephrine, which produces several compensatory mechanisms (Table 15–2). The beneficial effects of these mechanisms are an increase in venous return, an increase in CO, and an increase in O_2 delivery.

In response to shock states, the endocrine system is activated to increase **oxygen delivery** by increasing blood volume (Fig. 15–2). The hypothalamus releases adrenocorticotropic hormone (ACTH), which activates the adrenals to secrete aldosterone. Aldosterone causes sodium and water retention in efforts to increase the blood volume and blood pressure. Sodium and water retention stimulates the release of antidiuretic hormone (ADH), which increases reabsorption of water in the kidney tubules and increases blood volume. These hormones are released to preserve blood volume and conserve the amount of fluid the kidneys excrete.

CO must be augmented in shock to ensure adequate tissue perfusion. CO is proportional to venous return. To increase venous return, sodium and water are retained by aldosterone and ADH. In addition to these hormones, another mechanism, the

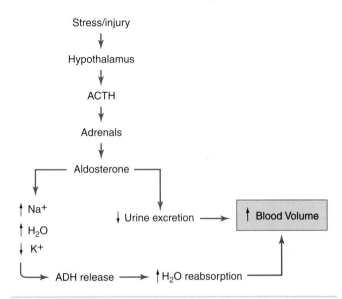

Figure 15–2 ■ ACTH, aldosterone, and ADH release.

renin–angiotensin–aldosterone cycle, is activated to increase blood volume and venous return. As a result of decreased blood flow to the kidneys, the juxtaglomerular cells in the kidneys excrete renin. Renin catalyzes angiotensinogen in the liver, which then converts to angiotensin I in the circulation. Once in the lungs, angiotensin I converts to angiotensin II, which is a potent vasoconstrictor. The vasoconstriction produced by angiotensin II increases blood pressure by increasing afterload. Angiotensin II is converted to angiotensin III, which stimulates the release of aldosterone. The renin–angiotensin–aldosterone cycle is depicted in Figure 15–3. The net effects of these hormonal mechanisms are increased blood pressure through vasoconstriction and increase in venous return through retention of sodium and water, and decreased urine output.

Compensatory mechanisms that occur in response to shock are designed to restore O_2 delivery by augmenting CO, redistributing blood flow, and restoring blood volume.

Progression of Shock

There are four stages of shock: initial, compensatory, progressive, and refractory. In the initial stage, decreased CO and decreased tissue perfusion are evident. Decreased O_2 delivery to cells results in anaerobic metabolism and lactic acidosis. In the compensatory stage, neuroendocrine responses are activated to restore CO and O_2 delivery. Clinical signs and symptoms are evident.

When compensatory mechanisms cannot restore homeostasis and if prompt and proper treatment has not been instituted, the third stage of shock can occur. Progressive shock results in major dysfunction of many organs. The continued low blood flow, poor tissue perfusion, inadequate O_2 delivery, and buildup of metabolic wastes over time lead to multiple organ dysfunction syndrome (MODS; see Module 16).

TABLE 15–2 Sympathetic Nervous System's Fight-or-Flight-Response

PHYSIOLOGIC RESPONSE	PHYSIOLOGIC RATIONALE
Increased heart rate	For rapid delivery of needed oxygen
Increased respiratory rate	To receive more oxygen and correct acidosis
Increased glycolysis	To increase availability of glucose for energy
Decreased urine output	To conserve fluid volume, return more blood volume to cardiovascular system to increase volume and blood pressure
Decreased blood flow to internal organs (e.g., kidneys, gastrointestinal tract, liver)	To allow more blood flow to more vital organs (e.g., heart and lungs)
Decreased intestinal peristalsis	Shunting of blood to vital organs, no need for digestion as body energy is redirected to lifesaving measures
Cool skin	Alpha receptors produce peripheral vasoconstriction to shunt blood to more vital organs
Diaphoresis	To release heat as a by-product of energy use

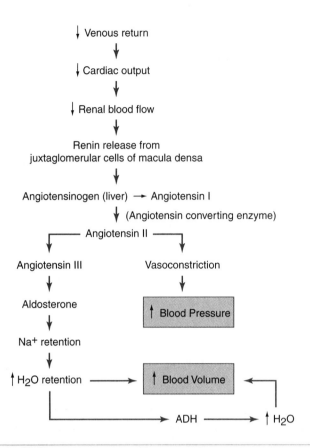

Figure 15–3 ■ Renin–angiotensin–aldosterone cycle.

The final stage of shock is the refractory stage. In this stage, the shock state is so profound and cell destruction is so severe that death is inevitable. The patient, although alive, has become refractory to conventional therapy. Profound hypotension occurs despite administration of potent vasoactive drugs. The patient remains hypoxemic despite O_2 therapy. A state of intractable circulatory failure leads to total body failure and death.

Not every patient progresses through all four stages. Often, the progression from one stage to the next is not obvious. If the shock state is assessed early and appropriate treatment is instituted, the progression of shock is halted, the O_2 supply-and-demand balance is restored, and the patient recovers.

In summary, compensatory mechanisms occur in response to shock in an attempt to prevent further deterioration and restore homeostasis. Complex neuroendocrine responses are triggered to overcome ineffective circulating blood volume. The hormones ACTH, aldosterone, and ADH are released to increase CO. The sympathetic nervous system releases a massive amount of norepinephrine, which produces multiorgan responses in an effort to sustain a life-threatening situation. The cardiovascular system tries to restore arterial blood pressure by augmenting CO through increased venous return. The renin–angiotensin–aldosterone cycle is initiated to enhance preload through increased venous return and increase afterload through vasoconstriction. When compensatory mechanisms cannot restore the system to homeostasis, shock progresses to a phase of continued inadequate tissue oxygenation. Cells die, metabolic wastes accumulate, and MODS occurs.

SECTION TWO REVIEW

1. Aldosterone increases blood volume by all of the following EXCEPT
   A. increasing sodium retention
   B. increasing water retention
   C. decreasing potassium retention
   D. increasing calcium retention
2. Angiotensin II
   A. is a vasoconstrictor
   B. is a vasodilator
   C. is released by ADH
   D. causes the release of ACTH
3. ACTH, aldosterone, and ADH
   A. sense alterations in pH and Pa_{CO_2}
   B. alert the hypothalamus to what could be a life-threatening situation
   C. conserve the amount of fluid excreted by the kidneys
   D. increase the heart rate for rapid delivery of oxygen

4. Norepinephrine produces which of the following compensatory mechanisms?
   A. decreased blood pressure
   B. increased intestinal peristalsis
   C. increased glycolysis
   D. decreased heart rate
5. Continued low blood flow, poor tissue perfusion, and inadequate oxygen delivery cause
   A. multisystem organ dysfunction
   B. the hypothalamus to release ACTH
   C. the release of renin from renal cells
   D. decreased urine output

Answers: 1. D, 2. A, 3. C, 4. C, 5. A

SECTION THREE: Clinical Findings Associated with Shock States

At the completion of this section, the learner will be able to list the clinical manifestations of each of the four functional shock states.

Clinical manifestations of all shock states are the result of inadequate O_2 delivery and the activation of compensatory mechanisms.

Traditional signs used to assess shock include blood pressure, heart rate, mentation, and urine output. However, these signs often underestimate the degree of physiologic abnormalities. Blood pressure is hard to assess because it is so individualized. A blood pressure of 90/60 mm Hg may be normotensive for one patient but hypotensive for another patient. There are many factors that cause tachycardia, including anxiety, pain, arrhythmia, and fever. Mentation may be hard to assess because of the presence of head injury, alcohol, drugs, or chronic diseases (e.g., Alzheimer's). Several factors may produce a false sense of security when adequate urine output is present (Boswell & Scalea, 2003). These can include the neuroendocrine response to shock, hyperglycemia, and diabetes insipidus. Research is ongoing, but evidence is mounting that shock states persist despite normalization of blood pressure, heart rate, and urine output (Boswell & Scalea, 2003).

Serum lactate levels can be used as an indirect measure of impaired oxygenation and shock. Normal serum lactate levels are less than 2 mMol/L. However, during shock states when there is impaired O_2 delivery to meet cellular O_2 demand, anaerobic metabolism occurs (see Module 14). The by-product of this is lactate. Hyperlactatemia can produce metabolic acidosis. Lactate levels indicate the degree of hypoperfusion (Boswell & Scalea, 2003). Patients whose lactate levels return to normal within 24 hours have increased survival rates and decreased occurrence of organ dysfunction (Boswell & Scalea, 2003).

Base deficit is the amount of base required to titrate 1 L of arterial blood to a normal pH. It is calculated from an arterial blood gas. Normal base deficit is $+3$ mMol to -3 mMol. A base deficit results from an imbalance between O_2 delivery and O_2 consumption producing a lactic acidosis secondary to anaerobic metabolism. Base deficit is classified as mild (-2 to -5), moderate (-6 to -14), and severe (less than -15). Ongoing or worsening base deficit may indicate further evaluation for an ongoing shock state.

A major focus in shock research has been in the evaluation of new technologies to assess the severity of shock states. These include gastric tonometry, infrared spectroscopy, sublingual capnography, and other noninvasive measurements (Boswell & Scalea, 2003).

Hypovolemic Shock States

In hypovolemic shock states that result from fluid loss, the signs and symptoms are related to the degree of volume depletion. The skin is cool, and capillary refill is poor. Depending on the amount of fluid volume lost, the blood pressure may be low, and orthostatic blood pressure changes may be noted. Tachycardia is evident, and urine output is low. Hemodynamically, as less volume is returned to the right atrium, the right atrial pressure (RAP) is low. As less fluid is delivered to the pulmonary vasculature and the left ventricle, pressures are low, as evidenced by a low pulmonary artery wedge pressure (PAWP), low pulmonary artery pressure (PAP), and low cardiac output (CO). The systemic vascular resistance (SVR) is elevated as vasoconstriction occurs in efforts to increase venous return and CO.

In neurogenic shock, signs and symptoms are related to the loss of sympathetic innervation. Persistent vasodilation produces a decreased SVR. Pooling of blood in dilated vessels results in diminished venous return, producing a lower RAP, PAP, PAWP, and CO. Heart rate (HR) is decreased as a result of parasympathetic innervation. Peripheral vasodilation produces warm skin. Hypothermia and absence of sweating below the level of the spinal cord injury may be present.

Severe anaphylactic shock frequently involves multiple organ systems of the body, but the most life threatening are those involving the cardiovascular and pulmonary systems. Anaphylactic shock can develop rapidly (5 to 30 min) or slowly (6 to 12 hrs) but follows a typical pattern of generalized itching followed by cutaneous flushing, urticaria, a fullness in the throat, anxiety, tightness in the chest, faintness, and loss of consciousness (Kemp & Lockey, 2002). Severe upper airway obstruction by edema can lead to asphyxia, whereas lower airway obstruction with wheezing and chest tightness is caused by bronchospasm (Kemp & Lockey, 2002).

A multitude of metabolic, hematologic, and hemodynamic abnormalities occur as a systemic response to the invasion of microorganisms in the bloodstream. These abnormalities are part of a complex syndrome that may ultimately culminate in septic shock. Early recognition and treatment of septic shock is crucial. Broad definitions of sepsis and septic shock assist in the early recognition and treatment of these disorders (Hollenberg, 2001). These definitions are summarized in Table 15–3.

Transport Shock States

Diminished oxygen-carrying capacity of the blood produces the clinical manifestations seen in transport shock states. In shock caused by anemia or hemorrhage, a low hematocrit and hemoglobin will be present. RAP and PAWP may be normal, depending on the patient's volume status.

Symptoms caused by carbon monoxide poisoning can be a result of exposure to low levels of carbon monoxide for prolonged periods or can arise from exposure to higher levels for a shorter duration (Weaver, 1999). Common symptoms of carbon monoxide poisoning include headache, malaise, nausea, difficulties with memory, and personality changes, as well as gross neurologic dysfunction (Weaver, 1999). An elevated carboxyhe-

TABLE 15–3 Definitions of Sepsis, Severe Sepsis, and Septic Shock

Sepsis

The systemic response to infection is manifested by two or more of the following conditions:

1. Temperature greater than 38°C or less than 36°C
2. Heart rate greater than 90 bpm
3. Respiratory rate greater than 20 breaths/min or $Paco_2$ greater than 32 mm Hg
4. White blood cell count greater than 12,000/mL or less than 4,000/mL or greater than 10 percent immature (band) forms

Severe sepsis

Sepsis associated with organ dysfunction, hypoperfusion, or hypotension. Hypoperfusion and perfusion abnormalities may include, but are not limited to, lactic acidosis, oliguria, or an acute alteration in mental status.

Septic shock

Sepsis associated with hypotension despite adequate fluid resuscitation along with the presence of perfusion abnormalities that may include, but are not limited to, lactic acidosis, oliguria, or an acute alteration in mental status.

moglobin level confirms carbon monoxide poisoning. Although carboxyhemoglobin levels may be greater than 70 percent, the carboxyhemoglobin level is not indicative of the level of neurological injury (Hampson et al., 2001).

Obstructive Shock States

The clinical manifestations of obstructive shock states are the result of a mechanical barrier to blood flow resulting in inadequate oxygen delivery.

Pulsus paradoxus is one of the classic signs of cardiac tamponade. Pulsus paradoxus is an exaggerated decrease (greater than 10 mm Hg) of the systolic blood pressure during inspiration. Other clinical manifestations of cardiac tamponade include distant heart sounds (muffled by the increased pericardial fluid) and a pericardial friction rub. In tamponade, RAP usually is elevated and is equaled by the PAWP. Beck's triad, consisting of elevated RAP, decreased blood pressure, and muffled heart sounds, may be present.

Increased pleural pressure as a result of a tension pneumothorax puts direct pressure on the heart, vena cava, and contralateral lung. As a result, there will be decreased breath sounds, tracheal deviation, and bradycardia. This results in poor ventilation, decreased venous return, and decreased CO.

Dyspnea is the most frequent symptom of pulmonary embolism, and tachypnea is the most frequent sign. The presence of pleuritic pain, cough, or hemoptysis suggests a small embolism near the pleura, and the presence of dyspnea, syncope, or cyanosis usually indicates a massive pulmonary embolism (Torbicki et al., 2000). The most frequent electrocardiographic abnormality is T wave inversion in the anterior leads (V_1 to V_3) and a right bundle brunch block (Torbicki et al., 2000). ABGs may be normal or indicate hypoxemia or hypercapnia. Perfusion lung scans, pulmonary angiography, spiral CT of the chest with contrast, or transthoracic echocardiography may be used in the diagnostic workup.

Cardiogenic Shock States

Clinical manifestations produced in cardiogenic shock states depend on whether heart failure is left sided or right sided.

Left ventricular failure produces clinical manifestations associated with hypoperfusion and pulmonary congestion, including dyspnea, bilateral rales (crackles), and distant heart sounds, and third or fourth heart sounds are usually present. The hemodynamic profile of cardiogenic shock includes an elevated PAWP (greater than 15 mm Hg), a low cardiac index (less than 2.2 L/min/m^2), and sustained systolic hypotension (less than 90 mm Hg for greater than 30 min) (Hollenberg, 2001).

Clinical manifestations of right ventricular failure are associated with systemic venous congestion. Peripheral edema may be evident. Lung sounds will be clear unless there is also left ventricular dysfunction. A split-second heart sound may be heard. This sound, produced by delayed closure of the tricuspid valve, indicates a distended right ventricle. The hemodynamic profile of right ventricular failure includes elevated RAPs in the presence of normal or low PAWP.

In summary, clinical manifestations associated with shock states are the result of impaired oxygenation and the compensatory mechanisms of the neuroendocrine and cardiovascular systems. In hypovolemic shock states that result from fluid loss, the signs and symptoms are related to the degree of volume depletion. In neurogenic shock, anaphylactic shock, and septic shock, signs and symptoms are related to vasodilation. A diminished supply of hemoglobin produces the clinical manifestations seen in transport shock states. The clinical manifestations of obstructive shock states are the result of a mechanical barrier to blood flow. Clinical manifestations of cardiogenic shock states depend on whether there is left or right ventricular failure. Left ventricular failure produces clinical manifestations associated with hypoperfusion and pulmonary congestion. Right ventricular failure produces signs associated with systemic venous congestion.

SECTION THREE REVIEW

1. The signs and symptoms of anaphylactic shock are
   A. related to the loss of sympathetic tone
   B. related to the release of chemical mediators
   C. decreased SVR, PAWP, and increased temperature
   D. decreased RAP, increased CO, and increased temperature

2. A low Hct and Hb will be present in shock caused by
   A. a pulmonary embolism
   B. cardiac tamponade
   C. anemia
   D. right ventricular failure

3. Mr. G was involved in a motor vehicle crash. He sustained a spinal cord injury. Which of the following are clinical manifestations of a spinal cord injury?
   A. increased heart rate, SVR, and RAP
   B. decreased heart rate, decreased SVR, and increased RAP

C. increased heart rate, increased SVR, and decreased RAP
   D. decreased heart rate, SVR, and RAP

4. Mr. T has hypovolemic shock. Which of the following clinical manifestations would be present?
   A. decreased SVR, decreased CO
   B. increased SVR, decreased CO
   C. decreased SVR, increased CO
   D. increased SVR, increased CO

5. Which of the following would characterize right-sided heart failure?
   A. RAP will be high and much higher than PAWP
   B. RAP will be low
   C. PAWP will be high and much higher than RAP
   D. RAP and PAWP will be greatly elevated

Answers: 1. B, 2. C, 3. D, 4. B, 5. A

SECTION FOUR: Treatment of Shock

At the completion of this section, the learner will be able to list the medical and nursing interventions used in the treatment of shock states that optimize oxygen delivery and decrease oxygen consumption. The primary goals of treatment are to identify and treat the underlying cause of shock, optimize oxygen delivery, and decrease oxygen consumption.

Interventions to Optimize Oxygen Delivery

Supplemental oxygen may be administered in an attempt to improve oxygen delivery to hypoxic tissues. For patients who are conscious, are spontaneously breathing, and have adequate arterial blood gases, oxygen delivered by nasal cannula or mask may be all that is necessary. However, in the unconscious patient or in the patient demonstrating respiratory distress, intubation and mechanical ventilation may be required.

Administration of IV fluids assists in restoring optimal tissue perfusion by restoring preload and increasing the cardiac output component of oxygen delivery. The fluid best suited for shock states remains controversial. Usually, a combination of crystalloids and colloids is administered. Crystalloid solutions (e.g., lactated Ringer's solution) restore interstitial and intravascular fluid volumes, and increase preload and cardiac output. Administration of colloids enhances the blood's oxygen-carrying capacity. Colloids have oncotic capabilities not inherent in crystalloids. Packed red blood cells are usually given to provide adequate hemoglobin concentration and to increase oxygen-carrying capacity. Blood may be given with crystalloids to main-

tain adequate circulatory volume. Inotropic medications may be necessary if volume administration is not sufficient to improve oxygenation.

Positive inotropic drugs increase contractility by stimulating the beta$_1$ receptors in the heart. Increased contraction results in increased stroke volume as the ventricles eject more completely. Inotropic drugs that increase cardiac output and enhance tissue perfusion include dopamine, dobutamine, and milrinone. Dopamine has both alpha- and beta-receptor effects. In moderate doses (greater than 5 mcg/kg/min), beta$_1$ receptors are activated, and cardiac output increases. Larger doses (greater than 10 mcg/kg/min) stimulate alpha receptors and increase blood pressure. Dobutamine selectively acts on beta$_1$ receptors to increase contractility and cardiac output. Dobutamine also decreases SVR. Milrinone is a phosphodiesterase inhibitor that increases contractility, reduces SVR, and results in improved cardiac output. All inotropic drugs must be used with caution because they increase myocardial oxygen consumption.

Vasoactive drugs act on the smooth muscle layer of blood vessels and affect preload and afterload (Module 14). These drugs are either vasoconstrictors or vasodilators. Vasoconstrictors, or vasopressors, mimic the sympathetic nervous system to increase blood flow to vital organs by increasing blood pressure and cardiac output. Vasopressors include epinephrine, norepinephrine, dopamine, and vasopressin. These drugs increase SVR and blood pressure and should be given only when the patient's volume status is adequate (as reflected by RAP or PAWP or both).

Afterload-reducing (vasodilating) drugs improve cardiac output and oxygen delivery. Peripheral arterial vasodilators (nitroprusside, nitroglycerine) decrease SVR. When afterload is decreased, stroke volume is improved. The ventricles have less resistance to overcome and eject blood with less force. These drugs decrease preload as well as afterload and therefore should be used with caution in shock. Afterload-reducing drugs should be given only to patients who have adequate fluid volume. The patient must be monitored carefully so that the blood pressure does not become so low that reflex tachycardia occurs and coronary perfusion suffers.

In most circumstances, a combination of drugs may be advantageous. Combining an inotropic drug with a vasodilating drug can maximize oxygen delivery by increasing contractility and decreasing afterload. Sympathomimetic drugs are temporary agents because they do not treat the underlying cause of shock. They have a relatively short duration of action and can be easily titrated to the patient's rapidly changing condition.

Placing the patient in Trendelenburg's position is a controversial intervention used for the treatment of hypotension. Trendelenburg's position may displace blood from the systemic venules and small veins into the right heart and increase stroke volume. However, Trendelenburg's position may also increase afterload to the left ventricle and decrease stroke volume. Further research is needed to evaluate the effects of Trendelenburg's position on stroke volume and blood pressure.

The patient's response to treatment must be assessed frequently for signs of improved oxygen delivery. Signs of improved oxygen delivery include improvements in cardiac index, urine output, and mean arterial pressure (Module 14).

Interventions to Decrease Oxygen Consumption

In addition to optimizing oxygen delivery, interventions also should include measures to decrease oxygen consumption. Interventions to decrease oxygen consumption should be directed toward decreasing total body work, decreasing pain and anxiety, and decreasing temperature (Module 14).

Decreasing total body work is an attempt to decrease oxygen demands of all tissues. Hyperventilation occurs in an effort to increase oxygen delivery to meet demands, but this requires a great deal of effort, and the patient can rapidly develop respiratory distress. Ventilation is ensured with intubation and mechanical ventilation. Mechanical ventilation also decreases the respiratory muscle oxygen demands. Decreasing oxygen consumption of voluntary muscles can be achieved with neuromuscular blocking agents such as pancuronium (Pavulon) or vecuronium (Norcuron). These drugs eliminate unnecessary muscle activity and allow oxygen to be redirected for use in involuntary muscles, such as the heart. For patients in which chemical paralysis is not desirable (e.g., patients with head injury), the use of propofol (Diprovan) may be ideal. Propofol quickly induces deep sedation and has a short half-life. When the drug is discontinued, the patient is arousable within minutes. An evaluation of mental status can be performed. When the drug is resumed, deep sedation is induced.

Pain and anxiety stimulate the sympathetic nervous system to release catecholamines. Catecholamines increase metabolic rate and oxygen consumption. Measures are taken to minimize pain and anxiety. Appropriate analgesics and anxiolytics are administered.

Hyperthermia increases metabolic demands and oxygen requirements. This is controlled with antipyretic drugs, such as acetaminophen, or physical cooling measures, such as a fan or cooling blanket.

Interventions to optimize oxygen delivery and minimize oxygen consumption are used for all patients in shock. Individualized interventions are initiated to treat the underlying cause of shock. These interventions are described briefly in the following paragraphs.

Hypovolemic Shock States

The treatment goal for hypovolemic shock states is to restore fluid volume. In hypovolemic shock, the source of the fluid loss is identified and controlled. Additional intravenous fluids (crystalloid or colloid) are administered. Assess for an improvement in heart rate, blood pressure, and urine output. If no response is noted, additional fluids may be administered.

The treatment goals for neurogenic shock (see Module 21) are to maintain stability of the spine and optimize oxygen delivery. Because of unopposed parasympathetic innervation, patients with complete, cervical spinal cord injuries have hypotension and bradycardia. Preload is restored with IV fluids or vasopressors. A slight bradycardia requires close monitoring. If a marked bradycardia occurs, medications to increase heart rate may be given.

The immediate goals for treatment of anaphylactic shock are to maintain an airway and to support blood pressure. Oxygen may be administered. Epinephrine (subcutaneous or intravenous routes) may be given to restore vascular tone and blood pressure. Hypotension is treated with IV fluids to restore intravascular volume. Antihistamines (diphenhydramine), H_2 histamine antagonists (ranitidine), bronchodilators (inhaled or IV), and steroids may be used (Kemp & Lockey, 2002).

"Surviving sepsis campaign guidelines," management guidelines for severe sepsis and septic shock, were developed to improve outcomes. These multi-disciplinary guidelines provide evidence-based recommendations for the care of patients with severe sepsis and septic shock (Dellinger et al., 2004). A summary of the guidelines is presented in the following paragraphs; however the reader is encouraged to review the full set of guidelines written by Dellinger and colleagues (2004) or to visit the Surviving Sepsis Campaign website.

A nursing priority should be to administer antibiotics within one hour of a physician's order. Initial fluid resuscitation (using colloid or crystalloids) is given until the RAP is 8–12 mm Hg, MAP greater than 65 mm Hg, urine output greater than 0.5 mL/kg/hr, or central or mixed venous oxygen saturation is greater than 70 percent. Administration of blood products and/or dobutamine may be required to achieve these goals. Fluids may be given at a rate of 500–1000 mL for crystalloids or 300–500 mL for colloids over 30 minutes; these doses may be repeated based on response of increases in urine output and blood pressure. Red blood cell transfusion is given only when Hb is less than 7 g/dL.

Vasopressors (norepinephrine or dopamine administered through a central line) may be administered to restore blood pressure even when hypovolemia has not yet been completely corrected. All patients receiving vasopressors should have an arterial catheter in place to monitor blood pressure. Vasopressin may be used to treat hypotension that does not respond to norepinephrine or dopamine. Corticosteroids may be given to patients with septic shock who, despite adequate fluid replacement, require vasopressor therapy to maintain adequate blood pressure. Historically, low-dose dopamine was used to increase renal perfusion and urine output. However, this practice is no longer recommended.

Administration of neuromuscular blocking agents is only used for the first few hours of mechanical ventilation. If they are used for longer periods, the depth of blockade is determined using train-of-four monitoring. Blood glucose levels are maintained to less than 150 mg/dL with continuous IV insulin infusion. Nutritional support should be provided using the enteral route. Prevention of deep vein thrombosis is accomplished with the administration of either low-dose unfractionated heparin or low-molecular weight heparin. Prevention of stress ulcer formation is accomplished with the administration of H_2 receptor inhibitors. Communication with the patient and family must include realistic treatment goals and likely outcomes. Decisions to limit support or withdrawal of support may be in the patient's best interest.

Evidence-Based Practice

- *Early goal-directed therapy provides significant benefits in patients with severe sepsis and septic shock. Early goal-directed therapy is defined as achieving the following parameters within 72 hours of diagnosis: RAP 8 to 12 mm Hg, MAP greater than 65 mm Hg and less than 90 mm Hg, central venous oxygen saturation greater than 70 percent (Rivers et al., 2001).*

- *During the first 6 hours of initial resuscitation of sepsis-induced hypoperfusion, the following parameters should be used as treatment goals: RAP 8 to 12 mm Hg, MAP greater than 65 mm Hg; urine output greater than 0.5 mL/kg/hr, SvO_2 less than 70 percent (Dellinger et al., 2004).*

- *To optimize identification of causative organisms of sepsis, at least two blood cultures should be obtained with at least one drawn percutaneously and one drawn through each vascular access device unless the device was recently (less than 48 hours) inserted (Dellinger et al., 2004).*

- *Intravenous antibiotics should be started within the first hour of diagnosis of severe sepsis after appropriate cultures have been obtained (Dellinger et al., 2004).*

- *Following stabilization of patients with severe sepsis, blood glucose should be maintained less than 150 mg/dL by the use of a continuous insulin infusion. Serum blood glucose should be monitored every 30 to 60 minutes initially; once the serum glucose stabilizes, serum glucose should be monitored on a regular basis (Dellinger et al., 2004).*

Research into the pathophysiologic processes involved in sepsis and septic shock has highlighted the role of the coagulation cascade. A key feature of this pathophysiology is microscopic clots that occlude blood flow to organs. Under normal circumstances, these clots are degraded by the body's fibrinolytic system. However, during septic shock, activated protein C (APC), a key component of fibrinolysis, is consumed at such a rate that clot dissolution is impeded (Schulman & Hare, 2003). APC not only plays a role in the coagulation cascade but it also has anti-inflammatory properties (Schulman & Hare, 2003). Repletion of the stores of APC shows promise in the treatment of septic shock (Bernard et al., 2001). Drotrecogin alfa is a recombinant APC that can be administered IV. Patients receiving drotrecogin alfa have a higher recovery rate from septic shock than those patients not receiving the drug (Dellinger, 2003). Patients at high risk of bleeding should not be treated with APC because bleeding is the most frequent and serious adverse event induced by this drug (Fourrier, 2004).

Transport Shock States

The treatment goal for transport shock states is to restore the oxygen-carrying capacity of red blood cells. For the treatment of anemia or hemorrhage, packed red blood cells may be administered in an effort to provide an adequate Hb concentration.

The treatment for carbon monoxide poisoning consists of the administration of high-fractional concentrations of supplemental oxygen. Data indicate that early, aggressive hyperbaric oxygen therapy may decrease the negative sequelae of carbon monoxide poisoning (Hampson et al., 2001). Serial carboxyhemoglobin levels should be monitored to evaluate patient response to treatment.

Obstructive Shock States

The treatment goal for obstructive shock states is to remove the mechanical barrier to blood flow. For a tension pneumothorax, trapped air is decompressed by a physician with the insertion of a 14-gauge needle or a chest tube. Needle pericardiocentesis may decompress the pericardium for cardiac tamponade. This decompression should improve the heart's pumping ability. If not, a thoracotomy may be required to surgically control and decompress the tamponade.

The cornerstone of management for pulmonary embolism is heparin because it prevents additional thrombi from forming and permits fibrinolysis to dissolve some of the clot (Torbicki et al., 2000). Inferior vena cava filters may be used in the presence of active hemorrhage or recurrent pulmonary embolism despite intensive prolonged anticoagulation (Torbicki et al., 2000). The use of thrombolytic therapy or surgical embolectomy may be necessary in the face of hemodynamic instability and shock (Torbicki et al., 2000).

Cardiogenic Shock States

The specific treatment for cardiogenic shock is based on the cardiac abnormality and whether the shock is caused by left-sided or right-sided heart failure. Nursing and medical interventions for patients in cardiogenic shock are directed toward decreasing myocardial oxygen demand and improving myocardial oxygen supply.

The initial management of the patient in cardiogenic shock may include fluid resuscitation (unless pulmonary edema is present), placement of central venous and arterial catheters, urinary catheterization, pulse oximetry, airway protection, correction of electrolyte abnormalities, and relief of pain and anxiety (Hollenberg, 2001).

Inotropic agents may be used in patients with normovolemia but inadequate tissue perfusion. Dobutamine can be used to improve myocardial contractility and increase cardiac output (Hollenberg, 2001). Hemodynamic monitoring using a pulmonary artery catheter permits serial measurements of CO, which allows titration of inotropic and vasopressor drugs to the minimum dose required to achieve therapeutic goals. Diuretics may be used to treat pulmonary congestion. Vasodilators may be used (after blood pressure has been stabilized) to decrease both preload and afterload. Further treatment may include thrombolytic therapy, an intra-aortic balloon pump, and revascularization (angioplasty or coronary artery bypass surgery).

Thrombolytic therapy reduces mortality rates in patients with acute myocardial infarction (MI), however, the benefits of this therapy in patients with cardiogenic shock are less certain. Thrombolytic therapy can reduce the likelihood of developing cardiogenic shock after initial presentation (Hollenberg, 2001). An intra-aortic balloon pump (IABP) reduces afterload and augments coronary perfusion, which increase cardiac output and improve coronary blood flow. The IABP is inserted into the femoral artery and advanced until it is in the descending thoracic aorta. The IABP is synchronized with the patient's heart rate. During ventricular diastole, the balloon inflates. With the balloon inflated, the blood distal to the balloon is forced back toward the aortic valve. This supplies the coronary arteries with additional oxygenated blood to meet myocardial oxygen needs.

Before ventricular systole, the balloon deflates, which decreases pressure in the aorta. This makes it easier for the left ventricle to contract and eject its stroke volume. In hospitals without direct angioplasty capabilities, stabilization with IABP and thrombolysis followed by transfer to a tertiary care facility may be the best treatment option (Hollenberg, 2001).

Mechanical revascularization for patients with cardiogenic shock caused by MI can be done. Direct percutaneous transluminal coronary angioplasty (PTCA) may be used to improve wall motion in the infarct area and increase perfusion of the infarct zone. In patients with cardiogenic shock who have either left main coronary artery or three vessel coronary disease, coronary artery bypass surgery may be performed (Hollenberg, 2001).

In the case of patients who present with advanced cardiac disease in which PTCA and bypass surgery is of no benefit, the use of left ventricular assist devices (LVAD) may be the only other option. There are three potential uses for LVADs. First, the LVAD may be used as a short-term mechanism to rest the injured myocardium, after which point it is removed from the patient (Bond et al., 2003). If the myocardium does not recover, the LVAD may be left in as a bridge to cardiac transplantation (Bond et al., 2003). Finally, in those patients who are not suitable for transplant, there are some LVADs approved for permanent use (Bond et al., 2003). The major risks of LVADs include infection, stroke, and device malfunction (Bond et al., 2003).

In summary, the primary goals of treatment for shock are to optimize oxygen delivery and decrease oxygen consumption. Interventions that optimize oxygen delivery include supplemental oxygen administration, restoration of intravascular fluid volume, administration of inotropic and vasoactive drugs, and Trendelenburg's position. Improved oxygen delivery should be assessed in terms of improved cardiac output, increased urine output, a decrease in heart rate, and an increase in blood pressure. Interventions that decrease oxygen consumption include decreasing total body work through adequate ventilation and neuromuscular blocking agents, minimizing pain and stress, and correcting hyperthermia. Further and more individualized interventions are directed at treating the underlying cause of shock for each of the four functional shock states.

SECTION FOUR REVIEW

You have been assigned to provide nursing care to Mr. J, a 74-year-old male with a diagnosis of septic shock. During the change-of-shift report, you are given the following information:

- Vital signs: blood pressure 70/42 mm Hg, pulse 140 bpm sinus tachycardia, respirations 38/minute, temperature 103°F
- Ventilator settings: SIMV 10, FiO_2 40 percent, tidal volume 350 mL, PEEP 5 cm H_2O
- Recent laboratory results: ABGs: pH 7.25, $PaCO_2$ 30, PaO_2 60, HCO_3 18, base deficit 8, Hct 27 percent, Hb 8 g/dL, Na 140 mEq/L, K 4.5 mEq/L
- Hemodynamic readings: MAP 51 mm Hg, RAP 3 mm Hg, PAP 18/8 mm Hg, PAWP 8 mm Hg, CO 4 L/min, SVR 356 dynes/sec/m^2
- IV fluids: D_5 and 1/2 NS plus 20 mEq KCl at 100 mL/hr
- Urine output past 8 hours: 160 mL/hr

As you walk to Mr. J.'s bedside, you note that he is pale and restless. He is lying in the semi-Fowler's position. Answer the following questions based on the information provided about Mr. J.

1. Which of the following would best increase Mr. J.'s cardiac output and restore preload?
   A. acetominophen
   B. O_2 therapy by nasal cannula
   C. low-dose dopamine
   D. LR at 200 mL/hr
2. Which of the following indicate that Mr. J.'s oxygen delivery is improving?
   A. pH 7.40
   B. RAP 1 mm Hg
   C. Hct 27 percent
   D. respiratory rate of 38/min
3. Which of the following indicates Mr. J. has increased oxygen consumption?
   A. sinus tachycardia
   B. temperature 103°F

C. respirations 38 per minute
   D. all of the above
4. Mr. J. may require vasopressors. Which of the following may be administered?
   A. norepinephrine
   B. dopamine
   C. dobutamine
   D. A and B are correct
5. The physician orders an antibiotic. The nurse must administer this drug within _____ hour(s) of the written order.
   A. one
   B. two
   C. four
   D. eight

Answers: 1. D, 2. A, 3. D, 4. D, 5. A

POSTTEST

1. Conditions common to all shock states are
   A. decreased blood pressure, heart rate, and urine output
   B. increased oxygen delivery with increased oxygen consumption
   C. impaired oxygen delivery with altered oxygen consumption
   D. decreased blood pressure, increased heart rate, and decreased urine output
2. Transport shock states have impaired oxygen delivery because
   A. a barrier impedes blood flow to tissues
   B. there is a loss of intravascular volume
   C. hemoglobin is unavailable to carry oxygen
   D. decreased sympathetic tone produces vasoconstriction
3. Vasodilation and maldistribution of circulating volume characterize
   A. anaphylactic shock
   B. septic shock
   C. neurogenic shock
   D. obstructive shock
4. ACTH and ADH
   A. cause sodium and water depletion
   B. are chemoreceptors that sense alterations in pH and Pa_{CO_2}
   C. release norepinephrine
   D. conserve blood volume by retaining sodium and water

5. The net effects of the renin-angiotensin-aldosterone cycle in compensatory shock are
   A. increased blood pressure through vasoconstriction
   B. increased venous return through retention of sodium and water
   C. increased urine output to eliminate fluid
   D. A and B are correct
6. Which of the following characterize the refractory stage of shock?
   A. decreased CO, decreased tissue perfusion
   B. release of neuroendocrine hormones to restore CO
   C. dysfunction of cardiac and renal systems
   D. profound hypotension despite administration of vasoactive drugs
7. Clinical signs of hypovolemic shock include
   A. cool skin, increased pulse, and low RAP
   B. warm skin, decreased pulse, and decreased CO
   C. cool skin, increased pulse, and increased CO
   D. warm skin, increased pulse, and low RAP
8. Systemic venous congestion is a manifestation of
   A. left ventricular failure
   B. right ventricular failure
   C. anaphylactic shock
   D. cardiac tamponade

9. Pulsus paradoxus is a classic sign of
   A. cardiac tamponade
   B. neurogenic shock
   C. carbon monoxide poisoning
   D. septic shock
10. Crystalloid solutions
   A. can increase the Hct by 2 to 3 percent
   B. are given to supplement Hb concentrations
   C. restore fluid volumes and increase preload
   D. possess oncotic capabilities
11. Afterload-reducing drugs
   A. increase blood pressure and CO
   B. restrict blood flow to internal organs

   C. produce vasodilation and improve SV
   D. produce vasoconstriction and increase myocardial oxygen consumption
12. According to the Surviving Sepsis Campaign Guidelines, patients who receive vasopressors should also receive
   A. vasodilators
   B. inotropic medications
   C. an arterial catheter to monitor blood pressure
   D. both A and B are correct

POSTTEST ANSWERS

Question	Answer	Section
1	C	One
2	C	One
3	B	One
4	D	Two
5	D	Two
6	D	Two

Question	Answer	Section
7	A	Three
8	B	Three
9	A	Three
10	C	Four
11	C	Four
12	C	Four

REFERENCES

Bernard, G. R. (2003). Clinical trials in sepsis: Research data II. In M. M. Levy & J. L. Vincent (Eds.), *Sepsis: Pathophysiological insight and current management* (pp. 65–72). Chicago, IL: Society of Critical Care Medicine.

Bernard, G. R., Vincent J. L., Laterre, P. F., et al. (2001). Efficacy and safety of recombinant human activated protein C for severe sepsis. *New England Journal of Medicine, 344,* 699–709.

Bond, A. E., Nelson, K., Germany, C. L., & Smart, A. N. (2003). The left ventricular assist device. *American Journal of Nursing, 103,* 32–40.

Boswell, S. A., & Scalea, T. M. (2003). Sublingual capnometry: An alternative to gastric tonometry for the management of shock resuscitation. *AACN Clinical Issues, 14,* 176–184.

Clochesy, J. M. (Ed.). (1998). *Essentials of critical care nursing* (p. 127). Rockville, MD: Aspen publishing.

Dellinger, R. P. (2003). Inflammation and coagulation: Implications for the septic patient. *Clinical Infectious Disease, 36,* 1259–1265.

Dellinger R. P., Carlet J. M., Masur H., et al. (2004). Surviving sepsis campaign guidelines for management of severe sepsis and septic shock. *Critical Care Medicine, 32,* 858–873.

Fourrier, F. (2004). Recombinant human activated protein C in the treatment of severe sepsis: An evidence-based review. *Critical Care Medicine, 32* [Suppl.], S534–S541.

Hampson, N. B., Mathieu, D., Piantadosi, C. A., et al. (2001). Carbon monoxide poisoning: Interpretation of randomized clinical trials and unresolved treatment issues. *Undersea and Hyperbaric Medicine, 28,* 157–164.

Hollenberg, S. M. (2001). Cardiogenic shock. *Critical Care Clinics, 17,* 391–410.

Kemp, S. F., & Lockey, R. F. (2002). Anaphylaxis: A review of causes and mechanisms. *Journal of Allergy and Clinical Immunology, 110,* 341–348.

Rice, V. (1991). Shock: A clinical syndrome. An update. Part 1. *Critical Care Nurse, 11*(4), 20–27.

Rivers, E., Nguyen B., Havstad S., et al. (2001). Early goal directed therapy in the treatment of severe sepsis and septic shock. *New England Journal of Medicine, 345,* 1368–1377.

Schulman, C. S., & Hare, K. (2003). New thoughts of sepsis: The unifier of critical care. *Dimensions of Critical Care Nursing, 22,* 20–30.

Torbicki, A., van Beek, E. J. R., Charbonnier, B., et al. (2000). Guidelines on diagnosis and management of acute pulmonary embolism. *European Heart Journal, 21,* 1301–1336.

Vincent, J., de Carvalho, F. B., & De Backer, D. (2002). Management of septic shock. *Annals Medicine, 34,* 606–613.

Weaver, K. L. (1999). Carbon dioxide poisoning. *Critical Care Clinics, 15,* 297–317.

MODULE 16

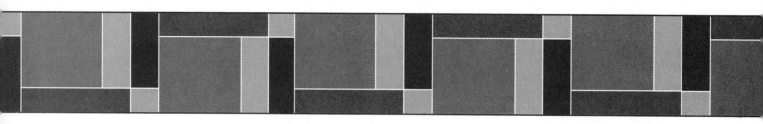

Multiple Organ Dysfunction Syndrome

Karen L. Johnson

OBJECTIVES Following completion of this module, the learner will be able to

1. State the physiologic changes that occur during the local inflammatory process.

2. Contrast the physiologic changes that occur with the local inflammatory response with those that occur with the systemic inflammatory response syndrome.

3. State four pathophysiologic changes that occur with multiple organ dysfunction syndrome.

4. Identify the seven most common organ systems that fail as a result of the SIRS process.

5. Describe the collaborative management of the patient with multiple organ dysfunction syndrome.

Multiple organ dysfunction syndrome (MODS) is a syndrome characterized by the progressive dysfunction of two or more organ systems. The clinical course of MODS typically results in prolonged hospital stays, during which potentially enormous resources are utilized. Despite the expenditure of significant time, resources, and technology, the mortality rate from MODS remains high. Through identification of risk factors and timely interventions, nurses can have an important role in detecting and preventing this highly lethal cascade of events.

This self-study module describes the local inflammatory response to injury (Section One), how the local response can progress to pathophysiologic changes associated with a systemic inflammatory response (Section Two), and the progression to multiple organ system dysfunction syndrome (Section Three). As pathophysiologic changes continue, organ involvement and dysfunction can occur remote from the initial site of injury (Section Four). Nursing management of the patient with MODS and organ dysfunction is presented in Section Five.

Each section includes a set of review questions to help the learner evaluate his or her understanding of the section's content before moving on to the next section. All Section Reviews and the module Pretest and Posttest include answers. It is suggested that the learner review those concepts answered incorrectly in the review questions before proceeding to the next section.

 PRETEST

1. Which of the following elicit the inflammatory response?
   A. mediators
   B. endotoxin
   C. bacteria
   D. heat

2. Which of the following cells are most important in the inflammatory process?
   A. neutrophils
   B. mast cells
   C. epithelial cells
   D. endothelial cells

3. Systemic inflammatory response syndrome (SIRS) can be characterized by all of the following EXCEPT
   A. temperature greater than 38°C (100°F)
   B. heart rate less than 80 beats per minute
   C. white blood cells greater than 12,000 cells/mm^3
   D. immature bands (greater than 10 percent)
4. A theory has emerged that suggests the SIRS response is rapidly followed by
   A. death
   B. septic shock
   C. mixed antagonistic response syndrome
   D. compensatory anti-inflammatory response syndrome
5. MODS is a progressive dysfunction of at least
   A. one organ
   B. two organ systems
   C. three organ systems
   D. four organ systems
6. Two forms of MODS are
   A. initial and progressive
   B. progressive and refractory
   C. local and systemic
   D. primary and secondary
7. Which of the following is essential to preventing mortality in MODS?
   A. early recognition and management of MODS
   B. strict aseptic technique
   C. preventing febrile states
   D. strict handwashing
8. Jaundice and coagulopathy characterize
   A. renal failure
   B. hematologic failure
   C. liver failure
   D. MODS

Pretest Answers:
1. A, 2. D, 3. B, 4. D, 5. B, 6. D, 7. A, 8. C

GLOSSARY

apoptosis   Programmed cell death.

cytopathic hypoxia   A pathologic state in which tissue hypoxia results from derangements in the cellular use of oxygen in the face of adequate oxygen delivery.

mediators   A broad category of bioactive substances that stimulate physiologic change in cells.

multiple organ dysfunction syndrome (MODS)   The presence of altered organ function in an acutely ill patient such that homeostasis cannot be maintained without intervention.

primary MODS   Organ dysfunction directly related to an organ insult.

secondary MODS   An abnormal and excessive inflammatory response as a consequence of the patient's response to a secondary insult.

sepsis   A subcategory of systemic inflammatory response syndrome.

systemic inflammatory response syndrome (SIRS)   A term used to describe a condition in which there is a systemic (rather than local) inflammatory process.

ABBREVIATIONS

ARDS	Acute respiratory distress syndrome	**MARS**	Mixed antagonistic response syndrome
CARS	Compensatory anti-inflammatory response syndrome	**MODS**	Multiple organ dysfunction syndrome
CO	Cardiac output	**Pao$_2$**	Partial pressure of oxygen in arterial blood
DIC	Disseminated intravascular coagulation	**PAR**	Pressure adjusted heart rate
Fio$_2$	Fraction of inspired oxygen	**RAP**	Right atrial pressure
GI	Gastrointestinal	**SIRS**	Systemic inflammatory response syndrome
HR	Heart rate	**WBC**	White blood cell
MAP	Mean arterial pressure		

TABLE 16–1 Functions of Endothelial Cells

Mediate vasomotor tone
Maintain vessel wall integrity
Control cellular and nutrient "traffic"
Regulate inflammatory and anti-inflammatory mediators
Participate in generating new blood vessels
Undergo apoptosis

SECTION ONE: The Endothelial Cell and Local Inflammatory Response

At the completion of this section, the learner will be able to state the physiologic changes that occur during the local inflammatory process.

An initiating event, such as an injury, invading organism, or ischemia, can trigger inflammation. The goal of a local inflammatory process is to limit the extent of injury and promote healing. Normally, the inflammatory process is contained within a local environment by a complex system of checks and balances. Mediators elicit the inflammatory response. **Mediators** are bioactive substances that stimulate physiologic changes in cells. They are released from endothelial cells.

Endothelial cells are not simply cells that line the inside of all blood vessels; they have many important functions (Aird, 2003) (Table 16–1). They are very active cells that are constantly sensing and responding to alterations in the local cell environment. They are activated by alterations in the local environment, such as minor trauma to blood vessels, transient bacteria, and stress. Endothelial cell activation is a normal adaptive response under physiologic conditions, but it also occurs in response to pathophysiologic conditions. When bacteria invade local tissues, endothelial cells are activated and release mediators. These mediators stimulate the inflammatory process, recruit white blood cells to the area, and promote localized clotting to contain the infection. During this process, endothelial cells undergo necrosis and **apoptosis,** or programmed cell death, as tissues are repaired.

The endothelium orchestrates this local physiologic response by promoting the adhesion and transmigration of white blood cells, altering local vasomotor tone, increasing permeability, inducing thrombin generation and fibrin formation, and triggering apoptosis (McCuskey et al., 1996). Normally, local and systemic negative feedback mechanisms maintain the response at local sites and dampen the response at more remote sites (Munford & Pugin, 2001).

How endothelial cells respond to alterations in the environment differ. The endothelium responds in ways that differ according to the host genetics, age, gender, nature of the pathogen, and location of the vascular bed (Aird, 2003). Endothelial cells can undergo intracellular structural changes in their cell membranes, cytoplasm, or nucleus (Vallet & Wiel, 2001). However, they more commonly undergo functional changes that include shifts in intracellular homeostatic balance, adhesion of certain cells (particularly white blood cells) to their cell membrane, altered vasomotor tone regulation, loss of barrier function, and apoptosis (Aird, 2003).

Containment of the localized inflammatory response limits further damage to the host and preserves the integrity of uninvolved endothelial cells. However, when the host response generalizes, it escapes the well-developed local checks and balances, resulting in an unregulated inflammatory response with widespread involvement of endothelial cells and a more generalized activation of inflammation and coagulation (Aird, 2003). This type of generalized response can lead to systemic inflammatory response syndrome (SIRS) and multiple organ dysfunction syndrome (MODS), which are discussed in the next sections.

In summary, an initiating event, such as an injury or invading organism, can trigger a localized inflammatory response. The response begins when these events activate endothelial cells that release mediators to stimulate the inflammatory process, recruit white blood cells, and promote localized clotting. During this process endothelial cells undergo necrosis and apoptosis. This inflammatory response occurs in a contained area to prevent further damage and to maintain the integrity of uninvolved endothelial cells. When the inflammatory response generalizes, it results in an unregulated inflammatory response characterized by inflammation and coagulation.

SECTION ONE REVIEW

1. A local inflammatory response can be initiated by all of the following EXCEPT
   A. injury
   B. ischemia
   C. bacteria
   D. biologically active mediators
2. Mediators stimulate the local inflammatory response. They are released from activated
   A. platelets
   B. endothelial cells
   C. epithelial cells
   D. bacteria
3. The endothelium orchestrates the local inflammatory response by all of the following EXCEPT
   A. decreasing capillary permeability
   B. promoting adhesion of white blood cells
   C. altering local vasomotor tone
   D. inducing thrombin generation

Answers: 1. D, 2. B, 3. A

SECTION TWO: Systemic Inflammatory Response Syndrome

At the completion of this section, the learner will be able to contrast the physiologic changes that occur with the local inflammatory response with those that occur with the systemic inflammatory response syndrome.

As discussed in Section One, localized inflammation is a physiologic defense mechanism that occurs in response to an injury, ischemia, or an invading pathogen. Containment of the localized inflammatory response limits further damage to the host and preserves the integrity of uninvolved endothelial cells. This response must be tightly controlled by the body at the local injury site or the response becomes overly activated, leading to an exaggerated, systemic response. When the local inflammatory response becomes generalized, a dysregulated inflammatory response occurs with widespread endothelial cell involvement and a more generalized activation of inflammation and coagulation (Aird, 2003).

The **systemic inflammatory response syndrome (SIRS)** is a term used to describe a condition in which there is a systemic (rather than local) inflammatory process. The initiating event may be caused by infection, trauma, major surgery, acute pancreatitis, or burns (Brun-Buisson, 2000). This systemic response is manifested by two or more conditions as listed in Table 16–2 (American College of Chest Physicians & Society of Critical Care Medicine, 1992).

TABLE 16–2 Definition of SIRS

Two or more of the following:
Temperature greater than 38°C or less than 36°C
Heart rate greater than 90 beats per min
Respiratory rate greater than 20 breaths/min or Paco$_2$ less than 32 mm Hg
White blood cell count greater than 12,000/mm^3 or less than 4,000/mm^3, or greater than 10 percent immature (band) forms

The term *SIRS* recognizes that in critical illness, clinical inflammation can arise from infectious and noninfectious stimuli. SIRS denotes systemic inflammation regardless of its cause. When the cause of SIRS is infection, the process is termed **sepsis.** The term *MODS* indicates that this complication is variable in what specific organ systems are involved and in the magnitude of physiologic derangement that occurs.

Some patients with infection, trauma, or surgery will have only mild SIRS and minor organ dysfunction that resolves rapidly (Jacobi, 2002), whereas others exhibit a massive inflammatory reaction and die from profound shock. The frequent association of MODS with sepsis, SIRS, acute respiratory distress syndrome (ARDS), and other inflammatory processes suggests there is a link to the complex pathophysiologic processes that are characteristic of SIRS (Balk, 2000). A theory has emerged that suggests that the SIRS response is rapidly followed in most patients by a compensatory anti-inflammatory response syndrome (CARS) (Balk, 2000). CARS occurs in an attempt to limit SIRS. The balance between proinflammatory (SIRS) and anti-inflammatory (CARS) has been referred to as the mixed antagonistic response syndrome (MARS). The balance is difficult to achieve and typically either proinflammatory or anti-inflammatory responses predominate. When there are excessive proinflammatory responses, organ dysfunction is likely to occur. When there is excessive anti-inflammatory response, the patient is at risk for secondary or opportunistic infections, which serve as additional insults to trigger the SIRS response (Balk, 2000; Bone et al., 1997).

In summary, SIRS is a systemic inflammatory response to an initiating event, such as trauma, infection, major surgery, burns, or pancreatitis. SIRS is manifested by at least two of the following: hypo/hyperthermia, tachypnea or hypercapnea, or leukopenia or leukocytosis. The pathogenesis of SIRS is linked with other inflammatory processes including sepsis, MODS, and ARDS. SIRS may be modulated by CARS. When excessive SIRS occurs, then MODS is more likely to occur. When excessive CARS occurs, secondary infections are more likely to occur.

SECTION TWO REVIEW

1. All of the following may cause SIRS EXCEPT
   A. obesity
   B. infection
   C. trauma
   D. major surgery
2. Your patient is assessed to have the following: temperature 39.5°C, heart rate 110 beats per minute, respiratory rate 12/min, WBC 15,000 cells/mm^3 with greater than 10 percent bands. This patient may have which of the following?
   A. MODS
   B. bacteremia

   C. SIRS
   D. a local inflammatory response
3. The pathogenesis of SIRS is
   A. not associated with MODS
   B. associated with MODS
   C. occurs in an attempt to limit CARS
   D. associated with an excessive anti-inflammatory response

Answers: 1. A, 2. C, 3. B

SECTION THREE: Multiple Organ Dysfunction Syndrome

At the completion of this section, the learner will be able to state four pathophysiologic changes that occur with MODS.

Multiple organ dysfunction syndrome (MODS), a complication of critical illness, is characterized by progressive (but potentially reversible) dysfunction of two or more organ systems and develops after an acute life-threatening disruption of systemic body homeostasis (Khadaroo & Marshall, 2002). Physiologic derangements of MODS occur as the result of an insult that initiates the inflammatory response. Although infection is the most common insult, numerous other stimuli have been implicated and are recognized as being risk factors for developing MODS. The pathophysiology of MODS is complex and not completely understood. It appears that MODS is the result of uncontrolled systemic infection (Offner & Moore, 2000).

MODS appears to follow two distinct pathways (Figure 16–1). **Primary MODS** occurs as the direct consequence of an initiating event. It occurs early and may be the direct consequence of injury, hemorrhage, or hypoxemia (Fry, 2000). Primary MODS is thought to be the result of inadequate oxygen delivery to cells and a failure of the microcirculation to remove metabolic end products. As progressively more cells die, organ dysfunction and failure occur. Acute tubular necrosis is an example of primary MODS. **Secondary MODS** is an event that occurs later in the patient's course, often weeks after the initial acute insult, and is thought to be secondary to SIRS (Fry, 2000). The initial insult is thought to prime the inflammatory response and a second insult reactivates it at an exaggerated level.

Risk factors for primary and secondary MODS have been identified. Risk factors for primary MODS include severity of injury, shock, or SIRS, and risk factors for secondary MODS include infection, transfusion, and multiple surgical operations (Offner & Moore, 2000). Advancing age and preexisting medical conditions have also been identified as host factors for MODS (Offner & Moore, 2000) (Table 16–3).

The pathophysiology of MODS is complex. Literally hundreds of biochemical and cellular abnormalities have been described. According to Marshall (2001), there are four prominent explanations for the pathologic changes that occur with MODS,

TABLE 16–3   Advancing Age and MODS

Those over 45 years of age have two to three times greater likelihood of developing MODS

Advancing age affects all organ systems

Worse outcome in elderly is attributed to presence of preexisting conditions (cirrhosis, ischemic heart disease, COPD, diabetes)

Advancing age decreases functional reserve and impairs stress response

including (1) uncontrolled systemic inflammation, (2) tissue hypoxia, (3) unregulated apoptosis, and (4) microvascular coagulopathy.

Uncontrolled Systemic Inflammation

Clinical evidence of systemic inflammation is evident in almost all patients with MODS (Marshall, 2001). A large number of proinflammatory mediators have been implicated in initiating and potentiating a systemic inflammatory response, but the mechanisms through which these mediators induce organ injury are not clear. Proinflammatory mediators can increase capillary permeability resulting in edema in organs such as the lungs (ARDS) or brain (altered sensorium) (Khadarro & Marshall, 2002). Proinflammatory mediators cause the release of nitric oxide from endothelial cells, which results in vasodilation. Neutrophils induce the release of oxygen radicals and proteolytic enzymes (Marshall, 2001). Neutrophils also potentiate increased vascular permeability.

Tissue Hypoxia

Decreased oxygen delivery or reduced cellular use of oxygen inhibits normal cell function. Current theories on the pathophysiology of MODS indicate that the common pathway to organ dysfunction is cellular hypoxia (Marshall, 2001). Even though the patient may appear clinically to have adequate oxygenation, regional tissue hypoxia may occur, particularly in the intestinal tract and brain. Tissue hypoxia may result from derangements in the cellular use of oxygen in the face of adequate oxygen delivery, a pathologic state termed **cytopathic hypoxia** (Schwartz et al., 1999).

Figure 16–1 ■ MODS pathways.

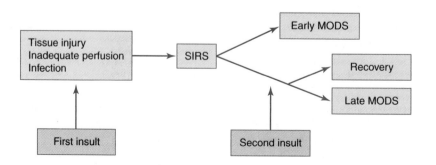

Unregulated Apoptosis

The controlled process of cellular death is called apoptosis. Derangements in the normal expression of apoptosis appear to be important in MODS. There appears to be an increase in apoptosis in some cell types (lymphocytes, gut epithelial cells) and delayed apoptosis with others (neutrophils) (Khadaroo & Marshall, 2002). In addition, excessive apoptosis occurs in certain organ systems, such as the liver, kidney, and heart (Marshall, 2001).

Microvascular Coagulopathy

The coagulopathy associated with MODS is biologically complex and intertwined with normal physiologic processes. The mechanisms that regulate inflammation are linked with those that control coagulation. Microvascular thrombosis is an important factor in the development of MODS.

Coagulation is initiated through tissue factor on the endothelial cell membrane. Tissue factor is released in response to the presence of endotoxin, or inflammatory cytokines (Marshall, 2001). Tissue factor activates factor VII of the extrinsic pathway of the coagulation cascade. The end result of the coagulation cascade is the formation of fibrin clots. The fibrin clot plays a critical role in hemostasis and localizing microorganisms. However, these microvascular clots impede blood flow and oxygen delivery to cells. This leads to the release of further inflammatory mediators. Anticoagulation mechanisms, such as those mediated by activated protein C, are impaired. Protein C is activated in the presence of thrombin that is bound to thrombomodulin. Activated protein C acts as a feedback messenger to inhibit further thrombin generation. In addition to its antithrombotic properties, activated protein C has anti-inflammatory and profibrinolytic properties (Ely et al., 2003). Clinical studies indicate that administration of activated protein C improves outcomes of patients with sepsis (Bernard et al., 2001b) (see Module 15). Drotrecogin alpha (activated), a recumbent form of human activated protein C, has been shown to decrease markers of coagulation and inflammation (Bernard et al., 2001a).

In summary, MODS appears to follow one of two pathways: primary MODS or secondary MODS. Primary MODs is the direct result of injury, hemorrhage, or hypoxemia. Secondary MODS occurs later in the course of acute illness and is thought to occur as a result of a "second hit," which activates SIRS. There are multiple risk factors for MODS including advancing age and preexisting medical conditions. The pathophysiology is complex, but it appears to occur as the result of uncontrolled systemic inflammation, tissue hypoxia, dysregulated apoptosis, and microvascular coagulopathy.

SECTION THREE REVIEW

1. MODS is characterized by the dysfunction of how many organ systems?
   A. one
   B. two or more
   C. three or more
   D. four or more
2. Primary MODS can occur in response to
   A. the insult itself
   B. secondary complications

   C. an exaggerated SIRS
   D. septic shock
3. Advancing age is a risk factor for developing MODS because the elderly
   A. don't have money to pay for services
   B. don't take antibiotics as prescribed
   C. have decreased functional reserve
   D. have increased functional reserve

Answers: 1. B, 2. A, 3. C

SECTION FOUR: Organ Involvement and Failure

At the completion of this section, the learner will be able to identify the seven most common organ systems that fail as a result of the SIRS process.

As the pathophysiologic changes, discussed in Section Three, continue, organ dysfunction continues. Organ dysfunction can occur far from the initial injury site as a result of SIRS. Mediators enable organ-to-organ interaction. Organ ischemia and cellular damage perpetuate SIRS, which perpetuates MODS. A vicious cycle develops. As each additional organ fails, mortality escalates.

Several different scoring systems and assessment tools have been proposed for the use of quantifying the extent of organ system dysfunction, but to date there has not been uniform acceptance of one tool over another. Most of the proposed tools use an assessment of seven major organ systems: respiratory, cardiovascular, neurologic, renal, hepatic, gastrointestinal, and hematologic. Most of the tools have been primarily used in clinical trials. Evaluation of disease severity involves assessment of several major organ systems for common indications of dysfunction in those organs.

The lungs are usually the first to show signs of dysfunction, and respiratory failure rapidly progresses to ARDS. The respiratory system is the main organ system affected in MODS (Offner

& Moore, 2000). Many conditions have been associated with ARDS either as a direct result of injury to the lung or as a result of a pulmonary response to a systemic insult. The most common direct, nonsurgical cause of ARDS is pneumonia (Lee & Angus, 2000). ARDS risk factors in the surgical patient and trauma patient include sepsis, major trauma, multiple transfusions, aspiration of gastric contents, pulmonary contusion, pneumonia, and smoke inhalation (Barie & Hydo, 2000). The lungs are particularly at risk for dysfunction because the pulmonary capillary bed acts as a filter that is exposed to cytokines, mediators, and activated neutrophils. This results in increased vascular permeability and interstitial edema, which impairs pulmonary gas exchange, inevitably resulting in respiratory failure and the need for mechanical ventilation.

The cardiovascular dysfunction of MODS includes abnormalities of cardiac function (hypotension unresponsive to fluid administration, dysrhythmias) and abnormalities of peripheral vascular function (increased capillary permeability, edema, alterations in regional blood flow) (Khadaroo & Marshall, 2002). Cardiovascular failure has been defined as a product of heart rate and the difference between mean arterial pressure and right atrial pressure (HR × [MAP-RAP]) (Khadaroo & Marshall, 2002). This formula, called the pressure adjusted heart rate (PAR), is analogous to the PaO_2/FIO_2 ratio with ARDS and is used as a measure of cardiovascular dysfunction in MODS. Increasing values of the PAR reflect worsening cardiovascular function.

Neurologic dysfunction is manifested in MODS as alterations in level of consciousness, confusion, and psychosis. There are many potential *causes* but the pathogenesis of these neurologic changes are controversial. They may occur as a result of hypoperfusion, microvascular coagulopathy, or cerebral ischemia (Barie & Hydo, 2000). Peripheral nervous system dysfunction presents as peripheral neuropathy and includes debility, muscle weakness, and atrophy (Barie & Hydo, 2000). Risk factors include prolonged sedation or therapeutic paralysis and bedrest, aminoglycoside therapy, malnutrition, electrolyte abnormalities, and muscle deconditioning from disuse and lack of exercise. Despite its limitations in the sedated and mechanically ventilated patient, the Glasgow Coma Scale is the most widely used measure of neurologic function.

The development of acute renal failure is multifactorial and can occur as the result of toxic or ischemic insults to renal tubular cells. Renal dysfunction tends to develop later in the course of MODS. Loss of renal function is evidenced by a rise in serum levels of substances normally excreted by the kidneys including creatinine, nitrogen, potassium, and drug metabolites. Regardless of the serum creatinine level, mortality appears to be lower when urine output is greater than 400 mL/day in an average sized adult (Barie & Hydo, 2000).

Hepatic failure involves progressive dysfunction in liver functions. Abnormalities of its synthesizing functions include low serum albumin, fibrinogen, and other clotting factors. Liver dysfunction typically manifests as high levels of serum bilirubin.

Gastrointestinal (GI) bleeding from acute stress ulceration of the stomach is not as common as it used to be. There are no reliable measures of GI function in MODS. There is subjective evidence of GI dysfunction with the development of an ileus or intolerance to enteral tube feedings (lack of absorption or diarrhea).

The most common hematologic dysfunction in MODS is thrombocytopenia secondary to increased consumption, sequestration of platelets in the vasculature, and impaired thrombopoesis as a result of bone marrow suppression (Khadaroo & Marshall, 2002). In its most severe form, the hematologic dysfunction of MODS is disseminated intravascular coagulation (DIC). DIC is characterized by widespread intravascular clotting with bleeding secondary to consumption of coagulation factors.

In summary, organ dysfunction can occur remote from the initial injury site because mediators enable organ-to-organ interaction. Organ ischemia and cellular damage perpetuate SIRS, which perpetuates MODS. Any organ system can manifest dysfunction, and seven of the most common organ systems were presented. As additional organs fail, mortality escalates.

SECTION FOUR REVIEW

1. Respiratory dysfunction is characterized by
   A. a high $PaCO_2$ with a high PaO_2
   B. excessive secretions
   C. rapid Kassmaul-like breathing
   D. a decrease in PaO_2/FIO_2 ratio
2. Which of the following reflect worsening cardiovascular function?
   A. a high cardiac output
   B. increasing PAR values
   C. increasing PaO_2/FIO_2
   D. tachycardia
3. A lower mortality in renal failure with MODS occurs when

A. urine output is greater than 400 mL/day
B. serum creatinine is greater than 4.0 mg/dL
C. neurologic function is maintained
D. hemodialysis is delayed until absolutely necessary

4. The most severe manifestation of hematologic dysfunction is
   A. anemia
   B. thrombocytopenia
   C. DIC
   D. jaundice

Answers: 1. D, 2. B, 3. A, 4. C

SECTION FIVE: Nursing Management of MODS

At the completion of this section, the learner will be able to describe the collaborative management of the patient with MODS.

In Section Four, the progression of SIRS to MODS was reviewed. An awareness of this natural progression may help the nurse to identify patients at risk and prevent the progression of SIRS to MODS. By being aware of SIRS and MODS criteria, nurses can promote early diagnosis and treatment. Early recognition and management of MODS is essential to prevent escalating mortality rates (Ely et al., 2003). A number of nursing measures can be used to assess and monitor patients for MODS.

Patients at risk for primary and secondary MODS should be identified (Section Three). The nurse should monitor vital signs indicative of SIRS including hypo/hyperthermia, tachycardia, tachypnea, and hypotension. Signs of organ dysfunction should be identified early.

Nurses play a vital role in preventing, recognizing, and managing patients with sepsis (Ely et al., 2003). Prevention of sepsis includes enforcement of infection control measures and measures to prevent nosocomial infections, including oral care, proper positioning (elevated head of bed during mechanical ventilation), turning, skin care, invasive catheter care, and wound care (Kleinpell, 2003).

In addition to providing comprehensive treatment of sepsis, including organ system support for patients with MODS,

Evidence-Based Practice

- *Bacterial colonization of the oropharynx is an important risk factor for ventilator associated pneumonia (Grap & Munro, 1997).*
- *The oral flora of critically ill patients is predominately gram-negative organisms that potentially cause ventilator associated pneumonia (Abele-Hom et al., 1997).*
- *The number of organisms present in oral cultures increases each day in patients who are intubated. Patients with ventilator-associated pneumonia have the same species in oral cultures as in tracheal aspirates (Munro et al., 2002).*
- *Chlorhexidine is effective in reducing respiratory infections in patients undergoing elective cardiac surgery when administration begins preoperatively (Houston et al., 2002).*
- *Kinetic therapy reduces ventilator-associated pneumonia in critically ill patients (Ahrens et al., 2004).*

monitoring and reporting responses to therapies are essential aspects of nursing care (Ely et al., 2003).

In summary, early recognition and management of MODS is essential. Patients at risk for developing primary and secondary MODS should be identified. Nurses play a vital role in preventing, recognizing, and managing patients with sepsis. Nursing interventions play a key role in preventing sepsis. Additional essential aspects of nursing care include comprehensive treatment of sepsis, organ support, and monitoring patient response to treatment.

SECTION FIVE REVIEW

1. Which of the following is essential to preventing mortality in MODS?
   A. early recognition and management of MODS
   B. administration of acetaminophen for febrile episodes
   C. prompt administration of aminoglycosides as ordered
   D. knowing how to operate a dialysis machine

2. Vital signs indicative of SIRS include all of the following EXCEPT
   A. hypothermia
   B. tachycardia
   C. hypertension
   D. tachypnea

Answers: 1. A, 2. C

POSTTEST

1. The goal of inflammation is to
   A. produce heat
   B. produce swelling
   C. kill bacteria
   D. limit the extent of injury and promote healing

2. Endogenous substances that stimulate physiologic and pathophysiologic changes are called
   A. endotoxins
   B. mediators
   C. white blood cells
   D. neurotransmitters

3. SIRS is an exaggerated systemic response to
   A. bacteria
   B. sepsis
   C. local inflammation
   D. endotoxins

4. Which of the following is a major etiologic factor in the development of MODS?
   A. SIRS
   B. ARDS
   C. DIC
   D. respiratory failure

5. MODS is characterized by progressive dysfunction of
   A. the immune system
   B. the inflammatory response
   C. the lungs and one other organ
   D. two or more organ systems

6. Secondary MODS occurs in response to
   A. sepsis
   B. SIRS
   C. renal failure
   D. cardiac arrest

7. A major contributor of the progression of SIRS to MODS is
   A. organ-to-organ communication
   B. renal failure

C. improper treatment of septic shock
D. inadequate perfusion

8. All of the following reflect organ dysfunction EXCEPT
   A. reduction in PaO_2/FIO_2
   B. increasing values of PAR
   C. increasing Glascow Coma Scale score
   D. high serum bilirubin

9. Prevention of sepsis includes all of the following EXCEPT
   A. proper oral care
   B. keeping patient supine with head of bed flat during mechanical ventilation
   C. invasive catheter care
   D. turning and skin care

10. Which of the following is essential to preventing mortality in MODS?
    A. administration of antipyretics early in the course of fever
    B. administration of oxygen
    C. titration of vasoactive drugs
    D. early recognition and management of MODS

POSTTEST ANSWERS

Question	Answer	Section	Question	Answer	Section
1	D	One	6	B	Three
2	B	One	7	A	Four
3	C	Two	8	C	Four
4	A	Two	9	B	Five
5	D	Three	10	D	Five

REFERENCES

Abele-Hom, M., Dauber, A., Bauernfeind A., et al. (1997). Decrease in nosocomial pneumonia in ventilated patients by selective oropharyngeal decontamination. *Intensive Care Medicine, 23,* 187–195.

Ahrens, T., Kollef, M., Stewart, J., et al. (2004). Effect of kinetic therapy on pulmonary complications. *American Journal of Critical Care, 13,* 376–383.

Aird, W. C. (2003). The role of the endothelium in severe sepsis and multiple organ dysfunction syndrome. *Blood, 101,* 3765–3777.

American College of Chest Physicians & Society of Critical Care Medicine. (1992). The AACP/SCCM consensus conference on sepsis and organ failure. *Chest, 101,* 1481–1483.

Balk, R. A. (2000). Pathogenesis and management of multiple organ dysfunction or failure in severe sepsis and septic shock. *Critical Care Clinics, 16,* 337–352.

Barie, P. S., & Hydo, L. J. (2000). Epidemiology, risk factors, and outcome of multiple organ dysfunction syndrome in surgical patients. In A. E. Baue, E. Faist, & D. E. Fry (Eds.), *Multiple organ failure: Pathophysiology, prevention, and therapy* (pp. 52–67). New York: Springer-Verlag.

Bernard, G. R., Ely, E. W., Wright, T. J., et al. (2001a). Safety and dose relationship of recombinant human activated protein C for coagulopathy in severe sepsis. *Critical Care Medicine, 29,* 2051–2059.

Bernard, G. R., Vincent, J. L., Laterr, P. F., et al. (2001b). Efficacy and safety of recombinant human activated protein C for severe sepsis. *New England Journal of Medicine, 344,* 699–709.

Bone, R. C., Grodzin, C. J., & Balk, R. A. (1997). Sepsis: A new hypothesis for pathogenesis of the disease process. *Chest, 112,* 235–243.

Brun-Buisson, C. (2000). The epidemiology of the systemic inflammatory response. *Intensive Care Medicine, 26,* 564–574.

Ely, E. W., Kleinpell, R. M., & Goyette, R. E. (2003). Advances in the understanding of clinical manifestations and therapy of severe sepsis: An update for critical care nurses. *American Journal of Critical Care, 12,* 120–133.

Fry, D. E. (2000). Systemic inflammatory response and multiple organ dysfunction syndrome: Biologic domino effect. In A. E. Baue, E. Faist, & D. E. Fry (Eds.), *Multiple organ failure: Pathophysiology, prevention, and therapy* (pp. 23–29). New York: Springer-Verlag.

Grap, M. J., & Munro, C. L. (1997). Ventilator associated pneumonia: Clinical significance and implications for nursing. *Heart and Lung, 26,* 419–429.

Houston, S., Hougland, P., Anderson, J. J., et al. (2002). Effectiveness of 0.12% chlorhexadine gluconate oral rinse in reducing prevalence of nosocomial pneumonia in patients undergoing heart surgery. *American Journal of Critical Care, 11,* 567–570.

Jacobi, J. (2002). Pathophysiology of sepsis. *American Journal of Health-System Pharmacy, 59*(suppl 1), S3–S8.

Khadaroo R. G., & Marshall, J. C. (2002). ARDS and multiple organ dysfunction syndrome. *Critical Care Clinics, 18,* 127–141.

Kleinpell, R. (2003). The role of critical care nursing in the assessment and management of the patient with severe sepsis. *Critical Care Nursing Quarterly, 15,* 27–34.

Lee, K., & Angus, D. C. (2000). Risk and setting for multiple organ failure in medical patients. In A. E. Baue, E. Faist, & D. E. Fry (Eds.), *Multiple organ failure: Pathophysiology, prevention, and therapy* (pp. 44–51). New York: Springer-Verlag.

Marshall, J. C. (2001). Inflammation, coagulopathy, and the pathogenesis of multiple organ dysfunction syndrome. *Critical Care Medicine, 29*(supple), S99–S106.

McCuskey, R. S., Urbaschek R., & Urbascheck, B. (1996). The microcirculation during endotoxemia. *Cardiovascular Research, 32,* 752–763.

Munford, R. S., & Pugin J. (2001). Normal responses to injury prevent systemic inflammation and can be immunosuppressive. *American Journal of Respiratory Critical Care Medicine, 163,* 316–321.

Munro, C. L., Grap, M. J., Hummel R., et al. (2002). Oral health status: Effect on ventilator associated pneumonia [abstract]. *American Journal of Critical Care, 11,* 280.

Offner, P. J., & Moore, E. E. (2000). Risk factors for MODS and pattern of organ failure following severe trauma. In, A. E. Baue, E. Faist, & D. E. Fry (Eds.), *Multiple organ failure: Pathophysiology, prevention, and therapy* (pp. 30–42). New York: Springer-Verlag.

Schwartz, D. R., Malhotra, A., & Fink, M. P. (1999). Cytopathic hypoxia in sepsis: An overview. *Sepsis, 2,* 279–289.

Vallet B., & Wiel, E. (2001). Endothelial cell dysfunction and coagulation. *Critical Care Medicine, 24,* S36–S41.

MODULE
17

Nursing Care of the Patient with Impaired Oxygenation

Karen L. Johnson

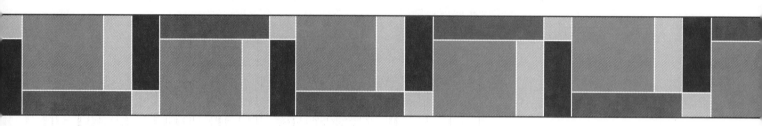

OBJECTIVES   Following completion of this module, the learner will be able to

1. Describe an appropriate database for a patient experiencing impaired oxygenation related to inflammation.

2. Discuss development of nursing diagnoses appropriate to patients with multiple organ dysfunction syndrome (MODS).

3. Explain the development of a plan of care for the patient with MODS.

4. Analyze outcomes of care in a patient with MODS.

This self-study module is designed to integrate the major points discussed in Modules 14, 15, and 16, as well as to assist the learner in clustering information to facilitate clinical application. Content is applied in an interactive learning style. Using a case study format, the learner is encouraged to identify nursing actions based on the assessment of a patient with impaired oxygenation. Consequences of selecting a particular action are discussed. Rationale for all answers is presented. The module ends with a brief summary of major points.

GLOSSARY

continuous arteriovenous hemofiltration (CAVH)   The use of a transmembrane pressure gradient to remove water, electrolytes, and small-to-medium-molecular-weight molecules from the vascular space. Blood enters the extracorporeal circuit by arterial access and returns by venous access. The patient's hydrostatic blood pressure drives the blood flow; no external pump is used.

extracorporeal membrane oxygenation (ECMO)   A process that uses a mechanical device to replace cardiac and lung function.

ABBREVIATIONS

ABG	Arterial blood gas	**CO**	Cardiac output
ARDS	Acute respiratory distress syndrome	**ECMO**	Extracorporeal membrane oxygenation
ATP	Adenosine triphosphate	**ED**	Emergency department
Bpm	Beats per minute	**ET**	Endotracheal tube
BUN	Blood urea nitrogen	**FIO$_2$**	Fraction of inspired oxygen
CAVH	Continuous arteriovenous hemofiltration	**HCO$_3$**	Bicarbonate
CI	Cardiac index	**Hct**	Hematocrit

Hgb	Hemoglobin
IV	Intravenous
MODS	Multiple organ dysfunction syndrome
O_2	Oxygen
PaO_2	Partial pressure of arterial oxygen
$PaCO_2$	Partial pressure of carbon dioxide in arterial blood
PAWP	Pulmonary artery wedge pressure
PEEP	Positive end-expiratory pressure

PERRLA	Pupils equal round reactive to light accommodation
RAP	Right atrial pressure
RBC	Red blood cell
SaO_2	Oxygen saturation of arterial blood
SIMV	Synchronized intermittent mandatory ventilation
SOB	Shortness of breath
SVR	Systemic vascular resistance
WBC	White blood cell

Case Study

A CASE OF IMPAIRED OXYGENATION

Mr. F. is admitted to your unit with a diagnosis of pneumonia. He presented to the emergency department (ED) after having 2 weeks of low-grade fever and chills. He complained of a cough. Mr. F. had completed 3 days of oral cephalosporin treatment given to him by a physician at an urgent care center. His chest x-ray showed bilateral pneumonia with greater involvement of the left lung than the right.

Initial Appraisal

On walking into the room, you note the following.

GENERAL APPEARANCE. Mr. F. is about 40 years of age. He appears as a "healthy," well-nourished man. He has well-developed arm muscles and dark skin from spending a lot of time outdoors. He is wearing glasses.

SIGNS OF DISTRESS. Mr. F. is diaphoretic and breathing rapidly. He is sitting upright and coughs frequently. Secretions are audible during coughing.

OTHER. You note an intravenous (IV) line in his right dorsal hand. Oxygen (O_2) is running at 2 L through a nasal cannula. A woman who identifies herself as his wife is in the room.

Focused Assessment

You quickly introduce yourself and immediately perform a rapid assessment, focusing on Mr. F.'s oxygenation. The results are as follows.

Mr. F. is restless but is oriented to person, place, and time. His respiratory rate is 30/min. Respirations are regular and shallow. He prefers to sit upright to ease his breathing. He is using accessory muscles in his neck while breathing, but no retractions are noted. Diffuse medium crackles are auscultated in the middle and lower lung fields bilaterally. S_1 and S_2 are auscultated without rub or murmur. His current blood pressure is 140/90 mm Hg, pulse is 110 beats per minute (bpm), and his temperature is 101.5°F (38.6°C) orally. He coughs up some white mucus.

QUESTION

What additional information could you obtain that would help you assess O_2 delivery?
- **A.** urine output
- **B.** arterial oxygen saturation
- **C.** mean arterial pressure
- **D.** sputum culture

ANSWER

The correct answer is B. To assess oxygenation, you must have information about Mr. F.'s O_2 delivery. This can easily be accomplished by application of a pulse oximeter. Knowing his urine output will help you assess whether he is receiving adequate blood flow to his kidneys, but adequate flow does not guarantee adequate oxygenation. Mean arterial pressure will tell you about afterload (the resistance that his heart must pump against). A sputum culture will provide information regarding the cause of his pneumonia. Arterial oxygen saturation is the ratio of oxygenated hemoglobin (Hgb) to total Hgb. More than 97 percent of all oxygen delivered to cells is delivered as oxyhemoglobin.

After the initial assessment you connect Mr. F. to the pulse oximeter. You look through his chart to see if any lab work was completed in the ED. You find the following:

CBC

WBC = 18,000/mL	(normal, 4,500 to 10,000/mL)
RBC = 5.33/10^6mL	(normal, 4.6 to 6.0/10^6mL)
Hgb = 15.3 g/dL	(normal, 13.5 to 17 g/dL)
Hct = 43.8 percent	(normal, 40 to 54 percent)
Platelets = 397,000/mL	(normal, 150,000 to 400,000/mL)

Electrolytes

Glucose = 95 mg/dL	(normal, 70 to 110 mg/dL)
BUN = 30 mg/dL	(normal, 5 to 25 mg/dL)
Creatinine = 0.9 mg/dL	(normal, 0.5 to 1.5 mg/dL)
Sodium = 139 mEq/L	(normal, 135 to 145 mEq/L)
Potassium = 4.6 mEq/L	(normal, 3.5 to 5.3 mEq/L)
Chloride = 110 mEq/L	(normal, 95 to 105 mEq/L)

Urine

Specific gravity = 1.030   (normal, 1.005 to 1.030)

Arterial Blood Gases

pH = 7.37   (normal, 7.35 to 7.45)
$Paco_2$ = 42 mm Hg   (normal, 35 to 45 mm Hg)
Pao_2 = 82 mm Hg   (normal, 75 to 100 mm Hg)
HCO_3 = 26 mEq/L   (normal, 24 to 28 mEq/L)
Sao_2 = 92 percent   (normal, 95 percent or greater)

QUESTION

Which of the following statements are true about Mr. F.'s condition?

A. he shows evidence of an infection
B. he is in respiratory acidosis
C. he may be dehydrated
D. he is anemic

ANSWER

In this case, both A and C are correct. Mr. F. shows signs of infection as evidenced by elevation in WBC count and fever. He may also be dehydrated as evidenced by hyperchloremia, elevated specific gravity, and elevated BUN in face of a normal creatinine. Although Mr. F.'s Sao_2 is low, he is compensating well and is not in respiratory acidosis because his pH is normal. His RBC and Hgb counts are normal, so he is not anemic.

You check the orders that have accompanied Mr. F. and find that he needs several things:

- IV D_5LR @ 200 mL/hr
- IV erythromycin 500 mg q6h
- Sputum culture
- Pulmonary function tests
- Acetaminophen 650 mg q4h PRN Temp greater than 38.5°C

QUESTION

Which of these orders should you implement first?

ANSWER

You should initiate the IV fluids and simultaneously hang the first dose of the IV erythromycin. These actions address both the dehydration and infection suggested by Mr. F.'s laboratory data, x-ray reading, and your assessment findings. Your actions will help promote oxygenation by increasing O_2 delivery through increased blood flow, improving pulmonary gas exchange by eliminating lung infiltrates, and increasing lung surface area for diffusion. If Mr. F. is dehydrated, it will be more difficult to obtain a sputum culture, plus it will take several days to obtain information from this test. The pulmonary function tests will require Mr. F.'s cooperation. In addition to being in minor distress, he is breathing too fast to perform these tests presently. Mr. F. is febrile. Fever increases O_2 consumption. Because Mr. F. already has impaired gas exchange from pneumonia and decreased O_2 delivery from dehydration, his fever should be treated with antipyretics as soon as the IV and antibiotic interventions have been initiated.

Focused Nursing History

Mr. F. started feeling poorly about 2 weeks ago. His shortness of breath has been increasing and 3 days ago he went to an urgent care center. After starting on cephalosporin, he initially felt better. Yesterday, his fever went up and his chills began. His cough prevents him from sleeping at night and eating as well as normal. Over-the-counter cough medicine has not relieved it. He occasionally brings up white, thick sputum.

He is allergic to penicillin, and nonsteroidal anti-inflammatory agents hurt his stomach. He denies smoking or using drugs. He has a history of gout and lumbar disc problems from a motor vehicle crash several years ago.

Systematic Bedside Assessment

You perform a head-to-toe assessment.

HEAD AND NECK. Mr. F. is tanned and it is difficult to assess for cyanosis. His mucous membranes are pink but dry. His lips are cracked. He has slight nasal flaring. His neck veins are full, not distended or flat.

CHEST. His pulmonary and cardiac exam is as previously stated.

ABDOMEN. His abdomen is slightly obese. Positive bowel sounds are auscultated in all quadrants. His abdomen is not tender on palpation. It is supple without rigidity.

PELVIS. Mr. F. voided 100 mL of clear, dark urine that smells strong. He denies any penile discharge or voiding discomfort.

EXTREMITIES. His skin turgor is adequate. He is warm and diaphoretic. No peripheral edema is noted. Sensation and motor function are present in all extremities. Peripheral pulses are palpated in all extremities.

POSTERIOR. He complains of slight tenderness on palpation of his lumbar–sacral area but says "it is normal." Posterior breath sounds are diminished greater in the left lower lung fields than in the right, with bilateral crackles.

Development of Nursing Diagnoses

CLUSTERING DATA. You have just completed your head-to-toe assessment and are ready to develop a problem list based on the subjective and objective data you have collected thus far. To cluster your data, you look for abnormalities found during your assessment. Mr. F.'s major symptom at this time is his labored breathing. This symptom can initiate your first cluster of critical clues.

CLUSTER 1

Subjective data. Patient complaining of shortness of breath (SOB) with greater breathing comfort sitting at 90 degrees. Malaise for 2 weeks. Increasing cough and fever for 3 days. Occasional white sputum produced. Has difficulty sleeping and eating because of cough. Symptoms not relieved with cough medicine or antibiotic.

Objective data. Labored, shallow respirations at 30/min. Some accessory muscle use. Diminished breath sounds in lower lung fields with left greater than right. Crackles auscultated bilaterally. Chest x-ray indicates bilateral pneumonia. Low Sao_2 on 2 L of O_2. Fever present.

QUESTION

Based on these data, which of the following nursing diagnoses would you select as being appropriate in planning Mr. F.'s plan of care?

   A. impaired gas exchange
   B. ineffective breathing pattern
   C. ineffective airway clearance
   D. all of the above

ANSWER

This is a tough question. The data supports only C at present. Because of Mr. F.'s increased production of secretions as a result of the inflammatory process and his inability to cough up these secretions consistently, pneumonia has developed. He may be fatigued from lack of sleep, and this may contribute to ineffective clearing of secretions. He is also dehydrated, which makes the secretions thicker. Because his ABGs are normal, he is not experiencing impaired gas exchange yet. He is at risk for this problem because of a decrease in lung surface area available for O_2 diffusion. His breathing pattern is effective at present to meet cellular oxygen needs but his Sao_2 is decreasing, suggesting that he may decompensate shortly.

   Desired patient outcomes for Mr. F. (evaluative criteria) would include

1. normal rate and depth of respirations
2. decreased SOB
3. improved breath sounds
4. improved Sao_2

CLUSTER 2

Subjective data. Patient complaining of increasing cough that prevents normal eating. The patient has had a fever for 3 days.

Objective data. Confirmed pneumonia on chest x-ray. Temperature 101.5°F. Respiratory rate 30/min. Urine dark and clear with strong odor. Specific gravity high normal. The patient is diaphoretic with full neck veins. Serum chloride 110 mEq/L. Mucous membranes are dry and lips are cracked. Pulse is 110 bpm.

   You make the nursing diagnosis of *high risk for fluid volume deficit* related to decreased oral intake and excessive fluid loss as a result of hyperventilation and diaphoresis. Because of Mr. F.'s inflammation, you realize that he is in a hypermetabolic state in an attempt to activate the immune response to limit the infection. Because a greater number of metabolic reactions are occurring, more heat is generated and more water is used. At present, his Hct and specific gravity are normal, suggesting that he is not dehydrated.

Developing the Plan of Care

The goals in Mr. F.'s plan of care are to (1) optimize his oxygenation, (2) promote his airway clearance, (3) provide adequate hydration, (4) maintain functioning alveoli, and (5) limit the infection. Nursing interventions consist of collaborative actions to fulfill orders written by the health care practitioner focused on treating the pathology and independent interventions aimed at treating Mr. F.'s responses to the pneumonia that are within the nursing scope of practice and can be initiated without a health care practitioner's order.

COLLABORATIVE INTERVENTIONS. The health care practitioner's orders may include the following:

1. **Pulmonary drug therapy.** Beta-adrenergic agents that promote bronchodilation may be ordered. These may be administered through nebulization or by metered-dose inhaler. Anticholinergic agents may also be used, such as ipratropium bromide. Steroids and xanthine derivatives (such as aminophylline) may be ordered. Oxygen will be administered until Mr. F. can maintain a normal Sao_2. Antibiotics will be started and changed as necessary based on the findings of sputum and blood cultures. An expectorant and mucolytic agent may be ordered to help liquefy Mr. F.'s mucus and assist him in clearing his airway. A cough suppressant may be ordered for nighttime use to facilitate sleeping.

2. **Laboratory and x-ray testing.** Of particular interest will be the results of a sputum culture and blood cultures. Blood cultures have not yet been ordered for Mr. F. They may be initiated on admission of the patient or in situations in which the patient does not respond to initial treatment. Pulmonary function tests may help determine the degree of volume change associated with the decreased lung surface area as a result of the infiltrates. Chest x-rays and ABGs will be monitored intermittently.

3. **Intravenous fluids.** Because of IV access for antibiotics and Mr. F.'s risk for dehydration, IVs have been ordered. The patency of this line should remain a nursing priority.

INDEPENDENT NURSING INTERVENTIONS

1. Assess for decreased respiratory function. Report
   - Respirations less than 8/min or greater than 30/min
   - Increasing dyspnea
   - A change in level of consciousness
   - A change in accessory muscle use
   - Decreasing Sao_2
2. Try to improve respiratory function:
   - Decrease patient's O_2 needs by relieving fever, pain, and anxiety
   - Promote position of comfort and prevent slumping to improve diaphragmatic excursion
   - Promote incentive spirometer use q2h
   - Perform nasotracheal suctioning as needed
   - Maintain O_2 therapy
   - Perform percussion and postural drainage q8h
3. Prevent dehydration:
   - Encourage oral fluids
   - Monitor BUN, Hct, urine output, fever

   Mr. F. initially improves and plans are made to discharge him. The night before his discharge, Mr. F.'s fever increased to 102.4°F (39°C). His oxygen saturation dropped to 82 percent. He became severely dyspneic. A stat chest x-ray was obtained and showed diffuse bilateral infiltrates. His arterial blood gas (ABG) on 2 L of O_2 was pH 7.45, $Paco_2$ 35, and Pao_2 44. Sao_2 was 82 percent. The decision was made to transfer Mr. F. to the intensive care unit.

Mr. F. is exhibiting acute respiratory distress syndrome (ARDS). The inflammatory process was initiated with the development of the infiltrates in the lung (evidence of neutrophil migration), the slightly elevated WBC count, and his fever. Damage has occurred to the alevolar–capillary membrane from the release of mediators. First, the capillary endothelium is injured, allowing fluid to enter the interstitial spaces; then, as osmotic pressure builds in the interstitium, fluid enters the alveoli, damaging type II cells that produce surfactant. The alveoli collapse, decreasing the surface area available for O_2 diffusion.

QUESTION

If Mr. F. is experiencing ARDS, why is he not in respiratory acidosis?

ANSWER

Mr. F. is exhibiting hypoxemia (Pao_2 44). He is probably hyperventilating, which is why his $Paco_2$ is borderline low and his pH is borderline for respiratory alkalosis. Eventually, the $Paco_2$ will increase as Mr. F. fatigues.

The sputum culture was negative, suggesting a viral form of pneumonia. Because Mr. F. was improving, additional diagnostic tests were not performed. Now, with his sudden deterioration, several orders are written:

1. 50 percent O_2 by simple face mask
2. Diagnostic bronchoscopy with lung biopsy
3. Blood cultures
4. Tuberculosis testing
5. Titers for *Mycoplasma, Pneumocystis,* Hantavirus, and *Legionella*
6. Ceftazidime 1 g IV q8h

QUESTION

Of the following orders, which should be implemented first?
   A. obtaining blood for the titers
   B. administering the heparin
   C. administering the ceftazidime
   D. administering the O_2

ANSWER

The correct answer is D. The O_2 should be given first. Inadequate O_2 to meet cellular demands will cause more inflammation and mediator release, thus greater alveoli damage.

Mr. F. continues to deteriorate in spite of receiving 50 percent O_2. He is now in respiratory acidosis (pH 7.3, $Paco_2$ 49, Pao_2 50). Because of his fatigue, he could not continue hyperventilating to compensate for his respiratory failure. He is intubated, and a pulmonary artery catheter is inserted. He receives lorazepam for sedation, and morphine sulfate for pain. His initial ventilator settings are tidal volume 700 mL, Fio_2 60 percent, synchronous intermittent mandatory ventilation (SIMV) mode, with 10 cm H_2O of positive end-expiratory pressure (PEEP) and 5 cm H_2O pressure support. His pulmonary artery pressures are 48/28 mm Hg, right atrial pressure (RAP) 10 mm Hg, pulmonary artery wedge pressure (PAWP) 14 mm Hg, cardiac output (CO) 15.3 L/min, and cardiac index (CI) 6.1 L/min.

Systematic Bedside Assessment

Once you have implemented the various stat activities for Mr. F., you begin a head-to-toe assessment.

HEAD AND NECK. Glasgow Coma Scale 11T. PERRLA at 5 mm. Orally intubated with #8 Fr tube. His jugular veins are full.

CHEST. Coarse crackles are present bilaterally. S_1 and S_2, no extra heart sounds are noted. A pulmonary arterial catheter is in place in the right subclavian vein. Dressing is dry and intact. Insertion site clean, no erythema.

ABDOMEN. No bowel sounds are auscultated. Abdomen is soft. No bruits auscultated.

PELVIS. A urinary catheter is present draining clear, dark amber urine. There is 50 mL for a 1-hour period.

EXTREMITIES. His skin is warm and dry. No peripheral edema is noted. Peripheral pulses are palpable.

POSTERIOR. No skin breakdown is noted. Scattered crackles are auscultated bilaterally throughout the posterior lung fields.

Development of Nursing Diagnoses

CLUSTERING DATA. The following data should be clustered based on abnormal findings.

CLUSTER 3

Subjective data. Denies pain, discomfort.

Objective data. Bilateral diffuse infiltrates on chest x-ray. Respiratory acidosis. Low oxygen saturation level. Crackles auscultated bilaterally. Failure to respond to antibiotic therapy.

Based on these data, the diagnosis of *impaired gas exchange* related to pulmonary alveoli membrane permeability and damage is appropriate. He is also at risk for ineffective airway clearance because of intubation, chemical paralysis, and increased secretion production. Mr. F. is also at risk for fluid volume excess related to noncardiac pulmonary edema (if the inflammatory process continues) and PEEP because PEEP may cause pulmonary hypertension, right heart failure, and decreased cardiac output.

Developing the Plan of Care

The goals in caring for a patient in ARDS are to (1) support tissue oxygenation, (2) prevent infection, and (3) treat the underlying cause. Interventions are both collaborative and independent.

COLLABORATIVE INTERVENTIONS

1. **Pulmonary drug therapy.** The same bronchodilator therapy may be used as discussed earlier in the case. Oxygen levels will be increased until the patient's Pao_2 level is 60 mm Hg. The goal is to keep the Fio_2 below 60 percent. Antibiotics or antiviral agents will be given and changed pending the results of the lung biopsy and titers.

2. **Ventilatory management.** Pressure support was added to decrease Mr. F.'s work of breathing. PEEP was added to prevent alveolar collapse and increase alveolar surface area available for pulmonary gas exchange. Depending on how Mr. F. responds to his current ventilatory setting, additional ventilatory modes may be instituted as protective lung strategies including low tidal volumes, inverse ratio, or pressure control modes.

3. **Cardiovascular drug therapy.** The aim is to optimize cardiac output without causing pulmonary edema so that peripheral tissue remains adequately oxygenated. Diuretics will be given if the PAWP increases, or IV fluids may be administered if the PAWP and CI decrease below normal.

Independent Nursing Interventions

Maintain Airway Patency

1. Suction endotracheal tube (ET) as needed; note color, amount, and consistency of secretions
2. Check ET tube placement
3. Change patient's position q2h
4. Assess breath sounds qh and PRN
5. Elevate head of bed 30 degrees

Maintain Hemodynamic Stability

1. Assess hemodynamic parameters
2. Monitor intake and output
3. Assess for signs of fluid overload (dependent edema, increased weight, increased crackles, increased RAP, decreased CI)
4. Assess for signs of decreased CI

Mr. F.'s lung biopsy shows interstitial pneumonia with marked diffuse alveolar damage. His titers are negative. His cultures fail to grow any specific organism. The reason for his ARDS is not known. His lactate level is 5.2 mMol/L. His glucose level increases to 320 mg/dL. Mr. F.'s BUN and creatinine elevate (70 and 2.8, respectively). His albumin level is 2.9 mg/dL. His WBC count is 25,100, whereas his hemoglobin is 7.5 and his hematocrit is 22.4 percent. Platelets are 86,000. His hemodynamic readings are PCWP 14 mm Hg, CO 14.2 L/min, CI 6 L/min. His systemic vascular resistance (SVR) is 907. Oxygen saturation is 92 percent on an FIO_2 of 1.00 and PEEP level of 15 cm H_2O. He is in metabolic acidosis but his latest ABGs have improved: pH 7.22, $PaCO_2$ 55, PaO_2 116, HCO_3 20. Oxygen saturation is 98 percent. His temperature is 99.1°F (37.2°C). The physician places Mr. F. on **extracorporeal membrane oxygenation (ECMO)** to remove carbon dioxide. He is started on **continuous arteriovenous hemofiltration (CAVH).** Mr. F. begins to bleed from his mouth, ET tube, and IV lines. You place a stat call to the physician.

Relating Mr. F.'s Symptoms to the Inflammatory Process

Mr. F. is probably in anaerobic metabolism as evidenced by high lactate levels. As the production of adenosine triphosphate (ATP) decreases, cell death occurs. Sodium passively enters the cell, water follows the sodium, and

eventually the ribosomes. The cell membrane ruptures and intracellular enzymes are released. Simultaneously, Mr. F.'s sympathetic nervous system is activated. This is why his CI is elevated and he is hyperglycemic. The fever is less than expected, given the elevated WBC count. Perhaps Mr. F. is unable to mount an adequate immune response. This is an ominous sign. Thus, Mr. F. has gone from dysfunction of one organ, the lungs, into a cascade of events producing dysfunction in multiple systems. He is experiencing MODS.

QUESTION

Mr. F.'s BUN and creatinine are elevated. Which of the following statements provides the best rationale for this elevation?

A. he is experiencing tubular cell necrosis from mediator destruction of the cell membrane and decreased renal blood flow
B. he is exhibiting nephrotoxicity from drugs
C. he is breaking down protein for glucose production
D. BUN and creatinine reflect the breakdown of RBCs due to his bleeding

ANSWER

The correct answer is A. As nephrons die, they release debris that form casts. These casts obstruct the renal tubules, decreasing the glomerular filtration rate. B may also be true in some patients with MODS. However, Mr. F. has not received aminoglycosides, the group of antibiotics most notorious for nephrotoxicity. Protein breakdown is occurring but this would not elevate the creatinine level, only the BUN. Destruction of RBCs produces bilirubin.

Systematic Bedside Assessment

As you await the call from the physician you complete a head-to-toe assessment.

HEAD AND NECK. Mr. F. is now in a chemically induced coma. There is blood in his ventilator tubing and some is oozing from his mouth.

CHEST. Coarse crackles are auscultated bilaterally with the ventilatory cycle. S_1 and S_2 are present. His apical rate is 116.

ABDOMEN. No bowel sounds are auscultated. His abdomen is distended.

PELVIS. He had 8,318 mL intake and 17,033 mL output via his CAVH in the past 24-hour period. No drainage is noted from the penis. His last bowel movement was loose and positive for blood.

EXTREMITIES. He has 3+ edema of both legs extending up to the shins. Pulses are palpable. Petechiae are noted on all extremities.

POSTERIOR. No skin breakdown is noted but there is redness in several areas along the vertebrae and the coccyx. Coarse crackles are auscultated bilaterally in the posterior lung fields.

Development of Nursing Diagnoses

CLUSTERING DATA. You cluster the major abnormal findings to derive the nursing diagnoses.

CLUSTER 1

Subjective data. None.

Objective data. Metabolic acidosis, elevated Paco₂ level. Coarse crackles bilaterally. Blood in the ET and ventilator tubing.

Based on these data you derive the nursing diagnoses of *impaired gas exchange, ineffective airway clearance,* and *high risk for aspiration.*

CLUSTER 2

Subjective data. None.

Objective data. Elevated CI. Sinus tachycardia. Decreased platelets. Bleeding from mouth, IV lines, ET, and in stool. Petechiae on all extremities.

QUESTION

Which of the following nursing diagnoses is most appropriate at this time?
- **A.** fluid volume excess
- **B.** alteration in tissue perfusion: cardiopulmonary
- **C.** fluid volume deficit
- **D.** decreased cardiac output

ANSWER

The correct answer is C. Mr. F. is actively losing blood. He may consume all his clotting factors and progress into hypovolemic shock. As a result of the inflammatory process, fluid shifts from vessels into the interstitial spaces and ultimately into the cells, and contributes to decreased circulating volume. Although B and D are appropriate nursing diagnoses at this time, C is the most appropriate. It is Mr. F.'s major problem. Fluid volume deficit is the cause of an alteration in tissue perfusion and decreased CO. Once fluid volume has been restored, tissue perfusion and CO will improve.

Clusters could be developed to support *altered tissue perfusion: Renal; high risk for impaired skin integrity: pressure ulcer;* and *altered nutrition: less than body protein–calorie requirements* (due to Mr. F.'s hypermetabolic state and need for glucose).

Developing the Plan of Care

COLLABORATIVE INTERVENTIONS

1. **Cardiovascular drug therapy.** As CO decreases secondary to pulmonary hypertension, dobutamine and nitroglycerin continuous infusions may be initiated. Dobutamine will augment contractility. Nitroglycerin will produce pulmonary venous vasodilation. This will decrease right heart afterload and augment right heart stroke volume.
2. **Maintaining oxygen supply.** Ventilatory settings will be adjusted to gradually decrease the FIo₂, PEEP, and pressure support as long as the Pao₂ remains above 60 mm Hg and the oxygen saturation is normal. ECMO may be used to remove carbon dioxide until Mr. F. is able to respond to the ventilator settings. Because of Mr. F.'s active bleeding, packed RBCs, fresh frozen plasma, and platelets will be administered to replace volume loss, proteins, and platelets.

INDEPENDENT INTERVENTIONS

1. **Decreasing oxygen demands.** The nurse must ensure that neuromuscular blockade is adequate to prevent any voluntary movement. This can be accomplished through train-of-four monitoring. Studies have shown patients can hear and remember events that occur during therapeutic paralysis. It is important that health care providers monitor their conversation at the bedside. Family should be encouraged to touch and talk with the patient. The nurse will continue to administer the neuromuscular blocking agent and sedative until Mr. F.'s metabolic demands decrease. Morphine decreases Mr. F.'s pain.
2. **Limiting the source of inflammation.** The nurse should maintain closed systems (such as in-line suction, capped IV ports). Proper suctioning can reduce Mr. F.'s risk of aspiration and promote his pulmonary hygiene. Turning and repositioning Mr. F. may prevent pressure ulcer formation and another site for infection. Careful skin and oral care prevents further bleeding and infection.
3. **Promoting nutrition.** Although they have not been ordered yet because of his active gastrointestinal (GI) bleeding, enteric feedings will be started when the bleeding stops. Enteral feeding maintains the intestinal mucosa and prevents disruption of the normal gut flora. Elevating the head of the bed, assuring tube patency and proper placement prior to feeding, and keeping the tube feeding infusing at the proper rate will help increase Mr. F.'s albumin level and protein stores. Sucralfate or an H₂ histamine blocker (ranitidine) may be used to prevent stress ulcer formation.
4. **Maintaining oxygen supply.** Proper ET tube suctioning will also promote oxygenation. Ensuring that the ventilator system operates correctly and that the patient remains connected are priorities.

Plan: Evaluation and Revision

Mr. F.'s treatment plan requires multiple revisions based on his changing status. His condition slowly improves. The following indicate progress. Mr. F. returns to a normal acid–base balance and the ECMO is discontinued. His blood glucose will return to normal as his metabolic state slows down. His protein stores will improve and his WBC count returns to normal. Mr. F.'s bleeding stops and his CO improves. As these events occur, renal function improves and the CAVH is discontinued. The last sign of progress is weaning from mechanical ventilation. This is the most difficult to accomplish because of Mr. F.'s alveoli damage, respiratory muscle wasting, and possible psychologic dependence on the ventilator.

Mr. F. did improve and was discharged to a rehabilitation facility after a 3-month hospital stay for the admitting diagnosis of pneumonia. Now, 1 year after his illness, Mr. F. has resumed full-time farming. Mr. F. is one of the lucky ones who survived MODS.

PART

5

Neurologic

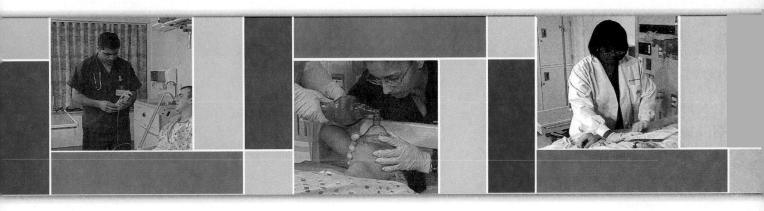

MODULE 18 | Determinants and Assessment of Cerebral Perfusion

MODULE 19 | Alterations in Cerebral Tissue Perfusion: Acute Brain Attack

MODULE 20 | Decreased Adaptive Capacity: Closed Head Injury

MODULE 21 | Sensory Perceptual Disorders

MODULE 22 | Nursing Care of the Patient with an Alteration in Cerebral Tissue Perfusion

18 Determinants and Assessment of Cerebral Tissue Perfusion

Karen L. Johnson

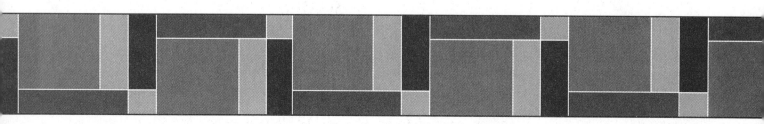

OBJECTIVES Following completion of this module, the learner will be able to

1. Explain cerebral blood flow.
   - Describe the relationship between cerebral oxygenation and metabolism.
   - Identify factors that affect cerebral oxygenation.
2. Define the Monro–Kellie hypothesis.
   - Explain the pathophysiologic mechanisms that produce increased intracranial pressure through alterations in brain volume, cerebral blood volume, and cerebrospinal fluid.
3. Calculate cerebral perfusion pressure based on mean arterial pressure and intracranial pressure.
4. Identify causes and effects of increases in brain volume, cerebral blood volume, and intracranial pressure.
5. State the components of an assessment of level of consciousness in terms of assessing arousal and content.
   - Compare and contrast components of the Glasgow Coma Scale.
   - Identify the components of an in-depth clinical neurological assessment that can be used to assess a patient with an altered level of consciousness.

- Compare and contrast normal and abnormal findings for the components of an in-depth neurological assessment.
- State the intracranial pressure monitoring types and systems, and discuss the advantages and disadvantages of each.
- Identify normal and abnormal intracranial pressure monitoring waveforms.
- Compare and contrast the more commonly performed diagnostic procedures used to diagnose conditions that cause impaired cerebral tissue perfusion and decreased intracranial adaptive capacity.

6. Identify collaborative interventions used to optimize cerebral tissue perfusion and oxygenation.
   - List the pharmacologic agents used in the treatment of increased intracranial pressure and identify the nursing implications of each.
   - Summarize nursing care priorities for patients receiving intracranial pressure monitoring.

This self-study module focuses on the physiologic and pathophysiologic processes involved in cerebral tissue perfusion. This module is composed of six sections, beginning with a brief review of anatomy and physiology pertinent to cerebral tissue perfusion. Section Two reviews pathophysiologic mechanisms that increase intracranial pressure. Section Three discusses how cerebral perfusion pressure is measured in the high-acuity setting. Section Four summarizes the causes and effects of decreased intracranial adaptive capacity. Section Five, "Assessment of Cerebral Tissue Perfusion," is a rather lengthy section because there are a wide variety of clinical assessment tools available to assess for impaired cerebral tis-

sue perfusion and decreased intracranial adaptive capacity. This section begins with bedside assessment tools available for the high-acuity nurse and ends with diagnostic procedures to aid in further diagnosis. The final section identifies collaborative interventions used to optimize cerebral tissue perfusion and improve intracranial adaptive capacity. Each section includes a set of review questions to help the learner evaluate his or her understanding of the section's content before moving on to the next section. All Section Reviews and the module Pretest and Posttest include answers. It is suggested that the learner review those concepts answered incorrectly in the review questions before proceeding to the next section.

PRETEST

1. Cerebral blood vessels dilate in response to
   A. increased serum oxygen
   B. increased serum carbon dioxide
   C. decreased serum oxygen
   D. decreased serum carbon dioxide

2. Pressure regulation is an autoregulatory mechanism whereby cerebral blood vessels constrict in response to
   A. systemic hypertension
   B. hypercarbia
   C. systemic hypotension
   D. hypoxia

3. Cerebral blood flow decreases with
   A. cerebral edema
   B. low cardiac output
   C. cerebral vasoconstriction
   D. all of the above

4. The Monro–Kellie hypothesis states that volume increases in the adult intracranial vault
   A. are initially well tolerated through compensatory mechanisms
   B. are tolerated well because of the flexibility of the cranial vault
   C. can be compensated for only by cerebrospinal fluid buffering techniques
   D. usually result in death because the vault is unable to accommodate increases in volume

5. Which of the following components of intracranial volume is displaced most easily and rapidly?
   A. brain volume
   B. cerebral blood volume
   C. CSF
   D. cranium

6. Flexion of the neck may cause elevations in intracranial volume by
   A. causing a decrease in venous outflow
   B. causing an increase in venous return
   C. causing cerebral vasodilation
   D. increasing venous outflow

7. What is the cerebral perfusion pressure if mean arterial pressure (MAP) = 95 mm Hg and intracranial pressure (ICP) = 15 mm Hg?
   A. 65 mm Hg
   B. 80 mm Hg
   C. 110 mm Hg
   D. 125 mm Hg

8. Normal cerebral perfusion pressure is
   A. highly individualized
   B. 50 to 80 mm Hg
   C. 80 to 100 mm Hg
   D. 100 to 120 mm Hg

9. Cerebral perfusion decreases when
   A. ICP is high
   B. MAP is low

C. ICP is the same as MAP
   D. all of the above

10. Cerebral edema is caused by
    A. an increase in cerebral blood volume
    B. an increase in brain volume
    C. an increase in CSF
    D. an increase in ICP

11. An accumulation of CSF is called
    A. herniation
    B. hydrocephalus
    C. cerebral edema
    D. intracranial hypertension

12. An increase in brain volume can result in
    A. herniation
    B. cerebral vasodilation
    C. autoregulation
    D. hydrocephalus

13. Your patient responds to stimuli and the Glasgow Coma Scale (GSC) is 15. What would be your initial assessment and your next action?
    A. level of responsiveness is intact; vital signs would be the next logical step
    B. level of responsiveness most probably not intact; an in-depth neurological assessment is required
    C. you are unable to completely evaluate the level of responsiveness and need more clinical data
    D. the patient demonstrates no cognitive deficits; pupillary assessment would be the next logical step

14. The most important component of the neurologic assessment is
    A. vital signs
    B. level of consciousness
    C. pupillary reactions
    D. protective reflexes

15. A unilaterally dilated pupil is indicative of
    A. atropine or atropine-like drugs
    B. a brainstem lesion
    C. opioid overdose
    D. cranial nerve lesion

16. The Glasgow Coma Scale assesses
    A. cognition
    B. speech patterns
    C. arousal
    D. problem-solving abilities

17. Mean arterial pressure should be maintained at more than _____ mm Hg to keep the cerebral perfusion pressure greater than _____ mm Hg.
    A. 90; 70
    B. 100; 80
    C. 50; 40
    D. 40; 80

18. A patient with a GCS less than _____ must have the airway secured.
    A. 9
    B. 10
    C. 13
    D. 15

19. Current guidelines recommend hyperventilation may be used to reduce ICP. What is the optimal range of $PaCO_2$?
    A. less than 25 mm Hg
    B. less than 35 mm Hg
    C. 35 to 45 mm Hg
    D. 45 to 55 mm Hg

20. Which of the following drugs may be used FIRST to reduce ICP?
    A. loop diuretics
    B. neuromuscular blocking agents
    C. barbituates
    D. analgesics

Pretest Answers: 1. B, 2. A, 3. D, 4. A, 5. C, 6. A, 7. B, 8. C, 9. D, 10. B, 11. B, 12. A, 13. C, 14. B, 15. D, 16. C, 17. A, 18. A, 19. C, 20. D

GLOSSARY

arousal The component of consciousness concerned with the ability of an individual simply to respond to environmental stimuli, such as opening the eyes to speech or turning the head toward a noise.

autoregulation The localized matching of cerebral blood flow with cerebral metabolism.

blood–brain barrier A network of cells and membranes that control brain volume and contents by controlling permeability.

cerebral blood flow (CBF) Blood flow to the brain is maintained at a constant rate by vasodilation of the vessels to increase the flow or vasoconstriction to decrease the flow.

cerebral blood volume The amount of blood in the cranial vault at any given point in time; occupies about 10 percent of the total intracranial volume.

cerebral perfusion pressure (CPP) An estimate of the adequacy of cerebral circulation. Perfusion pressure to the brain that is the difference between the mean systemic arterial pressure (arteries) and the mean intracranial pressure (reflecting veins). It is calculated as follows: **CPP = MAP − ICP.**

circle of Willis An area in the brain where carotid arteries and vertebral arteries unite to provide collateral blood flow to either side of the brain.

consciousness State of general awareness of oneself and the environment; made up of the components of arousal and content.

content The component of consciousness concerned with interpreting environmental stimuli; includes thinking, memory, problem solving, orientation, and speech.

Cushing's triad Vital sign changes that occur when ICP equals MAP and includes (1) increased systolic blood pressure, (2) decreased diastolic blood pressure, and (3) bradycardia.

decerebrate posturing Abnormal extension. Neck is extended with jaw clenched; arms pronate and extend straight out; feet are plantar flexed.

decorticate posturing Abnormal flexion. Upper arms move upward to the chest; elbows, wrists, and fingers flex; legs extend with internal rotation; feet flex.

doll's eye movements Oculocephalic reflex. Reflexive movements of the eyes in the opposite direction of head rotation.

expressive aphasia The inability to write or use language appropriately.

global aphasia The inability to use or understand language.

herniation A shifting or displacement of brain tissue, which causes pressure and traction on cerebral structures and produces clinical symptoms.

hydrocephalus A clinical syndrome caused by an increased production of cerebrospinal fluid that exceeds the absorption rate.

hyperemia A state in which cerebral blood flow is higher than cerebral metabolic needs; also known as "luxury perfusion."

intracranial pressure Pressure exerted by the cerebrospinal fluid within the ventricles of the brain; normal pressure is 0 to 15 mm Hg.

intracranial hypertension Increased intracranial pressure.

Monro–Kellie hypothesis A principle that states that the skull is a rigid vault filled with noncompressible contents: brain, blood, and cerebrospinal fluid; if any one component increases in volume, one or both remaining components must decrease in volume for overall volume to remain constant.

nystagmus Lateral tonic deviation of the eyes toward a stimulus.

otorrhea Drainage of fluid from the ear (usually CSF or blood).

receptive aphasia The inability to understand written or spoken words.

responsiveness A term synonymous with consciousness, which is a general state of awareness of oneself and the environment.

reticular activating system (RAS) A pathway of neurons and neuronal connections for transmission of sensory stimuli from the lower brainstem to the cerebral cortex; the anatomic basis of the arousal component of consciousness.

ABBREVIATIONS

CBF	Cerebral blood flow	**LP**	Lumbar puncture
CEO$_2$	Cerebral oxygen extraction	**MAP**	Mean arterial pressure
CPP	Cerebral perfusion pressure	**MRA**	Magnetic resonance angiography
CSF	Cerebrospinal fluid	**MRI**	Magnetic resonance imaging
CT	Computed tomography	**Pa$_{CO_2}$**	Partial pressure of carbon dioxide
EEG	Electroencephalography	**PCA**	Posterior cerebral artery
GCS	Glasgow Coma Scale	**PET**	Positron emission tomography
ICP	Intracranial pressure	**SPECT**	Single photon emission computed tomography
IVC	Intraventricular catheter	**TCD**	Transcranial doppler

SECTION ONE: Selective Anatomy and Physiology of Cerebral Tissue Perfusion

This section describes the anatomy and physiology pertinent to cerebral tissue perfusion. At the completion of this section, the learner will be able to explain cerebral blood flow, describe the relationship between cerebral oxygenation and metabolism, and identify factors that affect cerebral oxygenation.

Arterial Circulation

Cerebral arteries are structurally different from other arteries. They are thinner and more delicate and are, therefore, more susceptible to rupture with hypertension. The brain is supplied by two major pairs of arteries: the right and left internal carotid arteries and the right and left vertebral arteries (Fig. 18–1). Together their branches unite within the brain to form the **circle of Willis,** a connecting junction that provides collateral blood flow to either side of the brain. The internal carotids supply the retinas and the anterior two thirds of the cerebral hemispheres via its branches: the middle cerebrals, the anterior cerebral, and the anterior and posterior communicating arteries. The middle cerebral arteries are the largest branches of the internal carotids. They supply almost the entire lateral surface of the frontal, parietal, and temporal lobes; the underlying white matter; and the basal ganglia. These are the arteries most frequently involved with strokes. The anterior communicating artery connects the anterior cerebral arteries; and the posterior communicating arteries join the posterior cerebral arteries (PCAs) to complete the circle of Willis. The circle of Willis is protective because it is the primary collateral pathway when major cerebral vessels are occluded. For example, if the carotid artery is occluded, collateral flow may still be possible via the posterior communicating or anterior cerebral arteries to ischemic brain areas.

The vertebrobasilar system supplies the posterior portion of the cerebrum, cerebellum, and brainstem. The vertebral arteries originate from the subclavian arteries, enter the cranium, and, at the pontine-medullary level, join to form the single basilar artery. The vertebral arteries supply the lateral medulla and a portion of the cerebellum. The basilar artery supplies the pons and cerebellum. It divides at the junction of the pons and midbrain into the PCAs. The PCAs supply the midbrain, diencephalon (hypothalamus, subthalamus, thalamus), and inferior portion of the cerebrum. These major arteries are called conducting arteries and their small branches, called penetrating arteries, penetrate into the depths of the brain. Penetrating arteries are frequently involved in small lacunar or ministrokes.

Venous Circulation

The venous circulation is a low-pressure system, as compared with the arterial circulation, which is a high-pressure, high-resistance system. Craniospinal veins are valveless and drain by gravity, an important characteristic to remember when positioning patients with increased **intracranial pressure (ICP).** The dura mater contains venous sinuses that collect blood from the cerebral, meningeal, and diploic veins of the cranium and empty it into the internal jugular veins. These veins drain the cerebral hemispheres and to a lesser degree the brainstem and cerebellum. When intracranial pressure (ICP) increases, venous outflow from the brain decreases because the low-pressure veins are compressed.

Figure 18–1 ■ Major arteries serving the brain and the circle of Willis.

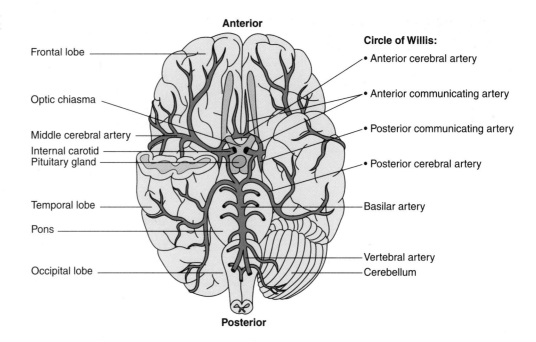

Anterior

Circle of Willis:
- Anterior cerebral artery
- Anterior communicating artery
- Posterior communicating artery
- Posterior cerebral artery
- Basilar artery
- Vertebral artery
- Cerebellum

Frontal lobe

Optic chiasma

Middle cerebral artery
Internal carotid
Pituitary gland

Temporal lobe

Pons

Occipital lobe

Posterior

Cerebral Oxygenation

The brain requires a continuous supply of glucose, oxygen, and substrates for energy because it cannot store oxygen and its glucose reserves last for only a few minutes. Cerebral metabolism varies regionally, with some areas of the brain being more metabolically active than others at any given time. **Cerebral blood flow (CBF),** or blood flow to the brain, varies regionally as well. The brain attempts to meet metabolic demands by locally increasing or decreasing CBF as needed. This localized matching of CBF with metabolism is achieved through the process of pressure **autoregulation.** Autoregulation enables cerebral arterioles to alter their blood flow within an average systemic arterial pressure limit (60 to 130 mm Hg in adults), to promote a constant blood supply to the brain regardless of systemic blood pressure fluctuations. When systemic blood pressure increases, cerebral arterioles constrict; when systemic blood pressure decreases, cerebral arterioles dilate, ensuring adequate cerebral perfusion. When CBF is inadequate to meet the brain's metabolic needs, a state of mismatching occurs, and ischemia results. Because the brain is unable to store oxygen or glucose, aerobic metabolism can no longer be supported and the brain is forced to switch to anaerobic metabolism. The end product of anaerobic metabolism is lactate (refer to Module 14). Lactate does not cross the blood–brain barrier; it accumulates, resulting in cerebral acidosis. Cerebral acidosis causes cerebral vasodilation, which upsets the state of equilibrium in the cranial vault.

The brain, through autoregulation, has the ability to maintain constant CBF with changes in body metabolism and in situations of altered acid–base balance. An increase in body metabolic rate (such as with fever or pain) increases CBF, whereas a decrease in body metabolic rate (as with sedation,

paralysis, or hypothermia) decreases CBF. Conditions that cause alkalosis (such as hypocapnia) produce cerebral vasoconstriction and a reduction of CBF. Conditions that cause acidosis (retention of CO_2, ischemia) produce cerebral vasodilation with an increase in CBF.

Because of the brain's attempt to match CBF with cerebral metabolism, CBF is an important variable when addressing cerebral oxygenation. Cerebral hypoxia occurs when CBF is too low to support cerebral metabolism. CBF decreases with cerebral edema, low cardiac output, or vasoconstriction. When CBF is higher than the metabolic needs of the brain, a state of **hyperemia** exists, also known as "luxury perfusion." Patients with this condition have progressive vasodilation, increased CBF, and eventual loss of autoregulation, all of which contribute to increased ICP. Both cerebral hypoxia and hyperemia have been described as pathophysiologic changes that occur following brain injury. Maintaining adequate cerebral oxygenation is of the utmost importance to support aerobic metabolism. Every effort should be made to avoid episodes of cerebral hypoxia or hypotension.

In summary, cerebral arteries are thin and delicate, which makes them more susceptible to rupture. The carotid and vertebral arteries form the circle of Willis. The circle of Willis is the primary collateral pathway when major cerebral vessels are occluded. The cerebral venous circulation is valveless and drains by gravity, mostly through the internal jugular veins. Cerebral oxygenation is maintained through a constant CBF through the process of autoregulation. Certain conditions affect CBF. When cerebral blood flow does not match cerebral metabolic needs, cerebral hypoxia or hyperemia can occur. Maintaining adequate cerebral oxygenation is of the utmost importance to support aerobic metabolism; episodes of hypoxia or hypotension must be avoided.

SECTION ONE REVIEW

1. Which of the following is protective because it is the primary collateral pathway when major cerebral vessels are occluded?
   A. circle of Willis
   B. left internal carotid artery
   C. right internal carotid artery
   D. middle cerebral artery
2. Cerebral arteries are more prone to rupture during hypertension because
   A. there are so many of them
   B. they have autoregulation
   C. they are thin and delicate
   D. they are not protected by skeletal muscles

3. Which of the following are TRUE statements about the venous circulation of the brain?
   A. craniospinal veins are valveless
   B. craniospinal veins drain by gravity
   C. the venous circulation is a low-pressure system
   D. all of the above
4. The localized matching of CBF with cerebral metabolism occurs through
   A. autoregulation
   B. anaerobic metabolism
   C. luxury perfusion
   D. CSF

Answers: 1. A, 2. C, 3. D, 4. A

SECTION TWO: Intracranial Pressure

At the completion of this section, the learner will be able to state the three components that define the Monro–Kellie hypothesis and explain the pathophysiologic mechanisms that produce increased intracranial pressure through alterations in brain volume, cerebral blood volume, and cerebrospinal fluid.

The intracranial vault is a rigid container within a limited space. The contents of the intracranial vault include the brain, cerebral blood volume, and cerebrospinal fluid. The volume of each component remains relatively stable (brain 80 percent; blood 10 percent, and CSF 10 percent). The **Monro–Kellie hypothesis** states that a change in volume of any one of these components must be accompanied by a reciprocal change in one or both of the other components. If this reciprocal change is not accomplished, the result is an increase in ICP.

Brain Volume

The brain volume is mainly water, and the majority of the water is intracellular. The brain volume remains constant through the **blood–brain barrier.** The blood–brain barrier, a network of cells and membranes in the brain capillaries, controls brain volume by regulating the solutes and water that attempt to cross it and enter the cerebral circulation. This barrier is selective in terms of membrane permeability and molecular size of the substance attempting to enter the cerebral circulation. It is permeable to water, oxygen, lipid-soluble compounds, and carbon dioxide and slightly permeable to the electrolytes. Most drugs do not cross the blood–brain barrier. This barrier is physically disrupted by trauma or functionally impaired by metabolic abnormalities, such as drug overdoses. Disruption of the barrier results in increased brain volume. Fluid escapes from the in-travascular space to the interstitial space of brain tissue, resulting in cerebral edema. According to the Monro–Kellie hypothesis, there is only so much room in the cranial vault and an increase in brain volume necessitates a decrease in either cerebral blood volume or CSF volume. (Under normal conditions, the brain cannot decrease its own size or displace itself). With the increase in brain volume, CSF or cerebral blood volume decrease to maintain normal ICP. If this does not occur, ICP continues to increase.

Cerebral Blood Volume

Cerebral blood volume is the amount of blood in the cranial vault at any point in time. Cerebral blood volume is maintained at a constant level through CBF. Recall from Section One that CBF is normally controlled by the process of pressure and chemical autoregulation. Conditions that affect cerebral blood flow and therefore cerebral blood volume are summarized in Table 18–1.

TABLE 18–1 Conditions That Affect Cerebral Blood Flow and Cerebral Blood Volume

INCREASED CEREBRAL BLOOD FLOW, INCREASED CEREBRAL BLOOD VOLUME	DECREASED CEREBRAL BLOOD FLOW, DECREASED CEREBRAL BLOOD VOLUME
Systemic hypotension	Systemic hypertension
Increase in body metabolic rate (fever, pain)	Decrease in body metabolic rate (sedation, paralysis, hypothermia)
Systemic acidosis (hypercapnia, ischemia)	Systemic alkalosis (hypocapnia)
	Cerebral edema
	Low cardiac output
Cerebral vasodilation	Cerebral vasoconstriction

Cerebrospinal Fluid

Cerebrospinal fluid (CSF) is the third component of intracranial volume. CSF circulates in the subarachnoid spaces and spinal cord and is reabsorbed into the venous system. Approximately 10 percent of the total intracranial volume is CSF, which accounts for about 150 mL of CSF at any given time. The functions of CSF are to (1) cushion and support the brain and spinal cord; (2) maintain a stable chemical milieu for the central nervous system; and (3) excrete toxic wastes, such as carbon dioxide, lactate, and hydrogen ions. The normal adult CSF pressure varies from 5 to 13 mm Hg, or 50 to 200 cm H_2O. Cerebrospinal fluid is similar to plasma content but has greater amounts of sodium, chloride, and magnesium. Potassium, glucose, and protein are lower in CSF than in plasma. This information is used to interpret CSF test results.

Of the three components in the cranial vault, CSF is displaced most easily and rapidly into the external jugular veins. This explains why a flexed neck or tight endotracheal tube ties obstructs, CSF outflow and increases ICP.

Intracranial Pressure

The combination of the three intracranial compartment volumes forms the total intracranial volume and ICP. ICP is measured in the CSF and is defined as the pressure exerted by the CSF within the ventricles of the brain. Normal ICP ranges from 0 to 15 mm Hg. ICP greater than 15 mm Hg for more than 5 minutes is considered abnormally elevated. Transient elevations in ICP greater than 15 mm Hg because of coughing or suctioning are normal if not sustained. ICP is dynamic. It fluctuates constantly in response to changes in respiratory rate, body position, and such activities as coughing and sneezing. Whereas ICP is a fluctuating phenomenon, intracranial volume is kept relatively stable and constant by reciprocal compensation, the principle outlined in the Monro–Kellie hypothesis. As this principle states, reciprocal compensation can occur in any one of the three compartments.

In summary, the Monro–Kellie hypothesis states that the cranial vault is rigid and fixed and is made up of three compartments: the brain, the cerebral blood volume, and CSF. Brain volume is controlled by the blood–brain barrier, and cerebral blood volume is controlled by CBF. Of the three compartments, CSF is displaced most easily and rapidly and is the first reciprocal response to increase in intracranial volume.

SECTION TWO REVIEW

1. According to the Monro–Kellie hypothesis, an increase in one intracranial compartment must be accompanied by a reciprocal
   A. decrease in another compartment
   B. increase in the blood–brain barrier
   C. decrease in the blood–brain barrier
   D. increase in another compartment
2. Which mechanism controls brain volume?
   A. cerebral blood flow
   B. displacement of CSF
   C. blood–brain barrier
   D. vasoconstriction

3. ICP remains relatively stable and, under normal conditions, it is usually less than
   A. 5 mm Hg
   B. 15 mm Hg
   C. 30 mm Hg
   D. 50 mm Hg
4. Normal adult CSF pressure in the supine position is
   A. 1 to 5 mm Hg
   B. 5 to 13 mm Hg
   C. 13 to 20 mm Hg
   D. 50 to 200 mm Hg

Answers: 1. A, 2. C, 3. B, 4. B

SECTION THREE: Cerebral Perfusion Pressure

At the completion of this section, the reader will be able to calculate a cerebral perfusion pressure based on mean arterial pressure and intracranial pressure.

Cerebral perfusion pressure (CPP) depends on cerebral blood flow (Section One) and intracranial pressure (Section Two). CPP is defined as the pressure gradient necessary to sup-ply adequate amounts of blood to the brain. It is the difference between mean arterial pressure (**MAP**) and ICP. Recall from Module 8 that MAP = [systolic BP + 2(diastolic BP)]/3. CPP is calculated using the following formula: CPP = MAP − ICP.

The normal CPP is 80 to 100 mm Hg. CPP must be greater than 70 mm Hg to ensure adequate cerebral oxygenation (Bullock, et al., 2000). Pressures above or below this will result in a loss of autoregulation and inadequate cerebral tissue oxygenation. Cerebral perfusion is decreased when ICP is high or MAP is low. Cerebral perfusion increases when ICP is low or MAP is high. If the ICP rises to the level of MAP, brain perfusion ceases and brain death results.

Calculate the CPP for the following scenario: The ICP is 10 mm Hg and the blood pressure is 120/80 mm Hg. Answer: The MAP is 93 (120 + 2 (80) = 280/3 = 93). The CPP in this situation would be 83 (93 − 10 = 83). CPP is within normal range.

Decreased CPP requires prompt recognition and treatment. Interventions for patients with decreased CPP include mechanisms to increase MAP and reduce ICP. Section Four discusses assessment of CPP and ICP. Section Five reviews interventions used to optimize CPP in the high-acuity patient.

In summary, CPP depends on MAP and ICP. CPP is calculated using the formula MAP − ICP. Normal CPP is 80 mm Hg. CPP decreases when MAP is low or ICP is high.

SECTION THREE REVIEW

1. CPP depends on all of the following EXCEPT
   A. cerebral blood volume
   B. brain volume
   C. CSF volume
   D. cerebral medullary regulation
2. CPP must be greater than _____ mm Hg to ensure adequate cerebral oxygenation.
   A. 70
   B. 60
   C. 50
   D. 40
3. Your patient's MAP is 80 mm Hg and the ICP is 15 mm Hg. What is the cerebral perfusion pressure?
   A. 50 mm Hg
   B. 65 mm Hg
   C. 95 mm Hg
   D. 110 mm Hg

Answers: 1. D, 2. A, 3. B

SECTION FOUR: Decreased Intracranial Adaptive Capacity

When intracranial mechanisms fail to compensate for increases in intracranial volume, ICP increases. The nursing diagnosis for this condition is *decreased intracranial adaptive capacity*. At the completion of this section, the reader will be able to identify causes and effects of increases in brain volume, cerebral blood volume, and CSF volume.

Several conditions can cause an elevation in ICP: (1) an increase in brain volume (cerebral edema, space-occupying lesions such as hematoma), (2) an increase in cerebral blood volume (hypercapnia, hypoxia), or (3) an increase in CSF. Increasing ICP impairs cerebral perfusion and oxygenation of brain cells. **Intracranial hypertension** is a sustained elevation in ICP and is potentially life threatening.

Increase in Brain Volume

Space-occupying lesions and cerebral edema are the primary processes that increase brain volume. Space-occupying lesions may be due to tumors, abscesses, hemorrhages (refer to Module 19), and hematomas (refer to Module 20). Cerebral edema is caused by an abnormal accumulation of fluid that increases brain tissue volume. It may occur in a localized area of the brain or it may occur throughout a more generalized area of the brain. Cerebral edema may occur after any type of insult to the head, including trauma, surgery, brain anoxia, or ischemia. Cerebral edema does not impair brain function until the edema increases ICP. When cerebral edema increases ICP, then cerebral perfusion decreases. The effect of increased brain volume depends on the rate of development. Slower-growing lesions, such as a chronic hematoma or slow-growing tumor, may be tolerated for a longer time period than an acute subdural hematoma, which develops at a faster rate.

A mass or edema that progresses and is uncompensated eventually results in a shifting of brain tissue, or **herniation,** and carries a grave prognosis. This process displaces brain tissue and exerts pressure or traction on cerebral structures. Herniation syndromes are described based on the end stage of the herniation (Table 18–2) and are depicted in Figure 18–2.

TABLE 18–2 Four Herniation Syndromes

Cingulate herniation	Lateral shift of brain tissue, usually as the result of a lesion in one of the cerebral hemispheres
Central or transtentorial herniation	Downward shift of one or both cerebral hemispheres, usually because of lesions in the frontal or parietal lobes
Uncal or lateral transtentorial herniation	Lateral and downward shift of brain tissue, usually the temporal lobe, as a result of lesions located most laterally, such as the middle fossa in the temporal lobe; this type of herniation causes compression of the oculomotor nerve, or cranial nerve III, evidenced by the classic sign of a unilaterally dilated pupil
Tonsillar herniation	Downward shift of brain tissue through the foramen magnum, which results in compression of the medulla and upper cervical spinal cord

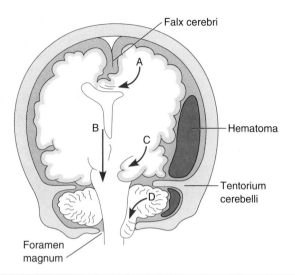

Figure 18–2 ■ Forms of brain herniation due to intracranial hypertension. *A,* Cingulate herniation occurs when the cingulate gyrus is compressed under the falx cerebri. *B,* Central herniation occurs when a centrally located lesion compresses central and midbrain structures. *C,* Lateral herniation occurs when a lesion at the side of the brain compresses the uncus or hippocampal gyrus. *D,* Tonsillar herniation occurs when the cerebellar tonsils are forced downward, compressing the medulla and top of the spinal cord.

Cerebral Blood Volume

Any systemic process that affects blood levels of carbon dioxide affects CBF, CPP, and cerebral blood volume. Therefore, conditions that produce hypercapnia and hypoxemia result in cerebral vasodilation and increased blood volume. These conditions may include chronic respiratory insufficiency, inadequate ventilation, hypoventilation, sedation by drugs, and insufficient supplemental oxygen. Cerebral blood volume increases with any process that impedes venous outflow. This includes anything that impedes jugular circulation, such as head/neck rotation or flexion, or endotracheal tube ties that are too tight or circumferential around the head and neck, Valsalva's maneuver, and use of positive end-expiratory pressure. A third cause of increased blood volume is loss of autoregulation. This regulatory mechanism becomes ineffective in states of ischemia, sustained elevations in ICP, and sustained states of hyperemia. When autoregulation is lost, the cerebral blood vessels passively dilate, and produce further increases in cerebral blood volume and ICP.

Cerebrospinal Fluid

CSF volume increases with increased production, obstructed circulation, or decreased absorption. This is a condition termed **hydrocephalus.** Obstruction to CSF can be caused by mass lesions or infection. Decreased absorption can result from a subarachnoid hemorrhage or meningitis. Hydrocephalus may be treated in one of two ways. If it is considered to be a permanent condition, a surgical shunt is placed; if it is considered temporary, a ventricular drain is inserted for intermittent or continuous drainage of CSF.

Table 18–3 summarizes the causes and effects of increased brain volume, cerebral blood volume and CSF. Keep in mind that uncompensated increases in brain or blood volume or CSF, if not treated result in herniation.

In summary, failure of intracranial mechanisms to compensate for increases in intracranial volume result in increased ICP and decreased intracranial adaptive capacity, and impair cerebral tissue perfusion and oxygenation. Space-occupying lesions and cerebral edema increase brain volume and result in herniation, which carries a grave prognosis. There are four herniation syndromes. Increased cerebral blood volume may be caused by increases in carbon dioxide levels, impaired venous outflow, or loss of autoregulation. Increases in CSF may be the result of increased production, obstructed circulation, or decreased absorption that results in hydrocephalus.

TABLE 18–3   Causes and Effects of Increases in Brain Volume, Cerebral Blood Volume, and CSF

COMPONENT	CAUSE	EFFECT
Brain volume	Space-occupying lesions	Herniation
	Cerebral edema	
Blood volume	Hypercapnia	Cerebral vasodilation
	Hypoxemia	Passive cerebral vessels
	Loss of autoregulation	
	Venous outflow obstruction	Increased cerebral blood volume
CSF	Obstruction	Hydrocephalus
	Decreased absorption	
	Increased production	

SECTION FOUR REVIEW

1. Which of the following conditions is NOT associated with increased intracranial volume?
   A. subdural hematoma
   B. hypotension
   C. subarachnoid hemorrhage
   D. meningioma

2. Which of the following is NOT a direct cause of increased CSF?
   A. meningitis
   B. hypoglycemia
   C. subarachnoid hemorrhage
   D. brain tumor

3. ICP can be increased by anything that
   A. increases intracranial volume
   B. results in high compliance
   C. results in low elastance
   D. decreases carbon dioxide levels
4. Accumulation of CSF results in
   A. herniation
   B. cerebral dilation
   C. hydrocephalus
   D. seizures

5. A downward shift of brain tissue through the foramen magnum which results in compression of the medulla and upper cervical spinal cord is called a
   A. cingulate herniation
   B. uncal transtentorial herniation
   C. lateral transtentorial herniation
   D. tonsillar herniation

Answers: 1. B, 2. B, 3. A, 4. C, 5. D

SECTION FIVE: Assessment of Cerebral Tissue Perfusion

Decreased CPP requires prompt recognition. This section reviews assessment techniques used for and abnormal findings associated with decreased cerebral tissue perfusion and decreased intracranial adaptive capacity. The first part of this section reviews pertinent physical assessment findings the high-acuity nurse must know in caring for patients with these nursing diagnoses. The types of systems used for ICP monitoring and nursing care for patients undergoing this monitoring are discussed. The last part of this section explains some common diagnostic procedures used to identify impaired cerebral tissue perfusion and decreased intracranial adaptive capacity. At the completion of this section, the learner will be able to (1) state the components of an assessment of level of consciousness in terms of assessing arousal and content; (2) compare and contrast components of the Glasgow Coma Scale; (3) identify the components of an in-depth clinical neurological assessment used to assess a patient with an altered level of consciousness; (4) compare and contrast normal and abnormal findings for the components of an in-depth neurological assessment; (5) state the intracranial pressure monitoring types and systems, and discuss the advantages and disadvantages of each; (6) identify normal and abnormal intracranial pressure monitoring waveforms; and (7) compare and contrast common diagnostic procedures used to diagnose conditions that cause impaired cerebral tissue perfusion and decreased intracranial adaptive capacity.

Level of Consciousness

Level of **consciousness** is the most important component of the neurologic assessment in the high-acuity patient. These assessments must be performed and documented in a reliable and consistent manner to provide an accurate transfer of information from clinician to clinician. Often a change in level of consciousness is the first sign of neurologic deterioration. In the high-acuity environment, assessment of level of consciousness is part of the recurring systems assessments made by the nurse.

The mnemonic "Vowel – TIPPS" is useful for remembering common etiologies for impaired consciousness:

Alcohol	**T**rauma
Epilepsy	**I**nfection
Insulin	**P**sych
Opiates	**P**oisons
Urates (renal failure)	**S**hock

There are two components of consciousness: arousal (alertness) and content (awareness).

Arousal

Assessment of the arousal component of consciousness involves an evaluation of the **reticular activating system. Arousal,** the lowest level of consciousness, centers on the patient's ability to respond to stimuli in an appropriate manner. Conditions that affect arousal do so by directly or indirectly depressing the brainstem structures and the reticular activating system. These conditions result in immediate loss of consciousness and produce coma. Any condition that impairs arousal will naturally impair content as well. Processes that impair arousal include mass lesions that destroy brainstem structures, compression of the brainstem by herniation, or any process that involves the brainstem and the cerebral hemispheres that is sufficient to produce a depressed level of consciousness. Labels, such as comatose, lethargic, and stuporous, should be avoided because they lend themselves to subjective interpretation.

The Glasgow Coma Scale (GCS) is the most frequently used assessment tool to identify changes in arousal. The scale assesses eye opening, verbal response, and best motor response to stimuli (Table 18–4). The best possible score is 15 and the lowest score is 3. A score less than 7 is consistent with a significant alteration in level of consciousness (coma state). Any deterioration in the GCS score is significant and requires immediate physician notification to allow for early intervention and prevent further neurologic compromise. Certain patient conditions prevent the use of the GCS. Patients with periorbital edema who are unable to open their eyes receive an eye opening response score of 1, which may or may not be valid. Motor deficits, such as hemiparesis or paraplegia, may be overlooked because the

TABLE 18–4 Glasgow Coma Scale

CATEGORY	SCORE	RESPONSE
Eye opening	4	Spontaneous—eyes open spontaneously without stimulation
	3	To speech—eyes open with verbal stimulation but not necessarily to command
	2	To pain—eyes open with noxious stimuli
	1	None—no eye opening regardless of stimulation
Verbal response	5	Oriented—accurate information about person, place, time, reason for hospitalization, and personal data
	4	Confused—answers not appropriate to question but correct use of language
	3	Inappropriate words—disorganized, random speech, no sustained conversation
	2	Incomprehensible sounds—moans, groans, and mumbles incomprehensibly
	1	None—no verbalization despite stimulation
Best motor response	6	Obeys commands—performs simple tasks on command; able to repeat performance
	5	Localizes to pain—organized attempt to localize and remove painful stimuli
	4	Withdraws from pain—withdraws extremity from source of painful stimuli
	3	Abnormal flexion—decorticate posturing spontaneously or in response to noxious stimuli
	2	Extension—decerebrate posturing spontaneously or in response to noxious stimuli
	1	None—no response to noxious stimuli; flaccid

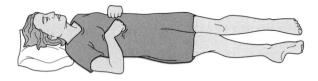

Figure 18–3A ■ Decorticate posturing. Upper arms move upward to the chest; elbows, wrists, and fingers flex; legs extend with internal rotation; feet flex.

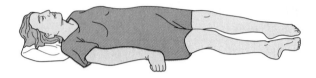

Figure 18–3B ■ Decerebrate posturing. Neck is extended with jaw clenched; arms pronate and extend straight out; feet are plantar flexed.

(Figure 18–3A). **Decerebrate posturing** (abnormal extension) indicates brainstem dysfunction and is a more ominous sign. With decerebrate posturing, the neck extends, the jaw clenches, arms pronate and extend straight out, and the feet plantar flex (Figure 18–3B).

Content

Assessment of the content component of consciousness is an evaluation of the cerebral hemispheres. **Content,** a higher level of functioning than arousal, centers on the patient's orientation to time, place, and person. The patient should respond to questions appropriately; any sign of disorientation may be the first indication of neurologic deterioration. Conditions that impair content do so by widely affecting the cerebral hemispheres. Alterations in content are manifested by cognitive deficits such as memory impairment, disorientation, impaired problem-solving abilities, and attentional deficits. The degree of cognitive deficit is related to the location and size of the lesion. Lesions that affect small areas of the hemispheres usually do not produce a significant depression in the level of consciousness. Hemispheric strokes and small intracerebral hematomas and contusions result in localized deficits. Conditions that diffusely affect the hemispheres cause a significant depression in the level of consciousness and may result in coma. Anoxia, ischemia, metabolic alterations, poisons, drugs, and psychiatric disturbances cause diffuse cerebral hemispheric dysfunction.

The content of consciousness is assessed by noting behavior. The patient should be assessed for orientation and should know his or her name, the date, and where she or he is. The patient is considered disoriented if unable to answer the questions correctly. Testing for orientation also assesses short-term memory. Orientation can be assessed only if the patient is able to respond verbally. After assessing orientation, the ability to follow commands is assessed. Ask the patient to perform such acts as sticking out the tongue or holding up two fingers. This not only

motor response scored is the best response elicited. Finally, it is impossible to evaluate a verbal response for patients who are intubated or have a tracheostomy; they also receive a score of 1, which may not be valid.

The first step is to determine what stimulus arouses the patient. First, address the patient by his name. If he does not respond, shake his arm or shoulder gently. If no response is elicited, proceed from light pain to deeper pain in an attempt to elicit a response. Always start with the least noxious stimulus and proceed to a more intense stimulus if necessary: shaking the arm, nailbed pressure, trapezius pinch. This assesses two things: (1) Is the patient responsive to verbal stimuli? and if not (2) Does the patient exhibit purposeful movement? Purposeful movement, such as removing the stimulus or withdrawing from the stimulus, indicates functioning of sensory pathways. Abnormal posturing in response to a noxious stimulus indicates a dysfunction of either the cerebral hemispheres or the brainstem. **Decorticate posturing** (abnormal flexion) indicates cerebral hemispheric dysfunction. In response to painful stimuli, the upper arms move up toward the chest with the elbows, wrists, and fingers. Flexed legs extend with internal rotation and the feet flex

helps determine whether the patient is awake enough to respond but also whether he or she is aware enough to interpret and carry out the commands. Next, behavioral changes are assessed by noting any restlessness, irritability, or combativeness. Such behavioral indicators can be caused by hypoxia, hypoglycemia, drug use, pain, or increased ICP. It is part of a nurse's role to notice and evaluate clues that may point to causes for changes in behavior. The last component of content that is assessed is verbal response. Assessment of speech provides information about the function of the relationship between the speech centers in the cerebrum and the cranial nerves, and can help localize the area of dysfunction. The patient's speech pattern is assessed for clarity. Is it clear or slurred and garbled? This may indicate drug use, metabolic disturbance, or cranial nerve injuries. Content of speech is assessed for use of appropriate or inappropriate words. Confused patients may use inappropriate words. Patients with cranial nerve dysfunction may give appropriate responses; however, the speech pattern may be slurred. Patients may experience receptive, expressive, or global aphasia. Inability to understand written or spoken words is **receptive aphasia.** Inability to write or use language appropriately is **expressive aphasia. Global aphasia** includes the inability to use or understand language.

In-Depth Clinical Assessment

Beyond the assessment of arousal and content, a more in-depth neurological assessment includes assessments of pupillary and oculomotor reactions, vital signs, and cranial nerve reflexes.

Pupillary and Oculomotor Reactions

Pupillary reactions provide information about the location of lesions. Pupils are assessed for size, symmetry, shape, and reaction to light. Pupil size is assessed using a standard pupil gauge (Fig. 18–4). Pupils should be equal in size. Abnormal pupil responses are shown in Figure 18–5. Nonreactive pupils in the midposition indicate damage to the midbrain (Fig. 18–5A). Pupils that are nonreactive to light and pinpoint indicate a pons lesion or opiate drug overdose (Fig. 18–5B). Pupils that are small but reactive to light may indicate a bilateral injury to the thalamus or hypothalamus or metabolic coma (Fig. 18–5C). A unilaterally dilated and fixed pupil may indicate compression of the oculomotor nerve (cranial nerve III) (Fig. 18–5D). Pupil changes are on the same side (ipsilateral) as the lesion. When both pupils are dilated and nonreactive (fixed), emergency action is required. This may be caused by severe anoxia or ischemia. Remember that certain drugs (atropine, epinephrine) can dilate the pupils (Fig. 18–5E).

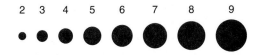

Figure 18–4 ■ Pupil gauge in millimeters.

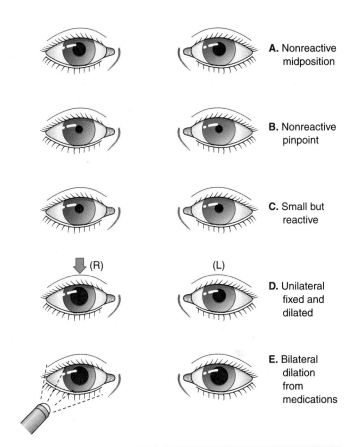

Figure 18–5 ■ Abnormal pupil responses.

A. Nonreactive midposition

B. Nonreactive pinpoint

C. Small but reactive

D. Unilateral fixed and dilated

E. Bilateral dilation from medications

Oculomotor Responses

Two reflexes used to determine brainstem integrity are the oculovestibular (caloric) and oculocephalic (doll's eyes) reflexes. Both reflexes involve cranial nerves III (oculomotor), IV (trochlear), VI (abducens), and VIII (acoustic). In the awake patient, it is easy to test these cranial nerves by asking the patient to perform a full range of eye movements. Asking the patient to look upward, downward, outward, inward, medially upward and outward, and laterally upward and outward demonstrates the full range of eye motion, also known as extraocular eye movements. Deficits in eye movements indicate a cranial nerve dysfunction of one or more of the previously mentioned cranial nerves. However, in the unresponsive patient, voluntary eye movement is lost and the patient is unable to perform extraocular eye movements. In this case, oculocephalic and oculovestibular responses are tested to evaluate eye movements.

In deteriorating levels of consciousness, spontaneous eye movements may be lost. Under normal conditions, both eyes move spontaneously in the same direction. Injury to the midbrain and pons impairs normal movement. **Doll's eye movements** (oculocephalic reflex) are reflexive movements of the eyes in the opposite direction of head rotation. This reflex is tested by holding the patient's eyes open and briskly turning the head from side to side, pausing at each side. If the patient has an intact brainstem, the examiner sees conjugate eye movement

Figure 18–6 ▪Doll's eye movements characteristic of altered level of consciousness.

Head in neutral position

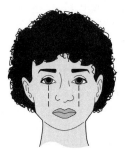

Eyes midline

Head rotated to patient's left

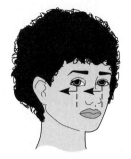

Doll's eyes present: Eyes move right in relation to head.

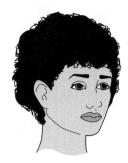

Doll's eyes absent: Eyes do not move in relation to head. Eyes remain in midposition.

opposite to the side the head is turned, known as "full doll's eyes" (Fig. 18–6). In cases of brainstem injury, the eyes will remain fixed in the midposition as the head is turned, and doll's eyes are absent. This test is contraindicated in patients whose cervical spine has not been cleared of injury.

Another reflex, oculovestibular reflex (cold caloric test) may be performed by a physician when determining brainstem function. Instilling cold water into the ear canal causes **nystagmus** (lateral tonic deviation of the eyes) toward the stimulus. This reflex is lost when brainstem function is lost. The oculovestibular reflex is a more sensitive indicator of brainstem function and central nervous system injury. Patients with an absent oculocephalic reflex have a normal oculovestibular reflex. Therefore, testing for the oculovestibular reflex always follows testing for the oculocephalic reflex. Testing the oculovestibular reflex is contraindicated if CSF or purulent drainage is leaking from the ear, or if there is perforation or a tear of the tympanic membrane.

Results of oculocephalic or oculovestibular testing are interpreted with caution because pharmacologic agents such as ototoxic drugs, neuromuscular blockers, and ethyl alcohol depress these reflexes.

Vital Signs

Routine parameters assessed in the high-acuity patient include respiratory rate and pattern, heart rate and rhythm, pulse oximetry, blood pressure, and temperature. Because the brainstem influences the cardiovascular and respiratory systems, changes in vital signs may indicate neurologic deterioration.

Respiratory pattern provides valuable information because it is correlated with the anatomic level of dysfunction. Respiratory rhythm and pattern are controlled by the medulla. Respirations are assessed for rate and rhythm and are counted for one full minute before stimulating the patient. Common abnormal respiratory patterns observed in neurologically impaired patients are discussed in the following paragraphs and depicted in Figure 18–7. As a nurse, remember that it is more important to

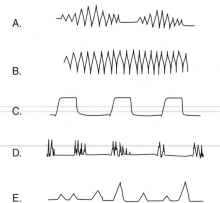

Figure 18–7 ▪Abnormal respiratory patterns. *A.* Cheyne-stokes pattern; *B.* Central neurogenic hyperventilation; *C.* Apeustic breathing; *D.* Cluster breathing; *E.* Ataxic breathing.

describe the pattern than to try to fit the patient's respiratory pattern into a category. If the patient is mechanically ventilated, it is difficult to observe these patterns, and it would be extremely detrimental to the patient to remove ventilatory support for the purpose of assessing abnormal patterns.

Cheyne–Stokes pattern indicates a bilateral lesion in the cerebral hemispheres, cerebellum, midbrain, or, in rare circumstances, upper pons and may be caused by cerebral infarction or metabolic diseases. This respiratory pattern is evidenced by a rhythmic waxing and waning in the depth of the respiration, followed by a period of apnea. *Central neurogenic hyperventilation* indicates a lesion in the low midbrain or upper pons and may be caused by infarction or ischemia of the midbrain or pons, anoxia, or tumors of the midbrain. This pattern is evidenced by respirations that have an increase in depth, are rapid (greater than 24), and are regular. *Apneustic breathing* indicates a lesion in the mid or low pons that may be caused by infarction of the pons or severe meningitis. This pattern is evidenced by prolonged inspiration, with a pause at the point where the respiration is at its peak, lasting for 2 to 3 seconds. This may alternate with an expiratory pause. *Cluster breathing* indicates a lesion in the low pons or upper medulla that may be caused by a tumor or infarction of the medulla. This pattern is described as clusters of irregular breathing with periods of apnea that occur at irregular intervals. *Ataxic breathing* indicates a lesion in the medulla that may be caused by a cerebellar or pons bleed, tumors of the cerebrum, or severe meningitis. These respirations are completely irregular, with deep and shallow random breaths and pauses. Remember that abnormal respiratory patterns also may be initiated by conditions such as acid-base and electrolyte imbalances, anxiety, pulmonary disease, or drugs, especially narcotics and anesthetic agents that depress the respiratory center.

The pulse is assessed for rate, rhythm, and quality. Increased heart rate may indicate poor cerebral oxygenation. Decreased heart rate is present in the late stages of increased ICP.

The medulla regulates blood pressure based on input from chemoreceptors and baroreceptors. Mean arterial pressure must be maintained at a sufficient level to produce adequate cerebral tissue perfusion when ICP is elevated. Cerebral trauma is rarely associated with hypotension. Quite the contrary. Cerebral trauma produces systemic hypertension. An important response to ischemia, known as the **Cushing's triad,** is a specific change in vital signs evidenced by (1) an increase in systolic blood pressure, (2) a decrease in diastolic blood pressure, and (3) bradycardia. This response is activated when ICP rises to a point where it equals or exceeds MAP.

The center for temperature regulation is in the hypothalamus. Injury to or dysfunction of the hypothalamus produces alterations in body temperature. Hypothermia occurs as a result of spinal shock, metabolic coma, drug overdose (especially depressants), and destructive lesions of the brainstem or hypothalamus. Hyperthermia occurs as a result of CNS infection, subarachnoid hemorrhage, hypothalamic lesions, or hemorrhage of the hypothalamus or brainstem. Temperature fluctuates widely and often exceeds 106°F. Hyperthermia is treated promptly because of the increased metabolic demands placed on the body and brain.

Cranial Nerve Reflexes

Cranial nerve reflexes are protective reflexes, and they indicate brainstem functioning. The unresponsive patient is assessed for these reflexes and if they are absent or decreased, measures must be taken to protect the patient from injury. The protective reflexes include (1) corneal reflex (blink), (2) gag reflex, (3) swallow reflex, and (4) cough reflex. The corneal reflex is assessed by touching the cornea, from the side, with a wisp of cotton. The eye blinks rapidly if the reflex is intact. The gag reflex is assessed by touching the posterior tongue with a tongue blade. If intact, the patient gags. The cough and gag reflexes can also be assessed while suctioning the intubated patient.

In summary, deterioration in function of the cerebral hemispheres results in changes in level of consciousness as evidenced by a decrease in GCS score, changes in pupillary and oculomotor responses, and changes in vital signs. Table 18–5 summarizes the manifestations of progressive deterioration of cerebral function. Assessment of these changes helps determine the extent of cerebral dysfunction. Early intervention at the sign of any of these changes may prevent further neurologic damage.

Intracranial Pressure Monitoring

ICP monitoring provides continuous data regarding the pressure within the cranial vault. The primary reasons for ICP monitoring are to assist in calculating and maintaining adequate CPP

TABLE 18–5   Manifestations of Progressive Deterioration in Brain Function

LEVEL OF CONSCIOUSNESS	PUPILLARY RESPONSE	OCULOMOTOR RESPONSES	MOTOR RESPONSES	BREATHING
Alert, oriented to time, place, person	Equal, round, reactive to light	Eyes move as head turns Caloric testing produces nystagmus	Purposeful movements; responds to commands	Regular rate, pattern
Responds to verbal stimuli; episodes of confusion, restlessness	Equal, round, reactive to light progressing to small, reactive	Roving eye movements	Purposeful movement in response to pain	Yawning, sighing
Requires continuous stimulation to rouse	Small reactive progressing to slowing response to light (sluggish)		Decorticate posturing	Cheyne–Stokes
Reflexive posturing to pain stimulus	Ipsilateral dilation; fixed (nonreactive)		Decerebrate posturing	Central neurologic hyperventilation
No response to stimuli	Bilateral dilation and fixation	No spontaneous eye movements; eyes fixed in mid-position with doll's eye No eye movements to cold caloric testing	Flaccidity	Cluster or ataxic breathing; apnea

Adapted from Lemone, P., & Burke, K. (2004). Medical surgical nursing: Critical thinking in client care, 3rd ed. [p. 1346]. Upper Saddle River, NJ: Prentice Hall.

and to permit early detection and treatment of increased ICP (Littlejohns & Bader, 2001). Continuous monitoring allows titration of therapies to maintain adequate tissue perfusion and thereby prevent ischemia. It enables the identification of impending brain herniation secondary to escalating ICP, determines the need for and impact of therapies, and predicts outcome. Patient selection is an important decision because not all patients with altered cerebral tissue perfusion require or are appropriate candidates for ICP monitoring. Current guidelines recommend that ICP monitoring may be appropriate for two situations: (1) patients with a GSC of 8 or less who also have abnormal findings on a head CT scan; or (2) patients with evidence of altered cerebral tissue perfusion, but who have a normal head CT scan, and have two or more of the following: age greater than 40 years, unilateral or bilateral motor posturing, or systolic blood pressure less than 90 mm Hg (Bullock et al., 2000).

Types of ICP Monitoring Devices

ICP monitoring is classified by the anatomic placement of the device. Basic monitoring systems include intraventricular catheters, subarachnoid screws, intraparenchymal catheters, and epidural probes (Fig. 18–8). Each system has advantages and disadvantages for monitoring ICP (Table 18–6).

Intraventricular monitoring, the gold standard for ICP monitoring, is used for both diagnostic and therapeutic purposes. This type of monitoring involves placing an intraventricular catheter (IVC) into the anterior horn of the lateral ventricle, preferably in the nondominant hemisphere. Diagnostically, it is the most reliable of the monitoring devices and provides precise and consistent waveforms. Therapeutically, CSF can be drained from the intraventricular cavity, thereby decreasing the CSF compartment and reducing ICP. Drainage of CSF can be continuous or intermittent. Continuous drainage is an open system whereby CSF automatically drains when the ICP exceeds a certain point. This point is determined by how high or low the drainage bag is placed above the foramen of Munro, which is the anatomic landmark for the lateral ventricle. Usually, this landmark is at the top of the outer ear. Intermittent drainage is a closed system that is opened for periodic drainage when the ICP exceeds a certain point, to be stipulated by the physician, but usually in the range of 20 to 25 mm Hg (Bullock et al., 2000). The IVC has several advantages. Because it is placed directly into the ventricle, it provides direct measurement of ICP and allows for drainage of CSF. However, the IVC is not risk free. It is the most invasive of the monitoring types and, therefore, carries the risk of infection. Because it is introduced directly into brain tissue, the risk of bleeding and destruction of neurons are factors that must be considered. Contraindications for placement of an IVC include patients

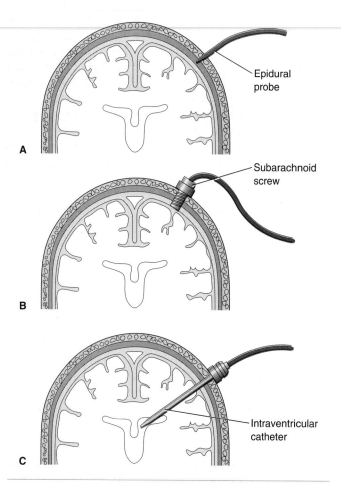

Figure 18–8 ■ Types of intracranial pressure monitoring devices *A,* Epidural probe. *B,* Subarachnoid screw. *C,* Intraventricular.

TABLE 18–6 Comparison of Monitoring Sites

SITE	ADVANTAGES	DISADVANTAGES
Intraventricular	Gold standard Allows for therapeutic intervention by drainage of CSF Direct measurement of CSF pressure Highly accurate	Most invasive; carries high risk for hemorrhage, infection Contraindicated with coagulopathies, or small, misshaped, or collapsed ventricles
Subarachnoid	Less invasive Easy placement Low risk of infection Useful if ventricles cannot be cannulated Able to sample CSF	Unable to drain CSF May become obstructed with bone or tissue Not as accurate as time progresses Needs frequent recalibration Unreliable at high ICPs
Intraparenchymal	Easy placement Low risk of infection Highly accurate	Unable to drain CSF Requires separate monitoring system Catheter fragile; may kink Cannot zero once in place Risk of hemorrhage, infection
Epidural probe	Easy placement Low risk of infection	Unable to drain CSF Cannot zero once in place Accuracy is variable

with coagulopathies, small or collapsed ventricles, or severe generalized cerebral edema.

An alternative to the IVC is the subarachnoid bolt or screw. This type of monitoring device is used in patients with small, collapsed, or shifted ventricles. The device is placed into the subdural or subarachnoid space and provides some of the same monitoring capabilities as the IVC, such as measurement of ICP and evaluation of waveforms, although the waveform is easily dampened because bits of bone and brain tissue may obstruct the tip of the bolt. Unlike the IVC, drainage of CSF is not possible because the ventricle is not cannulated.

Intraparenchymal monitoring devices are placed directly into the brain tissue via a bolt device, usually 1 cm below the subarachnoid space. These devices are easy to place, provide sharp and distinct waveforms, transmit accurate measurement of ICP, and carry a lower risk of infection. For these reasons, they are a desirable alternative to subarachnoid monitors. However, they are more costly, require a separate monitoring system, and do not have CSF drainage capabilities. A small fiber optic sensor can be placed through a burr hole and into the epidural space to monitor ICP. These catheters are easy to place and carry a low risk of infection. A major disadvantage of these catheters is that CSF cannot be drained.

ICP Waveforms

For all ICP monitoring devices, the catheters are connected to a monitoring system that converts pressure impulses (waveforms) into an electronic display on a bedside monitor, very much like hemodynamic monitoring. The waveform comes from pulsations that are transmitted in the brain from intracranial arteries and veins. The nurse must be able to recognize normal waveform patterns and identify dangerous signs and trends that indicate increased ICP. There are three peaks within each ICP waveform (Fig. 18–9). The first peak is P_1 which is referred to as the percussion wave. It has a sharp peak and it originates from pulsations of the choroid plexus. The second peak, P_2, reflects the compliance of brain tissue. If P_2 is as high or higher than P_1, a situation of decreased compliance is present. The third wave, P_3, is the dicrotic wave.

There are three types of ICP pressure waveform patterns: A waves, B waves, and C waves (Fig. 18–10). A waves, or plateau waves, are clinically significant. They typically occur when ICP is elevated. They are spikes of sharp increases in ICP that may be sustained in a plateau fashion for up to 20 minutes. Signs of neurologic deterioration may be seen with these waves (decreasing level of consciousness, pupillary changes, posturing). Plateau waves are significant, especially when the elevation in ICP decreases CPP. B waves often precede A waves. These waves are sharp oscillating waves. They occur every 30 seconds to 2 minutes. They are normal except when B waves elevate to an amplitude of greater than 15 mm Hg. This represents a state of low intracranial compliance. C waves are small rhythmic waves. They occur every 5 to 8 minutes and are normal. They vary with respiration and blood pressure.

Jugular Bulb Oximetry

Monitoring ICP and CPP provides an indirect assessment of cerebral tissue perfusion, but they do not indicate the adequacy of cerebral oxygenation. Measurement of cerebral oxygen saturation via jugular bulb oximetry (SjO_2) is used to assess the relationship between cerebral oxygen supply and demand. These catheters are similar to other mechanisms to monitor oxygenation such as pulse oximetry (SpO_2) and systemic mixed venous oxygen saturation (SvO_2). (Refer to Module 14). SjO_2 monitoring permits continuous measurement of cerebral venous oxygen saturation. The amount of oxygen extracted by cerebral tissue is reflected in the difference between the percentage of oxygen delivered to cerebral tissue (SaO_2 or SpO_2) and the percentage returning from cerebral tissue (SjO_2). Therefore, cerebral oxygen extraction (CEO_2) is $SpO_2 - SjO_2$. Normal CEO_2 is 30 percent. If

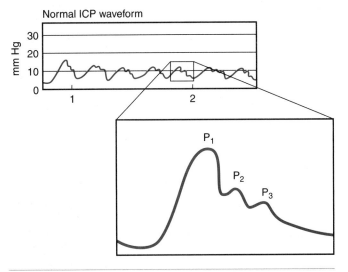

Figure 18–9 ■ Three points within each ICP waveform.

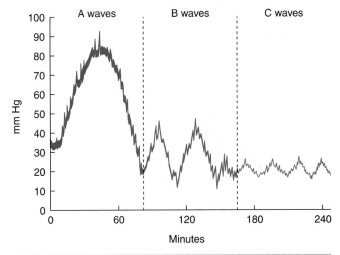

Figure 18–10 ■ A waves, spikes of sharp increases in ICP, are clinically significant; signs of neurologic deterioration may be present. B waves are oscillating waves that are normal except when elevated above 15 mm Hg. C waves are small rhythmic waves that are normal.

the brain is receiving less oxygen than it needs, it extracts more oxygen from the cerebral circulation and SjO_2 is lower. If CBF is higher than the brain requires, less oxygen will be extracted and the SjO_2 is higher. This information helps to determine therapies and interventions to improve cerebral oxygenation. The major advantage of using SjO_2 monitoring over simple ICP or CPP monitoring is that it can help determine if a given CPP is sufficient to satisfy cerebral metabolic demand.

Normal SjO_2 is 60 to 80 percent. SjO_2 less than 55 percent or CEO_2 greater than 40 percent reflect a state of oligemia; SjO_2 greater than 75 percent or CEO_2 less than 24 percent reflect a state of hyperemia or death of brain cells (dead tissue does not extract oxygen). If either hypoxia or hyperemia persists for more than 15 minutes, notify the physician (Kidd & Criddle, 2001).

The difference in the content of oxygen delivered to cerebral tissue and the content returned from cerebral tissue is calculated using the following formula:

$$\text{Cerebral } PaO_2 - PvO_2 = [(SaO_2 - SjO_2) \times 1.34 \times Hgb/100]$$

Normal cerebral $PaO_2 - PvO_2$ is 4 to 8 mL/dL. A narrow cerebral $PaO_2 - PvO_2$ (less than 4 mL/dL) is associated with hyperemia, whereas a wide cerebral $PaO_2 - PvO_2$ (greater than 9 mL/dL) is associated with oligemia.

The SjO_2 catheter is inserted by a physician in a similar manner to that of a central venous catheter. The fiber optic catheter is usually inserted into the right internal jugular vein because this vein drains a greater proportion of blood from the sagittal sinus than the left internal jugular and readings are more representative of global (versus local) brain oxygenation (Kidd & Criddle, 2001). After placement has been confirmed, the catheter is connected to a saline solution at a rate of 3 to 5 mL/hr. No other fluids or medications should be infused through this catheter. Further nursing care priorities for patients receiving this type of monitoring are reviewed in Section Six.

Evidence-Based Practice

- *ICP is lower and CPP is higher for a 30-degree backrest elevation than for a flat position in patients with closed-head injury (Winkleman, 2000).*

- *In neurologic intensive care unit patients, elevated body temperature is associated with longer ICU and hospital lengths of stay and worse outcome (Diringer et al., 2004).*

- *Hypoxic areas of injured brain may be less able to extract O_2 because of an increased gradient for O_2 diffusion (as a result of increased cerebral edema). Hypoxic cell death may not be solely a result of hypoperfusion, and the amount of ischemia in the injured brain may be underestimated using measures of cerebrovascular adequacy such as jugular oximetry (Menon et al., 2004).*

Diagnostic Procedures

Prompt and proper treatment of neurologic dysfunction is based on accurate and timely diagnosis. A variety of diagnostic tests are available. Some of the more commonly performed diagnostic tests will be reviewed.

Computed Tomography Scanning

Computerized tomography (CT) of the head is useful for detecting primary injuries, such as skull fractures, hematomas, and contusions; secondary injuries such as herniation, edema, and shifting of brain tissue secondary to swelling; and abscesses and tumors. The CT scan remains the initial procedure of choice in acute head injury because it is noninvasive, produces rapid results, is safe and painless, and reduces the need for more invasive procedures, such as angiograms. CT scans may be done with IV contrast to enhance visualization of vascular structures.

Magnetic Resonance Imaging

A magnetic resonance imaging (MRI) is superior to CT scanning. As with CT scanning, MRI can determine the anatomic location of a lesion. Additionally, MRI allows examination of the tissue itself, providing more anatomic detail than CT scanning. Therefore, detecting white matter shearing, infarction, and ischemic tissue is possible. MRI has the ability to detect pathologic processes at an earlier stage than is possible with a CT, and is therefore the procedure of choice for early diagnosis of cerebral infarction and brain tumors. MRI is the preferred diagnostic study for cervical spine imaging and evaluation of spinal cord injury. However, MRI has limitations that CT does not. Removal of all metal from the patient's body is essential because the MRI is a powerful magnet. Most dental fillings, prostheses, and internal clips do not prevent the patient from having an MRI, but specific questions and concerns must be directed to the neuroradiologist. Obtaining an MRI takes longer than a CT, and MRI provides a poor image of bone tissue. Therefore, a CT remains the procedure of choice when time is a factor, as with the unstable trauma patient or in the detection of spinal fractures.

Tomography

Diagnostic procedures using tomography involve IV injection and tracking of radionucleotides to evaluate cerebral blood flow. Two types are available: positron emission tomography (PET) and single photon emission computed tomography (SPECT). PET uses paired radiation sensitive detectors, whereas SPECT uses unpaired detectors. PET costs more than SPECT.

Transcranial Doppler

Transcranial doppler (TCD) is a noninvasive tool for measuring cerebral blood velocity in branches of the circle of Willis. TCD is governed by the underlying principle that velocity depends on the pressure gradient between the two ends of a vessel, the radius of the vessel, and blood viscosity. Therefore, changes in velocity may reflect either changes in CBF or in the diameter of a vessel. Diameter and flow do not always change in concert, so interpretation must be cautious. Low velocity may reflect low flow or arterial dilation; high velocity may indicate high flow or vessel constriction. TCD is ideal for use in the high-acuity environment because it is noninvasive and uses portable equipment. TCD is often used to monitor for cerebral vasospasm, intracranial lesions poststroke, and to detect cerebral blood flow changes associated with elevated ICP. TCD may be used during evaluation and determination of brain death.

Evoked Potentials

Evoked potentials are recordings of cerebral electrical impulses generated in response to visual, auditory, or somatosensory stimuli. Stimulation of the visual or auditory sensory organs or the peripheral nerves evokes an electrophysiologic response that is extracted from continuous electroencephalography (EEG) monitoring. Evoked potentials are used to detect lesions in the cerebral cortex or ascending pathways of the spinal cord, brainstem, and thalamus. This test is so sensitive that it detects lesions that cannot be detected with other clinical or laboratory tests. Visually evoked potentials are elicited by a flashing light or changing geometric pattern that stimulates the visual center in the occipital lobe. The delay, known as the degree of latency, correlates with disease severity. These are used to diagnose multiple sclerosis; Parkinson's disease; and lesions of the optic nerve, optic tract visual center, and eye. Auditorily evoked potentials are elicited by transmitting transient sounds, such as clicking noises, through earphones. They are useful to detect lesions in the central auditory pathway of the brainstem, identify lesions that result in hearing disorders, and assist in the diagnosis of acoustic tumors. Somatosensory-evoked potentials are elicited by the application of a peripheral stimulus. The response to this stimulus and the degree of latency is measured. These are used in the evaluation of spinal cord injury, to monitor spinal cord function during surgery and treatment of multiple sclerosis, and to assist in the evaluation of the location and extent of brain dysfunction after head injury. Testing for evoked potentials does not require an alert cooperative patient and is not affected by anesthesia or sedation. Evoked potentials may be useful in predicting coma outcome. They are also especially useful during therapeutically induced comas (such as barbiturate coma, Section Six) because the sensory pathways are not affected by barbiturates.

Electroencephalography

Electroencephalography (EEG) allows recording of the electrical activity of the brain using electrodes attached to the scalp. Abnormal voltage fluctuations indicate seizures or space-occupying lesions, cerebral infarct, altered consciousness, and brain death. For this test, electrodes are placed on the patient's head. Electrical impulses are detected and transferred to a device that interprets and converts the impulses into waveforms. Absence of electrical activity provides evidence for clinical determination of brain death. An EEG may detect seizure activity in the brain when seizures are not clinically apparent. However, abnormal EEG findings do not identify the cause of the abnormality. It is important to note that significant pathology can be present even in the face of a normal EEG. Continuous EEG may be used in some high-acuity units to monitor ICP, seizure activity, and cerebral ischemia.

Cerebral Angiography

Cerebral angiography involves the injection of contrast material into arteries to visualize intra- and extracranial circulation. An angiogram traces blood flow through the cerebrovascular circulation and allows visualization of the size and patency of these vessels. Results can diagnose arteriovenous malformations, aneurysms, carotid artery disease, vasospasm, and venous thrombosis. Although angiography is useful in the evaluation of cerebral vasculature, a major complication of the procedure is stroke caused from the dislogement of an atherosclerotic plaque.

Magnetic Resonance Angiography

Magnetic resonance angiography (MRA) combines MRI with angiography for noninvasive visualization of cerebral vasculature. MRA is useful in the evaluation of carotid artery disease and in the identification of intracranial aneurysms. MRA can be done with or without contrast.

Lumbar Puncture

For the lumbar puncture (LP) procedure, a needle is placed into the subarachnoid space, usually at the L4–L5 interspace. CSF is removed for laboratory analysis for the presence of blood or infection. Medications may also be administered by this route. This procedure is contraindicated in patients with increased ICP. Complications of LP include herniation of the brainstem, infection, and headache.

SECTION FIVE REVIEW

1. Findings from an initial assessment of a patient are as follows: Patient is awake; eyes are open and focusing; patient responds appropriately to verbal commands. Based on these findings, you could determine that
   A. the state of arousal is intact, but not content
   B. the state of content is intact, but not arousal
   C. arousal is intact; not enough data have been gathered to assess content completely
   D. content is intact; not enough data have been gathered to assess arousal

2. The Glasgow Coma Scale assesses
   A. cranial nerves
   B. abstract thinking
   C. arousal
   D. awareness
3. The Glasgow Coma Scale is useful because it
   A. is standardized
   B. evaluates the ability to interpret stimuli
   C. is subjective
   D. evaluates vital signs and pupil reactivity
4. A decorticate motor response indicates
   A. brainstem dysfunction
   B. the patient is close to death
   C. cerebral hemispheric dysfunction
   D. arousal is intact
5. Pupils that are bilaterally pinpoint and nonreactive to light indicate
   A. unilateral brain lesion
   B. metabolic coma
   C. herniation
   D. lesion in the pons
6. In cases of brainstem injury, doll's eye movements will
   A. remain fixed in the midposition as the head is turned
   B. conjugate opposite to the side the head is turned
   C. turn to the opposite side the head is turned
   D. turn to the same side the head is turned
7. The rhythmic waxing and waning in the depth of respiration followed by a period of apnea is referred to as
   A. central neurologic ventilation
   B. apneustic breathing
   C. Cheyne–Stokes breathing
   D. cluster breathing
8. Cushing's triad includes
   A. increase in systolic blood pressure
   B. decrease in diastolic blood pressure
   C. bradycardia
   D. all of the above

9. Which of the following ICP monitoring systems is the most accurate, reliable, and allows for drainage of CSF?
   A. intraventricular catheters
   B. intraparenchymal catheters
   C. subarachnoid bolt
   D. epidural catheters
10. Which of the following ICP waveforms occur when ICP is elevated and are considered to be clinically significant?
    A. P_1 waves
    B. A waves
    C. P_2 waves
    D. B waves
11. SjO_2 less than 55 percent or CEO_2 greater than 40 percent indicates
    A. adequate cerebral oxygenation
    B. hyperemia
    C. oligemia
    D. death of brain cells
12. CT, rather than MRI, scanning would be the procedure of choice for detecting
    A. white matter shearing
    B. the early stages of brain tumors
    C. cerebral infarction
    D. spinal fractures
13. PET scanning is useful for evaluating
    A. cerebral blood flow
    B. spinal fractures
    C. skull fractures
    D. anatomic location of a brain tumor
14. Evoked potentials
    A. is an invasive procedure
    B. is useful for imaging cellular metabolism
    C. is used in clinical research only
    D. evaluates a sensory response to a stimulus

Answers: 1. C, 2. C, 3. A, 4. C, 5. D, 6. A, 7. C, 8. D, 9. A, 10. B, 11. C, 12. D, 13. A, 14. D

SECTION SIX: Management of Decreased Cerebral Tissue Perfusion

At the completion of this section, the reader will be able to (1) identify collaborative interventions used to optimize cerebral tissue perfusion and oxygenation; (2) list the pharmacologic agents used in the treatment of increased ICP and identify the nursing implications of each; and (3) summarize nursing care priorities for patients receiving ICP monitoring.

Decreased cerebral tissue perfusion requires prompt recognition and treatment. Treatment is aimed at reducing one or more of the components of the cranial vault: blood volume, brain tissue volume, or CSF. A major goal is to identify and eliminate the cause of an elevation in these components. Interventions for patients with decreased cerebral tissue perfusion include mechanisms to increase MAP and reduce ICP.

Optimizing Cerebral Perfusion Pressure

Because CPP controls CBF, CPP is optimized by controlling blood pressure and temperature and promoting venous return. MAP is maintained at levels greater than 90 mm Hg so as to keep CPP greater than 70 mm Hg (Bullock et al., 2000). Pressures outside this range result in loss of autoregulation and inadequate CPP. CPP is maintained at 70 to 80 mm Hg with IV fluids to achieve euvolemia or slight hypervolemia to ensure adequate cerebral tissue perfusion. IV therapy and vasoactive agents enhance CPP and facilitate the delivery of oxygen to cerebral tissue (Littlejohns & Bader, 2001).

Temperature control is important because hyperthermia raises cerebral metabolism. Under conditions of increased cerebral metabolic rate, cerebral blood flow increases to meet tissue metabolic demands. To avoid an increased metabolic rate, hyperthermia must be prevented. Antipyretics and cooling blankets help to control body temperature. Severe injury/ischemia to the hypothalamus impairs thermoregulation and causes neurogenic (or central) fever, which does not respond to antipyretics.

Nursing care can promote venous return using body positioning. Unless the patient has a cervical spine injury, the head of the bed is elevated at least 30 degrees. This position avoids jugular compression, promotes venous drainage, and decreases, or at least controls, ICP. However, this practice has been questioned recently because it may place some patients at risk for cerebral ischemia caused by an increase in CPP. Therefore, the recent trend is to individualize head position based on nursing judgment. The nurse must assess the patient's response to position changes and determine which position maximizes CPP and minimizes ICP. Neck flexion, lateral head rotation, and hip flexion of greater than 90 degrees should be avoided because these positions cause venous congestion in the intracranial and abdominal compartments, which can increase ICP. The patient's body is turned as a unit; head, neck, trunk, and lower extremities are turned in unison to avoid head and neck rotation. Patients who are alert are assisted to move up in the bed. Asking patients to help by pushing with their legs initiates Valsalva's maneuver, which increases intrathoracic pressure and impedes venous return.

Optimizing Cerebral Oxygenation

Cerebral blood flow is an important variable to monitor with cerebral oxygenation, but more importantly, one must assess whether CBF matches cerebral metabolism. This can be determined by calculating cerebral $PaO_2 - PvO_2$.

Maintaining Ventilation

A patient with a GCS less than 9 who cannot maintain an airway or who remains hypoxemic must have an airway secured (Bullock et al., 2000). Hypoxia and hypercapnia are better controlled with mechanical ventilation. Hyperventilation reduces $PaCO_2$. A reduction in $PaCO_2$ produces vasoconstriction. Hyperventilation has been used to produce vasoconstriction of cerebral blood vessels. Standard practice for many years included using hyperventilation to keep the $PaCO_2$ less than 25 mm Hg. However, numerous studies indicated that blood flow is compromised during the first 24 hours after injury/ischemia (Gopinath et al.,

1999; Van den Brink et al., 2000). Current guidelines recommend that hyperventilation (to keep $PaCO_2$ less than or equal to 35 mm Hg) should be avoided during the first 24 hours because reduced blood flow compromises cerebral perfusion (Bullock et al., 2000). Futhermore, long-term hyperventilation ($PaCO_2$ less than or equal to 25 mm Hg) during the first 5 days (in the absence of increased ICP) should be avoided (Bullock et al., 2000). Patients are best maintained within a normal $PaCO_2$ range (35 to 45 mm Hg) because the level at which irreversible ischemia occurs has not been determined but the deleterious effects of continued hyperventilation are well documented (Littlejohns & Bader, 2001). Hyperventilation may be necessary for brief periods of time during periods of acute neurologic deterioration, but only after all other options have been instituted, and in this case, monitoring cerebral blood flow and jugular bulb oxygen saturation may be helpful in detecting periods of reduced cerebral tissue perfusion (Bullock et al., 2000).

Pharmacologic Therapy

Drug therapy is initiated for most patients with increased ICP to decrease intracranial volume, either by decreasing brain volume, decreasing CSF production, or decreasing the metabolic rate. Drug therapy includes osmotic diuretics, sedatives and paralytics, and barbiturates.

Osmotic Diuretics

Mannitol is effective in enhancing cerebral tissue perfusion and reducing ICP because it draws fluid from cerebral interstitial spaces (cerebral edema) into the vascular space. This reduces blood viscosity and increases cerebral blood flow and cerebral oxygen delivery. A bolus dose of 0.25 to 1.0 gm/kg is preferable to a continuous infusion (Bullock et al., 2000). Administration of mannitol requires the nurse to monitor the patient's serum osmolality. Serum osmolality is maintained at levels below 320 mMol to prevent acute renal failure (Bullock et al., 2000).

Sedatives and Paralytics

Pain and agitation increase metabolic rate, and result in increased ICP. Therefore, controlling pain and agitation are important nursing interventions. Opioid narcotics (morphine, fentanyl) are used for pain management. Benzodiazepines (midazolam, lorazepam) or sedative-hypnotics (propofol) are used for sedation. Propofol is used to decrease cerebral metabolic rate and to reduce ICP. However, at high doses propofol has hypotensive side-effects (Littlejohns & Bader, 2001). Although the use of sedatives and paralytics obscure the neurologic evaluation, the control of ICP outweighs the loss of the neurologic evaluation. Chemical paralysis (vecuronium [Norcuron], atracuronium [Tracrium]) are never used without the addition of a sedative. Agents such as pancuronium bromide (Pavulon) or vecuronium (Norcuron) do not have analgesic or sedating properties. Used alone, these agents will not blunt noxious stimuli that cause agitation and certainly will not block pain sensations. Paralytic agents are short acting, and the sedative of choice should be short acting as well to allow the nurse to periodically assess neurologic status. Particular attention is given to the patient when these medications are given because they may lower MAP and result in cerebral ischemia.

Barbiturates

Barbiturates are not a first-line therapy and generally are used to treat elevated ICP in patients with severe head injury that is not responsive to conventional therapies. Barbiturates decrease ICP by decreasing the metabolic rate, thereby reducing CBF, and reducing cerebral edema. High-dose barbiturate therapy may be considered in patients only after maximal conventional treatment of increased ICP has failed (Bullock et al., 2000). Commonly used barbiturates are pentobarbital and thiopental. Barbiturates also decrease cardiac output and blood pressure. It is essential that fluid status and blood pressure be monitored during administration of the drug. Continuous EEG is useful for titrating medication to a desired effect (Littlejohns & Bader, 2001). Barbiturate therapy is maintained until the ICP has been in the normal range for at least 24 hours and then the drug is tapered slowly over several days.

Nursing Care of Patients Receiving ICP or SjO₂ Monitoring

The focus of nursing care of the patient with an ICP monitoring device is on prevention of complications and maintenance of system integrity. Complications include those related to insertion, such as hemorrhage or hematoma formation; overdrainage of CSF; and infection, particularly with the IVC device. Patients with coagulopathies are at higher risk for hemorrhage or hematoma formation. Because a hemorrhage or hematoma is a space-occupying lesion, the patient's neurologic status must be carefully monitored before, during, and after insertion of the ICP monitoring device to detect neurologic deterioration. If an intraventricular device is inserted, the color of the CSF must be carefully observed. Pink-tinged or bloody CSF is an indication of bleeding.

The determination of when to drain CSF is important. Current guidelines recommend that ICP treatment is initiated at upper thresholds of 20 to 25 mm Hg. Interpretation and treatment are corroborated by frequent clinical examinations and CPP monitoring (Bullock et al., 2000). Clinical assessment and overall hemodynamic status are considered when the physician selects the appropriate ICP at which to initiate treatment (Littlejohns & Bader, 2001). It is imperative that the nurse clarify with the physician and receive orders that specify the ICP at which CSF drainage is initiated and terminated.

Overdrainage of CSF is a major complication of an intraventricular device, particularly an open system. To prevent overdrainage, the nurse observes unit standards for CSF drainage; accurately measures and positions the CSF drainage bag using the correct landmarks; and securely fastens the drainage bag at the prescribed level. Systems that are closed and periodically opened for therapeutic drainage require nursing interventions that are sound and clinically based. For this type of system, drainage is instituted when the ICP is consistently elevated. The keyword is *consistent*, rather than transient. Many factors transiently increase ICP including environmental stimuli, patient positioning, and nursing care activities. Once these stimuli are eliminated ICP may decrease to an acceptable level. If ICP remains elevated for several minutes, the appropriate nursing action is to institute CSF drainage.

The risk of infection is the greatest concern. Factors associated with infection are duration of ICP monitoring and type of device and system used. Sterile techniques must be absolutely observed during insertion of the ICP monitoring device. For fluid-filled systems, system integrity must be maintained. All connection points are checked to ensure that they are tight. Because fluid-filled systems require routine zero referencing and calibration, the risk of introducing pathogens into the system is increased. Care must be taken to rezero and recalibrate in an aseptic manner. The insertion site is inspected for signs of infection. The appearance of the insertion site and duration (in days) of the monitoring device placement is documented.

Troubleshooting and Maintenance of System Integrity

One of the most important nursing interventions is to gather, document, and report accurate data. Medical and nursing interventions are based on these data. Instituting interventions for data that are inaccurate negatively impact patient outcomes. It is the nurse's responsibility to ensure that ICP monitoring systems are intact and that data are accurate (Table 18–7). Accuracy is affected by a dampened, absent, or distorted waveform. Any interference, such as air bubbles within the system; kinked tubing; loose connections; or catheter occlusion from blood, brain, or bone tissue, produces a dampened waveform and inaccurate ICP readings. Technical malfunction within the external system also produces inaccurate data. Fiber optic cables are delicate and easily broken. If this occurs, the device must be removed and a new device inserted. Additionally, the internal transducer cannot be recalibrated. If significant drift is suspected and the data are suspect, the device must be replaced. When caring for patients with ICP monitoring technology, the nurse must have a clear understanding of the benefits and limitations of the system used, troubleshooting scenarios, and support from the manufacturer when needed (Littlejohns & Bader, 2001).

Just as with ICP monitoring, it is the nurse's responsibility to ensure data obtained from SjO₂ catheters are also accurate. A major limitation of these data is they are not reliable. Troubleshooting strategies, offered by Kidd and Criddle (2001), are summarized in Table 18–8.

TABLE 18–7 Troubleshooting System Integrity with ICP Monitors

PROBLEM	POTENTIAL SOURCE	ACTION
Dampened, absent, or distorted waveform	Catheter occlusion by blood, brain, or bone tissue	Systematically assess for problems
	Air bubbles in system	Remove air from system
	Loose connections	Tighten all connections
	Recalibration and zero referencing needed	Recalibrate and zero
	Kinked catheter or tubing	Examine tubing for kinks
	Technical problem with transducer/pressure module	Replace transducer or pressure module
	Fiber optic cables broken	Replace fiber optic device
	Dislodgement of catheter	Replace monitoring device
ICP values suspect	Recalibration and zero referencing needed	Recalibrate and zero if fluid-filled system, replace device if fiber optic
	Incorrect placement of catheter or transducer	Verify correct placement of external transducer
Leakage of fluid from tubing	Loosened connections	Tighten all connections

TABLE 18–8 Troubleshooting System Integrity with Sjo_2 Monitoring

PROBLEM	ACTION
Low light intensity	Monitor light intensity status indicator
	Flush catheter with 2 to 3 mL saline to remove debris from catheter tip
	Reposition patient's head to move catheter to area of more blood flow
	Notify physician if the light intensity monitor reading remains low
Questionable accuracy of reading	Upon catheter insertion and every 8 to 12 hours, confirm accuracy of catheter by sending a sample of mixed venous blood obtained from the Sjo_2 catheter to the lab for analysis
	If Sjo_2 readings are low, but light intensity indicator is within normal range, verify accuracy with a lab analysis
	A difference of more than 4 percent between oximetric readings and the results of blood gas analysis indicates the need to recalibrate the monitor

Providing a Safe and Protective Environment

The following nursing interventions are for patients with impaired content and are directed at protecting the patient from injury, reorienting, and creating a calm, safe environment. Patients with cognitive deficits become easily confused with external stimuli. Noise is kept to a minimum, information is presented simply and calmly, and the number of visitors at one time is limited. Keeping a dim light on at night and frequent checking by the nurse controls confusion caused by misperception of stimuli. Patients with cognitive deficits often attempt to get out of bed and may pull out IV lines and catheters. Interventions, such as keeping the bed in a low position, using siderails, and frequent checks, keeps the patient safe from harm. Frequent reorientation decreases confusion and disorientation.

In summary, ICP monitoring is an extremely useful adjunct in the care of the unresponsive patient but requires high-acuity, diligent nursing care. Various ICP monitoring devices and systems are available. The clinician must be familiar with the advantages and disadvantages specific to each device and system and should be aware of the potential complications associated with ICP monitoring. The nurse must have a working knowledge of each system and be able to recognize system inaccuracies.

SECTION SIX REVIEW

1. Mannitol acts to decrease ICP by
   A. decreasing CSF production
   B. preventing fluid absorption by cerebral cells
   C. reducing cerebral edema and blood viscosity
   D. decreasing the blood–brain barrier

2. Nursing interventions for patients with impaired content center around
   A. protection from injury
   B. maintaining the airway
   C. control of cerebral perfusion pressure
   D. drug therapy

3. One of the initial pharmacologic agents used to control ICP is a(n)
   A. fluid bolus
   B. vasodilator
   C. barbiturate
   D. osmotic diuretic

4. A patient's ICP is 22 mm Hg for more than 5 minutes. Your first action would be to
   A. recalibrate and zero the internal transducer
   B. immediately drain CSF until the desired ICP is obtained
   C. notify the physician immediately
   D. eliminate all stimuli and reposition the patient

Answers: 1. C, 2. A, 3. D, 4. D

POSTTEST

1. Hypoxemia and hypercapnia cause
   A. cerebral vasodilation
   B. decreased ICP
   C. cerebral vasoconstriction
   D. decreased CBF

2. Keeping the head and neck in alignment results in
   A. decreased venous outflow
   B. increased venous outflow
   C. increased intrathoracic pressure
   D. increased intra-abdominal pressure

3. As a compensatory mechanism, pressure regulation acts by constricting cerebral blood vessels in response to
   A. elevated blood levels of oxygen
   B. decreased blood levels of oxygen
   C. elevated systemic blood pressure
   D. decreased systemic blood pressure

4. The principle that explains reciprocal mechanisms involved in increased ICP is
   A. Monro–Kellie hypothesis
   B. cerebral perfusion formula
   C. autoregulation
   D. chemical regulation

5. When ICP increases, CSF is displaced into the
   A. external jugular veins
   B. blood–brain barrier
   C. spinal cord
   D. medulla

6. The blood–brain barrier is permeable to all of the following EXCEPT
   A. water
   B. oxygen
   C. lipid soluble compounds
   D. most drugs

7. Your patient's MAP is 100 mm Hg and ICP is 10 mm Hg. What is the CPP?
   A. 80 mm Hg
   B. 90 mm Hg
   C. 110 mm Hg
   D. 120 mm Hg

8. Cerebral perfusion pressure at or below _____ mm Hg will result in a loss of autoregulation and inadequate cerebral oxygenation.
   A. 70 mm Hg
   B. 60 mm Hg
   C. 50 mm Hg
   D. 40 mm Hg

9. What happens when ICP and MAP are equal?
   A. nothing; this is normal
   B. cerebral vasodilation
   C. CSF is displaced
   D. brain perfusion ceases

10. Which of the following disorders can produce an elevation in ICP?
    A. cerebral edema
    B. cerebral hematoma
    C. hydrocephalus
    D. all of the above

11. The net effect of a prolonged increase in ICP is
    A. impaired cerebral tissue perfusion
    B. cerebral vasodilation
    C. cerebral edema
    D. hydrocephalus

12. How does hypercapnia affect ICP?
    A. it impedes venous outflow
    B. it impairs autoregulation
    C. it results in cerebral vasodilation and increased blood volume
    D. it increases CSF production and increases ICP

13. Decorticate posturing
    A. is abnormal flexion and indicates cerebral hemispheric dysfunction
    B. is abnormal extension and indicates brainstem dysfunction
    C. is an ominous sign
    D. is when the arms are pronated and extended

14. Which of the following GCS scores is consistent with coma?
    A. 8
    B. 10

C. 12

D. 15

15. Cushing's triad is evidenced by

A. increase in systolic pressure

B. decrease in diastolic pressure

C. bradycardia

D. all of the above

16. Which of the following methods is the most accurate measure of ICP?

A. lumbar puncture

B. intraventricular catheters

C. epidural probe

D. subarchnoid screw

17. Normal SjO_2 is

A. 25 to 35 percent

B. 40 to 60 percent

C. 60 to 80 percent

D. greater than 90 percent

18. Which of the following can be used in high-acuity units to monitor ICP, seizure activity, and cerebral ischemia?

A. CT scan

B. MRI

C. PET

D. EEG

19. Which of the following measures may be instituted to maintain CPP at 70 to 80 mm Hg?

A. IV fluid

B. dopamine

C. phenylephrine

D. all of the above

20. When should hyperventilation be instituted to decrease ICP?

A. during the first 24 hours in ICU

B. during the first 5 days in ICU

C. when the $PaCO_2$ is 35 to 45 mm Hg

D. for brief periods of time during acute neurologic deterioration

21. When administering mannitol to a patient, the nurse should monitor which of the following lab tests?

A. serum osmolality

B. urine sodium

C. serum calcium

D. serum potassium

22. Continuous EEG monitoring is useful for patients who receive

A. mannitol

B. high-dose barbiturates

C. propofol

D. neuromuscular blocking agents

POSTTEST ANSWERS

Question	Answer	Section	Question	Answer	Section
1	A	One	12	C	Four
2	B	One	13	A	Five
3	C	One	14	A	Five
4	A	Two	15	D	Five
5	A	Two	16	B	Five
6	D	Two	17	C	Five
7	B	Three	18	D	Five
8	A	Three	19	D	Six
9	D	Three	20	D	Six
10	D	Four	21	A	Six
11	A	Four	22	B	Six

REFERENCES

Bullock, R., Chesnut, R. M., Clifton, G., et al. (2000). *Management and prognosis of severe traumatic brain injury.* New York: Brain Trauma Foundation and American Association of Neurological Surgeons.

Diringer, M. N., Reaven, N. L., Funk, S. E., et al. (2004). Elevated body temperature independently contributes to increased length of stay in neurologic intensive care unit patients. *Critical Care Medicine, 32,* 1489–1495.

Gopinath, S. P., Valadka, A. B., Uzura, M., & Robertson, C. S. (1999). Comparison of jugular venous oxygen saturation and brain tissue PO_2 as monitors of cerebral ischemia after head injury. *Critical Care Medicine, 27,* 2337–2345.

Kidd, K. C., & Criddle, L. (2001). Using jugular venous catheters in patients with traumatic brain injury. *Critical Care Nurse, 21*(6),16–24.

Littlejohns, L. R., & Bader, M. K. (2001). Guidelines for the management of severe head injury: Clinical applications and changes in practice. *Critical Care Nurse, 21*(6),48–65.

Menon, D. K., Coles, J. P., Gupta, A. K., et al. (2004). Diffusion limited oxygen delivery following head injury. *Critical Care Medicine, 32,* 1384–1390.

Van den Brink, W. A., van Santbrink, M., Steyerberg, E. W., et al. (2000). Brain oxygen tension in severe head injury. *Neurosurgery, 46,* 868–878.

Winkleman, C. (2000). Effect of backrest position on intracranial and cerebral perfusion pressures in traumatically brain injured adults. *American Journal of Critical Care, 9,* 373–383.

Alterations in Cerebral Tissue Perfusion: Acute Brain Attack

Humberto Zuniga, Karen L. Johnson, Amy Tarbay

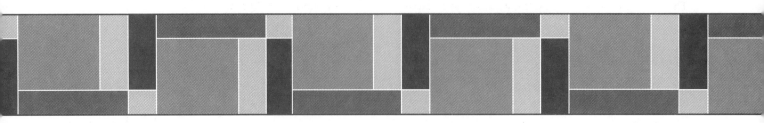

OBJECTIVES Following completion of this module, the learner will be able to

1. Define stroke.
   - Discuss the major classifications of stroke.
2. Explain the pathophysiology of stroke.
3. Identify the modifiable and nonmodifiable risk factors for stroke.
4. List the manifestations of stroke.
   - Explain the rationale of various diagnostic tests used in the evaluation of stroke.

5. Describe the implications of the medications used to treat patients who have had strokes.
   - Discuss the rationale for surgical interventions for management of stroke.
6. Discuss priority nursing interventions for the patient with an acute brain attack.

This self-study module is composed of six sections. Section One defines stroke and discusses the two major classifications of stroke (ischemic and hemorrhagic). Section Two explains the pathophysiology of stroke. Section Three presents the modifiable and nonmodifiable risk factors for stroke. Section Four presents the manifestations of stroke and the rationale for various diagnostic tests used in the evaluation of stroke. Section Five presents the medical management of stroke including pharmacological and surgical interventions as well as the

nursing diagnoses and management of the patient postoperatively. Section Six discusses the nursing challenges in caring for a patient with an acute brain attack in the acute care phase. Each section includes a set of review questions to help the learner evaluate his or her understanding of the section's content before moving on to the next section. All Section Reviews and the module Pretest and Posttest include answers. It is suggested that the learner review those concepts answered incorrectly in the review questions before proceeding to the next section.

 PRETEST

1. Stroke is an important cerebral vascular disorder because it
   A. is the second-leading cause of adult disability in North America
   B. is the third-leading cause of adult death in North America
   C. claims approximately 100,000 new victims each year in the United States
   D. is responsible for 500,000 deaths in the United States each year

2. The highest incidence of stroke is caused by
   A. atherothrombosis
   B. emboli
   C. primary intracerebral hemorrhage
   D. subarachnoid hemorrhage
3. A transient ischemic attack (TIA) is a(n)
   A. completed stroke
   B. stroke that extends beyond 24 hours but is reversible
   C. episode of focal neurologic deficit that resolves in a short period of time
   D. stroke that evolves over several days

4. The penumbra is
   A. caused by excessive intracellular sodium
   B. a band of minimally perfused cells around an infarcted region of cells
   C. a central core of dead or dying cells
   D. a region in the brain that controls speech

5. The most important modifiable risk factor for stroke is
   A. diabetes mellitus
   B. cardiac disease
   C. hypertension
   D. drug abuse

6. Mr. Dixon, age 65, is an African American with a history of atrial fibrillation. His blood pressure is 180/100 mm Hg. He weighs 200 pounds and is 5 ft 5 in. tall. His blood cholesterol is 290 mg/dL; he has drinking binges on weekends, and smokes one pack of cigarettes per day (for 30 years). How many modifiable stroke risk factors does Mr. Dixon have?
   A. 2   C. 6
   B. 4   D. 8

7. The most common manifestation of stroke is
   A. seizures
   B. loss of vision in one eye
   C. numbness and weakness involving the face and arm
   D. a sudden loss of memory

8. In the acute care phase, a focused neurologic assessment for the patient with a stroke should include tests for
   A. dysphagia
   B. hemianopsia
   C. hemiparesis
   D. all of the above

9. Computerized tomography should be performed as soon as possible after the patient presents to the emergency department because
   A. it improves patient outcome
   B. it can differentiate hemorrhagic from ischemic stroke
   C. if the patient loses consciousness, the test is invalid
   D. none of the above

10. Tissue plasminogen activator should be given
    A. within 3 hours of onset of ischemic stroke
    B. within 3 hours of onset of hemorrhagic stroke
    C. within 24 hours of onset of ischemic stroke
    D. within 24 hours of onset of hemorrhagic stroke

11. Which of the following interventional procedures has been successfully used to reverse neurologic deficits caused by atherosclerotic lesions of the cerebral arteries?
    A. aneurysm clipping
    B. embolization by arteriography
    C. cerebral angioplasty
    D. anticoagulant therapy

12. Which of the following statements is TRUE about seizures in the patient who has had a stroke?
    A. they commonly occur after the first month
    B. they occur regularly and frequently after a stroke
    C. because of the high incidence of poststroke seizures, anticonvulsant therapy is necessary

D. seizures are most likely to occur in the first 24 hours after a stroke

13. Surgical management of hemorrhagic strokes may include all of the following EXCEPT
    A. evacuation of the hematoma
    B. craniotomy
    C. aneurysm clipping
    D. carotid endarterectomy

14. Patients with subarachnoid hemorrhage are at risk for developing hyponatremia as a result of
    A. syndrome of inappropriate ADH secretion
    B. too much IV fluid given in the emergency department
    C. low sodium diets
    D. infusion of sodium chloride IV solutions

15. Which of the following characterize upper motor neuron lesions?
    A. muscle spasticity
    B. muscle hypertonicity
    C. abnormally brisk reflexes
    D. all of the above

16. Which of the following is a TRUE statement about drooling after a stroke?
    A. drooling rarely occurs after a stroke
    B. drooling signifies significant cerebellar dysfunction
    C. drooling is a clue that there may be swallowing problems
    D. drooling should not be tolerated in the immediate poststroke period

17. The term used to describe flaccid bladder is
    A. detrusor hyporeflexia
    B. detrusor hyperreflexia
    C. detrusor-sphincter dyssynergy
    D. none of the above

18. Which of the following interventions would be appropriate for the patient with diplopia?
    A. initiate aspiration precautions
    B. support the affected extremity during turning
    C. apply an eye patch to one eye
    D. talk loudly and slowly to the patient

19. Agnosia is
    A. the inability to recognize familiar sensory information
    B. a sign of Alzheimer's disease
    C. a sign of impending stroke
    D. the inability to swallow

20. Which of the following strategies should the nurse use to reinforce a positive body image after a stroke?
    A. use the terms *good side* and *bad side*
    B. use the terms *affected side* and *unaffected side*
    C. do not let the patient see him or herself in the mirror
    D. do not mention the hemiplegic extremities when a patient has hemiplegic neglect syndrome

Pretest Answers: 1. B, 2. A, 3. C, 4. B, 5. C, 6. C, 7. C, 8. D, 9. B, 10. A, 11. C, 12. D, 13. D, 14. A, 15. D, 16. C, 17. A, 18. C, 19. A, 20. B

GLOSSARY

agnosia   A perceptual impairment resulting in the failure to recognize familiar objects by the senses even though sensation is intact; types include tactile, visual, or auditory.

aneurysm   Thin-walled balloon-like outpouching of the arterial intima.

anosognosia   A severe form of neglect in which the patient fails to recognize his or her illness or paralysis.

aphasia   The inability to understand or use language; Wernicke's aphasia is the ability to receive auditory impulses but the inability to comprehend; Broca's aphasia is the use of inappropriate, uninhibited speech with an impaired memory for language; Global aphasia is a combination of Wernicke's and Broca's aphasia and is associated with a complete loss of comprehension and expression of speech.

apraxia   A perceptual and cognitive impairment resulting in an inability to perform movements voluntarily in the presence of intact motor power, sensation, or coordination; may move automatically but not purposefully; types include dressing, ideational, ideomotor, motor, and constructional.

ataxia   Impaired gait characterized by unsteadiness, poor balance, and lack of coordination (lesion site: cerebellum).

dysarthria   Impairment of the muscles that control speech.

dysphagia   Impaired swallowing.

dysphasia   Impaired capacity to interpret, formulate, or express meaningful language by speaking, writing, or gesturing (expressive or Broca's dysphasia); the inability to understand the written or spoken language (receptive or Wernicke's

dysphasia). There are mild to severe degrees of aphasia (literally no speech) as opposed to dysphasia (difficulty with speech) (lesion site: left dominant hemisphere).

flaccidity   Absence of muscle tone resulting in floppy, limp, flabby, hyporeflexic, nonfunctional limbs.

hemianopsia   Loss of the visual field of one or both eyes; the person with left hemianopsia cannot see objects in the left visual field.

hemiparesis   Weakness of one side of the body.

hemiplegia   Paralysis or loss of voluntary movement of one side of the body.

nuchal rigidity   Neck pain or stiffness.

paresthesias   Abnormal sensations, such as burning or tingling of the skin, often occurring during stroke recovery.

penumbra   An ischemic zone of viable, threatened tissue surrounding the brain infarct.

proprioception   Sensory awareness of the position of the body and its parts.

spasticity   A state of increased tone of a muscle resulting in a stiff muscle and continuous resistance to stretching.

stroke   A brain attack; an acute neurologic deficit that occurs when impaired blood flow to a localized area of the brain results in injury to brain tissue.

subluxation   Incomplete dislocation, most often seen in the shoulder joint following stroke.

transient ischemic attacks (TIAs)   Episodes of focal neurologic deficits that usually resolve in a few minutes or hours.

ABBREVIATIONS

ABG	Arterial blood gas	**ICP**	Intracranial pressure
ADH	Antidiuretic hormone	**IV**	Intravenous
CPP	Cerebral perfusion pressure	**ROM**	Range of motion
CSF	Cerebrospinal fluid	**rtPA**	Tissue plasminogen activator
CT	Computed tomography	**SAH**	Subarachnoid hemorrhage
DVT	Deep-vein thrombosis	**TIA**	Transient ischemic attack
ECG	Electrocardiogram		

SECTION ONE: Definition and Classifications of Strokes (Acute Brain Attacks)

At the completion of this section, the learner will be able to define stroke and discuss the major classifications of stroke.

Stroke is an acute neurologic deficit that occurs when impaired blood flow to a localized area of the brain results in injury to brain tissue. The term *brain attack* has been advocated to raise awareness of the need for rapid emergency treatment, similar to that with heart attack. Stroke is the third-leading cause of death in the United States and a leading cause of serious long-term disability (Brott & Bogousslavsky, 2000).

Major Classifications of Stroke

There are two major classifications of stroke: ischemic and hemorrhagic. Ischemic strokes occur when blood supply to a part of the brain is suddenly interrupted (thrombus or embolus). Hemorrhagic strokes occur when there is bleeding into brain tissue, such as that which occurs with head injury, aneurysms, arteriovenous malformations, or hypertension.

Ischemic strokes are caused by an interruption of cerebral blood flow by a thrombus or embolus. Interruption of cerebral blood flow can result in **transient ischemic attacks (TIAs).** A stroke may be preceded by a TIA similar to angina in a heart attack. TIAs are episodes of focal neurologic deficits that usually resolve in a few minutes or hours but are always completely resolved within 24 hours (Adams et al., 2003). Clinically, the patient may present with sudden unilateral dimness or partial loss of vision in one eye, weakness, numbness, tingling, severe headache, speechlessness, or unexplained dizziness. The symptoms are produced by inadequate perfusion to the brain. Inadequate perfusion can be caused by carotid stenosis (from atherosclerotic disease) or microemboli (from atherosclerotic plaques in major extracranial vessels). TIAs are warnings of an impending stroke and require immediate referral for treatment. The highest incidence for stroke occurs within the first few weeks after the TIA. The more frequently the TIAs occur, the higher the probability of stroke.

Atherosclerosis of cerebral arteries is the most common cause of ischemic stroke (Albers et al., 2001). Deposits of atherosclerotic plaque narrow vessel lumens and decrease cerebral blood flow. Plaque deposits in the intimal lining of arteries cause the internal elastic media to thin, weaken, expose the collagen layer, and create a "hole" in the vessel lining. Platelets become activated to adhere and aggregate in the tissue defect to "plug" the hole. Formation of a platelet plug initiates the coagulation cascade, which results in the formation of a stable fibrin clot. This clot may remain at the site, eventually getting large enough to completely occlude the vessel, or it may break off and become an embolus. *Thrombotic strokes* are more common in older persons and are frequently accompanied by evidence of atherosclerotic plaque deposits in the coronary heart or peripheral vasculature. Thrombotic strokes may occur at rest and are not associated with activity. Thrombotic strokes involving smaller vessels are referred to as *lacunar infarcts.* The infarcted areas leave behind small cavities (lacunae, or lakes). Lacunar infarcts occur in deep penetrating arteries in a single region of the brain. An *embolic stroke* is caused by a blood clot that travels from its original site and eventually becomes lodged in a vessel. Most emboli originate from a thrombus in the heart that develops with certain cardiac conditions (atrial fibrillation, rheumatic heart disease, recent myocardial infarction, or endocarditis). Emboli can also originate from rupture of atherosclerotic plaque. Embolic strokes, common in younger individuals, occur suddenly when the person is awake and active.

Intracranial hemorrhage, a type of hemorrhagic stroke, occurs when a cerebral blood vessel ruptures and blood accumulates in brain tissue. This results in compression of intracerebral contents, edema, and spasm of adjacent blood vessels. Hypertension is a common cause of intracranial hemorrhage. However, a variety of factors can also cause intracranial hemorrhage, including arteriovenous malformations, anticoagulant therapy, aneurysms, trauma, and erosions of blood vessels by tumors. Unlike ischemic strokes, which are preceded by TIAs, intracranial hemorrhage appears suddenly without warning (Ariesen et al., 2003). A spontaneous intracranial hemorrhage is the most common cause of a fatal stroke. There are several conditions that cause a cerebral blood vessel to rupture, including degenerative changes, which damage the elastic layer of the artery; developmental defects, which cause a poorly developed arterial wall; high blood flow areas, which cause hemodynamic stress; and hypertension, which accentuates any vascular weakness. Leakage of blood from **aneurysms** (thin-walled balloonlike outpouchings of the arterial intima) is usually found at arterial bifurcations (branchings) where blood velocity is higher and can be lethal with rupture. This type of stroke, usually a subarachnoid hemorrhage (SAH), develops suddenly without warning. The patient often complains of a sudden, severe unilateral headache—"the worst headache of my life"—neck pain or stiffness (**nuchal rigidity**) and vomiting. Meningeal irritation by blood produces the severe headache and other meningeal signs, such as photophobia (intolerance to light) and nuchal rigidity. Hypertension is common. The cerebrospinal fluid (CSF) is usually bloody because the aneurysm commonly ruptures in the subarachnoid space. Following a SAH a decrease in cerebral blood flow and transient loss of consciousness secondary to increased intracranial pressure (ICP) may occur.

Primary intracerebral hemorrhage usually involves bleeding directly into the brain parenchyma; it may occur as small (less than 3 cm) or large (greater than 3 cm) hemorrhages. Chronic hypertension, the major cause of these hemorrhages, produces gradual, degenerative changes in the small penetrating arteries, causing microaneurysms that burst with sudden increases in blood pressure.

In summary, stroke, or acute brain attack, is an acute neurologic deficit that occurs when impaired blood flow to a localized area of the brain results in injury to brain tissue. There are two major classifications of stroke: ischemic and hemorrhagic. Ischemic strokes are caused by an interruption of cerebral blood flow that results in a TIA, thrombotic stroke, or embolic stroke. Hemorrhagic strokes occur when a cerebral blood vessel ruptures and blood accumulates in or around brain tissue. Hypertension is a common cause of intracranial hemorrhage. Hemorrhagic strokes occur with subarachnoid hemorrhage or intracerebral hemorrhage. The major classifications of stroke, risk factors, and characteristics are summarized in Table 19–1.

TABLE 19–1 Major Strokes Compared

TYPE OF STROKE	AGE	RISK FACTORS	CHARACTERISTICS
Ischemic Stroke			
Thrombotic	Elders	Hypertension, smoking, high cholesterol, diabetes mellitus, atherosclerosis	May have TIAs Develop during sleep or on awakening May have mild headaches Predictable locations and symptoms Intermittent attacks and progression
Embolic	Adults of all ages	Cardiac abnormalities: Atrial fibrillation, valvular heart disease, carotid plaque or thrombosis	No warning, sudden attack Symptoms vary with attack Usually occur during daytime
Hemorrhagic Stroke			
Subarachnoid hemorrhage	Young, middle-aged adults	Ruptured aneurysms Arteriovenous malformations Brain tumors	Usually no warning, sudden attack Very severe headache, nausea/vomiting, photophobia Hypertension Decreasing level of consciousness
Primary intracerebral hemorrhage	Elders	Chronic hypertension Aneurysms Anticoagulant therapy	Usually no warning Gradual development Headache, nausea/vomiting, photophobia Hypertension Bloody CSF Decreased level of consciousness Motor-sensory deficit of face, arm, leg

SECTION ONE REVIEW

1. Mrs. Davis, age 33, had a brief (3-min) episode of heaviness in her right arm and inability to speak. Symptoms disappeared and function returned to normal. The category of brain attack she most likely experienced is a(n)
   A. subarachnoid hemorrhage
   B. TIA
   C. stroke
   D. heart attack

2. Which of the following are the major classifications of stroke?
   A. subarachnoid and intracranial hemorrhage
   B. thrombotic and embolic
   C. ischemic and hemorrhagic
   D. TIA and embolic

3. The most common cause of ischemic stroke is
   A. hypertension
   B. subarachnoid hemorrhage
   C. trauma
   D. atherosclerosis

4. Which of the following conditions are associated with emboli formation?
   A. myocardial infarction
   B. atrial fibrillation
   C. endocarditis
   D. all of the above

5. Which of the following appears suddenly and without warning?
   A. intracranial hemorrhage
   B. ischemic strokes
   C. TIAs
   D. none of the above; all strokes appear without warning.

Answers: 1. B, 2. C, 3. D, 4. D, 5. A

SECTION TWO: Pathophysiology of Stroke

At the completion of this section, the learner will be able to explain the pathophysiology of stroke.

Recall from Section One that a stroke is characterized by neurologic deficits that occur when cerebral blood flow is diminished as a result of ischemic or hemorrhagic cerebral vascular events. The majority of strokes result from ischemic infarction and inadequate blood flow (Albers et al., 2001). Atherosclerosis of cerebral arteries is a process similar to that found in cardiovascular arteries. Atherosclerosis and plaque formation result in narrowing or occlusion of arteries. The process of atherosclerosis results in plaque formation, which enhances platelet aggregation. Formation of a blood clot superimposed on atherosclerotic plaque causes significant stenosis of cerebral arteries. The most common sites for the atherosclerotic process to occur is at the bifurcation of the common carotid artery. An embolism results in a stroke when a clot, plaque, or platelet plug breaks off an atherosclerotic lesion, enters the circulation, and blocks an artery.

Diminished blood flow impairs oxygen delivery to neurons. Cerebral ischemia can be focal or global. Global ischemia is associated with a lack of collateral blood flow and irreversible brain damage (within minutes). With focal ischemia, some degree of collateral circulation remains, which allows for the survival of neurons and for reversal of neuronal damage after periods of ischemia. Because of the potential for recovery, focal ischemia is treatable.

Impaired oxygen delivery results in impaired cellular function because the cells do not have enough oxygen to generate energy (refer to Module 14). Without oxygen, the cellular sodium–potassium pumps fail. This results in increased intracellular concentrations of sodium, chloride, and calcium. Accumulation of these intracellular electrolytes is toxic to intracellular structures, particularly the mitochondria. Severe or prolonged ischemia leads to cellular death.

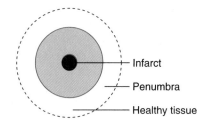

Figure 19–1 ■ Surrounding the infarcted zone is the penumbra. In this zone are neurons that are minimally perfused but still viable, and capable of responding to therapy. The goal of medical management is to limit the size of the infarct zone and reestablish perfusion to neurons in the penumbra zone.

In the evolution of a stroke there are usually two zones of affected neurons (Fig. 19–1). In the central zone are neurons that are infarcted and dead. They do not function and do not regain function. Surrounding the infarcted zone is a zone of neurons that are minimally perfused but not totally ischemic. This zone of neurons is called the **penumbra.** These neurons still function, although they are somewhat impaired. They remain viable and are capable of responding to therapy within a certain time frame. If perfusion to neurons in the penumbra is reestablished, the cells recover function. If perfusion is not reestablished, neurons in the penumbra die and the core of the nonfunctional neurons enlarges. Therefore, the fundamental goal of medical management is to restore cerebral blood flow and limit the size and extension of the infarcted zone (Brott & Bogousslavsky, 2000).

In summary, the majority of strokes result from ischemia caused by atherosclerotic lesions in cerebral blood vessels. Diminished blood flow results in neuronal dysfunction and cell death. There are two zones of affected neurons in the evolution of a stroke. The central zone is composed of infarcted neurons that do not regain function. The next zone is the penumbra. Cells in this zone are impaired, but still function and are capable of recovery. The goal of medical treatment is to limit the size of the central zone and reestablish perfusion to the neurons in the penumbra.

SECTION TWO REVIEW

1. Impaired cerebral oxygen delivery results in
   A. failure of sodium–potassium pumps
   B. aerobic metabolism
   C. immediate cell death
   D. none of the above
2. The penumbra is defined as the
   A. infarct zone
   B. zone of neurons that are minimally perfused
   C. zone of healthy neurons
   D. danger zone

3. The fundamental goal of medical management during cerebral ischemia is to
   A. limit sodium–potassium pumps
   B. promote anaerobic metabolism
   C. restore cerebral perfusion
   D. prevent clot formation

Answers: 1. A, 2. B, 3. C

SECTION THREE: Risk Factors for Stroke

Prevention of stroke includes identification and modification of risk factors. At the completion of this section, the learner will be able to explain the modifiable and nonmodifiable risk factors for stroke. Risk factors categorized as modifiable or nonmodifiable are summarized in Table 19–2.

Hypertension is an important modifiable risk factor for stroke and is implicated in both ischemic and hemorrhagic strokes. Both systolic and diastolic hypertension (greater than 140/95) are risk factors (Joint National Committee on Detection, Evaluation, and Treatment of High Blood Pressure, 2003). Reduction of both systolic and diastolic pressures in hypertensive individuals substantially reduces stroke risk (Albers et al., 1999). Hypotension, particularly in the elderly, may be a significant risk factor if the hypotensive episode is sudden and profound as may happen with the use of powerful antihypertensive agents, myocardial infarction, or bleeding. Dehydration also may dangerously lower blood pressure and decrease perfusion in the elderly, who already have an age-related decline in cerebral blood flow. Cardiac disease is another important modifiable risk factor for stroke. Individuals with cardiac disease such as coronary heart disease, congestive heart failure, left ventricular hypertrophy, or arrhythmias (specifically atrial fibrillation) have more than twice the stroke risk compared with those without cardiac disease (Bradberry & Fagan, 2002). Therefore, cardiovascular risk reduction must be implemented to reduce the risk of coronary heart disease and, in turn, stroke risk. Diabetes mellitus is a risk factor for ischemic stroke involving large and small vessels. An individual with a previous stroke has a high risk of developing a recurrent stroke. Dyslipidemia

is a risk factor for atherosclerosis in both the coronary and cerebral vascular beds. Hypercholesterolemia is, therefore, another modifiable risk factor for stroke. Multiple studies have shown that lipid-lowering drugs (statins) reduce risk of stroke in those with coronary artery disease and elevated total or low-density lipoprotein cholesterol (American Heart Association, 2004).

Cigarette smoking is a modifiable risk factor for stroke (Albers et al., 1999). Smoking causes increased fibrinogen, and platelet aggregation, as well as a reduction in high-density lipoproteins (Bradberry & Fagan, 2002). Cessation of smoking reduces the risk of stroke. The risk of stroke for women smokers is higher than that for men smokers, but the risk for all smokers decreases to that of nonsmokers 2 to 5 years after cessation (Bradberry & Fagan, 2002).

Nonmodifiable factors for stroke include age, gender, race, and genetic factors. Age is the single most important nonmodifiable risk factor for stroke; for each successive decade after 55 years, the stroke rate more than doubles (Heart and Stroke Facts, 2001). Men have a greater risk than women. African Americans, particularly males, have more hypertensive disease and more strokes than other races. Obesity, smoking, and diabetes mellitus are more prevalent among African Americans, which may account for their higher incidence of strokes (Sacco & Boden-Albala, 2001). Aging women sustain a large burden for stroke. While estrogen replacement therapy appears to have benefits for preventing stroke in animal studies, recent clinical trials do not support the use of estrogen replacement therapy for the prevention of vascular disease (Hurn & Brass, 2003). Although the specific gene has not been identified, there appears to be a genetic predisposition to stroke.

Despite our knowledge of the importance of reducing risk factors for stroke, control of these factors is still inadequate because of poor patient compliance and adherence to behavior modifications as well as decreased detection and treatment by health care providers (Albers et al., 1999). Further reductions in the risk of stroke require improvements in the ability to identify, modify, and manage cerebral vascular risk factors.

In summary, prevention of stroke begins with identification of modifiable and nonmodifiable risk factors. Modifiable risk factors include hypertension, hypotension, and dehydration in the elderly, coronary heart disease, dyslipidemia, hypercholesterolemia, and smoking. Elimination of these risk factors reduces the risk of stroke. Nonmodifiable risk factors include advancing age for both sexes, male gender, African American race, and family history of stroke. Nonmodifiable risk factors cannot be eliminated. Individuals with these risk factors must diligently eliminate modifiable risk factors in efforts to decrease the risk of stroke.

TABLE 19–2 Risk Factors for Stroke

MODIFIABLE	NONMODIFIABLE
Hypertension and hypotension	Age
Cardiac disease	Gender
Dysrhythmias (atrial fibrillation)	Race/ethnicity
Coagulopathies	Genetic factors
Diabetes mellitus	Prior stroke or heart attack
Drug abuse	
Cigarette smoking	
Excessive alcohol consumption	
Cocaine	
Physical inactivity	
Hypercholesterolemia	

SECTION THREE REVIEW

1. The most important modifiable risk factor for stroke is
   A. age
   B. hypertension
   C. atrial fibrillation
   D. diabetes mellitus
2. Which of the following modifiable risk factors are associated with increased risk of stroke?
   A. cigarette smoking
   B. heavy use of alcohol
   C. physical inactivity
   D. all of the above
3. The single most common nonmodifiable risk factor for stroke is
   A. advancing age
   B. race
   C. diabetes
   D. family history of stroke

Answers: 1. B, 2. D, 3. A

SECTION FOUR: Assessment and Diagnosis of Stroke

At the completion of this section, the learner will be able to list the manifestations of stroke and explain the rationale of various diagnostic tests used in the evaluation of stroke.

Manifestations of stroke vary according to the cerebral artery involved. About one third of patients who are having a stroke are aware of the symptoms; however, most bystanders are not knowledgeable about the signs of stroke (Brott & Bogousslavsky, 2000). The most common manifestation is numbness and weakness of the face and arm. Other manifestations may include difficulties with balance or speech and loss of vision in one eye. Symptoms are usually sudden at onset and one sided. The specific stroke signs depend on the specific vascular territory compromised according to Book (2002) as summarized in Table 19–3.

Manifestations that occur rapidly but progress slowly are typically associated with thrombotic strokes. Manifestations that appear suddenly and cause immediate neurologic deficits are typically associated with embolic strokes. The manifestations of hemorrhagic stroke also appear suddenly and depend on the location of the hemorrhage but may include headache, nausea/vomiting, seizures, **hemiplegia,** and loss of consciousness.

A patient thought to be having a stroke requires prompt triage. Accurate diagnosis is based on a complete history and a thorough physical assessment with a focused neurologic exam. The goal of the exam is to quickly determine whether the stroke is ischemic or hemorrhagic because they require different medical interventions. Important information to elicit includes any reports of recent medical or neurologic events (hemorrhage, surgery, trauma, myocardial infarction, or

TABLE 19–3 Signs and Symptoms of Stroke Related to Vascular Territory Compromised

VASCULAR TERRITORY COMPROMISED	SIGNS AND SYMPTOMS
Carotid ischemia	Monocular vision loss
	Aphasia (dominant hemisphere)
	Hemineglect (nondominant hemisphere)
	Contralateral sensory or motor loss
Vertebrobasilar ischemia	Ataxia
	Diplopia
	Hemianopsia
	Vertigo
	Cranial nerve defects
	Contralateral hemiplegia
	Sensory deficits

stroke) and medication history (antiplatelet or anticoagulant drugs). Particular attention is given to vital signs. An irregular heart rhythm may indicate atrial fibrillation. Hypertension increases the likelihood for intracranial hemorrhage. The focused neurologic assessment is key and includes tests for **dysphagia, hemianopsia, hemiparesis,** and other signs of focal injury (Brott & Bogousslavsky, 2000).

A focused clinical assessment of the patient is important to establish a baseline and to assist in diagnosis and prognosis in terms of survival and functional recovery. When a stroke is suspected, the ABCs (airway, breathing, and circulation) are assessed. Impaired airway clearance may result from hemiplegia, dysphagia, a weak cough reflex, and immobility. This places the patient at high risk for hypoxemia, pneumonia, and aspiration.

Continuous monitoring of breath sounds, breathing patterns, oxygen saturation, skin color, and arterial blood gases (ABGs) is important. The patient's ability to handle secretions is assessed. Intubation and mechanical ventilation are required for the patient who is comatose and has evidence of increased ICP. The patient may present with ineffective breathing patterns because of decreased level of responsiveness, aspiration, loss of protective reflexes, or a decrease in respiratory movements on the affected side. With inadequate ventilation, hypercapnia occurs, causing cerebral vasodilation. This, however, diverts blood from the penumbra and contributes to an extension of the infarct. To prevent hypercapnia, the nurse monitors rate and rhythm of breathing, ABGs, and level of consciousness. Cardiovascular assessment includes frequent monitoring of vital signs (particularly blood pressure and heart rate) until the patient is stable. The heart rhythm is assessed for dysrhythmias. Peripheral and carotid pulses are palpated. Continuous telemetry identifies abnormal cardiac rhythms.

There are several key physical assessment findings in patients who have had strokes that the nurse must recognize. If the patient is awake, the probability of a hemispheric stroke is high.

Lid ptosis and cranial nerve III (oculomotor) involvement suggest a posterior stroke may have occurred. Contralateral hemiparesis involving the face and limbs is indicative of a hemispheric (anterior or carotid) stroke. The nurse notes extremity position and assesses handgrips, arm drifts, and leg pushes for strength. The tone (**flaccidity** or **spasticity**) of the extremities is noted. Speech is assessed for incoherency, impropriety of speech content, and fluency. Orientation and the ability to follow commands is assessed. Loss of consciousness raises suspicion of a posterior (vertebrobasilar) stroke or a bilateral hemispheric stroke. During the physical assessment, the nurse is sensitive to cognitive and perceptual–visual–spatial deficits. Sensitivity to patient behavior manifesting as neglect or poor judgment choices is a key in assessment findings. Cranial nerve abnormalities (III to XII) reflect brainstem involvement or a vertebrobasilar stroke. Cranial nerve assessment helps the nurse establish a baseline against which to compare the patient's progress.

The National Institutes of Health Stroke Scale is widely used in the United States to assess neurologic outcome and degree of recovery (Table 19–4). The complete questionnaire with instructions is available on the Internet.

TABLE 19–4 National Institutes of Health Stroke Scale

TITLE	RESPONSES AND SCORES	TITLE	RESPONSES AND SCORES
Level of consciousness	0—Alert 1—Drowsy 2—Obtunded 3—Coma/unresponsive	Motor function (leg) a. Left b. Right	0—No drift 1—Drift before 5 seconds 2—Falls before 5 seconds 3—No effort against gravity 4—No movement
Orientation questions (two)	0—Answers both correctly 1—Answers one correctly	Limb ataxia	0—No ataxia 1—Ataxia in one limb 2—Ataxia in two limbs
Response to commands (two)	0—Performs both tasks correctly 1—Performs one task correctly	Sensory	0—No sensory loss 1—Mild sensory loss 2—Severe sensory loss
Gaze	0—Normal horizontal movements 1—Complete gaze palsy	Language	0—Normal 1—Mild aphasia 2—Severe aphasia 3—Mute or global aphasia
Visual fields	0—No visual field defect 1—Partial hemianopsia 2—Complete hemianopsia 3—Bilateral hemianopsia	Articulation	0—Normal 1—Mild dysarthria 2—Severe dysarthria
Facial movement	0—Normal 1—Minor facial weakness 2—Partial facial weakness 3—Complete unilateral palsy	Extinction or inattention	0—Absent 1—Mild (loss of one sensory modality) 2—Severe (loss of two modalities)
Motor function (arm) a. Left b. Right	0—No drift 1—Drift before 5 seconds 2—Falls before 5 seconds 3—No effort against gravity 4—No movement		

Note: This is a condensed version of the National Institutes of Health Stroke Scale. The actual form for recording the data contains detailed instructions for the use of the scale. The complete scale with instructions can be obtained from the National Institute of Neurological Disorders and Stroke.

The following tests or procedures are performed as soon as possible after arrival of the patient to the emergency department. Computerized tomography (CT) of the brain is performed urgently to differentiate hemorrhage from ischemic causes (Brott & Bogousslavsky, 2000). Arteriography of cerebral vessels evaluates vessel structures, vasospasm, or stenosis. Magnetic resonance imaging (with angiography) is used to diagnose lesions. Transcranial and extracranial, contrast-enhanced CT, and single-photon-emission CT may be used to establish the anatomical regions and structures involved and the cause of the infarction (Brott & Bogousslavsky, 2000). Lumbar puncture is done to detect blood in the cerebrospinal fluid if subarchnoid hemorrage (SAH) is suspected but not confirmed by CT scan. Transesophageal echocardiography detects cardiac and aortic causes of embolism. A 12-lead ECG is performed because cardiac abnormalities are prevalent among patients with stroke. A complete blood count, including platelets, prothrombin time, international normalized ratio, partial thromboplastin time, and fibrinogen, are evaluated to detect any coagulapathies and establish baselines for therapy. Serum electrolytes and blood glucose levels may be ordered to rule out other conditions that may mimic stroke, including hypoglycemia. Electrolyte imbalances are a source of cardiac dysrhythmias. Arterial blood gases, drug screen, and a serum alcohol level may be done if indicated by history to detect possible causes of stroke. Doppler ultrasonography and duplex imaging are emergency noninvasive tests that are done when carotid artery disease is suspected.

Priority nursing diagnoses in the acute care phase include (1) *altered cerebral tissue perfusion* related to interruption of arterial blood flow resulting from obstruction or rupture of vessels in an area of the brain causing possible increase in ICP and neurologic deficits; (2) *pain related to biological and physical* factors of pressure or irritation to pain-sensitive areas resulting from hemorrhagic stroke, cerebral infarction, or carotid artery occlusive stroke; and (3) *altered thought processes* related to physiological changes resulting from reduced cerebral blood flow causing impaired sensations and inaccurate interpretation of the environment.

In summary, manifestations of stroke vary according to the cerebral artery involved. It is important to quickly assess and determine whether the stroke is ischemic or hemorrhagic. This determination is based on a focused neurologic assessment and diagnostic tests. A focused clinical assessment of the patient with acute stroke is very important. The assessment begins with the ABCs to identify actual or potential life-threatening problems. Key physical assessment findings may include neuromuscular abnormalities as well as cognitive, perceptual–visual–spatial defects. Priority nursing diagnoses include *altered cerebral tissue perfusion, pain,* and *altered thought processes.*

SECTION FOUR REVIEW

1. The most common manifestation of stroke is
   A. numbness and weakness of the face and arm
   B. monocular vision loss
   C. aphasia
   D. hemineglect
2. Headache, nausea, vomiting, and seizures are common manifestations of
   A. thrombotic strokes
   B. embolic strokes
   C. hemorrhagic strokes
   D. TIAs
3. The diagnostic test that distinguishes cerebral hemorrhage from infarction during the first hours of stroke onset is

   A. duplex ultrasound
   B. transcranial doppler study
   C. CT scan
   D. electroencephalogram
4. Which of the following may be used to detect cardiac and aortic causes of embolism?
   A. CT scan
   B. MRI
   C. transesophageal echocardiography
   D. lumbar puncture

Answers: 1. A, 2. C, 3. C, 4. C

SECTION FIVE: Medical and Nursing Management

This section presents current guidelines on medical management of patients who have had strokes. At the completion of this section, the learner will be able to describe the implications of the medications used to treat patients who have had strokes and discuss the rationale for surgical interventions for management of stroke.

Medical Management of Strokes

Because most strokes are caused by an occlusion of a cerebral vessel, improvement and restoration of perfusion to the ischemic area is imperative. The concept of the penumbra is fundamental in treating ischemic strokes. Although a core of infarcted tissue is not salvageable, adjacent dysfunctional tissue is salvageable if circulation is promptly restored (Adams et al., 2003). Patients with acute ischemic stroke presenting to the emergency department within 48 hours of the onset of symptoms are given aspirin (160 to 325 mg/day) to reduce stroke mortality and decrease morbidity, provided contraindications, such as allergy and gastrointestinal bleeding, are absent and the patient has not or will not be treated with tissue plasminogen activator (Coull et al., 2003).

Intravenous tissue plasminogen activator (rtPA) is strongly recommended for carefully selected patients who can be treated within 3 hours of onset of ischemic stroke (Adams et al., 2003). The patient who receives this medication is usually admitted to an intensive care unit or stroke unit. A small dose is given as a bolus, and is followed by an IV infusion of the drug over an hour. During and after the infusion, the nurse performs frequent neurological assessments: every 15 minutes for the first 2 hours, every 30 minutes for the next 6 hours, and then every hour for 24 hours after treatment (Adams et al., 2003). If, during the infusion, the patient develops nausea, vomiting, severe headache, or acute hypertension, the infusion is discontinued and the physician is notified immediately (Adams et al., 2003). It is also important to monitor the patient's blood pressure during an infusion of rtPA: every 15 minutes for the first 2 hours, every 30 minutes for the next 6 hours, and then every hour for 24 hours after treatment (Adams et al., 2003). Antihypertensive medications are given as required. The placement of nasogastric tubes, bladder catheters, or intra-arterial catheters should be delayed (Adams et al., 2003).

The use of anticoagulant medications (heparin, low molecular weight heparin, heparinoid) for acute stroke care has been the subject of much debate. For many years, early anticoagulation was used frequently in the treatment of ischemic stroke. But this practice has changed substantially since the late 1990s because research has shown that it has not been effective (Broderick & Hacke, 2002). The administration of anticoagulants is currently contraindicated during the first 24 hours following treatment with rtPA (Adams et al., 2003). Administration of these medications increases the risk of serious bleeding complications. Present data indicate that the early administration of anticoagulants does not lower the risk of early recurrent stroke (Adams et al., 2003).

Much is known about the benefits of aspirin and antiplatelet drugs in patients with acute myocardial ischemia, but less is known about the use of these drugs in patients with cerebral ischemia. Recent research has evaluated the use of these antiplatelet drugs in the setting of acute stroke and additional research is in progress. Current recommendations, as summarized by Adams and colleagues (2003), are summarized in Table 19–5.

Seizures are most likely to occur within 24 hours of stroke; however, there is no evidence to support the use of prophylactic administration of anticonvulsants after stroke (Adams et al., 2003).

Cerebral angioplasty has been successfully used to reverse neurological deficits caused by atherosclerotic lesions in the cerebral arteries. This technique uses a balloon catheter to me-

TABLE 19–5 Current Recommendations of Antiplatelet Therapy and Ischemic Strokes

Aspirin should be given within 24 to 48 hours of stroke onset for most patients

The administration of aspirin, as an adjunct therapy, within 24 hours of the use of thrombolytic agents is NOT recommended

Aspirin should NOT be used as a substitute for other acute interventions (rtPA) for the treatment of acute ischemic stroke

No recommendation can be made about the urgent administration of other antiplatelet aggregating agents

chanically dilate vessels. Microballoon catheters are introduced via the femoral artery and directed to the major arteries at the base of the brain. Vascular stenting is an alternative to angioplasty. There are currently many different types of stents in various stages of clinical use and approval by the Federal Drug Administration. More clinical trials must be completed before widespread use can be recommended. Cerebral angiography carries the risks of intracerebral hemorrhage, injury to the vessel wall, and distal embolization. Following cerebral angioplasty or stenting, nursing assessments for neurologic and vital sign changes are done frequently until the patient is neurologically stable.

Surgical Management of Strokes

Cerebellar lesions are critical because a hemorrhage or infarction can rapidly become life threatening by compromising the brainstem. Emergency surgery is indicated for cerebellar infarction or hemorrhage with clinical evidence of brainstem compression and increased ICP, such as decreasing level of consciousness, restlessness, or cranial nerve palsies. The size of the hemorrhage or infarction is a critical variable in medical management. Patients with large hemorrhages or infarctions are more likely to have brainstem compression and urgent need for surgery.

Bleeding into the subarachnoid space, such as that which occurs with a ruptured aneurysm, requires immediate medical attention. Treatment, however, depends on the severity of neurological symptoms. Persons with no neurological deficits may only require cerebral arteriography and early surgery. The surgical procedure, performed within 72 hours of the bleed, is known as an "aneurysm clipping" and involves opening the cranium (craniotomy) and inserting a metal clip around the aneurysm to prevent rebleeding. Postoperative complications include cerebral vasospasm. Vasospasm decreases perfusion to brain tissue. Vasospasm is prevented and treated with "triple H therapy": hypervolemia, hypertension, and hemodilution. This combination of therapies is used to augment cerebral perfusion pressure CPP by raising systolic blood pressure, cardiac output, and intravascular volume to increase cerebral blood flow and minimize cerebral ischemia. Triple H therapy is maintained for the first few days postoperatively.

For ischemic cerebrovascular disease, surgery may be performed to prevent recurring cerebral infarcts and TIAs. The procedure is done to remove the source of the occlusion and to increase cerebral blood flow to the ischemic area. A carotid endarterectomy is a surgical procedure that is performed to remove atherosclerotic plaque. This procedure involves the removal of exposed occlusive atherosclerotic plaque from the carotid artery (Fig. 19–2). Postoperative nursing care for the patient who has a carotid endarterectomy, as summarized by Lemone and Burke (2004), is listed in Table 19–6.

In summary, most strokes are caused by an occlusion of a cerebral vessel. Improvement and restoration of perfusion to the ischemic area is imperative. Intravenous rtPA is recommended for treatment of ischemic stroke. Administration of anticoagulant medications is controversial. Cerebral angiography may be used to reverse neurological deficits caused by atherosclerotic lesions. This procedure, like all others, is associated with risks and, therefore, requires frequent nursing assessments of the patient after the procedure. Management of cerebellar lesions and subarachnoid hemorrhages require prompt surgical intervention. Triple H therapy is used to prevent and control cerebral vasospasm postoperatively for patients who have had

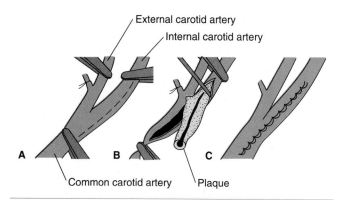

Figure 19–2 ■ Carotid endarterectomy. *A.* The occluded area is clamped off and an incision is made in the artery. B. Plaque is removed from the inner layer of the artery. *C.* To restore blood flow through the artery, the artery is sutured, or a graft is completed.

an aneurysm clipping. A carotid endarterectomy is performed to remove occlusive atherosclerotic plaque in the carotid arteries. Postoperative nursing assessments focus on early identification of complications and prevention of pressure/tension on the operative site.

TABLE 19–6 Nursing Care of the Patient after Carotid Endarterectomy

NURSING INTERVENTION	RATIONALE
Position patient on the unoperative side, with head of bed elevated 30 degrees	Elevation reduces operative site edema
Maintain head and neck alignment; avoid rotating, flexing, or hyperextending head	Proper alignment prevents additional tension or pressure on the operative side
Support the head during position change (teach patient to do the same)	Support prevents additional tension/stress on operative side; tension/stress may cause bleeding and hematoma formation
Nursing assessments focus on early identification of complications, including hemorrhage, respiratory distress, cranial nerve impairment, and alterations in blood pressure	The most common cause of respiratory problem is pressure on the trachea from hematoma formation
	Cranial nerves may be stretched during surgery, leading to temporary deficits in cranial nerve function; assess for facial drooping, tongue deviation, hoarseness, dysphagia, or loss of facial sensation
	Patients who have this procedure are at risk for developing unstable blood pressure as a result of denervation of the carotid sinus

SECTION FIVE REVIEW

1. Which of the following is fundamental to the current approach to the treatment of ischemic strokes?
   A. ischemic penumbra
   B. infarcted area
   C. cerebral edema
   D. cerebral perfusion pressure
2. During administration of rtPA, neurological assessments should be made every
   A. 12 hours   C. 1 hour
   B. 6 hours   D. 15 minutes

3. Which of the following statements is false about aspirin administration in cerebral ischemia?
   A. it should be given within 24 hours of thrombolytic agents
   B. it should not be given within 24 hours of thrombolytic agents
   C. it should not be used as a substitute for rtPA
   D. less is known about the use of this drug with cerebral ischemia

Answers: 1. A, 2. D, 3. A

SECTION SIX: Brain Attack: Nursing Challenges in the Acute Care Phase

In the high-acuity unit, care of the patient with a stroke focuses on prevention and treatment of complications that may be neurological (such as secondary hemorrhage, space-occupying edema, or seizures) or medical (infections, decubitus ulcers, deep-venous thrombosis, or pulmonary embolism) (Broderick & Hacke, 2002). At the completion of this section, the learner will be able to discuss priority nursing interventions for the patient with acute brain attack.

After having a stroke, the patient may be placed in a special high-acuity unit in the hospital—the stroke unit. A stroke unit is a hospital unit, or part of a hospital unit, staffed with a multidisciplinary team. The core disciplines of the team include experts from medicine, nursing, physiotherapy, occupational therapy, speech and language therapy, and social work. The acute stroke unit admits patients quickly and continues treatment for several days, until transfer to a rehabilitation or nursing facility, or to home (Broderick & Hacke, 2002).

Alteration in Tissue Perfusion

Altered tissue perfusion related to interruption of flow, venous stasis from inactivity is a priority nursing diagnosis for patients in the acute phase after a stroke. A serious threat to the hemiplegic stroke patient is a deep-vein thrombosis (DVT), which may lead to pulmonary embolus. Stroke patients are at high risk for DVT because of hemiplegia, loss of vasomotor tone, venous stasis, and edema in the paralyzed, flaccid limbs; and immobility. Dehydration places the patient at high risk for DVT. Hemiplegia or hemiparesis decreases muscle pump action for return of venous blood to the heart. Poor positioning (one extremity lying on another) or sitting for long periods in a chair can precipitate or exacerbate DVT. Subcutaneous unfractionated heparin, low-molecular-weight heparin, and heparinoids may be given for DVT prophylaxis for at-risk patients with ischemic stroke as well as other nonpharmacologic measures to prevent DVT (Coull et al., 2002). These include the following:

- Extremity elevation by raising the foot of the bed (to promote venous return to the heart)
- Intermittent pneumatic compression stockings (to increase blood flow velocity, reduce venous stasis, and stimulate fibrinolytic activity)
- Continuous passive motion devices (to increase muscle and venous valvular action)
- Elastic support hose (to increase blood flow velocity and reduce edema and venous distention)

Impaired Physical Mobility

Impaired physical mobility is related to motor and sensory deficits, particularly hemiplegia and impaired balance, changes in postural tone, and disinhibition of primitive reflex activity.

Rehabilitation begins early after a stroke in an effort to increase independence. A multidisciplinary effort is required (Broderick & Hacke, 2002). Physical therapists assess motor function, plan exercise programs, and provide splints to prevent contractures. Occupational therapists assess, provide a plan of therapy, and evaluate sensory and cognitive problems that interfere with functional independence. The physiatrist is a physician responsible for diagnosing and treating rehabilitative problems, such as spasticity and **subluxations.**

Following a stroke, cerebral shock may occur, causing hypotonicity or flaccid hemiplegia. During cerebral shock, a state of temporary disruption of neural transmission and integration processes occurs. When a stroke causes hemiplegia, initially the patient is flaccid; later, tone is palpated in affected limb muscles and spasticity begins, with some resistance to movement. Spasticity results when reflex activity is released from cerebral inhibition after damage to the motor system. This spasticity is associated with an upper motor neuron lesion because the frontal cortex (motor centers) and/or corticospinal (voluntary motor) tracts are interrupted. Muscle spasticity, hypertonicity, resistance to passive stretch in joints, and abnormally brisk reflexes characterize upper motor neuron lesions. The patient can present with mild hemiparesis to severe hemiplegia, quadriplegia, **ataxia,** or involuntary movements depending on the stroke site.

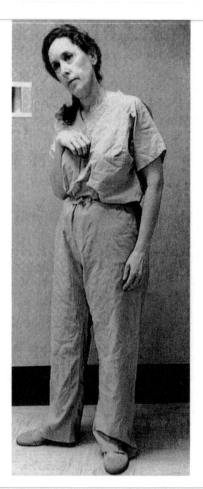

Figure 19–3 ■ The hemiparetic posture.

Poststroke spasticity (excessive muscle tone) affects the antigravity muscles. In the lower limbs, these are the knee extensors and plantar flexors of the foot. In the upper limbs, these are the elbow flexors and wrist and finger flexors. The patient assumes a spastic "hemiparetic posture," with the neck and trunk tilted toward the hemiparetic side; the shoulder pulled down and back; the elbow, wrist, and fingers flexed; and the arm adducted (Fig. 19–3). The lower limb is extended, with the hip internally rotated and adducted, and the foot plantar is flexed with supination, inversion, and flexed toes. Because flexor muscles are stronger in the arms and extensors stronger in the legs, the patient is prone to flexion contractures in the upper extremity and extension contractures in the lower extremities.

Maintaining functional abilities in the acute phase after stroke is important. Active and/or passive range of motion (ROM) exercises performed at least three or four times a day prevent contractures. Proper body alignment is important to prevent contractures. The patient is placed in positions that neutralize the abnormal hemiparetic posture. When lying supine, the head and spine are straight and the entire affected arm is elevated on pillows with the hand and fingers extended in a functional position, preferably with the palm up. A folded towel is placed under the affected shoulder so that both shoulders are symmetrical. A firm roll along the lateral aspect of the hip and thigh neutralizes the tendency of the affected leg to rotate externally. If positioned on the affected side, the patient's body is rotated slightly less than 90 degrees to rest on the shoulder blade rather than directly on the shoulder, to avoid the body's weight on the paralyzed arm or leg. The affected arm is extended perpendicular to the body, and the leg slightly flexed (Fig. 19–4). When positioned on the unaffected side, the patient's body is rotated more than 90 degrees with the affected shoulder forward, extremities beyond midline, the affected arm extended and elevated on pillows, and the affected leg functionally flexed

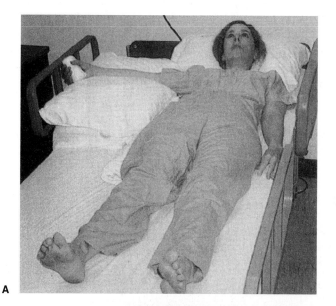

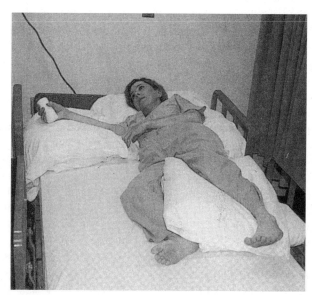

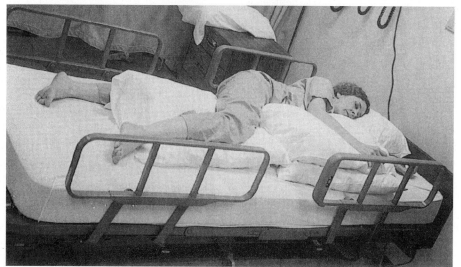

Figure 19–4 ■ Positioning the stroke patient. **A.** Lying on back. **B.** Lying on affected side. **C.** Lying on the unaffected side.

and elevated on pillows. When eating in the upright position, the affected arm is elevated on a pillow to maintain proper body alignment. During turning, avoid pulling on the affected arm because this may produce subluxation of the shoulder joint. Tennis shoes help to prevent contractures in the flaccid stage but tend to stimulate more spasticity in the hyperreflexic stages. Hard rolls or inflatable splints are used to maintain functional hand and arm position and are applied, particularly at night. Correct positioning by abduction and external rotation of the shoulder prevents shoulder pain.

Ambulation and Activities of Daily Living

The patient is ready to ambulate when there is evidence of leg strength, some balance, and **proprioception.** Muscle tone is assessed regularly, and the patient is not asked to do an activity with the disabled limb until muscle tone is restored. Traditional slings are avoided because they reinforce the abnormal posture of the spastic flexed arm and adduction, and promote shoulder contractures. The affected arm is handled gently to avoid subluxation of the shoulder joint and is supported with pillows.

Potential Alteration in Nutrition

Dysphagia, absent or diminished gag reflexes, facial paralysis, perceptual and cognitive deficits, hemiplegia (particularly affecting the dominant hand), an inability to perform bilateral hand tasks, and immobility all contribute to undernutrition. Absent gag reflexes and facial paralysis limit chewing and swallowing movements and increase the risk for aspiration. Perceptual deficits, such as impaired depth perception, agnosias, apraxias, hemianopsia, or neglect, may produce injury during eating.

The hypermetabolic stress response initiated by the brain attack results in hyperglycemia as well as decreased intake. Thus, metabolic demands become greater at a time when oral intake is often acutely restricted. Clinically, the patient may manifest a decrease in serum protein leading to a compromised immune state, weight loss, muscle weakness and atrophy, increased risk of pressure ulcers, higher morbidity and mortality, and a prolonged hospital stay. In well-nourished patients nutritional support is started if no oral intake is anticipated for greater than 5 days. If the patient is malnourished on admission, as defined by a greater than 10 percent weight loss before critical illness, nutritional support is initiated promptly (Evans-Stoner & Mullen, 2001).

The patient is assessed for the ability to bring food to the mouth, handle utensils, see all the food on the tray, and successfully chew and swallow food and liquids, with no pocketing in the affected cheek. Early and rapid evaluation of swallowing is done as soon as possible (Broderick & Hacke, 2002). In addition, the patient is assessed for (1) cognitive ability to feed self, (2) drooling (a clue to swallowing problems) or difficulty swallowing liquids or foods, (3) continuous clearing of the throat or coughing while eating, and (4) appropriate positioning during eating. Dysphagia, or difficulty in swallowing, is usually caused by lesions involving cranial nerves V (trigeminal), VII (facial), IX (glossopharyngeal), X (vagus), XI (accessory), and XII (hypoglossal). Dysphagia is suspected when these signs appear: food put in the mouth causes the patient to choke, drool, have poor lip closure, engage in food pocketing, or have asymmetry of the mouth or a protruded tongue; food in the back of the throat causes the patient to choke, aspirate or have nasal regurgitation, become weak, or develop a hoarse voice; and food passing through the esophagus causes the patient to regurgitate.

Evidence-Based Practice

- *Stroke patients treated with rtPA who remain normotensive for the first 6 hours after treatment are unlikely to have subsequent hypertension (Aiyagari et al., 2004).*

- *Routine measurement of the length of the QT interval on ECG in patients with subarachnoid hemorrhage may help detect predisposition to potentially lethal tachyarrhythmias, particularly if the patient also has a low serum potassium (Sommargren, 2002).*

- *Eating difficulties following stroke mainly arise in the area of manipulating food on the plate, manipulating food in the mouth, and swallowing (Jacobson et al., 2000).*

- *Stroke survivors can benefit from counseling on participation in physical activity and exercise training (Thompson et al., 2003).*

- *Among patients with acute stroke, early hospital discharge with home-based rehabilitation (4 weeks of physical therapy, occupational therapy, speech therapy, dietary consultation, nursing care) results in better health and integration into the community (Mayo et al., 2000).*

- *Aggressive rehabilitation beyond the usual 6-month period increases aerobic capacity and sensorimotor function (Mack et al., 2001).*

- *Physical activity and exercise training recommendations for stroke survivors should be viewed as one component of a comprehensive stroke and cardiovascular risk-reduction program (Gordon et al., 2004).*

Alteration in Elimination

Alteration in elimination may be related to impaired mobility, cognitive impairment, aphasia, and preexisting elimination problems. Elimination problems most frequently encountered in the stroke patient are as follows (Table 19–7):

- Detrusor muscle hyporeflexia (flaccid bladder)
- Detrusor muscle hyperreflexia (uninhibited or spastic bladder)
- Detrusor muscle–sphincter dyssynergy (unsynchronized detrusor and sphincter muscles producing urinary retention)

Patients with detrusor hyporeflexia have large-capacity, flaccid bladders with overflow incontinence. Indwelling Foley catheters should be inserted as soon as possible after the stroke (Broderick & Hacke, 2002). After the acute phase of the injury

TABLE 19–7 Neurogenic Bladder Types in the Acute Stroke Patient

BLADDER TYPE	FEATURES	LESION SITE	EFFECTS ON PATIENT	NURSING APPROACH
Detrusor hyporeflexia	Flaccid (large capacity)	Above the pons	Overflow incontinence Distended bladder High urine residual volumes	Montior intake and output Observe for overdistention Intermittent catheterization Keep urine volume less than 400 mL
Detrusor hyperreflexia (uninhibited)	Spastic (small capacity)	Cerebral cortex, internal capsule, basal ganglia	Urinary frequency, urgency Bladder contractions/spasms Nocturia Low-volume voidings Incontinence (unable to reach toilet in time)	Voiding schedule every 2 hours or longer Monitor intake, output Encourage fluids Limit caffeine and evening fluids Upright position to void Antispasmotics may be prescribed
Detrusor–sphincter dyssynergy (noncoordinated)	Spastic bladder and external sphincter that contract simultaneously (small capacity)	Pons, and pathways between pons and above sacral spinal cord	Small, frequent, or no voids Sensation of bladder fullness Dribbling, overflow incontinence High urine residual volumes Dysuria	Consistent fluid intake Time voiding schedule Possibly intermittent catheterization within 5 minutes of voidings Observe for overdistention symptoms Keep residuals less than 75 mL Monitor intake, output

has passed, the Foley is removed, the nurse monitors intake and output, and uses an intermittent catheterization program every 4 hours to ensure that the urine volume does not exceed 400 mL. For patients with bladder hyperreflexia, a voiding schedule is established with the patient and family based on previous patterns of voiding. When possible, diapers should be avoided.

Constipation is more common after stroke, probably because of age-related hypotonicity of the bowel, a decrease in roughage and fluid intake, immobility, the inability to communicate the need to defecate, and medications such as diuretics. Straining during defecation can cause hypertension. To promote adequate bowel elimination, a convenient pattern is established after assessing former and current bowel patterns. Information related to fluids and foods that normally elicit bowel movements and patient preferences in roughage foods is elicited. Stool softeners and suppositories are used to establish a regular pattern, as well as gastrointestinal reflexes when establishing an optimal toileting time (e.g., after meals). Daily assessment and outcome criteria are established for bowel elimination based on the individual's pattern.

Sensory Alterations

Sensation and skin integrity may be altered in the stroke patient as related to loss of sense of touch, pressure, temperature and sensation, or motor or vascular tone loss. Lesions in the parietal cortex or its afferent pathways produce a loss of primary sensations or **paresthesias,** placing the patient at risk for burns, bruises, and other forms of injury. Impaired tactile sensation affects motor activity because sensory feedback is limited. It also affects perception because sensory information needed for interpretation and integration is limited. Loss of proprioception or position sense may lead to falls. Loss of vision and hearing causes injury, social isolation, and impaired learning. A nursing priority is to protect the patient from injury.

The nurse protects the cornea by taping the eyelid shut and administers prescribed artificial tears or lubricants to prevent drying and corneal ulceration. For the diplopic patient, an eyepatch applied to one eye and alternated every 3 to 4 hours while the patient is awake permits a clear image. Avoiding extremes in heat and cold to desensitized areas is also important to prevent injury. Gentle handling of patients when transferring from bed to wheelchair and teaching the patient and family environmental hazards to avoid in the home are essential aspects of care for patients with altered sensations. When transferring from bed to wheelchair, the neglected or hemiplegic part must be supported and protected.

In the acute stages of stroke, the patient is prone to develop pressure ulcers because of sensory, motor, or vascular tone loss as well as incontinence, parietal neglect, and spasticity. The patient with a hemisensory deficit or hemiplegia cannot change positions. In addition, if nutrition is poor, the skin tissue is likely to break down in the immobile patient. Perceptual deficits compound the problem, particularly parietal neglect, when portions of the body are ignored.

To protect the patient from injury and to maintain skin integrity in hemiplegics or those who are experiencing neglect or denial, the nurse must alert the patient and family to the deficit and hazards. This includes teaching them to inspect the skin with mirrors; to observe the skin for adequate capillary refill, pallor, and hyperemia; and to avoid pressure on the area should these appear. The patient is repositioned at least every 2 hours and the skin is inspected with each reposition. The turning schedule is revised based on patient tolerance and skin integrity.

Perceptual hemineglect is a disorder of attention causing an inability to integrate and use perceptions in the contralateral side or space. The patient fails to respond to stimuli presented to the side contralateral to the brain lesion; therefore, that side is ignored but can be used if attention is drawn to it. Right brain damage produces this syndrome. Hemineglect is seen alone or in combination with **anosognosia** and left homonymous hemianopsia (hemineglect syndrome).

Nurses can assist a person with hemineglect syndrome by increasing the patient's awareness of the surroundings and by alleviating apprehension as to the source of the problem. When homonymous hemianopsia is present, initially the nurse compensates for the patient and approaches the patient from the unaffected side, positions the patient so that the intact visual field is toward the action, arranges personal items within the field of vision, and teaches the patient to scan the environment by turning the head vertically and horizontally. As the patient's apprehension decreases, the nurse stimulates the patient by placing personal items toward the affected side to encourage awareness of and attention to that side. This is accomplished by positioning so that the eyes are facing the affected side and by teaching the patient to handle, position, exercise, bathe, and dress the affected extremities with the patient's unaffected arm. Denial of illness usually resolves as the patient recovers.

Agnosia is a cortical impairment that results in the inability to recognize or interpret familiar sensory information although there is no impairment of sensory input or dementia. The agnosias can be tactile, visual, or auditory (Table 19–8). Tactile agnosia (astereognosia) is the inability to recognize objects by touch although tactile sensation is present. Visual agnosia is the inability to recognize or name familiar objects or faces although visual acuity is intact (e.g., the patient is unable to recognize utensils, toothbrush, clothes, or photographs). Auditory agnosia is the inability to recognize familiar sounds, such as a doorbell, telephone, horn, gun, or siren. When assessing for agnosias, ask the patient to name objects and cite their purpose. Ask the patient to identify objects in the hands or to identify sounds, music, or songs with his or her eyes closed. When deficits are found, a referral is made to an occupational therapist (OT) who evaluates and establishes a rehabilitative program.

Apraxia is the inability to carry out a purposeful movement although movement, coordination, and sensation are intact. There are several types of apraxias, which are summarized in Table 19–9. To assess for motor apraxia, the nurse observes the ability to initiate responses to motor commands, such as "Brush your teeth . . . comb your hair . . . put on your gown." Ideomotor apraxias is assessed by asking the patient to carry out a complex command, such as writing or drinking from a cup. The nurse notes the patient's ability to do spontaneous simple acts. Ideational apraxia is assessed by observing the patient's ability to perform spontaneous acts or acts on command, such as writing. The patient with ideational apraxia is unable to conceptualize the act and cannot perform a spontaneous act. Asking the patient to copy or draw a clock or daisy, or to build three-dimensional designs, such as a house or block, are used to assess the patient with constructional apraxia. Asking the patient to put on or remove a shirt, gown, or robe assesses dressing apraxia.

The effectiveness of therapy for ideomotor and ideational apraxia is uncertain. For ideomotor and ideational apraxia, the components of a motor sequence leading up to the entire activity need to be broken down and taught in simple terms, speaking slowly with clear directions. The patient with dressing apraxia is assisted by the use of labels to distinguish right and left, back from front, right and wrong side, or by color-coding garments. For all apraxic patients, repetition, consistency, avoidance of distractions, and visual motor coordination exercises are useful.

TABLE 19–8 Agnosias

TYPE	LESION SITE
Tactile	Either parietal lobe
Visual	Temporal–occipital lobe of either hemisphere
Auditory	Temporal lobe in dominant hemisphere

TABLE 19–9 Apraxias

TYPE	LESION SITE
Motor: Memory deficit for motor sequences affecting only upper limbs, although muscle and sensory function are intact	Frontal lobes
Ideomotor: Inability to perform a motor act on command even though the patient understands the act and has muscle and sensory function; can perform spontaneous, simple, isolated acts but not complex acts, such as writing or dressing	Left dominant parietal lobe
Ideational: Inability to perform activities automatically or on command	Left dominant parietal lobe
Constructional: Inability to copy, draw, or construct designs in two or three dimensions on command or spontaneously	Occipitoparietal cortices
Dressing: Inability to dress self because of a disorder in body schema, unilateral neglect, and/or spatial relations	Usually nondominant (right) parietal–occipital area

Impaired Communication

Patients with left hemispheric dysfunction caused by middle cerebral artery involvement experience aphasia/dysphasia if the speech centers or their pathways are involved in the lesion. Aphasia/dysphasia is a disorder of linguistic processing in which there is a disruption of translating thought to language. Literally, **aphasia** means a total inability to understand or formulate language. Language comprehension, speech expression, or writing ability may be lost. **Dysphasia** is difficulty with comprehending, speaking, or writing.

In Wernicke's aphasia, the patient receives auditory impulses but is unable to comprehend them. It is a receptive aphasia characterized by fluent, well-articulated speech with intact tone but inappropriate speech content that is unintelligible because of poor word choices. The patient makes up new words. Reading and speech comprehension, repetition of speech, and naming of objects is impaired. The patient is unable to write coherently. Motor deficits are seldom seen in these patients because the lesion is in the left temporal lobe. The goal of therapy for patients with Wernicke's aphasia is to develop an awareness of the language problem and to increase comprehension. Removing extraneous sounds and distractions, such as the television or radio, assist in getting the person's attention. The patient and nurse use nonverbal behavior to enhance communication. Keeping the conversation on one defined subject with one question at a time and avoiding multiple choices when communicating is helpful.

Broca's aphasia is an expressive aphasia characterized by nonfluent, telegraphic speech with outbursts of profanity, uninhibited speech, and word-finding difficulty, which reflects impaired memory for language. The patient uses nouns or phrases with pauses between words, and lacks grammar. An awareness of speech errors is present and speech production is labored and frustrating. A poor capacity for repetition and difficulty naming objects exists although recognition of objects is present. Oddly, these patients can sing fluently because musical ability is intact in the nondominant hemisphere. Comprehension is usually intact and responses are appropriate. Reading comprehension is variable and writing ability is impaired, possibly because an associated right hemiparesis or hemiplegia is often found in these patients because Broca's area is located adjacent to the primary motor centers in the frontal lobe. The goal for the patient with Broca's aphasia is to establish reliable language output to express needs. This may be accomplished initially by asking the patient "yes–no" questions.

Global aphasia is a combination of Broca's and Wernicke's aphasia with an almost complete loss of comprehension and expression of speech. The lesion involves the frontal and temporal lobes. The patient has nonfluent speech and an inability to express his or her ideas in speech or writing. The goal for the patient with global aphasia is to improve the ability to communicate. The patient is taught to enhance communication with nonverbal gestures and facial expressions. The measures cited for both Wernicke's and Broca's aphasias are applicable with these patients as well.

Dysarthria is an impairment of the muscles that control speech. Hemispheric or brainstem strokes produce dysarthria, which is characterized by slurred, muffled, or indistinct speech. If the basal ganglia or cerebellum are involved, uncoordinated, slow, monotonal speech results. Language comprehension and formulation are intact unless the patient also has an aphasia. The goal of therapy is to strengthen the speech muscles in order to speak more clearly and fluently. Encouraging the person to enunciate one word at a time, particularly consonants, and increasing voice volume when it is low helps.

High Risk for Ineffective Patient and Family Coping

Patients and their families are faced with multiple psychosocial stressors. The potential for ineffective coping is related to abrupt change in lifestyle, loss of roles, dependency, and economic insecurity. The inability to cope with abrupt and severe changes in body function or image, lifestyle changes, fears of becoming a burden on the family, dependency, and economic insecurity with loss of the breadwinner role provide ample and valid reasons for ineffective coping. In addition, the family may have to assume new roles as care providers and relinquish jobs and salaries. They may be overwhelmed with medical bills or faced with nursing home placement of their loved one and subsequent guilt. Fears of another stroke as well as inability to care for the patient at home create more stress. Dominant hemispheric stroke patients, in addition, are prone to severe depression because of their awareness of their deficits. Other causes for ineffective coping are the emotional and cognitive impairments following a stroke. Emotional lability with inappropriate crying, laughing, or euphoria, or socially inappropriate behavior with an inability to interpret social cues of communication, create stress for both the patient and family. Uninhibited behavior with outbursts of profanities or abrupt or impulsive behavior provides additional sources of stress. Confusion and bewilderment may compound the problem. In terms of impaired cognition, there may be delayed processing, diminished learning and reasoning ability, and a short attention span. Memory deficits vary with the hemispheric involvement. If the nondominant hemisphere is involved, a memory deficit for performance may be seen; if the dominant hemisphere is involved, a memory deficit for language, word-finding difficulty, and naming problems surface. In addition, there are hemispheric differences in judgment. Patients with lesions in the left hemisphere are slow, cautious, and underestimate their abilities. In contrast, patients with right hemispheric lesions may be prone to injury because they overestimate their abilities.

To assist the patient in coping effectively, the nurse provides appropriate information to alleviate fears and strengthen support systems. Clergy, friends, and family support groups may help assist the patient in coping and may provide comfort for both the patient and the family. Informing the patient that most recovery takes up to 6 months and some recovery of function even longer may be helpful in preventing unrealistic expectations for recovery.

If inappropriate crying or laughter occurs, divert the patient's attention from the behavior to stop it. Provide feedback in a matter-of-fact way when behavior is inappropriate. Avoid nagging, angry, or punitive responses. Be patient and gently slow down impulsive behavior.

A positive body image is reinforced when one focuses on the function that is left and not on that which is lost. Speak positively about the remainder of body functions. Use terms such as *affected* and *unaffected* rather than *good* and *bad* side. Reinforce independence early by involving the patient in decisions about care. Teach the family to do the same related to family roles and care.

For the patient and family, multidisciplinary referrals may be necessary. Social workers, home health nurses, dieticians, occupational therapists, physiatrists, support groups, and voluntary and governmental agencies (e.g., Medicare) provide assistance. The American Heart Association and the National Stroke Association provide free and low-cost literature on stroke care developed by experts. These referral groups and services are essential for the functional recovery and provide invaluable assistance in restoring the patient to a functional or complete recovery.

In summary, nursing care of the patient with a stroke during the acute phase of recovery is extremely challenging. Impaired physical mobility is related to motor and sensory deficits, particularly hemiplegia and impaired balance, changes in postural tone, and disinhibition of primitive reflex activity. To increase independence, rehabilitation must begin as early as possible following stroke and requires a multidisciplinary effort. Dysphagia, diminished or absent gag reflexes, facial paralysis, perceptual and cognitive deficits, hemiplegia, an inability to perform bilateral hand tasks, and immobility all contribute to undernutrition. Alteration in elimination may be related to impaired mobility, cognitive impairment, aphasia, and preexisting elimination problems. Neurogenic bladder conditions may be present and require astute nursing care. Constipation is common. Impaired sensation and skin integrity related to loss of touch, pressure, temperature and sensation or motor or vascular tone loss are all possibilities. Nursing interventions must address patient safety. The patient with a stroke may experience a variety of visual–spatial–perceptual deficits. The nurse in the high-acuity setting recognizes these deficits and plans nursing care accordingly.

SECTION SIX REVIEW

1. Correct positioning of the hemiplegic patient is described in which of the following statements?
   A. unaffected side: the patient's body is at 90 degrees with the affected arm flexed and elevated on a pillow
   B. supine: the head is midline and in neutral position with the arms at the side
   C. affected side: the patient's body is rotated laterally less than 90 degrees with the affected arm extended and elevated on pillows and the affected leg slightly flexed on pillows
   D. affected side: the patient's body is at 90 degrees with a pillow between the legs and the arm extended and elevated on pillows.

2. All of the following are causes of undernutrition in stroke patients EXCEPT
   A. dysphagia
   B. hemiplegia
   C. perceptual deficits
   D. hypometabolic state

3. Which of the following is true of elimination problems in acute stroke patients?
   A. bowel incontinence is common
   B. indwelling urinary catheters are useful for patients with hyperreflexic bladders
   C. incontinence is usually stress related
   D. scheduled voiding programs can promote continence

4. Which of the following is true regarding the hemineglect syndrome seen in stroke patients?
   A. it usually occurs in dominant strokes
   B. it is accompanied by left homonymous hemianopsia
   C. the patient is paralyzed on one side of his or her body
   D. the patient has insight into the cause of the impairment

5. MB, age 30, had an embolic stroke involving her left frontal and parietal lobes. She follows commands, has difficulty naming objects, blurts out profanities on occasion, and speaks in words and phrases in nonfluent speech. Her communication impairment most likely is
   A. Wernicke's aphasia
   B. global aphasia
   C. Broca's aphasia
   D. dysarthria

6. Which of the following is not a potential stressor for patients with acute brain attacks?
   A. changes in body image
   B. independence
   C. fears of becoming a burden to the family
   D. role modification

Answers: 1. C, 2. D, 3. D, 4. B, 5. C, 6. B

POSTTEST

1. Which of the following statements is true about stroke?
   A. stroke is an acute neurologic deficit
   B. stroke occurs in a localized area of the brain
   C. stroke occurs as a result of impaired blood flow
   D. all of the above

2. WJ is a 79-year-old man who presents to the emergency department with the following symptoms: partial loss of vision in one eye, and numbness, tingling, and weakness of the left arm. These symptoms usually last 15 to 30 minutes and then go away. WJ most likely has
   A. a cerebellar brain tumor
   B. hyponatremia
   C. TIAs
   D. subarachnoid hemorrhage

3. Which of the following cardiac conditions places patients at risk for developing an embolic stroke?
   A. carotid stenosis
   B. recent myocardial infarction
   C. ventricular hypertrophy
   D. pulmonary artery stenosis

4. A penumbra is defined as
   A. an infarct to brain cells
   B. a band of minimally perfused brain cells
   C. an aura that preceeds onset of stroke
   D. an inability to recognize familiar objects

5. Impaired oxygen delivery to brain cells results in
   A. intracellular accumulation of sodium
   B. failure of sodium–potassium pumps
   C. mitochondrial injury
   D. all of the above

JC is an 82-year-old African American man with a history of hypertension, type I diabetes, and a stroke (2 years ago). He smokes cigarettes and admits to being a "couch potato."

6. How many modifiable risk factors for stroke does JC have?
   A. one
   B. two
   C. three
   D. four

7. How many nonmodifiable risk factors for stroke does JC have?
   A. two
   B. four
   C. six
   D. eight

8. What is the role of lipid-lowering drugs (statins) in preventing strokes?
   A. they prevent heart disease, not stroke
   B. they must be instituted at the first sign of a TIA
   C. they may reduce the risk of ischemic strokes
   D. they are actually harmful to patients at high risk for stroke

9. PE is a 79-year-old female who presents to the emergency department with monocular vision loss, aphasia, and hemineglect. These signs and symptoms are typical of patients with
   A. carotid ischemia
   B. vertebrobasilar ischemia
   C. cranial nerve defects
   D. subarachnoid hemorrhage

10. To evaluate contralateral hemiparesis, the nurse would
    A. have the patient swallow
    B. ask the patient, "who is the president of the United States?"
    C. examine the flaccidity and spasticity of bilateral extremities
    D. give the patient the Snellen eye chart for a vision examination

11. One of the first priorities in the evaluation of a patient who has had a stroke is to determine whether the stroke was caused by ischemia or hemorrhage. Which of the following diagnostic tests helps to differentiate these causes?
    A. lumbar puncture
    B. electrocardiogram
    C. transcranial doppler ultrasonography
    D. CT scan

12. TP is receiving an infusion of rtPA for treatment of acute ischemic stroke. In which of the following situations would it be most appropriate to emergently discontinue the infusion?
    A. if the patient develops a severe headache, acute hypertension, and vomiting
    B. if the patient's blood pressure elevates to 180/100
    C. if the patient required placement of a nasogastric tube
    D. if the patient developed atrial fibrillation

13. Which of the following is a false statement about aspirin administration?
    A. it should be given within 24 hours of thrombolytic therapy
    B. it should not be given within 24 hours of thrombolytic therapy
    C. it should not be used as a substitute for rtPA
    D. less is known about the use of aspirin with cerebral ischemia

14. A carotid endarterectomy is a surgical procedure to remove
    A. an embolism
    B. atherosclerotic plaque
    C. a carotid artery
    D. a subarchnoid hemorrhage

15. The patient with SAH is at risk for developing which of the following complications?
    A. cerebral vasospasm
    B. hypertension
    C. respiratory arrest
    D. cor pulmonale

16. Dysphagia usually involves which of the following cranial nerves?
   A. I, II, III, IV, V, VI
   B. III, IV, V, VI, VII, VIII
   C. V, VII, IX, X, XI, XII
   D. II, III, V, VII, IX, X

17. The most common type of incontinence in acute stroke patients is produced by
   A. bladder hyperreflexia (spasticitiy)
   B. bladder hyporeflexia (flaccidity)
   C. detrusor–sphincter dyssynergy
   D. stress

18. Mrs. J, age 40, is an acute stroke patient with hemiplegia and parietal neglect following a stroke. She is at risk for decubitus ulcers for all of the following reasons EXCEPT
   A. she has a loss of vasomotor tone
   B. she ignores her left side
   C. she has venous stasis of her affected limbs
   D. she has dysphagia

19. The nurse assists Mrs. J by
   A. teaching her to inspect her skin for pallor or redness with a mirror
   B. turning her every 4 hours
   C. avoiding reference to her neglected side
   D. massaging her legs every 4 hours

20. Which of the following assessments would not be used in the assessment of MC, age 30, for visual–perceptual deficits following an acute stroke?
   A. ask her to draw a clock
   B. observe her dietary tray after meals
   C. ask her to read a page
   D. ask her to sing a song

POSTTEST ANSWERS

Question	Answer	Section	Question	Answer	Section
1	D	One	11	D	Four
2	C	One	12	A	Five
3	B	One	13	A	Five
4	B	Two	14	B	Five
5	D	Two	15	A	Five
6	D	Three	16	C	Six
7	B	Three	17	A	Six
8	C	Three	18	D	Six
9	A	Four	19	A	Six
10	C	Four	20	D	Six

REFERENCES

Adams, R. J., Chimowitz, M. I., Alpert, J. S., et al. (2003). Coronary risk evaluation in patients with transient ischemic attack and ischemic stroke. *Circulation, 108*, 1278–1290.

Aiyagari, V., Gujjar, A., Zazulia, A., et al. (2004). Hourly blood pressure monitoring after tissue plasminogen activator for ischemic stroke: Does every one need it? *Stroke, 35*, 2326–2330.

Albers, G. W., Amarenco, P., Easton, J. D., Sacco, R. L., & Teal, P. (2001). Antithrombotic and thrombolytic therapy for ischemic stroke. *Chest, 119*, 300S–320S.

Albers, G. W., Hart, R. G., Lutsep, H. L., Newell, D. W., & Sacco, R. L. (1999). Supplement to the guidelines for the management of transient ischemic attacks. *Stroke, 30*, 2505–2511.

American Heart Association. (2004). Statins after ischemic stroke and transient ischemic attacks. American Heart Association Science Advisory and Coordinating Committee. *Stroke, 35*, 1023.

Ariesen, M. L., Claus, M. D., Rinkel, G. J. E., & Algra, A. (2003). Risk factors for intracerebral hemorrhage in the general population: A systematic review. *Stroke, 34*, 2060–2066.

Book, D. (2002). Disorders of brain function. In C. M. Porth (Ed.), *Pathophysiology: Concepts of altered health states* (6th ed., pp. 1159–1199). Philadelphia: Lippincott Williams Wilkens.

Bradberry, J. C., & Fagan, S. C. (2002). Stroke. In J. T. DiPiro, R. L. Talbert, G. C. Lee, et al. (Eds.), *Pharmacotherapy: A pathophysiologic approach* (5th ed., pp. 375–394). New York: McGraw Hill.

Broderick, J. P., & Hacke, W. (2002). Treatment of acute ischemic stroke: Part II: Neuroprotection and medical management. *Circulation, 106*, 1736–1740.

Brott, T., & Bogousslavsky, J. (2000). Treatment of acute ischemic stroke. *New England Journal of Medicine, 343*, 710–722.

Coull, B. M., Williams, L. S., Goldstein, L. B., et al. (2002). Anticoagulants and antiplatelet agents in acute ischemic stroke. *Stroke, 33*, 1934–1942.

Evans-Stoner, N., & Mullen, J. L. (2001). Nutritional therapy. In P. N. Lanken (Ed.), *The intensive care manual* (pp. 153–154). Philadelphia: W. B. Saunders.

Gordon, N. F., Gluanick, M., Costa, F., et al. (2004). Physical activity and exercise recommendations for stroke survivors: American Heart Association Scientific Statement. *Stroke, 35*, 1229–1239.

Heart and Stroke Facts. (2001). *2001 statistical supplement.* Dallas: American Heart Association.

Hurn, P. D., & Brass, L. M. (2003). Estrogen and stroke: A balanced analysis. *Stroke, 34,* 338–341.

Jacobson, C., Axelsson, K., Osterlind, P. O., et al. (2000). How people with stroke and healthy older people experience the eating process. *Journal of Clinical Nursing 9,* 255–264.

Joint National Committee on Detection, Evaluation, and Treatment of High Blood Pressure. (2003). *The seventh report of the Joint National Committee on Detection, Evaluation, and Treatment of High Blood Pressure* (JNC VII).

Lemone, P., & Burke, K. (2004). Nursing care of clients with cerebrovascular and spinal cord disorders. In P. Lemone & K. Burke (Eds.), *Medical surgical nursing: Critical thinking in client care* (3rd ed., pp. 1306–1344). Upper Saddle River, NJ: Prentice Hall.

Mack, R. F., Smith, G. V., Dobrovolyny, C. L., et al. (2001). Treadmill training improves fitness reserve in chronic stroke patients. *American Journal of Physical and Medical Rehabilitation, 82,* 879–884.

Mayo, N. E., Wood-Dauphinee, S., Cole, R., et al. (2000). There's no place like home: An evaluation of early supported discharge for stroke. *Stroke, 31,*1016–1023.

Sacco, R. L., & Boden-Albala, B. (2001). Stroke risk factors: Identification and modification. In M. Fisher (Ed.), *Stroke therapy* (2nd ed., pp. 1–17). Boston: Butterworth, Heinemann.

Sommargren, C. E. (2002). Electrocardiographic abnormalities in patients with subarachnoid hemorrhage. *American Journal of Critical Care, 11,* 48–56.

Thompson, P. D., Buchner, D., Pina, I., et al. (2003). Exercise and physical activity in the prevention and treatment of atherosclerotic cardiovascular disease: A statement from the council on clinical cardiology. *Circulation, 107,* 3109–3116.

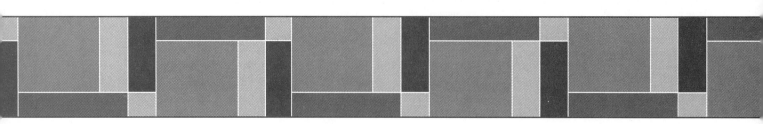

MODULE

20 Decreased Adaptive Capacity: Closed-Head Injury

Adam DaDeppo

OBJECTIVES Following the completion of this module, the learner will be able to

1. List the three primary mechanisms of injury associated with closed-head injury.

   ■ Describe the four types of skull fractures that can occur with injury to the head, and interventions.

2. Differentiate between focal and diffuse brain injuries.

   ■ Identify medical and nursing interventions for the treatment of focal and diffuse brain injuries.

3. Explain the pathophysiology of secondary brain injury.

   ■ Recognize current medical and nursing interventions for the treatment of secondary injury.

4. Identify four complications associated with closed-head injury.

   ■ Discuss medical and nursing interventions for the treatment of complications associated with closed-head injury.

   ■ Define the criteria used to diagnose brain death.

This module focuses on closed-head injury: the mechanisms of injury, pathophysiological changes that accompany such injuries, and a review of the medical and nursing care high-acuity patients with these injuries require. This module is composed of four sections. Section One introduces the reader to mechanisms of injury and skull fractures associated with head trauma. Section Two discusses the different types of primary brain injury and the medical and nursing interventions used to treat these injuries. Section Three reviews the pathophysiology and consequences of secondary brain injury and how secondary brain injury can be prevented. Section Four discusses complications associated with closed-head injury, medical and nursing interventions, and introduces the reader to the criteria used to diagnose brain death.

All section reviews and the module pretest and posttest include answers. It is suggested that the learner review those concepts answered incorrectly in the review questions before proceeding to the next section.

 PRETEST

1. Which of the following is NOT a mechanism of closed-head injury associated with trauma to the head?
   A. rotational
   B. diffuse
   C. acceleration/deceleration
   D. penetrating

2. Which of the following fractures are most commonly associated with an increased risk of infection?
   A. linear skull fracture
   B. open skull fracture
   C. basilar skull fracture
   D. depressed skull fracture

3. Battle's sign, raccoon eyes, and otorrhea are all common physical assessment findings associated with
   A. linear fractures
   B. depressed skull fractures
   C. open skull fractures
   D. basilar skull fractures

4. Which of the following is NOT an example of focal brain injury?
   A. concussion
   B. subdural hematoma
   C. subarachnoid hemorrhage
   D. epidural hematoma

5. Which focal brain injury has acute, subacute, and chronic stages?
  A. subdural hematoma
  B. intracerebral hematoma
  C. epidural hematoma
  D. subarachnoid hematoma

6. Which of the following is NOT a cause of secondary brain injury?
  A. ischemia
  B. cerebral swelling
  C. axonal shearing
  D. inflammation

7. Which of the following is NOT a nursing intervention to prevent secondary injury?
  A. completing multiple-patient care activities at once to decrease patient stimulation
  B. maintaining neck alignment
  C. keeping the patient's hip flexion at less than 90 degrees
  D. preoxygenating patients prior to suctioning

8. Diabetes insipidus is the result of
  A. increased production of antidiuretic hormone
  B. decreased production of antidiuretic hormone
  C. elevated blood glucose
  D. hypoglycemia

9. Treatment of SIADH includes
  A. fluid restriction
  B. fluid resuscitation
  C. replacement of sodium with salt tabs and intravenous saline
  D. administration of vasopressin

10. Cushing's triad includes all of the following signs EXCEPT
  A. tachycardia
  B. hypertension
  C. bradycardia
  D. irregular breathing pattern

Pretest Answers:
1. B, 2. B, 3. D, 4. A, 5. A, 6. C, 7. A, 8. B, 9. A, 10. C

GLOSSARY

brain death   Irreversible cessation of all brain function, including brainstem function.

cerebral hematoma   Cerebral injury associated with accumulation of blood in the cranial vault.

concussion   Mild traumatic brain injury caused by blunt trauma to the head.

diffuse axonal injury (DAI)   Injury that occurs when shearing forces disrupt the structure of neurons and their nearby blood vessels.

diffuse injury   Injury that occurs in several areas of the brain.

epidural hematoma (EDH)   Bleeding in the space between the dura mater and the skull.

focal injury   Injury that occurs in a well-defined area of the brain.

intracerebral hematoma (ICH)   Accumulation of blood in the parenchyma of brain tissue.

otorrhea   CSF leakage from the ear.

primary injury   Neurons sustain direct injury from an offending event.

rhinorrhea   CSF leakage through the nose.

secondary injury   Injury that occurs in response to direct injury.

subarachnoid hematoma (SAH)   Accumulation of blood between the arachnoid layer of the meninges and the brain.

subdural hematoma (SDH)   Accumulation of blood between dura and arachnoid layers of the meninges.

ABBREVIATIONS

ADH	Antidiuretic hormone	**ICP**	Intracranial pressure
CHI	Closed-head injury	**ICU**	Intensive care unit
CPP	Cerebral perfusion pressure	**IV**	Intravenous
CSF	Cerebrospinal fluid	**IVC**	Intraventricular catheter
CSW	Cerebral salt wasting	**MRI**	Magnetic resonance imaging
CT	Computerized tomography	**MTBI**	Mild traumatic brain injury
DAI	Diffuse axonal injury	**Paco₂**	Partial pressure of oxygen in arterial blood
DDAVP	Desmopressin	**PbtO₂**	Local brain tissue oxygen content
DI	Diabetes insipidus	**SAH**	Subarachnoid hematoma
EDH	Epidural hematoma	**SDH**	Subdural hematoma
ICH	Intracerebral hematoma	**SIADH**	Syndrome of inappropriate antidiuretic hormone

SECTION ONE: Mechanisms of Injury and Skull Fractures

At the completion of this section, the learner will be able to list the three primary mechanisms of injury associated with closed-head injury and describe the four types of skull fractures that can occur with injury to the head.

Mechanism of Injury

Closed-head injury (CHI) is a diagnosis with a wide-ranging degree of severity. In its simplest form, CHI is represented by concussion. At the other end of the spectrum is severe CHI, which occurs with epidural hematoma and diffuse axonal injury, both of which are associated with a high mortality. Understanding the mechanism of injury associated with closed-head injury is essential to assessment and management of patients with these injuries. There are three primary mechanisms of injury associated with CHI: acceleration/deceleration, rotational, and penetrating.

The most common mechanism of CHI is the result of acceleration and deceleration forces. *Acceleration injury* occurs when the stationary brain is suddenly and rapidly moved in one direction along a linear path (Fig. 20–1). This type of injury is seen in victims of assault who have been hit in the head with a fist or bat. The sudden acceleration causes brain injury at the site of impact. *Deceleration injury* occurs when the brain stops rapidly in the cranial vault. As the skull ceases movement, the brain continues to move until it hits the skull. The force of deceleration causes injury at the site of impact with the skull. An example of this is the victim of a fall. The rapid deceleration of the person's head hitting the ground results in a deceleration injury of the brain as it hits the bony wall of the cranium. Acceleration and deceleration injuries can occur together, as can be seen in a coup–contrecoup injury. Coup injury affects the cerebral tissue directly under the point of impact. Contrecoup injury occurs in a line directly opposite the point of impact.

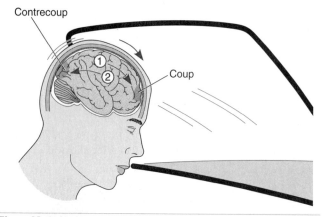

Contrecoup

Coup

Figure 20–1 ■ Coup–contrecoup head injury. 1) Following the initial (acceleration) injury (coup), 2) the brain rebounds within the skull and sustains additional (deceleration) injury (contrecoup) in the opposite part of the brain.

Rotational injury occurs when the force impacting the head transfers energy to the brain in a nonlinear fashion resulting in shearing forces being exerted throughout the brain. An example of this type of mechanism is in boxing. When a boxer is punched in the side of the head the force causes rapid rotational movement of the head and its contents, which causes tearing of the axons in the brain.

Penetrating injury occurs when a foreign object invades the brain. The penetrating object may be a bullet, knife, or a falling object. The penetrating object may pass completely through the brain and exit on the opposite side or it may bounce around the cranium causing multiple areas of injury. As well as the obvious injury, some projectiles, such as bullets, may cause additional injury from shock waves transmitted throughout the brain.

Skull Fractures

There are four types of skull fractures that can occur with injury to the head: linear, depressed, open, and basilar skull fractures. All types indicate substantial force has been absorbed by the skull and underlying brain tissue injury may be present.

Linear skull fractures are associated with minor traumatic injury. They are not typically obvious to the naked eye and are usually discovered during a head computerized tomography (CT) scan. Linear skull fractures are not life threatening and are allowed to heal over time without surgical intervention.

As the force of impact increases, depressed skull fractures may occur. Depressed skull fractures may be visible and palpable. The fracture itself may tear the underlying meninges of the brain and extend into brain tissue. Clearly, with such force to cause the skull to lose its shape, the probability of substantial cerebral injury is high. Medical interventions include surgical repair of the fracture and meninges and the evacuation of any hematomas beneath the fracture. Nursing interventions focus on frequent neurological assessments and pain management. The nurse must be cautious when administering pain medications to patients with head injuries. The presence of narcotics may obscure the neurological exam and make it difficult during an assessment to differentiate changes in mental status as a result of the actual injury from changes caused by the narcotic.

Open skull fractures are depressed skull fractures accompanied by a scalp laceration. These fractures are of particular concern because of the risk of infection associated with exposure of the dura to a contaminated environment. Medical interventions include surgical repair and debridement of the contaminated wound. Nursing care is focused on neurological assessment, pain management, and administration of antibiotics to prevent infection.

Basilar skull fractures, another common sequelae of high-impact head injury, are fractures of one of the bones that make up the base of the skull. Assessment findings associated with a basilar skull fracture may include the presence of periorbital ecchymosis ("raccoon eyes"), mastoid ecchymosis ("Battle's sign"), otorrhea, rhinorrhea, or facial nerve paralysis. Careful physical assessment of drainage from the nares and ear canals must be performed to detect the presence of cerebral spinal fluid (CSF) drainage. CSF drainage indicates the meninges are torn. CSF may leak through the nose (**rhinorrhea**) or through the ear (**otorrhea**). Any drainage from the ear or nose should be tested for the presence of glucose with a glucose reagent strip. Clear drainage that tests positive for glucose indicates the fluid is CSF.

Medical management of this condition includes allowing the CSF to drain and the dura to close on its own. If the injury does not heal itself within the first 1 to 2 weeks postinjury, surgical repair may be necessary. Nursing priorities include neurological assessment, pain management, and monitoring the patient for signs and symptoms of infection associated with the disrupted meningeal layer. All dressings should be changed with aseptic technique in an effort to reduce the possibility of an infection. Sterile cotton gauzes are placed in the ear or under the nose. Dressings are changed when wet because moisture facilitates the movement of microorganisms and predisposes the patient to infection.

In summary, closed-head injury is a diagnosis with a wide-ranging degree of severity. The three primary mechanisms of injury associated with CHI include acceleration/deceleration, rotational, and penetrating. Understanding the mechanism of injury is essential to assessment and management of patients with these injuries. There are four types of skull fractures that can occur with injury to the head: linear, depressed, open, and basilar skull fractures. All types indicate substantial force has been absorbed by the skull and underlying brain tissue may be present.

SECTION ONE REVIEW

1. Acceleration/deceleration injuries are the result of impact following
   A. rotational movement of the brain in the skull
   B. penetrating trauma
   C. linear movement of the brain in the skull
   D. none of the above
2. Which of the following mechanisms of injury commonly results in the tearing of axons in the brain?
   A. rotational injury
   B. acceleration injury
   C. deceleration injury
   D. penetrating injury

3. The administration of narcotics to a patient with a closed-head injury
   A. will make the pain worse
   B. may mask neurological changes in the patient
   C. allows the injury to heal quicker
   D. is a priority nursing intervention
4. Raccoon eyes are an assessment finding typically associated with what type of skull fracture?
   A. linear fractures
   B. depressed fractures
   C. open fractures
   D. basilar fractures

Answers: 1. C, 2. A, 3. B, 4. D

SECTION TWO: Focal and Diffuse Head Injuries

At the completion of this section, the learner will be able to differentiate between focal and diffuse injuries and identify medical and nursing interventions for the treatment of focal and diffuse brain injuries.

Closed-head injury takes on two distinct forms: focal or diffuse. **Focal injuries** occur in a well-defined area of the brain and may be the result of hematomas. **Diffuse injuries** occur in several areas of the brain and may occur with concussion and diffuse axonal injury.

Focal Head Injuries: Cerebral Hematomas

Cerebral hematomas represent a group of focal cerebral injuries associated with the accumulation of blood in the cranial vault. Hematomas occur as the result of injury to a cerebral vein or artery. There are several types of cerebral hematomas; each are named according to its location within the layers of the meninges: epidural hematoma, subdural hematoma, subarachnoid hematoma, and intracerebral hematoma (Fig. 20–2). With high-impact injury, two or more different types of cerebral hematomas may occur.

An **epidural hematoma** (**EDH**) occurs in the space between the dura mater and the skull (Fig. 20–2). High impact to the temporal areas of the brain can induce an EDH. When the force of the impact is transferred to the brain, small arteries are sheared. This results in an accumulation of blood between the skull and the dura mater. People with these injuries may have a brief loss of consciousness immediately following the injury, followed by an episode of being alert and oriented, and then a loss of consciousness again. This scenario is the classical presentation of EDH, but it is important to remember that not all patients with EDH will present with these symptoms. A fixed and dilated pupil on the same side as the impact area may be

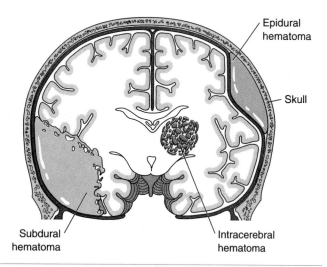

Figure 20–2 ■ Three types of hematomas: epidural hematoma, subdural hematoma, and intracerebral hematoma.

present. Because an artery is most often the source of the hematoma, the rapid accumulation of blood makes it essential to identify and treat these injuries quickly before intracranial pressure (ICP) reaches a critical point.

Medical management of the EDH involves surgical evacuation of the hematoma with possible placement of an ICP monitor. These patients may be admitted to the ICU for frequent neurological checks and ICP monitoring. Nursing care associated with EDH focuses on diligent neurological assessment. The nurse must look for sudden changes in level of consciousness and for the presence of a fixed and dilated pupil on the side of injury. These findings suggest bleeding has recurred and represents an emergent medical situation.

Subdural hematoma (SDH) is the accumulation of blood between the dura and the arachnoid layers of the meninges (Fig. 20–2). In contrast to EDH, SDH usually develops secondary to venous injury. This results in a slower onset of symptoms. SDH is categorized by the time between when the injury took place and the development of neurological changes. The three categories of SDH are acute (less than 48 hours from injury), subacute (48 hours to 2 weeks), and chronic (greater than 2 weeks from injury) (Davis, 2000). Assessment findings are determined by the rate of blood accumulation in the subdural space. Manifestations of acute SDH include drowsiness, headache, confusion, slowed thinking, or agitation. Because the expansion of the hematoma is over a longer period of time with subacute SDH, neurological deterioration may not occur for days or weeks. Clinical manifestations of chronic SDH are vague and often attributed to other conditions. The patient may complain of headache, lethargy, absent-mindedness, and vomiting. Other more serious symptoms may be present, including seizures, stiff neck, pupil changes, or hemiparesis.

Medical management of SDH involves surgical evacuation of the hematoma and possible placement of a subdural drain, which may remain in place for a few days postoperatively. As with EDH, nursing priorities for SDH include monitoring level of consciousness and performing regular and frequent focused neurological assessments.

Subarachnoid hematoma (SAH) is the accumulation of blood between the arachnoid layer of the meninges and the brain. Additional accumulation of blood results in blood leaking into the CSF. Patients with this type of hematoma may manifest nuchal rigidity (neck stiffness) (Roth & Farls, 2000).

Medical management of SAH includes placement of an intraventricular catheter (IVC) to permit drainage of bloody CSF and to monitor ICP. Priority nursing care includes monitoring neurological status and ICP, paying particular attention to the quantity and color of the CSF drainage from the IVC.

Intracerebral hematoma (ICH) is the accumulation of blood in the parenchyma of brain tissue (Fig. 20–2). ICHs result from uncontrolled hypertension, ruptured aneurysm, or trauma with a high-impact blow to the head. Manifestations vary according to the location of the hematoma and may include headache along with decreasing level of consciousness, dilation of one pupil, and hemiplegia. Surgical evacuation of the ICH is usually not possible because the hematoma is deep within brain tissue. Medical management includes management of ICP and cerebral perfusion pressure (CPP) (refer to Module 18).

Diffuse Head Injuries

Concussion, classified as mild traumatic brain injury (MTBI), is caused by blunt trauma to the head. Signs of MTBI include a transient period of unconsciousness (lasting up to 20 minutes) and a Glasgow Coma Scale score of 13 to 15, and signs of neurological deficits (e.g., unilateral weakness, pupillary abnormalities) are usually absent (Cushman et al., 2001). Although the term *MTBI* implies a relatively benign injury, the injury can have devastating effects including the inability to function at preinjury levels.

On presentation to the emergency department the patient may report having amnesia about the event that caused the injury. The patient may report headache, dizziness, vertigo, nausea, vomiting, slurred speech, or confusion. Patients who report any of these symptoms will require a CT scan of the head for further evaluation.

Nursing care for the patient with MTBI in the acute care phase includes diligent and frequent neurological assessments and pain management. Discharge planning must begin early because some patients require rehabilitation services. Almost half of patients with MTBI will develop postconcussive syndromes that include symptoms similar to those on presentation to the emergency department. These symptoms may continue for 3 months or more after injury (Cushman et al., 2001).

Diffuse axonal injury (DAI) occurs when shearing forces disrupt the structure of neurons and their nearby blood vessels, often as a result of rotational forces on the brain. DAI is typically associated with high-speed acceleration/deceleration injury that occurs with motor vehicle crashes. DAI is associated with widespread shearing of axons in the white matter. DAI can range from mild to severe. Patients with DAI are usually in a coma. Mild DAI can result in a comatose state lasting hours to days. In more severe DAI the prognosis is poor: death or a persistent vegetative state.

Although they are difficult to assess on a CT scan, the presence of multiple small hemorrhages is strongly suggestive of DAI. The use of magnetic resonance imaging (MRI) may provide a more conclusive diagnosis. The outcome of the patient with DAI is unpredictable. Patients may have minimal neurological damage or may remain in a permanent vegetative state (Marik et al., 2002). Medical and nursing interventions to lower ICP, increase CPP, and stabilize vital signs all contribute to an improved outcome.

In summary, closed-head injury takes on two distinct forms: focal or diffuse. Focal injuries occur in well-defined areas of the brain and diffuse injuries occur in several areas of the brain. Cerebral hematomas, a group of focal cerebral injuries, include EDH, SDH, SAH, and ICH. Patients with EDH may require surgical evacuation of the hematoma and possible placement of an ICP monitor. Patients with SDH may require surgical evacuation of the hematoma and placement of a subdural drain. Patients with SAH may require placement of a IVC to drain CSF and to monitor ICP. Surgical evacuation of ICH is usually not possible. Medical management includes management of ICP and CPP. Priority nursing care for patients with cerebral hematomas focuses on diligent neurological assessments and monitoring for signs of increasing ICP.

Diffuse head injury includes MTBI and DAI. MTBI, although a relatively minor injury, is associated with long-term symptoms. DAI results in a coma that can last hours to years. The patient's recovery from this injury is unpredictable.

SECTION TWO REVIEW

1. A brief loss of consciousness followed by a period of being alert and oriented, and then a loss of consciousness again, is a typical presentation for which of the following?
   A. SDH
   B. EDH
   C. ICH
   D. SAH
2. Accumulation of blood within the parenchyma of brain tissue is called a(n)
   A. ICH
   B. SAH
   C. EDH
   D. SDH

3. Management of ICH may include all of the following EXCEPT
   A. placement of an IVC
   B. frequent neurological assessments
   C. emergent surgical evacuation
   D. maximizing CPP
4. Presence of dizziness, headache, and confusion for long periods of time after concussion is
   A. always expected
   B. known as postconcussive syndrome
   C. caused by taking too much pain medication
   D. the result of something other than the concussion

Answers: 1. B, 2. A, 3. C, 4. B

SECTION THREE: Secondary Injury

At the completion of this section, the learner will be able to explain the pathophysiology of secondary brain injury and recognize current medical and nursing interventions for the prevention of secondary brain injury.

Primary injury occurs when neurons sustain direct injury from the offending event. For example, a person involved in a motor vehicle crash hits her or his head on the dashboard resulting in DAI. The primary injury in this case is the shearing of the axons. **Secondary injury** occurs in response to primary injury. There are four causes of secondary injury: ischemia, neuronal death, cerebral swelling, and inflammation (Littlejohns et al., 2003). Medical and nursing interventions are directed at preventing these causes of secondary injury in order to maximize positive patient outcomes.

Many of the traditional methods to prevent secondary injury target the reduction of ICP and the improvement of CPP, thus minimizing ischemic injury to the brain. The Brain Trauma Foundation guidelines (2003) recommend maintaining a CPP greater than 60 mm Hg to reduce secondary injury. Medical interventions, such as osmotic diuretics, hypertonic saline, hypothermia, and, at times, hyperventilation, are used alone or in combination to help achieve this recommended CPP. Ongoing research on the assessment and management of secondary brain injuries includes new methods for measuring cerebral perfusion, new drugs that reduce cerebral swelling and ischemia, drugs that limit the release of inflammatory mediators and cell death, and surgical interventions to treat intractable intracerebral hypertension.

The advent of cerebral tissue oxygen monitoring is reshaping current thoughts on management of brain injury. Clinicians now have the ability to measure local brain tissue oxygen content (PbtO$_2$). The measurement of this new parameter is achieved using a fiber optic monitoring device, which is inserted into the white matter of the brain (Littlejohns et al., 2003). PbtO$_2$ levels less than 15 mm Hg have been associated with poor outcomes including death (Littlejohns et al., 2003). Therefore, current practice indicates maintaining PbtO$_2$ levels greater than 20 mm Hg (Littlejohns et al., 2003).

Hypertonic saline has been shown to prevent secondary injury. Hypertonic saline has several effects on injured brain tissue. This medication causes reduction of cerebral edema by creating an osmotic gradient that promotes passage of intracellular fluid from swollen neuronal cells into the vasculature. Hypertonic saline also possesses hemodynamic, vasoregulatory, and anti-inflammatory properties that help reduce secondary injury (Doyle et al., 2001). Nurses caring for patients receiving hypertonic saline must pay careful attention to the patient's serum sodium levels and serum osmolarity because extreme elevations in these values may result in neurological injury and renal failure.

Medical intervention for the treatment of ICP refractory to all other medical interventions may include the use of high-dose barbiturates. This intervention induces a comatose state and significantly decreases cerebral oxygen requirements. Surgical intervention for the treatment of ICP refractory to conventional medical interventions may include decompressive craniotomy (Jaeger et al., 2003). Decompressive craniotomy is a surgical procedure where a portion of skull is removed to allow more space for the injured brain to expand during the acute phase of injury (Fig. 20–3). By opening the cranial vault, ICP is reduced and ischemia prevented. Not all patients are candidates for this form of aggressive treatment.

Nursing interventions to reduce secondary injury focus on preventing complications associated with CHI and minimizing ICP. Astute nursing assessments are required, especially during routine care, such as bathing and suctioning, to evaluate the patient's response to interventions. Although relatively benign in nature, simply touching the patient to wash his or her face can be enough stimulation to elevate ICP and compromise cerebral blood flow and oxygenation. In order to avoid unnecessary elevations of ICP, nursing activities are spaced apart to allow recovery time for the patient (Yanko & Mitcho, 2001). The patient's neck is kept in proper alignment (no flexion or rotation) and hip flexion is kept at less than 90 degrees to allow for proper venous return and prevention of elevated ICP (Yanko & Mitcho, 2001). Elevating the head of the bed to 30 degrees reduces ICP without compromising CPP and may decrease the risk of pneumonia (Marik et al., 2002). Because hyperthermia increases cerebral metabolic rate and increases cerebral oxygen requirements, antipyretics or cooling measures are used to reduce body temperature. Finally, when suctioning patients, the nurse preoxygenates the patient and limits passage time of the suction catheter to 10 seconds or less (LeJeune & Howard-Fain, 2002).

There are a number of interventions that prevent ischemia of neuronal tissue. Although not all have been scientifically proven to provide long-term benefits, the importance of monitoring the patient and providing the best possible medical and nursing care improves outcomes in this population.

In summary, secondary injury occurs in response to primary injury. Causes of secondary injury include ischemia, neuronal death, cerebral swelling, and inflammation. Medical and nursing interventions are directed at preventing these causes of secondary injury. Reducing ICP and improving CPP minimize ischemic injury. Local brain tissue oxygen content can be monitored with a fiber optic monitoring device. Hypertonic saline may prevent cerebral swelling. Decompressive craniotomy may be required for the treatment of ICP refractory to conventional medical therapy.

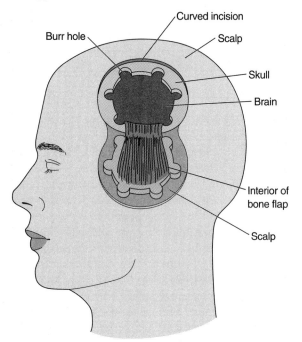

Figure 20–3 ■ In a craniotomy, a portion of the skull and overlying scalp is removed to allow access to the brain.

Curved incision
Burr hole
Scalp
Skull
Brain
Interior of bone flap
Scalp

Evidence-Based Practice

■ *Patients in the acute care phase after a head injury who are heavily sedated when receiving endotracheal suctioning have fewer detrimental effects on ICP, CPP, and cerebral oxygenation than patients with a head injury who are not heavily sedated and cough and move during the suctioning procedure (Gemma et al., 2002).*

■ *Elevation of the head of the bed 30 degrees in patients with severe closed-head injury leads to consistent reduction of ICP and improvement in CPP (Ng et al., 2004).*

■ *A concentrated effort by nursing staff to reduce environmental stimuli at preset discrete intervals ("quiet time protocol") increases the likelihood of sleep for patients in the neurocritical care unit (Olsen et al., 2001).*

■ *During the acute care phase, family members of patients with severe traumatic brain injury need to know information, need consistent information, need involvement, and need to make sense of the experience (Bond et al., 2003).*

SECTION THREE REVIEW

1. A nursing intervention to reduce secondary injury is
   A. maintaining CPP less than 60 mm Hg
   B. spacing out patient care activities
   C. vigorous suctioning of the patient
   D. keeping the patient flat at all times
2. Secondary injury is caused by
   A. hypoxia and ischemia
   B. cerebral swelling
   C. inflammation of cerebral tissue
   D. all of the above
3. Decompressive craniotomy
   A. is appropriate for all patients with secondary injury
   B. is used to treat intractable ICP elevation in some patients

C. will reduce CPP
D. will increase ICP
4. Hypertonic saline has all of the following properties EXCEPT that it
   A. decreases ICP
   B. increases CPP
   C. increases cellular swelling
   D. decreases cellular inflammation

Answers: 1. B, 2. D, 3. B, 4. C

SECTION FOUR: Complications Associated with Closed-Head Injury

At the completion of this section, the learner will be able to identify four complications associated with CHI, discuss medical and nursing interventions for the treatment of complications associated with CHI, and define the criteria used to diagnose brain death.

A significant number of complications occur as a result of closed-head injury. Four complications that commonly occur in high-acuity patients with CHI include diabetes insipidus, syndrome of inappropriate antidiuretic hormone, cerebral salt wasting, and herniation.

Diabetes Insipidus

Diabetes insipidus (DI) is a condition associated with improper water balance. Water balance is maintained in the body in part because of the secretion of antidiuretic hormone (ADH) by the posterior pituitary gland. Normally ADH is secreted to prevent diuresis and loss of urine in times of physiologic stress (such as hypotension). However, CHI may result in pressure on the pituitary gland and loss of ADH secretion. Loss of ADH secretion results in diuresis. Any patient with CHI and increased ICP is at risk of developing DI. The earliest signs of DI include large amounts of pale, clear "waterlike" urine and hypotension. The classic diagnostic profile of DI includes the production of large amounts (greater than 200 mL/hr) of dilute (specific gravity less than 1.005) urine with an associated increase in serum sodium (greater than 145mEq/L). Treatment of DI involves aggressive replacement of intravascular volume with intravenous (IV) fluids and the administration of synthetic ADH. Administration of ADH may be either in the form of a vasopressin infusion or

desmopressin (DDAVP) either IV, subcutaneous, or intranasal (Holcomb, 2002). Indications of improvement are decreased urine output and increased specific gravity.

Syndrome of Inappropriate Antidiuresis Hormone

Syndrome of inappropriate antidiuretic hormone (SIADH) increases total body water because excess ADH secretion results in retention of water. The classic profile of SIADH includes the production of small amounts (less than 400 mL/day) of concentrated (specific gravity greater than 1.020) urine with an associated decrease in serum sodium (dilutional hyponatremia). The presence of this hypoosmolar state results in cellular swelling, systemically and intracerebrally (Yanko & Mitcho, 2001). Cerebral swelling increases ICP and leads to secondary injury. Treatment of SIADH involves restricting fluid intake to prevent further dilution of the serum (Palmer, 2000). Nursing interventions for the patient with SIADH include monitoring intake and output, neurologic status, and enforcement of fluid restriction.

Cerebral Salt Wasting

Cerebral salt wasting (CSW) is similar to SIADH because patients present with a low serum sodium and a low serum and urine osmolality. However, whereas SIADH represents a state of fluid overload, CSW is a state of hypovolemia. The mechanism of CSW is not well understood, but the end result is the loss of sodium into the urine causing water to follow. It is important to differentiate CSW from SIADH because restricting fluid in the CSW patient, who is already volume depleted, can lead to disastrous results. The patient with CSW is treated with salt

TABLE 20–1 DI, SIADH, and CSW: Complications of Closed-Head Injury

COMPLICATION	PATHOPHYSIOLOGY	URINE OUTPUT	SPECIFIC GRAVITY	SERUM SODIUM
DI	No ADH secretion leads to fluid volume deficit	Diuresis	Low	High
SIADH	Excess ADH secretion leads to fluid volume excess	Oliguria	High	Low
CSW	Mechanism unknown leads to fluid volume deficit	Diuresis	Low	Low

replacement via IV saline and oral salt tablets. CSW tends to correct itself over the course of 3 to 4 weeks (Palmer, 2000). Table 20–1 compares DI, SIADH, and CSW.

Herniation

Herniation is a catastrophic complication of CHI. As ICP increases and the space occupying the skull becomes filled with edematous brain tissue, the brain is forced to move from its normal position in the cranial vault to the space in the spinal column, which can accommodate its new size. The way in which the brain herniates depends on the type of injury. Two common types are cingulated and central herniation (Fig. 20–4). Cingulate herniation occurs when one hemisphere of the brain is forced across the falx cerebri (the portion of the dura separating the hemispheres) into the space occupied by the contralateral hemisphere. This usually occurs as a result of accumulation of blood on one side of the brain as seen with SDH. Central herniation occurs when cerebral swelling forces both hemispheres to be displaced downward across the tentorium (the separation between the cerebrum and the cerebellum and medulla). Herniation of either type is devastating as increased pressure is placed on the medulla where basic functions needed to sustain life are

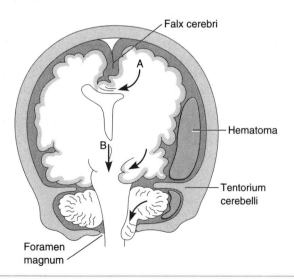

Figure 20–4 ■ Forms of brain herniation as a result of intracranial hypertension. *A.* Cingulate herniation occurs when the cingulate gyrus is compressed under the falx cerebri. *B.* Central herniation occurs when a centrally located lesion compresses central and midbrain structures.

located. The nurse should expect to see drastic neurological changes as well as alterations in vital signs. The classic vital sign changes seen are called *Cushing's triad.* This triad consists of bradycardia, severe hypertension with a widened pulse pressure, and irregular breathing. Signs of impending death include loss of the body's ability to maintain adequate blood pressure, profound bradycardia, and loss of basic neurological functioning (fixed and dilated pupils, absence of cough/gag reflex).

Brain Death

Brain death is an irreversible cessation of all brain function, including brainstem function. The evolution of CHI to brain death can be both long and, at times, unexpected. Some patients may arrive in the ICU for something as simple as frequent neurological exams following a concussion and then decline rapidly as a missed or new injury develops. Other patients may survive for weeks as health care providers battle increased ICP and associated injuries, only to succumb to total cerebral infarct. Brain death is suspected when there is no evidence of brainstem function for up to 24 hours in a patient with a normal temperature who is not under any influence of depressant drugs or alcohol.

The diagnosis of brain death is made using several different methods. Ultimately, the physician must be able to document coma, absence of brainstem reflexes, and apnea (Wijdicks, 2001). Spontaneous respiratory effort is absent and apnea is present. The apnea test is performed by taking the patient off the ventilator, allowing the $Paco_2$ to rise above 60 mm Hg. If the brainstem is functional, this high level of $Paco_2$ should stimulate respiration. Pupils are fixed and dilated. Ocular responses to head turning and cold caloric stimulation are absent (see Module 18). The electroencephalogram demonstrates absence of brain activity with flat (isoelectric) waves. An angiogram reveals no cerebral blood flow. Motor and reflex movements are absent. However, it is also not unusual for the body to continue to exhibit signs of movement even after brain death has been established. The movements represent spinal reflexes only, and their significance must be explained to family members. The nurse caring for the brain dead patient needs to be able to provide support to the family with emotional reassurance and to provide a spiritual advisor on request.

In summary, four complications that commonly occur in high-acuity patients with CHI include DI, SIADH, CSW, and herniation. DI is associated with the lack of ADH secretion which results in diuresis, fluid volume deficit, and a high serum sodium. Treaments include DDAVP and administration of IV fluids. SIADH is associated with excess ADH secretion which results in oliguria, fluid volume overload, and a low serum sodium. Treatment includes fluid restriction. Although the pathophysiologic mechanisms that cause CSW are not well understood, this condition results in fluid volume deficit, diuresis, and a low serum sodium. Treatment includes salt replacement with IV saline or oral salt tablets. Herniation, a catastrophic complication of CHI, is recognized by the presence of Cushing's triad. The evolution of brain death can be both long and, at times, unexpected. The diagnosis includes the following signs: coma, absence of brainstem reflexes, and apnea.

SECTION FOUR REVIEW

1. Treatment of DI includes
   A. massive fluid resuscitation
   B. fluid restriction
   C. administration of vasopressin
   D. A and C
2. SIADH is treated with
   A. fluid restriction
   B. fluid resuscitation
   C. salt restriction
   D. salt replacement
3. CSW is treated with
   A. fluid restriction
   B. adminstration of vasopressin
   C. salt restriction
   D. salt replacement
4. The single most important indicator of progression of brain injury is/are
   A. change in mental status exam
   B. changes in vital signs
   C. elevation of ICP
   D. reduced CPP

Answers: 1. A, 2. A, 3. D, 4. A

POSTTEST

All 10 module Posttest questions relate to Mr. A. You are the nurse caring for him. He is admitted to the emergency department following an assault with a baseball bat.

1. An MRI shows the presence of DAI. What is the most likely mechanism of injury for Mr. A?
   A. acceleration
   B. deceleration
   C. rotational
   D. penetrating
2. Mr. A's Glasgow Coma Scale decreases by 1 point, and he develops a fixed and dilated pupil. Which of the following interventions would you do FIRST?
   A. reassess the patient in 15 minutes
   B. call the physician immediately
   C. prepare the patient for a CT scan
   D. inform the family of these changes
3. You notice the presence of clear fluid draining from Mr. A's ears and nose. It is found to be CSF. With what type of skull fracture is CSF drainage most commonly associated?
   A. linear
   B. open skull fracture
   C. depressed skull fracture
   D. basilar skull fracture
4. Several hours after admission to the unit, you walk into Mr. A's room and find he is lethargic, confused, mumbling his speech, and very difficult to arouse. What may be the cause(s) of these changes in his level of consciousness?
   A. decreased ICP
   B. worsening brain injury
   C. Mr. A is simply tired
   D. A and B
5. Mr. A is rushed to a CT scan where it is revealed he has an expanding EDH. He is taken to the operating room to have it evacuated and returns to the ICU ventilated and with an IVC in place. What is the minimal CPP Mr. A should have?
   A. greater than 50 mm Hg
   B. greater than 60 mm Hg
   C. greater than 70 mm Hg
   D. greater than 80 mm Hg
6. Mr. A's ICP increases. Before calling the neurosurgeon you decide to try to decrease the ICP with nursing interventions. Which of the following would NOT decrease ICP?
   A. keep the patient supine with the head of bed flat
   B. preoxygenate Mr. A before suctioning
   C. realign Mr. A's neck
   D. elevate the head of the bed 30 degrees

7. The nursing interventions fail to decrease the ICP. The neurosurgeon is called. What orders might the nurse anticipate the neurosurgeon to give?
   A. prepare Mr. A for the operating room for emergent decompressive craniotomy
   B. hypertonic saline IV bolus
   C. hypotonic saline IV bolus
   D. DDAVP

8. Mr. A continues to have elevated ICP and now is putting out nearly a liter an hour of pale urine. Mr. A is diagnosed with DI. What is the pathophysiological cause of DI?
   A. too much ADH
   B. loss of sodium
   C. retention of sodium
   D. not enough ADH

9. Mr. A has an abrupt hypertension, bradycardia, and an irregular breathing pattern. These signs are indicative of
   A. pain
   B. anxiety
   C. impending herniation
   D. cardiac arrest

10. Which of the following is NOT a criteria for brain death?
   A. spontaneous breathing
   B. apnea
   C. presence of coma
   D. loss of brainstem reflexes

POSTTEST ANSWERS

Question	Answer	Section
1	C	One
2	B	Two
3	D	One
4	B	One
5	B	Three

Question	Answer	Section
6	A	Three
7	B	Three
8	D	Four
9	C	Four
10	A	Four

REFERENCES

Bond, A. E., Draiger, C. R., Mandleco, B., et al. (2003). Needs of family members of patients with severe traumatic brain injury: Implications for evidenced based practice. *Critical Care Nurse, 23*, 63–72.

Brain Trauma Foundation. (2003). Update notice. Guidelines for the management of severe traumatic brain injury: Cerebral perfusion pressure. Available at: *http://www2.braintrauma.org/guidelines/*. Accessed September 3, 2003.

Cushman, J. G., Agarwal, N., Fabian, T. C., et al. (2001). Practice management guidelines for the management of mild traumatic brain injury: The EAST practice management guidelines work group. *Journal of Trauma Injury Infection and Personal Care, 51*, 1016–1026.

Davis, A. E. (2000). Mechanisms of traumatic brain injury: Biomechanical, structural, and cellular considerations. *Critical Care Nurse Quarterly, 23*(3), 1–13.

Doyle, J. A., Davis, D. P., & Hoyt, D. B. (2001). The use of hypertonic saline in the treatment of traumatic brain injury. *Journal of Trauma Injury Infection and Personal Care, 50*, 367–383.

Gemma, M., Tommasino, C., & Cerri, M., et al. (2002). Intracranial effects of endotracheal suctioning in the acute phase of head injury. *Journal of Neurosurgical Anesthesiology, 14*, 50–54.

Holcomb, S. S. (2002). Diabetes insipidus. *Dimensions of Critical Care Nursing, 21*, 94–97.

Jaeger, M., Soehle, M., & Meixensberger, J. (2003). Effects of decompressive craniectomy on brain tissue oxygen in patients with intracranial hypertension. *Journal of Neurology, Neurosurgery, and Psychiatry, 74*, 513–515.

LeJeune, G. M., & Howard-Fain, T. (2002). Nursing assessment and management of patients with head injuries. *Dimensions of Critical Care Nursing, 21*, 226–227.

Littlejohns, L. R., Bader, M. K., & March, K. (2003). Brain tissue oxygen monitoring in severe brain injury, I. *Critical Care Nurse, 23*, 17–25.

Marik, P. E., Varon, J., & Trask, T. (2002). Management of head trauma. *Chest, 122*, 699–711.

Ng, I., Lim, J., & Wong, W. B. (2004). Effects of head posture on cerebral hemodynamics: Its influence on intracranial pressure, cerebral perfusion pressure, and cerebral oxygenation. *Journal of Neurosurgery, 54*, 593–597.

Olsen, D. M., Borel, C. O., Laskowitz, D. T., et al. (2001). Quiet time: A nursing intervention to promote sleep in the neurocritical care unit. *American Journal of Critical Care, 10*, 74–78.

Palmer, B. F. (2000). Hyponatremia in a neurosurgical patient: Syndrome of inappropriate antidiuretic hormone secretion versus cerebral salt wasting. *Nephrology Dialysis Transplantation, 15*, 262–268.

Roth, P., & Farls, K. (2000). Pathophysiology of traumatic brain injury. *Critical Care Nurse Quarterly, 23*(3), 14–25.

Wijdicks, E. F. (2001). Current concepts: The diagnosis of brain death. *New England Journal of Medicine, 344*, 1215–1221.

Yanko, J. R., & Mitcho, K. (2001). Acute care management of severe traumatic brain injuries. *Critical Care Nurse Quarterly, 23*(4), 1–23.

Sensory Perceptual Disorders

MODULE

21

Karen L. Johnson, Kathy Hausman

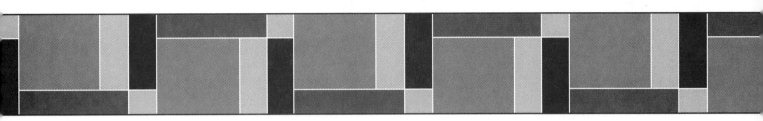

OBJECTIVES Following completion of this module, the learner will be able to

1. Explain anatomic features of the spinal cord and vertebrae.
   - Define unstable spinal cord injury.
   - Compare and contrast the functions of the gray matter and white matter of the spinal cord.
2. Differentiate complete versus incomplete spinal cord injury.
   - Define paraplegia, quadraplegia, and tetraplegia.
   - Discuss the results of damage to upper and lower motor neurons.
   - Explain the mechanisms of injury for primary injury and the pathophysiology of secondary spinal cord injury.
3. Describe diagnostic tests frequently used to identify the type and severity of spinal cord injury.
   - Discuss physical assessment techniques for assessing motor, sensory, and reflex activity in patients with SCI.
   - Differentiate spinal shock from neurogenic shock.
4. Discuss surgical and manual stabilization techniques used for spinal cord injuries.
   - State the indications for and controversies with the use of methylprednisolone after spinal cord injury.
5. Identify priority nursing assessments and interventions for the patient with a spinal cord injury in the acute care phase of recovery.
   - Discuss priority nursing assessments and interventions to identify and prevent complications after spinal cord injury in the acute care phase of recovery.
   - Define seizure and epilepsy.
6. State the manifestations of simple partial seizure, complex partial seizure, absence generalized seizure, and tonic-clonic generalized seizure.
   - Discuss the nursing and pharmacologic management of seizure disorders.

This self-study module was developed as a teaching guide for nurses caring for patients with sensory perceptual disorders. Disorders selected for this module include spinal cord injury and seizure disorders. Successful completion of this module will help the reader prepare to care for patients with these disorders in a high-acuity environment.

The module is composed of six sections. Section One reviews the spinal cord anatomy and physiology. Section Two discusses the mechanisms of injury to the spinal cord and the sequelae of those injuries on sensory and motor function. Section Three explains the diagnostic procedures used in the evaluation of spinal cord injury and the key nursing assessments that must be made for patients with spinal cord injuries. Section Four introduces the reader to the surgical and manual stabiliza-

tion techniques used in spinal cord injuries and the nursing implications of these therapeutic modalities, and Section Five identifies the important nursing interventions and assessments for care of the patient with a spinal cord injury in the acute care phase. Section Six reviews seizure disorders, key assessments, and pharmacologic and nursing management of patients with these disorders.

Each section includes a set of review questions to help the learner evaluate his or her understanding of the section's content before moving on to the next section. All Section Reviews and the module Pretest and Posttest include answers. It is suggested that the learner review those concepts answered incorrectly in the review questions before proceeding to the next section.

PRETEST

1. MW has a stable C5 spinal cord injury. Which of the following statements is true about this injury?
   A. the vertebrae are unable to support the injured area
   B. the vertebral and ligamentous structures are able to support and protect the injured area
   C. two of the columns are damaged
   D. ligamentous structures are unable to support the injured area

2. In order to bear weight, vertebral bodies
   A. increase in size as they descend
   B. decrease in size as they descend
   C. consist of a body and an arch
   D. are fused to one another

3. Which region of the spinal cord is most susceptible to injury?
   A. cervical   C. lumbar
   B. thoracic   D. sacral

4. Diving accidents typically result in damage to which region of the spinal cord?
   A. cervical
   B. thoracic
   C. lumbar
   D. sacral

5. Secondary injury to the spinal cord occurs from
   A. improper movement of the patient
   B. the forces producing a closed-head injury
   C. biochemical processes that destroy neurons
   D. small hemorrhages in spinal gray matter

6. The presence of perineal reflexes indicate
   A. priapism
   B. intact bulbocavernosus reflex
   C. upper motor neuron injury
   D. bowel and bladder training may be feasible

7. Swimmer's position x-ray may be used to diagnose
   A. a spinal cord tumor
   B. C7-T1 injuries
   C. C1-C2 injuries
   D. vascular disruptions to the cord

8. Sensation that begins at or above the nipple line is associated with what dermatomes?
   A. C5   C. T4
   B. C7   D. L1

9. Gardner-Wells tongs are inserted to stabilize a cervical spine. This device requires all of the following EXCEPT
   A. screws implanted in the skull
   B. weights
   C. part of the head to be shaved
   D. bone grafting

10. Timely spinal alignment and stability
    A. maximizes cord recovery
    B. minimizes additional damage
    C. prevents late deformity
    D. all of the above

11. Which of the following statements would you use to prepare a patient with a SCI for placement of Gardner-Wells tongs?
    A. "A wrench will be placed on your chest."
    B. "Two screws will be implanted in your skull."
    C. "You will feel pain but not pressure."
    D. "Four pins will be inserted into your skull."

12. The rehabilitation potential of a person with an L1–L5 injury is
    A. independent eating; independent bathing; independent mobility with the use of knee, ankle, and foot orthoses
    B. independent eating, independent bathing, electric wheelchair
    C. independent eating, minor assistance with bathing, manual wheelchair
    D. independent eating, independent bathing, manual wheelchair

13. Autonomic dysreflexia is a health emergency because
    A. airway spasm occurs
    B. severe vasoconstriction occurs
    C. spasticity produces joint immobility
    D. hypoxia results from regurgitation

14. Suctioning may produce which of the following in the SCI patient?
    A. airway spasm
    B. bradycardia
    C. hypertension
    D. vomiting

15. TB is a 32-year-old man with a closed-head injury. His Glasgow Coma Scale is 15. Suddenly, he becomes unresponsive, his eyes are open, and he has a blank stare on his face. He has no motor movement. You suspect he has had what type of seizure?
    A. ictal seizure
    B. complex partial seizure
    C. absence seizure
    D. status epilepticus

16. While a patient is receiving anticonvulsant therapy, it is important to assess
    A. cardiac rhythm
    B. pulse oximetry
    C. serum drug levels
    D. serum potassium

17. A complication that may occur during a seizure is
    A. aspiration
    B. apnea
    C. head injury
    D. all of the above

Pretest Answers:

1. B, 2. A, 3. A, 4. A, 5. C, 6. D, 7. B, 8. C, 9. D, 10. D, 11. B, 12. A, 13. B, 14. B, 15. C, 16. C, 17. D

GLOSSARY

absence seizure   Characterized by a blank stare, loss of consciousness, and a sudden onset of no motor movement.

autonomic dysreflexia   Potentially life-threatening complication following spinal cord injury caused by excessive sympathetic nervous system stimulation that produces extreme vasoconstriction and hypertension.

complete spinal cord injury   Traumatic disruption that completely transects the spinal cord resulting in loss of sensation and motor transmission to areas below the region of injury.

dermatome   A cutaneous section of the body innervated by a spinal or cranial nerve.

dysesthetic pain   Central pain arising from the spinal cord; referred to as "phantom pain."

epilepsy   Term used to denote a condition of reoccurring seizures. Also called seizure disorder.

flaccid paralysis   Damage to lower motor neurons producing loss of both voluntary and involuntary movement.

generalized seizure   Type of seizure where there is loss of consciousness; involves deep brain structures of both hemispheres.

Incomplete spinal cord injury   Traumatic disruption of part of the spinal cord with some motor or sensory transmission below the level of injury.

neurogenic shock   Condition that occurs with an injury above T6; manifested by hypotension, bradycardia, decreased cardiac output, and inability to sweat below the level of the injury.

paraplegia   Injury to the thoracolumbar region of the spine causing loss of motor function in the lower extremities.

partial seizure   Involves the activation of only a restricted part of one hemisphere of the brain; no loss of consciousness.

poikilothermia   Loss of internal temperature control whereby the patient assumes the temperature of the environment.

postictal period   Phase following a tonic-clonic seizure; patient remains unconscious but is relaxed and breathing quietly.

priapism   Persistent penile erection produced by reflex activity.

primary injury   Neurologic damage that occurs at the moment of impact.

proprioception   The ability to determine spatial position; knowing where the body or a body part is positioned in space.

quadriplegia   Injury to cervical or thoracic regions of the spinal cord that may result in impaired function of the arms, trunk, legs, and pelvic organs; also known as tetraplegia.

secondary injury   Complex biochemical processes that occur within minutes of injury and can last for days to weeks.

seizure   An excessive, uncontrolled discharge of electrical activity from the brain.

somatosensory-evoked potentials (SEPs)   Stimulation of pain and touch to peripheral nerves to determine whether a response is elicited by the cerebral cortex.

spastic paralysis   Damage to upper motor neurons resulting in the inability to carry out a skilled movement.

spinal shock   A condition that occurs within 60 minutes after spinal cord injury. Manifested by hypotension, bradycardia, flaccid paralysis, absence of muscle contractions, and bowel and bladder dysfunction.

status epilepticus   A neurological emergency, defined as a continuing series of seizures without recovery or regaining consciousness between attacks.

tetraplegia   Injury to cervical or thoracic regions of the spinal cord that may result in impaired function of the arms, trunk, legs, and pelvic organs; also known as quadriplegia.

tonic-clonic seizure   A type of generalized seizure characterized by a tonic phase, which is a loss of consciousness, apnea, and sharp rhythmic contractions of the extremities, followed by the clonic phase, which is characterized by hyperventilation and alternating contraction and relaxation of muscles.

unstable spinal injury   An injury to two or more of the spinal columns; vertebral and ligamentous structures are unable to support and protect the injured area.

ABBREVIATIONS

C	Cervical vertebrae (C1–C7)	SCI	Spinal cord injury
CT	Computed tomography	SEPs	Somatosensory-evoked potentials
L	Lumbar vertebrae (L1–L5)	T	Thoracic vertebrae (T1–T12)
MRI	Magnetic resonance imaging		

SECTION ONE: Spinal Cord Anatomy and Physiology

At the completion of this section, the learner will be able to explain anatomic features of the spinal cord and vertebrae, define unstable spinal cord injury, and compare and contrast the functions of the gray matter and white matter of the spinal cord.

Spinal Cord Anatomy

The spine is composed of 33 individual and fused vertebrae. There are 7 cervical (C), 12 thoracic (T), and 5 lumbar (L) vertebrae. The sacral and coccygeal vertebrae are fused in the adult. Each vertebrae consists of a body (anterior) and an arch (posterior) (Fig 21–1). The arch section is composed of two pedicles that attach the arch to the body and two laminae that form the roof of the arch. The spinous process is located at the rear of the vertebrae. In order to bear additional weight, vertebral bodies increase in size as they descend.

The spine is conceptualized as having three columns: an anterior column that includes the anterior part of the vertebral body, a middle column that houses the posterior wall of the vertebral body, and a posterior column that includes the vertebral arch (Fig. 21–1). If two or more of these columns are damaged, the injury is considered to be unstable. **Unstable spinal injury** exists when the vertebral and ligamentous structures are unable to support and protect the injured area.

The spinal cord runs through the center of the vertebral column through the spinal canal (Fig. 21–1). It starts at the foramen magnum of the brain and ends at the first or second lumbar vertebra (Fig. 21–2). In the cervical region, the cord receives afferent impulses from the upper and lower extremities. The end of the cord contains reflex centers for bowel, bladder, and sexual function. The C1–C7 spinal nerves exit above the correspondingly numbered vertebrae. The C8 spinal nerve exits below the C7 vertebrae. The spinal nerves of T1 and below exit below the correspondingly numbered vertebrae. The spinal nerves join complex networks after leaving the cord to innervate parts of the body.

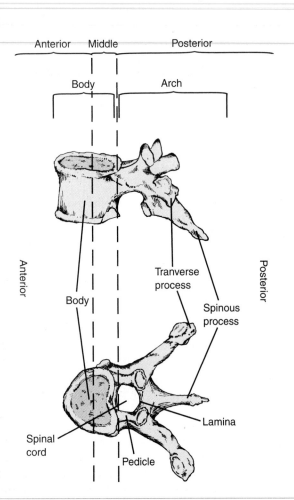

Figure 21–1 ■ A lateral view and cross-section of a vertebra.

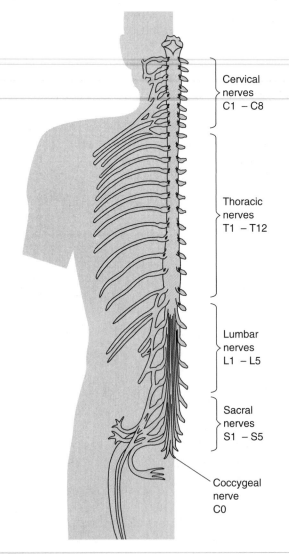

Figure 21–2 ■ Distribution of spinal nerves.

The main blood supply to the spinal cord is provided by the anterior spinal artery and the posterior spinal arteries. Any disruption in this vascular supply may damage the cord without direct physical trauma.

Neuronal Function

The spinal cord consists of an outer region of white matter and an inner region of gray matter. The gray matter helps transmit motor activity from the brain to the body. It also serves as a "relay" station for sensory messages from the body to the brain. In the first thoracic through the second lumbar section of the cord, the gray matter gives rise to the sympathetic nervous system. Activation of the thoracic section gray matter stimulates the sympathetic nervous system to increase perfusion and ventilation, and decrease elimination and digestion.

The white matter of the spinal cord consists of insulated nerve fibers that function as transmission cables (tracts). The three major tracts are the corticospinal, spinothalamic, and posterior column tracts for touch, vibration, and position sense, respectively. The corticospinal tract originates in the brain and crosses over in the brainstem to innervate the opposite side of the body. It transmits motor activity. The spinothalamic tract originates in the spinal cord, where it crosses over within two segments of entry into the cord and ascends to the thalamus in the brain. It transmits pain and temperature. The posterior horn contains axons from the peripheral sensory neurons.

The parasympathetic nervous system originates in a group of neurons located in the brainstem and in a group located between the second and fourth sacral segments of the cord. Parasympathetic stimulation produces specific responses that assist elimination and digestion, among other functions. Damage to specific regions of the cord may produce alterations in either sympathetic or parasympathetic function.

In summary, the spine is composed of cervical, thoracic, and lumbar vertebrae. The spine is conceptualized as having three columns. If two or more of these columns are damaged, the injury is considered to be unstable because the vertebrae and ligaments cannot support or protect the injured area. The spinal cord runs through the center of the vertebrae in the spinal canal. It consists of an outer region of white matter and an inner region of gray matter. Each has important functions.

SECTION ONE REVIEW

1. M.S. has been diagnosed with an unstable spinal injury. This means
   A. she has injured the reflex center for bowel function
   B. the vertebral structures are unable to support the injured area
   C. multiple spinal fractures are present
   D. the main blood supply to the spinal cord is disrupted
2. The spinal cord is located in the
   A. spinal canal
   B. spinous process
   C. plexus
   D. body of vertebrae

3. The end of the spinal cord contains reflex centers for
   A. bowel function
   B. bladder function
   C. sexual function
   D. all of the above
4. Activation of the thoracic section gray matter stimulates the
   A. sympathetic nervous system
   B. parasympathetic nervous system
   C. brainstem
   D. spinothalamic tract

Answers: 1. B, 2. A, 3. D, 4. A

SECTION TWO: Spinal Cord Injury

At the completion of this section, the learner will be able to differentiate complete versus incomplete spinal cord injury; define paraplegia, quadraplegia, and tetraplegia; discuss the results of damage to upper and lower motor neurons; and explain the mechanisms of injury for primary injury and the pathophysiology of secondary spinal cord injury.

Approximately 14,000 individuals in the United States sustain a permanent spinal cord injury (SCI) each year (American Association of Neurological Surgeons, 2002). The most frequent injuries occur in the cervical region (more than 52 percent of all cases) and thoracic region (more than 30 percent of all cases) (Hickey, 2003). Violence and fall-related SCIs have increased, whereas SCIs from motor vehicle crashes and sports have decreased. Respiratory complications are the most frequent cause of death. Prognosis is poorest for individuals over the age of 50 with complete lesions at the time of injury.

Spinal cord injury may be described as **complete spinal cord injury** (loss of all voluntary motor and sensory function below the level of injury) caused by transection of the spinal cord or **incomplete spinal cord injury** (preservation of some sensory or motor function below the level of injury because of partial transection of the spinal cord). The injury is identified by vertebral level. For example, a C5 SCI is at the fifth cervical vertebrae. About 60 percent of patients admitted to high-acuity units have incomplete SCI and 59 percent of these develop significant recovery of function; however, of those who have complete SCI only 3 percent develop significant recovery within 24 hours postinjury (Karlet, 2001).

Complete Spinal Cord Injury

Complete spinal cord injury results in one of two conditions: **paraplegia** or **quadriplegia** (also referred to as **tetraplegia**). Paraplegia is the result of injury to the thoracolumbar region (T2 to L1) (Fig. 21–2) causing loss of motor and sensory function of the lower extremities. Upper extremity function remains intact. Quadriplegia is the result of injury to cervical or thoracic regions (C1 to T1) (Fig. 21–2). Muscle function depends on the specific segments involved but impaired function of the arms, trunk, legs, and pelvic organs may occur.

Incomplete Spinal Cord Injury

Types of incomplete spinal cord injuries are described in Table 21–1. Note that with these syndromes each has evidence of partially interrupted motor and sensory pathways. The alterations in function that occur as the result of a spinal cord injury vary greatly depending on the amount of tissue damage and the level of injury.

Upper and Lower Motor Neuron Injuries

Spinal cord injury damages upper or lower motor neurons. Motor neurons are functional units that carry motor impulses. *Upper motor neurons* are located in the cerebral cortex, thalamus, brainstem, and corticospinal tracts and are responsible for voluntary movement. Damage to an upper motor neuron pathway results in loss of cerebral control over reflex activity below the lesion level. Upper motor neurons may become hyperactive to local stimuli, producing **spastic paralysis** (the inability to carry out a skilled movement). *Lower motor neurons* originate in the spinal cord and form spinal nerves outside the cord. They transmit from target organs to the spinal cord, where they synapse with another lower motor neuron to transmit back to the same target organ. Lower motor neurons create reflex arcs and involuntary responses. Damage to lower motor neurons produces **flaccid paralysis** (loss of both voluntary and involuntary movement).

Mechanisms of Injury

Like closed-head injuries (Module 20), spinal cord injuries occur as a result of primary and secondary injury. **Primary injury** is the neurologic damage that occurs at the moment of impact. Primary spinal cord injuries are caused by violent motions of the head and trunk, fracture or dislocation of the vertebral column, and blunt or penetrating trauma. **Secondary injury** refers to the complex biochemical processes that occur within minutes of injury and can last for days to weeks. Secondary injury occurs as a result of vascular injury to the cord from arterial or venous disruption causing bleeding, edema, and hypoxia of the spinal cord. Associated factors, such as the position of the person's head, neck, and trunk at the time of injury, and the magnitude and duration of the injuring force, affect vertebral injury.

Primary Spinal Cord Injuries

Primary injury to the spinal cord occurs when excessive force is applied to the spinal cord. Mechanisms of injury include hyperflexion, hyperextension, rotation, and axial loading. hyperflexion injury is most often caused by a sudden deceleration of the motion of the head (head-on collision). This forcible bending forward dislocates anterior vertebrae, tears posterior ligaments, and compresses the cord (Fig. 21–3A). The spinal column is unstable because torn posterior muscles and ligaments cannot support the spinal column. Hyperextension injuries are caused by a forward and backward motion of the head (rear-end collisions, diving accidents). With this injury, the anterior ligaments are torn and the spinal cord is stretched (Fig. 21–3B). A mild form of hyperextension injury is the whiplash injury. Rotation injury is caused by severe rotation of the neck causing a tearing of the posterior ligaments and rotation of the spinal column (nonbelted person in a car hit broadside). Axial loading injury, or compression fracture, is caused by a vertical force along the spinal cord. This vertical force fractures vertebral bodies that

TABLE 21–1 Incomplete Spinal Cord Injury Syndromes

SYNDROME	FUNCTIONS LOST	FUNCTIONS PRESENT
Anterior cord	Motor, pain, temperature and touch	Proprioception, vibration
Brown–Séquard	Loss of voluntary motor movement on same side as injury; loss of pain, temperature, sensation on the opposite side	Side of the body with the best motor control has little or no sensation
Central cord	Motor, sensory deficit in upper extremities	Motor, sensory pathways in lower extremities; some bladder, bowel function
Anterior cord	Motor function, loss of pain and sensation below level of injury	Senses of position, pressure, vibration

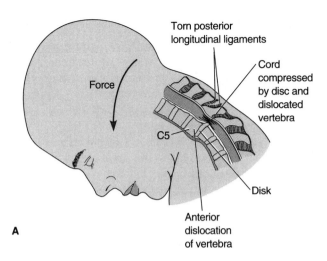

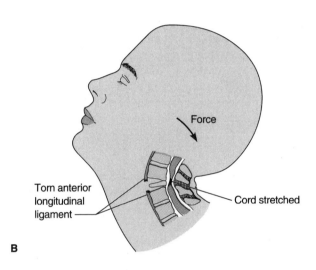

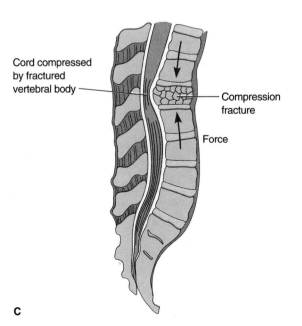

Figure 21–3 ■ Mechanisms of spinal cord injury. *A.* Hyperflexion injury. *B.* Hyperextension injury. *C.* Compression fracture.

send bony fragments into the spinal cord (Fig. 21–3C). Compression fractures typically occur with diving into shallow water or jumping from tall heights and landing on the feet or buttocks.

Cervical Injuries

The cervical region is the most vulnerable region of the spine because of its poor stability. Complete cord injuries at the C1 or C2 level are often fatal. Hyperflexion injuries of the cervical spine, especially C5 to C6, are associated with rapid deceleration. C4 and C5 damage frequently occurs from diving accidents.

Thoracic and Lumbar Injuries

Great force is needed to produce T1 through T10 injuries because of the stability of the rib cage. The most common site of thoracic spinal injury is located at the T12–L1 junction. Flexion may occur with compression of the anterior aspects of the vertebrae. A fall onto the upper back can produce flexion along with rotation. Thoracic region injuries may result from vertical compression forces experienced during a fall onto the buttocks or feet. A patient with calcaneus fractures of the feet should be suspected of having thoracic vertebral or cord damage. The same forces producing thoracic injuries may be responsible for lumbar injuries. Violent flexion of the lumbar spine may occur with wearing a lap belt without a shoulder restraint (e.g., middle passenger in the rear seat) in a motor vehicle crash.

Nontraumatic Etiologies

Several conditions may produce narrowing of the spinal canal and subsequent SCI. Degenerative changes as a result of osteoarthritis in the spine predispose a person to hyperextension injuries. Ankylosing spondylitis (calcification of ligaments and soft tissue) and rheumatoid arthritis (inflammation causing osteoporosis and decreased mobility) are two precipitating causes of SCI. Space-occupying lesions (abscesses and solid tumors) may produce spinal cord compression. Lymphoma and multiple myeloma are two oncologic conditions associated with bone metastases. The first sign of spinal cord compression from tumor growth is usually a constant, dull, back pain aggravated by coughing or sneezing. Leg weakness, urinary retention, and sexual dysfunction may also develop.

In some regions where deep sea diving is a recreational activity, spinal cord injury may result from gas bubbles in the vertebral venous system (a form of decompression sickness). Because the spinal cord receives a high rate of blood flow, venous stasis secondary to bubble formation obstructs flow.

Secondary Spinal Cord Injuries

The 24-hour period immediately following SCI involves a series of pathophysiologic processes that contributes to secondary spinal cord injuries. These processes include: ischemia, an increase in intracellular calcium, and inflammation (Dubendorf,

1999). These processes cause cellular membrane destruction and are very similar to secondary injuries associated with closed-head injury (Module 20). Knowledge of the pathophysiology of these secondary processes has led to research focused on inhibiting secondary injury processes and preserving functional neurons (Dubendorf, 1999).

Ischemia. Blood flow to the spinal cord decreases immediately on injury as a result of hypotension and vasospasm induced thrombosis. Thrombi in the microcirculation impede blood flow. Elevated interstitial pressure related to edema further impairs perfusion to the cord. Vasoconstrictive substances, such as norepinephrine, are released postinjury, contributing to decreased circulation and cellular perfusion. The zone of ischemia can spread if perfusion to the cord is not restored.

Elevated Intracellular Calcium. Calcium ions accumulate in injured cells, causing a breakdown of intracellular protein and phospholipids. Demyelination and destruction of the cell membrane occur when these substances are broken down. The breakdown of phospholipids releases fatty acids. The fatty acids produce arachadonic acid, which ultimately produces leukotrienes and prostaglandins, mediators in the inflammatory process. Eicosanoids, prostaglandins, and mediators contribute to cellular membrane damage. Once the cell membrane is damaged, neuronal death occurs.

Inflammatory Processes. Leukocytes infiltrate the injured area immediately postinjury. The inflammatory process is another factor in edema formation, further decreasing blood supply to the injured area. As the cord swells within the bony vertebrae, edema moves up and down the cord. A patient may exhibit symptoms as a result of the edema and not the initial injury. For example, a patient with a C4 injury may have edema up to the C2 level. Because edema can extend the level of injury for several cord segments above and below the affected level, the extent of injury may not be determined for several days, until after the cord edema has resolved.

In summary, SCI is described as complete or incomplete. Complete SCI results in paraplegia or quadraplegia. Incomplete SCI results in one of several syndromes of varying motor and sensory deficits. Damage to upper motor neurons results in spastic paralysis. Damage to lower motor neurons results in flaccid paralysis. Spinal cord injuries occur as a result of primary and secondary processes. Primary mechanisms of injury include hyperflexion, hyperextension, rotation, and axial loading. Secondary mechanisms of injury occur as a result of ischemia, increased intracellular calcium, and inflammation.

SECTION TWO REVIEW

1. DW has been diagnosed with anterior cord syndrome. This syndrome represents
   A. an upper motor neuron problem
   B. a lower motor neuron problem
   C. the best prognosis for recovery
   D. an incomplete cord syndrome
2. Damage to upper motor neurons can produce
   A. quadraplegia
   B. spastic paralysis
   C. flaccid paralysis
   D. paraplegia
3. Whiplash is a mild form of which of the following primary injuries to the spinal cord?
   A. hyperflexion
   B. axial loading
   C. hyperextension
   D. rotation
4. Which region of the spine is most vulnerable to injury?
   A. cervical
   B. thoracic
   C. lumbar
   D. sacral
5. The events contributing to secondary injury of the spinal cord include all of the following EXCEPT
   A. ischemia
   B. increased intracellular calcium
   C. hypertension
   D. inflammation

Answers: 1. D, 2. B, 3. C, 4. A, 5. C

SECTION THREE: Assessment and Diagnosis of Spinal Cord Injury

At the completion of this section, the learner will be able to describe diagnostic tests frequently used to identify the type and severity of SCI; discuss physical assessment techniques for assessing motor, sensory, and reflex activity in patients with SCI; and differentiate spinal shock from neurogenic shock.

The diagnosis of SCI begins with a detailed history of events surrounding the incident, radiographic studies of the spine, and an assessment of sensory and motor function. Frequently, diagnostic testing of the SCI patient is completed in the emergency department. In situations in which SCI is suspected later in the hospitalization, diagnostic testing may be initiated in the high-acuity setting. Therefore, the nurse should be aware of the types of tests ordered and the information they provide in order to prepare the patient and family. Spinal cord injury is frequently associated with closed-head injury. Therefore, the health care professional assumes that an unconscious patient has an SCI until it is ruled out. SCI should also be suspected in a patient with maxillofacial injury and clavicle or upper rib fractures.

Patients with acute cervical SCI are admitted to an ICU for close monitoring of cardiac, respiratory, and hemodynamic function (American Association of Neurological Surgeons, 2002).

Radiographs

Radiographic assessment documents the level of injury and provides information regarding the stability of the cord injury. As soon as the patient is stabilized (airway, breathing, and circulation), x-rays of the spine are obtained. Not everyone with a potential neck injury needs an x-ray, only those who have changes in level of consciousness as a result of injury, alcohol, or drugs who cannot complain of neck tenderness or those who complain of neck tenderness and have some obvious symptoms (American Association of Neurological Surgeons, 2002). Anterior and posterior views of the spine may be ordered. An x-ray that is taken with the patient's mouth open is needed to visualize C1-2 and the odontoid process. Another specialized view or position, called the swimmer's position, is needed to visualize C7 to T1. To obtain this view, the physician or specially trained nurse pulls the patient's shoulders downward toward the foot of the bed (Hickey, 2003).

Computed Tomography Scan

A computed tomography (CT) scan may be ordered after completion of x-rays if the spine is not well visualized or there are suspicious findings. A CT scan provides superior visualization of bony structures of the spine and identifies spinal fractures. The CT scan is more accurate for detecting posterior and central column injuries as well as cord impingement. If radiopaque contrast is used, the nurse must question the patient about dye and seafood allergies and any underlying kidney disease.

Magnetic Resonance Imaging

Magnetic resonance imaging (MRI) identifies injuries to the spinal cord, ligaments, and disks. It is also used to detect tumors and vascular disruptions in the spinal cord.

Somatosensory-Evoked Potentials

Somatosensory-evoked potentials (SEPs) are used to establish a functional prognosis after resolution of spinal cord edema. In an extremity below the level of injury, a peripheral nerve is stimulated. The response of the cerebral cortex to this stimulation (evoked potential) is recorded using scalp electrodes. In complete SCI, SEPs are absent because the stimulus is not transmitted to the cortex.

Physical Assessment

Accurate assessment of motor, sensory, and reflex function is important for several reasons: to assist in diagnosis of the lesion, to provide a baseline with which to compare effectiveness of treatment, and to determine realistic functional goals. The American Spinal Injury Association (ASIA) Standard Neurological Classification of SCI assessment form is used to document sensory and motor function (Fig. 21–4). This scale remains the most frequently used tool to evaluate both acute and long-term progress (Barker & Saulino, 2002). Serial neurologic exams are performed hourly for at least the first 24 hours after SCI (Hedger, 2002).

Motor Assessment

Motor strength varies based on preinjury characteristics including gender, fitness level, and age. Voluntary movement requires both upper and lower motor neuron activity. Motor activity is assessed for strength. The examiner begins at the head and moves toward the toes (Karlet, 2001). Initially, the examiner starts with eliminating gravity (for example, the wrist is propped on a pillow and placed through flexion and extension). Next, movement against gravity is assessed (pillow removed and the arm dangles off the bed during flexion and extension). Finally, the patient's range of movement against resistance (examiner's hand) is noted. Each side is evaluated and compared. Flexion and extension of the joints are assessed.

Sensory Assessment

The most important data to collect in the sensory examination is the exact point on the patient where normal sensation is present. The sensory assessment begins by moving from the lower to upper body regions because it is easier for the patient to recognize the onset of a sensory stimulus rather than cessation of a stimulus (Karlet, 2001).

Sensation is tested along **dermatomes.** A dermatome is a section of the body innervated by a particular spinal (or cranial) nerve (Fig. 21–5). A cotton swab is used to assess sensation (spinothalamic tract function). A pin prick is used to assess pain (posterior column function). The patient's eyes are closed. The examination begins distal and moves proximal (that is, up the neurologically intact area). Position sense (**proprioception**) is tested by moving the big toes and thumbs up and down and asking the patient to confirm the direction. The areas where sensation and pain are present are marked and dated on a dermatome diagram similar to that shown in Figure 21–5. Table 21–2 shows the relationship between nerve root and innervated area.

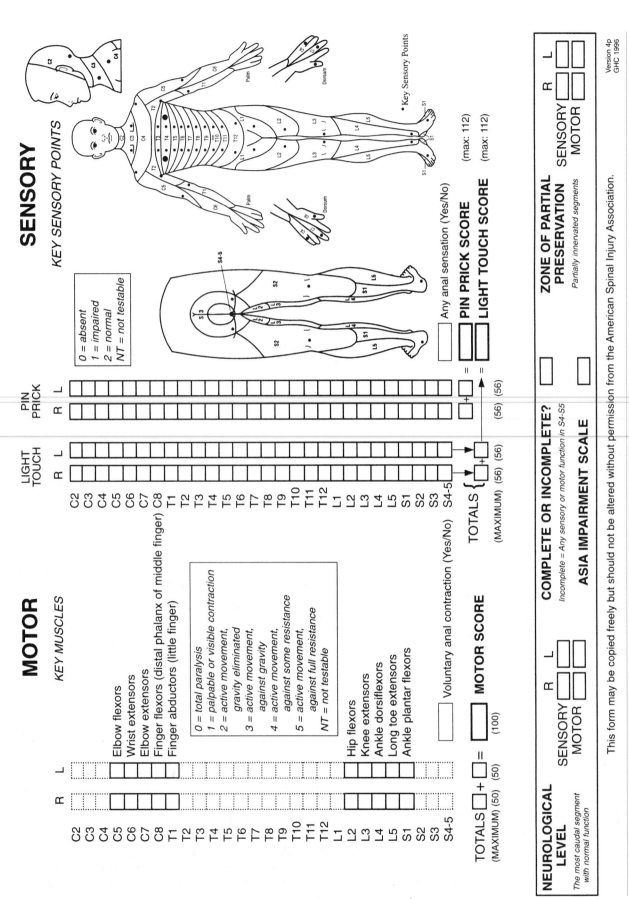

Figure 21–4 ■ Standard neurological classification of spinal cord injury.

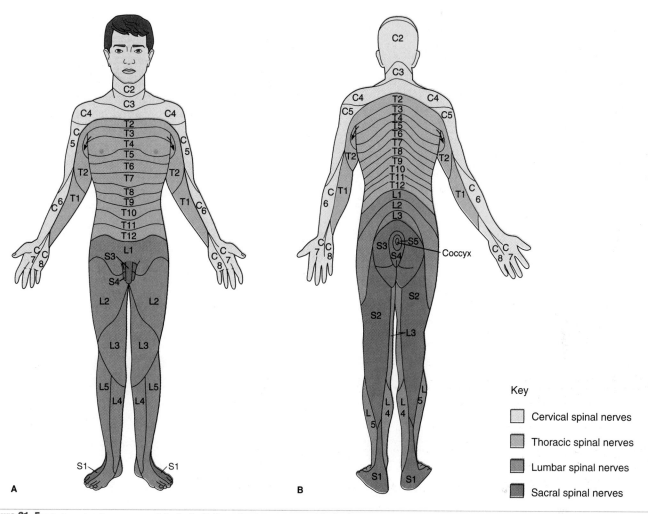

Figure 21–5 ■ *A.* Anterior dermatomes of the body. *B.* Posterior dermatomes of the body.

TABLE 21–2 Relationship Between Nerve Root and Innervated Area for Sensory Testing

NERVE ROOT	INNERVATED AREA
C5	Upper lateral arm
C6	Posterior aspect of thumb
C7	Posterior aspect of middle finger
C8	Posterior aspect of little finger
T4	Nipple line
T10	Umbilicus
L1	Groin
L2	Anterior thigh
S1	Sole of the foot
S3, S4, S5	Perianal

TABLE 21–3 Deep Tendon Reflexes and Their Neural Source of Origin

DEEP TENDON REFLEX	NEURAL ORIGIN
Biceps	C5
Supinator	C6
Triceps	C7
Knee (patellar)	L3
Ankle (Achilles)	S1

Reflex Activity

The presence of deep tendon reflexes (Table 21–3) below the level of injury indicates an incomplete lesion. The presence of perineal reflexes indicates that bowel and bladder training may be feasible. **Priapism** (persistent penile erection) may be present in males. The anal wink reflex is initiated by a pin prick in the perianal area. A visual external anal sphincter contraction will occur if the reflex is present. The bulbocavernosus reflex is initiated by placing a gloved finger in the patient's rectum and tugging on the penis or the clitoris. The rectal sphincter will contract if the reflex is present. The presence of the anal wink and bulbocavernosus reflexes indicate that the injury is an upper motor neuron injury.

Assessing for Shock States

It is important to assess the patient for the presence of spinal shock and neurogenic shock.

Spinal Shock

Spinal shock occurs within 30 to 60 minutes after injury; however, it may take several hours to become clinically apparent. It is manifested by hypotension, bradycardia, flaccid paralysis, absence of muscle contractions, and bowel and bladder dysfunction. This syndrome may last 7 to 20 days postinjury (Karlet, 2001) and resolves spontaneously. Treatment is symptomatic. The end of this period is seen with the return of some reflexes, spasticity, and increased muscle tone. It is difficult to classify a spinal cord injury accurately until spinal shock has resolved.

Neurogenic Shock

Neurogenic shock occurs in patients with an injury above T6. The loss of sympathetic control from the brainstem and higher centers allows the parasympathetic output to go unchecked. Consequently, the patient experiences hypotension, bradycardia, decreased cardiac output, and loss of the ability to sweat below the level of the lesion.

In summary, the diagnosis of SCI begins with a detailed history surrounding the event, radiographic studies of the spine, and assessment of sensory and motor function. Radiographs may include x-rays, CT, and/or MRI scans. SEPs establish functional prognosis after SCI. Sensory and motor function are assessed and documented using the ASIA Neurologic Classification. Bilateral motor assessments are made. Sensation is tested along dermatomes. The presence of deep tendon reflexes below the level of injury indicates an incomplete lesion. Spinal shock occurs within 60 minutes after injury. SCI cannot be accurately classified until spinal shock resolves. Neurogenic shock occurs as the result of unopposed parasympathetic innervation.

SECTION THREE REVIEW

1. MF has been admitted with a diagnosis of a possible C7 compression injury. A CT scan with contrast of the cervical spine is ordered for MF. The nurse should
   A. remove all metal objects
   B. supply in-line mobilization of the neck
   C. ask if MF is allergic to seafood or radiopaque dye
   D. prep MF's neck with povidone–iodine solution
2. Two days later a SEP test is used to help establish a functional prognosis. MF did not have any SEPs during the test. This means
   A. the SCI is complete
   B. the SCI is unstable
   C. an upper motor neuron lesion is present
   D. a lower motor neuron injury is present
3. Which of the following scales is the most frequently used tool to evaluate acute and long-term progress after SCI?
   A. Glasgow Coma Scale
   B. NIH Scale

C. ASIA Standard Neurological Classification
   D. CT scan
4. The exact point on the patient where normal sensation is present is assessed with
   A. testing along dermatomes
   B. MRI
   C. proprioception
   D. SEPs
5. Hypoperfusion, bradycardia, and flaccid paralysis are signs of
   A. priapism
   B. autonomic dysreflexia
   C. neurogenic shock
   D. spinal shock

Answers: 1. C, 2. A, 3. C, 4. A, 5. D

SECTION FOUR: Stabilization and Management of Spinal Cord Injury in the Acute Care Phase

At the completion of this section, the learner will be able to discuss surgical and manual stabilization techniques used in SCI, and to state the indications for and controversies with the use of methylprednisolone after SCI.

Stablization of the Spinal Cord

Timely spinal cord alignment and stabilization maximize cord recovery, minimize additional damage, and prevent late deformity. The spinal cord is stabilized using surgical or manual techniques. Stabilization in the high-acuity unit includes bedrest with log rolling maneuvers, and a hard cervical collar until the spine has been stabilized with surgery or traction.

Surgical Stabilization

There is great controversy concerning the need for surgical stabilization of SCI. Even those who advocate surgical management debate the optimal time at which surgery is conducted postinjury (Papadopoulos, 2003). The best advantage to surgical stabilization is that it affords earlier mobilization and thus decreases complications attributed to immobility (e.g., pulmonary emboli). Spinal segments are fused during surgery. Spinal canal decompression is accomplished. Rods are inserted to stabilize thoracic spinal injuries. External traction may be required postoperatively. Special braces, such as the Jewett orthosis, may be used postoperatively to maintain hyperextension when the patient is not supine. Surgery is reserved for patients not sufficiently aligned with manual stabilization.

Manual Stabilization

The spinal cord may be immobilized through the use of manual fixation devices including tongs, halos, and braces.

Skull Tongs. Tong devices, such as Gardner-Wells or Vinke cervical tongs, may be used initially to reduce a fracture (Fig. 21–6). Screws are implanted into the patient's skull a few inches above the ear using a local anesthetic. The patient feels pressure but not pain. Sequential weights are added to these devices. Ten pounds of traction is applied if an injury but no fracture is present. If a

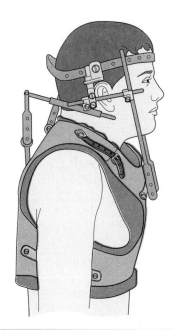

Figure 21–7 ■ The halo external fixation device.

fracture is present, 5 pounds per interspace beginning with C1 to the level of lesion is applied. Muscle relaxants promote the efficacy of the traction.

Halo Device. The halo device is an external fixation device (Fig. 21–7). It keeps the spine aligned and prevents flexion, extension, and rotational movement of the head and neck, and allows for early mobilization. The device is secured with four pins inserted in the skull—two in the frontal lobe and two in the occipital bone. The halo ring is attached to a rigid plastic vest. Patients in these devices require special nursing responsibilities, which are summarized in Table 21–4.

Braces

A hard cervical collar and a molded plastic body jacket (clam shell) brace may be sufficient for stabilization of some injuries. Braces, such as the Jewett orthosis, are most frequently used with thoracic and lumbar spine injuries.

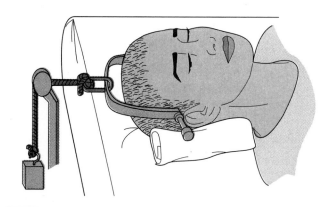

Figure 21–6 ■ Cervical traction may be applied by several methods, including Gardner-Wells tongs.

TABLE 21–4 Nursing Care of the Patient in a Halo Vest

INTERVENTION	RATIONALE
1. Tape a halo vest wrench on the front of the vest.	The fixation device must be taken off to remove the vest to expose the chest in the event CPR is required.
2. Inspect pins and traction bars for loose pins.	It is a nursing responsibility to maintain the integrity of the external system.
3. Do not pull the vest's struts to move or position the patient.	This can disrupt the integrity of the device and potentially damage the cord.
4. Assess motor function and sensation every 2 to 4 hours.	Early identification of neurologic deficits can be made.
5. Perform pin care per unit protocol and monitor pin sites for signs of infection.	Organisms can enter through the pin insertion sites.
6. Turn every 2 hours, inspect skin around vest edges.	Prevent skin breakdown.

TABLE 21–5 Methods, Indications, Goals and Lengths of Therapy, and Precautions of Various Spine Immobilization Techniques

METHODS	INDICATIONS	GOAL OF THERAPY	LENGTH OF THERAPY	PRECAUTIONS
Cervical spine				
Hard cervical collar (short term) Philadelphia collar and Stif-neck collar	Prehospital immobilization Uncleared c-spine	Preevaluation, presumptive	Less than 48 hours	Ensure good collar fit Skin care Decubitus ulcers
Hard cervical collar (long term) Miami-J collar and Aspen collar	Stable c-spine fracture Ligamentous injury	Hasten healing, diminish pain	8–12 weeks	Ensure good collar fit Worn continuously—provide second collar for washing Meticulous skin care
Soft cervical collar	Cervical strain, whiplash	Symptom management	Varies, depending on symptom severity	Limit use to avoid dependence (e.g., nighttime, riding in car only)
Cervical traction				
Gardner-Wells tongs	Unstable maligned c-spine fracture, dislocation, or ligamentous injury	Cervical reduction Bridge to operative therapy	Varies	Pin site care and assessment Reposition patient every 2 hours
Halo vest	Unstable c-spine fracture, dislocation, or ligamentous injury	Definitive cervical immobilization	8–12 weeks	Pin site assessment and care Decubitus ulcers beneath vest
Four poster or Yale brace	Stable c-spine injuries or adjunct to surgery for unstable c-spine injuries	Hasten healing, diminish pain	8–12 weeks	
Thoracic or lumbar spine				
Hyperextension cast and thoraco–lumbar support orthotic (clam-shell or tortoise-shell brace)	Stable thoracic or lumbar spine column fractures; anterior compression fracture with <40% loss of height; burst fractures with no neurologic deficit, <50% vertebral body involvement, <30% canal compromise, angulation <20°	Hasten healing, diminish pain After spinal decompressive and stabilization surgery for support and comfort	8–12 weeks	Requires custom fit Meticulous skin care
Elastic thoraco–lumbar supports	Minor compression fractures or transverse process fractures Lumbar strain	Symptom management	Varies, depending on symptom severity	

From Logan © 1999, Principles of Practice for the Acute Care Nurse Practitioner, reprinted by permission of Prentice Hall Inc., Upper Saddle River, NJ.

Whether surgical or mechanical stabilization of the spine is used, the goals are the same: to align and stabilize the spine, minimize additional damage, and prevent late deformity. The methods, indications, goals and lengths of therapy, and precautions of various spine immobilization techniques are summarized in Table 21–5

Methylprednisolone

Methylprednisolone, administered post-SCI, may decrease free fatty acid production, inhibit phospholipid breakdown, and reduce infiltration of leukocytes (Hickey, 2003). By these actions, secondary injury to the spinal cord is prevented because blood flow to the cord is improved and mediators of the inflammatory process are not released. Studies have shown that patients who receive methylprednisolone after SCI have a reduction in secondary injury to the spinal cord and that methylprednisolone

has a profound effect on functional level (Dyson-Hudson & Stein, 1999). National Acute Spinal Cord Injury studies suggest that secondary injury may be diminished if methylprednisolone is initiated within 8 hours of injury with an initial bolus of 30 mg/kg, followed by a continuous infusion of 5.4 mg/kg/hr over 23 to 48 hours (Bracke et al., 1997).

Currently considerable controversy exists on the use of methylprednisolone for the management of spinal cord injury in the acute care phase. The use of this therapy must be weighed against its potential adverse reactions including gastric ulceration, electrolyte imbalances, and delayed wound healing (American Association of Neurological Surgeons, 2002).

In summary, timely spinal cord alignment and stabilization maximizes functional recovery and minimizes complications. Surgical stabilization allows for early mobilization, but is only required for patients not sufficiently aligned with manual stabilization. Manual stabilization is accomplished with tongs, halos, or braces. Each requires specialized nursing care.

SECTION FOUR REVIEW

1. BR is admitted to the unit with an unstable T2 SCI. The physician will place cervical traction in 6 hours. What is a priority nursing intervention?
   A. administer pain medications as ordered
   B. place a hard cervical collar and perform log rolling maneuvers
   C. shave and prep BR's head
   D. place a wrench at BR's bedside
2. The best advantage to surgical stabilization is that it
   A. decreases complications attributed to immobility
   B. secures the spine better than cervical tongs
   C. is cheaper
   D. is available to all patients with SCI
3. Which of the following is a priority nursing intervention for the patient with a halo vest?
   A. place an appropriate wrench on or near the patient
   B. maintain the hard neck collar

C. log roll the patient
D. add sequential weights

4. Which of the following statements is TRUE about the use of methylprednisolone for SCI?
   A. it must be given to all patients within 6 hours of injury
   B. it is now considered to be contraindicated in all patients with SCI
   C. it is considered to be a treatment option
   D. high doses are better than low doses

Answers: 1. B, 2. A, 3. A, 4. C

SECTION FIVE: High-Acuity Nursing Care of the Patient with a Spinal Cord Injury

At the completion of this section, the learner will be able to identify priority nursing assessments and interventions for the patient with a spinal cord injury in the acute care phase of recovery and discuss priority nursing assessments and interventions to identify and prevent complications postinjury in the acute care phase of recovery.

Impaired Gas Exchange, Ineffective Breathing Patterns

As with any high-acuity patient, the nurse begins the patient assessment using the ABCs. The patient's airway and breathing may be compromised, particularly with a cervical cord injury. Patients with C1–C2 injuries will require mechanical ventilation because of loss of phrenic nerve ennervation to the diaphragm. Those with injuries to C3–C5 will have varying degrees of diaphragm paralysis and need some ventilatory support. They may be able to be weaned from mechanical ventilation. Injuries below C6 have varying degrees of impaired intercostal and abdominal muscle function. Patients with these injuries experience compromise in respiratory protective reflexes, including coughing and sneezing.

Patients with SCI, especially cervical injuries, have a high incidence of pulmonary complications, including pneumonia, atelectasis, and respiratory failure; and respiratory failure is the leading cause of death in patients with SCI (Lanig & Peterson, 2000). According to Cook (2003), the goals of respiratory management in the patient with SCI are to (1) prevent secondary neural damage, (2) prevent hypoxemia, (3) prevent and treat atelectasis, (4) maximize alveolar ventilation, and (5) maximize pulmonary hygiene for impaired cough and secretion clearance. Patients with SCI require close monitoring of respiratory drive, ventilation, ability to cough, pulse oximetry, and arterial blood gases (Karlet, 2001).

The respiratory management goals are achieved through aggressive respiratory therapy, and careful monitoring to identify and promptly treat actual and potential respiratory problems. Humidified oxygen is administered via nasal cannula or face mask. The patient is taught to use an incentive spirometer and assisted with "quad" coughing. Quad coughing is the use of pillows to push against the abdomen to increase intra-abdominal pressure to cough. When assisted coughing is used, bronchodilators and mucolytics are beneficial in mobilizing secretions to gain maximal benefit from the cough (Lanig & Peterson, 2000).

Chest physiotherapy may be done depending on the patient's ability to tolerate this procedure and the level and extent of injury. The decision to suction the patient should be based on assessment findings because this procedure may stimulate the vasovagal response and lead to bradycardia. Mobilization of secretions is best obtained with frequent turning and position changes. However, this may not be possible because of the patient's injury and the use of traction devices. The nurse should collaborate with the health care team to determine if the use of a specialized bed is warranted for the patient with a spinal cord injury.

Decreased Cardiac Output

The patient with SCI is at high risk for developing decreased cardiac output related to orthostatic hypotension, spinal and neurogenic shock, venous pooling, emboli, and bradycardia. In the acute care phase, invasive and noninvasive monitoring may be used to closely monitor cardiac output. Cardiac monitoring allows for early detection of bradycardia which is a constant threat because of unopposed vagal stimulation of the heart. Patients with a SCI are at risk for developing bradycardia and even asystole during endotracheal tube manipulation, suctioning, or insertion of a nasogastric tube (Karlet, 2001). Atropine should be at the bedside at all times (Hedger, 2002; Karlet, 2001). All sensitive patients should be premedicated with atropine before high-risk procedures (Karlet, 2001).

Techniques to monitor preload (see Module 9) may be required. Judicious use of IV fluids is required when treating hypotension because too much fluid can precipitate pulmonary edema. Inotropic and/or vasopressor support may be required to maintain adequate cardiac output and tissue perfusion. In patients with SCI, it may be difficult to keep the systolic blood pressure over 90 mm Hg. Therefore, the aim of therapy is to maintain adequate tissue perfusion, not an absolute pressure (Karlet, 2001). However, a systolic blood pressure less than 90 mm Hg is detrimental because it causes hypoperfusion to the cord and, therefore, current guidelines recommend that MAP should be maintained 85 to 90 mm Hg for the first 7 days post-SCI (American Association of Neurological Surgeons, 2002).

Altered Urinary Elimination and Constipation

The degree of bladder dysfunction depends on the location and completeness of the SCI. SCI removes the ability of the pontine micturation center and higher centers in the brain to inhibit, control, or coordinate the activity (Siroky, 2002). Patients with complete quadraplegia are typically unaware of bladder activity except through ancillary clues (sweating, chills). For the first few days post-SCI, an indwelling urinary catheter is used. After this initial phase, the catheter is removed and an intermittent catheterization schedule is instituted. Overdistension of the bladder must be prevented. After the acute care phase, the patient is taught self-catheterization. Constipation and fecal impaction are major problems.

Cervical or high thoracic injuries cause reflex bowel—the patient does not feel the urge to defecate, but the anal–rectal reflex remains intact (Gibson, 2003). A bowel care program is employed including laxatives and stool softeners and appropriate fluid and fiber intake. A bowel training program to regulate fecal elimination is instituted in patients with upper motor neuron injuries. Patients with lower motor neuron injuries lose the defecation reflex and are not able to succeed in bowel retraining.

Ineffective Thermoregulation

Interruption in communication between the spinal cord and the hypothalamus results in loss of temperature control (**poikilothermia**). This condition is dangerous because the patient's body temperature depends on the temperature of the environment. This problem resolves once spinal shock ends and peripheral reflex activity returns. Hyperthermia then becomes a problem because loss of sympathetic control of the sweat glands below the level of the lesion prohibits sweating as temperature rises. The patient may need to be kept warm with passive warming devices. However, when these devices are used, the patient is monitored carefully to avoid thermal injury to insensitive skin (Karlet, 2001).

Imbalanced Nutrition

In the initial phase of recovery, paralytic ileus is common. A nasogastric tube prevents gastric distention. A nutrition consult is initiated as soon as possible to help ensure the patient's nutritional needs are met. In the acute care phase, patients with SCI are hypermetabolic (American Association of Neurological Surgeons, 2002). They are at risk for receiving less nutrition than their bodies' requirements because of interruption of bowel innervation, limited ability to feed self, anorexia from lack of taste sensation, and depression. The type of diet patients receive depends on their level of consciousness and the severity of associated injuries. Nursing care includes monitoring intake, changes in the patient's weight, assessing electrolyte balance, and administering total parenteral nutrition, or enteral feedings as ordered. In some cases, dysphagia is problematic. Thickening food to allow formation of a food bolus is helpful.

Self-Care Deficits

Baseline and ongoing motor, sensory, and reflex assessment provide information about the patient's neurological progress. Rehabilitative goals are set and independence (to the degree possible) of the patient encouraged early. Bowel and bladder routines are initiated and ambulation supported as necessary. Table 21–6 outlines functional goals appropriate for the patient, based on level of SCI.

Preventing Complications

Complications associated with SCI (Fig. 21–8) can be classified into three broad categories related to changes in mobility, perfusion, and reflex activity.

Complications Related to a Change in Mobility

Skin Integrity. Several factors contribute to skin breakdown in the patient with a SCI. Sensory and motor impairment results in areas of the skin being subjected to prolonged periods of pres-

TABLE 21–6 Functional Status Based on Level of SCI

LEVEL	EATING	DRESSING	BATHING	BOWEL/BLADDER	MOBILITY
C1–C4	Dependent	Dependent	Dependent	Dependent	Electric wheelchair with breath, head, or shoulder controls; requires ventilatory support (partial or full)
C5	Independent with aids	Major assistance with aids	Wheelchair shower with major assistance	Major assistance with aids	Electric wheelchair with adapted hand controls
C6	Independent with aids	Minor assistance with aids	Independent in wheelchair shower	Independent with aids	Independent in manual wheelchair with hand controls; can use some manual wheelchair types
C7	Independent	Independent with aids	Independent wheelchair shower or tub with bath board	Independent with aids	Independent in manual wheelchair with hand controls
C8–T1	Independent	Independent	Independent in tub with bath boards	Independent with aids	Independent in manual wheelchair
T2–T12	Independent	Independent	Independent	Independent with aids	Independent in manual wheelchair
L1–L5	Independent	Independent	Independent	Independent	Optional use of knee, ankle, or foot orthoses
S1–S5	Independent	Independent	Independent	Independent	Independent with or without ankle or foot orthoses

sure. The patient is unable to feel the discomfort or pain from pressure and is unable to change position independently. In addition to the usual areas of pressure development (sacrum, heels) the patient's ears, ankles, and occipital area of the head need to be assessed for early indications of the development of pressure ulcers. Moisture exposure from bladder or bowel incontinence, or sweating, also contributes to pressure ulcer formation. Frequent positioning, specialized beds, and foot and heel protectors help minimize this risk.

Decreased Joint Mobility. This complication is preventable. The tendency to remain in one position for extended periods is greater when one is dependent on someone else to initiate movement. Spasticity may contribute to this problem by exaggerating responses to movement. The higher the level of the lesion, the greater the spasticity. Spasms can be used positively to enable use of some assistive devices. Deformity and contracture develop if joint mobility is not maintained through range of motion.

Deep-Vein Thrombosis (DVT). Peripheral vasodilation in conjunction with decreased muscle function encourages venous stasis and potential formation of deep-vein thrombosis. A dislodged thrombus leads to a potentially life-threatening pulmonary emboli. Patients with SCI need to have DVT prophylaxis as soon as possible after injury (Karlet, 2001). Current guidelines recommend low molecular weight heparin, adjusted dose heparin, or low dose heparin and pneumatic compression stockings (American Association of Neurological Surgeons, 2002).

Heterotopic Ossification. Ectopic bone formation (overgrowth of bone) occurs below the SCI, further restricting joint mobility. The cause of this phenomenon is unknown.

Complications Related to Abnormal Perfusion

Autonomic Dysreflexia. **Autonomic dysreflexia,** a potentially life-threatening complication, occurs when a stimulus triggers excessive sympathetic nervous system activation below the level of the SCI. Systemic vasoconstriction results, producing sweating, anxiety, headache, blurred vision, and hypertension. The most serious danger of autonomic dysreflexia is severe hypertension (systolic blood pressure greater than 200 mm Hg), which can trigger cerebral hemorrhage and stroke, myocardial infarction, or seizures. The parasympathetic nervous system compensates for this reaction by producing massive vasodilation above the level of the lesion and bradycardia (heart rate less than 40 beats per minute). However, this compensation is inadequate because it affects only the neurologically intact section of the body, whereas the sympathetic reaction affects the total body. This phenomenon occurs after spinal shock has resolved, usually within the first 6 months of injury. However, autonomic dysreflexia remains a potential problem throughout the patient's life. Therefore, both family and patient are taught how to recognize and treat the condition. It is more prevalent in lesions at and above T6. Numerous factors produce autonomic dysreflexia; the most frequent factors are summarized in Box 21–1. While the search for the stimulus that triggered the sympathetic response is conducted, antihypertensive agents are administered.

Box 21–1 Factors that Produce Autonomic Dysreflexia

- Bladder distention/spasm
- Bowel impaction
- Stimulation of anal reflex
- Labor
- Temperature change
- Ingrown toenails
- Tight, irritating clothes
- Urinary tract infection
- Decubiti
- Pain

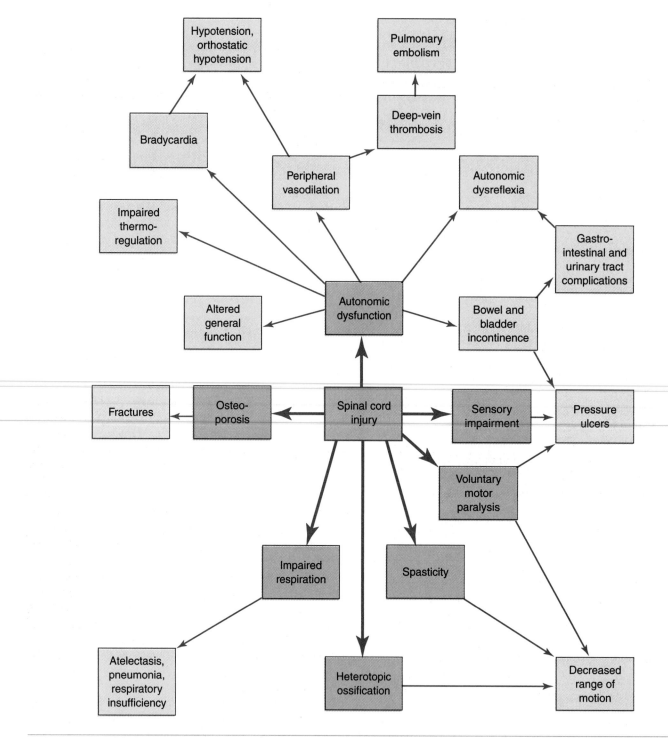

Figure 21-8 ■ Schematic representation of the physical effects of spinal cord injury. *(From Somers, M. [1992]. Spinal cord injury: Functional rehabilitation. Norwalk, CT: Appleton & Lange.)*

Orthostatic Hypotension. Chronic peripheral vasodilation causes orthostatic hypotension, particularly for patients with injuries at T6 or above (Gibson, 2003). This factor in combination with a quick position change results in a loss of consciousness. Therefore, initial attempts to mobilize the patient are done slowly. Gradually raise the head of bed, and assess patient tolerance to these position changes. Feet are dangled on the side of the bed prior to movement out of bed to a chair.

Complications Related to Abnormal Reflex Activity

Bladder Dysfunction. Despite improved methods of treatment, urinary tract infection (UTI) is the second-leading cause of death in the patient with SCI (Siroky, 2002). Incontinence, reflux, development of stones, and neuronal obstruction increase the risk for UTI. Intermittent catheterization when compared to indwelling catheters reduces the risk of infection and is the preferred method of bladder drainage in this patient population, but it too is associated with risks, including urethral trauma, urethral strictures, and hematuria (Siroky, 2002). The use of condom catheters in male patients is associated with infection rates similar to intermittent catheterization, but this method does not guarantee proper drainage of the bladder and may itself be the source of obstruction (Siroky, 2002). Although daily changes of the catheter is standard practice, there is no evidence to support this practice. Chronic use of the same drainage bag predisposes colonization of the drainage bag and retrograde introduction of bacteria into the anterior urethra (Siroky, 2002). UTIs are often preceeded by colonization of bowel bacteria on genitalia, perineum, and the urethra; therefore, strategies to prevent UTIs must include good perineal hygiene (Siroky, 2002).

Bowel Dysfunction. Anticholinergic agents, vitamins, iron supplements, and opioids increase the risk of constipation, ileus, and fecal impaction in the patient with SCI (Gibson, 2003).

Sexual Dysfunction. Although it may not be a priority in the acute care phase post-SCI, the patient or partner may ask questions about sexual function after an injury to the spinal cord. Sexual function is still possible for all patients with SCI. Men may have reflexogenic erections, but very few men are able to ejaculate (Gibson, 2003). Fatherhood is a possibility because ejaculation can be stimulated and the sperm used to inseminate the partner. Men should be referred at some point to a urologist for information on new erectile and fertility treatments.

Approximately 50 to 70 percent of women with SCI are able to have an orgasm (Gibson, 2003). Menses may be disrupted for several months postinjury, but after menses return, pregnancy is still possible. The major risk these pregnant women face is autonomic dysreflexia that can occur during labor and delivery.

Evidence-Based Practice

- *Every step of the recovery process after SCI gives patients energy and direction for the future. Nurses need the skills to foster hope and enable recently spinal cord injured patients to look forward beyond the immediate situation and direct their energies appropriately (Lohne & Severinsson, 2004).*

- *Bladder filling sensation is present to some degree in incomplete SCI patients (especially with lesions below T10). When present, this sensation can prevent early emptying attempts, unnecessary catheterizations, and overdistention episodes (Ersoz & Akyuz, 2004).*

- *Urethral flora is a significant source for the development of urinary infections in SCI injury patients (Levendoglu et al., 2004).*

- *Venous thromboembolism is more likely to develop in SCI patients who are older, obese, and have flaccid paralysis or cancer. These patients should receive vigorous prophylaxis against venous thromboembolism (Green et al., 2003).*

Psychosocial Issues

Spinal cord injury changes the independent individual into a more dependent person. In the initial acute care phases, patients with SCI experience severe dependency, profound distress, and social isolation (Lohne, 2001). Recent nursing research has demonstrated these patients often have feelings of dispair that may dominate feelings of hope (Lohne & Severinsson, 2004). Therefore, patients tend to focus on the present concrete daily routines to avoid the unpleasant sensations of disappointment and uncertainty about the future (Lohne & Severinsson, 2004). Adaptation depends on personality, coping styles, and life experiences. Self-esteem, body image, and role performance are affected. Emotions may include fear of death, fear of living, anger, denial, and hopelessness. Educational level, employment status, income, and social support systems are factors associated with postinjury quality of life. The nurse encourages verbalization of feelings, and encourages the patient to take an active role in self-care activities and health care decisions. The family is included in these discussions. Referral to a local support group or professional counseling is also helpful.

Dysesthetic pain (referred to as phantom or central pain) is frequently experienced. This pain is described as a burning, stabbing pain aggravated by movement. It occurs within 1 year of injury and is more prevalent in paraplegic patients. Amitriptyline (Elavil), carbamazepine (Tegretol), and gabapentin (Neurontin) may be administered to relieve this pain. Tricyclic antidepressants (e.g., amitriptyline) increase the availability of serotonin.

Table 21–7 summarizes nursing care appropriate in the acute care phase for the patient with a spinal cord injury.

TABLE 21-7 High-Acuity Nursing Care of the Patient with a Spinal Cord Injury

NURSING DIAGNOSIS	EVALUATIVE CRITERIA	INTERVENTIONS
Ineffective airway clearance, impaired gas exchange, ineffective breathing patterns R/T diaphragm muscle paralysis	Normal ABGs Clear breath sounds Normal temperature Clear sputum Vital capacity 60 to 75 mL/kg Pulse oximetry greater than 90 percent	Assess respiratory rate and pattern, chest expansion, and breath sounds Quad assist cough Suction as needed Deep breaths, incentive spirometer Chest percussion Reposition frequently Administer oxygen therapy as ordered
Decreased cardiac output R/T impaired vasomotor tone	Heart rate greater than 50 beats/min Systolic blood pressure greater than 80 mm Hg Normal mentation All extremities warm with capillary refill less than 4 secs; 4+ pulses	Monitor vital signs Cardiac monitoring Assess intake and output Administer fluids, vasopressors as ordered Slowly elevate head of bed to prevent orthostatic hypotension
Risk for aspiration R/T paralytic ileus, loss of protective cough reflex	No emesis Clear breath sounds Normal temperature	Maintain patency of nasogastric tube Administer histamine blockers, proton pump inhibitors
Impaired urinary elimination R/T impaired reflex function	Less than 400 mL residual urine after voiding	Assess for bladder distention Begin intermittent catheterization when intake is less than 2 L/day
Impaired bowel elimination R/T impaired reflex function	Regular bowel elimination pattern of soft stool	Record bowel movements Adhere to bowel elimination schedule Administer stool softener
Risk for impaired skin integrity R/T decreased mobility, impaired bowel/bladder function	No evidence of skin breakdown	Determine need for specialized bed Turn frequently and regularly Inspect bed for foreign objects
Impaired adjustment, anxiety	Able to express feelings, concerns	Support patient and family Make appropriate referrals (social worker, chaplain)

SECTION FIVE REVIEW

1. Which of the following SCIs require long-term mechanical ventilation?
   A. C1-C2
   B. C6-C7
   C. T1-T5
   D. all patients with SCI require long-term mechanical ventilation

2. The main cause of complications or deaths post-SCI are related to
   A. sepsis
   B. respiratory complications
   C. autonomic dysreflexia
   D. bradycardia

3. TR is admitted to your unit with a C8 SCI. Which of the following statements is true about his recovery after this injury?
   A. he will be independent with eating
   B. he will be independent with dressing
   C. he will be independent in a manual wheelchair
   D. all of the above

4. Which of the following signs indicate autonomic dysreflexia?
   A. heart rate 60 beats per minute
   B. blood pressure 220/120
   C. priaprism
   D. poikilothermia

5. To prevent orthostatic hypotension, the nurse
   A. gradually increases the head of bed
   B. administers dopamine prn as ordered
   C. administers antihypertensives prn as ordered
   D. prevents constipation

6. AB has a T1 SCI. His wife asks you if they will ever have sexual relations again. What is the most appropriate response?
   A. he will never be able to have an erection
   B. he can have an erection, but he will be infertile
   C. sexual function is still possible
   D. they will never have sexual relations again

Answers: 1. A, 2. B, 3. D, 4. B, 5. A, 6. C

SECTION SIX: Seizure Disorders

At the completion of this section, the learner will be able to define seizure and epilepsy; state the manifestations of simple partial seizure, complex partial seizure, absence generalized seizure, and tonic-clonic generalized seizure and discuss the nursing and pharmacologic management of seizure disorders.

A **seizure** is an excessive, uncontrolled discharge of electrical activity from the brain. **Epilepsy** (or seizure disorder) is the term used to denote a condition of reoccurring seizures. People with epilepsy have intermittent seizures that occur over days, weeks, or years. In high acuity patients, seizures may occur as a result of an acute febrile state, or a metabolic disorder such as hypoglycemia or syndrome inappropriate antidiuretic hormone (refer to Module 20), as a result of a pathological process (infection, brain tumors, cerebral circulation alterations, or head trauma). In general, seizures are classified based on the clinical location of onset: partial (focal or local) and generalized.

Partial Seizures

Seizures are classified into those that only affect part of the brain and those that affect a generalized area of the brain. **Partial seizures** involve the activation of a restricted part of one hemisphere of the brain. Partial seizures are further classified as simple partial seizures if there is no impairment of consciousness during the seizure or complex partial seizure if there is impaired consciousness.

Manifestations of a simple partial seizure depend on the activated area of the brain. Patients may experience alterations in motor or sensory function. Motor alterations occur as a result of activation of a portion of the motor cortex of the brain, which causes muscle contractions on the contralateral side of the body. This typically occurs in the face or a hand. The motor activity may be confined to one area or it may spread to adjacent muscles. A seizure that begins in one area and spreads sequentially to adjacent muscles is called a Jacksonian seizure. Multisystem alterations occur when there are disruptions in the autonomic nervous system during partial or generalized seizure activity, such as hypotension or hypertension, tachycardia or bradycardia, and urinary or bowel incontinence.

A complex partial seizure is characterized by impaired consciousness and repetitive activities (lip smacking). It may be several hours after the seizure before the patient regains full consciousness, and patients typically experience amnesia.

Generalized Seizures

Generalized seizures involve deep brain structures on both hemispheres. There are two major types of generalized seizures: absence (non-convulsive) and tonic-clonic (convulsive). Absence seizures are characterized by a blank stare, impaired consciousness, and cessation of movement of brief duration. If preceded by an aura (a sensation that often involves visual, taste, or olfactory hallucinations) a tonic-clonic seizure is classified as a partial onset generalized seizure. When there is no aura, a tonic-clonic seizure is classified as generalized. The patient then loses consciousness, falls to the ground, and sharp rhythmic muscle contractions occur. This is known as the tonic phase (Fig. 21–9A). Muscles are rigid, neck is hyperextended, and all extremities are extended. Incontinence of urine or feces can occur. Breathing ceases and cyanosis may develop—depending on how long the apnea is, typically 10 to 15 seconds. The clonic phase is characterized by the return of breathing—in fact the patient is now hyperventilating. Muscles contract and relax (Fig. 21–9B). This phase gradually subsides. The

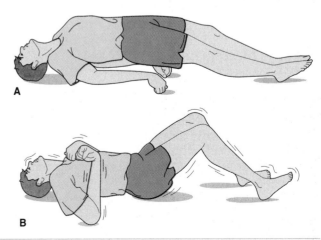

Figure 21–9 ■ Tonic-clonic seizures. *A.* Tonic phase. *B.* Clonic phase.

entire tonic-clonic seizure typically lasts about a minute. The phase following the clonic phase is known as the **postictal period.** During this time the patient remains unconscious but is relaxed and breathing quietly. The patient gradually regains consciousness but has amnesia. Confusion, disorientation, fatigue, and headaches may also occur. The real danger to patients who have these types of seizures is the risk of injury when they lose consciousness in the tonic phase. That means whatever the patient is doing at the time ceases: driving a car, walking down stairs, sitting on the toilet, and so on. Patients with these types of seizures are at risk for injury when they fall during the tonic phase.

Status Epilepticus

Status epilepticus is a neurological emergency with potentially lethal consequences if left untreated or if treatment is delayed. It is defined as a continuous series of seizures without recovery or regaining consciousness between attacks. It occurs as a result of untreated or inadequately treated seizures and most commonly occurs from abrupt cessation of pharmacologic treatment. The continuous series of seizures causes ischemic brain damage because of impaired respirations, producing anoxia. Therefore, immediate control of the seizures and maintaining a patent airway are critical interventions.

Pharmacologic Management

Anticonvulsant therapy reduces or controls seizure activity, but it does not cure a seizure disorder. Drug therapy is based on the type of seizure and is introduced in gradually increasing doses until a therapeutic drug level is achieved. Several drugs may be tried before the most effective drug is identified. Some common anticonvulsants include phenytoin, phenobarbital, and carbamazepine. Serum drug levels are monitored to ensure therapeutic levels are reached—not toxic levels. If the patient remains seizure free for 2 years and has a normal electroencephalogram, therapy may be discontinued. Cessation of the drug is titrated in decreasing doses.

Nursing Management

The goals of nursing management of the patient with seizures are to protect the patient from injury, to control the seizure, and to provide patient and family teaching. Any patient with the potential for seizure activity is placed on seizure precautions which include padding the bedrails, keeping the bedrails up, placing suction equipment at the bedside, and keeping the bed in the lowest position.

Observation and documentation of the events surrounding the seizure that are important to identify include the type of

TABLE 21–8   What to Note and Document about a Seizure Event

- Time seizure began and ended
- Patient status before the seizure
- Description of the seizure
    - Type of motor movement
    - Parts of the body involved
- Level of consciousness before, during, and after the seizure
- Pupil response and pupil deviation
- Was the patient incontinent or diaphoretic?
- Any complication during the seizure
    - Apnea or cyanosis?
- Vital signs after the seizure including pulse oximetry
- Postictal status
    - Sensory and motor status
    - Neurological sign
    - Behavior such as confusion, headache, drowsiness

seizure and the patient's response to the interventions (Table 21–8). Level of consciousness immediately before, during, and after the seizure is recorded. The time elapsed between the onset and cessation of seizure activity; the type of motor activity; and any complications, such as aspiration or apnea, are also noted. The nurse has an important role in educating the patient and family in the management of seizure disorders. Teaching includes medication protocols (including side effects and adverse reactions), recognizing seizure activity, activity restrictions, and acute management.

Care of the patient includes ensuring appropriate IV access. An infusion bag of normal saline is readily available. Medications may include lorazepam (Ativan) or diazepam (Valium) to stop the motor movement. A complication of the administration of diazepam is respiratory depression, which may necessitate intubation and mechanical ventilation. Patients who receive phenytoin require cardiac monitoring to detect arrhythmias.

Nursing care includes all of the previously discussed information regarding seizure management. In addition, the patient's vital signs and pulse oximetry are obtained. Oxygen is administered and the patient is suctioned as needed. Blood is obtained for glucose levels, electrolytes, and therapeutic levels of anticonvulsants.

In summary, seizures are classified as partial or generalized. Partial seizures may be simple or complex. Generalized seizures involve a loss of consciousness and can be either absence or tonic-clonic seizures. Status epilepticus is a neurological emergency. Seizures cannot be cured, but they can be managed with pharmacologic therapy. Anticonvulsants are used for acute and long-term management. Acute nursing management includes protecting the patient from injury and observing and documenting the seizure activity.

SECTION SIX REVIEW

1. You are the nurse caring for TY who has a closed-head injury. He has a GCS of 5. While giving him a bath, you note rhythmic contractions in his left hand. These contractions sequentially spread up his left arm. This seizure is called
   A. simple partial seizure
   B. complex partial seizure
   C. petit mal seizure
   D. tonic-clonic seizure
2. Which of the following drugs may be used as an anticonvulsant?
   A. phenytoin
   B. phenobarbital
   C. carbamazepine
   D. all of the above
3. An important nursing implication for patients experiencing seizure activity is
   A. the potential for aspiration
   B. restraining the patient until the seizure has abated
   C. the drug of choice for seizure control is mannitol
   D. checking the pupils for size, reactivity, and symmetry at 1-minute intervals until the seizure activity has stopped

Answers: 1. A, 2. D, 3. A

POSTTEST

1. A diagnosis of unstable SCI is made based on
   A. disruption of two or more of the spinal columns
   B. degree of sensory involvement
   C. presence of associated hemodynamic changes
   D. degree of flaccid paralysis present
2. The corticospinal tract originates in the brain and innervates the
   A. peripheral sensory neurons
   B. opposite side of the body
   C. parasympathetic nervous system
   D. sympathetic nervous system
3. A lower motor neuron lesion results in
   A. permanent loss of bladder function
   B. flaccid paralysis
   C. contralateral motor effects
   D. spastic paralysis
4. Which of the following is an example of an incomplete spinal cord injury?
   A. paraplegia
   B. quadraplegia
   C. tetraplegia
   D. Brown-Sequard syndrome
5. A sudden deceleration of the head in a head-on collision can produce which of the following injuries to the spinal cord?
   A. hyperflexion
   B. hyperextension
   C. rotation
   D. axial loading
6. Which of the following radiographic tests may be needed to diagnose a ligament injury?
   A. lateral x-ray
   B. CT scan
   C. MRI
   D. SEP
7. Moving the big toe up and down and asking the patient to confirm the direction assesses
   A. priapism
   B. proprioception
   C. dermatomes
   D. sensation
8. A spinal cord injury cannot be accurately classified until the resolution of
   A. spinal shock
   B. neurogenic shock
   C. autonomic dysreflexia
   D. priapism
9. Which of the following is not an external fixation device used for stabilizing a SCI?
   A. halo device
   B. Gardner-Wells tongs
   C. Vinke cervical tongs
   D. cervical rods
10. Which of the following is an external fixation device that is secured with four pins inserted into the skull?
    A. Gardner-Wells tongs
    B. halo device
    C. clam shell
    D. Jewett orthosis

11. Which of the following interventions is contraindicated for the patient in a halo vest?
    A. pull the vest's struts to move the patient up in bed
    B. inspect the pins for security
    C. perform pin care per unit protocol
    D. turn the patient every 2 hours
12. The patient with a SCI is at risk for developing decreased cardiac output related to
    A. orthostatic hypertension
    B. neurogenic shock
    C. venous pooling
    D. all of the above
13. Which of the following statements accurately describes autonomic dysreflexia?
    A. it is a spastic disorder limiting mobility
    B. it is a cardiovascular problem produced by decreased cardiac output secondary to bradycardia
    C. it is a vasoconstrictive problem produced by excessive sympathetic nervous system stimulation
    D. it is a parasympathetic nervous system problem resulting from unopposed vasodilation
14. When assessing a patient's ability to cope with a SCI, which of the following is the most important factor to assess?
    A. income
    B. education
    C. age
    D. social support system
15. What typically happens after a tonic-clonic seizure? The patient
    A. is incontinent
    B. fully regains consciousness
    C. remains unconscious, is relaxed, and breathing quietly
    D. hyperventilates
16. Anticonvulsant therapy is typically discontinued when
    A. the patient is seizure free for 2 years
    B. the patient is seizure free for 1 year
    C. the EKG is normal
    D. serum drug levels have reached a therapeutic level
17. Which of the following nursing interventions is important when caring for a patient with a seizure disorder?
    A. pad the bedrails
    B. keep the bedrails up
    C. keep the bed in the lowest position
    D. all of the above

POSTTEST ANSWERS

Question	Answer	Section
1	A	One
2	B	One
3	B	Two
4	D	Two
5	A	Two
6	C	Three
7	B	Three
8	A	Three
9	D	Four

Question	Answer	Section
10	B	Four
11	A	Four
12	D	Five
13	C	Five
14	D	Five
15	C	Six
16	A	Six
17	D	Six

REFERENCES

American Association of Neurological Surgeons. (2002). Guidelines for the management of acute cervical spine injury. *Neurosurgery, 50*(3, suppl), S1–S84.

Barker, E., & Saulino, M. (2002). First ever guidelines for spinal cord injury. *RN, 65*(10), 32–37.

Bracke, M. B., Shepard, M. J., Holford, T. R., et al. (1997). Administration of methylprednisolone for 24–48 hours or triliazid mesylate for 48 hours in the treatment of acute spinal cord injury: Results of the third National Acute Spinal Cord Injury Randomized Clinical Trial. *JAMA: Journal of the American Medical Association, 277*, 1597–1604.

Cook, N. (2003). Respiratory care in spinal cord injury with associated traumatic brain injury: Bridging the gap in critical care nursing interventions. *Intensive & Critical Care Nursing, 19*(3), 143–53.

Dubendorf, P. (1999). Spinal cord injury pathophysiology. *Critical Care Nurse Quarterly, 22*(2), 31–39.

Dyson-Hudson, T. A., & Stein, A. B. (1999). Acute management of traumatic cervical spine injury. *Mount Sinai Journal of Medicine, 66*, 170–178.

Ersoz, M., & Akyuz, M. (2004). Bladder filling sensation in patients with spinal cord injury and the potential for sensory dependent bladder emptying. *Spinal Cord, 42*, 110–116.

Gibson, K. L. (2003). Caring for a patient who lives with a spinal cord injury. *Nursing, 33*(7), 36–41.

Green, D., Hartwig, D., Chen, D., et al. (2003). Spinal cord injury risk assessment for thromboembolism. *American Journal of Physical Medicine and Rehabilitation, 82,* 950–956.

Hedger, A. (2002). Action stat: Spinal cord injury. *Nursing, 32*(12), 96.

Hickey, J. V. (2003). *Neurological and neurosurgical nursing.* Philadelphia: Lippincott Williams & Wilkins.

Karlet, M. C. (2001). Acute management of the patient with spinal cord injury. *International Journal of Trauma Nursing, 7*(2), 43–8.

Lanig, I. S., & Peterson, W. (2000). The respiratory system in spinal cord injury. *Physical Medicine and Rehabilitation Clinics of North America, 11*(1), 29–43.

Levendoglu, F., Ugurlu, H., Uzerbil, U. M., et al. (2004). Urethral cultures in patients with spinal cord injury. *Spinal Cord, 42,* 106–109.

Lohne, V. (2001). Hope in spinal cord injury patients: A literature review related to nursing. *Journal of Neuroscience Nursing, 33*(6), 317–326.

Lohne, V., & Severinsson, E. (2004). Hope during the first few months after acute spinal cord injury. *Journal of Advanced Nursing, 47,* 279–286.

Papadopoulos, S. M. (2003). Emergent treatment of acute spinal cord injuries: Current treatment. *Barrows Quarterly, 19*(3), 24–27.

Siroky, M. B. (2002). Pathogenesis of bacteriuria and infection in the spinal cord injured patient. *American Journal of Medicine, 113,* 67S–79S.

MODULE

22 Nursing Care of the Patient with an Alteration in Cerebral Tissue Perfusion

Karen L. Johnson, Pamela Stinson Kidd

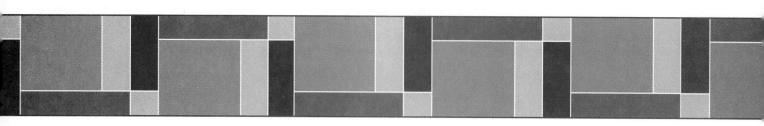

> **OBJECTIVES**   Following completion of this module, the learner will be able to
>
> 1. Describe appropriate nursing assessment data to collect for a patient experiencing a change in consciousness.
> 2. Identify relationships among patient symptoms, clinical signs, and pathophysiology for a patient experiencing a brain attack.
> 3. Cluster assessment data to formulate nursing diagnoses associated with brain attack.
> 4. Identify priorities in care for a patient with brain attack.
> 5. Explain rationale for nursing actions that prevent complications associated with brain attack.

Module 22 is designed to integrate the major points discussed in Modules 18 and 19. This module summarizes relationships between key concepts and assists the learner in clustering information to facilitate clinical application. Content is applied in an interactive learning style. The learner is encouraged to identify nursing actions based on an assessment of a patient in a case study format. Consequences of selecting a particular action are discussed and the rationale for correct actions is presented. The last part focuses on nursing challenges in caring for a patient with an acute brain attack in the acute care phase.

GLOSSARY

aphasia   Total inability to understand or formulate language.
computed tomography (CT)   Directed use of x-ray beams to determine the presence of normal versus abnormal anatomic structures through computerized measurement of the attenuation of the beams based on density of structures.

dysarthria   Impairment of the muscles that control speech.
dysphasia   Difficulty comprehending, speaking, or writing.

ABBREVIATIONS

aPTT	Activated partial thromboplastin time	**DVT**	Deep-vein thrombosis
BUN	Blood urea nitrogen	**ECG**	Electrocardiogram
CBC	Complete blood count	**ED**	Emergency department
CHI	Closed-head injury	**EEG**	Electroencephalogram
CT	Computed tomography	**GCS**	Glasgow Coma Scale

ICU	Intensive care unit
INR	International normalized ratio
IV	Intravenous
LOC	Level of consciousness
LP	Lumbar puncture
MVC	Motor vehicle crash
O_2	Oxygen

PT	Prothrombin time
rtPA	Tissue plasminogen activator
SpO_2	Saturation of oxygen in arterial blood as measured by a pulse oximeter
SIADH	Syndrome of inappropriate antidiuretic hormone
TIA	Transient ischemic attack

Case Study

A CASE OF ALTERED CEREBRAL TISSUE PERFUSION

E.C. is brought to the emergency department (ED) after being involved in a minor motor vehicle crash (MVC). She was alert and oriented at the scene, according to the person who was involved in the crash with her, but as the police officer was completing the crash report, E.C. became disoriented, her speech became slurred, and she was unable to walk because of "weakness in her legs." An ambulance was called and she was transported to the ED.

Initial Appraisal

You are on duty in the ED when E.C. arrives. E.C. received O_2 in route through a nonrebreather mask. She has an intravenous (IV) line in place with lactated Ringer's infusing at a keep-vein-open rate. Her vital signs are blood pressure 164/100, pulse rate 76 (irregular), temperature 98°F. SpO_2 is 92 percent. The police officer is asking for a blood alcohol level to be drawn because of her behavior at the scene.

Focused Assessment

You proceed with your nursing assessment. She responds to questions, but you cannot always tell what she is saying because of her slurred speech. She denies chest or back pain. She can spontaneously move her left extremities but not her right extremities. Her pupils are unequal in dilation (left greater than right), but both are reactive to light. Her Glasgow Coma Scale (GCS) score is 14. You place her on the cardiac monitor and she is in atrial fibrillation. The O_2 is continued at 100 percent by way of nonrebreather mask. Her breath sounds are clear. There are no extra heart sounds but she does have a pulse deficit (apical rate is greater than peripheral pulse rate).

Focused Nursing History

Meanwhile, E.C.'s family arrives. They tell you that she has been in good health. She is 74 years old and weighs 170 pounds. She has a history of hypertension and type II diabetes mellitus. She has been recently treated for an irregular heartbeat. The family does not know the exact names of the medications E.C. is taking. They are looking for her purse in hopes the medications are inside. As far as they know, she does not have any medication allergies. They say she has no history of alcohol abuse. She had what the family describes as "ministrokes" about 2 years ago without residual neurologic deficit. At this point, it may be necessary to place a call to E.C.'s primary physician to get an accurate medical history.

QUESTION

Based on the assessment data you collected thus far, which of the following factors could be the source of E.C.'s neurological symptoms?

A. alcohol
B. closed-head injury
C. irregular heartbeat
D. brain attack
E. hypoglycemia
F. hyperglycemia
G. use of anticoagulant medications
H. hypertension

ANSWER

Factors that should be considered are (B) closed-head injury, (C) irregular heartbeat, (D) brain attack, (E) hypoglycemia, (F) hyperglycemia, and (G) use of anticoagulant medications.

CLOSED-HEAD INJURY. You check the prehospital run sheet or speak with the police officer to determine whether E.C. was wearing a seat belt, to discover the estimated speed at the time of the crash, and to find out about the damage to the vehicle. These factors interact in determining severity of injury. In this case, E.C. was restrained, the crash occurred at an intersection at an estimated 30 miles per hour, and the major damage was to the passenger side of the vehicle. The windshield was not broken; she was not ejected. Therefore, the likelihood of a closed-head injury (CHI) is low.

IRREGULAR HEARTBEAT. E.C. is currently in atrial fibrillation. This means her atria are not completely emptying with each contraction. Therefore, as blood pools in the atria, emboli can form and, if ejected, through the aorta, can produce a brain attack. Her medication history is important. An irregular heartbeat may not be problematic if she is anticoagulated. Her family informs you that she was recently treated for this irregular heartbeat. Because the irregular rhythm continues, you question whether she was taking the medication appropriately or if she is experiencing an acute cardiac event (such as a conduction disorder, conduction block, or myocardial ischemia). The fact that she has no chest or back pain, no extra heart sounds, breath sounds are clear, and a pulse deficit supports the atrial fibrillation rhythm and the fact that left ventricular dysfunction has not occurred as a result of a primary cardiac event. However, to be certain, a 12-lead electrocardiogram (ECG) is obtained.

BRAIN ATTACK. E.C. has several modifiable risk factors for stroke. She is obese, and has a history of diabetes mellitus, hypertension, and irregular heartbeat. The new onset of the irregular heartbeat may have been the final precipitating factor to producing a thrombus. Her age is a nonmodifiable risk factor for stroke. She may have experienced transient ischemic attacks (TIAs) based on her family's description. You ask her family if E.C.'s parents or siblings have had strokes because this is another nonmodifiable risk factor.

HYPOGLYCEMIA. The likelihood of hypo- or hyperglycemia to the degree that it produces a change in level of consciousness (LOC) is less in type II diabetics than in type I diabetics. However, if E.C. took her oral hypoglycemic drug inappropriately (assuming she is on this type of medication) and she did not eat prior to the MVC, these factors combined with the stress of being involved in an MVC may have produced hypoglycemia. However, her sensory and motor symptoms are unilateral. She is alert. She is not diaphoretic. Therefore, hypoglycemia is considered as a possible cause and a bedside glucose measurement obtained, but it is less likely than other precipitating causes already discussed.

HYPERGLYCEMIA. E.C. is not flushed. She is not diaphoretic. She does not have symptoms of diabetic ketoacidosis (Kussmaul respirations, uremia, loss of consciousness). Hyperglycemia is an unlikely cause of her symptoms but, as stated previously, because of her history of type II diabetes, a bedside glucose measurement is obtained.

USE OF ANTICOAGULANT MEDICATIONS. Elderly patients are more likely to experience subdural hematomas as a form of CHI because of less pliable vessels and more space between the dura and the skull. This risk is greater if the patient is anticoagulated. It would be helpful to discover the medications E.C. is taking to determine whether she is taking any anticoagulants. You also try to determine E.C.'s use of aspirin and nonsteroidal anti-inflammatory agents as over-the-counter drugs.

The following diagnostic tests are ordered:

- Noncontrast computed tomography (CT) of the brain
- Cerebral angiography
- Complete blood count (CBC)
- Chest x-ray
- Comprehensive metabolic profile
- Platelet count

- Prothrombin time (PT)
- Activated partial thromboplastin time (aPTT)
- International normalized ratio (INR)
- ECG

Quick Review

What is the rationale for ordering these tests on E.C.?

CT OF THE BRAIN. Recall from Module 19, patients thought to be having a stroke require prompt triage. The goal is to quickly determine whether the stroke is ischemic or hemorrhagic. A CT of the brain is performed urgently to differentiate hemorrhagic from ischemic causes.

CEREBRAL ANGIOGRAPHY. The cereberal angiography procedure evaluates vessel structures, vasospasm, or stenosis.

CBC. A CBC provides the baseline measurement of hemoglobin and hematocrit. Although she was restrained and appears to have no acute injuries from the MVC, it is possible, though not likely, that internal bleeding may be present.

CHEST X-RAY. A chest x-ray will rule out congestive heart failure, aortic aneurysm, or pulmonary malignancy that could complicate treatment.

COMPREHENSIVE METABOLIC PROFILE. A comprehensive metabolic profile assesses electrolyte levels, liver enzymes, glucose level, and renal function. Hypo- or hyperkalemia can contribute to an irregular heartbeat. Liver and renal function are important to assess prior to administration of anticoagulants. Hyperglycemia (if acute) can increase lactic acid production and contribute to greater brain damage with ischemia.

PLATELET COUNT, PT, aPTT, AND INR LEVELS. These labs detect any coagulopathies and establish baselines for therapy.

ECG. An ECG detects myocardial ischemia. A myocardial infarction alters the tissue plasminogen activator (rtPA) administration procedure (see Module 19).

QUESTION

The physician did not order an electroencephalogram (EEG) or lumbar puncture (LP). Do you think you should call the physician and ask her whether these tests were overlooked? Or is there a good reason why these tests may not have been ordered?

ANSWER

These tests may not need to be ordered. An LP helps diagnose increased intracranial pressure and subarachnoid hemorrhage. E.C.'s GCS score is 14. Her pupils are reactive to light. She has a history that supports a gradual onset of symptoms. Her sensory and motor symptoms are unilateral and more consistent with an ischemic, rather than a hemorrhagic, stroke. An EEG will not give any additional information that will alter treatment. An EEG is helpful in diagnosing seizure activity. She did not experience a seizure today and has a negative history for seizures. Seizure activity is more consistent with a hemorrhagic stroke.

The results of some of the diagnostic tests are back. E.C.'s CBC and platelets are normal. Her PT, aPTT, and INR are at the high end of normal values. Her glucose is 140 mg/dL. Electrolytes are normal. Liver enzymes, blood urea nitrogen (BUN), and creatinine are normal. The chest x-ray shows a slightly enlarged heart without pulmonary edema. The CT scan reveals an increased density on the left, indicating infarction. There is no evidence of hemorrhage. Her ECG is negative for ischemia. She remains in an atrial rhythm and tachycardic.

QUESTION

It has now been 3 hours since the onset of E.C.'s symptoms. Is she a candidate for rtPA administration?

ANSWER

This is a difficult question. Her stroke could be the result of emboli (from atrial fibrillation) or thrombosis (from her history of TIAs, diabetes, and obesity). Both are classified as ischemic in nature and therefore she is technically eligible for treatment with rtPA. The exact onset of E.C.'s symptoms is known. She could receive rtPA because it is within the 3-hour timeline. However, we are not sure that she meets all of the screening criteria. Although her PT and aPTT are normal now, she may have taken large doses of nonsteroidal anti-inflammatory drugs or aspirin, which could precipitate bleeding post rtPA administration. More importantly, the CT scan shows evidence of infarction or necrosis even though it was less than 3 hours from the onset of symptoms. Because of these factors, the physician decides not to administer rtPA.

Development of Nursing Diagnoses

E.C. continues to receive 100 percent O_2. She received 325 mg of aspirin. Her IV fluids are changed to 0.45 NS at 60 mL/hr. A urinary catheter is placed, with an immediate output of 350 mL. She receives a loading dose of digitalis IV. She is admitted to the high-acuity unit to monitor for post-stroke complications. The next priority is to develop a plan of care based on the data collected.

CLUSTER 1

Subjective data. History of TIAs, diabetes, obesity, acute onset of slurred speech, unilateral weakness; denies chest or back pain.

Objective data. GCS score on arrival is 14. Pupils unequal but reactive to light. Weakness in right extremities. CT scan shows left cerebral infarction. ECG shows atrial fibrillation. Hyperglycemic.

Cluster 2

Subjective data. History of irregular heartbeat; denies chest or back pain.

Objective data. Pulse deficit, no extra heart sounds, breath sounds clear, chest x-ray and ECG consistent with slight cardiomegaly without acute cardiac ischemia or pulmonary edema. Spo_2 adequate.

All of the following nursing diagnoses apply to E.C.:

Alteration in cerebral tissue perfusion
Alteration in urinary elimination
Impaired physical mobility
Impaired verbal communication
Risk for ineffective airway clearance
Risk for decreased cardiac output
Altered peripheral tissue perfusion
Risk for fluid volume imbalance
Risk for ineffective individual coping
Risk for ineffective family coping
Risk for injury
Unilateral neglect
Risk for impaired skin integrity
Risk for impaired swallowing
Bathing/hygiene self-care deficit
Dressing/grooming self-care deficit
Risk for altered nutrition

QUESTION

Based on the three clusters of assessment data, which nursing diagnoses should be the priority focus during the high-acuity nursing phase?

ANSWER

Alteration in cerebral tissue perfusion (supported by cluster 1)
Risk for decreased cardiac output (supported by cluster 2)
Independent nursing interventions in the high-acuity phase should focus on the preceding nursing diagnoses.

ALTERED CEREBRAL TISSUE PERFUSION. As you recall from the pathophysiology of a stroke, cerebral edema occurs secondary to cellular membrane destruction and intracellular contents moving into the interstitial space. Ischemia begins this process. It is critical to assess minor changes in neurological status in order to prevent additional ischemia. Changes in LOC, pupillary reaction, and sensory and motor function are signs of cerebral edema and increased intracranial pressure, as well as damaged neurons. Enhancing cerebral oxygenation through maintenance of airway patency, supplemental oxygen, and elevation of the head of the bed all help cerebral perfusion.

RISK FOR DECREASED CARDIAC OUTPUT. The nurse promotes cardiac output by maintaining blood pressure and heart rate within an acceptable range. Medications are used to support these vital signs (i.e., calcium channel blocking agents such as verapamil, cardiac glycosides such as digitalis; see collaborative nursing interventions in the next section). A change in LOC may indicate a change in cardiac output and not a primary cerebral event. Promoting oxygenation decreases myocardial ischemia and prevents angina.

ALTERED PERIPHERAL TISSUE PERFUSION, IMPAIRED SKIN INTEGRITY. Sensory changes in the affected extremities and altered mobility put E.C. at risk for pressure ulcers. Vascular tone is disrupted to the extremity, encouraging pooling of blood and supporting the development of deep-vein thrombosis (DVT) and pressure ulcers. E.C. must be repositioned every 2 hours. E.C. is reminded to shift her weight with her unaffected arm once she is not on bedrest. Assess the skin for pallor, pulses, temperature, and capillary refill. Assess for the presence of Homan's sign in both lower extremities.

Later, when E.C. is less acute, the risk of increased intracranial pressure is low, and the risk of additional strokes is minimized, nursing care expands to address the following nursing diagnoses.

RISK FOR INJURY. The components for normal balance are vision, proprioception, and vestibular function, and at least two of these must be intact to adequately maintain balance. Poststroke postural asymmetry, leaning or falling to the hemiparetic side, and the inability to use protective righting reflexes when the center of gravity is displaced contribute to injury.

IMPAIRED PHYSICAL MOBILITY. Proper body alignment is important to prevent contractures. This would include supporting E.C.'s shoulders to prevent adduction. Use trochanter rolls to prevent hip rotation as well as foot supports. Her fingers and hands should be placed in anatomical alignment.

Active or passive ROM exercises performed three to four times daily prevents contractures and loss of muscle strength. E.C. is taught to exercise the affected extremities by using the unaffected arm to move the affected extremities. E.C. is encouraged to use the affected arm in bathing, eating, and grooming.

RISK FOR INEFFECTIVE INDIVIDUAL COPING AND INEFFECTIVE FAMILY COPING. Depression frequently occurs poststroke. Appropriate information is provided so that E.C. understands treatment goals and probabilities of outcomes. Clergy, friends, family members, and support groups are encouraged to provide comfort and support. To maximize E.C.'s independence, she is involved in decision making and activities of daily living.

IMPAIRED VERBAL COMMUNICATION. E.C.'s stroke involves her left hemisphere, the center for speech and language in 95 percent of people. Thus, she may experience **aphasia** and **dysphasia.** She is already experiencing **dysarthria** as evidenced by her slurred speech. Speak slowly, praise any attempt she makes to communicate, and help her to use gestures, facial expressions, and visual/tactile communication boards.

RISK FOR ALTERED URINARY ELIMINATION. Without a more definitive description of the type of stroke E.C. has experienced, it is impossible to anticipate the exact voiding problems she may have. However, once the urinary catheter is removed, she may experience functional incontinence because of difficulty getting to the bathroom and performing toileting in a timely manner as a result of change in mobility and balance. She may not be able to verbally convey the need to go to the bathroom. Developing a schedule wherein the nurse consistently assesses E.C.'s need to void and provides her with an opportunity to void will help her regain bladder control.

Collaborative Nursing Interventions

HYPERGLYCEMIA CONTROL. Insulin may be ordered if E.C.'s blood sugar continues to rise. Oral hypoglycemic agents may also be used.

ATRIAL FIBRILLATION CONTROL AND DVT PREVENTION. Beta blockers may be administered in addition to digitalis. Low molecular weight heparin may be administered to prevent DVT and to inhibit clot propagation. Coumadin will be started prior to hospital discharge.

ADMINISTRATION OF IV FLUIDS. The IV fluid E.C. is receiving is her only source of fluid intake at the present time. If secondary damage to the pituitary gland or hypothalamus occurs as a result of cerebral edema or extension of the stroke, syndrome of inappropriate antidiuretic hormone (SIADH) may result. If SIADH occurs, fluids need to be restricted. At the present time E.C.'s stroke is ischemic in nature and relatively confined according to the CT scan. Thus, the probability of SIADH is low. In her case, prevention of dehydration is paramount because dehydration promotes increased blood viscosity and a greater likelihood of thrombosis.

DESIRED PATIENT OUTCOMES IN THE HIGH-ACUITY PHASE. Desired patient outcomes for patients in the high-acuity phase poststroke are (1) intracranial pressure within normal limits as evidenced by no change in neurologic status, no vomiting, and no headache; (2) blood pressure and heart rate in expected range, no new dysrhythmia, and no angina; (3) peripheral pulses remain strong and symmetrical, no peripheral edema, skin color normal without streaks, and temperature of extremities warm and symmetrical.

Summary

In summary, this module has focused on the nursing care of the brain attack patient during the high-acuity phase. For the purposes of the case presented, potential injuries from the MVC were not explored because injury is the focus of other modules.

Rather, assessment of the patient with a suspected brain attack, diagnostic tests, and nursing diagnoses and interventions were presented.

PART
6
Metabolic

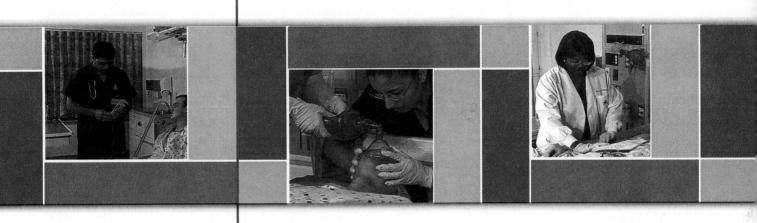

MODULE 23 | Metabolic Responses to Stress

MODULE 24 | Acute Hematologic Dysfunction

MODULE 25 | Altered Immune Function

MODULE 26 | Organ Transplantation

MODULE 27 | Altered Glucose Metabolism

MODULE 28 | Acute Renal Dysfunction

MODULE 29 | Nursing Care of the Patient with Altered Metabolic Function

Metabolic Responses to Stress

Valerie Sabol, Theresa Loan

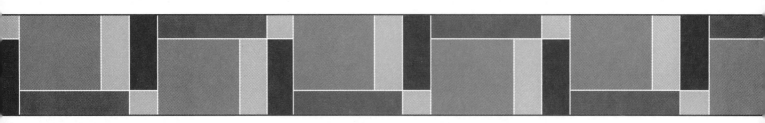

OBJECTIVES   Following completion of this module, the learner will be able to

1. Describe normal nutrition.
2. Explain basic normal metabolism.
3. Describe the focused nutritional/metabolic assessment.
4. Recognize the typical metabolic alterations in the high-acuity/critically ill patient.
5. Describe the major nutritional alterations associated with specific disease states.

6. Describe the enteral methods used to provide nutrition for the high-acuity patient, including potential complications.
7. Discuss the parenteral methods used to provide nutrition for the high-acuity ill patient, including potential complications.

This self-study module focuses on the metabolic responses that occur in the high-acuity patient. The module is composed of seven sections. Section One describes the concept of nutrition, including macronutrients—carbohydrates, proteins, and lipids. Section Two provides an overview of normal metabolism. Section Three explains the interpretation of physiologic and laboratory data pertinent to nutritional assessment of the high-acuity patient. Common metabolic alterations encountered in high-acuity patients are discussed in Section Four, whereas Section Five presents an

overview of nutritional needs of patients with specific disease processes. The module concludes with a discussion of methods of nutrient delivery in Sections Six and Seven. Each section includes a set of review questions to help the learner evaluate his or her understanding of the section's content before moving on to the next section. All Section Reviews and the module Pretest and Posttest include answers. It is suggested that the learner review those concepts answered incorrectly in the review questions before proceeding to the next section.

 PRETEST

1. The metabolic stress response is the result of
   A. psychologic stress
   B. overexertion from exercise
   C. injured tissue in the body
   D. hyperventilation
2. The two phases of the metabolic stress response are
   A. ebb phase and catabolic phase
   B. ebb phase and flow phase

   C. ebb phase and recovery phase
   D. flow phase and recovery phase
3. Hypermetabolism refers to
   A. an elevated metabolic rate
   B. the breakdown of total body protein
   C. elevated serum insulin levels
   D. increased immunoglobulins

4. Hypercatabolism refers to
   A. an elevated metabolic rate
   B. the breakdown of total body protein
   C. elevated serum insulin levels
   D. increased immunoglobulins

5. Enteral nutrition has many advantages over total parenteral nutrition (TPN), including the fact that it (choose all that apply)
   1. reduces risk for bacterial translocation
   2. provides central venous access
   3. maintains gut morphology and function
   4. is less costly
   A. 2 and 4
   B. 1, 3, and 4
   C. 2 and 3
   D. 1, 2, and 3

6. Which nutrient does a person's body use as the "preferred" energy source?
   A. intact proteins
   B. amino acids
   C. carbohydrates
   D. lipids

7. Feeding tube occlusion is a potential mechanical complication of enteral feedings. Possible causes of occlusion include (choose all that apply)
   1. viscous formulas
   2. lack of proper flushing
   3. food coloring
   4. medications
   A. 2, 3, and 4
   B. 1 and 2
   C. 1, 2, and 4
   D. 3 and 4

8. Which condition is a complication associated with intragastric tube feeding?
   A. nosocomial pneumonia
   B. bacterial translocation
   C. stress ulcer
   D. metabolic acidosis

9. Total parenteral nutrition is indicated when
   A. adequate amounts of nutrients cannot be delivered through the gastrointestinal tract
   B. the patient is hypermetabolic
   C. bowel sounds are not audible
   D. the hypercatabolic patient is not able to eat for 3 days

10. Total parenteral nutrition with glucose concentration greater than 10 percent should be administered through a
    A. nasoenteric feeding tube
    B. peripheral vein
    C. surgically placed jejunal feeding tube
    D. central vein

11. Catheter-related sepsis is a potentially lethal complication of total parenteral nutrition and is primarily caused by
    A. a malpositioned catheter or guidewire during the central line insertion
    B. lack of sterility during central line placement and inadequate maintenance of the line
    C. inadvertent puncture or laceration of the subclavian or carotid artery
    D. puncture or laceration of the vein on insertion of the needle/catheter

12. Mechanical complications of TPN consist of (choose all that apply)
    1. air embolism
    2. catheter fracture
    3. pneumothorax
    4. CRS
    A. 2 and 3
    B. 1, 3, and 4
    C. 3 and 4
    D. 1, 2, and 3

13. What nursing action would you undertake first when a patient receiving tube feeding develops diarrhea?
    A. stop the tube feeding
    B. send a stool specimen for *Clostridium difficile* cytotoxin analysis
    C. check liquid medications for sorbitol content
    D. dilute the tube feeding

14. Nutritional goals for the patient with pulmonary failure include (choose all that apply)
    1. higher sodium content
    2. lower protein content
    3. lower carbohydrate content
    4. higher fat content
    A. 2, 3, and 4
    B. 1, 2, and 3
    C. 2 and 3
    D. 1 and 4

15. A high-acuity patient with acute renal failure may experience abnormalities in (choose all that apply)
    1. protein catabolism
    2. fluid and electrolytes
    3. fat absorption and digestion
    4. increased carbon dioxide levels
    A. 1 and 2
    B. 2, 3, and 4
    C. 3 and 4
    D. 1, 2, and 3

Pretest Answers:
1. C, 2. B, 3. A, 4. B, 5. B, 6. C, 7. C, 8. A, 9. A, 10. D,
11. B, 12. D, 13. C, 14. A, 15. A

GLOSSARY

anabolism A constructive metabolic process whereby simple molecules are converted into more complex molecules.

anergy Lack of immune response.

cachexia Observable wasting of body mass caused by malnutrition.

catabolism Process by which complex nutrients are converted into more basic elements, such as glucose, fatty acids, and amino acids.

catheter-related sepsis (CRS) A potentially lethal complication of total parenteral nutrition (TPN); microorganisms are introduced through the TPN catheter, eventually causing a systemic infection (sepsis).

direct calorimetry Measurement of the body's heat production while the individual is isolated in a chamber or room specifically equipped for this purpose.

ebb phase The first phase of the metabolic stress response, characterized by reduced systemic circulation, decreased metabolic rate, gluconeogenesis, glycogenolysis, and hyperglycemia, and persisting for 24 to 48 hours.

energy The ability to do work; synonymous with calories; most common sources are carbohydrates and fats.

enteral nutrition Nutrition delivered into the gastrointestinal tract through a feeding tube; it is a lactose-free, nutritionally complete formula composed of protein, carbohydrates, fats, electrolytes, vitamins, and minerals.

flow phase The second phase of the metabolic stress response, characterized by hypermetabolism, hypercatabolism, increased nitrogen losses, gluconeogenesis, and hyperglycemia.

gluconeogenesis Formation of glucose from protein and fat stores in the body; seen in the ebb phase and flow phase.

glycogenolysis Conversion of glycogen into glucose in the body tissues; seen only in the ebb phase.

Harris–Benedict equation Estimates caloric requirements of a resting, fasting, unstressed individual based on the individual's height, weight, age, and sex; expressed in kilocalories.

hypercatabolism Breakdown of total body protein; skeletal muscle protein is used initially for conversion to glucose through gluconeogenesis; visceral (organ) protein is used after skeletal muscle protein; occurs in the flow phase of the metabolic stress response.

hypermetabolism An increased metabolic rate in response to a major bodily insult requiring increased quantities of oxygen and nutrients to meet the increased metabolic needs; occurs in the flow phase of the metabolic stress response.

indirect calorimetry A technique of estimating an individual's metabolic or energy expenditure through the measurement of oxygen consumed ($\dot{V}O_2$) and carbon dioxide produced ($\dot{V}CO_2$); can also calculate respiratory quotient (RQ).

kwashiorkor A state of malnutrition in which there is a prolonged deficiency for absence of protein in the presence of adequate carbohydrate intake.

macronutrients Carbohydrates, lipids (fats), and proteins.

malnutrition A state of poor nutrition that arises from a lack of meeting the body's minimum nutritional requirements of carbohydrates, proteins, lipids, and other essential nutrients; may be caused by anorexia, poor diet, or malabsorption of nutrients in the gastrointestinal tract.

marasmus A state of malnutrition in which there is inadequate intake of protein and calories and generalized wasting is evident.

metabolic stress response A well-defined pattern of metabolic and physiologic responses that occur as the result of injured tissue in the body.

micronutrients Electrolytes, vitamins, minerals, and trace elements.

nitrogen A basic unit of protein (amino acid) breakdown; excreted primarily in urine in the form of urea; a 24-hour urinary urea nitrogen (UUN) measures nitrogen losses for a 24-hour period.

nutrients Elements and compounds required for growth and maintenance of life; consist of macro- and micronutrients.

nutrition A complex process by which an organism takes in and uses food substrates for the purpose of providing energy for growth, maintenance, and repair; nutrition involves ingestion, digestion, absorption, and metabolism.

respiratory quotient (RQ) A ratio of carbon dioxide ($\dot{V}CO_2$) to oxygen consumed ($\dot{V}O_2$); provides information about fuel composition used by the body; $\dot{V}CO_2$ and $\dot{V}O_2$ are obtained from an indirect calorimetry study.

total parenteral nutrition (TPN) A nutritionally complete, IV-delivered solution composed of protein, carbohydrate, fat, electrolytes, vitamins, and trace elements; TPN with a glucose concentration of greater than 10 percent is administered through a central vein.

ABBREVIATIONS

AAA	Aromatic amino acid	**BCAA**	Branched-chain amino acid
Alk phos	(ALP) Alkaline phosphatase; previously SGOT	**BMR**	Basal metabolic rate
ALT	Amino alanine transferase	**BUN**	Blood urea nitrogen
AST	Aspartate aminotransferase; previously SGPT	**CNS**	Central nervous system
ATP	Adenosine triphosphate	**CPB**	Cardiopulmonary bypass

CRS	Catheter-related sepsis		RFS	Refeeding syndrome
IDPN	Intradialytic parenteral nutrition		RQ	Respiratory quotient
kcal	Kilocalories		SIRS	Systemic inflammatory response syndrome
MODS	Multiple organ dysfunction syndrome		TLC	Total lymphocyte count
NAD*	Nicotinic acid dehydrogenase		TPN	Total parenteral nutrition
NPO	Nothing by mouth		UUN	Urine urea nitrogen
PEM	Protein–energy malnutrition		$\dot{V}CO_2$	Carbon dioxide produced
pHi	Intramucosal pH		$\dot{V}O_2$	Oxygen consumed
REE	Resting energy expenditure			

SECTION ONE: Nutrition

At the completion of this section, the learner will be able to describe the primary functions of carbohydrates, lipids, and proteins, and the nutritional needs of the high-acuity patient.

Nutrition is a complex process by which an organism takes in and uses food substrates for the purpose of providing energy for growth, maintenance, and repair. Nutrition involves ingestion, digestion, absorption, and metabolism. **Nutrients** are the elements and compounds necessary for the nutrition process.

Nutrients as an Energy Source

Nutrients are divided into two basic categories. **Macronutrients** consist of carbohydrates, proteins, and lipids (fats). Vitamins (fat soluble and water soluble), minerals, and trace elements are called **micronutrients.** Adequate intake of both macronutrients and micronutrients is essential to restore health and to promote healing in the high-acuity patient (Pleuss, 2002).

Carbohydrates

Carbohydrates are the desired fuel source for most tissues and are necessary to supply energy for the most basic cellular functions. Heat produced during the oxidation of carbohydrates is used to maintain body temperature. Carbohydrates are introduced into the body in various forms of sugars or starches, all of which are converted to glucose. Excess glucose not needed for cellular activities is stored as glycogen in the liver and muscle cells. This process is called **gluconeogenesis.** Stored glycogen can then be reconverted to glucose to maintain blood glucose levels within a relatively steady range. Also, during times of physiologic stress, glycogen can be metabolized into glucose to provide an immediate fuel source. This utilization of glycogen is called **glycogenolysis.**

Glucose metabolism is regulated by the two hormones, insulin and glucagon. Insulin is necessary for transport of glucose into cells. Under normal circumstances, ingestion or infusion of glucose causes an increase in insulin release from the beta cells of the pancreas. This process is altered during periods of physiologic stress, leading to hyperglycemia. Hyperglycemia, typical of the body's stress response, is discussed further in Section Four.

Glucagon, secreted by the alpha cells of the pancreas, is released in response to falling blood glucose levels. This event then stimulates conversion of stored glycogen into glucose. Stored glycogen is also released in response to increased levels of epinephrine, norepinephrine, vasopressin, and angiotensin II. These hormones are immediately released during physiologic stress. Glycogen stores are used rapidly in the high-acuity patient who experiences intense and/or prolonged physiologic stress, such as occurs with surgery, trauma, or infection. Excess glucose is converted to lipids and stored for later conversion back into glucose when energy is needed.

Approximately 25 percent of the body's glucose supply is consumed by the brain and nervous system. The brain's capacity to store glucose is extremely limited, so maintenance of blood glucose levels within a narrow range is essential for preservation of central nervous system (CNS) functioning. Although the brain can use ketone bodies (derived from fat metabolism) as a fuel source, this does not supply enough energy for the brain to maintain its essential cellular functions (Carroll & Curtis, 2002).

Adequate carbohydrate intake prevents proteins from being used as a fuel source. Proteins can provide energy, but this use is not beneficial to overall well-being because proteins are primarily needed for other cellular functions. Carbohydrates supply 4 kilocalories (kcal) of energy for each gram ingested. Approximately 50 percent of calories consumed should be in the form of carbohydrates.

Proteins

Proteins are composed of various combinations of amino acids and contain **nitrogen** in addition to carbon, hydrogen, and oxygen. Formation of proteins requires metabolism of carbohydrates and lipids. Proteins serve many complex functions at the cell membrane and are essential for formation and maintenance of all cells, tissues, and organs. Proteins also play a role in many of the body's transport mechanisms, such as transmission of nerve impulses. Proteins are considered building blocks because they contribute to the structure of muscles, organs, antibodies, enzymes, and hormones. Maintenance of osmotic pressure and appropriate blood pH also depend on an adequate protein supply. Proteins are categorized according to their location in the body:

■ Visceral proteins are found within internal organs. Prealbumin, albumin, and transferrin (plasma proteins) are frequently measured in laboratory tests as indicators of protein status as well as overall nutritional status.

■ Somatic proteins are found in accessory and skeletal muscles.

Protein synthesis and degradation is an ongoing process. Under usual circumstances, the overall content of proteins in the body is relatively steady; however, under stress conditions, protein catabolism is increased. In the high-acuity patient, inadequate protein intake can quickly lead to malnutrition, prolonged wound healing, diminished resistance to infection, and even death. Like carbohydrate metabolism, protein metabolism is influenced by hormones. Protein synthesis is enhanced by growth hormone. Conversely, synthesis is diminished when insulin levels decrease.

When carbohydrate availability is not adequate to meet the body's energy requirements, proteins are broken down into their amino acid components. Ketoacids, by-products of amino acid metabolism, can then be further metabolized in the Krebs cycle to produce glucose needed for cellular energy. Proteins supply 4 kcal of energy per gram. Average, healthy adults require about 15 to 20 percent of their nutrient intake as proteins. This amount increases considerably under conditions of physiologic stress. Protein malnutrition leads to atrophy of the gut mucosa and is a factor in the development of bacterial translocation (discussed in Section Four, "Alterations in the GI Tract").

Impairment of skin integrity, delayed wound healing, and loss of skeletal muscle mass result from protein malnutrition.

Lipids

Lipids are also referred to as fats. At the cellular level, lipids contribute to the structure of the membrane. Lipids are the primary source of fuel reserve and are readily stored as triglycerides, phospholipids, and cholesterol for later use as a fuel source. A portion of the triglyceride molecule can be used for glucose metabolism. Lipids provide 9 kcal of energy per gram, more calories than any other nutrient. Functionally, lipids are similar to carbohydrates because their availability as a fuel source can save proteins from being broken down for energy.

As with the other macronutrients, insulin influences lipid synthesis and reserves. Insulin is needed for the transport of glucose into fat cells. Only small quantities of stored fat are found in the circulating blood. Most fat is stored in adipose tissue and the liver. The liver can produce lipids from glucose or amino acids, a process called lipogenesis. This occurs when there are more carbohydrates present than required for energy or for glycogen storage in the liver. Under normal conditions, lipogenesis predominates. During stress, lipolytic metabolism predominates, which increases the availability of fatty acids for adenosine triphosphate (ATP) and energy (Guyton & Hall, 2000).

Lipids are a source of essential vitamins and aid the absorption of the fat-soluble vitamins A, D, E, and K. Stored lipids provide insulation for the body in the form of subcutaneous fat and provide structural protection for some organs such as the kidneys. The American Heart Association guidelines recommend consumption of no more than 30 percent of the total diet as fats. Fat intake in the United States, however, generally exceeds this recommendation, being approximately 34 percent fat (Dwyer, 2001). Table 23–1 summarizes information on the macronutrients.

TABLE 23–1 Summary of Macronutrients

NUTRIENT	CALORIC VALUE (KCAL/GRAM)	PERCENT OF RECOMMENDED TOTAL DAILY INTAKE	GENERAL FUNCTIONS
Carbohydrates Basic unit: glucose	Enteral: 4 IV: 3.4	About 50	• Maintenance of body temperature • Supply energy for basic cell functions
Proteins Basic unit: amino acids	4	15–20	• Many complex functions at cell membrane • Essential for formation and maintenance of all cells, tissues, and organs • Contribute to structure of muscles, organs, antibodies, enzymes, and hormones • Important role in transport mechanisms • Important in maintenance of osmotic pressure and blood pH
Lipids (fats) Basic unit: fatty acids	9	No more than 30	• Primary source of fuel reserve • Body insulation • Structural protection for some organs (e.g., kidneys)

Nutrients as Immune Function Support

The intake of nutrition via the gastrointestinal (GI) tract helps maintain tissue integrity and supports the bowel's immune function. In the high-acuity patient, concern for the proper functioning of the gut is often overlooked until there is an overt problem such as vomiting, bleeding, or diarrhea. The GI tract is primarily thought of as the body region involved with digestion and absorption of nutrients. Of equal importance are the significant immune functions served by the gut (Dwyer, 2001).

The organs of the GI tract essentially are hollow vessels that accept and process food. Specialized cells throughout the tract participate in secretion of digestive substances and absorption of nutrients. The GI tract is structured with four distinct cellular layers:

1. **Serosa**—the outermost layer, with a surface epithelial layer and connective tissue
2. **Muscularis propria**—contains perpendicular layers of smooth muscle responsible for peristalsis
3. **Submucosa**—connective tissue and highly vascular with lymph system and nerves
4. **Mucosa**—the innermost layer, the site of intestinal immune activities, secretion of digestive substances, and nutrient absorption. The mucosa forms a protective barrier between highly contaminated GI contents and the sterile interior of the abdomen (Johnson & Gerwin, 2001).

Normal Digestion

Digestion begins with intake of food into the mouth and proceeds through the stomach where gastric juice (containing hydrochloric acid) mixes with the food. The acid medium of the stomach is an immune mechanism that discourages bacterial growth in the area. The major activities of digestion, however, occur in the small intestine. The small intestine is about 20 feet (61 m) long and consists of three sections: the duodenum, the jejunum, and the ileum. The surface area is more extensive because of fingerlike projections of the mucosal layer, called villi. Reabsorption of water and gastric juices occurs mainly in the large intestine. The GI system is presented in detail in Module 30, "Acute Gastrointestinal Dysfunction."

In summary, adequate intake of both macronutrients and micronutrients is essential to restore health and to promote healing in the high-acuity patient. Carbohydrates are the desired fuel source for most tissues and are necessary to supply energy for the most basic cellular functions. Proteins are considered building blocks because they contribute to the structure of muscles, organs, antibodies, enzymes, and hormones. Lipids are the primary source of fuel reserve and are readily stored as triglycerides, phospholipids, and cholesterol for later use as a fuel source. The intake of nutrients via the gastrointestinal (GI) tract helps maintain tissue integrity and supports the bowel's immune function.

SECTION ONE REVIEW

1. Glucose metabolism is regulated by which two hormones?
   A. epinephrine and norepinephrine
   B. glycogen and glucagon
   C. insulin and vasopressin
   D. glucagon and insulin
2. Which nutrient provides the greatest amount of calories per volume?
   A. carbohydrates
   B. fats
   C. visceral proteins
   D. somatic proteins
3. Which organ is most dependent on maintenance of normal blood glucose levels?
   A. heart
   B. lungs
   C. kidney
   D. brain
4. Maintenance of appropriate osmotic pressure depends on which nutrient?
   A. complex carbohydrates
   B. simple sugars
   C. proteins
   D. fats

Answers: 1. D, 2. B, 3. D, 4. C

SECTION TWO: Metabolism

At the completion of this section, the learner will be able to explain basic normal metabolism.

The energy required to maintain life is generated by chemical processes involving transformation of nutrients and occurring throughout the body. Collectively, these processes are called *metabolism*, which means state of change. Metabolism is further described as anabolic, catabolic, aerobic, or anaerobic.

Anabolism and Catabolism

Anabolism is a constructive metabolic process whereby simple molecules are converted into molecules that are more complex. It involves synthesis of cell components and contributes to tissue building. Anabolic events require energy. **Catabolism** is the process by which complex nutrients are converted into more basic elements such as glucose, fatty acids, and amino acids. Catabolism occurs when energy is required. Anabolism and catabolism are ongoing processes and under normal circumstances occur simultaneously to varying degrees. When a person is faced with a serious acute or chronic illness, catabolism may exceed anabolism and sometimes threaten survival. Anabolic and catabolic processes both require enzyme catalysts. Substances acted on by enzymes are called *substrates;* therefore, nutrients are called substrates because enzymatic processes are required for their use as fuel (Pleuss, 2002).

Aerobic and Anaerobic Metabolism

Production of energy is a highly organized process. Nutrients are transformed into energy for immediate use or for storage inside the cell mitochondria for later use. Energy is used or stored in the form of ATP. Energy is generated from two distinct physiologic pathways—aerobic and anaerobic.

Aerobic Metabolism

The cell mitochondria are the sites of aerobic metabolism. When oxygen is adequate, oxidation of nutrients (carbohydrates, lipids, and proteins) occurs in the mitochondria. Pyruvate, which is produced by glycolysis, moves into the mitochondria to be processed in the Krebs (citric acid) cycle, ultimately forming end products of carbon dioxide and water. Carbon dioxide and water normally are harmless and easily excreted from the body; however, excess retention of either of these substances can result in acid–base and/or fluid excess problems. Figure 23–1 shows a simplified concept of the aerobic (oxidative) pathway.

Anaerobic Metabolism

Not all cells contain mitochondria, so not all are capable of aerobic metabolism. Cells without mitochondria receive their energy by the oxidation of glucose to pyruvate, which is then converted to ATP. The process of glucose oxidation in the cytoplasm is called *glycolysis.* Under circumstances in which there is decreased or delayed oxygen delivery to the cells (even those containing mitochondria), glycolysis is used for energy production and is referred to as anaerobic metabolism.

Nicotinic acid dehydrogenase (NAD^+), an oxygen-reducing coenzyme, is required for anaerobic glycolysis. Maintaining adequate levels of NAD^+ depends on oxygen. When the supply of oxygen is inadequate, the energy of glucose can be released by the process of anaerobic glycolysis. During the anaerobic process, pyruvate is converted to lactic acid by NAD^+, which is then free to participate in further energy synthesis. Most body cells can use lactic acid as an energy source temporarily; however, the brain and nervous system have extremely limited capabilities to extract lactic acid as a fuel source. Figure 23–2 shows a simplified concept of the anaerobic (glycolytic) pathway.

The anaerobic metabolic pathway is inefficient as an energy source but is reversible with the reestablishment of an adequate oxygen supply. Anaerobic metabolism is partially a compensatory mechanism that allows energy production to proceed whenever energy demands exceed the oxygen supply, such as during exercise. Anaerobic metabolism, however, is intended only to be temporary and cannot sustain life indefinitely. High-acuity patients are at increased risk of developing anaerobic metabolism because of periods of severe or sustained decreases in oxygen delivery to the tissues. Serum lactic acid levels serve as an indicator of the severity and duration of anaerobic metabolism (Pleuss, 2002).

Energy

The ability to do work is called **energy.** Heat is generated in the conversion of nutrients to energy. Energy is measured in units called *calories,* which is the amount of energy needed to raise the temperature of 1 g of water by 1° Centigrade. Because a calorie is such a minute quantity, energy measurement within the body is usually described in terms of a kilocalorie (1,000 calories). A kilocalorie (kcal), then, is the amount of energy required to increase the temperature of 1 kg (1,000 g) of water by 1° Centigrade.

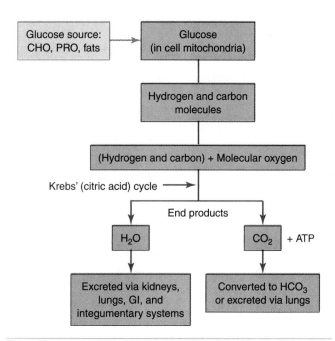

Figure 23–1 ■ Simplified illustration of aerobic (oxidative) pathway. More than 90 percent of metabolism occurs using the aerobic pathway. The end products of water and carbon dioxide are normally eliminated readily from the body.

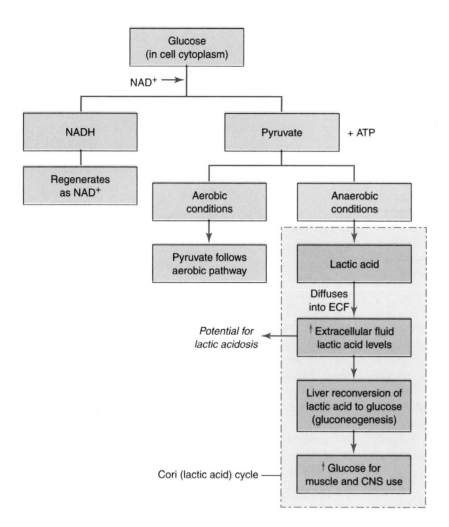

Figure 23–2 ■ Simplified illustration of anaerobic (glycolytic) pathway. The anaerobic pathway is reversible when oxygen becomes available. Severe anaerobic conditions, such as cardiac arrest or shock, can lead to lactic acidosis.

The majority of energy needed by the body (about 40 percent) is used to maintain ion gradients across cell membranes. Synthesis of proteins and central nervous system functions each require about 20 percent of the energy expenditure. Other essential functions such as oxidation of nutrients, breathing, and cardiac pumping consume the rest of the energy expenditure. Physical activities require an even greater amount of energy above that required to maintain normal homeostatic mechanisms in a resting state.

In summary, normal metabolism requires an adequate supply of nutrients and oxygen. Inadequate oxygen intake, such as may occur in high-acuity patients, leads to anaerobic metabolism. Anaerobic metabolism has limited capabilities to sustain life; therefore, provision of an adequate oxygen supply is a priority in caring for such patients.

SECTION TWO REVIEW

1. Catabolism is best described as
   A. metabolism occurring in the absence of oxygen
   B. metabolism occurring in the presence of oxygen
   C. breakdown of complex nutrients into more basic nutrients
   D. building of cells and tissues from nutrients

2. Which lab test is frequently used as an indicator of anaerobic metabolism?
   A. total lymphocyte count
   B. lactic acid
   C. arterial blood gas
   D. blood urea nitrogen

3. Which part of the cell is the site of aerobic metabolism?
   A. mitochondria
   B. cell membrane
   C. cytoplasm
   D. nucleus

4. High-acuity patients are at risk for significant anaerobic metabolism because of
   A. NPO status
   B. increased energy requirement
   C. severe or sustained decrease in oxygen delivery
   D. fluid volume overload

Answers: 1. C, 2. B, 3. A, 4. C

SECTION THREE: Nutritional/Metabolic Assessment

At the completion of this section, the learner will be able to describe the focused nutritional/metabolic assessment.

When dealing with the high-acuity patient, the history may be difficult to obtain; it often requires obtaining a patient history from family members. Assessing the patient's nutritional/metabolic status provides the nurse with information that is essential to the development of a comprehensive nursing care plan. Assessment data helps identify the patient's current nutrition/metabolic status, provides baseline data with which to compare the effectiveness of therapies, and identifies patients who may be at risk for complications related to their nutritional status. General components of the nutritional history include the following:

- History of food and fluid intake
- Barriers to normal food consumption
- Alterations in gastrointestinal anatomy
- Recent weight changes

The patient's metabolic status is pertinent to everything else that he or she may be experiencing; therefore, an understanding of the laboratory and physiologic tests commonly used to assess the patient's overall metabolic/nutritional status is essential to providing safe, efficient nursing care.

Laboratory Data

Common laboratory tests used to assess nutritional/metabolic status include albumin, prealbumin, transferrin, total lymphocyte count (TLC), and serum electrolytes. Serum electrolytes are presented in detail in Module 3. Serum albumin, prealbumin, and transferrin are indicators of visceral protein status. Below-normal levels of these plasma proteins indicate that muscle has been catabolized for energy, which can result in serious multisystem complications.

Albumin

The plasma protein albumin is the major protein produced in the liver. Normal levels of albumin are crucial for maintenance of intravascular volume because of its influence on blood osmotic pressure. Albumin is frequently measured in high-acuity patients and is often used by clinicians as a primary indicator of overall nutritional status. Low albumin levels coincide with increased occurrence of clinical complications and poor patient outcomes; however, this value must be interpreted cautiously. Albumin has a 21-day half-life and is dispersed throughout many sites, factors that make it of little value for assessing nutritional status in an acute situation. Albumin, therefore, should not be used as an indicator to detect early malnutrition or effectiveness of nutrition support. Below-normal albumin values may be detected in patients with liver or renal disease even when protein intake is adequate. In patients who receive fluid resuscitation, low serum albumin values are likely to be dilutional and not an accurate indicator of the actual albumin level. The greatest utility of albumin is in tracking long-term changes in protein status.

Prealbumin

Prealbumin aids transport of thyroxine in the plasma and is the carrier for retinol-binding protein. The half-life of prealbumin is 24 to 48 hours with a small body pool. It is considered a more reliable indicator of acute changes in catabolism than serum albumin. Prealbumin is technically easy and inexpensive to measure in the laboratory. It is not influenced by hydration, renal, or liver status to the same extent as albumin. Periodic monitoring of prealbumin provides an indication of the effectiveness of nutrition support and the overall catabolic state. Upward trending of prealbumin levels indicates improvement in the overall anabolism.

Transferrin

Transferrin is a plasma protein that binds with and transports iron to cells. Transferrin may be more useful than albumin for tracking responses to nutritional therapies because its half-life is 8 to 10 days. Accuracy of transferrin as a nutritional indicator depends on the patient's underlying iron level. Use of transferrin as an indicator of adequacy of nutrition in the high-acuity patient may be limited because of other blood-related factors, such as blood loss anemia or blood transfusions.

Nitrogen Balance

In the high-acuity patient, nitrogen balance may be evaluated as an indicator of protein status. Simply defined, nitrogen balance

TABLE 23–2 Calculating Nitrogen Balance

Nitrogen balance = nitrogen in − (nitrogen out + 4 g/day)

Nitrogen in = g of protein received during the 24 hours of UUN collection, divided by the constant 6.25

Nitrogen out = g of protein excreted in the urine as measured by the UUN plus insensible loss, estimated at 4 g

TABLE 23–3 Laboratory Tests To Assess Nutritional Status

TEST	NORMAL VALUE
Blood urea nitrogen (BUN)	5–25 mg/dL
Serum creatinine	0.5–1.5 mg/dL
Albumin	3.5–5.0 g/dL
Prealbumin	17–40.6 mg/mL
Transferrin	200–430 mg/dL

Data from Gianino, S., & St. John, R. E. (1993). Nutritional assessment of the patient in the intensive care unit. Critical Care Clinics of North America, 5, *1–16.*

is the difference between nitrogen output and nitrogen intake. Calculation of nitrogen balance first requires collection of a 24-hour urine specimen with an accurate account of urinary output during the collection time. Because nitrogen is a component of protein, it also is necessary to know the patient's protein intake during the time of the urine urea nitrogen (UUN) collection. Nitrogen balance is easy to calculate once the UUN is reported by the laboratory. Table 23–2 provides the equations needed to calculate nitrogen balance.

The major disadvantage of using the UUN level to assess protein need is that it is not valid in renal failure. Urinary nitrogen output is expected to be low in renal failure because the kidneys are unable to excrete nitrogen wastes. The UUN is used to calculate the amount of protein needed. For a patient who is stressed and catabolic, the goal of protein administration should be to provide a positive nitrogen balance.

Total Lymphocyte Count

Many cells of the immune system, such as antibodies and lymphocytes, contain a significant amount of protein. Proper functioning of the immune system depends on an adequate total protein level. Measurement of the TLC provides some quantification of the effect of protein loss on immune system functioning. The TLC is an easily obtained indicator of overall immune status and adequacy of protein. This indicator is considered most reliable when white blood cell and lymphocyte counts are relatively stable; therefore, a TLC should be interpreted with caution in the high-acuity patient experiencing hypermetabolism or infections.

The TLC should be about 20 to 40 percent of the total white blood cell (WBC) count. Although there are many disease states and treatments that affect immunocompetence, poor nutrition is a major contributor to immunosuppression. Malnutrition causes immunosuppression by depressing neutrophil chemotaxis and total lymphocyte count. It also delays hypersensitivity reactivity and may cause complete **anergy** to antigen skin testing. A total lymphocyte count of less than 1,500 mm³ is indicative of impaired immune functioning. Total lymphocyte count can be calculated using the following formula:

$$TLC = \frac{\% \text{ lymphocytes} \times WBC}{100}$$

Table 23–3 provides a summary of laboratory values pertinent to the nutritional/metabolic assessment of the high-acuity patient.

Anergy Screen

Cell-mediated immunity is one of the body's defense mechanisms that is most affected by malnutrition. Delayed cutaneous hypersensitivity screening, also referred to as skin testing, is a simple method for evaluating cell-mediated immunity status. A test dose of a known antigen, such as tuberculin, *Candida*, mumps, or *Trichophyton*, is administered intradermally. The individual's ability to respond to this immunologic challenge is evaluated 24 and 48 hours after administration. If cellular immunity is intact, an induration of 2 to 5 mm should be observed at the injection site. If no skin reaction occurs, the patient is considered to be anergic, which means that cellular immunity has been negatively affected by malnutrition (Porth, 2002).

Physiologic Data

Oxygen consumption ($\dot{V}o_2$) and energy expenditure are indicators of the metabolic state. Oxygen consumption is the amount of oxygen used by the tissues, measured in mL/m²/min. Oxygen consumption in a healthy individual ranges from 150 to 300 mL/m²/min. Consumption of oxygen by the tissues requires energy; therefore, oxygen consumption is associated with energy expenditure. Any situation that increases tissue's oxygen requirement also causes an increase in energy expenditure. Fever, shivering, pain, increases in environmental temperature, and physical activity are common sources of increased oxygen consumption and energy expenditure. The nurse should attempt to minimize these factors in the high-acuity patient.

Energy expenditure is the amount of kilocalories being burned. Normal values are established based on gender, height, weight, age, and activity level. An average-sized adult with an estimated average oxygen consumption of 200 mL/m²/min is considered to have an energy expenditure of 1,440 kcal/day (Ahrens & Rutherford, 1993).

Oxygen consumption and energy expenditure can be assessed by various methods. In-depth discussion of energy expenditure is beyond the scope of this text, but a basic understanding of the measurement is beneficial to the nurse caring for the high-acuity patient.

Normally, the body extracts about 25 percent of the oxygen available from arterial blood for consumption by the tissues. This equates to about 250 mL/m^2/min of oxygen. After gas exchange occurs at the capillary bed, about 750 mL/m^2/min of oxygen is returned to the venous blood, which makes the normal oxygen saturation of venous blood (Svo_2) about 75 percent. Oxygen consumption can increase considerably in the high-acuity patient; therefore, close monitoring of Svo_2 can provide important data regarding tissue oxygen consumption in this patient population. Svo_2 can be continuously monitored at the bedside using a special thermodilution fiber optic catheter.

Energy Expenditure

An estimation of energy expenditure can be derived from arterial and venous blood gases or by measurement of gas exhalation using calorimetry.

Harris–Benedict equation. Several equations are used to estimate an individual's resting energy expenditure (REE), but the **Harris–Benedict equation** is one of the more commonly used formulas. This equation states that the REE should be the same for persons of the same gender, age, weight, and height with the same activity level. The Harris–Benedict equation for both genders is as follows:

Male: 66 + (13.7 × weight [kg])
+ (5.0 (height [cm]) − (6.8 × age)
Female: 655 + (9.6 × weight [kg])
+ (1.8 × height [cm]) − (4.7 × age)

This formula was developed in 1919 using 100 normal resting subjects; therefore, the total must be adjusted for the presence of stress factors, such as elevated body temperature, activity, disease processes, and trauma (Harris & Benedict, 1919). Some of the more commonly encountered conditions and their stress factors are listed in Table 23–4. The following is an example of use of the Harris–Benedict equation to estimate daily caloric need:

> If a patient with multiple trauma was estimated by the Harris–Benedict equation to have an energy expenditure of 2,000, this figure would be multiplied by 1.1 to 1.5 to obtain an energy expenditure of 2,200 to 3,000. This patient would require 2,200 to 3,000 nonprotein kilocalories per day.

The Harris–Benedict equation assumes that the patient is within the range of ideal weight relative to height. Ideal weight for adult males and females is 100 pounds for a height of 5 feet. For males, the weight allowance is 6 pounds for every inch above 5 feet. For females, the ideal weight allowance is 5 pounds for every inch above 5 feet. For patients above their ideal weight, a calculation is made for an adjusted weight to be used in the

TABLE 23–4 Harris–Benedict Equation and Stress Factors

CLINICAL CONDITION	STRESS FACTOR
Well-nourished, unstressed	1.0
Maintenance	1.0–1.2
Surgery	
Minor	1.2
Major	1.2–1.5
Cancer	1.0–1.5
Sepsis (acute phase)	
Hypotensive	0.5
Normotensive	1.2–1.7
Sepsis (recovery)	1.0
Multiple trauma (acute phase)	
Hypotensive	0.8–1.0
Normotensive	1.1–1.5
Multiple trauma (recovery)	1.0–1.2
Burned (before skin graft)	
0–20 percent body surface area (BSA)	1.2–1.5
20–40 percent BSA	1.5–2.0
Greater than 40 percent BSA	1.8–2.5
Burned (after graft)	1.0–1.3

From Schlichtig, R., & Ayres, T. S. (1988). Nutritional support of the critically ill. *Chicago: Year Book Medical Publishers.*

Harris–Benedict equation. Adjusted weight is obtained from the following calculation:

Adjusted weight = Actual weight − Ideal weight × 0.25
+ Ideal weight

Calorimetry. Measurement of energy expenditure can also be accomplished by direct or indirect calorimetry. **Direct calorimetry** measures whole body heat production while the individual is isolated in a chamber or a room specifically equipped for this purpose, which makes it highly impractical for clinical application. **Indirect calorimetry** offers a practical approach to bedside measurement of energy expenditure, oxygen consumption, and nutrient oxidation. An indirect calorimeter is also called a "metabolic cart." This portable unit (about the size of a portable cardiac monitor) estimates the REE by measurement of respiratory gas exchange.

The procedure, which takes 15 to 20 minutes, can be performed on patients receiving mechanical ventilation or breathing room air. The metabolic cart estimates energy expenditure by comparing the amount of oxygen consumed with carbon dioxide produced. In the high-acuity patient, the energy expenditure obtained by indirect calorimetry may be multiplied by 1.1 to 1.2. Because the measurement of the energy expenditure occurs only over a relatively brief period, not a 24-hour day, this multiplication is done to account for possible changes in the patient's activity or body temperature during a 24-hour period.

The **respiratory quotient (RQ)** is another valuable parameter provided by indirect calorimetry. The RQ is the ratio of carbon dioxide produced to oxygen consumed. The normal value of 0.82 to 0.85 indicates that the individual is using about an equal amount of carbohydrates, fats, and proteins for energy. The greater the amount of glucose being used, the higher the RQ; thus, an RQ above 0.85 indicates that the patient is receiving too much carbohydrate. Because glucose breaks down to carbon dioxide, excess carbohydrate intake can be harmful to the high-acuity patient and can lead to carbon dioxide retention. Retention of carbon dioxide can increase the work of breathing and, subsequently, can fatigue the high-acuity patient and potentially impair weaning from mechanical ventilation.

Oxygen Consumption

Oxygen consumption can be measured by indirect calorimetry or calculated using the Fick equation. Indirect calorimetry provides a value obtained from a minute-to-minute value averaged over the length of the testing procedure, usually 15 to 20 minutes. Because indirect calorimetry is not available in all facilities, the Fick method can offer an acceptable substitute if the nurse is attentive to drawing the blood over a 30-second time frame while avoiding introduction of air bubbles into the blood specimen. The Fick method (Table 23–5) requires blood gas analysis

TABLE 23–5 Fick Equation for Oxygen Consumption

$$\dot{V}_{O_2} = (Ca_{O_2} - Cv_{O_2}) \times CO \times 10$$

Where: $\dot{V}_{O_2}$ is tissue oxygen uptake; CO is cardiac output; Ca_{O_2} is arterial oxygen content (hemoglobin $\times$ 1.34 $\times$ arterial oxygen saturation [decimal]); and Cv_{O_2} is mixed venous oxygen content (hemoglobin $\times$ 1.34 $\times$ venous oxygen saturation [decimal])

of arterial and venous blood. There are two disadvantages of using the Fick method: (1) It represents the oxygen consumption for only one moment in time; and (2) errors in calculation of the cardiac output can occur, which alters the accuracy of the oxygen consumption value obtained. A more detailed description of oxygen consumption is provided in Module 14, " Determinants and Assessment of Oxygenation."

In summary, assessment of the patient's nutritional/metabolic status provides the nurse with information that is essential to development of a comprehensive nursing care plan. Common laboratory tests used to assess nutritional/metabolic status include serum electrolytes, albumin, prealbumin, transferrin, and total lymphocyte count (TLC). Prealbumin is a more reliable indicator of acute changes in catabolism than serum albumin. Energy expenditure can be estimated, derived by calculation from arterial and venous blood gases, or by measurement of gas exhalation using calorimetry. Oxygen consumption ($\dot{V}_{O_2}$) and energy expenditure are indicators of the patient's metabolic state.

SECTION THREE REVIEW

1. Which lab value is the best indicator of current nutritional status?
   A. prealbumin
   B. albumin
   C. transferrin
   D. BUN
2. What information is obtained by indirect calorimetry?
   A. amount of protein needed
   B. kilocalories being used
   C. body fat composition
   D. condition of immune system
3. Which laboratory test is an indicator of the patient's daily protein need?
   A. UUN
   B. BUN

   C. hemoglobin
   D. albumin
4. Which condition makes the 24-hour urine urea nitrogen test an invalid indicator of protein breakdown?
   A. diabetes mellitus
   B. liver failure
   C. renal failure
   D. hypercatabolism

Answers: 1. A, 2. B, 3. A, 4. C

Metabolic Alterations in the High-Acuity Patient

At the completion of this section, the learner will be able to recognize the typical metabolic alterations occurring in the high-acuity ill patient.

Alterations in the GI Tract

When a patient has undergone surgical alteration of the GI tract, it is essential that the nurse is aware of the precise anatomic changes. Surgical intervention in the tract can alter the digestive and absorptive functions, which greatly affects the patient's clinical status and nutritional needs. Mucosal cells have a high-energy requirement; thus, they depend on a steady supply of nutrients and oxygen to maintain proper functioning. This also means that the mucosa is highly susceptible to hypoxia and diminished tissue perfusion. Interruption of oxygen and nutrient supply can cause death of mucosal cells followed by mucosal atrophy. The mucosal cells perform an important barrier function between the interior of the gastrointestinal tract, which contains many potentially toxic or pathogenic substances, and the sterile environment of the peritoneal cavity. When this barrier is interrupted, gut bacteria may cross the mucosal layer into the lymphatics, blood vessels, or even into the free peritoneal cavity, a process called bacterial translocation (Howard, 2001).

Nutrition in the High-Acuity Patient

High-acuity patients may experience high levels of stress and starvation because of their severe illnesses. Increased stress and a state of starvation both significantly alter metabolism. Older adults or those with chronic illness may be in a starvation or semistarvation state at the time of an injury or acute illness. These patients need to be rapidly identified because their already-compromised nutritional/metabolic state complicates any acute disease state they are experiencing. Starvation can also develop in hospitalized patients as a nosocomial problem. Most high-acuity patients have a greatly increased need for nutrients and calories because of the stress response. Patients who receive no nutrients for several days can easily develop starvation. Because many high-acuity patients are unable to take nourishment by mouth as a result of decreased consciousness or treatments, such as intubation or sedation, provision of nutrition by alternate means is a nursing priority.

Before proceeding with this section, it is necessary to understand the following terms:

Starvation—a clinical condition that occurs when nutrient intake, particularly calories and protein, is unable to meet the body's energy demands.

Hypometabolism—a clinical condition in which the basal metabolic rate (BMR) is less than expected in an individual relative to age, gender, weight, height, and activity.
Hypermetabolism—a clinical condition in which nutrients are metabolized at an increasing rate to supply the energy needed to support immune functions and tissue repair.
Hypercatabolism—the acceleration of protein breakdown for use as a fuel source. The degree of hypercatabolism can be assessed by measurement of urinary nitrogen loss (24-hour UUN).

Malnutrition

Malnutrition is a state of poor nutrition that arises from a lack of meeting the body's minimum nutritional requirements of carbohydrates, proteins, lipids, and other essential nutrients. It can be caused by anorexia, poor diet, or malabsorption of nutrients in the gastrointestinal tract. Malnutrition in hospitalized patients is associated with increased length of stay, complications, and increased morbidity and mortality. The incidence of malnutrition in hospitalized patients is as high as 30 to 50 percent (Dwyer, 2001). Severe and ongoing malnutrition leads to a more advanced state of compromise called starvation.

Starvation

Starvation exists on a continuum of increasing severity that continues until either it is relieved by restoration of adequate nutritional intake or the person dies. Starvation occurs when an individual does not receive adequate nutrition to meet the body's nutritional demands. Starvation can occur in as little as a week, which makes provision of sufficient nutrition a priority in the high-acuity patient. Starvation, a severe condition of malnutrition, is generally described as two types—marasmus and kwashiorkor. Both conditions are also referred to as protein–energy malnutrition.

Marasmus develops when there is inadequate intake of calories and protein and generalized body wasting is evident. Adult marasmus can progress until there are severe losses of fat and protein stores and the patient appears cachetic. Marasmus is often associated with altered gastrointestinal functioning or prolonged periods of anorexia. Immune system integrity often remains intact at this stage. Adult marasmus coupled with the occurrence of a physiologic insult, such as surgery, injury, or infection, leads to a more severe hypoalbuminemiemia (low serum albumin) malnutrition. Skeletal and visceral protein mass deteriorates further. At this stage immune function is impaired. If allowed to progress, eventually the patient progresses to an adult kwashiorkor-like syndrome.

Prolonged deficiency or absence of protein, in the presence of adequate carbohydrate intake, leads to **kwashiorkor.** In this condition, stores of fat and skeletal muscle protein are preserved; however, there is ongoing breakdown of visceral proteins, such as serum albumin and immunoglobulins (antibodies).

Edema is an easily recognizable symptom of kwashiorkor and may mask the muscle-wasting process. Generalized edema results from a decrease in the serum albumin, which lowers the intravascular colloidal osmotic pressure. This allows water to leak from the circulating blood volume into the extracellular spaces. Marasmus and kwashiorkor occur in varying intensities.

One of the first responses to inadequate nutrient intake is the individual's voluntary limitation of physical activity. In the hospitalized high-acuity patient, physical activity may already be minimal relative to the clinical condition. The body attempts to compensate for the inadequate nutritional intake by decreasing release of catecholamines and thyroid hormone. The result is an involuntary decrease in the BMR, which is the same as resting energy expenditure.

Stored carbohydrate is an insignificant factor during starvation because only about 1,200 kcal of energy is stored as carbohydrate at any given time. For the average-sized adult, at rest, 1,200 kcal is less than 1 day's caloric need. Protein is metabolized to provide a fuel source when carbohydrate intake is inadequate, but the rate of protein turnover is also diminished during starvation. When a fasting situation exists, the amount of protein in the muscles is usually sufficient to meet the brain's energy requirements for about 2 weeks. After about 2 weeks of starvation, the body switches to using fat as the main fuel source. Ketone bodies, which are by-products of fatty acid metabolism, replace glucose as the fuel source for the brain; however, the brain cannot extract enough energy from ketone bodies to meet its energy needs, and an undesirable state of anaerobic metabolism is established in the brain. Survival is linked to the amount of stored fat. Theoretically, an obese person should survive longer than a nonobese person during prolonged states of starvation. Fat stores will last about 60 to 75 days in an adult with ideal body weight.

Weight loss accompanies inadequate nutrient supply; however, weight loss reaches a plateau as physical activity and basal metabolism rate decline. As protein is burned for energy, cell death occurs as a result of inadequate protein for cellular repair and synthesis. Cell death also contributes to potassium losses. The fluid constituents of the destroyed cells are shifted to the extracellular volume; thus, generalized edema may be evident. Edema also occurs as a result of water and sodium conservation. Intravascular fluid volume losses are most prominent during the first 2 weeks of fasting and add to hemodynamic instability. Loss of bone mass occurs only in the most severe starvation conditions.

Metabolic Stress Response

The **metabolic responses** to physiologic stress, such as surgery, trauma, or infection, are fairly predictable. Two distinct phases of this response have been identified. The initial phase is called the **ebb phase,** which lasts about 24 hours after the occurrence of tissue injury. The ebb phase is followed by the **flow phase.**

The duration of the flow phase is highly variable and is associated with the patient's clinical condition.

Ebb Phase

The individual's metabolic rate is likely to be initially unchanged or slightly decreased during the first 24 hours after injury. Exceptions to this are patients with burns and severe head injury (Glasgow Coma Scale score of 8 or less). A slightly hypothermic body temperature may be observed secondary to decreased oxygen consumption. Increases in blood glucose and lactate levels are common.

Alterations in both carbohydrate and lipid metabolism are observed in the ebb phase. Glucose production is increased after injury in an attempt to provide energy for wound healing. Increased release of hormones, such as epinephrine, glucagon, and cortisol, stimulates conversion of glycogen stores to glucose. Decreased production of insulin along with insulin resistance in peripheral tissues contributes to hyperglycemia following injury.

Controversy exists regarding the utility of providing nutrition during the ebb phase. Arguments that the instillation of nutrients into the GI tract immediately after injury could divert blood flow from the major organs, thereby promoting hemodynamic instability, have not been well supported. Recent studies have observed beneficial effects, such as decreases in the hypermetabolic response, when enteral feeding is initiated within the first 24 hours after injury.

Fat stores are mobilized to contribute to energy needs. As fats are oxidized, fatty acids are produced and contribute to increases in lactate levels. Lactate levels increase as anaerobic metabolism occurs in injured, ischemic tissues. The increasing quantity of lactate is converted to glucose in the liver, thereby increasing hyperglycemia (Porth, 2002).

Flow Phase

The onset of the flow phase begins about 24 to 36 hours following the physiologic insult. The flow phase is characterized by increased oxygen and calorie demands to provide for wound healing. Typical symptoms of the flow phase include the onset of tachycardia, tachypnea, increased cardiac output, and fever. **Hypercatabolism** is prominent as stored protein is metabolized to help meet the sudden increase in oxygen consumption and energy expenditure. Increased oxygen consumption and energy expenditure along with hypercatabolism comprise the clinical condition known as **hypermetabolism.**

Hyperglycemia is frequently observed after tissue injury. Glucose production is increased in response to increased energy demands. The immediate release of catecholamines at the time of injury stimulates the liver to increase glucose production, and insulin production and utilization are altered. Resistance to insulin in the peripheral tissues contributes to higher levels of blood glucose, but the primary cause of hyperglycemia is increased gluconeogenesis. Administration of insulin may be ineffective in controlling elevated glucose levels during the metabolic stress response.

Patient prognosis worsens as hypermetabolism persists. Individuals experiencing tissue trauma (from any etiology) usually have a decreased capacity to take nutrition; therefore, they depend on their caregivers to provide appropriate nutrient intake. Patients with tissue trauma experience a reduced ability to use carbohydrates, proteins, and lipids, another factor that contributes to malnutrition in the high-acuity patient.

The peak of the hypermetabolic response usually occurs 3 to 4 days following the initiating event (e.g., surgery, trauma, or infection). In the patient without complications, the hypermetabolic stress response usually lasts 7 to 10 days; however, the hypermetabolic high-acuity patient is rarely without complications. Exacerbation of the hypermetabolic response occurs with repeated episodes of tissue ischemia, localized infections, or septicemia. The metabolic alterations occurring with hypermetabolism and hypercatabolism can be a vicious cycle leading to further clinical deterioration if the patient does not receive adequate metabolic/nutritional support within the first few days of the precipitating event. Table 23–6 provides a synopsis of the metabolic differences between starvation and the hypermetabolic stress response.

Refeeding Syndrome

Refeeding Syndrome (RFS) refers to a nutritional complication associated with reinitiating nutritional support in a person who is significantly or chronically malnourished. Even though the patient may be in a catabolic state with depleted nutritional stores, many serum electrolytes remain at a normal steady state because of renal compensatory mechanisms. During periods of starvation, stored fat becomes the body's primary fuel source; however, once refeeding is initiated with large glucose and pro-

tein loads, the pancreas is stimulated to release more insulin. The increased insulin causes an increased uptake of glucose and other electrolytes, such as phosphorus, potassium, and magnesium, into the cells. Sudden shifts of serum concentrations of phosphorus and other electrolytes places the patient at risk for potentially life-threatening respiratory and cardiac muscle dysfunction and failure and neurologic symptoms (Marinella, 2003). In fact, the hallmark of refeeding syndrome is severe hypophosphatemia (Crook et al., 2001). The patient requires intravenous phosphorus replacement as well as scheduled doses of phosphorus via the gastrointestinal tract (if access is available). Other characteristics of refeeding syndrome include hyperglycemia, hypokalemia, hypomagnesemia, hyponatremia, and fluid shifts. Patients who are at particular risk for developing RFS include those with cancer cachexia, chronic alcoholism, and anorexia nervosa. Urinary losses of electrolytes, such as sodium, potassium, and phosphorus, begin as soon as 48 hours without nutrient intake.

Identification of individuals at risk for refeeding syndrome is the main preventive step. In patients with the potential to develop refeeding syndrome, feeding should begin slowly. Caloric intake should not be more than 1.2 times the patient's resting energy expenditure (as calculated by the Harris–Benedict equation or measured by indirect calorimetry). Increases of feeding to the target level may need to occur over several days to minimize the sudden and severe electrolyte changes attributable to rapid refeeding in the starved patient.

In summary, patients who experience tissue injury will experience alterations in their metabolic processes to some extent. In some circumstances, the patient succumbs not to the initial traumatic event, but to the metabolic sequelae. The nurse's ability to identify accurately those patients with alterations in metabolism is essential to achievement of positive patient outcomes. The nurse has two primary objectives in caring for the patient with altered metabolism: (1) delivery of optimal nutrition and (2) provision of optimal oxygenation.

TABLE 23–6 Comparison Between Starvation and Hypermetabolism

	STARVATION	HYPERMETABOLISM
Metabolic goal	Preservation of lean body mass	Repair of injured tissue
Metabolic rate	Decreased	Increased
Energy needs	Decreased	Increased
Fuel source	Primarily fat (stored glycogen depleted within 24 hours)	Mixed
Protein metabolism	Decreased synthesis	Decreased synthesis
	Decreased catabolism	Increased catabolism
	Decreased ureagenesis	Increased ureagenesis
	Decreased UUN	Increased UUN
Carbohydrate metabolism	Decreased gluconeogenesis (stored glycogen depleted within 24 hours)	Increased gluconeogenesis Hyperglycemia
Fat metabolism	Increased ketones	Increased compared to normal; ketones decreased compared to starvation

SECTION FOUR REVIEW

1. Which condition is characteristic of the flow phase of the metabolic stress response?
   A. conservation of protein
   B. hypothermia
   C. increased energy expenditure
   D. hypoglycemia
2. Which condition places an individual at risk for refeeding syndrome?
   A. diabetes
   B. NPO status for 7 days
   C. excess fat intake
   D. obesity
3. The metabolic rate would be expected to decrease in
   A. flow phase metabolic stress response
   B. starvation
   C. hyperglycemic stress response
   D. hyperthermia
4. During NPO status, the average-sized adult has enough stored carbohydrate to supply energy needs for
   A. 1 day
   B. 1 week
   C. 48 hours
   D. 3 days

Answers: 1. C, 2. B, 3. B, 4. A

SECTION FIVE: Nutritional Alterations in Specific Disease States

At the completion of this section, the learner will be able to describe the major nutritional alterations associated with specific disease states.

Specific nutritional alterations occur in hepatic failure, pulmonary failure, acute and chronic renal failure, cardiac failure, gut failure, burns, and traumatic brain injury, all of which require more specialized nutritional regimens.

Hepatic Failure

Hepatic failure can be caused by cirrhosis, hepatitis, acetaminophen toxicity, or total parenteral nutrition. The liver plays a vital role in nutrition and metabolism. Major metabolic functions of the liver include synthesis and excretion of plasma proteins; synthesis of bile acids; conversion of ammonia to urea; storage of fat-soluble vitamins; maintenance of adequate coagulation; and metabolism of carbohydrates, proteins, and lipids.

The liver plays a key role in metabolism of carbohydrates, the body's preferred energy source. The liver converts complex carbohydrates to simple sugars (glucose) that can be used for immediate energy needs or stored for later use. Excess carbohydrate is converted to glycogen and stored in the liver as energy reserves for later use. During times of physiologic stress, when energy needs rapidly accelerate, the liver converts stored glycogen back to glucose. When glycogen stores are depleted, the liver then converts protein and stored fat (triglycerides) to glucose as an energy source.

All plasma proteins, except gamma globulins and immunoglobulins, are produced in the liver. Most of the circulating plasma proteins are also secreted by the liver, including albumin, prealbumin, and transferrin. Decreased serum albumin is a major indicator of severe liver dysfunction; however, with a long half-life of 14 to 21 days, decreased serum albumin is not immediately evident.

The liver is the primary site for lipid synthesis and degradation. Excess carbohydrate is converted to triglycerides by the liver. Triglycerides are then stored in adipose tissue deposits as a reserve energy source. Cholesterol, phospholipids, and lipoproteins, which are also produced by the liver, are necessary for cell wall integrity and transmission of nerve impulses.

Nutritional alterations associated with hepatic failure include hyperglycemia, hypercatabolism, hyponatremia (usually dilutional), and impaired fat metabolism. Hyperglycemia is caused by decreased pancreatic production of insulin and insulin resistance in the peripheral muscles. Reduced nutrient intake as a result of general malaise, nausea, vomiting, and/or diarrhea can result in hypercatabolism. Coagulopathy and gastrointestinal varices often complicate feeding tube placement because of the increased potential for bleeding. Progressive malnutrition leads to increased breakdown of skeletal muscle with release of branched-chain amino acids (BCAAs) and aromatic amino acids (AAAs). In some patients, impaired hepatic metabolism results in excessive uptake of AAA by the central nervous system, which may contribute to encephalopathy, a characteristic of the later stages of hepatic failure.

Impaired fat metabolism is also a factor in hypercatabolism. Lipids stored as triglycerides in adipose deposits are not metabolized normally because of diminished production of ketone bodies. Increasing triglyceride levels are associated with hepatic failure. Renal failure combined with hepatic failure is often an indicator of poor outcome. With renal failure, dialysis is often indicated to treat elevated blood urea nitrogen (BUN) levels, which can be worsened by excessive protein intake or accumulation of free blood within the gastrointestinal tract, which breaks down into nitrogen.

Energy expenditure is typically increased in high-acuity patients with hepatic failure; therefore, they require high carbohydrate intake, normal to moderate protein intake, but low fat intake. Excessive fat intake can contribute to progressive liver dysfunction with accumulation of fatty deposits in the liver cells. Because of the numerous metabolic alterations associated with hepatic failure, overfeeding is just as detrimental as underfeeding. This type of high-acuity patient particularly benefits from having energy expenditure measured by indirect calorimetry.

The amount and type of protein intake appropriate for patients with hepatic failure remains somewhat controversial. Because hypermetabolism and hypercatabolism are often present, protein may be provided in amounts of about 1.0 to 1.4 g/kg. If the patient is experiencing hepatic encephalopathy, protein intake may be slightly more restricted. Excessive protein dosing contributes to an accumulation of serum ammonia and aromatic amino acids, which lead to hepatic encephalopathy. Ammonia, which crosses the blood–brain barrier, is toxic to brain cells. Aromatic amino acids are hypothesized to interfere with normal neurotransmitter activity in the central nervous system, causing sedation. Nutritional products that contain about 50 percent of their protein source as branched-chain amino acids may be beneficial to mental status in some patients. Fluid and electrolyte imbalance and infection are causes of hepatic encephalopathy, which should be corrected before initiating feeding with significant amounts of branched-chain amino acids (Porth, 2002).

Pulmonary Failure

Malnutrition is common among high-acuity patients with pulmonary failure. Nutritional needs of pulmonary failure patients are similar to other hypermetabolic, hypercatabolic patients. Energy expenditure increases with work of breathing, whereas food intake declines because of fatigue and dyspnea. In the absence of adequate calorie and protein intake, the respiratory muscles are catabolized to meet acute energy requirements. As protein deficiency progresses, decreased intravascular oncotic pressure leads to pulmonary edema.

Carbon dioxide is produced when carbohydrates, lipids, and proteins are metabolized for energy. The largest quantity of carbon dioxide is released by carbohydrates. Excessive carbohydrate and overall calorie intake may contribute to increased carbon dioxide levels in some patients. A carbohydrate intake of about 50 percent of total calories is generally recommended for patients with carbon dioxide retention, with the remaining 50 percent divided between proteins and lipids (Dwyer, 2001). Elevations in carbon dioxide may clinically present as an increased respiratory rate, bounding pulse, ruddy face, and drowsiness.

Phosphorus levels should be closely monitored in patients with impaired gas exchange. Phosphorus is a component of 2,3-diphosphoglycerate (2,3-DPG), which facilitates oxygen transport. Low levels of 2,3-DPG diminishes hemoglobin's ability to release oxygen to the tissues. Elevated levels of 2,3-DPG lowers hemoglobin's affinity for oxygen, thereby contributing to impaired gas exchange. Low phosphorus causes decreased contractility of the diaphragmatic muscles and promotes abnormal breathing patterns. Ventilator weaning should not be attempted in patients with a low phosphorus level.

Excessive protein intake increases minute ventilation, respiratory rate, and oxygen demand. Nitrogen balance, blood urea nitrogen, and creatinine should be monitored frequently to individualize protein dosing (see Section Three for details). Sodium and fluid restriction may be indicated for patients with pulmonary edema.

Acute Renal Failure

Metabolic alterations of acute renal failure include hypercatabolism, hypermetabolism, volume overload, and abnormal electrolytes and trace elements. Inadequate nutritional intake, loss of nutrients in dialysate, and underlying comorbid conditions contribute to hypermetabolic and hypercatabolic responses. Serum levels of potassium, phosphorus, and magnesium are usually elevated as a result of catabolism of lean body mass and decreased electrolyte excretion by the kidneys. Volume overload is a major concern during the oliguric phase of acute renal failure.

When acute renal failure is due to fluid volume deficit, kidney function may return without dialysis. In this situation, nutrition support, especially protein intake, may be restricted because of elevated BUN. Acute renal failure often accompanies other physiologic conditions that produce significant increases in energy expenditure. Provision of nutrition support may contribute to volume overload and accumulation of metabolic waste, such as BUN. In some patients, dialysis may need to be performed to permit adequate nutrition support.

Protein dosing varies depending on whether the patient is receiving some form of dialysis. In the absence of dialysis, daily protein intake will be restricted to about 0.75 to 0.90 g/kg. When dialysis is used, protein intake can be liberalized to about 1.2 to 1.5 g/kg.

Specialty renal formulas are available, which contain little or no electrolytes and low protein. The protein content is low in most of these formulas so that protein needs to be added to the formula even when the patient is protein restricted. Many patients can be maintained on regular enteral formulas that have lower protein content. Specialty renal formulas may be reserved for use in patients who have elevated electrolytes. Patients with acute renal failure require close monitoring of their fluid and electrolyte status. Nutritional goals will fluctuate relative to changes in the patient's underlying condition and dialysis therapy.

Chronic Renal Failure

In patients undergoing long-term hemodialysis, morbidity and mortality are higher among those who are malnourished. Until recently, the trend in nutrition care in this population has been to treat malnutrition if it developed rather than focusing on prevention. Chronic renal failure predisposes a person to multiple gastrointestinal problems attributable to uremia, including anorexia, nausea, and delayed gastric emptying. Anorexia may be related to unappetizing and restricted diets. Nutrients are also lost into the dialysate bath. Weight loss with resultant decrease in lean body mass is common. Serum albumin levels are inversely correlated with morbidity and mortality.

During the past 20 years, an ongoing debate has questioned the benefit of parenteral nutrition administered during the typical 3- to 4-hour dialysis period. Intradialytic parenteral nutrition (IDPN) is easy to deliver via the dialysis machine, but research has not validated its usefulness in the acute care setting. To date, studies devoted to IDPN have been hampered by small sample sizes, inconsistent methods and analyses, and a lack of nutritional assessment prior to initiation of IDPN. For this reason, research has not produced a consensus opinion regarding the benefit of this costly and potentially risky nutritional therapy.

One of the most serious risks of IDPN is the large glucose load delivered in a short period. Generally, a liter of IDPN, containing 250 g of glucose, is administered over 3 to 4 hours. Blood glucose levels can rise dramatically during this interval. Usually, this amount of glucose in a total parenteral nutrition (TPN) solution is delivered over nearly a 24-hour period. Patients receiving IDPN need to have their blood glucose monitored frequently during the dialysis period as well as for a few hours after therapy. Extremely high values of blood glucose have been observed in patients within the first few hours after receiving IDPN.

Cardiac Failure

Protein–energy malnutrition (PEM) is relatively common in hospitalized patients, with an incidence as high as 25 to 50 percent. Although it was once believed that the heart was spared from the muscle-wasting effects of malnutrition, this has been negated. Loss of muscle mass results in decreased cardiac pumping effectiveness. Cardiac **cachexia** is a specific type of PEM that develops with persistent circulatory failure. As cardiac failure continues, tissues become increasingly deprived of oxygen. This is essentially a form of tissue injury, and hypermetabolism is observed. The patient experiences the scope of the hypermetabolic response as described in Section Four. Muscle proteins and stored fat are used for energy with resultant loss of lean body mass. With a vicious cycle effect, cachexia contributes to the progression of cardiac failure.

Nosocomial cardiac cachexia develops postoperatively in adequately nourished patients when surgical complications prevent them from oral intake. Malnutrition develops in days or weeks in patients who are not receiving appropriate nutritional support. For surgical patients with cardiac disease, nutrition support should be started within 3 to 5 days if they do not have optimal intake.

Nutritional needs of all high-acuity patients with cardiac disease should be closely monitored. Nutritional intake can have a negative effect on hemodynamics in some patients. Oxygen consumption increases with food intake. For patients who have meals, the postprandial elevation of oxygen consumption can be significant enough to cause hemodynamic instability. The presence of food in the gastrointestinal tract results in greater blood flow through the splanchnic circulation. This increased blood volume is obtained by shunting blood from other vital organs, such as the myocardium, kidneys, and/or brain; therefore, among patients who can eat, intake should be limited to frequent, small amounts of food. For patients who require enteral or parenteral nutrition support, continuous infusion of the formula may be beneficial to regulate the thermogenic effect of the nutrients; however, nutrition delivery is generally dictated by individualized tolerance, and, in the case of enteral tube feeding, location of the tip of the feeding tube.

Anorexia is a frequently observed characteristic in patients with cardiac failure. Dyspnea, fatigue, and unappetizing restricted oral diets contribute to lack of appetite. Cardiac contractility is impaired by low levels of many of the electrolytes. Thiamine deficiency leads to vasodilation of the peripheral blood vessels, producing high-output failure. Cardiomyopathy can be attributed to selenium deficiency in patients receiving long-term total parenteral nutrition.

Balanced nutrient intake is important for all patients, but particularly so for patients with potential or actual alterations of oxygenation. Hospitalized patients receiving only intravenous glucose have a significant increase in their respiratory quotient. An RQ value near 1.00 is indicative of significantly increased carbon dioxide production.

Gut Failure

Inadequate intestinal perfusion produces increased gut permeability and facilitates bacterial translocation from the bowel into the peritoneal cavity, lymph, and portal circulations. Bacterial translocation is now accepted as a major etiology of sepsis in hospitalized patients. Intestinal ischemia is a recognized adverse effect of cardiopulmonary bypass (CPB), and, although the incidence of ischemia related to CPB is low, mortality is relatively high.

Regional assessment of splanchnic circulation can be performed indirectly by gastric tonometry, which measures the pH of the gastric mucosa. The value of the gastric intramucosal P_{CO_2} is obtained by aspiration of a fluid sample via a specially designed nasogastric tube (gastric tonometer). An arterial blood gas supply is obtained at the same time as the gastric sample. The bicarbonate value of the blood and the P_{CO_2} value of the gastric sample are placed into the Henderson–Hasselbach equation. The final value is called the intramucosal pH (pHi). If the result is acidic, the assumption is that circulation to the splanchnic organs is compromised. Values of gastric intramucosal pH have been observed to change prior to changes in more traditional assessments of tissue oxygenation, such as oxygen delivery, oxygen consumption, and mixed venous PO_2 (Marshall & West, 2004).

Burns

Burn patients are among those with the highest expected energy, protein, and fluid needs. The extent of the hypermetabolic response is related to the severity of the burn. Energy expenditure typically increases from 2 to 2.5 times above the individual's resting value. However, energy demands seem to reach a peak with a 50 percent burn. Burns greater than 50 percent severity are observed to have less intense energy expenditure. The exact nature of this decrease in the hypermetabolic alterations is thought to be a result of the body's inability to respond to such a dramatic insult as a greater-than-50-percent burn injury.

Elevated energy expenditure may persist longer in the burn patient than in patients with other types of tissue injuries. Alteration of the temperature-regulation mechanism increases core temperature, which is responsible for the dramatic elevation of energy expenditure. Decreases in the patient's energy needs will be noticed when skin grafting is done or when there is regeneration of epithelium. As with other types of injuries, hypermetabolism reoccurs with repeated infections or additional insults, such as multiple organ dysfunction syndrome.

As with any extensive wounds, vitamin supplementation is beneficial for healing and maintenance of overall immune function. Vitamins A, B complex, and C, along with zinc, support wound healing. Dosage recommendations vary, but the general intent for supplementation is to treat or prevent micronutrient deficiencies.

Burn patients are expected to have massive fluid losses because the skin serves as a barrier against evaporative water loss. Protocols for calculating fluid resuscitation are found in various sources including Advanced Trauma Life Support guidelines for the burn patient.

The body's temperature-regulation mechanism is altered in the burn patient. Increased skin cooling as a result of accelerated evaporation was once considered to be the cause of the extreme elevation of energy expenditure, but this was not supported experimentally. Increase in the core temperature is viewed as the causative factor of the dramatic elevation of energy expenditure in burn patients. Blunting of the hypermetabolic response is observed when nutrient intake is initiated within the first few hours after injury (EAST Practice Management Guidelines Work Group, 2001).

Traumatic Brain Injury

Second only to burns, traumatic brain injury causes the most extreme hypermetabolic and hypercatabolic responses. Energy expenditure is highest in patients with fever, seizure activity, and decerebrate/decorticate muscle posturing. As with any tissue injury, the sympathetic nervous system stimulates release of corticosteroids from the adrenal medulla, catecholamines, and glucagon. Increases of these hormones are responsible for conversion of glycogen to glucose for energy. Glucagon acts on the liver to convert amino acids into glucose while stored fat is also converted into glucose. Decreased insulin release from the pancreas combined with rapid conversion of stored nutrients into glucose results in hyperglycemia. Hyperglycemia has been identified as a significant predictor of outcome from head injury (Rovlias & Kotsou, 2000).

The extent of hypermetabolism in head-injured patients is inversely correlated with the Glasgow Coma Score. Such accelerated catabolic rate and increased nitrogen losses associated with acute traumatic brain injury and acute spinal cord injury are consistent sequelae to major trauma (American Association of Neurological Surgeons and the Congress of Neurological Surgeons, 2001). Hypercatabolism is prominent with traumatic brain injury. The exact mechanism of significant urinary nitrogen losses is unclear. Immobility, decreased nitrogen efficiency, steroid administration, and decreased nutrient intake have all been suggested as causative factors.

The brain is the organ with the highest oxygen consumption. When oxygen demand exceeds supply, cardiac output is increased along with the amount of oxygen that the brain extracts from the blood. When oxygen demand surpasses supply, hypoxemia occurs. The brain tries to compensate for the hypoxemia by increasing blood flow and, therefore, oxygen delivery to the brain; however, this compensatory response contributes to the increased intracranial pressure that is the hallmark of head injury. Hypoxemia leads to anaerobic metabolism in the brain tissue. Lactic acid, an end product of anaerobic metabolism, cannot adequately supply the brain's energy needs (Guyton & Hall, 2000).

Treatment for refractory intracranial hypertension sometimes includes pentobarbital-induced coma, which lowers overall oxygen consumption. Clinicians are sometimes hesitant to attempt enteral feeding in these patients because of gastroparesis and the belief that enteral feeding will not be absorbed because of the effects of pentobarbital. Even though gastrointestinal motility is greatly diminished, absorption of nutrients by the small bowel is usually maintained.

Those patients with a decreased level of consciousness or who have a poor cough or gag reflex are at increased risk for pulmonary aspiration. Therefore, placement of a postpyloric small-bore feeding tube using a blind approach is often preferred, but success seems to be related to clinician experience and gastric motility. Endoscopic feeding tube placement may be necessary. Enteral feeding during drug-induced coma is efficacious and well tolerated by many patients, thus limiting the need for parenteral nutrition.

In summary, nutrition plays a major role in the care of the high-acuity patient. Specific disease states or clinical conditions produce alterations in normal metabolism. The nurse should be familiar with the nutritional/metabolic alterations that may occur with common disease states to permit early intervention. Nutritional/metabolic therapies should be appropriately individualized to avoid potential metabolic complications.

SECTION FIVE REVIEW

1. A high-acuity patient with hepatic failure may typically experience (choose all that apply)
   1. breakdown of skeletal muscle protein
   2. diminished fat use
   3. dilutional hyponatremia
   4. increased carbon dioxide levels
   A. 2, 3, and 4
   B. 1, 3, and 4
   C. 2 and 3
   D. 1, 2, and 3
2. Nutritional goals for the patient experiencing pulmonary failure includes (choose all that apply)
   1. higher sodium content
   2. lower protein content
   3. lower carbohydrate content
   4. higher fat content
   A. 2, 3, and 4
   B. 1, 2, and 3
   C. 1, 3, and 4
   D. 2 and 3

3. A high-acuity patient with acute renal failure may typically experience abnormalities in (choose all that apply)
   1. protein catabolism
   2. fluid and electrolyte levels
   3. metabolic rate
   4. glucose levels
   A. 1, 3, and 4
   B. 2, 3, and 4
   C. 2 and 3
   D. 1, 2, and 3
4. The purpose for supplementing nutritional intake with vitamins A, B complex, and C, as well as zinc, is to
   A. promote red blood cell count
   B. promote wound healing
   C. lower BUN level
   D. lower cholesterol

Answers: 1. D, 2. A, 3. D, 4. B

SECTION SIX: Methods of Enteral Nutrition

At the completion of this section, the learner will be able to describe the benefits and potential complications of enteral nutrition, explain the rationale for gastric versus postpyloric feeding, and identify barriers to providing optimal enteral nutrition to the high-acuity patient.

Criteria for Selection of Enteral Nutrition

Nutrition support should be provided via the enteral route in patients with a functional gastrointestinal tract. Unless there is known traumatic disruption or chronic malabsorptive disease, it is generally assumed that the gastrointestinal tract is capable of absorption of nutrients, fluids, and electrolytes. Patients with a high-acuity illness or injury, who are unable to consume oral nutrition, will require a feeding tube. Selection of the specific type of enteral feeding is based on the following criteria: (1) gastrointestinal integrity and function, (2) baseline nutritional status, and (3) illness severity and possible duration.

Gastrointestinal Integrity and Function

When assessing a patient's GI function, first consider if the patient will be able to eat within 3 to 5 days. If so, nutritional support may not be indicated. If the patient is expected to be unable to eat for this time period or longer, he or she will require placement of a feeding tube. The specific type of feeding

Evidence-Based Practice

- *Critically ill obese patients receiving enteral feedings may do as well with hypocaloric nutrition (less than 20 kcal/kg) as with eucaloric nutrition (20 kcal/kg or greater) when protein levels are maintained (Dickerson et al., 2002).*
- *Use of enteric nutrition resulted in a significantly decreased incidence of infectious complications when compared to parenteral nutrition. In addition, parenteral nutrition was associated with increased hyperglycemia (Gramlich et al., 2004).*
- *Use of nasogastric feedings in postoperative patients with ventilator-associated pneumonia (VAP) was associated with a higher mortality rate from all causes than in postoperative patients who did not receive enteric feedings (Bullock et al., 2004).*
- *Use of an evidence-based nutrition management protocol shortened the duration on mechanical ventilation and reduced mortality risk (Barr et al., 2004).*

tube placed is related to the anticipated time of recovery, the patient's level of consciousness, the patient's comfort, and cost effectiveness.

Illness Severity and Possible Duration

Energy expenditure, calorie, and protein requirements increase with the severity of illness. The hypermetabolism of the metabolic stress response can persist for extended periods in the presence of physiologic complications, such as extensive wounds or sepsis. Advances in the understanding of the metabolic stress response and the immunologic functions of the gut have led to a greater appreciation for the need to provide nutrition support to the high-acuity patient early during the course of illness or injury (Dwyer, 2001).

Timing of Nutrition Support

Providing nutrition early in the course of illness or injury is a treatment priority. Numerous randomized clinical trials among general surgical patients indicate that early provision of **enteral nutrition** facilitates wound healing. Randomized clinical trials examining the effect of early versus delayed enteral feeding on infectious morbidity in trauma patients have produced contradictory findings. Although studies have shown no significant differences in mortality, meta-analysis supports the benefit of early initial enteral tube feeding in acutely ill patients (Marik & Zaloga, 2001).

Readiness for enteral feeding should not be determined by the presence of bowel sounds. Active bowel sounds have been used as a criteria to initiate feeding, but there is no scientific evidence to support this practice. Bowel sounds are a poor indicator of small bowel motility and nutrient absorption. Bowel sounds result from air being taken into the stomach and passing through the intestinal tract. Many interventions such as nasogastric suctioning, sedation, and nothing-by-mouth (NPO) status prevent the normal passage of air through the GI tract. Therefore, waiting for bowel sounds places the patient at undue risk for malnutrition.

Benefits of Enteral Nutrition

A major benefit of enteral nutrition is that it helps maintain gut barrier function. Reductions in gut barrier function are associated with increased bacterial translocation, systemic inflammatory response syndrome (SIRS), and multiple organ dysfunction syndrome (MODS). In animal models, fasting is associated with increased translocation of bacteria from the GI tract into mesenteric lymph nodes, portal circulation, and the peritoneal cavity (Dwyer, 2001). Other major benefits include

1. Maintenance of gut immunologic function
2. More physiologic than parenteral nutrition
3. Possible decrease in severity of metabolic stress response
4. More cost effective than parenteral nutrition
5. Decreased risks of infectious complications
6. Enhancement of wound healing

Although invasive, feeding tube insertion has less inherent risk of mechanical and infectious complications than central venous line insertion for TPN administration. The cost of enteral formulas is about 10 to 20 percent of the daily cost of TPN. Even the most expensive specialty enteral formulas do not equal the cost of providing TPN.

Common Contraindications to Enteral Nutrition

Contraindications to enteral nutrition have diminished as its safety and efficacy has been demonstrated in many types of high-acuity patients. Contraindications include

1. Massive gastrointestinal hemorrhage
2. Distal gastrointestinal fistula (high output)
3. Severe malabsorption
4. Total distal small bowel obstruction
5. Inability to place a feeding tube because of a mechanical obstruction (such as a tumor)
6. Intractable diarrhea

Many patients who were once thought to require TPN are now often successfully fed via the enteral route. Enteral nutrition can be provided to patients with gastrointestinal fistulas if the tube can be positioned distal to the site of the fistula.

Criteria for Selection of Nutritional Support

Selection of the type of nutritional support is based on the following criteria: (1) GI function, (2) baseline nutritional status, and (3) present catabolic state and possible duration.

Gastrointestinal Function

When determining a patient's GI function, first consider whether the patient will be able to eat solid food within 2 to 3 days. If so, nutritional support may not be instituted. If the patient is unable or unwilling to ingest sufficient nutrients normally by mouth and has a relatively functional GI tract, the preferred route of nutritional support is enteral.

Baseline Nutritional Status

Baseline nutritional status is an important determinant for deciding when and what type of nutritional support to initiate. Clinical studies indicate that severely malnourished patients have a greater risk of developing complications and mortality. High-acuity patients should be fed as early as possible, particularly if they are malnourished.

Present Catabolic State and Possible Duration

For the high-acuity patient who is highly catabolic (nitrogen loss greater than 15 to 20 g/day), nutritional support should be initiated as soon as possible after arrival in the critical care unit.

The goal is to minimize further breakdown of the skeletal muscle and visceral protein stores. Numerous enteral formulas are available. Choosing the appropriate formula for the high-acuity patient is based on the energy and protein requirements of the patient, the underlying disease state or organ function, intestinal absorptive and digestive function, and fluid requirements. Commonly used are the lactose-free, nutritionally complete formulas that contain a mixture of carbohydrates, fats, protein, trace elements, and vitamins. Feedings are supplied in varying osmolalities and range in caloric density from 1.0 to 2.0 kcal/mL. A number of Silastic or polyurethane, weighted, or nonweighted small-bore (8 to 12 Fr) feeding tubes are available for enteral patients; endoscopic or surgical placement of a gastric or jejunal feeding tube may be preferable.

Feeding Tube Placement

Enteral feeding access can be achieved by a variety of methods that include blind placement of a small-bore feeding tube, radiologic-assisted placement, percutaneous placement of a gastrostomy and/or jejunostomy, or surgical placement of a gastrostomy or jejunostomy. The small-bore feeding tube is the least invasive and most economical device for delivery of enteral nutrition. This polyurethane weighted or nonweighted tube can be used for gastric or transpyloric feeding.

Successful postpyloric placement of the feeding tube via the nasal or oral cavity requires clinician skill, tube design, patient positioning, and, oftentimes, use of prokinetic medications. Passage of the feeding tube from the stomach into the small bowel is associated with upper gastrointestinal motility. Motor function of the upper GI tract is altered in critically ill patients; those on mechanical ventilation; and those with chronic conditions, such as diabetes mellitus, vagotomy, and intestinal pseudo-obstruction (Guyton & Hall, 2000). Repeated attempts to position the feeding tube postpyloric can cause patient discomfort and delay of feeding. Repeated abdominal x-rays to verify tube position and clinician time contribute to increased cost.

Gastric versus Postpyloric Feeding

One of the ongoing controversies of nutrition support is whether high-acuity patients should be fed by means of intragastric or postpyloric feeding. In situations when repeated blind attempts to place the feeding tube postpyloric delays onset of feeding, it may be beneficial to initiate gastric feeding with a more concentrated formula at a low hourly rate in some patients. Delayed gastric emptying (gastroparesis) associated with critical illness is a primary reason for preference of feeding into the small bowel instead of the stomach. Some clinicians believe that transpyloric feeding decreases the risk of aspiration, but that belief is not supported by the literature. The documented benefits of transpyloric feeding include less interruption of feeding and, therefore, higher nutritional intake and lower incidence of pneumonia in some groups (Howard, 2001).

Increased gastric colonization of gram-negative bacilli has been reported in mechanically ventilated critically ill patients receiving intragastric feeding. The normal high acidity of gastric contents protects against gastric colonization. Histamine type 2 blockers and enteral formulas both elevate the intragastric pH, reducing the protection usually provided by higher gastric acid against gram-negative colonization. Colonization of gastric gram-negative bacilli leads to nosocomial pneumonia. Aspiration is the major mechanism for entry of bacteria into the lungs and contributes to development of nosocomial pneumonia. The risk of pulmonary aspiration of tube feeding is increased by medications, such as theophylline, dopamine, anticholinergics, calcium channel blockers, and meperidine, that cause relaxation of the lower esophageal sphincter.

Patients with postpyloric feeding tube placement are likely to receive more of their prescribed nutritional intake compared to gastric feeding. Gastric feedings are interrupted for instillation of medications, vomiting, formula retention, and abdominal distention. Postpyloric tube feedings do not need to be interrupted when medications are delivered into the stomach via a nasogastric tube. Enteral feeding is held for an hour before and after phenytoin (Dilantin) as a precaution against drug–nutrient interaction, regardless of site of administration.

Complications of Enteral Nutrition

Complications of enteral feedings are classified under five categories: gastrointestinal, nutritional, mechanical, metabolic, and infectious. Table 23–7 lists potential enteral complications, possible causes, and suggested treatment.

In summary, enteral feedings are the preferred route of nutritional support in the high-acuity patient who cannot or will not ingest sufficient nutrients by mouth but has a functioning gastrointestinal tract. Enteral feedings have many advantages over parenteral feedings. Commonly used enteral feedings are lactose-free, nutritionally complete formulas that contain a mixture of carbohydrates, fats, protein, trace elements, and vitamins. Enteral feedings are delivered preferably to the small bowel via a nasoenteric feeding tube. Potential complications of enteral feedings are categorized under gastrointestinal, nutritional, mechanical, metabolic, and infectious complications. There are various causes for these potential complications. Diagnostic, pharmacologic, and dietary treatments are suggested for these potential complications.

TABLE 23–7 Complications of Enteral Nutrition

COMPLICATION	POSSIBLE CAUSE	SUGGESTED TREATMENT
Gastrointestinal		
Nausea/vomiting	Hyperosmolar feeding	Start isotonic feeding
	Rapid infusion rate	Start feedings slowly and advance as tolerated
	Obstruction	Reassess gastrointestinal function
	Delayed gastric emptying	Prokinetic agent (metoclopramide, erythromycin) to increase gastric empty-ing: Feed distal to pylorus
	Contaminated solution or infusion set	Hang canned formula for no longer than manufacturer's recommendation; hang prepared formulas no longer than 4 hours; change container and infusion set every 24 hours; use good handwashing technique before handling formulas
Diarrhea	Antibiotics may alter intestinal flora causing bacteria overgrowth: *Clostridium difficile* infection and pseudomembranous colitis	Send stool specimens for culture and sensitivity, white blood cell count, ova, parasites, and *Clostridium difficile* cytotoxin. Flexible sigmoidoscopy provides a faster and more reliable diagnosis than stool studies; treatment of choice for *Clostridium difficile* toxin is IV/PO metronidazole (Flagyl) or IV vancomycin; hold any antidiarrheal agents until infectious source is ruled out
	Liquid medications containing sorbitol or other concentrated sugar base have a laxative effect (common cause of diarrhea in patients receiv-ing liquid medications)	Crush tablet form of medication if possible
Nutritional		
Malnutrition	Malnutrition associated with loss of microvilli, villous brush border enzymes, and subsequent reduction in intestinal absorptive surface area	Supply elemental diet to improve absorption; elemental diets are for digestive disorders requiring a more easily digested, absorbed diet
Hypoalbuminemia	Hypoalbuminemia is associated with lack of in-travascular osmotic pressure required to draw nutrients across intestinal epithelium, thus compromising absorption	Poor tolerance is evident in patients with serum albumin less than 2.5 mg/dL; benefit of albumin administration should outweigh cost and potential complications
	Protein-losing enteropathy	Semielemental formula
Mechanical		
Feeding tube occlusion	Medications lack of proper flushing; viscous formulas	Irrigate feeding tube with 30 to 50 mL warm water every 4 hours, after medication administration, after checking residuals (gastric)
		Alternate positive/negative pressure with syringe to dislodge clot
		Warm water, juices, or colas have been cited as agents to dissolve clots
		Do not attempt to dislodge clots with stylet; may cause esophageal/gastric mucosal perforations; *prevention* is key
Metabolic		
Hypoglycemia	Sudden cessation of feeding	Provide supplemental glucose
Hyperglycemia	Stress response, diabetic or glucose intolerance	Usually resolves as stress is alleviated; initiate feedings slowly; monitor blood glucose every 6 hours
Electrolyte imbalance	Dilutional states (dehydration or fluid overload)	Monitor fluid status; monitor electrolytes and replace as needed
		Replace fluid and electrolytes as needed
	Excess losses (diarrhea, fistula, nasogastric drainage, ascites)	
	Disease states (renal/liver failure)	Provide appropriate organ failure formula
Infectious		
Aspiration pneumonia	High-risk patients include comatose, weak, debilitated	Elevate head of bed at least 30 degrees; feed into small bowel distal to pylorus
	Patients with tracheostomies or intubated pa-tients; patients with neuromuscular disorders	Add food coloring to feeding to detect for aspiration
		Check residuals every 4 hours if feeding into stomach

SECTION SIX REVIEW

1. Which condition is associated with intragastric feeding?
   A. nosocomial pneumonia
   B. stress ulcer
   C. accelerated gastric emptying
   D. diarrhea
2. The severely malnourished patient has a greater risk of developing complications and eventual death. These severely malnourished patients should be fed
   A. whenever oral intake is possible
   B. after recovery from the acute illness
   C. as early as possible
   D. never
3. A patient has a relatively functioning gastrointestinal tract but is unable to take adequate nutrients by mouth. What is the best method for administering nutritional support to this patient?
   A. nasoenteric feedings
   B. oral diet
   C. withholding nutrition
   D. TPN
4. Enteral nutrition has many advantages over TPN, including (choose all that apply)
   1. less risk of bacterial translocation
   2. providing central venous access
   3. maintaining gut morphology and function
   4. less costly
   A. 1 and 2
   B. 1, 3, and 4
   C. 2, 3, and 4
   D. 1, 2, and 3
5. Enteral feedings are preferably delivered to the _____ via a nasoenteric feeding tube.
   A. oral cavity
   B. gastric mucosa
   C. small bowel
   D. large bowel
6. The categories of potential complications of enteral feedings include (choose all that apply)
   1. gastrointestinal
   2. intravenous
   3. metabolic
   4. mechanical

A. 2, 3, and 4
B. 1, 3, and 4
C. 2 and 3
D. 1, 2, and 3

7. Diarrhea may occur from enteral feedings, but the more common cause is antibiotics. Antibiotics can alter intestinal flora, causing bacterial overgrowth (*Clostridium difficile* infection and pseudomembranous colitis). The suggested treatment includes (choose all that apply)
   1. send stool specimens for testing
   2. perform flexible sigmoidoscopy
   3. administer antidiarrheal agents
   4. administer metronidazole (Flagyl) or vancomycin
   A. 2 and 4
   B. 2, 3, and 4
   C. 1, 2, and 4
   D. 1, 2, and 3
8. Possible causes of an occluded feeding include (choose all that apply)
   1. elemental diet
   2. lack of proper flushing
   3. medications
   4. viscous formulas
   A. 2, 3, and 4
   B. 1, 2, and 3
   C. 3 and 4
   D. 2 and 3
9. Which one of the following factors is an advantage of transpyloric feeding?
   A. less likely to cause diarrhea
   B. prevents tube feeding aspiration
   C. prevents stress ulcers
   D. patients receive more tube feeding compared to intragastric route

Answers: 1. A, 2. C, 3. A, 4. B, 5. C, 6. B, 7. C, 8. A, 9. D

SECTION SEVEN: Methods of Total Parenteral Nutrition

At the completion of this section, the learner will be able to discuss the parenteral methods used to provide nutrition for the high-acuity/critically ill patient, including potential complications.

Total parenteral nutrition (TPN) is a nutritionally complete, intravenous-delivered solution composed of amino acids (protein), dextrose (carbohydrate), lipids (fats), electrolytes, vitamins, and trace elements. TPN with greater than 10 percent glucose must be delivered through a central line to allow mixing of blood to decrease the vessel irritation associated with the increased osmolarity of the TPN solution. Glucose concentrations of 10 percent or less can be delivered via a peripheral vein, as peripheral parenteral nutrition (PPN). Solutions are designed to meet the individual energy and protein needs of a patient based on the clinical condition, underlying disease states, and organ function.

TPN is indicated when nutrition cannot be delivered through the GI tract. Conditions appropriate for TPN include total bowel obstruction, mechanical obstruction, gut-versus-host disease, some cases of severe acute pancreatitis, acute bowel inflammation producing persistent diarrhea, or some cases of short bowel syndrome. Patient refusal to have a feeding tube placed does not necessitate nutrition support with TPN.

TPN is contraindicated in those patients with a functioning, usable GI tract capable of absorption of adequate nutrients, when sole dependence is anticipated to be less than 5 days, when aggressive support is not warranted, and when the risks of TPN outweigh the potential benefits.

Multilumen catheters are commonly used. These catheters allow for one central venous access, with multiple ports for hemodynamic monitoring and fluid/medication delivery without risk of drug incompatibility. To minimize the risk of line infections, one part of multilumen catheters should be dedicated for TPN administration.

Complications of Total Parenteral Nutrition

Complications from TPN fall under three classifications: infectious, metabolic, and mechanical.

Infectious Complications

Catheter-related sepsis (CRS) is a potentially lethal complication, particularly in the high-acuity population. Review of the literature reveals that the primary causes of CRS are as follows:

1. Lack of sterility during placement of central lines
2. Inadequate precautions taken with maintenance of the central line (i.e., changing tubings, dressings, bags)

Clinical signs and symptoms of CRS are as follows:

- Erythema, swelling, tenderness, or purulent drainage from the catheter site
- Leukocytosis
- Sudden temperature elevation that should resolve on catheter removal
- Sudden glucose intolerance that may occur up to 12 hours before temperature elevation
- Bacteremia/septicemia/septic shock

Prompt evaluation and identification of the source of septicemia is important. Pancultures (urine, sputum, and two sets of peripheral blood cultures) should be obtained. Additionally, on removal, the tip of the catheter should be cut (with sterile scissors) and sent for culture. If a catheter tip culture results in growth of more than 15 colonies, this most likely indicates the source of infection. Infected catheters may result from migration of bacteria from a contaminated solution, bacteremia, administration set, catheter, or infected skin tract. Antimicrobial therapy should be initiated.

Prevention is the key. To avoid contamination of the catheter, maintain dry, sterile, and intact dressings at all times; prepare the junction of administration sets with povidone–iodine (unless contraindicated by a patient allergy); minimize the number of entries into the system; and always use meticulous technique with all aspects of catheter care (Rombeau & Rolandelli, 2001).

Metabolic Complications

Metabolic complications of TPN are similar to those of enteral nutrition. Refer to Section Six for metabolic complications, possible causes, and suggested treatment.

Other possible metabolic derangements caused by TPN are prerenal azotemia and hepatic dysfunction. Prerenal azotemia is caused by overaggressive protein administration and is aggravated by underlying dehydration. Presenting signs and symptoms include an elevated serum BUN, serum sodium, and clinical signs of dehydration. If the condition is not corrected, the patient may develop progressive lethargy and possibly coma. Close monitoring of body weight, fluid balance, and adequate protein intake is important in preventing this complication.

Hepatic dysfunction can occur secondary to the macronutrient concentrations in TPN solutions, particularly excessive glucose concentrations. Steatohepatitis (or fatty liver) may be reflected in elevated serum liver function tests (including aspartate aminotransferase [AST], amino alanine transferase [ALT], alkaline phosphatase [Alk phos; ALP], and possibly bilirubin levels) during the course of TPN and usually return to normal spontaneously when the infusion is stopped.

Mechanical Complications

Mechanical complications include pneumothorax, catheter fracture, subclavian/carotid artery puncture, air embolism, and dysrhythmias. All may be a result of the central venous catheter insertion.

Pneumothorax, the most common mechanical complication, is caused by the puncture or laceration of the pleura on insertion of the needle/catheter. Air enters into the pleural space, with partial or complete collapse of the lung. Most pneumothoraces produce symptoms, although some are totally asymptomatic. In general, the larger the collapse, the more pronounced the symptoms. Commonly seen are shortness of breath, restlessness, dyspnea, hypoxia, and chest pain radiating to the back. Treatment depends on the severity of the collapse and respiratory compromise. Moderate to large collapse will require a chest tube to restore negative pressure within the chest cavity.

Catheter fracture and occlusion are other mechanical complications that can occur. Fractures or breakage of the catheter can result from reduced pliability over time. Occlusion can occur from lodging of the catheter tip against the vessel wall or from being physiologically "pinched" between the clavicle and first rib. Other occlusions can occur from fibrin buildup, blood or lipid deposition, and drug precipitates. Another type of occlusion, known as "withdrawal occlusion," is an occlusion that allows infusion of a solution but prevents blood withdrawal.

Inadvertent puncture or laceration of the subclavian or carotid arteries is indicated by a flashback of arterial blood in the syringe, pulsatile blood flow, bleeding from the catheter site or development of a large hematoma, and hypotension. Treatment involves withdrawing the syringe/catheter and applying direct pressure to the site until bleeding ceases.

Air embolism may occur whenever the central venous system is open to air. Signs and symptoms vary with the amount of air pulled into the venous system but may include respiratory distress, tachycardia, hypotension, sudden cardiovascular collapse, neurologic deficits, or cardiac arrest. Immediate action is required. Occlude the catheter nearest to the entry site of the skin. Place the patient on the left side and in the Trendelenburg position. This allows an air embolus to float into the right ventricle of the heart, away from the pulmonary artery. Prevention is the key. Always use Luer-Lock or other secure connectors and air-eliminating filters on central line tubings.

Dysrhythmias during central venous insertions are the result of a malpositioned catheter or guidewire. The result may be atrial, junctional, or ventricular dysrhythmias, which may cause decreased cardiac output, decreased blood pressure, or loss of consciousness. Appropriate intervention is to withdraw the catheter or guidewire partially. If the dysrhythmia continues, an antiarrhythmic may be required.

In summary, the nurse, as the member of the health care team who is in constant contact with the patient, is in a significant position to manage individual nutritional/metabolic therapies, support energy and oxygen needs, and prevent complications related to the numerous metabolic complications that occur with tissue injury. With an increasing emphasis on providing therapies that are beneficial yet cost saving, the nurse is in a pivotal position to evaluate the appropriateness and effectiveness of nutritional therapies in the high-acuity patient. Nurses are ideally suited to design and implement research protocols related to the metabolic needs of the high-acuity patient.

SECTION SEVEN REVIEW

1. TPN is indicated when
   A. adequate amounts of nutrients can be delivered through the GI tract
   B. adequate amounts of nutrients cannot be delivered through the GI tract
   C. a functioning, usable gastrointestinal tract is capable of absorption of adequate nutrients
   D. aggressive nutritional support is not warranted
2. TPN with a greater than 10 percent glucose should be administered through a
   A. nasoenteric feeding tube
   B. peripheral vein
   C. surgically placed jejunal feeding tube
   D. central vein
3. Which of the following factors can lead to prerenal azotemia in the patient receiving TPN?
   A. excessive protein administration
   B. excessive carbohydrate administration
   C. excessive fluid administration
   D. excessive lipid administration
4. CRS is a potentially lethal complication of TPN and is caused primarily by
   A. a malpositioned catheter or guidewire during the central line insertion
   B. lack of sterility during central line placement and inadequate maintenance of the line
   C. inadvertent puncture or laceration of the subclavian or carotid artery
   D. puncture or laceration of the vein on insertion of the needle/catheter
5. Hypoglycemia is a potential metabolic complication of TPN and results from
   A. gluconeogenesis
   B. glucose intolerance
   C. sudden cessation of feeding
   D. insulin resistance
6. Mechanical complications of TPN consist of (choose all that apply)
   1. air embolism
   2. hydrothorax
   3. pneumothorax
   4. CRS
   A. 2 and 3
   B. 1, 3, and 4
   C. 2, 3, and 4
   D. 1, 2, and 3

Answers: 1. B, 2. D, 3. A, 4. B, 5. C, 6. D

POSTTEST

1. Which organ plays a major role in lipogenesis?
   A. spleen
   B. pancreas
   C. liver
   D. gallbladder

2. Which one of the following substances is the body's preferred energy source?
   A. proteins
   B. lipids
   C. carbohydrates
   D. amino acids

3. A high-acuity patient with hepatic failure may experience (choose all that apply)
   1. breakdown of skeletal muscle protein
   2. diminished fat use
   3. hyponatremia
   4. increased carbon dioxide levels
   A. 1 and 2
   B. 1, 3, and 4
   C. 2 and 3
   D. 1, 2, and 3

4. Nutritional goals for the pulmonary failure patient include (choose all that apply)
   1. higher sodium content
   2. lower protein content
   3. lower carbohydrate content
   4. higher fat content
   A. 2, 3, and 4
   B. 1, 2, and 3
   C. 1, 3, and 4
   D. 2 and 4

5. For the high-acuity patient with acute renal failure, which of the following nutritional therapies is appropriate for the patient undergoing hemodialysis?
   A. protein intake should be restricted to about 0.75 to 0.90 g/kg/day
   B. protein intake should be liberalized to about 1.2 to 1.5 g/kg/day

   C. carbohydrate intake should be limited to less than 50 percent of total nutrition
   D. lipid intake should not exceed 20 percent of total nutrition

6. A patient has a functioning GI tract but is unable to take adequate nutrients by mouth. What is the BEST method for administering nutritional support to this patient?
   A. nasoenteric feedings
   B. oral diet
   C. withholding nutrition
   D. TPN

7. The absence of a skin reaction after cutaneous administration of an anergy screen indicates
   A. the normal response
   B. that the patient's cellular immunity has been negatively affected by malnutrition
   C. that the patient is adequately nourished
   D. that the patient's cellular immunity is intact

8. The primary rationale for postpyloric feeding is that it
   A. prevents aspiration of tube feeding
   B. negates the need for a nasogastric tube
   C. promotes greater amount of nutritional intake in patients likely to have delayed gastric emptying
   D. facilitates bolus feeding

9. TPN is appropriate for use in patients with
   A. liver failure and nausea
   B. nonresectable gastric tumor that prevents passage of enteral feeding tube
   C. chronic pancreatitis
   D. hyperemesis gravidarum

10. Which laboratory finding is indicative of refeeding syndrome?
    A. hypophosphatemia
    B. hypoglycemia
    C. hyperkalemia
    D. hypernatremia

POSTTEST ANSWERS

Question	Answer	Section
1	C	Two
2	C	Two
3	D	Five
4	A	Five
5	B	Five

Question	Answer	Section
6	A	Six
7	B	Three
8	C	Six
9	B	Seven
10	A	Four

REFERENCES

Ahrens, T. S., & Rutherford, K. (1993). *Essentials of oxygenation.* Boston: Jones & Bartlett.

American Association of Neurological Surgeons and the Congress of Neurological Surgeons. (2001). The section on disorders of the spine and peripheral nerves: Nutritional support after spinal cord injury. Available: *http://www.spineuniverse.com/pdf/traumaguide/11.pdf.* Accessed April 28, 2004.

Barr, J., Hecht, M., Flavin, K. E., Khorana, A., & Gould, M. K. (2004). Outcomes in critically ill patients before and after the implementation of an evidence-based nutritional management protocol. *Chest, 125*(4), 1446–1458.

Bullock, T. K., Waltrip, T. J., Price, S. A., & Galandiuk, S. (2004). A retrospective study of nosocomial pneumonia in postoperative patients shows a higher mortality rate in patients receiving nasogastric tube feeding. *American Surgery, 70*(9), 822–827.

Carroll, E. W., & Curtis, R. L. (2002). Organization and control of neural function. In C. M. Porth (Ed.), *Pathophysiology: Concepts of altered health states* (6th ed., pp. 1043–1089). Philadelphia: Lippincott Williams & Wilkins.

Crook, H. A., Hally, V., & Panteli, J. V. (2001). The importance of refeeding syndrome. *Nutrition, 17*(7/8), 632–637.

Dickerson, R. N., Boschert, K., Kudsk, K. A., & Brown, R. O. (2002). Hypocaloric enteral tube feeding in critically ill obese patients. *Nutrition, 18*(3), 241–247.

Dwyer, J. (2001). Nutritional requirements and dietary assessment. In E. Braunwald, A. S. Fauci, D. L. Kasper, S. L. Hauser, D. L. Longo, & J. L. Jameson (Eds.), *Harrison's principles of internal medicine* (15th ed., pp. 451–454). New York: McGraw-Hill Medical Publishing Division.

EAST Practice Management Guidelines Work Group. (2001). *Practice management guidelines for nutritional support of the trauma patient.* Allentown, PA: Eastern Association for the Surgery of Trauma (EAST).

Gillies, D., O'Riordan, E., Carr, D., O'Brien, I., Frost, J., & Gunning, R. (2003). Integrative literature reviews and meta-analyses: Central venous catheter dressings: a systematic review. *Journal of Advanced Nursing, 44*(6), 623–633.

Gramlich, L., Kichian, K., Pinilla, J., Rodych, N. J., Dhaliwal, R., & Heyland, D. K. (2004). Does enteral nutrition compared to parenteral nutrition result in better outcomes in critically ill adult patients? A systematic review of the literature. *Nutrition, 20*(10), 483–489.

Guyton, A. C., & Hall, J. E. (Eds.). (2000). *Metabolism of carbohydrates, and the formation of adenosine triphosphate. Textbook of medical physiology* (10th ed.). Philadelphia: W. B. Saunders.

Harris, J. A., & Benedict, F. G. (1919). *A biometric study of basal metabolism in man.* Washington, DC: Carnegie Institute of Washington, Publ. no. 279.

Howard, L. (2001). Enteral and parenteral nutrition therapy. In E. Braunwald, A. S. Fauci, D. L. Kasper, S. L. Hauser, D. L. Longo, & J. L. Jameson (Eds.), *Harrison's principles of internal medicine* (15th ed.). New York: McGraw-Hill Medical Publishing Division.

Johnson, L. R., & Gerwin, T. A. (2001). *Gastrointestinal physiology* (2nd ed.). St. Louis: C. V. Mosby.

Marik, P. E., & Zaloga, G. P. (2001). Early enteral nutrition in acutely ill patients: A systematic review. *Critical Care Medicine, 29*(12), 2264–2270.

Marinella, M. A. (2003). The refeeding syndrome and hypophosphatemia. *Nutrition Reviews, 61*(9), 320–323.

Marshall, A. P., & West, S. H. (2004). Gastric tonometery and monitoring gastrointestinal perfusion: Using research to support nursing practice. *Nursing in Critical Care, 9*(3), 123.

Pleuss, J. (2002). Alterations in nutritional status. In C. M. Porth (Ed.), *Pathophysiology: Concepts of altered health status* (6th ed., pp. 209–229). Philadelphia: Lippincott Williams & Wilkins.

Porth, C. M. (2002). Alterations in the immune response. In C. M. Porth (Ed.), *Pathophysiology: Concepts of altered health states* (6th ed., pp. 357–377). Philadelphia: Lippincott Williams & Wilkins

Robertson, C. S., Clifton, G. L., & Grossman, R. G. (1984). Oxygen utilization and cardiovascular function in head-injured patients. *Neurosurgery, 15,* 307–313.

Rombeau, J., & Rolandelli, R.: (2001). *Clinical nutrition: Parenteral nutrition* (3rd ed.). Philadelphia: W. B. Saunders.

Rovlias, A., & Kotsou, S. (2000). The influence of hyperglycemia on neurological outcome in patients with severe head injury. *Neurosurgery, 46*(2), 335–342.

ADDITIONAL READINGS

American Society for Parenteral and Enteral Nutrition, Board of Directors. (2002). Guidelines for the use of parenteral and enteral nutrition in adult and pediatric patients. *Journal of Parenteral & Enteral Nutrition, 26*(1 suppl), 1SA–138SA.

Guenter, P. (2001). Tubefeeding administration. In P. Guenter & M. Silkrowski (Eds.), *Tube feeding: Practical guidelines and nursing protocols.* Gaithersburg, MD: Aspen.

Riggs, J. E. (2002). Neurologic manifestations of electrolyte disturbances. *Neurologic Clinics, 20*(1), 227–239.

MODULE 24

Acute Hematologic Dysfunction

Susan Bohnenkamp, Kathleen Dorman Wagner

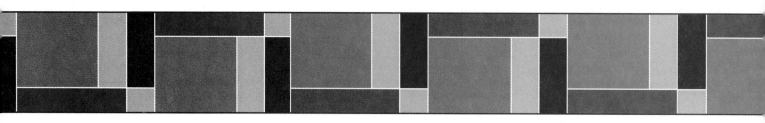

OBJECTIVES Following completion of this module, the learner will be able to

1. Describe the anatomic components and physiologic functions of the blood.

2. Discuss the assessment and diagnosis of hematologic disorders.

3. Describe the etiology, pathophysiology, clinical manifestations, and management of red cell disorders.

4. Discuss the etiology, pathophysiology, clinical manifestations, and management of white cell disorders.

5. Describe the etiology, pathophysiology, clinical manifestations, and management of thrombocytopenia and disseminated intravascular coagulation (DIC).

6. Discuss the nursing implications appropriate to managing the care of patients experiencing acute hematologic dysfunction.

This self-study module presents the physiologic and pathophysiologic processes involved in acute hematologic dysfunction and management of the patient who is experiencing one or several blood cell abnormalities. The module is composed of six sections. Section One is a review of the anatomy and physiology of the blood. Section Two provides an overview of the assessment and diagnosis of hematologic problems. Sections Three through Five describe specific hematologic disorders, including disorders of red cells (anemia and polycythemia), white cells (neutropenia and leukemia), and platelets

(hemostasis). Included in the hemostasis section is an overview of disseminated intravascular coagulation (DIC). Finally, Section Six provides a brief discussion of the nursing implications that commonly apply to patients with hematologic problems. Each section includes a set of review questions to help the learner evaluate her or his understanding of the section's content before moving on to the next section. All Section Reviews and the module Pretest and Posttest include answers. It is suggested that the learner review those concepts answered incorrectly in the review questions before proceeding to the next section.

 PRETEST

1. Adequate iron is a crucial part of hemoglobin because
   A. it cements the hemoglobin chain together
   B. it facilitates the release of oxygen to the tissues
   C. the heme molecule attaches to it to make a chain
   D. the oxygen molecule attaches to it
2. The process by which circulating neutrophils and macrophages squeeze out of a capillary to migrate to the site of injury is called
   A. diapedesis
   B. chemotaxis

   C. margination
   D. translocation
3. Platelets are not actually cells. They are _____ from _____ in the bone marrow.
   A. granules; leukocytes
   B. lysosomes; erythrocytes
   C. cell fragments; megakaryocytes
   D. secretions; plasma cells

4. An elevated reticulocyte count in the presence of anemia indicates that the
   A. RBCs are being destroyed prematurely
   B. bone marrow is depressed
   C. RBCs are being sequestered in the spleen
   D. bone marrow is functioning correctly

5. Hematocrit is best defined as a measurement of
   A. weight
   B. concentration
   C. volume
   D. dehydration

6. When a shift to the left occurs in the neutrophil count, it refers to a(n)
   A. elevated band level
   B. decreased band level
   C. elevated seg level
   D. decreased seg level

7. The bone discomfort associated with anemia is usually caused by
   A. inflammation of the bone
   B. decreased oxygen in the bone marrow
   C. irritation of nerves in the bone marrow
   D. increased hematopoietic activity in bone marrow

8. The most common form of anemia found worldwide is/are
   A. megaloblastic anemias
   B. iron-deficiency anemia
   C. aplastic anemia
   D. blood loss anemia

9. The definitive treatment for aplastic anemia in younger patients is
   A. blood transfusions
   B. antibiotic therapy
   C. immunosuppressant therapy
   D. bone marrow transplant

10. The most common cause of blood loss anemia is
    A. alcohol abuse
    B. menorrhagia
    C. surgery
    D. gastrointestinal bleeding

11. When severe neutropenia is present, the primary symptom of infection may be
    A. pus formation
    B. fever
    C. local edema
    D. local erythema

12. About 70 percent of acute lymphocytic leukemia (ALL) cases involve proliferation of immature
    A. B cells
    B. T cells
    C. plasma cells
    D. megakaryocytes

13. The major characteristic of chronic lymphocytic leukemia (CLL) is the presence of _____ mature lymphocytes.

A. larger-than-normal
B. fewer-than-normal
C. irregularly shaped
D. abnormally small

14. The MOST common cause of death in adults with acute leukemia is
    A. hemorrhage
    B. infection
    C. tissue hypoxia
    D. brain infiltration

15. A "complete remission" is obtained when there are no leukemic cells in the
    A. lymph nodes and bone marrow
    B. lymph nodes and peripheral blood
    C. bone marrow and brain
    D. bone marrow and peripheral blood

16. The initial treatment of the acute leukemias is
    A. surgery
    B. chemotherapy
    C. radiation therapy
    D. bone marrow transplant

17. Treatment of CLL is usually initiated
    A. when the WBC count is greater than 100,000
    B. when the hemoglobin is less then 6
    C. at stage III or IV of disease
    D. at the time of diagnosis

18. The typical bleeding pattern of thrombocytopenia involves bleeding into the
    A. joints
    B. peritoneum
    C. internal organs
    D. skin and mucous membranes

19. The major treatment of idiopathic thrombocytopenia purpura is
    A. alkylating chemotherapy
    B. platelet transfusions
    C. corticosteroid therapy
    D. bone marrow transplant

20. The activity intolerance created by some of the hematologic disorders is specifically related to a(n)
    A. intravascular fluid volume loss
    B. O_2 supply-and-demand imbalance
    C. decreased systemic blood flow
    D. inadequate secondary defenses

21. A nursing diagnosis that commonly addresses tissue hypoxia associated with hematologic disorders includes
    A. fatigue
    B. pain
    C. risk for infection
    D. decreased cardiac output

Pretest Answers:

1. D, 2. A, 3. C, 4. D, 5. B, 6. A, 7. D, 8. B, 9. D, 10. C,
11. B, 12. A, 13. D, 14. B, 15. D, 16. B, 17. C, 18. D, 19. C,
20. B, 21. A

GLOSSARY

ablation   Elimination or removal.

anemia   A condition in which there is decreased numbers of RBCs, decreased hemoglobin, or decreased hematocrit.

band (stab)   An immature neutrophil.

bandemia   Elevated serum band (immature neutrophil) level.

cell differentiation   Development of specific cell functions through a maturation process.

chemotaxis   Directional migration of leukocytes to the site of injury or inflammation.

committed stem cell   A pluripotential stem cell that has committed its development to either the myeloid or lymphoid cell line.

D-dimer   A protein that is released into the circulation during the breakdown of fibrin blood clots.

diapedesis   The movement of WBCs through an intact vessel wall using ameboid movement.

erythrocytes   Red blood cells; part of the hematopoietic stem cell line; produced in the bone marrow.

granulocyte   A type of blood cell with granules located in the cytoplasm.

hemolytic anemia   Breakdown (pathologic destruction) of red blood cells.

hemostasis   Stoppage of bleeding; stagnation of blood flow.

hypochromic   The abnormal pale coloring of RBCs, indicating reduced hemoglobin content.

macrocytic   Abnormally large RBC.

macrophages   Mature monocytes; large phagocytes.

margination   The movement and adhering of circulating WBCs to the capillary wall in preparation for shifting out of the vessel to move to the site of injury.

mean corpuscular hemoglobin (MCH)   A measurement of the average weight (concentration) of hemoglobin in red blood cells.

mean corpuscular hemoglobin concentration (MCHC)   The ratio of hemoglobin weight to erythrocyte volume.

mean corpuscular volume (MCV)   A measurement of the size (volume) of RBCs.

microcytic   Abnormally small RBC.

neutropenia   Abnormally low number of neutrophils.

neutrophils   Segmented granulocytes of the myeloid cell line.

normochromic   The normal coloring of RBCs, indicating normal hemoglobin content.

normocytic   Normal-sized cells.

platelet factor 4   A protein located in the platelet alpha granules.

pluripotential hematopoietic stem cells (PHSC)   Stem cells produced in the bone marrow that have the potential to become erythrocytes, leukocytes, or thrombocytes.

polycythemia   Abnormally elevated red blood cell mass.

polymorphonuclear   The presence of multiple nuclei in a cell (e.g., segmented neutrophils).

pseudopods   Fingerlike projections.

reticulocytes   Immature RBCs.

reticuloendothelial system   A group of cells found throughout the body that are capable of ingesting particles; cells include macrophages, reticular cells, and other tissue macrophages.

Rh incompatibility   Rh (for rhesus) factor is an antigen found on red blood cells. Not all humans have this antigen present. Rh positive indicates it is present, while Rh negative indicates that it is not. A reaction, or incompatibility, occurs when a person with Rh negative blood receives a transfusion of Rh positive blood.

segmented cells (segs)   Mature neutrophils.

thrombosis   Intravascular aggregation of cells creating a blood clot.

ABBREVIATIONS

ABO	Refers to the A, B, O blood types	**Hct**	Hematocrit
ALL	Acute lymphocytic leukemia	**Hgb**	Hemoglobin
AML	Acute myelogenous (myelocytic) leukemia	**HLA**	Histocompatibility antigen
ATG	Antithymocyte globulin	**HTLV-1**	Human T cell leukemia virus type 1
CBC	Complete blood count	**IF**	Intrinsic factor
CLL	Chronic lymphocytic leukemia	**IgG**	Immunoglobulin G
CML	Chronic myelongenous (myelocytic) leukemia	**IgM**	Immunoglobulin M
DIC	Disseminated intravascular coagulation	**ITP**	Idiopathic thrombocytopenia purpura
DNA	Deoxyribonucleic acid	**IVIG**	Intravenous immune globulin
ESR	Erythrocyte sedimentation rate	**MCH**	Mean corpuscular hemoglobin
G-CSF	Granulocyte-colony stimulating factor	**MCHC**	Mean corpuscular hemoglobin concentration
GM-CSF	Granulocyte macrophage-colony stimulating factor	**mcL**	Microliter

MCV	Mean corpuscular volume	**RBC**	Red blood cell
Ph¹	Philadelphia chromosome	**RDW**	Red blood cell (R) distribution width
PHSC	Pluripotential hematopoietic stem cell	**SLE**	Systemic lupus erythematosus
PMN	Polymorphonuclear neutrophil	**WBC**	White blood cell
Rh	Rhesus		

SECTION ONE: Anatomy and Physiology of the Blood

At the completion of this section, the learner will be able to describe the anatomic components and physiologic functions of the blood.

Blood is composed of plasma, plasma proteins, and blood cells. Blood transports oxygen, glucose, hormones, electrolytes, and cell wastes. The adult body contains about 5 L of blood. Plasma is a clear fluid that remains after cells have been removed. Plasma makes up 55 percent of the whole blood volume. The remaining 45 percent of the whole blood volume is composed of cells (Gould, 2002). The anatomic components of blood and their physiologic functions are summarized in Figure 24–1.

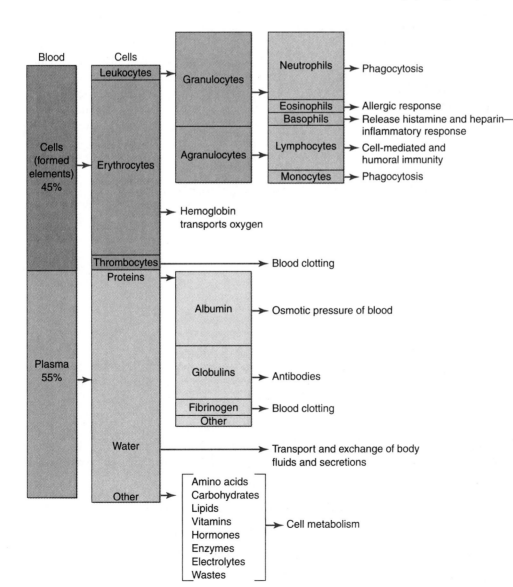

Figure 24–1 ■ Components of blood and their functions. (*Reprinted from Gould, B. (2002). Pathophysiology for the health professionals, (2nd ed., p. 234. Copyright 2002, with permission from Elsevier.*)

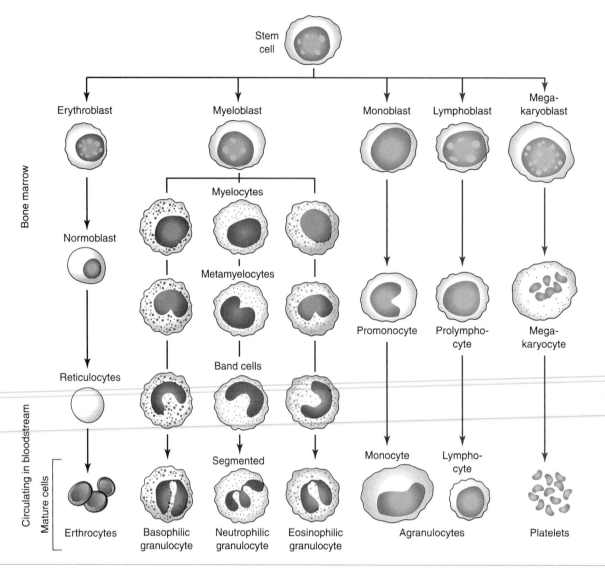

Figure 24–2 ▪ Simplified illustration of blood cell lineage. Committed cell proliferation follows either the myeloid cell line or the lymphoid cell line. Cells become increasingly differentiated as they move down the cell line toward maturity. *(Adapted from Chabner, D. E. [2001]. The language of medicine, (6th ed., p. 467) with permission from Elsevier.)*

Blood cells include **erythrocytes** (red blood cells), leukocytes (white blood cells), and thrombocytes (platelets). All three types of blood cells develop from the same stem cells, called **pluripotential hematopoietic stem cells (PHSC)**, which reside in the bone marrow. Once appropriately induced to reproduce a particular type of blood cell, the pluripotential stem cell divides. During PHSC division, one cell may remain as a PHSC, whereas the other becomes a **committed stem cell** of either the myeloid or lymphoid cell line (Fig. 24–2). This means that the newly committed cell begins to mature down a particular cell development pathway of cell growth and differentiation. The term **cell differentiation** refers to the matu-

ration process that a cell undergoes. It begins as an immature, undifferentiated cell with no specific functions and ultimately becomes a mature, well-differentiated cell with specific cell functions. The cell maturation process requires special proteins, called growth inducers and differentiation inducers. Factors external to the bone marrow trigger the formation of these special proteins. For example, chronic hypoxia induces secretion of erythropoietin, a growth factor that increases production of erythrocytes (Gould, 2002; Guyton & Hall, 1997). Table 24–1 provides a summary of normal blood cell ranges and common causes of abnormal complete blood count (CBC) results.

TABLE 24–1 Hematologic Causes for Abnormal CBC Results in Adults

TYPE	REFERENCE VALUE	DECREASED LEVEL	ELEVATED LEVEL
Red Blood Cells (RBCs)			
RBC count (mcL)	Adult: M: 4.5–6.0 Fe: 4.0–5.0 Elderly: M: 3.7–6.0 Fe: 4.0–5.0	Hemorrhage Anemias Hemodilution (overhydration)	Hemoconcentration (dehydration) Polycythemia vera
Hgb (g/dL)	Adult: M: 13.5–18.0 Fe: 12.0–16.0 Elderly: M: 11.0–17.0 Fe: 11.5–16.0	Anemias: Iron deficiency, aplastic, hemocytic Acute blood loss Hemodilution	Hemoconcentration (dehydration) Polycythemia vera
Hct (%)	Adult: M: 40–54 Fe: 36–41 Elderly: M: 38–42 Fe: 38–41	Anemias: Aplastic, hemolytic, folic acid deficiency, pernicious, sickle cell	Hemoconcentration (dehydration) Polycythemia vera
MCV (mcm^3)	Adult: 80–98 Elderly: M: 74–110 Fe: 78–100	Microcytic anemia: Iron deficiency	Macrocytic anemias Aplastic Hemolytic Pernicious
MCH (pg)	Adult: 27–31 Elderly: M: 24–33 Fe: 23–34	Microcytic, hypochromic anemia	Macrocytic anemias
MCHC (%)	Adult: 32–36 Elderly: M: 28–36 Fe: 30–36	Microcytic, hypochromic anemia Thalassemia	
RDW (Coulter S)	11.5–14.5		Anemias: Iron deficiency, folic acid deficiency, pernicious, sickle cell
White Blood Cells (WBC) with Differential			
WBC count (mcL)	Adult: 5,000–10,000 Elderly: M: 4,200–16,000 Fe: 3,100–10,000	Anemias: Aplastic, pernicious	Anemias: Hemolytic, sickle cell
Neutrophils (%)	Adult: 50–70 Elderly: 45–75	Anemias: Aplastic, folic acid deficiency, iron deficiency	Anemia: Acquired hemolytic
Basophils (%)	Adult: 0.5–1.0		Anemia: Acquired hemolytic
Lymphocytes (%)	Adult: 25–35 Elderly, Ave: 30	Anemia: Aplastic	
Monocytes (%)	Adult: 4–6 Elderly, Ave: 10	Anemias: Aplastic, iron deficiency, folic acid deficiency	Anemias: Sickle cell, hemolytic
Platelets			
Platelet count (mcL)	Adult: 150,000–400,000	Idiopathic thrombocytopenia purpura, leukemias, anemias, disseminated intravascular coagulation (DIC)	Polycythemia vera Acute blood loss

Kee, J. L. (2002). Laboratory and diagnostic tests with nursing implications. *Adapted by permission of Pearson Education, Inc. Upper Saddle River, NJ.*

Erythrocytes

When compared to the total numbers of white cells and platelets, red blood cells (RBCs) or erythrocytes are by far the most plentiful of the blood cells. This quantity difference becomes readily apparent when looking at the laboratory blood cell counts: RBCs are measured in million per microliter (mcL), whereas white blood cells (WBCs) and platelets are measured in cells per mcL. RBCs have a relatively long life span of approximately 120 days.

The Roles of Erythropoietin and Vitamins B$_{12}$ and Folic Acid

Erythrocyte production is tightly regulated. The purpose of erythrocytes is oxygen transport; thus, regulation is based on the level of tissue oxygenation, which is a function of tissue demand and oxygen transport. Erythrocyte production is regulated by *erythropoietin*, a circulating hormone that is primarily produced by the kidneys (about 90 percent). It is believed that erythropoietin may be produced in the renal tubular cells. The renal tubular cells are major consumers of oxygen that are particularly sensitive to lowering oxygen levels. Erythropoietin is a critical part of an erythrocyte production feedback loop (Fig. 24–3). Two vitamins, B$_{12}$ and folic acid, are essential to the maturation of erythrocytes for normal development of deoxyribonucleic acid (DNA). When an inadequate amount of either vitamin exists, it interferes with normal cell nucleus development and reproduction.

Hemoglobin

Hemoglobin is sometimes referred to as the respiratory protein because its function is to transport oxygen. As its name suggests, hemoglobin has two components—heme (nonprotein) and

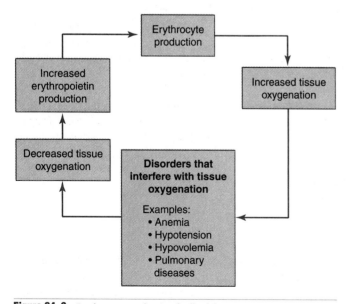

Figure 24–3 ■ Erythrocyte production feedback loop.

globin (protein). One heme molecule contains one iron atom and one oxygen molecule. The oxygen molecule (O$_2$) located in hemoglobin is attached only to the single iron atom in the molecule; thus, when there is deficient iron in the body (e.g., iron-deficiency anemia), the oxygen-carrying capacity is significantly reduced. A heme molecule joins with a polypeptide chain to form a hemoglobin chain. It takes four hemoglobin chains, linked together, to form one hemoglobin molecule. In a normal adult male, there are about 15 g of hemoglobin in every 100 mL of blood. Each gram of hemoglobin can bind with a maximum of about 1.34 mL of oxygen. Normally, the hemoglobin in 100 mL of blood (if fully saturated with oxygen) can bind with 20 mL of oxygen. Oxygen combines with hemoglobin loosely and reversibly. This means that oxygen can be loaded up on the hemoglobin, transported to the tissues, and then released from the hemoglobin to diffuse across the capillary membrane into the tissues.

Leukocytes

The environment in which we live is not a sterile one. We are exposed to potentially disease-producing organisms (pathogens) on a daily basis. It is through the strong protective mechanisms of the immune system that we are able to survive such constant pathogen exposure. The leukocytes (WBCs) are the circulating cells of the immune system. Although their quantities are limited, they are an extremely quick and powerful defense system. This section focuses on neutrophils and briefly discusses monocytes. Lymphocytes are presented in detail in Sections Four and Five of Module 25, "Altered Immune Function."

Neutrophils

Neutrophils, eosinophils, basophils, and monocytes have a common origin, the myelocyte. Neutrophils, eosinophils, and basophils are all *polymorphonuclear granulocytes.* The term **polymorphonuclear** refers to the presence of multiple nuclei and explains why they are commonly referred to as *polys* or *polymorphonuclear neutrophils* (**PMNs**). Neutrophils significantly outnumber all of the other types of leukocytes, comprising 50 to 70 percent of the total leukocyte (WBC) count (Kee, 2002). The myelocyte cell lineage is illustrated in Figure 24–2.

The term **granulocyte** refers to cells with granules located within the cytoplasm. The granules contain special enzymes that break down foreign and other substances. Neutrophils mature in the bone marrow and stay in reserve in the marrow for about 5 days before being sent into the general circulation (Knoop, 2003; Parslow, 1994). Once released from the bone marrow, they have a brief life span of only 6 to 8 hours; thus, they must be reproduced at an extremely fast rate to keep up with the rapid turnover.

Neutrophils are the immune system's first line of defense in the presence of an acute infection or inflammation. They are first at the scene, within 90 minutes of an injury event (Gould, 2002; Sommers, 1998). Neutrophils are responsible for the formation of pus. As neutrophils die, their degrading enzymes are released, causing breakdown and liquefaction of local cells as well as foreign substances. This forms pus, a thin liquid residue that is an important indicator of inflammation. Pus is an important consideration in the presence of neutropenia and will be discussed in more detail later in the module.

Basophils and Eosinophils

Basophils are from the same cell line as mast cells and, like mast cells, their granules contain histamine and heparin, which are released during an allergic reaction. Basophil degranulation results in vasodilation, spasm of smooth muscle, and increased vascular permeability. During a severe allergic response, basophils are capable of triggering anaphylactic shock (Turgeon, 1999). Whereas basophils increase the inflammatory response, eosinophils play an important role in quieting the response. The homeostatic role of eosinophils seeks to control and localize inflammation. This is accomplished through suppression of the reactivity of inflamed tissue and by reversing the activities of basophils and mast cells (Turgeon, 1999). Eosinophils may act on foreign proteins during an antibody-antigen allergic response by releasing chemical mediators or enzymes that detoxify the offending foreign protein (Gaspard, 2005).

Monocytes

Monocytes are large, single-nucleus phagocytes that provide the second line of defense. They act as long-term backup for neutrophils, arriving at the scene within about 5 hours of the event. Monocytes and neutrophils become the predominant cell types at the site of injury within 48 hours of the precipitating event (Gould, 2002; Sommers, 1998). Monocytes live much longer than neutrophils, with a life span of 4 to 5 days. Monocytes circulate in the blood for about a day before taking up residence in a tissue, becoming tissue macrophages (histiocytes) (Gould, 2002). Tissue macrophages can remain in a fixed position within the tissue for months or years until they are required to protect the tissue through their phagocytic functions.

Circulating monocytes are immature immune cells that do not actively participate in defense. Monocytes undergo maturational changes once they move into the tissues (Gould, 2002; Guyton & Hall, 1997). During the maturation process, they enlarge by up to fivefold and develop a large number of lysosomes in their cytoplasm. Lysosomes provide a digestive system that can digest nutrients, bacteria, or other particles that are brought into the cell. Once they have matured, the monocytes are called **macrophages,** which are powerful phagocytes.

Migration Properties of Neutrophils and Macrophages

Circulating neutrophils and monocytes require some means of recognizing where they are needed, and then they must be able to transfer from circulation to the site of injury. The process by which they do this involves multiple steps, including margina-

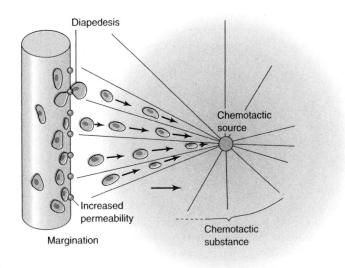

Figure 24–4 ■ Movement of leukocytes to injury site. Movement of neutrophils by the process of chemotaxis toward an area of tissue damage. *(Reprinted from Guyton, A. C., & Hall, J. E. (2002) Human physiology and mechanisms of disease, (6th ed., p. 282.) Copyright 2002, with permission from Elsevier.)*

tion, diapedesis, migration, and chemotaxis. Soon after initiation of the inflammatory response, the capillary endothelium becomes more permeable, allowing fluid to escape into the inflamed or injured area. The loss of fluid locally results in increased blood viscosity and increased concentration of cells in the local capillaries. When tissue becomes inflamed, a variety of chemicals, including chemical mediators and cytokines, are released at the site of injury (Gould, 2002; Sommers, 1998). These chemical substances cause alterations of local capillary endothelial cells and stimulate leukocytes to increase their release of adhesion molecules. **Margination** occurs as circulating leukocytes begin to accumulate and adhere to the capillary wall. Once the cells have adhered to the capillary wall, they develop **pseudopods** (fingerlike projections) and squeeze out of the capillary using ameboid movement, a process called **diapedesis.** Once the leukocyte is outside the capillary, it requires guidance to move to the correct location. This is accomplished through **chemotaxis,** "the directional migration of white blood cells (WBCs) along a concentration gradient of chemotactic factors, which are substances that attract leukocytes to the site of inflammation" (Lewis, 2000, p. 191). The leukocytes then follow the signal, traveling by ameboid action to the site. Figure 24–4 illustrates this concept.

Platelets

The hematologic system is sometimes referred to as a fluid organ. Correct functioning of an organ requires that its borders remain intact. The blood vessel walls constitute the hematologic system's borders. Vascular integrity is maintained through two closely interwoven mechanisms, hemostasis and blood coagulation. Discussion here will focus on the cellular component of hemostasis, the thrombocytes (platelets).

Platelets are not actually cells. They are tiny cell fragments composed of cytoplasm that are shed from megakaryocytes in the bone marrow. Mazur (1998) explains that the mechanism by which shedding occurs is not well understood. One theory suggests that mature megakaryocytes may transform in response to some unknown signal, forming spiderlike projections called *proplatelets*. These tiny proplatelets break off from the megakaryocyte as a result of a shearing force when they encounter blood flow in the bone marrow sinusoids. The normal platelet count in an adult is 150,000 to 400,000/mcL (Kee, 2002). Platelet production is closely regulated by thrombopoietin, which is primarily produced by the liver. Certain cytokines (e.g., interleukin-3) are also known to stimulate the production of platelets using different mechanisms (Gould, 2002; Mazur, 1998). Mature platelets survive for 8 to 10 days, with about two thirds being in the circulation at all times and the remaining one third being stored in the spleen. The stored platelets are continuously exchanging with circulating platelets (Gould, 2002).

The Hemostatic Function of Platelets

Hemostasis is defined as prevention of blood loss. Platelets play a crucial role in hemostasis by creating a platelet plug to seal off leaking vessels (Guyton & Hall, 1997). The internal structures of platelets also contain a variety of coagulation-related proteins and enzymes that interact with the coagulation process. Under normal circumstances, platelets circulate freely throughout the vascular system as smooth, disk-shaped particles. When vessel endothelial injury occurs, special activating factors, such as thrombin and platelet-activating factor, stimulate platelet hemostatic activities. On activation, the platelets undergo significant changes including adhesion and aggregation. Parise et al. (2001) and Turgeon (1999) explain

that within 1 to 2 minutes after vascular integrity is lost, platelets begin to adhere to the collagen fibers of the damaged subendothelium. To do this, they rapidly reshape themselves, developing pseudopods along the vessel's endothelial surface. As the platelets accumulate, they begin to aggregate or clump together and eventually form a cohesive mass, called a *platelet plug*. Once the platelet plug is formed, it is stabilized and consolidated by fibrinogen, eventually forming a fibrin clot. Platelet plugs are particularly effective in rapid repair of small vascular leaks.

In summary, the major solid components of the blood include erythrocytes, leukocytes, and platelets (thrombocytes). All of these cells come from the same pluripotential stem cell but take different committed pathways to maturation. Erythrocytes provide an effective oxygen transport system. Adequate production of healthy erythrocytes requires erythropoietin and vitamins B_{12} and folic acid. Hemoglobin, the major component of the erythrocyte, is the actual oxygen carrier. Hemoglobin requires iron as an integral part of its molecular structure. Leukocytes are the circulating cells of the immune system. There are five different types of leukocytes: neutrophils, monocytes, lymphocytes, eosinophils, and basophils. Each one plays a unique role in providing immune defense. Neutrophils are small, powerful, granulated polymorphonuclear cells that are the first line of defense. Basophils, like mast cells, contain granules that, when activated, release histamine and heparin. Eosinophils are homeostatic cells that help control the inflammatory response. Monocytes, on activation as macrophages, provide the second line of defense. Neutrophils and monocytes are able to leave the vascular system and move to a site of inflammation or infection through the mechanisms of margination, diapedesis, migration, and chemotaxis. Platelets are tiny cell fragments that protect the body's vascular integrity. They are an integral part of the hemostatic and coagulation functions. Their major activity is the sealing of tears in the blood vessels, thus stopping bleeding. Table 24–1 provides a summary of the normal serum values of the blood cells.

SECTION ONE REVIEW

1. On appropriate stimulation, pluripotential hematopoietic stem cells divide and create a
   A. RBC
   B. WBC
   C. committed stem cell
   D. megakaryocyte

2. The purpose of the erythrocyte is
   A. oxygen transport
   B. nutrient transport
   C. hemostasis
   D. protection

3. Adequate iron is a crucial part of hemoglobin because
   A. it cements the hemoglobin chain together
   B. it facilitates the release of oxygen to the tissues
   C. the heme molecule attaches to it to make a chain
   D. the oxygen molecule attaches to it

4. The primary purpose of granules located in the granulocyte, such as a neutrophil, is to
   A. detect the presence of infection
   B. break down foreign substances
   C. stimulate the production of monocytes
   D. initiate ameboid cell movement

5. To actively participate in phagocytic activities, monocytes must mature into
   A. neutrophils
   B. lysosomes
   C. cytokines
   D. macrophages
6. The process by which circulating neutrophils and macrophages are able to squeeze out of a capillary to go to the site of injury is called
   A. diapedesis
   B. chemotaxis
   C. margination
   D. translocation
7. Platelets are not actually cells, they are _____ from _____ in the bone marrow.
   A. granules; leukocytes
   B. lysosomes; erythrocytes
   C. cell fragments; megakaryocytes
   D. secretions; plasma cells

Answers: 1. C, 2. A, 3. D, 4. B, 5. D, 6. A, 7. C

SECTION TWO: Assessment and Diagnosis

At the completion of this section, the learner will be able to discuss the assessment and diagnosis of hematologic disorders.

Learning some basic information about laboratory tests that evaluate blood cells can assist the nurse in gaining a better understanding of the patient's condition and cause of clinical manifestations. It can also assist the nurse in developing an effective plan of care based on this understanding. A proactive knowledge of such tests may alert the nurse to potential complications so that preventative measures can be taken in a timely manner.

Evaluation of Erythrocytes

Basic information about the size, shape, and concentration of erythrocytes is easily obtained by performing peripheral blood smears. Tests that are commonly used to evaluate erythrocytes include reticulocyte count, mean corpuscular volume (MCV), total RBC count, hemoglobin and hematocrit, and evaluation of erythrocyte color. Table 24–2 provides a summary of the red blood cell indices.

Reticulocyte Count

Reticulocytes are immature erythrocytes that are easily detected and measured. Under normal circumstances, only about 1 percent of circulating erythrocytes are reticulocytes that have entered the circulation to replace dying mature erythrocytes. There are two general reasons why the reticulocyte count rises: (1) an increase in circulating reticulocytes or (2) a reduction in circulating red cells. A common type of reticulocyte count is the "corrected" count that corrects for the presence of anemia. The corrected reticulocyte count is calculated as follows:

$$\% \text{ reticulocytes} \times \frac{\text{Hct (patient)}}{\text{Hct (normal)}}$$

Obtaining a corrected reticulocyte count helps differentiate between types of anemia. An elevation (greater than 1.5 percent) occurs when the bone marrow is stimulated by erythropoietin to produce more reticulocytes. As a result of erythropoietin stimulation, reticulocytes are produced and released from the bone marrow at a faster rate. An elevated reticulocyte count is present in types of anemia where the bone marrow is functioning normally (e.g., blood loss and extrinsic hemolytic anemias). A reduced reticulocyte count suggests that the bone marrow is unable to respond to the increased demand (e.g., aplastic anemia, bone marrow depression or failure).

TABLE 24–2   Red Blood Cell Indices

RED BLOOD CELL COUNT	BASIS	DESCRIPTION
Mean corpuscular volume (MCV)	Red blood cell size	Microcytic = small size—Iron deficiency anemia and thalassemia
		Normocytic = normal size—Anemia of chronic disease
		Macrocytic = large size—Pernicious and folic acid anemia
Mean corpuscular hemoglobin (MCH)	Weight	Indicates the weight of hemoglobin
Mean corpuscular hemoglobin concentration (MCHC)	Hemoglobin concentration	Indicates the hemoglobin concentration per unit volume of RBCs
RBC distribution width (RDW)	Size difference	RDW is the measurement of the width of the distribution curve on a histogram. An elevated RDW indicates iron deficiency, folic acid deficiency, and vitamin B_{12} deficiency anemias.

Data from Kee, J. L. (2002). Laboratory and diagnostic tests with nursing implications. Adapted by permission of Pearson Education, Inc., Upper Saddle River, NJ.

Mean Corpuscular Volume

Kee (2002) explains that measurement of **mean corpuscular volume (MCV)** evaluates the size (volume) of the RBCs. Using MCV criteria, anemias can be divided into three categories: microcytic, normocytic, and macrocytic. A low MCV value indicates the presence of **microcytic** RBCs, which are smaller than normal in size and are present in such conditions as iron deficiency anemia and thalassemia. **Normocytic** RBCs are normal in size and are present in blood loss anemia, renal insufficiency, and early iron-deficiency anemia. **Macrocytic** RBCs are larger than normal in size and are found in conditions such as vitamin B_{12} or folate deficiency and drug-induced anemias. Anemias associated with chronic illness are generally either microcytic or normocytic.

Mean corpuscular hemoglobin (MCH) and **mean corpuscular hemoglobin concentration (MCHC)** are frequently measured with MCV; however, they provide little additional information that is not found in the MCV because MCH values parallel MCV values (Kee, 2002; Rose & Berliner, 1998). The MCH measures the average weight (concentration) of hemoglobin in red blood cells. MCHC is the hemoglobin concentration per unit volume of RBCs (Kee, 2002).

Total RBC Count

The healthy adult has between 4 million and 6 million/mcL × 10^{12} red blood cells (Kee, 2002). Men normally have higher RBC counts than women or children. Abnormally low levels (erythrocytopenia) are associated with specific anemias (e.g., blood loss, chronic renal failure), alcoholic cirrhosis, and other conditions. Abnormally high levels (erythrocytosis) may be seen in posthemorrhage states, leukemias, sickle cell and hemolytic anemias, and other conditions.

Hemoglobin and Hematocrit

Hemoglobin (HGB).   Hemoglobin has been discussed in the previous section. Higher-than-normal Hgb levels may result from hemoconcentration (e.g., dehydration), polycythemia (primary or secondary, discussed later in this section), and severe burns. Lower-than-normal levels may result from certain anemias (e.g., aplastic, iron deficiency), hemorrhage, hepatic cirrhosis, leukemias, and many other conditions (Kee, 2002). Table 24–3 summarizes the severity of anemia based on hemoglobin levels.

Hematocrit (HCT).   The hematocrit is a concentration measurement. It is the volume (in milliliters) of packed red blood cells in 100 mL of blood and is stated as a percentage. An elevated hematocrit suggests dehydration situations (e.g., severe diarrhea or hypovolemia), polycythemia vera, secondary polycythemia (as seen with late chronic obstructive pulmonary disease [COPD]), and other problems. A lower-than-normal hematocrit is most commonly associated with leukemias and anemias (Kee, 2002).

TABLE 24–3   Severity of Anemia Based on Hemoglobin Level

SEVERITY	HEMOGLOBIN LEVEL	COMMON MANIFESTATIONS
Mild	10–14 g/dL	Asymptomatic usually
		Cardiopulmonary: None, or may have mild palpitations or dyspnea on exertion
Moderate	6–10 g/dL	May be asymptomatic if slow onset or patient is sedentary
		Cardiopulmonary: Dyspnea, increased palpitations
		Other: Fatigue
Severe	Less than 6 g/dL	Symptomatic at rest or with activity
		Cardiopulmonary: Tachycardia, increased blood pressure, tachypnea, dyspnea, orthopnea, congestive heart failure, myocardial infarction
		Other: Bone pain, pallor, vertigo, headache, decreased activity tolerance

Data from O'Mara, A. M., & Whedon, M. B. (2000). Nursing management: Hematologic problems. In S. M. Lewis, M. M. Heitkemper, & S. R. Dirksen (Eds.), Medical–surgical nursing: Assessment and management of clinical problems, (5th ed.) St. Louis: C.V. Mosby. With permission from Elsevier.

Evaluation of Erythrocyte Color

Laboratory descriptions of erythrocytes as well as descriptions of erythrocytes in anemias usually include the descriptive terms, hypochromic or normochromic. Normally, the color of the biconcave disk-shaped RBC is pinkish-red in color in the outer two thirds of the disk and very pale in the center third (called the *central pallor*). This 2:1 (dark-to-light) ratio gives the RBC its "healthy" appearance, reflecting the presence of adequate levels of hemoglobin. The normal color appearance is called **normochromic.** In certain anemia types, the 2:1 ratio is lost, and the central pallor extends beyond its one-third border. This extended pallor gives the RBC a pale, or **hypochromic,** appearance. Hypochromic RBCs are most commonly seen in iron-deficiency anemia. Color alterations can also reflect cell immaturity, if the immature RBC has not yet taken in all of its hemoglobin.

Red Cell Mass

Red cell mass, also called red cell volume, is used to make a differential diagnosis of polycythemia. To perform this serum test, the patient has about 25 mL of blood drawn. The blood sample is radiolabeled with chromium (Cr-51) and a known quantity of the labeled blood is then reinjected into the patient's bloodstream. After about 1 hour, a second blood specimen is obtained. The second sample is then appropriately prepared and the circulating blood volume can be calculated. Patients with polycythemia have an abnormally high circulating red cell mass.

Red Cell Distribution Width

The red cell distribution width (RDW) is a recent addition to erythrocyte laboratory tests. According to Kee (2002), it is an index of RBC size variation and is calculated using a histogram. The normal RDW range is 11.5 to 14.5 percent. An elevated level (greater than 14.5 percent) has been associated with anemias caused by deficiencies in folic acid, B_{12}, or iron; and hemolysis. Although it maintains an independent relationship with MCV, the RDW is often used in comparison with MCV values. The RDW value is an earlier indicator of nutritional deficiencies than the MCV value. Comparisons of the two tests can also help distinguish among types of anemia. For example, iron-deficiency anemia results in a high RDW and a normal to low MCV, and anemia associated with chronic disease results in a normal RDW and a normal to low MCV.

Erythrocyte Sedimentation Rate (ESR)

Although the erythrocyte sedimentation rate (ESR) is not part of the CBC count, it is of interest to the high-acuity patient. The ESR is commonly referred to as "sed rate" or "sedimentation rate." It is "the rate at which red blood cells (RBCs) settle in unclotted blood in millimeters per hour (mm/hr)" (Kee, 2002, p. 164). ESR is a nonspecific screening measure of inflammation or infection; however, elevated levels also result from a variety of other problems. When ESR is abnormal, more specific diagnostic testing is indicated for making a differential diagnosis. ESR is measured in millimeters per hour (mm/hr) and the normal range changes with aging. In patients younger than 50, the normal range in males is zero to 15 mm/hr and it is zero to 20 in females; in patients older than 50, the normal range in males is zero to 20 and it is zero to 30 in females (Kee, 2002). Abnormally high ESR is associated with acute myocardial infarction, cancer, hepatitis, and rheumatic-type problems, such as rheumatic fever or rheumatoid arthritis. Abnormally low levels may be seen in patients with congestive heart failure, angina pectoris, or polycythemia vera (Kee, 2002).

Evaluation of Leukocytes

Although a simple WBC count is often adequate for general screening purposes, it is insufficient for gaining an in-depth understanding of the patient's infectious or inflammatory status. This information is obtained through the WBC differential count. The differential cell count breaks out the constituent cells of the WBCs: neutrophils (immature and mature), monocytes, eosinophils, and basophils.

Neutrophils

Neutrophils are measured in the serum as a percentage of maturity versus immaturity. The mature neutrophils, called **segmented cells** or **segs** (referring to a segmented nucleus), normally constitute about 50 to 70 percent of the total WBC count (Kee, 2002). Immature neutrophils, called **bands** or **stabs** (referring to the band- or horseshoe-shaped nucleus), normally make up 5 percent or less of the total WBC count (Kee, 2002). When called into action, neutrophils are produced at a faster rate by the bone marrow to meet the new demand. During periods of extremely high neutrophil production (e.g., severe infection), the bone marrow releases immature neutrophils. The elevated band level (**bandemia**) is referred to as a "shift to the left." The neutrophil count increases (neutrophilia) in response to inflammatory disorders (including cancer), bacterial infections, and tissue necrosis (Gould, 2002; Sommers, 1998). An abnormally low neutrophil count (neutropenia) can occur under circumstances involving increased destruction or decreased production. Neutropenia is discussed in detail in Section Four.

Monocytes

Monocytes comprise about 4 to 6 percent of the total WBC count (Kee, 2002). Elevated levels of monocytes (monocytosis) are associated with chronic infections (e.g., bacterial endocarditis and tuberculosis), rickettsial diseases (e.g., malaria), and inflammatory bowel disease. Monocytosis is also seen in acute and chronic monocytic leukemia (CML). Two examples of disorders with low levels of monocytes are aplastic anemia and hairy cell leukemia (Lichtman, 2001)

Eosinophils

Eosinophils comprise 1 to 3 percent of the total WBC count (Kee, 2002). The eosinophil count increases during many types of allergic responses (e.g., asthma and drug reactions) and parasitic infections. It also increases with certain types of neoplastic disorders, such as Hodgkin's disease. The eosinophil count decreases with elevated steroid levels of endogenous or exogenous origin.

Basophils

Basophils comprise 0.4 to 1 percent of the total WBC count (Kee, 2002). Basophilia (elevated basophil count) may be caused by a myeloproliferative disease such as leukemia, an allergy or inflammation, or an infection. Basophilopenia (lower than normal basophil count) may be caused by elevated levels of glucocorticoids, hyperthyroidism, ovulation, and hypersensitivity reactions (Galli et al., 2002).

Bone Marrow Biopsy

The bone marrow biopsy is used to rule out, confirm, or make a differential diagnosis of a disorder involving the bone marrow. It is often performed after suspicious cells are found in the peripheral blood. The biopsy is usually performed by needle aspiration and is usually taken from the iliac crest in an adult. The bone marrow is examined for the presence, number, and type of abnormal cells, or the absence of normal cells.

In summary, there are many measurements available to evaluate blood cells. This section provided an overview of some of the major tests used to evaluate the bone marrow, erythrocytes, and leukocytes. Tests that evaluate erythrocytes include the reticulocyte count, MCV, MCH, MCHC, total red cell count, hemoglobin, and hematocrit. Tests that evaluate leukocytes include the WBC count with or without the differential cell count. The differential is a more valuable test because it separates out and measures the relative values of each of the WBC component cells, including neutrophils, monocytes, eosinophils, and basophils. The bone marrow biopsy is performed to confirm a diagnosis or to evaluate the severity of a hematologic problem.

SECTION TWO REVIEW

1. An elevated reticulocyte count in the presence of anemia indicates that the
   A. red blood cells are being destroyed prematurely
   B. bone marrow is depressed
   C. red blood cells are to be sequestered in the spleen
   D. bone marrow is functioning correctly
2. An example of a condition that is associated with microcytic red blood cells (a low MCV) is
   A. aplastic anemia
   B. vitamin B$_{12}$ deficiency anemia
   C. iron-deficiency anemia
   D. blood loss anemia
3. A higher-than-normal hemoglobin level can result from
   A. dehydration
   B. aplastic anemia
   C. hepatic cirrhosis
   D. leukemia
4. Segmented neutrophils normally make up _____ percent of the total WBC count.

   A. 20 to 35
   B. 35 to 50
   C. 50 to 70
   D. 65 to 80
5. When a shift to the left occurs in the neutrophil count, it refers to a(n)
   A. elevated band level
   B. decreased band level
   C. elevated seg level
   D. decreased seg level
6. An elevated monocyte (monocytosis) level is associated with
   A. early bacterial infection
   B. aplastic anemia
   C. hemolytic anemia
   D. chronic infections

Answers: 1. D, 2. C, 3. A, 4. C, 5. A, 6. D

SECTION THREE: Red Blood Cell Disorders

At the completion of this section, the learner will be able to describe the etiology, pathophysiology, clinical manifestations, and management of red blood cell disorders.

Red blood cell disorders can be divided into two general groups: problems of too few RBCs (anemia) and problems of too many RBCs (polycythemia).

Anemia

The term **anemia** literally means "without blood." Its definition, however, refers to a reduction of or dysfunction in erythrocytes (RBCs). It can be clinically expressed in terms of a reduced RBC, hematocrit, or hemoglobin count. Anemia is not a disease; rather, it is an important sign of some underlying disorder.

Clinical Manifestations

Regardless of the cause, the clinical manifestations of anemia are primarily attributable to one dysfunction—*impaired oxygen transport.* Additional manifestations may be present, related to the rate of onset of the anemia, the hematocrit level, and the underlying cause (Rose & Berliner, 1998; Blackwell & Hendrix, 2001).

Tissue Hypoxia Manifestations

Impaired oxygen transport causes tissue hypoxia. Compensatory mechanisms in response to tissue hypoxia result in tachycardia and tachypnea, and contribute to bone pain that may develop as a result of increased hematopoietic activity in the bone marrow. Other hypoxia-related manifestations include fatigue, exercise intolerance, dyspnea, orthopnea, inability to concentrate, vertigo, irritability, anorexia, and others.

Rate of Onset

The speed with which the anemia occurs is an important factor in determining the severity of symptoms. When a mild-to-moderate anemia develops slowly, the person often remains asymptomatic as long as the body is not stressed (increasing oxygen demand). Given a slow enough onset, a person may remain relatively asymptomatic (if sedentary) with a hemoglobin as low as 6 or 7 g/dL (Blackwell & Hendrix, 2001; Turgeon, 1999). When the onset of anemia is rapid (e.g., severe hemorrhage), there is insufficient time for adequate compensatory mechanisms to activate, which can potentially result in severe hypoxemia and tissue ischemia.

Underlying Cause

The patient's clinical manifestations usually reflect both the underlying disorder and the anemia. For example, a person with end-stage renal failure will have symptoms related to anemia plus symptoms resulting from severe renal dysfunction. Some of the anemias also have their own unique manifestations. For example, sickle cell anemia (sickle cell disease) has many unique symptoms related to microvascular occlusion. One type of anemia (aplastic) is part of a pancytopenia problem (involving two or more blood cell types). If pancytopenia is present, the patient will also develop the clinical manifestations of deficiencies in the other cell types.

Categories of Anemias

There are different ways that the experts categorize anemias. The mechanism by which the anemia occurs is a particularly useful category system. There are three mechanisms: decreased RBC production, increased RBC destruction, and increased blood loss (Fig. 24–5). This section focuses on acute anemias that are particularly found in the high-acuity patient.

Decreased RBC Production

In Section One, RBC proliferation was presented as a tightly regulated and sequential maturation process in the bone marrow. Under certain circumstances, however, RBC proliferation becomes depressed. This can result from inadequate intake or absorption of certain vitamins or minerals, particularly iron (iron-deficiency [microcytic] anemia), vitamin B_{12}, and folic

acid (both are megaloblastic macrocytic anemias). It can also result from bone marrow depression secondary to chemotherapy, infection, or primary failure (aplastic anemia).

Iron-Deficiency Anemia. Iron-deficiency anemia is the most common form of anemia found worldwide. Iron deficiency is caused by inadequate dietary intake, increased demand for iron, or increased loss of iron (e.g., acute or chronic bleeding or menstrual blood loss). Because iron is the atom that oxygen attaches to on the hemoglobin molecule, its lack thereof directly alters the oxygen-carrying capacity of the hemoglobin. Laboratory analysis of RBCs in iron-deficiency anemia will show RBCs that are microcytic and hypochromic and have a decreased MCV and MCHC. The RBC membrane often becomes fragile, making it more susceptible to damage (Gould, 2002). The underlying cause for the iron-deficiency anemia must be identified and iron supplementation may be required. Oral forms of iron should be given with food to avoid upset stomach. Liquid iron may stain teeth and, therefore, a straw should be used for ingestion of the medication (Gould, 2002). The intravenous forms of iron may cause anaphylaxis.

Megaloblastic Anemias. The term *megaloblastic* refers to the large size of the RBCs. These cells typically have large, immature nuclei with fairly mature cytoplasm (Gould, 2002; Rose & Berliner, 1998). Vitamins B_{12} (cobalamin) and folic acid are essential components of RBC development. Vitamin B_{12} deficiency most commonly occurs under two circumstances: (1) through inadequate dietary intake and (2) through malabsorption, such as seen with loss of intrinsic factor (IF), a glycoprotein that is produced by the parietal cells in the fundus of the stomach. When vitamin B_{12} enters the stomach, it forms a stable *IF–cobalamin complex*. In this form, it travels through the gastrointestinal system to the ileum, where it is reabsorbed (Turgeon, 1999; Fairbanks & Beutler, 2001). Loss of intrinsic factor from any cause (e.g., autoantibodies) leads to vitamin B_{12}–deficiency anemia (pernicious anemia). Folic acid is also necessary in RBC development. Folic acid deficiency is most

Figure 24–5 ■ Classification of anemias.

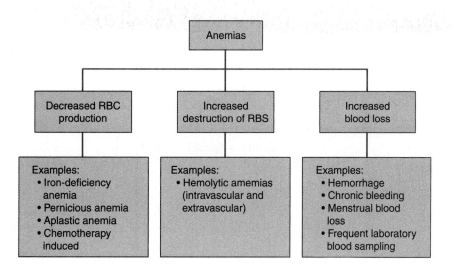

commonly caused by inadequate intake. Laboratory analysis of RBCs associated with megaloblastic anemias shows the presence of megaloblastic RBCs (macro-ovalocytes), a low RBC count, and low hemoglobin. Common characteristics are weakness, beefy red tongue, and systemic signs of anemia. Megaloblastic anemias are most commonly seen as chronic forms of anemia. Lack of vitamin B_{12} causes demyelination of the peripheral nerves that progresses to the spinal cord. Sensory fibers are affected first, then the motor fibers. The entire process may be irreversible (Gould, 2002). Treatment of the cause and supplemental vitamin B_{12} may prevent cardiac stress and neurological damage.

Acquired Aplastic Anemia. Aplastic anemia, a hypoproliferative form of anemia, is characterized by a decrease in production of blood cells from bone marrow failure (Gould, 2002). It has two peak incidence periods: a major peak in young adults (ages 20 to 25) and a lesser peak in the elderly (ages 60 to 65) (Andreoli et al., 1997; Gould, 2002). In the high-acuity patient, it may be seen as part of bone marrow depression or failure secondary to some acquired (extrinsic) mechanism, such as a viral, drug, radiation, or autoimmunity mechanism. When the etiology remains unknown, it is referred to as *idiopathic* aplastic anemia. Because the entire bone marrow is usually compromised, it results in a pancytopenia. Fatty tissue replaces the normal hematopoietic tissue in the bone marrow.

Etiology. In cases in which causation has been adequately established, aplastic anemia has been associated with

- Benzene
- Drugs (e.g., chloramphenicol, phenylbutazone, gold salts, phenytoin, and cytotoxic chemotherapeutic agents)
- Infections (rare; e.g., Epstein–Barr virus, hepatitis B and C)
- Ionizing radiation

Pathophysiology. Aplastic anemia develops when damaged or impaired stem cells inhibit red blood cell production (Gould, 2002). Aplastic anemia varies widely in severity, from mild to severe. The prognosis is based on the severity of the disease (Andreoli et al., 1997; Gould, 2002). Severe aplastic anemia is a relentless disease with rare spontaneous remissions. If left untreated, the prognosis is poor, with most patients dying within 6 months of onset. Even with effective treatment, life expectancy is often only a few years.

Treatment. The treatment for aplastic anemia focuses on three general areas: supportive, immunosuppressive, and bone marrow replacement. Supportive therapy includes blood transfusions to replace RBCs and platelets, and antibiotic therapy to protect from infection. Immunosuppressive therapy frequently consists of antithymocyte globulin (ATG) or a combination of ATG, steroids, and/or cyclosporine. These drugs are used when bone marrow transplantation is not planned. Bone marrow transplantation is the definitive treatment for aplastic anemia in younger patients. If the patient is a candi-

date for bone marrow transplantation, blood transfusions will be limited, with no transfusions coming from potential marrow donors. This helps reduce the risk of hypersensitivity reactions and potential bone marrow rejection.

Increased Destruction of RBCs

The term **hemolytic anemia** refers to anemias that are caused by premature destruction of red blood cells, either intravascularly or within the **reticuloendothelial system** (Gould, 2002; Rose & Berliner, 1998). Hemolytic anemia can result from intrinsic (e.g., congenital) problems or, more commonly, from extrinsic problems. The high-acuity patient is much more at risk for acquired (extrinsic) problems. Acquired hemolytic anemia is often categorized by the condition or agent that causes the destruction, including immune disorders, drugs, infectious agents, physical agents, and conditions associated with microangiopathy.

Immune Disorders. Premature destruction of RBCs by the immune system is a major cause of hemolytic anemia. Antibodies or complement (or sometimes both) coat the red blood cell membrane, causing premature death of the cell. The antibodies can be autoimmune induced, isoimmune induced, or drug induced (e.g., sulfonamides). Autoimmune-induced hemolytic anemia (AIHA) results from production of autoantibodies against the person's own red blood cells. The cause is unknown, but it is theorized that the autoimmune reaction may at times result from an infectious agent, such as infectious mononucleosis (Gould, 2002; Turgeon, 1999). Isoimmune-induced hemolytic anemia is primarily seen in two situations. It most commonly results from **ABO** blood type incompatibility between mother and baby. It can also result from **Rh incompatibility** in newborn infants.

Drugs. Drug-induced hemolytic anemia can damage and prematurely destroy RBCs by several mechanisms:

- Attachment of the drug or immune complexes to RBC membranes
- Production of autoantibodies (usually **IgM**) (Turgeon, 1999)

Examples of drugs that are known to cause drug-induced hemolytic anemia include alpha-methyldopa and sulfonamides. Fortunately, RBC destruction caused by drugs is often transient, ending when the agent is removed; thus, rapid recognition of the offending agent with rapid withdrawal is the priority action in initiating treatment.

Infectious Agents. Infectious agents have a variety of mechanisms by which they destroy RBCs. Some bacteria produce toxins and other substances that hemolyze cells, for example, *Clostridium perfringens* infections. Malaria is a protozoan infectious disease in which the protozoa enters the RBC and begins reproducing. Eventually, the RBC ruptures, and the disease spreads to other RBCs.

Physical Agents. RBCs are exposed to high temperatures in severe burn injury. Heat is a physical agent that makes RBCs fragile and causes them to fragment (called *schistocytes*). The fragmented cells are filtered out by the spleen and serum RBC levels drop significantly (Turgeon, 1999).

Conditions Associated with Microangiopathy. Microangiopathic hemolytic anemia involves the fragmentation of RBCs as they move through damaged small blood vessels (Rose and Berliner, 1998). Microangiopathy occurs in such conditions as disseminated intravascular coagulation (DIC), thrombotic thrombocytopenic purpura (TTP), and malignant hypertension; it has also been observed in pregnancy complications (e.g., HELLP syndrome and eclampsia). It can also result from damage caused by administration of certain drugs (e.g., cyclosporine and mitomycin-c). The schistocytes are easily found on peripheral blood smears. In addition, RBC fragmentation caused by artificial heart valve trauma is sometimes classified under this category.

Increased Blood Loss

Anemia caused by blood loss is a common problem. Blood loss can be acute (rapid onset) or chronic (slow, insidious onset), and can involve gross or occult bleeding. These two sets of factors largely determine the patient's clinical presentation. This discussion is confined to acute blood loss, which is more prevalent in high acuity patients.

Acute Blood Loss Anemia

Trauma is a major cause of acute blood loss. It is also associated with surgery and acute gastrointestinal (GI) bleeding. The clinical manifestations of acute blood loss are usually more severe than those associated with chronic blood loss because of the inability of the body to muster sufficient compensatory mechanisms in an acute situation. Hillman and Hershko (2001) and Turgeon (1999) suggest that less than 20 percent of total blood volume lost (less than 1 L in an adult) often remains asymptomatic. Blood loss of more than 20 percent significantly reduces total blood volume, producing cardiovascular changes. A blood loss of more than 30 percent (greater than 1.5 L) is associated with decreased blood pressure at rest and increased restlessness, and a loss of more than 40 percent (greater than 2 L) produces hypovolemic shock (discussed in detail in Module 15, "Shock States"). Acute GI bleeding is presented in detail in Module 30, "Acute Gastrointestinal Dysfunction."

During acute bleeding, early laboratory studies are deceptive. Hemoglobin and hematocrit do not initially reflect anemia because plasma as well as cells are equally lost. As bleeding continues, fluid begins to shift from the extravascular spaces into the intravascular space. This fluid shift causes dilution of the remaining blood cells. In addition, as fluid resuscitation is initiated, the intravascular space is loaded with fluids, which further increases the dilutional effect. The end result is a significant reduction in serum hemoglobin and hematocrit. The full extent of the bleed cannot be evaluated using Hgb and Hct values until 48 to 72 hours after the acute bleed. There is an elevation of the reticulocyte count within several days of the bleeding event as the bone marrow begins to produce and release the immature RBCs at a rapid rate. The anemia resulting from acute bleeding is typically described as normocytic and normochromic.

Polycythemia

Polycythemia refers to the production and presence of an abnormally high number of red blood cells. There are two major forms of polycythemia: primary and secondary. This section provides a brief overview of primary polycythemia and focuses on secondary polycythemia, which is more commonly seen in the high-acuity patient.

Primary Polycythemia

Primary polycythemia, called *polycythemia vera,* is a rare, clonal myeloproliferative disease involving the pluripotential hematopoietic stem cell (PHSC). All cells in the myeloid cell line are usually affected, including erythrocytes, leukocytes, and thrombocytes. It involves excessive production of all three cell types but the degree of RBC proliferation is particularly striking. Polycythemia vera is a chronic disease that exists on a continuum from mild to severe but tends to worsen over many years. It is a disorder of older age and affects more men than women. The cause is unknown but certain risk factors have been identified, such as chemical exposure and unclear genetic influences. The disease is characterized by a significant increase in the RBC mass, an elevated hematocrit, hypervolemia, increased viscosity of the blood, and splenomegaly from pooling of RBCs. Because RBC proliferation is the most extreme, the major clinical manifestations revolve around this characteristic. In general, the most significant complications associated with polycythemia vera include an increased risk for thromboses and infarction that may affect the extremities, liver, kidneys, brain or heart.

Secondary Polycythemia

Secondary polycythemia, or *erythrocytosis,* is not a disease; rather, it is a symptom of some underlying pathology or environmental factor. In the high-acuity patient, secondary polycythemia frequently occurs as an appropriate compensatory response to chronic tissue hypoxia. Compensatory secondary polycythemia can result from environmental factors (e.g., living at a high altitude), from chronic cardiac or pulmonary diseases (e.g., congenital heart disease or COPD), and from smoking. In the presence of chronic tissue hypoxia, the kidneys produce more erythropoietin, which then stimulates the bone marrow to produce more RBCs (erythrocytosis). The elevated RBC count results in increased oxygen-carrying capacity of the blood and ultimately, increased oxygen to the tissues (Beutler, 2001; Rose & Berliner, 1998; Turgeon, 1999).

Clinical Manifestations. The clinical manifestations of secondary polycythemia can be attributed to three underlying problems:

1. Increased red blood cell count
2. Increased viscosity of the blood
3. Increased blood volume

A significant increase in red blood cell mass increases the thickness (viscosity) of the blood as well as the blood volume. The end result of these events is sluggish or stagnant blood flow, particularly in the microcirculation. Laboratory studies reflect these events as well. Hypertension and thrombosis are complications that result from blood hyperviscosity. These complications may be manifested as a stroke, peripheral vascular disease, or ischemic heart disease (Beutler, 2001; Rose & Berliner, 1998). Treatment focuses on eliminating or reducing the underlying problem. Phlebotomy is frequently performed to maintain a hematocrit of less than 45 percent, which reduces the risk of complications (Beutler, 2001; Shulman, 1998).

In summary, anemias can be divided into three general categories based on the cause, including decreased RBC production, increased RBC destruction, and increased blood loss. Anemias that result from decreased RBC production include nutritional deficiencies and aplastic anemias. Iron-deficiency anemia is the most common type of anemia worldwide. Aplastic anemia usually involves all blood cell types (pancytopenia) and, in severe cases, has a high mortality rate. Acquired hemolytic anemias cause premature RBC destruction, which may be related to immune, infectious agents, physical agents, and microangiopathic conditions. Blood loss anemia cannot be accurately measured until 2 to 3 days following the bleed, when fluid shifts have stabilized. Acute bleeding is generally more symptomatic because of the inability to muster adequate compensatory mechanisms with rapid fluid volume loss. Polycythemia refers to excessive red blood cells. It can occur as a malignant disease called polycythemia vera, a rare myeloproliferative disease. This form involves hyperproliferation of all myeloid cell lines. In the high-acuity patient, polycythemia most frequently results from chronic tissue hypoxia. Clinical manifestations and complications develop from increased RBCs, increased blood viscosity, and increased blood volume.

SECTION THREE REVIEW

1. The clinical manifestations of the anemias are primarily attributable to
   A. decreased cardiac output
   B. impaired oxygen transport
   C. decreased blood volume
   D. impaired bone marrow function
2. The severity of symptoms associated with anemia largely depends on the
   A. type of anemia
   B. total blood volume
   C. speed with which it develops
   D. degree of bone marrow involvement
3. The most common form of anemia found worldwide is
   A. megaloblastic anemias
   B. iron-deficiency anemia
   C. aplastic anemia
   D. blood loss anemia
4. Loss of intrinsic factor (IF) causes development of which form of anemia?
   A. megaloblastic
   B. hemolytic
   C. aplastic
   D. iron-deficiency
5. The form of anemia that usually involves pancytopenia is
   A. aplastic
   B. hemolytic

C. megaloblastic
D. iron-deficiency
6. The definitive treatment for aplastic anemia in younger patients is
   A. blood transfusions
   B. antibiotic therapy
   C. immunosuppressant therapy
   D. bone marrow transplant
7. The most common etiology of hemolytic anemia is
   A. infectious agents
   B. immune disorder
   C. physical agents
   D. microangiopathy
8. The most common cause of acute blood loss anemia is
   A. alcohol abuse
   B. menorrhagia
   C. trauma
   D. GI bleeding
9. The underlying cause of secondary polycythemia is
   A. chronic tissue hypoxia
   B. myeloproliferative disease
   C. depletion of erythropoiesis
   D. chronic obstructive pulmonary disease

Answers: 1. B, 2. C, 3. B, 4. A, 5. A, 6. D, 7. B, 8. C, 9. A

SECTION FOUR: White Cell Disorders

At the completion of this section, the learner will be able to discuss the etiology, pathophysiology, clinical manifestations, and management of white cell disorders.

Neutropenia

Neutropenia (granulocytopenia) refers to an abnormally low level of neutrophils. Neutropenia is not a disease; rather, it is an important symptom of some other underlying problem. High-acuity patients are at risk for developing neutropenia related to the severity of their illnesses. Neutropenia exists when the neutrophil count drops below 50 percent of the total WBC count. It is commonly defined as a neutrophil count of less than 2,000 cells/mcL. A neutrophil count below 1,000/mcL places the neutropenic person at a high risk for developing an infection, and a count below 500/mcL is considered life threatening (Andreoli et al., 1997; Knoop, 2003)—the lower the neutrophil count, the higher the risk. The absolute neutrophil count (ANC) equals the number of white blood cells multiplied by the sum of the percentage of segmented neutrophils plus the percentage of band neutrophils (**ANC = WBC × [segs + bands]**). Neutropenia can be intrinsic (rare) or acquired. Acquired neutropenia is associated with premature destruction and decreased production of neutrophils. Table 24–4 is the National Cancer Institute's grading system of neutropenia.

Premature Destruction

Premature death of neutrophils is most commonly associated with drugs. Certain drugs (e.g., antibiotics) can cause development of drug–antibody immune complexes, which then attach to the neutrophils. Neutropenia can also result from an isolated autoimmune process, or as a complication of another autoimmune disorder, such as systemic lupus erythematosus (SLE). In addition, the spleen is capable of entrapping neutrophils and destroying them; this sometimes occurs with disorders associated with splenomegaly.

Decreased Production

Decreased production of neutrophils can occur by direct injury to the bone marrow (e.g., aplastic anemia), by overcrowding of normal bone marrow components from infiltration of malignant cells (e.g., leukemia), or bone marrow suppression by cancer chemotherapy or irradiation. It can also result from severe nutritional deficits (e.g., starvation), and vitamin B_{12} or folate deficiency.

Clinical Manifestations

Neutropenia causes altered responses to inflammation and infection because neutrophils are the first line of internal defense against infection and play a crucial part in the inflammatory process. The patient who develops neutropenia is at risk for infection. The source of the infection is often from normal flora because the body is host to a variety of pathogens, both externally and internally. Under normal circumstances, these pathogens remain harmless, but in conditions such as neutropenia, they can invade the body and cause serious, sometimes life-threatening infections.

The clinical manifestations associated with infection are altered to the degree that the neutrophil count is compromised. In mild cases of neutropenia, a fairly normal inflammatory response to infection occurs. The person may exhibit typical manifestations: fever, chills, malaise, and formation of exudate, adventitious breath sounds (e.g., pneumonia), but perhaps to a lesser degree. In more severe cases of neutropenia, however, the inflammatory response becomes significantly depressed. A moderate fever may become the primary symptom—often no higher than 100.5°F (38.1°C). Formation of pus may occur later in the infection or not at all if severe neutropenia is present. Febrile neutropenia is a life-threatening event and must be treated as soon as possible (Byars, 2003).

Treatment

Early discovery and aggressive treatment of the underlying cause of the neutropenia is imperative. Investigation of the cause may include antibody or bone marrow testing, or discontinuing drugs. Empiric antibiotic therapy is often initiated, with close attention being placed on monitoring for secondary infections. G-CSF (granulocyte-colony stimulating factor) or **GM-CSF** (granulocyte macrophage-colony stimulating factor) may be administered to try to stimulate the bone marrow to increase production of neutrophils (Byars, 2003). Nursing management of the immunosuppressed patient is discussed in Module 25.

Leukemia

Leukemia and bone marrow transplant patients are frequently seen in the intensive care units. Leukemia is included in this module as an oncologic prototype to lay a foundation for

TABLE 24–4   National Cancer Institute Neutropenia Grading Scale

GRADE	ABSOLUTE NEUTROPHIL COUNT (ANC) (/MM³)	INFECTION RISK
1	Less than 2,000	Slight
2	Less than 1,500	Minimal
3	Less than 1,000	Moderate
4	Less than 500	Severe

Data from National Cancer Institute. (1999). National Institutes of Health.

discussion of hematologic issues that are common with many types of cancers.

Leukemia is a malignant process in which there is a transformation of hematopoietic cells, causing unregulated clonal growth (Gould, 2002; Shulman, 1998). Leukemias are categorized as being either acute or chronic. The acute leukemias are characterized by aggressive proliferation of immature lymphoid or myeloid blast cells. Refer to Figure 24–2 to view the early stage of blast cells in cell development. Chronic leukemias, however, are characterized by production of mature, differentiated cells of either lymphoid or myeloid lineage. Chronic leukemias have a more insidious long-term clinical course than the acute leukemias.

Leukemia involves an uncontrolled production of malignant cells in the bone marrow that suppresses and replaces the normal cells, which leads to progressive pancytopenia. In untreated acute leukemia, the patient rapidly succumbs to complications of pancytopenia, particularly infection or hemorrhage (Gould, 2002; Shulman, 1998). The acute leukemias are also associated with infiltration into other tissues, such as the gums, spleen, central nervous system, and lymph nodes, thereby creating clinical manifestations specific to each affected tissue. Diagnosis of the exact type of leukemia can be difficult. The blast cells are sometimes so primitive that it initially may be difficult to determine whether the malignant cell clones are of myelocytic or lymphocytic origin (Gould, 2002).

Causes

The exact causes of leukemia are unknown. It is believed that there may be multiple factors involved in the development of each of the different leukemias, including environmental and genetic factors. There is an increased incidence of leukemia with chromosomal abnormalities, for example, children with Down syndrome. In several types of leukemia, a chromosomal abnormality has been isolated called the Philadelphia chromosome (Ph[1]), which involves the translocation between the long arms of chromosomes 22 and 9 (Caudell, 1998; Gould, 2002; Shulman, 1998). Certain chemical and drug exposures are associated with development of leukemia (e.g., benzene, chloramphenicol, and some antineoplastic agents). Radiation exposure provides an environmental hazard such as occurs in nuclear disasters or following radiation treatment for previous malignancies. Although human viruses are suspected as a potential cause of leukemia, only one has been established: human T cell leukemia virus type I (HTLV-1) (O'Mara & Whedon, 2000).

Acute Leukemias

There are two forms of acute leukemia: acute lymphocytic (lymphoblastic) leukemia and acute myelogenous leukemia.

Acute Lymphocytic (Lymphoblastic) Leukemia. Acute lymphocytic leukemia (ALL) is primarily a disease of childhood. For children under the age of 15, ALL accounts for one fourth of all cancers and 76 percent of all leukemias (Ching-Hon, 2001).

Acute lymphocytic leukemia is associated with proliferation of immature lymphoblasts from the B cell lineage (about 70 percent of ALL cases) or, less commonly, the T cell lineage (Ching-Hon, 2001; Shulman, 1998). The leukemic cells fail to mature or differentiate any further than the stage at which they are produced; therefore, they cannot carry on normal immune functions.

Laboratory findings typically found in acute lymphocytic leukemia include leukocytosis that is usually not severe. According to Turgeon (1999) and Ching-Hon (2001), the peripheral blood contains almost all lymphoblasts and lymphocytes. Anemia and thrombocytopenia are common, but the cells are normal mature erythrocytes and platelets to the extent that they are present at all. Somewhat immature neutrophils may be present in the peripheral blood.

Acute Myelogenous (Myelocytic) Leukemia. Acute myelogenous leukemia (AML) is most commonly seen in the adult population, with about one half of cases occurring over the age of 60 (Caudell, 1998). Acute myelogenous leukemia is characterized by proliferation of malignant blast cells from the myeloid stem cell lineage (Lichtman & Liesveld, 2001a; Shulman, 1998). The proliferation can involve any or all of the cells in the myeloid lineage (erythroblasts, megakaryoblasts, monoblasts, or myeloblasts). Blast cells are not programmed to die; thus, malignant blast clones can produce malignant cells indefinitely (Lichtman & Liesveld, 2001a; Shulman, 1998). Cells rapidly accumulate in the bone marrow and then infiltrate into other tissues.

Laboratory findings consistent with AML include the presence of thrombocytopenia and anemia. Leukocytosis is commonly noted, usually accompanied by neutropenia. An examination of peripheral blood and the bone marrow shows a predominance of myeloblastic cells. Auer rods may be present in the cytoplasm of the myeloblasts.

Chronic Leukemias

There are two forms of chronic leukemia: chronic lymphocytic leukemia and chronic myelogenous leukemia.

Chronic Lymphocytic Leukemia. According to Turgeon (1999), chronic lymphocytic leukemia (CLL) is primarily a disease of middle-age to older adults (more than 50 years old), and it is more commonly seen in males than females. It has a variable life expectancy, ranging from 2 to 10 years, with some patients surviving for 30 years or more. Death commonly results from infection, but many persons with CLL die of unrelated causes. About one third of persons with CLL eventually develop hemolytic anemia of autoimmune etiology. Chronic lymphocytic leukemia is almost always B cell type. The major characteristic of CLL is the presence of smaller-than-normal mature lymphocytes in the peripheral blood and bone marrow. These cells can often be found in the spleen and lymph nodes, causing splenomegaly and lymphadenopathy. The small CLL lymphocytes often are not fully functional as immune cells, causing *hypogammaglobulinemia,* which means abnormally low levels of gamma globulin in the blood. When present, the person with

CLL is immunodeficient and at increased risk for development of infection.

Laboratory findings consistent with chronic lymphocytic leukemia include anemia and thrombocytopenia. These two conditions are further aggravated if autoantibodies develop, causing premature cell destruction. Existing granulocytes, thrombocytes, and erythrocytes appear normal. Diagnostic criteria for CLL include a lymphocyte count of 10,000 cells/mcL or greater and the presence of at least 40 percent lymphocytes in the bone marrow (Andreoli et al., 1997; Kipps, 2001). About one third of persons with CLL have a leukocyte count of greater than 100,000 cells/mcL. A sample of the peripheral blood usually shows between 80 and 90 percent small leukocytes (Kipps, 2001; Turgeon, 1999). The bone marrow is infiltrated with leukemic cells.

Chronic Myelogenous (Myelocytic) Leukemia. Chronic myelogenous leukemia (CML), a type of myeloproliferative disease, is primarily a disease of adults but occurs at all ages. More males than females are affected, and in 5 to 10 percent of cases, there is a history of high-radiation exposure (Lichtman & Liesveld, 2001b; Turgeon, 1999). Chronic myelogenous leukemia is directly linked to the Ph[1] chromosome abnormality. CML, like AML, involves hyperproliferation of myelocytic stem cells; thus, it involves all of the cell types in the myelocyte lineage. This translocation results in the transfer of the Ableson (Abl) oncogene to an area on chromosome 22 called the breakpoint cluster region (bcr). The fused bcr-Abl gene and the production of an abnormal tyrosine kinase protein may be found in CML. Chronic myelogenous leukemia is characterized by the predominance of excessive numbers of mature and immature myelocytic cells. It is a slow-onset, slowly progressive disease. The course of CML typically runs in phases: chronic, accelerated, and acute (blast).

During the *chronic phase,* the patient has leukocytosis, but the neutrophils and thrombocytes are usually normal. It is during this phase that the diagnosis is usually made. The patient typically presents with marked thrombocytosis and splenomegaly. The chronic phase is usually treatable and the patient remains asymptomatic. Without treatment, the chronic phase lasts from 2 to 4 years (O'Mara & Whedon, 2000). With treatment, this phase may last 5 or more years.

The *accelerated phase* begins with the onset of increased signs and symptoms. It usually occurs with or without treatment; however, treatment during the chronic phase can significantly delay onset of the accelerated phase. Eventually, most persons with CML develop resistance to therapy, heralding in the accelerated phase. The accelerated phase generally ends in an *acute (blast transformation) phase,* when the patient's leukemia changes from chronic to acute. The acute phase is characterized by the onset of a "blast crisis" in which the blast cells are no longer able to differentiate into their more mature forms, resulting in blast cell domination in the bone marrow and peripheral blood. In most cases, the blast crisis reflects a transformation that is similar to AML; however, in about 20 percent of cases, there is a

transformation of lymphocytes, with subsequent ALL-type findings (Lichtman & Liesveld, 2001b; Shulman, 1998; Timmerman, 1998). The blast crisis is typically resistant to treatment and usually ends in death within a few months.

Laboratory findings consistent with CML depend on the phase of the disease. Overall, however, CML is characterized by extreme leukocytosis and the existence of any combination of mature and immature myelogenous cells in the bone marrow and blood. The total leukocyte count may exceed 300,000, placing the patient at high risk for leukostasis problems (Lichtman & Liesveld, 2001b; Turgeon, 1999). Anemia and thrombocytosis are often present early in the disease, although thrombocytopenia is possible.

Clinical Manifestations of Leukemia

The initial clinical presentation of a person at the onset of acute leukemia is often dramatic, with complaints of fevers and headache. Other common presenting symptoms include infection, bleeding, and malaise (Gould, 2002; Turgeon, 1999). The major clinical manifestations of the leukemias can be categorized into two groups: those that are caused by pancytopenia and those that are caused by expansion and infiltration of malignant cells into other tissues. Table 24–5 provides a summary of manifestations.

TABLE 24–5 Clinical Manifestations of Leukemia

CATEGORY	COMMON CLINICAL MANIFESTATIONS
Pancytopenia	Leukopenia (immunodeficiency)
	• Frequent infections
	• Fever
	Thrombocytopenia (bleeding tendencies)
	• Epistaxis, bleeding gums
	• Petechiae and ecchymosis
	Erythrocytopenia (anemia)
	• Pale mucous membranes
	• Fatigue, activity intolerance, malaise
	• Intolerance to cold
	• Tachycardia, tachypnea
Malignant Cell Expansion	Bone
	• Bone tenderness or pain
	Vascular system
	• Leukocytosis and leukostasis
	• Impaired circulation (particularly brain and/or lungs)
Infiltration	CNS
	• Headache, nausea, and vomiting
	• Seizures, coma
	• Papilledema, cranial nerve palsies
	Liver and spleen
	• Hepatomegaly and splenomegaly
	• Abdominal discomfort
	• Worsening thrombocytopenia/pancytopenia

Pancytopenia Manifestations.   As the red blood cell count decreases, the person with leukemia becomes increasingly anemic, demonstrating all of the manifestations of that problem. As the normal leukocyte count decreases, the patient becomes immunodeficient and becomes increasingly at risk for infections; however, the typical clinical picture associated with infection may be diminished or absent. Infection is the most common cause of death (about 70 percent) in adults with acute leukemia (Gould, 2002; Turgeon, 1999). Fever is commonly noted related to infection and increased metabolism of the malignant cells (Caudell, 1998; Gould, 2002). Finally, as platelet numbers decrease, the patient develops bleeding problems, particularly petechiae and ecchymosis on the skin, as well as epistaxis and bleeding gums.

Malignant Cell Expansion and Infiltration Manifestations. As the malignant cells proliferate in the bone marrow, their expanding volume increases the pressure inside the bone. The increased pressure causes bone tenderness or pain. Malignant cells can infiltrate into the central nervous system (CNS), leading to multiple CNS-related manifestations, such as nausea and vomiting, headache, seizures, coma, papilledema, and possible cranial nerve palsies (Caudell, 1998; Gould, 2002). Infiltration of malignant cells into the spleen and liver gives rise to splenomegaly and hepatomegaly, which can cause general abdominal discomfort and worsening pancytopenia, particularly thrombocytopenia (Caudell, 1998). The extreme degree of leukocytosis (greater than 100,000) associated with some types of leukemia (e.g., AML) can precipitate a severe complication called *leukostasis.* Small, thin-walled capillaries become dilated and congested with rigid leukemic (blast) cells, causing impaired circulation. The lungs and the brain are the two organs most commonly involved. The primary pulmonary manifestation is dyspnea. CNS manifestations include confusion, visual problems, and headache.

Diagnosis and Treatment

Diagnosis of leukemia requires bone marrow aspiration with analysis of the cells. It is critical that the leukemic cells be identified and characterized for planning of correct treatment. Identification is accomplished by immunophenotyping and molecular analysis (cytogenetics). When either AML or ALL is diagnosed, or if the myeloblast count is greater than 100,000, the situation is considered a medical emergency. Once identified, leukostasis is treated with leukophoresis followed by chemotherapy (Andreoli et al., 1997; Lichtman & Liesveld, 2001a). Leukemias are classified or staged to aid in diagnosis and treatment. Several classification and staging systems have been developed over the years to aid in diagnosis and treatment. For example, the French–American–British (FAB) classification system was developed to differentiate acute leukemias by morphology (Table 24–6).

Acute Leukemia Treatment.   According to Ching-Hon (2001) and Andreoli et al. (1997), there are two major goals underlying the treatment plan for the acute leukemias: to destroy the ma-

TABLE 24–6 French–American–British (FAB) Classification of Acute Leukemia

Acute myelocytic leukemia (AML)	M_1: AML, undifferentiated
	M_2: AML, differentiated (myeloblasts and promyelocytes predominate)
	M_3: Acute promyelocytic leukemia; promyelocytes
	M_4: Acute myelomonocytic leukemia; monocytes and myelogenous cells predominate
	M_5: Acute monocytic leukemia; monocytes predominate
	M_6: Erythroleukemia; predominance of erythroid and granulocyte precursors
	M_7: Megakaryotic leukemia; predominance of megakaryoblasts (large and small)
Acute lymphocytic leukemia (ALL)	L_1: Homogeneous; predominance of one cell type, primarily small cells; childhood type
	L_2: Heterogeneous; cells larger than L_1, adult type
	L_3: Large cells (Burkitt-like); homogenous, large cells

Data from Turgeon, M. L. (1999). Clinical hematology: Theory and procedures, 3rd ed. Philadelphia: Lippincott Williams & Wilkins; Andreoli, T. E., Carpenter, C. C., Bennett, J. C., & Plum, F. (1997). Disorders of the hematopoietic stem cell. In T. E. Andreoli et al. (Eds.), Cecil's essentials of medicine, (4th ed.) Philadelphia: W. B. Saunders.

lignant cells and to produce complete remission. This is achieved through aggressive chemotherapy, which may require multiple courses of treatment that may last for 2 years (Andreoli et al., 1997; Ching-Hon, 2001).

The initial phase of chemotherapy is referred to as *induction,* which lasts for approximately 1 week. Patients may stay in the hospital for about a month until the blood counts increase and it is safe for the patient to be discharged home. While in the hospital, many patients are on intravenous antibiotics and receive blood products to support the patients through the therapy. Induction in the AML patient may include cytosine arabinoside and a drug from the anthracycline group. Chemotherapy induction in the ALL patient usually requires a combination drug approach and may include prednisone, L-asparaginase, vincristine, and others. Induction therapy aims at creating a state of complete remission—no leukemic cells in the bone marrow or peripheral blood. Induction therapy produces complete remission in about 75 percent of AML patients younger than 60 years of age. Long-term remission is less common in adults than in children. In children with ALL, induction is associated with complete remission for more than 5 years in about 90 percent of cases.

Induction therapy may be followed by *consolidation* chemotherapy, which aims to solidify the remission and eliminate any remaining leukemic cells. It frequently includes the same chemotherapeutic agents used during induction but at lower doses and for shorter durations.

The final phase of chemotherapy is called *maintenance* chemotherapy, which is primarily required for treatment of ALL. During this phase, the patient with ALL may have intrathecal prophylactic treatment of the CNS and possibly brain radiation. In AML, monoclonal antibodies may be used if the tumor is positive for CD33 antigen (Lichtman & Liesveld, 2001a). Bone marrow transplant may be the curative treatment of choice, particularly in patients with AML or relapsed ALL. The best results come from a well-matched family donor.

Chronic Leukemia Treatment. Treatment of CLL may be reserved until the person moves into the advanced stages (III and IV) of the disease, develops pancytopenia, and/or becomes symptomatic. CML is incurable and therapy is aimed at palliation (Kipps, 2001). Chemotherapy is the usual initial form of therapy, often using a combination of an alkylating agent (e.g., chlorambucil) and corticosteroids (e.g., prednisone) (Kipps, 2001; Salmon & Sartorelli, 1998). A newer chemotherapeutic agent, fludarabine, may be used as initial therapy in the presence of advanced stage CLL. Fludarabine has been shown to significantly reduce tumor size and possibly induce a complete remission in 70 percent of cases in which conventional chemotherapy has only brought about partial remission (Andreoli et al., 1997; Kipps, 2001). Partial remission exists when no malignant cells are found in the peripheral blood but some can be found on examination of the bone marrow. Radiation therapy may be used to reduce the size of bulky masses in the lymph nodes or spleen. Splenectomy may be performed if autoimmunity develops. Antibiotic therapy is ordered as necessary to treat infections.

Lichtman and Liesveld (2001b) explain that treatment of CML typically begins during the chronic phase and focuses on reduction of the leukocyte count and splenomegaly. Antimetabolite therapy (e.g., hydroxyurea and busulfan) is frequently ordered to accomplish these tasks. Although antimetabolite therapy can prolong the chronic phase, it does not prevent progression into the acceleration phase. Alpha-interferon has improved the prognosis associated with CML. Alpha-interferon, administered subcutaneously, has been found to decrease the number of bone marrow cells with the Ph[1] chromosome and increase the number of normal clone cells. Imatinib mesylate (Gleevec) acts as a specific inhibitor of the bcr-Abl tyrosine kinase. Gleevec is taken orally and may be given in the chronic, accelerated, or acute phases of a patient with Philadelphia chromosome positive CML (Leukemia and Lymphoma Society, 2002). Bone marrow transplant is the only curative therapy. The best results come from a sibling donor who is HLA matched.

Oncologic Treatment Crises (Oncologic Emergencies)

Oncologic treatment often includes drug regimens that can be toxic to organs, cause severe immunosuppression, and overwhelm the body's homeostasis mechanisms in a variety of ways. Many of these iatrogenic problems are considered life threatening, thus medical emergencies. It is important, then, to have a basic understanding of these crises. The following overview highlights some of the more common oncologic

treatment crises. Table 24–7 provides a summary of clinical findings and risk factors for development of the various oncologic crises discussed.

Organ Toxicities

Multiple cancer chemotherapeutic agents are known to include organ toxicity as major adverse effects of therapy; thus, effective treatment of the cancer may severely injure one or more organs as a result of that therapy.

Cardiac Toxicity. Some cardiac toxic effects that have been associated with cancer treatments are arrhythmias, cardiac ischemia, congestive heart failure, pericardial disease, and shock. Antineoplastic medications have been reported to cause certain arrhythmias. Paclitaxel may cause an asymptomatic bradyarrhythmia or ventricular tachycardia. Interleukin 2 (biotherapy) has been reported to cause ventricular tachycardia. Cardiac ischemia may occur with the administration of 5-FU, an antimetabolite chemotherapy medication. The incidence of congestive heart failure (CHF) and cardiomyopathy caused by anthracyclines depends on the cumulative dose of the drug. Alkylating agents such as Cytoxan used for bone marrow **ablation** are known to cause severe myocarditis and exudative pericarditis. Radiation may affect any structure of the heart, such as the myocardium or pericardium (Stanholtz, 2001).

Pulmonary Toxicity. Pulmonary toxicities from cancer treatment include acute respiratory distress syndrome (ARDS), interstitial lung disease, radiation pneumonitis and fibrosis, and pulmonary veno-occlusive disease. ARDS may be caused by all-trans retinoic acid, a drug used to treat acute promyelocytic leukemia. The syndrome of fever and respiratory distress includes weight gain, pleural and pericardial effusions, pulmonary infiltrates, hypotension, renal insufficiency, and hyperbilirubinemia. Treatment for the syndrome is high-dose steroids. Bleomycin is known for causing pulmonary fibrosis but can also cause ARDS related to high FIO_2 injury (Stanholtz, 2001). Interstitial lung disease may be caused by cancer treatment. Toxicity may be caused by any dosage of drug and may appear months after treatment. Treatment includes discontinuing the drug and administering corticosteroids (Stanholtz, 2001). Radiation pneumonitis and fibrosis are related to the volume of lung irradiated and the dose of radiation received. In the acute phase, the patient presents with dyspnea and cough, which may advance to respiratory failure ARDS. The latent phase occurs after symptoms have resolved. Corticosteroids may be of benefit during acute radiation pneumonitis but of no benefit in the treatment of radiation fibrosis (Stanholtz, 2001).

Pulmonary veno-occlusive disease may be a complication of antineoplastic treatment using bleomycin, mitomycin-C, and bone marrow transplant drug regimens. The symptoms include dyspnea, hypoxia, respiratory failure, and pulmonary hypertension. Prognosis for pulmonary veno-occlusive disease is poor. Treatment includes discontinuing the offending drugs and administration of vasodilator therapy (Stanholtz, 2001).

TABLE 24–7   Summary of Oncologic Treatment Crises (Oncologic Emergencies)

	MANIFESTATIONS	RISK FACTORS
Organ Toxicities		
Cardiac	Cardiac dysrhythmias Cardiac ischemia Congestive heart failure, shock Pericardial disease	Paclitaxel Interleukin 2 5-FU Cytoxan
Pulmonary	Acute respiratory distress syndrome (ARDS) Interstitial lung disease Radiation pneumonitis and fibrosis Pulmonary veno-occlusive disease	All-trans retinoic acid (ATRA) Radiation therapy Bleomycin Combination therapy: Bleomycin and mitomycin-C
Liver	Decreased liver function: Elevated liver enzymes (ALT, AST, Alk Phos), bilirubin Decreased serum albumin and protein Bleeding tendencies Jaundice	L-asparaginase Antimetabolite agents Interferon Retinoic acid
Other Crises		

Sepsis	Altered vital signs:
	    HR greater than 125/min
	    RR greater than 30/min
	    SBP less than 90 mm Hg
	    Temperature less than 35°C or greater than 40°C
	        (in immunosuppressed state—temperature 38°C or
	        greater [100.4°F or greater])
	Altered mental status
		Immunosuppressed states
		Exposure to pathogens (e.g., bacteria, viruses, and fungi)

Tumor lysis syndrome	Elevated serum:
	    Uric acid, phosphorus, potassium
	Abnormally low serum:
	    Calcium
	Possible renal failure
		Advanced stage cancer
		Elevated LDH
		Chemotherapy

Hypercalcemia	Weight loss Fatigue Muscle weakness	Bony metastases Hyperparathyroidism
Spinal cord compression	Back pain Motor weakness Sensory deficits	Systemic cancer Tumor(s) of vertebrae, usually thoracic spine
Superior vena cava syndrome	Hoarseness, cough, dyspnea Edema of face, arm, or neck Erythema of face	Primary intrathoracic cancer Bronchogenic cancer Metastatic cancers of breast or testicles
Neutropenic enterocolitis	Severe neutropenia (less than 1,000 cells/mm^3) Fever Right upper quadrant (RUQ) abdominal pain and abdominal distention Diarrhea (bloody or watery) Nausea and vomiting	Severe immunosuppressed states Use of myelotoxic chemotherapy agents
Hemorrhagic cystitis	Hematuria Bladder hemorrhage	Chemotherapy and/or bladder radiation
Hypersensitivity reactions	Pruritus Dyspnea Agitation	Antineoplastic agents L-asparaginase Taxanes Biological agents

Data from Stanholtz, C. (2001). Acute life threatening toxicity of cancer treatment. In J. S. Groeger (Ed.), Critical care clinics: Oncology and critical care *(pp. 483–502). Philadelphia: W. B. Saunders; and Vasudeva, R., & Leong, K. (2002). Neutropenic enterocolitis. E-medicine.*

Liver Toxicity. Hepatotoxicity has been associated with blood and bone marrow transplantation and certain chemotherapeutic drugs. Because the liver is the primary source of drug metabolism, it is at high risk for toxicity problems with cancer chemotherapy agents, which can be extremely toxic. L-asparaginase and antimetabolite medications are particularly associated with liver damage. In addition, interferon and retinoic acid have been reported to cause hepatotoxicity (Stanholtz, 2001). Hepatotoxicity may initially present as decreased liver function, which may be noted first as abnormal liver profile laboratory results. Treatment may require dose reduction or discontinuance of a particular offending agent.

Other Oncologic Treatment Crises

While chemotherapeutic agents and radiation directly injure organs, other treatment-related complications cause injury more indirectly, either during or after completion of therapy. Some of the more common treatment-induced crises include sepsis, tumor lysis syndrome, hypercalemia, spinal cord compression, superior vena cava syndrome, neutropenic enterocolitis, hemorrhagic cystitis, and drug-induced hypersensitivity reactions. The remainder of this section provides a brief overview of these crises.

Sepsis. Patients receiving cancer treatment have a greater risk of acquiring opportunistic infections resulting from therapy-induced immunosuppression. Leukemic and blood or marrow transplant patients are at high risk when their marrow has been ablated. Low virulent agents may cause a life-threatening infection in the immunosuppressed patient. To complicate the care of the immunosuppressed patient, the patient could develop multiple infections. The neutropenic patient is predisposed to bacteria, viruses, and fungi. Herpes simplex virus can reactivate when the neutrophil count is decreased; therefore acyclovir may be ordered prophylactically or for treatment of the herpes virus. Fungi are common causes of infections in the second and third weeks of neutropenia, particularly candidemia and aspergillosis. Disseminated fungal infections may lead to life-threatening infections and may not respond to the standard treatment of amphotericin B. Patients with bacteremia are placed on intravenous antibiotics, which should continue at least until the neutrophil count is above 500 cells/mm^3. Renal function should be monitored before and during treatment with antifungal agents. Treatment may be changed to the newer liposomal preparations of amphotericin to protect renal function.

Tumor Lysis Syndrome. Tumor lysis syndrome (TLS) is usually associated with treatment for leukemia and lymphoma but may be associated with other types of cancer. As cancer treatment destroys tumor cells, the intracellular metabolites from the destroyed cells spill out into the circulation at a rate that exceeds the kidneys' ability to excrete them, causing potentially life-threatening elevations in serum levels of metabolites (Escalante et al., 2004). Common clinical findings include hyperuricemia, hyperphosphatemia, hyperkalemia, and hypocalcemia. Unless properly treated, TLS can result in renal failure and possible death of the patient. Treatment of TLS includes intravenous hydration and loop diuretics. Allopurinol is used to decrease uric acid levels and protect the kidneys. A renal consult should be obtained if there is significant renal impairment. Hemodialysis is an effective treatment to rid the body of the excess metabolites (Kapoor & Chan, 2001).

Hypercalcemia. The most common cancer-related metabolic emergency is hypercalcemia, in which there is an increased bone resorption by osteoclasts and decreased renal excretion

of calcium. The clinical manifestations may include nausea, vomiting, anorexia, abdominal pain, polyuria, weakness, fatigue, seizures, and coma. Severe hypercalcemia may cause complete heart block and cardiac arrest. The treatment for hypercalcemia includes volume expansion with normal saline to improve renal function and decrease calcium resorption. Bisphosphonates, such as pamidronate and etidronate, inhibit osteoclastic activity and bone resorption. Calcitonin decreases calcium by inhibiting bone resorption and increasing renal excretion. Corticosteroids are used to treat calcitrol-induced hypercalcemia. Dialysis may be needed if the patient is unable to tolerate volume expansion. Treatment for the cancer is the ultimate treatment for malignancy-associated hypercalcemia (Kapoor & Chan, 2001).

Spinal Cord Compression. Oncology patients who have back pain should be evaluated for possible spinal cord compression (SCC). Tumors may cause SCC through direct extension or by metastatic disease in the vertebral column. Edema and diminished blood supply to the spinal cord can lead to paresis and paralysis. Symptoms may include pain, motor weakness, and sensory deficit. Treatment options for SCC may include surgery, chemotherapy, radiation, and medications. A laminectomy or spinal fusion may be required when the symptoms are rapidly progressing or if the tumor is resistant to radiation. The patient with slowly progressing symptoms can be treated with radiation. Corticosteroids are given to decrease spinal cord edema.

Superior Vena Cava Syndrome. Malignant disease is the most common cause of superior vena cava (SVC) syndrome, which causes compression of the superior vena cava and engorgement of the upper trunk. If the development of SVC syndrome is gradual, then collateral circulation will have time to develop. If the development is rapid, then interventions are required to maintain an open airway and cardiac output. Radiation is first-line therapy and should decrease the edema and venous distention. Chemotherapy may be used to treat SVC syndrome depending on the tumor being treated. If a thrombosis caused the SVC syndrome, then heparin therapy may be ordered. An expandable wire stent may be placed into the obstructed portion of the SVC.

Neutropenic Enterocolitis. Neutropenic enterocolitis (necrotizing enteritis or ileocecal syndrome) is a necrotizing process that affects the bowel of immunosuppressed patients, most commonly leukemic patients. The pathogenesis of neutropenic enterocolitis in unknown but is associated with a neutrophil count of less than 1,000 cells/mm^3. The mucosal layer of the small and large intestines becomes inflamed, injured, and ulcerated. The patient's severely immunosuppressed state allows bacterial invasion of the damaged mucosal layer that can eventually result in transmural intestinal wall damage, perforation, and possible peritonitis (Vasudeva & Leong, 2002). Risk factors for development include chemotherapy, myeloproliferative neoplasms, and bone marrow or solid organ transplant, among others. Symptoms are fever, abdominal pain, and diarrhea.

Plain radiographic films are nonspecific but may show gas in the cecum, colonic distention, pneumatosis, ascites, and small bowel distention. CT scans show thickening of the bowel wall. Treatment in mild cases is conservative, whereas severe cases may require surgery (Stanholtz, 2001).

Hemorrhagic Cystitis. Chemotherapy and radiation can cause severe bladder irritation that results in acute bladder hemorrhage. Two chemotherapy agents, cyclophosphamide and ifosfamide, produce a liver metabolite, acrolein, which is a urotoxin. Preventive therapy may include mesna (sodium 2-mercaptoethanesulfonate), which binds with acrolein to prevent bladder problems. Treatment for hemorrhagic cystitis includes evacuating any clots and continuing continuous bladder irrigation until the bleeding has stopped. A cystoscopy may be performed to evaluate the bleeding further. In severe cases a hypogastric artery embolization, open cystotomy, or a total cystectomy may be required (Stanholtz, 2001).

Hypersensitivity Reactions. Certain cancer chemotherapy agents are known to cause a hypersensitivity reaction, particularly L-asparaginase, taxanes, and biological agents. With some drugs, such as L-asparaginase, the chances of a hypersensitivity reaction increase with each dose. Common manifestations of a reaction include pruritus, dyspnea, and agitation. Prophylactic administration of dexamethasone, diphenhydramine, and an H2-antagonist decreases the incidence of a hypersensitivity reaction. Most reactions occur within the first 10 minutes of therapy and resolve when the drug infusion has been discontinued. If the reaction is severe, the use of antihistamines, fluids, or vasopressors may be required (Stanholtz, 2001).

Biological agents (e.g., interferon and interleukin) and monoclonal antibodies (e.g., muromonab-CD3) also cause hypersensitivity reactions. Interferon and interleukin generally cause flu-like symptoms and rash; however, the exact reaction may vary dependent on the dose and administration route. Interleukin can cause a severe reaction that includes hypotension and capillary leak syndrome. Monoclonal antibodies, particularly muromonab-CD3, can cause a syndrome of hypersensitivity reaction-related symptoms called cytokine release syndrome (CRS). This syndrome develops with the first or second drug dose and then decreases with each subsequent dose. Usually CRS causes fever, headache, chills, and rigors but can potentially trigger a severe life-threatening anaphylaxis-like reaction. Prophylactic therapy may include acetaminophen, methylprednisolone, and an antihistamine. Monoclonal antibodies and CRS are discussed in more detail in Module 26: Organ Transplantation.

In summary, this section has presented major disorders of the white blood cells. Neutropenia, abnormally low levels of neutrophils, can be caused by premature destruction (e.g., immune reaction) or decreased production (e.g., aplastic anemia, leukemia). Neutropenia causes an altered response to inflammation and infection. The leukemias consist of a group of disorders that are characterized by uncontrolled growth of malignantly transformed blood cells in the bone marrow. There are four types of leukemias, including acute lymphocytic leukemia (ALL), acute myelogenous leukemia (AML), chronic lymphocytic leukemia (CLL), and chronic myelogenous leukemia (CML). The clinical manifestations of the leukemias are divided into two general groups: those resulting from pancytopenia (anemia, leukopenia, and thrombocytopenia) and those resulting from malignant cell expansion and infiltration. Diagnosis of leukemia requires review of the peripheral blood followed by immunophenotyping and cytogenetic analysis of the bone marrow. Cancer chemotherapy is capable of causing harm to organs while it is destroying the cancerous lesions. Toxicity of the heart, lungs, and liver was briefly described. Other potential complications of cancer treatment include sepsis, tumor lysis syndrome, hypercalcemia, spinal cord compression, superior vena cava syndrome, neutropenic enterocolitis hemorrhagic cystitis, and hypersensitivity reactions. Many of these complications are considered medical emergencies; thus, it is critical that they be recognized and treated rapidly.

SECTION FOUR REVIEW

1. A neutrophil count of less than _____ cells/mcL places the patient at high risk for development of an acute infection.
   A. 500
   B. 1,500
   C. 2,000
   D. 2,500
2. The most common cause of premature destruction of neutrophils is
   A. environmental toxins
   B. autoimmune disorder
   C. drug–antibody reaction
   D. bacterial infection

3. When severe neutropenia is present, the primary symptom of infection may be
   A. pus formation
   B. fever
   C. local edema
   D. local erythema
4. The myelocytic leukemias differ from lymphocytic leukemias in that both forms of myelocytic leukemias involve
   A. more than one type of blood cell
   B. a predominance of mature blood cells
   C. red blood cells
   D. plasma cell proliferation

5. In general, the cause of death in the patient who has untreated acute leukemia is
   A. infection
   B. tissue hypoxia
   C. pancytopenia
   D. hemorrhage
6. About 70 percent of ALL cases involve proliferation of immature
   A. B cells
   B. T cells
   C. plasma cells
   D. megakaryocytes
7. The presence of Auer rods in the cytoplasm is primarily found in which type of leukemia?
   A. ALL
   B. AML
   C. CLL
   D. CML
8. CML is associated with a *blast crisis,* which is best described as occurring when the
   A. disorder transforms into acute leukemia
   B. blast cells obstruct the circulation
   C. bone marrow completely fails
   D. blast cells infiltrate the brain
9. The most common cause of death in adults with acute leukemia is
   A. hemorrhage
   B. infection
   C. tissue hypoxia
   D. brain infiltration
10. The term *leukostasis* refers to
    A. infiltration of brain and lungs by blast cells
    B. inability of leukocytes to move out of bone marrow
    C. loss of vision or stroke caused by stagnant blood flow
    D. impaired circulation as a result of capillary congestion by blast cells
11. A "complete remission" is obtained when there are no leukemic cells in the
    A. lymph nodes and bone marrow
    B. lymph nodes and peripheral blood
    C. bone marrow and lymph nodes
    D. bone marrow and peripheral blood
12. The initial treatment of acute leukemias is
    A. surgery
    B. chemotherapy
    C. radiation therapy
    D. bone marrow transplant
13. Treatment of ALL may include "maintenance" therapy, which commonly includes
    A. intrathecal chemotherapy
    B. total body irradiation
    C. bone marrow transplantation
    D. corticosteroid therapy
14. Use of alpha-interferon in the treatment of CML has been found to
    A. prolong the acceleration phase
    B. put patients in complete remission
    C. decrease the number of normal clonal cells
    D. decrease the number of Ph^1 chromosome cells

Answers: 1. A, 2. C, 3. B, 4. A, 5. C, 6. A, 7. B, 8. A, 9. B, 10. D, 11. D, 12. B, 13. A, 14. D

SECTION FIVE: Hemostasis Disorders

At the completion of this section, the learner will be able to describe the etiology, pathophysiology, clinical manifestations, and management of thrombocytopenia and acute disseminated intravascular coagulation (DIC).

This section focuses on platelets, the cellular component of hemostasis. Discussion is specific to disorders associated with abnormally low levels of platelets—thrombocytopenia. It also provides a brief overview of DIC.

Thrombocytopenia

Thrombocytopenia is clinically defined as a platelet count of less than 150,000 cells/mcL. The major complication of thrombocy-topenia is bleeding. The bleeding associated with thrombocy-topenia is different from bleeding caused by other coagulo-pathies. Thrombocytopenia typically manifests itself as petechiae and purpura on the skin and mucous membranes. Epistaxis is a common finding of patients that have severe thrombocytope-nia. Two important assessments of epistaxis are the length of time required to stop the epistaxis and the involvement of one or both nostrils. Epistaxis in one nostril is probably caused by a local vascular abnormality rather than thrombocytopenia. Co-agulopathies caused by missing or abnormal coagulation factors tend to cause internal bleeding. Thrombocytopenia is usually not a life-threatening condition unless severe (less than 10,000 to 20,000 cells/mcL); however, the underlying disorder that is causing it may be serious or life-threatening (Howell & Roth-man, 2001). Thrombocytopenia can be intrinsic (e.g., a heredi-tary disorder) or acquired. This section focuses on acquired types of thrombocytopenia.

Causes of Thrombocytopenia

Four general conditions cause thrombocytopenia, including decreased production, increased destruction, utilization, and problems with distribution (George & Rizvi, 2001; Turgeon, 1999). In addition, the commonly used anticoagulant heparin can cause a potentially life-threatening condition called heparin-induced thrombocytopenia (HIT).

Problems of Decreased Production. Any problem that injures the bone marrow can result in a temporary or permanent reduction in megakaryocytes, for example, chemicals, drugs, and irradiation. A thorough drug history is important because many drugs may affect platelet number and function. Nonprescription drugs, such as aspirin; nonsteroidal anti-inflammatory drugs; and herbal supplements may affect platelet function and bleeding time (Howell & Rothman, 2001). Production can also be decreased by problems with thrombopoiesis, as is seen with megaloblastic anemia.

Problems of Increased Destruction. George and Rizvi (2001) and Turgeon (1999) explain that destruction of platelets can result from several types of immune reactions. Certain drugs (e.g., quinidine, heroin, and morphine) and substances (e.g., snake venom) can destroy platelets. The mechanism of destruction is generally a drug antibody–platelet antigen response, or complement activation. Platelets can also be destroyed when they attach to antigen–antibody immune complexes. This is seen with certain types of bacterial sepsis. A second immune mechanism involves the attachment of a bacterial antigen to platelets, forming an antigen–platelet complex. The complex activates formation of antibodies, which then coat the complex, destroying the platelet. This has been shown to occur with a specific form of malaria (*Plasmodium falciparum*). A third immune mechanism is direct destruction of platelets by antibodies of autoimmune origin. The autoimmune problem can occur in the neonate because of maternal platelet autoantibodies.

Problems of Increased Utilization. Increased platelet consumption most commonly results from idiopathic (immunologic) thrombocytopenia purpura (ITP). ITP is more common in children than adults. In adults, it is most commonly found in young women as a chronic disorder of autoimmune origin, with formation of platelet autoantibodies (usually Immunoglobulin G[IgG]), and it sometimes develops in conjunction with SLE. Characteristics of ITP include a normal bone marrow with a low platelet count, absence of splenomegaly, and no identifiable cause of thrombocytopenia. Ruling out all other possible etiologies of thrombocytopenia is the major diagnostic criterion. The clinical manifestations of ITP are typical of any thrombocytopenia, including petechiae, purpura, bleeding gums, epistaxis, and menorrhagia. Less common findings include gastrointestinal bleeding and hematuria, which are considered symptoms that are more serious. Treatment includes oral glucocorticoids (e.g., prednisone) and possibly immunoglobulin for acute bleeding management. Intravenous immune globulin (IVIG) is given if the thrombocytopenia is refractory to steroids, causing active bleeding, or requires a rapid increase in the platelet count. After the administration of IVIG the platelet count should increase within 3 to 5 days (Howell & Rothman, 2001). The spleen is a major destroyer of the antibody-coated platelets and splenectomy is usually recommended for patients who either do not respond to corticosteroid therapy or who cannot be maintained on low doses. Platelet transfusions are not generally required unless the patient is hemorrhaging.

Problems of Platelet Distribution. In the presence of splenomegaly, the spleen can hold vast numbers of platelets, which significantly reduces the numbers in the circulating blood. The total number of platelets may increase by two to three times normal to compensate for those pooled in the spleen. Disorders associated with this problem include cirrhosis (posthepatic or alcoholic), leukemias, lymphomas, and others (Howell & Rothman, 2001; Turgeon, 1999).

Heparin-Induced Thrombocytopenia (HIT). According to Howell and Rothman (2001), heparin is the most significant cause of life-threatening thrombocytopenia. About 3 percent of patients receiving intravenous heparin develop a transient form of mild-to-moderate thrombocytopenia. In a small percentage of patients, however, the decreased platelet count can drop as low as 20,000/mcL, causing a severe heparin-induced thrombocytopenia. Antibodies in the patient's serum bind to a complex formed by heparin and a component of platelets (**platelet factor 4**). These antibody–heparin/platelet complexes activate platelets, causing them to aggregate and release their granular contents. Platelet aggregation can result in thromboembolism (*paradoxical thromboembolism*) or arterial thrombosis (*white clot syndrome*) (George & Rizvi, 2001; Owen & Webster, 1998). Platelet aggregation can also result in thrombocytopenia, rather than **thrombosis,** if the platelets are removed by the reticuloendothelial system. Patients who are receiving heparin therapy should have their platelet count monitored on a regular basis. Recognition of this syndrome is extremely important as the risk of thromboemboli is high. Treatment usually consists of discontinuing the heparin and initiating an oral anticoagulation therapy until the platelet count normalizes (Howell & Rothman, 2001). Heparin use is contraindicated in patients who have a history of severe heparin-induced thrombocytopenia.

Acute Disseminated Intravascular Coagulation

Acute disseminated intravascular coagulation (DIC) is a complication of some underlying acute condition rather than a disease in itself. DIC is a coagulation paradox involving excessive clotting (with depletion of clotting factors) followed by excessive bleeding. The development of DIC is a critical setback for the patient for two reasons: (1) It significantly increases mortality, and (2) correction of the precipitating cause(s) does not

TABLE 24–8   Major Risk Factors for Development of Acute DIC

Most common
  Sepsis (particularly gram-negative)
  Severe trauma or burns
  Shock (any type)
  Abruptio placenta
Other
  ABO incompatibility blood transfusion reaction
  Severe liver disease
  Disseminated cancer or leukemia

always halt the DIC process (Toh & Denis, 2003). DIC can be acute or chronic. Chronic DIC most commonly is associated with metastatic cancers, dead fetus syndrome, and aortic aneurysm, whereas acute DIC is most often triggered by severe acute pathology. Table 24–8 lists some of the more common risk factors for development of acute DIC. The widespread deleterious effects of DIC can result in multiple organ dysfunction syndrome (MODS).

The Coagulation Cascade and DIC

To understand DIC, it is important to have a basic knowledge of the coagulation pathways. The two basic pathways are extrinsic and intrinsic. The extrinsic pathway is activated by damage to the endothelial lining of a blood vessel, which triggers the development of a clot by the release of thromboplastin. The intrinsic pathway is activated by a vascular injury that exposes subendothelial tissue to direct contact with the bloodstream. When factor XII comes into direct contact with the exposed tissue the coagulation cascade continues until a clot is formed (Geiter, 2003). The normal clot formation cascade maintains homeostasis by balancing stimulating and inhibiting factors (Geiter, 2003).

Disseminated intravascular coagulation is caused by overstimulation of the normal coagulation cascade (Geiter, 2003; Owen & Webster, 1998; Seigsohn, 2001). An underlying pathology (e.g., sepsis) stimulates cytokines, such as interleukins and tumor necrosis factor, and activates the clotting cascade. Platelet activation, clot formation, and fibrinolysis are three important homeostatic activities in the normal coagulation process but also are an integral part of the pathology of DIC.

Platelet Activation. When the coagulation cascade is activated, platelets change form from smooth to spiny shaped and become sticky, making them capable of attaching to the damaged endothelial cells or lining. The adherence of the platelets to the vessel wall begins a process of degranulation. Granules containing mediators (serotonin, histamine, adenosine diphosphate, and thromboxane A2) are released from the cytoplasm of the platelets (Geiter, 2003). Vasoconstriction caused by serotonin and histamine limits blood loss while the clot is formed. Adenosine diphosphate (ADP) is the precursor to ATP and is released by platelets during degranulation, which causes increased adherence of nearby platelets. The clot size becomes larger and causes platelets to begin degranulation, increasing chemical mediators. Thromboxane A2 effects clot formation by platelet degradation and vasoconstriction, which leads to release of more chemical mediators. Prostacyclin is released from the damaged endothelial cells, which counteracts the effect of thromboxane A2, ADP, serotonin, and histamine. This action normally limits (and localizes) vasoconstriction and degranulation. In the presence of DIC, platelets collect throughout the microcirculation and, eventually, the platelet supply becomes exhausted.

Clot Formation. The coagulation cascade converts prothrombin to thrombin, which then converts fibrinogen to fibrin and stimulates platelet aggregation. Antithrombins, such as protein S and protein C, are chemical mediators that block the effects of thrombin. Fibrin binds the platelets, white blood cells, and red blood cells when a clot is formed and functions to stabilize the clot (Geiter, 2003). In DIC, the amount of thrombin becomes excessive and increases clot formation in the microcirculation.

Fibrinolysis. When the coagulation cascade is stimulated, tissue plasminogen activator (tPA) dissolves the clot by activating plasminogen to convert to plasmin (Geiter, 2003). The plasmin digests fibrinogen and fibrin in clots and in the circulation. DIC is a coagulation paradox—the blood is coagulating at the same time that clots are being dissolved, which results in bleeding from the consumption of platelets and coagulation factors or tissue ischemia from occlusive microthrombi. Figure 24–6 provides an illustration of the sequence of events involved in DIC.

Clinical Findings of DIC

Actual clinical manifestations reflect the volume of blood being lost and organ-related manifestations. Bleeding is often the first and most obvious sign of DIC. Extensive ischemic organ dysfunction can result from microthrombi formation, for example, renal ischemia may result from microthrombosis of the afferent glomerular arterioles or from hypotension related to acute tubular necrosis. The lungs may develop a range of problems from mild (transient hypoxemia) to severe (ARDS or hemorrhage). The cerebral vasculature is at risk for ischemic problems or hemorrhage; thus, changes in mental status are monitored closely. Infectious disease and prolonged hypotension contribute to hepatocellular dysfunction which results in jaundice as bilirubin levels increase. Finally, shock is a possible complication resulting from either DIC or from the underlying pathology (Seigsohn, 2001). Table 24–9 summarizes some of the more common clinical findings associated with DIC.

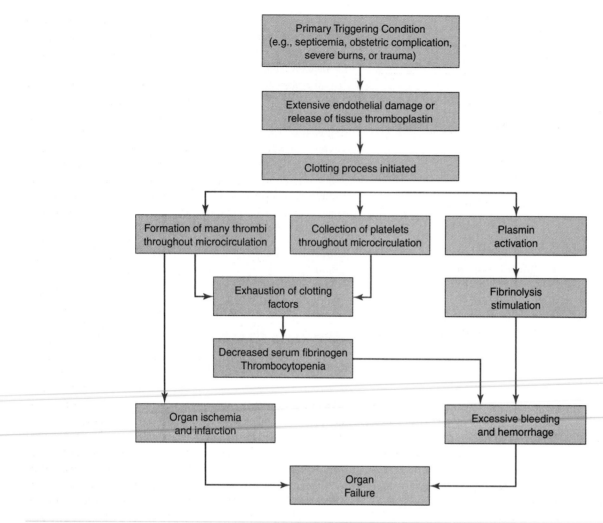

Figure 24–6 ■ Disseminated intravascular coagulation sequence of events. *(Adapted from Gould, B. [2002]. Pathophysiology for the health professions, (2nd ed., p. 252). Copyright 2002, with permission from Elsevier.)*

Laboratory Studies

Diagnosis of DIC requires close examination of the patient's entire clinical condition and all laboratory results. Laboratory tests can assist the clinician in distinguishing acute from chronic DIC. The underlying disease may also affect the lab values so the tests should be repeated every 6 to 8 hours. In acute DIC the patients are critically ill. The laboratory tests should include a platelet count, prothrombin time (PT), activated partial thromboplastin time (aPTT), **D-dimer,** thrombin time (TT), fibrinogen level, fibrinogen degradation products (FDP), and a blood film to check for fragmented red cells. Table 24–10 summarizes the adult DIC coagulation laboratory screening tests. In most cases, there may be changes of three or more parameters plus a decreased platelet count (Seigsohn, 2001).

Treatment

Treating the underlying disease is imperative to correct DIC and restore the patient's vital functions. Volume replacement and correction of hypotension improve blood flow. Instituting supportive measures for the pulmonary, cardiac, and renal systems improve oxygenation, cardiac output, and fluid and electrolyte balance. Blood components, such as platelets, cryoprecipitate, and fresh-frozen plasma, should be administered if the patient is depleted of hemostatic factors, bleeding, and preparing for surgery. Thrombocytopenia should be treated with the administration of platelets to increase the platelet count to greater than 50,000. Hypofibrinogenemia should be treated by giving 8 to 10 units of cryoprecipitate. Fresh-frozen plasma may be ordered if the patient is depleted of coagulation factors. Replacement ther-

TABLE 24–9   Clinical Manifestations of DIC

BASIS OF FINDINGS	CLINICAL MANIFESTATIONS
Bleeding related	Superficial bleeding
	Petechiae, ecchymoses
	Bleeding/continuous oozing from arterial lines, catheters, and injured tissues
	Internal bleeding
	GI tract, lungs, and CNS (potentially life threatening)
Microthrombosis related	Superficial
	Cyanosis/ischemia of fingers, nose, and ears
	Signs of organ ischemia/dysfunction
	Renal: Oliguria/anuria, azotemia, hematuria
	Pulmonary: Transient hypoxemia, pulmonary hemorrhage, ARDS
	CNS: Delirium, coma, cerebral hemorrhage
	Hepatic: Jaundice

Data from Seigsohn, U. (2001). Disseminated intravascular coagulation. In E. Beuther, M. A. Lichtman, B. S. Coller, T. J. Kipps. & U. Seligsohn (Eds.), Williams hematology, (6th ed., pp. 1677–1695). New York: McGraw Hill.

apy should be evaluated every 8 hours after reviewing the platelet count, PT, aPTT, and fibrinogen level (Seigsohn, 2001). In most cases of acute DIC, heparin administration has not shown a reduction in mortality but may aggravate bleeding. Administration of heparin is beneficial in some categories of chronic DIC, for example, metastatic carcinoma, dead fetus syndrome, and aortic aneurysm. Patients with acute DIC may respond to heparin therapy if they have not responded to blood component therapy or when thrombosis threatens to cause irreversible tissue injury. Antithrombin-III concentrate, an inhibitor of coagulation, has been used to treat patients with DIC.

Clinical trials using antithrombin-III for treatment of DIC have shown some beneficial effects (e.g., improved laboratory parameters, decreased duration of DIC, and improved organ function) but not a reduction in mortality (Levi, 2004).

In summary, thrombocytopenia is an abnormally low platelet count. It results in bleeding problems, primarily of the skin and mucous membranes. Acquired thrombocytopenia is associated with four major underlying mechanisms: (1) decreased production (e.g., bone marrow injury or decreased production of thrombopoiesis); (2) increased platelet destruction, which usually involves an antigen–antibody immune reaction that destroys the platelets, but can also result from an autoimmune problem; (3) increased platelet utilization, which is associated with acute bleeding or DIC; and (4) increased pooling of platelets in the spleen in the presence of splenomegaly. In addition, the anticoagulant heparin may produce a potentially life-threatening form of thrombocytopenia called heparin-induced thrombocytopenia (HIT). Acute disseminated intravascular coagulation (DIC) is a complication of some underlying acute pathology rather than a disease in itself. DIC is caused by overstimulation of the normal coagulation cascade. Platelet activation, clot formation, and fibrinolysis are three important homeostatic activities in the normal coagulation process but also an integral part of the pathology of DIC. Actual clinical manifestations reflect the volume of blood being lost and organ-related manifestations. Diagnosis of DIC requires close examination of the patient's entire clinical condition and all laboratory results. Management of DIC centers on treatment of the underlying condition and fluid volume replacement. Support of the cardiovascular and coagulation systems as they become damaged is done to prevent further complications. Nursing management focuses on protection of the patient, prevention of further injury, and pain management. Health professionals need to monitor the patient's lab values and assess for DIC symptoms (Geiter, 2003).

TABLE 24–10   Adult DIC Screening Tests

TEST	NORMAL VALUE	SUGGESTIVE OF DIC	OTHER
Bleeding time	1–6 min	Greater than 6 min	Useful in determining abnormal function of platelets
Platelet count	150,000–400,000	Less than 150,000	Increased destruction of platelets
PT	11–15 sec	Greater than 15 sec	Tests anticoagulant therapy
aPTT	60–70 sec	Greater than 60 sec	Detecting clotting factors and platelet disorders
Factor 1: Fibrinogen	200–400 mg/dL	Less than 100 mg/dL	A deficiency of fibrinogen results in bleeding
Fibrin degradation product (FDP)	2–10 mcg/dL	Greater than 10 mg/dL	Increased FDP usually indicative of DIC caused by severe injury or trauma
D-dimer	Negative for D-dimer fragments	Greater than 250 mg/dL	Confirms presence of FDP

Adapted from Kee, J. L. (2002). Laboratory and diagnostic tests with nursing implications, (6th ed., p. 735). Upper Saddle River, NJ: Prentice Hall. With permission.

SECTION FIVE REVIEW

1. Thrombocytopenia is clinically defined as a platelet count of less than
   A. 50,000
   B. 100,000
   C. 150,000
   D. 200,000

2. The typical bleeding pattern of thrombocytopenia involves bleeding into the
   A. joints
   B. peritoneum
   C. internal organs
   D. skin and mucous membranes

3. An example of decreased platelet production caused by a reduction in thrombopoiesis is
   A. megablastic anemia
   B. hemolytic anemia
   C. sequestration of platelets in spleen
   D. idiopathic thrombocytopenia purpura

4. The most common mechanism of platelet destruction by drugs is
   A. autoimmune reaction
   B. drug antibody–platelet antigen reaction
   C. antigen–antibody immune complex reaction
   D. direct toxic effect

5. Idiopathic thrombocytopenia purpura is believed to be
   A. of autoimmune origin
   B. caused by a drug reaction
   C. closely associated with splenomegaly
   D. of antibody–antigen immune complex origin

6. The major treatment of idiopathic thrombocytopenia purpura is
   A. alkylating chemotherapy
   B. platelet transfusions

C. corticosteroid therapy
D. bone marrow transplant

7. The paradoxical thromboembolism associated with heparin-induced thrombocytopenia (HIT) is caused by
   A. platelet aggregation
   B. heparin–platelet complexes
   C. accumulation of leukocytes
   D. red blood cell aggregation

8. Which statement is correct regarding disseminated intravascular coagulation (DIC)?
   A. vessels become occluded because of vasospasm
   B. clot formation uses up all available platelets
   C. DIC is a disease that causes acute myocardial infarction
   D. DIC is caused only by activation of the intrinsic pathway

9. In the presence of DIC, what happens to platelets?
   A. they lose their adherence qualities
   B. they massively collect in the spleen, destroying it
   C. they do not take part in the coagulation cascade
   D. they collect throughout the microcirculation, exhausting the supply

10. DIC is called a coagulation paradox because
    A. platelets are being destroyed while fibrinolysis is occurring
    B. coagulation factors are being produced at the same rate as platelets
    C. blood is coagulating at the same time that clots are being dissolved
    D. thrombin is excessively produced while platelet production is decreased

Answers: 1. C, 2. D, 3. A, 4. B, 5. A, 6. C, 7. A, 8. B, 9. D, 10. C

SECTION SIX: Nursing Implications

At the completion of this section, the learner will be able to describe the nursing implications appropriate to managing the care of patients experiencing acute hematologic dysfunction.

This section provides an overview of nursing considerations, including a focused nursing history and assessment, as well as some of the more common nursing diagnoses that may apply to individuals experiencing the hematologic problems described in this module. Many of the nursing diagnoses included in this section are presented in more detail in other modules in the text.

The Focused Nursing Database

The Focused Nursing History

Obtaining a thorough nursing history is essential because many hematologic problems are linked to health conditions and behaviors, recent illnesses, environmental/occupational exposure, or heredity. The patient's family history may suggest possible hereditary problems, such as sickle cell anemia or hemophilia. Information on the patient's residential or occupational environment may give clues to possible exposures to toxic substances, such as benzene, that have been associated with aplastic anemia. A dietary history can indicate a risk for nutritional-related problems, such as iron-deficiency anemia. Obtaining information regarding the patient's medical history and prescription and nonprescription drug use may indicate a risk for such problems as hemolytic anemia (Gould, 2002).

The Focused Nursing Assessment

Focused Neurologic Assessment. The neurologic status of the patient can change related to tissue hypoxia, bleeding, or leukemic cell infiltration. The nurse's neurologic assessment may include level of consciousness (LOC), pupillary checks, cranial nerve assessment, and monitoring for increased intracranial pressure. The patient's state of consciousness is a sensitive indicator of tissue oxygenation; thus, in the presence of severe anemia (an oxygen transport problem), LOC should be closely monitored. Cranial bleeding may manifest itself as headache, weakness, altered LOC, pupillary changes, altered cranial nerve functions, or symptoms of increased intracranial pressure. Patients suffering from leukemia may develop leukostasis, which is associated with impaired circulation caused by a massive circulating blast cell count (Caudell, 1998; Gould, 2002). CNS manifestations of leukostasis include severe headache and confusion.

Focused Cardiopulmonary Assessment. Hematologic problems can cause significant alterations in the hemodynamic and oxygenation status of the high-acuity patient. In the presence of anemia, infection, or bleeding, the nurse can anticipate development of compensatory vital signs, such as tachycardia, tachypnea, and changes in blood pressure. Blood pressure may rise with oxygenation problems or may fall, associated with hypovolemia from bleeding. The patient may develop dyspnea or orthopnea associated with tissue hypoxia. Sputum should be checked for occult blood in patients with bleeding problems. If the hematologic problem causes increased risk for hemorrhage, vital signs and hemodynamic parameters should be monitored closely for hypovolemic shock.

Focused Gastrointestinal Assessment. Hepatomegaly and splenomegaly are associated with several hematologic disorders; thus, the nurse may want to palpate for their presence. Patients with bleeding disorders should have all gastrointestinal secretions closely monitored for occult or gross bleeding. Intestinal bleeding is also associated with cramping, diarrhea, and melena.

Focused Renal Assessment. Patients with bleeding problems should have their urine routinely tested for occult blood. If hemoglobin is free in the urine, hemoglobinuria develops, which its characteristically port wine colored-urine.

Focused Integumentary Assessment. In the patient with anemia, monitoring the skin, nailbeds, and mucous membranes for the presence and degree of cyanosis is important. If the patient develops thrombocytopenia, the skin and mucous membranes should be examined for petechiae, purpura, and ecchymoses. Patients experiencing hemolytic anemia should be

monitored for jaundice because of excessive bilirubin from RBC destruction. The jaundice may also be accompanied by pruritus.

The Nursing Plan of Care

There are no North American Nursing Diagnosis Association (NANDA)–approved nursing diagnoses that directly address anemia, polycythemia, leukopenia, or thrombocytopenia. A plan of care is developed around the manifestations and complications associated with each disorder. These can be divided into five major underlying problems:

1. Tissue hypoxia
2. Hypertension
3. Stasis of blood flow
4. Infection
5. Bleeding

Tissue Hypoxia. Impaired oxygen transport associated with the anemias causes varying degrees of tissue hypoxia, depending on the severity of the anemia. Many of the clinical manifestations associated with tissue hypoxia are addressed as nursing diagnoses, such as

- *Fatigue* related to decreased energy production
- *Activity intolerance* related to oxygen supply-and-demand imbalance
- *Altered tissue perfusion* related to decreased oxygen-carrying capacity of the blood
- *Ineffective breathing pattern* related to decreased energy, fatigue
- *Risk for injury* related to tissue hypoxia
- *Pain* related to tissue hypoxia

Potential complications associated with tissue hypoxia include organ ischemia and infarction.

Hypertension. Hypertension is a common finding in polycythemia related to increased intravascular volume and increased RBC mass. Ulrich and Canale (2001) suggest that two nursing diagnoses commonly apply to hypertension:

- *Altered tissue perfusion*
- *Pain: headache*

Potential complications associated with hypertension include stroke, heart failure or myocardial infarction, renal dysfunction, and others.

Stasis of Blood Flow. Stagnant blood flow is particularly associated with polycythemia (extreme erythrocytosis) and leukemia (extreme leukocytosis). The major nursing diagnosis that addresses this problem is *altered tissue perfusion* related to decreased systemic blood flow (venous stasis). Stasis of blood flow places the patient at risk for thrombus and thromboembolism complications.

Infection. Hematologic problems that particularly place the patient at risk for the complication of infection include aplastic anemia, neutropenia, and the leukemias. The collaborative nursing diagnosis that addresses infection is *risk for infection* related to inadequate secondary defenses. The degree of infection largely depends on the severity of the leukopenia. The management of neutropenia includes strategies to avoid infections. The patient's own defense system is not working correctly, so it is extremely important to do meticulous central line and mouth care. The patient and health care providers need to wash their hands frequently. Invasive techniques or therapies, such as Foley catheters, should be avoided because they may allow bacteria to enter the body. The patient should be encouraged to shower to decrease the number of microbes on the body. Regular use of incentive spirometry and increased activity also protect the patient against infection. Constipation, which causes microbes to stay in the bowel longer than normal, should be prevented. The nurse should also educate the patient and family regarding the importance of not allowing anyone who is ill with any potentially communicable disease (e.g., cold virus, flu, chicken pox, etc.) into the patient's room.

Bleeding. The bleeding related to decreased platelet count (thrombocytopenia) is primarily caused by aplastic anemia, leukemia, and chemotherapy. Nursing diagnoses that apply to excessive bleeding include *fluid volume deficit* related to intravascular fluid volume loss and *decreased cardiac output* related to decreased intravascular volume. The nurse should maintain fluid balance with IV fluids and transfusions as per physicians' orders. Precautions should be instituted to avoid any patient falls or trauma that may cause bleeding. The nurse should notify the physician if the patient develops confusion or a headache.

In summary, this section provided a brief overview of some of the typical nursing diagnoses that might apply to patients with hematologic problems. The nursing diagnoses were categorized by five major underlying problems associated with the hematologic disorders discussed in this module, including tissue hypoxia, hypertension, stasis of blood flow, infection, and bleeding.

SECTION SIX REVIEW

1. Which of the following causes the neurologic manifestations associated with anemia?
   A. leukostasis
   B. bleeding
   C. tissue hypoxia
   D. increased intracranial pressure
2. The compensatory vital sign changes associated with anemia, infection, and bleeding result in
   A. elevated temperature
   B. increased heart rate
   C. decreased respiratory rate
   D. decreased blood pressure
3. A nursing diagnosis that commonly addresses tissue hypoxia associated with hematologic disorders includes
   A. fatigue
   B. pain
   C. risk for infection
   D. decreased cardiac output

4. *Altered tissue perfusion* related to decreased systemic blood flow is a nursing diagnosis that addresses which of the following underlying problems in polycythemia vera?
   A. tissue hypoxia
   B. infection
   C. bleeding
   D. hypertension
5. The activity intolerance created by some of the hematologic disorders is specifically related to
   A. intravascular fluid volume loss
   B. O_2 supply and demand imbalance
   C. decreased systemic blood flow
   D. inadequate secondary defenses

Answers: 1. C, 2. B, 3. A, 4. D, 5. B

 ## POSTTEST

Questions 1 through 7 pertain to the following case: Robin T, a 24-year-old woman, is brought to a local walk-in clinic by her husband with complaints of severe fatigue, recurrent respiratory infections accompanied by high fevers, and intermittent episodes of epistaxis. Petechiae and purpura are noted on her trunk and arms. Her history is negative for exposure to toxins, and she takes no medications other than occasional non-steroidal anti-inflammatory drugs (NSAIDs) for headache. Blood work is drawn and shows pancytopenia, with a reticulocyte count of 30,000/mcL, neutrophil count of 1,000/mcL, and platelet count of 60,000/mcL. She is diagnosed as having idiopathic aplastic anemia.

1. Her low reticulocyte count suggests
   A. overproduction of RBCs in bone marrow
   B. microcytic, hypochromic RBCs
   C. bone marrow depression or failure
   D. RBCs are being rapidly hemolyzed
2. Her current hemoglobin is 5 g/dL. Which of the following descriptions is most consistent with this level of anemia?
   A. asymptomatic at rest
   B. dyspnea and palpitations
   C. spontaneous epistaxis
   D. intermittent high fevers
3. Robin's neutrophil count is most likely the cause of
   A. recurrent infections
   B. severe fatigue
   C. intermittent epistaxis
   D. petechiae and purpura

Robin complains of activity intolerance, an inability to concentrate, and orthopnea. Her heart rate is 106/min and respirations are 24 to 26/min.

4. Which of the following underlying problems best explains these manifestations?
   A. slow internal bleeding
   B. chronic infection
   C. tissue hypoxia
   D. increased bone marrow activity
5. An aspiration bone marrow biopsy is taken. In the presence of aplastic anemia, the bone marrow should consist of
   A. immature cells
   B. plasma cells
   C. normal tissue
   D. fatty tissue
6. The definitive treatment for aplastic anemia in younger patients is
   A. transfusions of RBCs and platelets
   B. bone marrow transplant
   C. immunosuppressive therapy
   D. supportive therapy
7. If Robin is not a candidate for bone marrow transplantation, her supportive treatment regimen will include
   A. radiation therapy
   B. immunosuppressive therapy
   C. alpha-interferon
   D. vitamin B_{12} injections

Questions 8 through 11 pertain to the following case: Joey P, 3 years old, is brought into the pediatric clinic by his mother. He has a high fever associated with a persistent respiratory infection that has been treated multiple times with antibiotic therapy. His mother states that he is no longer able to play with his siblings but lies on the floor or in a chair for most of the day. The nurse notes petechiae on Joey's trunk and arms. He has had several episodes of epistaxis and bleeding gums that are difficult to control. A complete blood count (CBC) shows a pancytopenia present. Following further blood work, a diagnosis of acute lymphoblastic leukemia (ALL) is made.

8. The pancytopenia associated with Joey's leukemia is caused by which problem of the bone marrow?
   A. crowding out of normal cells
   B. bone marrow failure
   C. proliferation of fatty tissue
   D. hemolysis by antigen–antibody complexes
9. Which of the following statements best reflects leukemic cell maturation?
   A. they mature at an accelerated rate
   B. they differentiate slower than normal cells
   C. they differentiate in an unpredictable manner
   D. they do not mature beyond the stage at which they are produced
10. Joey's leukocyte count climbs to 105,000/mcL. He develops dyspnea, confusion, and severe headache. These manifestations are most consistent with which complication of leukemia?
    A. leukostasis
    B. severe neutropenia
    C. CNS infiltration
    D. bone marrow failure
11. Joey is now receiving "consolidation" chemotherapy. The goal of this drug regimen is best described as
    A. production of a complete remission
    B. halting all bone marrow cell production
    C. elimination of leukemic cells from the CNS
    D. solidification of remission/elimination of remaining leukemic cells

[end of scenario]

12. Common clinical manifestations of thrombocytopenia include
    A. internal hemorrhage
    B. corneal hemorrhage
    C. purpura on mucous membranes
    D. altered level of consciousness, headache
13. Disseminated intravascular coagulation is said to be a coagulation paradox because
    A. coagulation and bleeding are occurring simultaneously
    B. the intrinsic and extrinsic coagulation pathways are both stimulated
    C. coagulation occurs throughout the vascular system
    D. a coagulation problem can result in multiple-organ failure
14. The nurse is working with a trauma patient. During the assessment, the nurse notes blood oozing around the patient's arterial and internal jugular central lines. Fresh bleeding is also noted on the patient's facial injuries and an old puncture wound. Labs are drawn, showing the

following: platelet count, 45,000; PTT, 82 seconds; fibrin degradation product (FDP), 14 mcg/dL; and D-dimer, 300 ng/mL. Which statement is correct regarding these data?

A. they are suspicious of aplastic anemia

B. they are suggestive of idiopathic thrombocytopenia purpura

C. the clinical picture suggests onset of sepsis

D. the clinical picture strongly suggests DIC

15. When performing a cardiopulmonary assessment on a patient with a problem of hematologic function, the nurse should focus on the patient's

A. urine output

B. lung sounds

C. vital signs

D. level of consciousness

16. The nurse is developing a list of nursing diagnoses appropriate to a patient with aplastic anemia. The nursing diagnosis that best reflects impaired oxygen transport would be

A. risk for infection

B. activity intolerance

C. fluid volume deficit

D. decreased cardiac output

POSTTEST ANSWERS

Question	Answer	Section
1	C	Two
2	B	Two
3	A	Two
4	C	Three
5	D	Three
6	B	Three
7	B	Three
8	A	Four

Question	Answer	Section
9	D	Four
10	A	Four
11	D	Four
12	C	Five
13	A	Five
14	D	Five
15	C	Six
16	B	Six

REFERENCES

Andreoli, T. E., Carpenter, C. C., Bennett, J. C., & Plum, F. (1997). Disorders of the hematopoietic stem cell. In T. E. Andreoli, C. C. Carpenter, J. C. Bennett, & F. Plum (Eds.), *Cecil's essentials of medicine* (4th ed., pp. 358–380). Philadelphia: W. B. Saunders.

Beutler, E. (2001). Polycythemia. In E. Beutler, M. A. Lichtman, B. S. Coller, T. J. Kipps, & U. Seligsohn (Eds.), *Williams hematology* (6th ed., pp. 689–702). New York: McGraw Hill.

Blackwell, S., & Hendrix, P. C. (2001). Common anemias. *Clinician Reviews, 11*(3), 53–64.

Byars, L. (2003). Neutropenia risk assessment and management in the ambulatory care setting. *Oncology Supportive Care Quarterly, 1*(1), 27–39.

Caudell, K. A. (1998). Disorders of white blood cells and lymphoid tissues. In C. M. Porth (Ed.), *Pathophysiology: Concepts of altered health states* (5th ed., pp. 151–164). Philadelphia: J. B. Lippincott.

Ching-Hon, P. (2001). Acute lymphoblastic leukemia. In E. Beutler, M. A. Lichtman, B. S. Coller, T. J. Kipps, & U. Seligsohn (Eds.), *Williams hematology* (6th ed., pp. 1141–1162). New York: McGraw Hill.

Erslev, A. J. (2001). Clinical manifestations and classification of erythrocyte disorders. In E. Beutler, M. A. Lichtman, B. S. Coller, T. J. Kipps, & U. Seligsohn (Eds.), *Williams hematology* (6th ed., pp. 369–375). New York: McGraw Hill.

Escalante, C. P., Manzullo, E., & Bonin, S. R. (2003). Oncologic emergencies and paraneoplastic syndromes. In R. Pazdur, L. R. Coia, W. J. Hoskins, & L. D. Wagman (Eds.), *Cancer management: A multidisciplinary approach* (7th ed., pp. 959–982). Huntington, NY: Publisher Research & Representation, Inc.

Fairbanks, V. F., & Beutler, E. (2001). Iron deficiency. In E. Beutler, M. A. Lichtman, B. S. Coller, T. J. Kipps, & U. Seligsohn (Eds.), *Williams hematology* (6th ed., pp. 447–470). New York: McGraw Hill.

Galli, S. J., Metcalfe, D. D., & Dvorak, A. M. (2002). Basophils and mast calls and their disorders. In E. Beutler, M. A. Lichtman, B. S. Coller, T. J. Kipps, & U. Seligsohn (Eds.), *Williams hematology* (6th ed., pp. 801–815). New York: McGraw Hill.

Gaspard, K. J. (1998). The red blood cell and alterations in oxygen transport. In C. M. Porth (Ed.), *Pathophysiology: Concepts of altered health states* (5th ed., pp. 133–149). Philadelphia: Lippincott Williams & Wilkins.

Gaspard, K. J. (2005). Hematopoietic system. In C. M. Porth (Ed.), *Pathophysiology: Concepts of altered health states* (7th ed., pp. 279–285). Philadelphia: Lippincott Williams & Wilkins.

Geiter, H. (2003). Disseminated intravascular coagulopathy. *Dimensions of Critical Care Nursing, 22*(3), 108–114.

George, J. W., & Rizvi, M. A. (2001). Thrombocytopenia. In E. Beutler, M. A. Lichtman, B. S. Coller, T. J. Kipps, & U. Seligsohn (Eds.), *Williams hematology* (6th ed., pp. 1495–1540). New York: McGraw Hill.

Gould, B. (2002). *Pathophysiology for the health professions* (2nd ed.). Philadelphia: W. B. Saunders.

Guyton, A. C., & Hall, J. E. (1997). *Human physiology and mechanisms of disease* (6th ed.). Philadelphia: W. B. Saunders.

Hillman, R. S., & Hershko, C. (2001). Acute blood loss anemia. In E. Beutler, M. A. Lichtman, B. S. Coller, T. J. Kipps, & U. Seligsohn (Eds.), *Williams hematology* (6th ed., pp. 677–682). New York: McGraw Hill.

Howell, C. J., & Rothman, J. (2001). The etiology of thrombocytopenia. *Dimensions of Critical Care Nursing, 20*(4), 10–16.

Kapoor, M., & Chan, G. Z. (2001). Fluid and electrolyte abnormality. In J. S. Groeger (Ed.), *Critical care clinics: Oncology and critical care* (pp. 503–529). Philadelphia, W. B. Saunders.

Kee, J. L. (2002). *Laboratory and diagnostic tests with nursing implications* (6th ed.). Upper Saddle River, NJ: Prentice Hall.

Kipps, T. J. (2001). Chronic lymphocytic leukemia and related disease. In E. Beutler, M. A. Lichtman, B. S. Coller, T. J. Kipps, & U. Seligsohn (Eds.), *Williams hematology* (6th ed., pp. 1163–1194). New York: McGraw Hill.

Knoop, T. (2003). Myelosuppression related to the treatment of cancer. *Oncology Supportive Care Quarterly, 1*(3), 6–25.

Krimmel, T. (2003). Disseminated intravascular coagulation. *Clinical Journal of Oncology Nursing, 7*(4), 479–481.

Leukemia and Lymphoma Society. (2002). *Gleevec: A targeted therapy for chronic myelogenous leukemia.* New York: The Leukemia and Lymphoma Society.

Levi, M. (2004). Current understanding of disseminated intravascular coagulation, *British Journal of Haematology, 124,* 567–576.

Lewis, S. M. (2000). Nursing management: Inflammation and infection. In S. M. Lewis, M. M. Heitkemper, & S. R. Dirksen (Eds.), *Medical–surgical nursing: Assessment and management of clinical problems* (5th ed., pp. 189–211). St. Louis: C. V. Mosby.

Lichtman, M. A. (2001). Classification and clinical manifestations of disorders of monocytes and macrophages. In E. Beutler, M. A. Lichtman, B. S. Coller, T. J. Kipps, & U. Seligsohn (Eds.), *Williams hematology* (6th ed., pp. 877–880). New York: McGraw Hill.

Lichtman, M. A., & Liesveld, J. L. (2001a). Acute myelogenous leukemia. In E. Beutler, M. A. Lichtman, B. S. Coller, T. J. Kipps, & U. Seligsohn (Eds.), *Williams hematology* (6th ed., pp. 1047–1084). New York: McGraw Hill.

Lichtman, M. A., & Liesveld J. L. (2001b). Chronic myelogenous leukemia and related disorders. In E. Beutler, M. A. Lichtman, B. S. Coller, T. J. Kipps, & U. Seligsohn (Eds.), *Williams hematology* (6th ed., pp. 1085–1124). New York: McGraw Hill.

Mazur, E. M. (1998). Platelets. In F. J. Schiffman (Ed.), *Hematologic pathophysiology* (pp. 123–160). Philadelphia: Lippincott-Raven.

NCI. (1999). Grading scale on neutropenia. National Cancer Institute. Available at: *www.nci.nih.gov.* Accessed March 11, 2005.

O'Mara, A. M., & Whedon, M. B. (2000). Nursing management: Hematologic problems. In S. M. Lewis, M. M. Heitkemper, & S. R. Dirksen (Eds.), *Medical–surgical nursing: Assessment and management of clinical problems* (5th ed., pp. 736–789). St. Louis: C. V. Mosby.

Owen, D. C., & Webster, J. S. (1998). Hematology disorders. In M. R. Kinney, S. B. Dunbar, J. A. Brooks-Brunn, N. Molter, & J. M. Vitello-Cicciu (Eds.), *AACN's clinical reference for critical care nursing* (4th ed., pp. 897–914). St. Louis: C. V. Mosby.

Parise, L. V., Smyth, S. S., & Coller, B. S. (2001). Platelet morphology, biochemistry, and function. In E. Beutler, M. A. Lichtman, B. S. Coller, T. J. Kipps, & U. Seligsohn (Eds.), *Williams hematology* (6th ed., pp. 1357–1408). New York: McGraw Hill.

Parslow, T. G. (1994). The phagocytes: Neutrophils and macrophages. In D. P. Stites, A. I. Terr, & T. G. Parslow (Eds.), *Basic and clinical immunology* (8th ed., pp. 9–21). Norwalk, CT: Appleton & Lange.

Rose, M. G., & Berliner, N. (1998). Red blood cells. In F. J. Schiffman (Ed.), *Hematologic pathophysiology* (pp. 49–96). Philadelphia: Lippincott-Raven.

Salmon, S. E., & Sartorelli, A. C. (1998). Cancer chemotherapy. In B. G. Katzung (Ed.), *Basic and clinical pharmacology* (7th ed., pp. 881–915). Norwalk, CT: Appleton & Lange.

Seigsohn, U. (2001). Disseminated intravascular coagulation. In E. Beutler, M. A. Lichtman, B. S. Coller, T. J. Kipps, & U. Seligsohn (Eds.), *Williams hematology* (6th ed., pp. 1677–1695). New York: McGraw Hill.

Shulman, L. N. (1998). Hematologic malignancies. In F. J. Schiffman (Ed.), *Hematologic pathophysiology* (pp. 291–317). Philadelphia: Lippincott-Raven.

Sommers, C. (1998). Immunity and inflammation. In C. M. Porth (Ed.), *Pathophysiology: Concepts of altered health states* (5th ed., pp. 189–212). Philadelphia: Lippincott Williams & Wilkins.

Stanholtz, C. (2001). Acute life-threatening toxicity of cancer treatment. In J. S. Groeger (Ed.), *Critical care clinics: Oncology and critical care* (pp. 483–502). Philadelphia: W. B. Saunders.

Timmerman, P. (1998). Common hematological disorder. In C. M. Hudak, B. M. Gallo, & P. G. Morton (Eds.), *Critical care nursing: A holistic approach* (7th ed., pp. 933–949). Philadelphia: J. B. Lippincott.

Toh, C. H., & Denis, M. (2003). Disseminated in travascular coagulation: Old disease new hope. *British Medical Journal, 327* (7421), 974–978.

Turgeon, M. L. (1999). *Clinical hematology: Theory and procedures* (3rd ed.). Philadelphia: Lippincott Williams & Wilkins.

Ulrich, S. P., & Canale, S. W. (2001). *Medical–surgical nursing care planning guides* (5th ed.). Philadelphia: W. B. Saunders.

Vasudeva, R., & Leong, K. (2002). Neutropenic enterocolitis. *E-medicine.* Available at: *http://www.emedicine.com/med/topic2658.htm.* Accessed November 4, 2004.

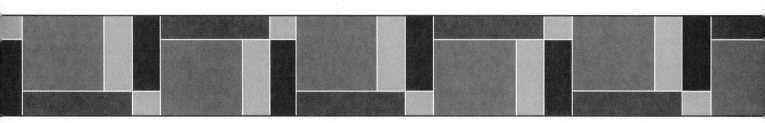

OBJECTIVES   Following completion of this module, the learner will be able to

1. Cite the location and functional role of organs and tissues primarily involved in the immune response.

2. Contrast the nature of natural immunity and acquired (active and passive) immunity.

3. Describe the characteristics of antigens and antigen–antibody responses.

4. Discuss the nature and primary function of cellular components of the immune system.

5. Describe mechanisms of specific immunity (humoral and cell mediated) and mechanisms of nonspecific immunity.

6. Explain the theoretical concepts for the occurrence of types I, II, III, and IV immunoglobulin hypersensitivity and autoimmune disorders.

7. Describe the effects of aging, malnutrition, trauma, and stress related to the functions of the adult immune system.

8. Characterize immunodeficiency and describe the human immunodeficiency virus (HIV) and acquired immunodeficiency syndrome (AIDS) and treatment.

9. Discuss nursing considerations pertinent to the assessment and care of the immunocompromised patient.

With respect to normal physiologic functioning, the immune system serves to protect the body from foreign invaders. These invaders might be disease-producing pathogenic microorganisms (also called pathogens) or abnormal cells, such as cancer cells. However, the immune system is actually the body's third and slowest line of defense against such invasion. An intact skin tissue provides the first line of defense, creating a physical barrier between the internal environment of the body and the external environment surrounding it. If, however, an invading organism or other foreign agent manages to get past this barrier, the inflammatory response is initiated, whereby invading agents are neutralized or destroyed. Failing that mechanism of protection, the immune system is alerted for action. This module is devoted to the structure and function of the immune system, with particular emphasis on the acutely ill adult.

Section One discusses the location and function of specialized cells and organs of the immune system. Particular organs and tissues are described in their relationship to immunity. The emphasis of Section Two is the primary characteristics of active and passive immunity. Section Three presents the learner with

characteristics and outcomes of antigen–antibody activity. Section Four addresses with more detail the origin and function of the various cellular components of the immune system, including T cells, B cells, and macrophages. Section Five discusses the nature of immune mechanisms, including cell-mediated and humoral immunity, phagocytosis, and the role of interferon. Section Six explores the pathogenesis of hypersensitivity reactions and the notion of autoimmune disorders. Section Seven summarizes the impacts of aging, malnutrition, stress, and trauma on the immune system. Human immunodeficiency virus (HIV) is addressed in Section Eight with regard to the nature of the virus, its transmission and growth, and attempts toward treatment. Finally, Section Nine discusses nursing considerations pertinent to care of the immunocompromised patient.

Each section includes a set of review questions to help the learner evaluate his or her understanding of the section's content. All Section Reviews and the module Pretest and Posttest include answers. It is suggested that the learner review those concepts answered incorrectly in the review questions before proceeding to the next section.

PRETEST

1. Which type of tissue or cell is primarily responsible for T cell differentiation?
   A. bursa equivalent
   B. thymus
   C. stem cells
   D. lymph nodes

2. The bursa equivalent is thought to be located in the
   A. spleen
   B. Peyer's patches
   C. bone marrow
   D. thymus

3. Nonspecific immune response involves
   A. recognition of a particular antigen
   B. production of antibodies
   C. recognition of nonself
   D. T cell differentiation

4. A child who first has chicken pox and then is immune from that disease in the future is said to have
   A. active acquired immunity
   B. passive acquired immunity
   C. natural immunity
   D. species-specific immunity

5. An individual whose antibody titer is greater than the preestablished level of immunity is said to
   A. demonstrate immunity from the disease in question
   B. require reimmunization
   C. demonstrate a specific antigen–antibody complex
   D. transmit the disease as a carrier

6. HLA antigen is located on which site?
   A. the gamma globulin protein fraction
   B. the erythrocytes
   C. chromosome 6
   D. the RNA chains

7. Which type of cell is responsible for direct antigen attack and destruction?
   A. helper T cell
   B. killer T cell
   C. suppressor B cell
   D. memory B cell

8. Macrophages are primarily responsible for
   A. interfering with the immune response
   B. protecting against local mucosal invasion of bacteria
   C. triggering the complement system
   D. carrying the antigen to B cells and T cells

9. Humoral immunity is best characterized by
   A. the development of antibodies from B cells
   B. the recognition of self and nonself
   C. specific recognition and memory of antigens
   D. differentiation of cellular function known as killer, helper, and suppressor cells

10. Which immunoglobulin comprises about 75 percent of the total immunoglobulins in the healthy human body?
    A. IgA
    B. IgE
    C. IgG
    D. IgM

11. Which immunoglobulin affords the body local protection at the mucosal level against invading organisms?
    A. IgA
    B. IgG
    C. IgD
    D. IgE

12. An example of therapeutically eliciting the primary and secondary response patterns of humoral immunity is
    A. exposure to chicken pox and subsequent immunity
    B. tetanus vaccine and booster vaccines
    C. interferon treatment for malignancy
    D. transference of killer T cells from donor to recipient

13. The results of a true type I hypersensitivity response are caused by
    A. a histamine precursor causing anaphylaxis
    B. antigen–IgE–mast cell interaction
    C. antigen–antibody complexes deposited in vessel walls
    D. massive numbers of destroyed red blood cells (RBCs)

14. What characterizes the concept of autoimmune disease?
    A. recognition of self as foreign
    B. exacerbation and death
    C. accelerated production of killer T cells
    D. immunosuppression and altered cortisol levels

15. Which statement BEST characterizes HIV disease?
    A. symptoms result from opportunistic pathology
    B. clinical manifestations are of a characteristic and predictable sequence
    C. the HIV virus invades cells primarily through the bloodstream
    D. individuals who test positive for the HIV virus are carriers and considered contagious

16. Which fluid is known to be a mode of transmission for the acquired immune deficiency syndrome (AIDS) virus?
    A. tears
    B. perspiration
    C. plasma
    D. saliva

17. What is the function of zinc in the competent immune system?
    A. it is required for normal function of lymphocytes
    B. zinc protects B cells from being destroyed by macrophages
    C. T cells require zinc for production of gamma globulin
    D. macrophages are composed primarily of zinc

18. What effect does the normal aging process have on the immune system?
    A. B cell function in general is particularly depressed
    B. the immune system becomes hypervigilant to invading organisms with increasing age
    C. autoantibodies begin to diminish with increasing age
    D. T cells begin to deteriorate in functioning

19. In the acutely ill adult, which nutritional loss to the body is a critical factor in immune system integrity?
    A. protein
    B. vitamin C
    C. complex carbohydrate chains
    D. iron
20. Decreased levels of neutrophils are associated with
    A. stress
    B. bone marrow depression
    C. infectious conditions
    D. tissue necrosis

21. The most important clinical manifestation associated with infection in an immunocompromised patient is
    A. elevated WBC
    B. local inflammation
    C. fever
    D. pain

Pretest Answers:
1. B, 2. C, 3. C, 4. A, 5. A, 6. C, 7. B, 8. D, 9. A, 10. C, 11. A, 12. B, 13. B, 14. A, 15. A, 16. C, 17. A, 18. D, 19. A, 20. B, 21. C

GLOSSARY

acquired immunity, active   Immunity resulting from exposure to a specific antigen and subsequent formation and programming of antibodies; may be produced from having the disease or by injection of the weakened organism (vaccination).

acquired immunity, passive   Temporary immunity provided by injection of sera containing antibodies, placental crossover, or mother's milk.

allergic response   A hypersensitivity reaction of antigen–antibody activity in response to a specific substance that in nonsensitive people in similar amounts produces no effect.

alpha-fetoprotein (AFP)   An antigen produced normally during fetal development by the yolk sac and the liver. It is also found in serum of patients with cirrhosis, and testicular and some liver cancers. This antigen is an example of low immunogenicity and does not evoke an immune response.

antigenic determinant site   Sites on antigens that interact with specific immune cells to bind in lock-and-key fashion; the binding elicits the immune response.

antigens   Coded materials that allow the body to distinguish tissue as "nonself" or "self" and are generally capable of eliciting immune responses; antigens that do not evoke immune responses include tumor-associated antigens such as CEA, AFP, and PSA.

Arthus vasculitis reaction   A severe local inflammatory reaction to an antigen; one example of a type III antigen–antibody hypersensitivity reaction.

autoimmunity   A destructive response in which the immune system recognizes self as foreign and begins to destroy the body's own cells and tissues.

B lymphocytes (B cells)   Lymphocytes primarily responsible for antibody production on exposure to a specific antigen; the primary cells in humoral immunity.

bursa equivalent   Tissue thought to be located in the bone marrow, primarily responsible for differentiating lymphocytes into B cells for humoral immunity.

carcinoembryonic antigen (CEA)   An antigen found in the bloodstream of patients with colon, lung, breast, and pancreatic tumors; this antigen is an example of an antigen that is not immunogenic.

CD markers   Refers to "clusters of differentiation" cell surface antigen markings on lymphocytes. All T cells express the CD3 marker, and all B cells express the CD19 marker. Subsets of T cells and B cells are distinguished and recognizable by these markings (e.g., helper T cells, or T4 cells, are specifically marked as CD4).

cell-mediated immunity   A type of protection against invading antigens characterized by surveillance and direct attack of foreign material; the primary effector cell is the T lymphocyte.

chemotaxis   The migration of phagocytes toward the site of infection via a chemical attraction.

complement system   A progressive, sequential cascade of events produced by substances found naturally in the circulating sera; components of the system must be triggered individually and cause cellular lysis of antigens.

cytokines   A collective term referring to chemical messengers primarily produced by leukocytes that activate other components of the immune system. Cytokines produced by B cell and T cell lymphocytes are called lymphokines; those produced by macrophages are called monokines. Examples include tumor necrosis factor (TNF), interferons (INF), and interleukin (IL).

histocompatibility antigens (human leukocyte antigens [HLA])   Genetically determined surface antigens found in all nucleated cells in the body; one's own HLA antigens are substances that the body recognizes as self.

humoral immunity   The type of protection against foreign antigens provided by antibody formation from B lymphocytes.

hypersensitivity   An exaggerated response of the immune system to an antigen or antigens otherwise considered nonpathogenic; an allergy to a certain substance is an example of a hypersensitivity reaction.

immunity   A normal adaptive response to the external environment; it functions to protect the body from disease by means of both resistance to offending organisms and attack on offending organisms.

immunodeficiency state   A general term referring to a state of deficient immune activity.

immunodeficiency, primary   Failure of either T cell or B cell function or both, resulting from embryonic or congenital lack of development of such organs as the thymus.

immunodeficiency, secondary (acquired)   A deficiency of T cells or B cells or both resulting from illnesses, chemotherapy, radiation therapy, or a direct pathogenic attack on the immune system.

immunogenicity/immunogenic   Capable of evoking an immune response; in varying degrees, antigens are immunogenic; some antigens do not evoke an immune response (e.g., CEA, AFP).

immunoglobulins (Ig)   The product of plasma cells in the humoral immune response following exposure to a specific antigen; the five classes of immunoglobulins are IgA, IgD, IgE, IgG, and IgM; antibodies.

innate immunity   Immunologic activity that is relatively nonspecific and generally prevents infection. Components include the skin and mucous membranes; chemical cytolytic substances produced by the body; and cellular types including monocytes, macrophages, eosinophils, neutrophils, and natural killer cells.

interferons   A cytokine involved in signaling between cells of the immune system and in protection against viral infections.

interleukins   Cytokines involved in signaling between cells of the immune system.

lymphokines   Substances produced by T cells that influence the function of macrophages and inflammatory cells.

macrophage   A monocyte that ingests and digests antigens, then carries the antigen to the T cells and B cells; the link between the immune response and the inflammatory response.

major histocompatibility complex (MHC)   A group of genes located on the sixth chromosome; responsible for coding histocompatibility antigens.

mast cells   Large granule-containing tissue cells that are located in connective tissue throughout the body.

natural immunity   A type of species-specific immunity with which one is born.

natural killer (NK) cells   Leukocytes containing lethal substances that kill on contact when released. NK cells are neither T cells nor B cells in structure but contribute to cell-mediated immunity through nonspecific attack. They are incapable of developing immunologic memory and are particularly effective against viruses.

opsonins   Factors that provide binding sites for attachment of macrophages or neutrophils to the antigen; composed of IgG immunoglobulin and C3b, a fragment of the complement system.

pathogens   Disease-producing microorganisms.

plasma cells   The result of the transformation of mature B cells in response to exposure to a specific antigen; primary cell to produce or secrete antibodies (immunoglobulins).

primary response   The initial humoral response to antigen exposure; characterized by a latency period during which the antigen is recognized as nonself and identified specifically, following which antibodies are formed in response to the antigen makeup.

rejection phenomenon   Attempted destruction of transplanted tissue at the cellular level by the host's immune system.

reticuloendothelial system   Refers to a group of immune cells and tissues, including monocytes, macrophages, and certain specialized endothelial cells; also known as the monocyte–macrophage system.

secondary response   The humoral response to subsequent exposures to the same antigen; immune response is heightened, and antibody formation is triggered more quickly than in the primary response.

T lymphocytes (T cells)   Lymphocytes primarily responsible for direct attack and destruction of invading antigens and for primary cell-mediated immunity.

thymus   Organ in the mediastinum primarily responsible for differentiating lymphocytes into various types of T cells for cell-mediated immunity.

tumor-associated antigen   A particular antigen that distinguishes normal cells from abnormally transformed cells.

ABBREVIATIONS

ABO	Refers to the ABO blood group system
AFP	Alpha-fetoprotein
AIDS	Acquired immune deficiency syndrome
AZT	Azidothymidine
B cells	Bursa cells
CD marker	Surface antigen marker
CEA	Carcinoembryonic antigen
ELISA	Enzyme-linked immunosorbent assay
HIV	Human immunodeficiency virus
HLA	Human leukocyte antigen
HTLV	Human T cell lymphotropic virus
Ig	Immunoglobulin
IL	Interleukin
IL-1	Interleukin-1
IL-2	Interleukin-2
INF	Interferon

mcg	Microgram
MHC	Major histocompatibility complex
NK cells	Natural killer cells
PCP	Pneumocystis carinii pneumonia
PCR	Polymerase chain reaction

RES	Reticuloendothelial system
SCID	Severe combined immune deficiencies
SLE	Systemic lupus erythematosus
T cells	Thymus cells
TNF	Tumor necrosis factor

SECTION ONE: Role of the Immune System in Body Defense

At the completion of this section, the learner will be able to cite the location and functional role of organs and tissues primarily involved in the immune response.

Acting as a surveillance mechanism, the immune system monitors the internal environment of the body for foreign agents. It is a complex system of organs and cells capable of distinguishing self from nonself, remembering previous invaders, and reacting according to needs as they arise. The primary lymphoid organs are the bone marrow and the thymus, which are the major sites of lymphocyte development. The secondary lymphoid organs include the tonsils and adenoids, lymph nodes, spleen, and other lymphoid tissue. Cellular and humoral immune responses occur in the secondary lymphoid organs. The spleen responds to primary blood borne antigens, whereas the lymph nodes respond to antigens circulating in the lymph system. The tonsils respond to antigens, which enter through the mucosal barriers (Lydyard & Grossi, 2001). Contributing to the immune response are lymphoid tissues in nonlymphoid organs (such as the intestinal tissue), and circulating immune cells, such as T cells, B cells, and phagocytes. The circulating immune cells are discussed further in Section Four. Figure 25–1 shows primary organs and lymph tissue sites as well as the sites of T cell and B cell differentiation.

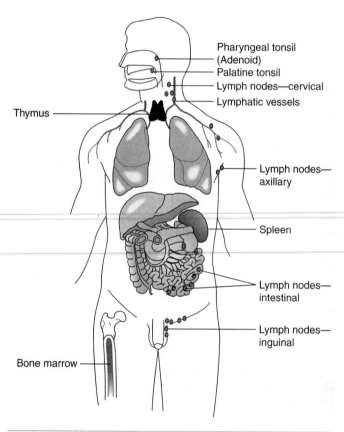

Figure 25–1 ■ Major lymphoid organs and tissues in the immune system. *(Reprinted from Gould, B. E. (2002). Pathophysiology for the health professions (2nd ed., page 36). Copyright 2002, with permission from Elsevier.)*

The Thymus

The **thymus** is a flat, lobed organ located in the neck below the thyroid and extending into the upper thorax behind the sternum. Each lobe is arranged into lobules and then divided into an outer cortex and an inner medulla. The outer cortex contains the majority of immature proliferating thymocytes, whereas the more mature cells are found in the medulla. The epithelial cells throughout the lobules play a role in the differentiation of the bone marrow-derived prethymic cells and the mature T lymphocytes (Lydyard & Grossi, 2001). Reaching its peak size at puberty, the thymus diminishes in size and composition steadily until it is hardly distinguishable in adulthood. Its lymphoid tissue is gradually replaced by adipose tissue over a person's lifetime.

The primary function of the thymus is the development of the immune system. During embryonic life, most lymphocytes develop from stem cells in the bone marrow and travel to the thymus after birth to be marked as T cells (T, of thymus origin). During extrauterine life, the role of the thymus is to differentiate lymphocytes into various types of T cells. In this process, the thymus alters the surface antigens of these cells, which gives them their identity as T cells, a specialized lymphocyte. Mature, differentiated lymphocytes are released into the bloodstream, and they relocate in peripheral lymph tissue, such as lymph nodes, tonsils, intestines, and spleen, where they await a call to action in body defense.

Bursa Equivalent

Much like the thymus in T cell maturation, the **bursa equivalent** in the bone marrow differentiates lymphocytes into B cells (B, of bursa origin). Prior to birth, B cells develop from fetal liver tissue beginning at 8 to 9 weeks of gestation. Later, B cell production shifts to the bone marrow, where it continues throughout life. Once released, these immature B cells migrate to the peripheral lymph tissue (lymph nodes, spleen, and tonsils), where they mature and await the body's need for defense against foreign agents. The majority of B cells do not reach the circulation but undergo a process of programmed cell death (Lydyard & Grossi, 2001).

Lymph System

The blood is filtered continuously by the lymph system. The lymph nodes actually serve two purposes for the body: They act as a filtering system for foreign materials, and they serve as a reservoir for the specialized immunologic T cells and B cells. Peripherally, the serous portion of the blood (excluding platelets, red blood cells, and large proteins) diffuses from the capillaries into the peripheral lymph channels, where it is progressively filtered and then returned to the cardiovascular system. Lymph ducts carry the serous fluid through lymph nodes, where it is filtered. It may be useful to think of a lymph node as a sponge, where the meshwork serves as a surface on which antigens and other foreign materials are arrested and destroyed or neutralized. Large clusters of lymph nodes are found in the axillae, groin, thorax, abdomen, and neck. With many infectious processes, these nodes become enlarged as their activity increases and defense cells proliferate. T cells are most abundant here, although B cells can be found also.

Spleen

The spleen is a small organ about the size of a fist in the left upper quadrant of the abdomen. It is protected by the ninth, tenth, and eleventh ribs and, thus, usually it is nonpalpable. The spleen serves three functions, only one of which is actually immune related. First, it is the site for the destruction of injured and worn out red blood cells. Second, it is a reservoir for B cells, although T cells also are found there. Third, it serves as a storage site for blood, which is released from distended vessels in times of demand.

The tonsils, Peyer's patches in the intestine, and the appendix are quite similar in function and structure to the lymph nodes and the spleen. The tonsils, like the thymus, diminish in size after childhood and, unless inflamed, are difficult to distinguish from surrounding tissue in the posterior pharynx.

In summary, the ability to produce and maintain an intact immune system requires the interaction of the thymus, bursa equivalent, lymph nodes, spleen, and tonsils as well as lymphoid tissue in nonlymphoid organs, such as the intestines. Although much of the immune system is well in place before birth, ongoing processes of marking and maturation of cells are critical to adequate functioning for nonspecific immune responses and specific antigen–antibody reactions to occur.

SECTION ONE REVIEW

1. Which type of cell or tissue is primarily responsible for T cell differentiation?
   A. bursa equivalent
   B. thymus gland
   C. stem cells
   D. lymph nodes
2. As a person ages, thymus gland lymphoid tissue is slowly replaced by
   A. Peyer's patches
   B. stem cells
   C. bursa cells
   D. adipose tissue
3. The bursa equivalent is thought to be located in the
   A. spleen
   B. Peyer's patches
   C. bone marrow
   D. thymus

4. A major function of the lymph nodes is to
   A. filter foreign substances
   B. destroy worn out red blood cells
   C. produce lymphocytes
   D. produce stem cells
5. Which function is correct regarding the spleen?
   A. it destroys worn out white blood cells
   B. it filters out foreign materials
   C. it produces the hormone thymosin
   D. it is a reservoir for B cells

Answers: 1. B, 2. D, 3. C, 4. A, 5. D,

SECTION TWO: Characteristics of the Immune System

At the completion of this section, the learner will be able to contrast the nature of natural immunity and acquired (active and passive) immunity. **Immunity** is a normal adaptive response to the external environment. It functions to protect the body from disease by both resistance to offending organisms and attack on offending organisms. Immunity can be either natural (innate) or acquired.

Natural (Innate) Immunity

Natural immunity is species specific; that is, human beings are immune to a variety of diseases to which certain animals are susceptible, and vice versa. For example, human beings are not vulnerable to feline leukemia, and cats are not susceptible to human immunodeficiency virus (HIV).

Natural immunity is innate; human beings are born with specific immunities. This **innate immunity** is relatively nonspecific and provides primary protection against infection with cells that are incapable of developing long-term memory. Natural resistance to a particular infectious agent is not improved with repeated exposure to the agent. Natural immunity includes physical barriers to disease by means of the skin and mucous membranes, and natural chemical barriers found in the gastrointestinal tract, respiratory tract, and genitourinary structures. Specialized leukocyte cells that provide innate immunity include monocytes, macrophages, eosinophils, and **natural killer (NK) cells.** NK cells are instrumental in surveillance functions and provide antiviral activity on contact (Male, 2001).

Acquired/Adaptive Immunity

Acquired immunity is a highly integrated adaptive process that is antigen specific. Resistance to a particular infectious agent is significantly improved with repeated exposure to specialized cells that have been differentiated into long-term memory cells. This adaptive immunity includes certain monocytes and macrophages, and T lymphocytes (T cells) and B lymphocytes (B cells) (Male, 2001).

Acquired immunity can be either active or passive. **Active acquired immunity** is developed on exposure to an antigen, such as the chicken pox virus, during which time antibodies are programmed to protect the body from illness with future exposures. These antibodies are quite specific, often providing lifetime immunity against another attack of the same antigen. Inoculation provides another means for development of active immunity through exposure to a specific antigen by introduction of a vaccine. Such vaccines as those for smallpox and polio provide a lifetime force of antibody protection without an actual illness occurring. Active immunity following exposure to a specific antigen does not provide immediate protection but develops over a period of days. However, the programming of specific antibodies provides heightened protection with subsequent exposures within a matter of minutes or hours.

Passive acquired immunity is a temporary immunity involving the transfer of antibodies from one individual to another or from some other source (laboratory cultures, other animals) to an individual. An infant receives passive immunity both in utero and from breast milk. A neonate does not yet have a mature immune system capable of efficient development of antibodies in response to invading agents. Passive immunity can be transferred also through vaccination either of antiserum, such as rabies; an antitoxin, such as tetanus; or as gamma globulin, which contains a variety of antibodies.

Both passive and active immunity create levels of antibodies circulating in the body. Many of these levels can be monitored by venipuncture blood tests to determine full immunity to a particular disease. The result of testing the level of a particular antibody is called the *antibody titer*. The titer of the specific antibody is compared with a preestablished level thought to guarantee immunity. If the individual's titer is found to be lower than the preestablished norm, he or she may require repeated immunization with the vaccine. An example of such a process is the increased scrutiny of individuals regarding their immune status to rubella.

In summary, there is ongoing interaction between the body and the environment as substances known as antigens come in contact with the immune system. The body has several avenues by which it might protect itself against foreign antigens. First, a natural immunity occurs normally and is species specific. Second, the healthy body is able to respond to antigenic stimulation and produce its own antibodies that continue to circulate long after the antigen is destroyed, in some cases for a lifetime. Finally, antibodies may be transferred to the body by injection or through the common maternal–fetal circulation and breast milk. Table 25–1 summarizes information on active and passive immunity.

TABLE 25–1   Types of Immunity

TYPE	SUMMARY

Natural (innate)	Species specific
	Present at birth
	Does not increase with repeated exposures
	Barriers
	    Physical (e.g., skin, mucous membranes)
	    Chemical (e.g., gastric acid)
	Immune cells involved: monocytes//macrophages, eosinophils, natural killer (NK) cells

Acquired/adaptive	Antigen specific
	Not present at birth
	Increased resistance with repeated exposures
	Immune cells involved: certain monocytes/macrophages, T cells and B cells
	Active
	    Exposure to antigen (e.g., chicken pox, inoculation)
	    Provides life-time immunity
	Passive
	    Temporary
	    Transfer of antibodies (e.g., mother–fetus, mother–baby via breast milk)
	    Vaccination (e.g., tetanus, gamma globulin)

SECTION THREE: Antigens and Antigen–Antibody Response

At the completion of this section, the learner will be able to describe characteristics of antigens and antigen–antibody responses.

Antigens

Antigens are substances that are capable of triggering an immune response if they can be recognized by a B cell antibody or T cell (Male, 2001). The immune response can involve either humoral or cellular components of the immune system but commonly involves both. The degree to which an antigen stimulates an immune response is referred to as its **immunogenicity** or its **immunogenic nature** and is influenced by factors such as physical and chemical properties of the antigen, the relative foreignness of the antigen, and the person's genetic makeup. Antigens may be either foreign to the body or be important self-markers or tumor markers.

Foreign Antigens

Some foreign-body antigens are capable of causing disease and are called **pathogens** or pathogenic antigens. Many bacteria, viruses, parasites, and other microorganisms are pathogenic antigens, such as *Staphylococcus aureus,* Mycobacterium tuberculosis, herpes simplex, and HIV. Other antigens, such as vaccines, are foreign to the body but are not pathogenic microorganisms. Vaccines induce a protective immunologic response by introducing either viruses or bacteria that are killed, treated, or attenuated (selectively altered). These vaccines are incapable of inducing a disease state but effectively stimulate a mild immune response as a protective mechanism against similar live microorganisms.

A second example of a nonpathogenic antigen is a transplanted heart or kidney. The cells making up the tissues of these organs are not disease producing but are recognized by the body as being foreign (nonself); thus, the transplanted organ can pre-cipitate an immune reaction. Although the immune system is certainly capable of distinguishing self from nonself in its natural state, it is not able to determine that a foreign material is acceptable even if that material is beneficial to the well-being of the body as a whole. This is the scenario that occurs in organ transplant rejection. Organ transplant rejection is discussed in detail in Module 26, "Organ Transplantation."

Histocompatibility Antigens

In addition to foreign materials being antigens, all nucleated cells in the body contain surface antigens, which are proteins found on the surface of a cell. These proteins distinguish an individual's tissue (self) from tissue of other persons (nonself). Surface antigens are genetically determined and are referred to as **histocompatibility antigens** or **human leukocyte antigens (HLA)**. The HLA proteins are coded by a group of genes called the **major histocompatibility complex (MHC)** located on the sixth chromosome. Histocompatibility antigens are presented in detail in Module 26, "Organ Transplantation."

Tumor-Associated Antigens

Some human tumors have been found to display particular antigens (**tumor-associated antigens**) that distinguish normal cells from abnormally transformed cells. Identification of tumor-associated antigens has progressed rapidly with technological advances in tumor immunology. Tumor-associated antigens typically do not evoke an immune response (low immunogenicity), perhaps because they are recognized as self from early development during embryonic and fetal stages. Although many of these antigens occur naturally in small quantities, an elevation of the particular antigen type can be helpful in detecting potentially abnormal cells and tracking progression of disease or regression of disease following treatment (Gould, 2002). For example, **carcinoembryonic antigen (CEA)** has been found to be elevated in a variety of adenocarcinomas of the colon, lung, breast, and pancreas; **alpha-fetoprotein (AFP)** is frequently elevated in patients with testicular and hepatic cancer; and serum elevations of prostate-specific antigen (PSA) have been found in occurrences of prostatic cancer (Gould, 2002). Serum elevations of tumor-associated antigens are also possible with several non-malignant disease states. Success in identifying and characterizing tumor-specific antigens that are not found in other disease states or on other host cells has been less successful to date.

Antigenic Determinants

Antigens have several specific sites, called **antigenic determinant sites,** which interact with immune cells to elicit the immune response. These sites are quite specific in configuration, requiring a specific structure of the immunoglobulin molecule or antibody. The binding of antigen to antibody occurs at spe-

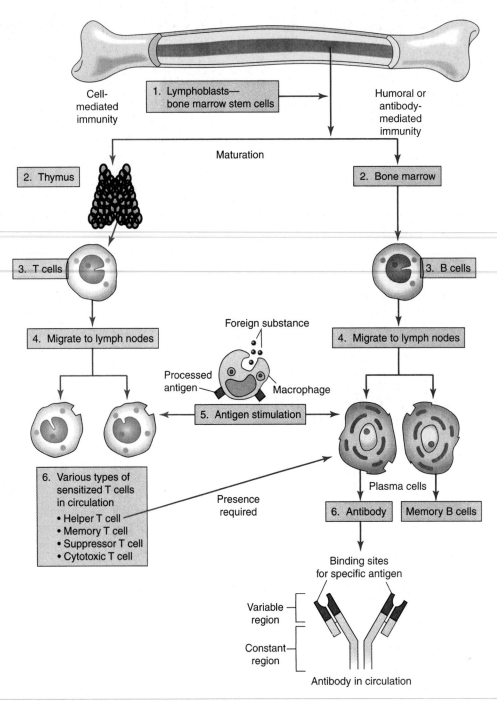

Figure 25–2 ■ Cellular and humoral immunities. *(Reprinted from Gould, B.E. (2002).* Pathophysiology for the health professions *(2nd ed., p. 38). Copyright 2002, with permission from Elsevier.)*

cific receptor sites and is similar to the notion of a lock and key. Some molecules are so small that they cannot act as antigens until they attach to larger molecules or carriers. The immune response recognizes the antigens, and destroys and eliminates them. When the antigen is eliminated, the immune system is turned off (Male, 2001). Figure 25–2 illustrates how the immune system responds (cellular and humoral immunities) to a specific antigen.

Immune Responsiveness

Immune responsiveness may be either specific or nonspecific. A specific response requires the recognition of a particular antigen and involves the production and action of a programmed antibody for that antigen. Normally, an antibody circulates in the bloodstream until it encounters an appropriate antigen to which it can bind. Such binding results in antigen–antibody complexes, or immune complexes. The process of binding is such that the antibody binds to specifically conformed antigenic determinant sites on the antigen, which effectively prevent the antigen from binding with receptors on host cells. The overall effect is protection of the host from antigen infection or penetration.

An antigen–antibody reaction can have several consequences for the invading agent. The reaction can cause agglutination (clumping of the cells), neutralization of the antigen toxin (e.g., a bacterial toxin), cell lysis (destruction of the antigen), enhanced phagocytosis of the antigen by other cells, opsonization, or activation of the complement system.

A nonspecific response requires only the recognition of the invader as being nonself, or foreign, but does not involve a particular antibody. A nonspecific immunologic response might involve the complement system, interferons, natural killer cells, and phagocytosis. These mechanisms of immunity are discussed in Section Five.

Antigen Entry Site

The entry site of an antigen is an important consideration. Many enzymes and other secretions are important components as defense mechanisms. Some antigens are destroyed before they cross into the bloodstream. For example, some antigens are readily destroyed or neutralized by salivary and other digestive enzymes in the gastrointestinal tract, rendering them incapable of causing disease. Other antigens are not affected by these enzymes and can proliferate rapidly, creating pathologic states. The site of entrance also determines the strength or virulence of the antigen. For example, an antigen that is neutralized by digestive enzymes in the gastrointestinal tract might be quite virulent if entering the body through the genitourinary tract or the respiratory tract where digestive enzymes are not normally found.

In summary, the antigen–antibody phenomenon is the cornerstone for much of the body's protective immune system. Both antigens and antibodies have particular configurations that allow them to bind to one another. Once an antibody binds with an antigen, the antigen is no longer capable of binding with the host cell. The effect of binding may result in agglutination of the offending antigen neutralization, cell lysis (destruction), enhanced phagocytosis, opsonization, or activation of the complement system. Which effect occurs depends on the class of antibody and the nature of the antigen.

SECTION THREE REVIEW

1. A nonspecific immune response involves
   A. T cell differentiation
   B. production of antibody
   C. recognition of nonself
   D. recognition of a particular antigen
2. HLA antigens are located on
   A. RNA chains
   B. erythrocytes
   C. chromosome 6
   D. the gamma globulin protein fraction
3. Specific sites on antigens that interact with immune cells to elicit the immune response are called
   A. antigenic determinants
   B. surface cells
   C. human leukocyte antigens
   D. histocompatibility complexes
4. Antigens that precipitate disease states are called
   A. immunoglobulins
   B. pathogens
   C. human leukocyte antigens
   D. histocompatibility antigens
5. Which statements regarding the entry site of an antigen are correct? (choose all that apply)
   1. saliva in the mouth destroys many antigens
   2. digestive enzymes neutralize many antigens
   3. site of entry helps determine virulence of the antigen
   4. entry location does not determine strength of the antigen
   A. 2, 3, and 4
   B. 1, 3, and 4
   C. 2 and 3
   D. 1, 2, and 3

Answers: 1. C, 2. C, 3. A, 4. B, 5. D

SECTION FOUR: Cells of the Immune Response

At the completion of this section, the learner will be able to discuss the nature and primary function of cellular components of the immune system.

There are three major types of immune cells involved in the immune response to foreign material: the T cell, the B cell, and the macrophage. Each of these cell types carries a distinct responsibility and contributes to the integrity of the body as a whole. Figure 25–3 provides an illustration of the principal components of the immune system.

T Lymphocytes

The **T lymphocytes** (also referred to as **T cells** or T lymphs) provide cell-mediated immunity, which is discussed in a later section. T cells have a life expectancy of several years. They are marked by the thymus with specific surface antigens that characterize them and distinguish them from B cells. The T cells represent approximately 70 to 80 percent of the total lymphocyte count.

Subsets of mature T cells are identified by a nomenclature referred to as clusters of differentiation (CD). These clusters are actually surface antigens commonly known as **CD markers.** For example, helper T cells (T4 cells) bear a CD4 marker; suppressor T cells and killer/cytotoxic T cells (T8 cells) carry a CD8 marker. Approximately 70 percent of mature T cells carry the CD4 marker, and 30 percent carry the CD8 marker.

There are several different types of T cells. The type 1 T helper cells interact with the mononuclear phagocytes and assist in the destruction of pathogens. The type 2 T helper cells interact with the B cells and assist the B cells in division and production of antibodies. The T cytotoxic cells are responsible for the destruction and lysis of the infected host cells. T cells act in one

of two ways: They either release soluble proteins (cytokines) or have cell-to-cell interactions (Male, 2001).

B Lymphocytes

The **B lymphocytes** (**B cells**) are the larger of the lymphocyte cells and have a much shorter life span than the T cells. They mature with exposure to an antigen. Immature B cells are stored in the bone marrow, the lymph nodes, and other lymphatic tissue. They are also found circulating in the bloodstream. It is the B lymphocytes that are primarily responsible for antibody production. Following exposure to an antigen, mature B cells transform into plasma cells, which then secrete antibodies called **immunoglobulins** (**Ig**). Each plasma cell is specialized to produce only one type of antibody. Several types of antibodies have been identified, and each is active within a given course of events in the immune response. Immunoglobulins are identified as IgA, IgD, IgE, IgG, or IgM. They are discussed in Section Five.

Monocyte–Macrophage System

The monocyte–macrophage system, also known as the **reticuloendothelial system,** refers to a group of immune cells and tissues, including monocytes, macrophages (mobile and fixed tissue), and certain endothelial cells found in the spleen, bone marrow, and lymph nodes (Guyton & Hall, 1997). Monocytes are not active phagocytes; that is, they require activation by the immune system to become macrophages, which are powerful phagocytes. There are two types of macrophages: mobile and fixed. Mobile macrophages circulate in the blood supply and migrate out of the vessels into the tissues when required through the process of chemotaxis. Fixed macrophages, on leaving the circulation, affix

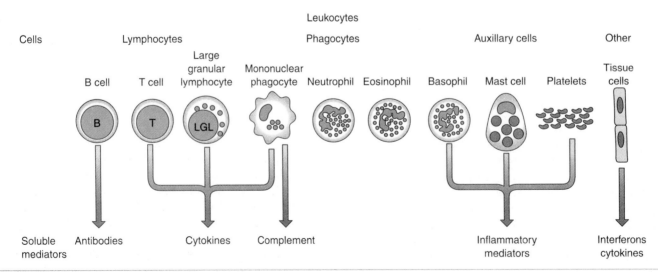

Figure 25–3 ■ Main cells and molecules involved in the immune system. *(Reprinted from Platts-Mills, T. (2001). Hypersensitivity type I. In I. Roitt, J. Brostoff, & D. Male (Eds.),* Immunology, *(6th ed., p. 323). Copyright 2001, with permission from Elsevier.)*

themselves to tissues and remain there, waiting for pathogens to appear. When needed, fixed macrophages are able to break away from the tissue to initiate phagocytic activity. Common examples of fixed macrophages include the Kupffer's cells in the liver and the type I alveolar cells in the lungs. They play important roles in protecting the organs against pathogens (e.g., bacteria or viruses, sloughing tissue or foreign particles) (Guyton & Hall, 1997).

The **macrophage** participates in the immune response by processing the antigen and presenting it in such a way as to increase its recognition and reaction by the B cells and T cells. By means of phagocytosis, the macrophage ingests and digests the antigen; in the process, the altered antigen is released through the macrophage cell membrane, where it attaches to receptor sites on the surface of the macrophage. It is at these receptor sites that the interaction takes place with the invading antigen and T cells. In its function as an antigen-presenting cell (APC), the macrophage is primarily responsible for carrying antigens to the lymph tissue, where the B cells and T cells reside. The macrophage is a critical factor in the immune response to both the T cells and the B cells and is considered the link between the inflammatory response and the specific resistance of antibody production and cell mediation by its production of interleukins. The liver, lungs, and lymph nodes contain macrophages because these areas encounter many antigens (Gould, 2002).

Immune Mediators: Cytokines

Cells of the immune system are regulated by chemical messengers, collectively known as **cytokines** or immune mediators, which serve to activate components of the immune system. B cells and T cells produce **lymphokines** (a type of cytokine). Of particular interest are interleukin (IL), tumor necrosis factor (TNF), and interferons (INF). Interferons are important in limiting the spread of viral infections by inducing a state of antiviral resistance. **Interleukins** are produced mainly by the T cells and are involved in directing cells to divide and differentiate. Colony-stimulating factors (CSF) are involved in the division and differentiation of bone marrow stem cells. The different colony-stimulating factors influence the proportion of different cell types that are produced. For example, tumor necrosis factor is important in mediating inflammation and cytotoxic reactions (Male, 2001).

In summary, T cells, B cells, and macrophages work together to maintain the integrity of the body against invading antigens. It is the macrophage, however, that plays the important role of preparing the antigen for the T lymphocytes and B lymphocytes. Without adequate macrophage support, the remaining cellular components of the immune system would be severely impaired.

SECTION FOUR REVIEW

1. Which type of immune cell is responsible for direct antigen attack and destruction?
   A. helper T cell
   B. killer T cell
   C. suppressor B cell
   D. memory B cell
2. A major responsibility of the B lymphocytes is
   A. phagocytosis
   B. direct attack on antigens

   C. helper T cell function
   D. antibody production
3. Macrophages are primarily responsible for
   A. interfering with the immune response
   B. protecting against local mucosal invasion of bacteria
   C. triggering the complement system
   D. carrying the antigen to B cells and T cells

Answers: 1. B, 2. D, 3. D

SECTION FIVE: Mechanisms of Immunity

At the completion of this section, the learner will be able to describe mechanisms of specific immunity (humoral and cell mediated) and mechanisms of nonspecific immunity.

The immune system can be described as providing two types of specific immunity. Humoral immunity is based on the activity and characteristics of the B lymphocyte. Cell-mediated immunity is based on the role of the T lymphocyte. In contrast, the nonspecific immune response is initiated solely on the recognition of foreign material being nonself antigens and not on their particular identity.

Specific Immunity

Humoral Immunity

Humoral immunity consists of the activity of the B lymphocytes. These lymphocytes mature with exposure to an antigen, develop into **plasma cells,** and produce specific antibodies, or immunoglobulins. Each plasma cell is capable of producing only one type of antibody and thus becomes committed to producing antibodies only to a specific antigen. Each plasma cell then produces identical cells capable of continuing production of antibodies in response to a particular antigen. Some of the offspring of a particular plasma cell continue to produce

TABLE 25–2   Immunoglobulins in Adults

IMMUNOGLOBULIN (PERCENTAGE OF TOTAL IG)	TOTALS (MG/DL EXCEPT IGE)	DESCRIPTION
Total Ig	900–2,200	
IgG (80 percent)	650–1,700	Function: Antibacterial and antiviral activities
		Produced on secondary exposure to an antigen
IgA (15 percent)	70–100	Function: Protection of mucous membrane from invading pathogens
		Location: Secretions (respiratory, gastrointestinal, genitourinary tracts, saliva and tears)
IgM (4 percent)	40–350	Function: Primary immunity
		Produced within 48 to 72 hours following presentation of antigen
IgD (0.2 percent)	0–8	Function: Unknown
IgE (0.0002 percent U/mL)	Less than 40 U/mL	Levels elevate during hypersensitivity reactions

Data from Kee, J. L. (2002). Laboratory and diagnostic tests with nursing implications, 6th ed. Upper Saddle River, NJ: Prentice Hall. Adapted with permission.

antibodies, whereas other cells of that set become memory cells for the particular antigen.

The immunoglobulins are in the globulin fraction of the plasma protein. Each has a distinct amino acid chain that creates its specificity to react with a particular antigen. Because of this basic protein matrix of antibodies, the nutritional status of the individual in general and the protein status in particular are critical to an actively functioning immune system. Five classes of immunoglobulins have been identified (Table 25–2). The plasma cell becomes the producer of immunoglobulin. Each of the five types plays a particular role in the immune response.

The most common immunoglobulin is IgG. It comprises approximately 80 percent of the immunoglobulins and is found circulating in body fluids. It is the only immunoglobulin that is known to cross the placental barrier and is responsible for protecting the newborn during the first few months of life. IgG contains several types of antibodies, including antiviral, antibacterial, and antitoxin. It also activates the complement system. IgG can be administered as passive immunity via inoculation.

IgA comprises approximately 15 percent of the total immunoglobulins. It is found in large quantities in secretory body fluids, such as tears; saliva; breast milk; and vaginal, bronchial, and intestinal secretions. IgA is produced by B cells in Peyer's patches, tonsils, and other lymph tissue. IgA affords the body a more local protection against invading organisms. The foreign material might well encounter the IgA antibody long before it encounters the IgG antibody. IgA provides protection at the mucosal level of invasion, whereas IgG provides protection more systemically from the position of circulating body fluids.

Smaller amounts of other immunoglobulins play roles in the immunity processes. IgM is instrumental in forming natural antibodies (e.g., for ABO blood antigens). It occurs early in the immune response to most antigens and is also important in activating the complement system. Comprising only 0.0002 percent of the total immunoglobulins, the function of IgE seems to be most prevalent in allergic and hypersensitivity reactions involving the mast cells. The function of IgD is uncertain at the present time, although it may be involved in B cell maturation.

Humoral Response Patterns. Humoral immunity—the recognition of antigens and the production of specific antibodies—occurs with a primary and secondary response pattern (Fig. 25–4). During the **primary response,** there is a latency period before the antibody can be detected in the serum. This delay may be 48 to 72 hours after exposure. It represents the time needed for the antigen to be recognized as nonself and specifically identified, and following which antibodies are formed in response to the antigen's particular molecular makeup. After this latency period, a blood/serum test should reflect the level of antibody to a particular antigen and the degree of immune response. This level of antibody is called the *antibody titer.* The antibody titer normally continues to rise for about 10 days to 2 weeks. The peak of the titer generally occurs during recovery from most infectious diseases.

The **secondary response** occurs with subsequent exposures to the same antigen. It is during this time that the memory cells of the plasma cell clones recognize the antigen almost immediately and initiate the immune response with heightened antibody formation. If a titer were to be drawn at this exposure, the antibody titer would be higher than that of the primary exposure. The follow-up booster regimen of many vaccines, such as tetanus, takes advantage of this secondary response and boosts the titer of specific antibodies to a level that will prevent the disease from occurring. This is the rationale for administering a tetanus booster within 24 hours of a new puncture wound.

Cell-Mediated Immunity

Cell-mediated immunity is based on the activity and characteristics of the T cell. During this portion of the immune response,

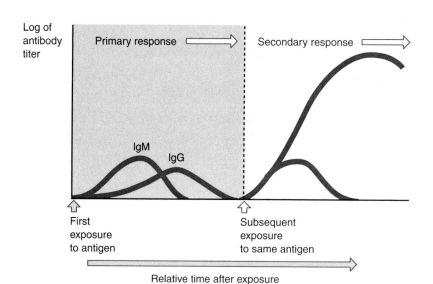

Figure 25–4 ■ Primary and secondary responses of humoral immunity to the same antigen. The introduction of an antigen induces a response dominated by two classes of immunoglobulins: IgM and IgG. IgM predominates in the primary response, with some IgG appearing later. After the host's immune system is primed, another challenge with the same antigen induces the secondary response, in which some IgM and large amounts of IgG are produced. *(Reprinted from McCance, K., & Huether, S. (1998). Pathophysiology: The biologic basis for disease in adults and children (3rd ed., p. 177). Copyright 1998 with permission from Elsevier.)*

the T cell and macrophage predominate, creating a direct attack on invading antigens. T cell immunity provides protection from intracellular organisms (such as viruses, fungi, and parasites), cancer cells, and foreign tissue. It is the T cell that is also responsible for much of the **rejection phenomenon** of transplanted organs and grafts. It is, however, one of the body's primary surveillance and attack mechanisms for protection from growth of malignant cells.

Unfortunately, T cell protection is not readily transferred from one individual to another, as humoral protection is. Cell-mediated immunity depends heavily on thymus and lymph node integrity as well as a nutritionally healthy body.

Complement System

The **complement system** is an immune mechanism that resembles the blood coagulation cascade in that, once initiated, it progresses through several sequential stages, each contributing to the immune response and resulting in cellular destruction or cytolysis. The precursors to the complement pathways are normally circulating in the bloodstream. They are activated only by specific agents, such as IgG and IgM. The complement system is instrumental in facilitating phagocytosis by making antigens more susceptible to digestion, lysis of antigen cell membranes, and attraction of phagocytes to the invading antigen.

Nonspecific Immunity

Phagocytosis

Phagocytosis is a nonspecific immune response whereby invading foreign materials or injured cells are ingested and destroyed by phagocytic cells. Both neutrophils and macrophages are instrumental cellular components to this immune mechanism.

Phagocytosis involves **chemotaxis,** the chemical attraction of phagocytic cells to antigens, as well as the engulfing of antigens for purposes of destruction or neutralization. A process known as opsonization modifies the antigen, making it more susceptible to phagocytosis. Two circulating factors enhance the opsonization process. The IgG immunoglobulin and C3b, a fragment of the complement system, are called **opsonins** and provide binding sites for attachment of macrophages or neutrophils to the antigen.

Interferons

The **interferons** also play an important but nonspecific role in the immune response. Interferons serve as the first-line defense in the protection of the body against viruses and other intracellular pathogens. Antiviral interferons inhibit the synthesis of viral protein in their reproduction without inhibiting the host's protein synthesis in normal cell reproduction. Immune interferons are known to be one of the strongest activators of macrophage activity. Interferons are lymphokines originating from CD8 and some CD4 T cells and NK cells. Although they are pathogen nonspecific, they are species specific; thus, animal interferons offer little, if any, protection for human beings as vaccines. There is growing interest in the possible role of interferons as cell growth regulators in the study of malignant tumor control.

In summary, to maintain a total surveillance function, the immune system must be diverse enough to provide protection from foreign agents with a variety of immune mechanisms. Specific immune response mechanisms include humoral immunity with the formation of antibodies (immunoglobulins) and cell-mediated immunity with its direct-attacking T cells. Nonspecific protection is provided with phagocytes and interferons, which recognize nonself as being foreign but do not specifically program themselves for each individual antigen.

SECTION SIX: Pathogenesis of Hypersensitivity and Autoimmunity

At the completion of this section, the learner will be able to explain the theoretical concepts of the occurrence of types I, II, III, and IV immunoglobulin hypersensitivity and autoimmune disorders.

Although several types of hypersensitivity reactions are recognized as immune responses, only those particularly associated with the acutely ill adult are discussed here. Some immune responses can cause an excessive or inappropriate reaction referred to as **hypersensitivity** (Platts-Mills, 2001). Historically, hypersensitivity disorders have been described as immediate or delayed reactions based on time from exposure to symptom appearance. Since 1962, hypersensitivity disorders have been commonly described as types I, II, III, and IV (Fig. 25–5). Of these four recognized categories, types I, II, and III involve humoral immunity and specific immunoglobulins. Type IV, however, is a cell-mediated response. Many hypersensitivity responses manifest themselves with mild to moderately distressful symptoms, such as watery eyes, sneezing, and nasal congestion. Strong hypersensitivity responses, however, are capable of triggering a severe response, for example, anaphylactic shock response, severe transfusion reaction, or allergic asthma response.

Immunoglobulin Hypersensitivity

Type I Response

The type I hypersensitivity response is often called the **allergic response** and involves an interaction between IgE and mast

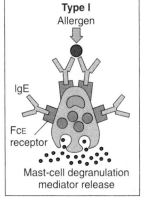
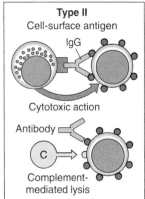
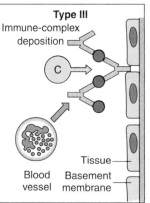
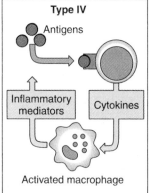

Figure 25–5 ■ Four types of hypersensitivity reaction. *(Reprinted from Roitt, I., Brostoff, J., & Male, D. (2001). Immunology. (6th ed.). Copyright 2001, with permission from Elsevier.)*

cells. **Mast cells** are large granule-containing tissue cells that are located in connective tissue throughout the body. The heaviest concentration of mast cells is in the skin and mucous membranes (e.g., gastrointestinal, genitourinary, and respiratory tracts), which places them in close proximity to where antigens are most likely to appear (Porth, 2002). Mast cells contain potent mediators, such as histamine, heparin, and bradykinin; and chemotactic factors. When stimulated, the mediators and chemotactic factors trigger strong vascular, smooth muscle, hematologic, and other activities. A type I response involves a sensitization (priming) phase and subsequent exposure. When a person initially encounters an allergen–antigen (e.g., pollen), IgE attaches itself to mast cells (e.g., pollen would involve mast cells in the respiratory tract). The person's mast cells are now primed for an allergic response. With repeated exposure to the same allergen–antigen, the allergic response (antigen–IgE–mast cell) interaction is triggered, causing degradation of the mast cells and release of mediators and chemotactic factors—and the person becomes symptomatic.

Allergic asthma and allergic rhinitis (hay fever) are especially noteworthy examples of a type I response. In allergic asthma, the chemical mediators cause smooth muscle constriction in the bronchioles and histamine release results in edema of the bronchial tissues. The combination of bronchiolar constriction and bronchial edema, when severe, may require emergency treatment to prevent death by asphyxiation. Antihistamines may be used to block the effect of histamine release, but corticosteroids often are administered to suppress the entire immune response. A severe type I allergic response can develop rapidly and may prove fatal if not interrupted. There is little if any involvement of T lymphocytes in this process.

Altered Immunocompetence: Anaphylaxis. Although IgE antibodies are primarily responsible for a type I hypersensitivity reaction, causing the atopic disorders of allergic rhinitis, latex allergies, and asthma, they are also responsible for the occurrence of anaphylaxis. Anaphylaxis is a severe type I hypersensitivity response caused by the massive release of chemical mediators and other substances. Systemic anaphylaxis occurs immediately—within minutes—and simultaneously in multiple organs in response to an allergen capable of stimulating the immune system. Most commonly, the causative allergens are food, drugs, or insect venom. Of significance is that the reaction lacks a genetic predisposition and may be fatal in response to prior sensitization to a minute amount of allergen.

Anaphylaxis typically involves the cardiovascular, respiratory, cutaneous, and gastrointestinal systems. IgE antibodies interact with mast cells triggering the release of histamine, which, because of its potent vasodilator effect, causes widespread edema and vascular congestion. Smooth muscle and vascular beds are affected. Histamine's potent vasodilator effect causes increased capillary permeability and leaking, smooth muscle contraction, and bronchial constriction. Complement is also a causative factor and further stimulates histamine release as well as a widespread inflammatory response. *Anaphylactic shock* is the extreme result of this histamine-related generalized vasodilation and increased vascular permeability causing rapid loss of plasma into interstitial spaces. This shift of fluid causes hypovolemic shock with profound hypotension, decreased cardiac output, myocardial ischemia, and widespread organ death. Figure 25–6 illustrates the effects of anaphylaxis. Anaphylactic shock is presented in more detail in Module 15, "Shock States."

Urticaria or hives are the result of histamine release from the IgE–mast cell interaction in which receptors in cutaneous blood vessels cause the characteristic redness and swelling. Urticaria alone is not life threatening but heralds the presence of an anaphylactic response. Assessment should include examining the patient for the potential risk of upper airway edema with asphyxiation and the risk of irreversible shock. Gastrointestinal involvement is related to smooth muscle contraction and edema of the mucosa resulting in cramplike pain, nausea, and diarrhea. Similar responses can occur within the uterus, causing cramplike pelvic pain and a risk of spontaneous abortion.

Treatment must be instituted immediately and includes epinephrine (intravenous, intramuscular, or subcutaneous depending on the intensity). Laryngeal edema may require tracheostomy when edema precludes endotracheal airway placement. Oxygen and injectable antihistamines should be administered. The patient should be kept warm if shock is suspected. Glucocorticoids may be used for severe or prolonged reactions because they reduce the immune response and stabilize the vascular system. Other symptoms, such as gastrointestinal cramping and urticaria, respond well to antihistamines. After the patient has fully recovered, diagnostic skin testing may be ordered to identify the offending allergen.

Type II Response

A type II hypersensitivity response is referred to as a cytotoxic reaction. The immunoglobulins IgM and IgG react directly with cell surface antigens, activating the complement system, and producing direct injury to the cell surface. Cellular membranes are disrupted, and target cells such as erythrocytes (red blood cells [RBCs]), thrombocytes (platelets), and leukocytes (white blood cells [WBCs]), are destroyed. Transfusion reactions are one example of this type of hypersensitivity. Other examples include Rh incompatibility in the neonate, drug reaction induced hemolytic anemia, and hyperthyroidism caused by Graves' disease.

Altered Immunocompetence: Transfusion Reaction. The type II hypersensitivity response can be characterized by describing a transfusion reaction, which is a type of hemolytic reaction. Preexisting antibodies in the recipient's serum typically target and attach to the erythrocytes (RBC) of the transfusing donor blood. As the immune system is activated, macrophages destroy the donor RBCs, which allows hemoglobin to escape into the circulation. The released hemoglobin flows through the circulation and is filtered through the glomeruli of the kidneys. This event creates a high risk of oliguria and renal shutdown because obstruction by

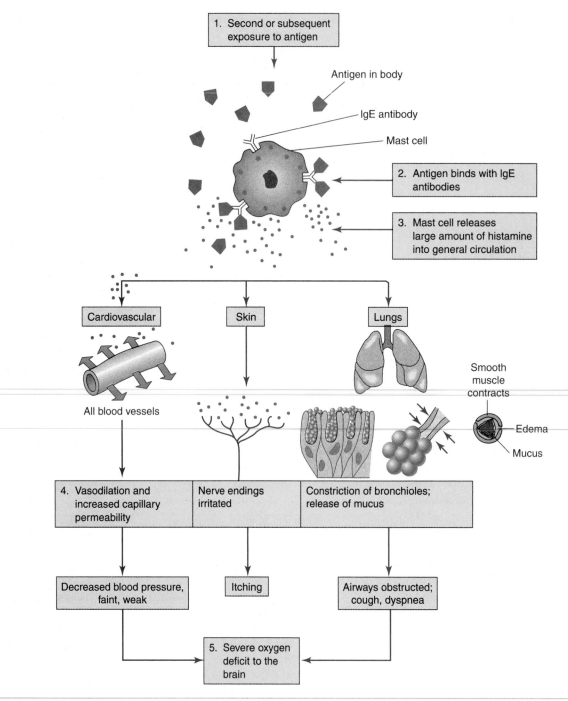

Figure 25–6 ■ The effects of anaphylaxis *(Reprinted from Gould, B.E. (2002).* Pathophysiology for the health professions *(2nd ed., page 46). Copyright 2002, with permission from Elsevier.)*

hemoglobin fragments reduces renal tubular blood flow. Symptoms of a hemolytic transfusion reaction are caused by ABO surface antigen incompatibility and are likely to occur in the first 2 to 5 minutes of the transfusion. Evidence of the reaction includes the sensation of heat and redness at the infusion site, nausea, headache, back pain, chills, fever, and a sense of chest heaviness with difficulty breathing. Tachycardia, hypotension, and death can follow if the transfusion is not interrupted and treatment begun to reestablish cardiovascular stability.

Type III Response

The type III reaction is an example of an immune complex reaction involving antigen–antibody complexes with IgG and IgM. Type III reactions are characterized by deposits of antigen–antibody complexes in the epithelial lining of blood vessels, the kidneys, joints, skin, and other organs, rather than direct cell surface damage as in type II reactions. An acute inflammatory reaction begins as the complement system is initiated by the immune complex, and vessels become occluded with edema, hemorrhage, clotting, and accumulation of neutrophils, causing localized tissue necrosis. Type III reactions may be associated with infections, such as hepatitis B and bacterial endocarditis, malignancies, drug therapy, and autoimmune disease.

Altered Immunocompetence: Vasculitis and Organ Damage. One example of the type III reaction is the **Arthus vasculitis reaction.** Although it may be considered transient and treatable in some body systems, in the case of a graft tissue rejection, the graft may become necrotic from the vasculitis and fail to recover. The Arthus reaction also may occur in other parts of the body unrelated to graft rejection, such as the alveoli, gastrointestinal tract, and skin, from fungal antigens, gluten intolerance, and drug therapy. Type III responses are also responsible for lung, joint, and skin damage in autoimmune disorders, such as systemic lupus erythematosus (SLE) and kidney damage in glomerulonephritis.

Type IV Response

Cell-mediated type IV hypersensitivity is a delayed response involving primarily the T lymphocytes, with no antibody activity. Tissue destruction is its hallmark, most notably through direct cellular destruction by T cell toxins, lysosomal enzymes, or phagocytosis following activation by the release of cytokines and lymphokines.

Altered Immunocompetence: Graft and Organ Transplant Rejection. Local reaction to a type IV response can also be demonstrated in the induration of a positive tuberculin test or contact dermatitis, such as poison ivy, and perhaps latex allergies. Clinical examples include graft or organ transplant rejection in which the HLA antigen is the principal target (graft-versus-host and host-versus-graft diseases). Immunosuppressive drugs, such as azathioprine (Imuran) and cyclosporin (Sandimmune), are given to delay or lessen this acute rejection phenomenon. (Refer to Module 26, "Organ Transplantation," for a more in-depth discussion of transplant complications.)

Autoimmune Disorders

For reasons yet unknown, the immune system occasionally begins to recognize self as foreign. With the usual physiologic actions, the immune system can set out to destroy self. Just as it cannot distinguish beneficial foreign material from destructive foreign material in the transplant phenomenon, the system recognizes self as foreign and initiates a destructive response in autoimmune diseases. **Autoimmunity** is intolerance to one's own body tissue that can involve abnormal activity of B cells, T cells, or the complement system. Characteristic of most autoimmune disorders is B cell hyperactivity. Viruses can contribute to autoimmunity by causing proliferation or destruction of lymphocytes. Many diseases are now attributed to such an autoimmune response, and many others are suspected. Table 25–3 provides a list of common autoimmune diseases. Immunodeficiency or immunosuppression may be a therapeutic goal in treating autoimmune disorders. Immune-mediated tissue damage may be suppressed through drug-induced, radiation-induced, or surgically induced immunodeficiency.

In summary, hypersensitivity is an exaggerated or inappropriate immune response to an antigen that results in harm to the body. The allergic response is one type of hypersensitivity reaction and commonly involves an antigen from the environment otherwise considered to be nonpathogenic and not intrinsically harmful to most persons. This section described the four types of hypersensitivity responses, type I, II, III, and IV, and gave examples of each. Finally, the concept of autoimmunity was briefly addressed, in which the immune system becomes self-destructive. To date, no mechanism is known to prevent the abnormal responses of autoimmunity.

TABLE 25–3   Common Autoimmune Diseases

Respiratory	**Neuromuscular**
Goodpasture's disease	Multiple sclerosis
Gastrointestinal	Cardiomyopathy
Ulcerative colitis	Myasthenia gravis
Crohn's disease	Rheumatic fever
Pernicious anemia	**Connective tissue**
Endocrine	Systemic lupus erythematosus
Graves' disease (hyperthyroidism)	Scleroderma (progressive
Type 1 diabetes mellitus	systemic sclerosis)
Addison's disease	Rheumatoid arthritis
Partial pituitary deficiency	Ankylosing spondylitis
Renal	**Hematologic**
Immune-complex glomerulonephritis	Autoimmune hemolytic anemia
	Autoimmune thrombocytopenic purpura

SECTION SIX REVIEW

1. The results of a true type I hypersensitivity response are the result of
   A. a histamine precursor causing anaphylaxis
   B. antigen–IgE–mast cell interaction
   C. antigen–antibody complexes deposited in vessel walls
   D. massive numbers of destroyed red blood cells

2. Type III hypersensitivity reactions are often characterized by
   A. specific target cells
   B. widespread multiorgan involvement
   C. rapidly progressing symptoms
   D. relatively low-risk patterns
3. Which statement is correct regarding type IV cell-mediated hypersensitivity responses?
   A. it involves primarily antibody activity
   B. it does not harm body tissues
   C. T cell activity is responsible
   D. it directly interacts with cell surface antigens

4. Disorders thought to be autoimmune in etiology include (choose all that apply)
   1. chronic bronchitis
   2. ulcerative colitis
   3. pernicious anemia
   4. diabetes mellitus (type 1)
   A. 2, 3, and 4
   B. 1, 3, and 4
   C. 1, 2, and 3
   D. 2 and 4

Answers: 1. B, 2. B, 3. C, 4. A

SECTION SEVEN: Aging, Malnutrition, Stress, Trauma, and the Immune System

At the completion of this section, the learner will be able to describe the effects of aging, malnutrition, stress, and trauma related to the function of the adult immune system.

Aging

The functionality of the immune system declines with age. The thymus gland, where T lymphocytes mature and differentiate, begins to atrophy early in life and continues to shrink until a person reaches middle age. Although T lymphocytes continue to be produced, their maturation and differentiation into the various functional T cells (e.g., T helper cells) decreases. This places the older patient at higher risk for increased frequency and severity of infections accompanied by a decreased ability to resolve the infection. Macrophages continue to function throughout life; however, the length of time it takes them to clear the pathogens significantly increases with age. The ability of the immune system to discriminate between antigens that are "self" from those that are "nonself" declines with aging, which increases the incidence of autoimmune diseases by middle age and older. In addition, the immune system also becomes significantly less efficient at recognizing and destroying mutated (tumor) cells, which at least partially accounts for the increased incidence of cancer in the older adult. B lymphocyte response to antigens declines in cell numbers and efficacy with aging. Production of the immunoglobulin IgM decreases; however, production of IgA and IgG increases, possibly related to autoantibody responses to self-antigens.

Malnutrition

Although nutritional deficiencies can occur at any age, the older adult, particularly the frail elderly, are at particular risk.

Many factors can contribute to the development of malnutrition in this patient population, including decreased appetite, loss of social supports, decreased accessibility to grocery stores, impaired functional status, and others. The possibility of malnutrition should be considered by the nurse whenever an acutely ill older adult is admitted because it can have a profound impact on the immune system, thus, on the patient's prognosis. Basic components of calorie and protein intake play key roles in the formation and integrity of T cells and immunoglobulins (antibodies). Malnutrition contributes to immunocompromise by causing impaired response of lymphocytes to pathogens, to vaccines, and to components of defense, such as the complement and macrophage functions (Gould, 2002). Zinc plays a major role in the structure and function of both B cells and T cells and in collagen synthesis for wound healing. As a cofactor, zinc is required for the normal function of lymphocytes in their production of enzymes. Although zinc deficiencies do not normally occur with regular eating habits, there can be significant loss through the gastrointestinal tract with malabsorption syndrome or inflammatory bowel disease. It also can be lost through the skin in burn victims. Several vitamins serve as cofactors in enzyme production and, in malnutrition states, affect the function of both T cells and B cells. These vitamins include A, E, pyridoxine, folic acid, and pantothenic acid.

Malnutrition is also believed to contribute to sepsis as the malnourished gut becomes atrophied and more permeable to bacteria following trauma. When bacteria seep out of the gut, immune system mediators are released and trigger systemic lymphocyte activity. TNF, a major immune mediator, is primarily responsible for precipitating multiple organ dysfunction syndrome. Early enteral feedings, which prevent gut atrophy in the acutely ill patient, are also instrumental in preventing sepsis, excess circulating immune mediators, and subsequent multiple organ dysfunction in the critically ill patient (Gould, 2002). Multiple organ dysfunction syndrome is presented in more depth in Module 16, "Multiple Organ Dysfunction Syndrome."

Stress

Stress affects the immune system primarily through the effects of cortisol. During periods of stress, either physical or psychological, the adrenal glands produce more cortisol in response to needs based on increased metabolism, but cortisol has a direct suppressing effect on the immune system. Normally, when an antigen enters the body, a series of reactions takes place. The antigen is recognized as nonself, and it is presented to T cells by macrophages. The macrophages secrete interleukin-1 (IL-1), which activates helper T cells, and these helper T cells produce interleukin-2 (IL-2), which stimulates more T cell production. Finally, B cells may be stimulated to program antibodies to the antigen. Cortisol inhibits the production of IL-1 and IL-2, thus decreasing the T cell response and the subsequent B cell response.

Trauma

Trauma, both intentional (such as surgery) and unintentional (such as burns, motor vehicle crashes, and falls) suppresses T cell and B cell function. Trauma can cause cellular dysfunction, characterized by decreased chemotactic and phagocytic activities and decreased antibody and lymphocyte levels (Gould, 2002). Impaired T cell activity and depressed lymphokines have been linked to multiple organ dysfunction and poor clinical outcomes in the trauma patient (Gould, 2002; Puyana et al., 1998). Although the degree of immunosuppression directly correlates with the severity of the injury, the cause for such changes is not fully understood. Additionally, medications can suppress the immune response. Among these are glucocorticoids, general anesthetic agents, and cytoxic drugs.

The immune system is complex and is highly sensitive to changes in the body. Trauma, burns, hemorrhage, blood transfusions, and surgery/anesthesia all contribute to immunosuppression (Gould, 2002). Immune consequences of trauma most likely are related to neurohormonal stress responses and altered cytokine/immune mediator activity. Hypovolemic shock has been found to decrease antigen-specific antibody production, cellular immunity, and macrophage function for approximately 2 weeks following hemorrhage (Gould, 2002). The critically ill trauma patient enters the intensive care unit immunosuppressed from the outset because of a stress response to the injury, hemorrhage, and shock. Subsequent malnutrition, organ dysfunction, hypoxia, and multiple invasive procedures all create a potential scenario of vulnerability to virulent nosocomial pathogens.

In summary, aging, malnutrition, stress, and trauma play a significant role in immunosuppression, seemingly just when the body is in acute need of protection against invading pathogens. The aging patient is more susceptible to infection because of age-related decline in immune function. Malnutrition is a relatively common problem in the high acuity patient population, and its presence significantly impairs the immune system, which is largely protein based. Stress alters immune system function primarily through the effects of cortisol, an adrenocortical hormone that is secreted in greater amounts during periods of stress. Cortisol inhibits the production of IL-1 and IL-2, which ultimately reduces T cell and B cell responses. Finally, severe trauma is known to suppress both T cell and B cell function. The combined influences of aging, malnutrition, stress, and trauma are potentially devastating to the body's immune system, which can cause potentially life-threatening complications such as severe infection, inability to heal, and multiple organ dysfunction syndrome (MODS).

SECTION SEVEN REVIEW

1. What is the function of zinc in the competent immune system?
   A. it is required for normal lymphocyte function
   B. it protects B cells from being destroyed by macrophages
   C. T cells require zinc for production of gamma globulin
   D. macrophages are composed primarily of zinc
2. What effect does the normal aging process have on the immune system?
   A. B cell function in general is particularly depressed
   B. T cells begin to deteriorate in functioning
   C. autoantibodies begin to diminish with increasing age
   D. the immune system becomes hypervigilant to invading organisms

3. In the acutely ill adult, which of the following nutritional losses is a critical factor in immune system integrity?
   A. iron
   B. vitamin C
   C. complex carbohydrate chains
   D. protein
4. Stress primarily affects the immune system through the effects of
   A. lymphokines
   B. interleukin
   C. cortisol
   D. epinephrine

Answers: 1. A, 2. B, 3. D, 4. C

HIV Disease: A Manifestation of Immunodeficiency

At the completion of this section, the learner will be able to characterize immunodeficiency and describe the human immunodeficiency virus (HIV) and acquired immune deficiency syndrome (AIDS) and treatment.

Assuming that the immune system and its component parts are intact and functioning normally, one might expect reasonable protection against invading microorganisms, pathogens, and foreign material. Even in such a case, the body often cannot overcome a pathogenic process. The immune system can be subject to inadequate development, disease, and injury from illness or treatments that can result in deficient immune activity. Such a situation is called an **immunodeficiency state.**

Primary Immunodeficiency

Characteristics of **primary immunodeficiency** may vary widely depending on the basic etiology. Immunodeficiency results from a loss of function of one or more components of the immune system. The problem may be acute or chronic. Primary deficiencies involve a failure somewhere in the system (e.g., bone marrow or thymus). Most primary states of immunodeficiency are the result of embryonic anomaly, genetic predisposition, or congenital failure of the system to develop, thus occurring almost exclusively in infants and toddlers. For example, T cells may fail to develop because of some embryonic anomaly or genetic code. DiGeorge syndrome is an example of a congenital thymic aplasia or hypoplasia in which there are greatly decreased levels of T cells because of partial lack of a thymus. B cell deficiency also may develop from embryonic dysfunction or developmental delay of an infant's immune system, which results in lowered levels of immunoglobulins. A condition in which immunoglobulins are almost totally absent from the circulation is known as agammaglobulinemia.

In some instances, both B cells and T cells are affected, as in severe combined immune deficiencies (SCID). In SCID, the bone marrow stem cells for lymphocyte development may be absent. Affected children spend a good portion of their short lives in an environment of total protection from any antigen.

Secondary Immunodeficiency

Secondary (acquired) immunodeficiency refers to loss of the immune response and may occur at any age. The causes include infection, splenectomy, malnutrition, liver disease, use of immunosuppressive drugs in patients with organ transplants, and chemotherapy and radiation for cancer treatment. For example, the patient with Hodgkin's disease, a malignancy of the lymphatic tissue, might well suffer from subsequent immun-

odeficiency following malignant invasion of lymph tissue. Prolonged corticosteroid (acquired) therapy suppresses the adrenal glands through the negative feedback loop (immunosuppression). Eventually, suppression of the immune system creates a state of immunodeficiency caused by atrophy of lymphoid tissue, decreased antibody formation, decreased development of cell-mediated immunity, and impaired phagocytosis. Finally, immunosuppressive drugs, such as azathioprine (Imuran) and cyclosporine, are administered for the purpose of suppressing the immune response to transplanted organs and grafts.

Human beings can become immune deficient from a direct attack on the immune system by pathogens. When such a situation exists, it is known as acquired immunodeficiency. Acquired immunodeficiency is not primary in that it is not genetically transmitted, nor is it embryonic in the sense of lymphoid tissue failing to develop adequately. It is a secondary form of immunodeficiency because it was caused by another disease or therapy.

Human Immunodeficiency Virus (HIV) and Acquired Immunodeficiency Disease Syndrome (AIDS)

Human immunodeficiency virus (HIV)/Acquired Immunodeficiency Disease Syndrome (AIDS) is the most common disease associated with secondary (acquired) immunodeficiency. The remainder of this section provides a broad overview of HIV/AIDS including cellular manifestations characterizing HIV disease, epidemiology and transmission, viral invasion, phases of infection, screening, clinical manifestations, AIDS in special populations, and treatment approaches.

Cellular Manifestations Characterizing HIV Disease

The immune deficiency characterizing HIV disease is manifested by markedly depressed T lymphocyte functioning, with a reduction of helper T4 cells (CD4), impaired killer T cell activity, and increased suppressor T cells (T8). By selectively invading and infecting T cells, the virus damages the very cell whose function it is to orchestrate the identification and destruction of the virus as antigen. Other cells with the same molecular makeup and surface markers might also become infected. Eventually, the individual's supply of functional T cells becomes depleted. In a person with a competent immune system, the number of T4 lymphocytes ranges from 600 to 1,200 cells/mcL, whereas the patient with HIV might have zero to 500 cells/mcL T4 cells. The humoral response in producing antibodies is less directly affected by the HIV virus. B cell production does not seem to be decreased, but the induction and regulation of the humoral response may be affected by the lack of T cell regulators (e.g., T4 cell helpers and T8 cell suppressors).

Epidemiology and Transmission of the HIV Virus

The first populations generally thought to be the major contributors to the current HIV epidemic in the United States were homosexuals and persons using intravenous (IV) drugs while sharing used needles. Studies now show that the disease has become widely disseminated to include heterosexual groups and all races and ethnic groups represented in the United States. The greatest increase of HIV infection is occurring in women, with heterosexual men and women contracting the disease at about equal rates. The mode of transmission is predominantly by infected blood and body secretions, generally excluding saliva and tears. The most common modes of transmission are sexual contact, administration of contaminated blood and blood products, contaminated needles, and mother to fetus, although blood transfusions of whole blood, packed cells, and fresh frozen plasma are most unlikely to be the cause of transmission with the sophisticated crossmatching and antibody screening measures in use today. Individuals needing specific blood components (such as factor VIII and frequent plasma replacement) may be at more risk because of the large numbers of donors needed to produce adequate quantities of these components. The risk of acquiring the virus increases with the number of potential carriers involved, just as multiple sexual contacts create higher risk. The HIV virus is fragile, is easily destroyed by chemical disinfectants, and cannot survive outside the body.

Viral Invasion

HIV, formerly known as the human T cell lymphotropic virus (HTLV-III), is a lentivirus of the retrovirus family, carrying genetic information in ribonucleic acid (RNA) rather than in deoxyribonucleic acid (DNA). The virus infects the T lymphocyte by binding to it at the CD4$^+$ T cell receptor site and penetrating the T cell membrane. Through an enzyme called reverse transcriptase, the HIV RNA is copied as a double-stranded DNA and inserted into the host cell chromosome where noninfectious, immature viral proteins are formed. When the T cell is activated to reproduce, such as with other viral infections or stresses, its genetic information is programmed to produce more of the infectious HIV virus, and the number of functional T cells diminishes rapidly. Viral load and CD4$^+$ T cell counts are reflective of viral activity and disease progression. Unfortunately, reverse transcriptase is highly error-prone and may produce multiple mutations during each replication of the HIV virus. The AIDS patient could have hundreds of viral mutations to transmit. Most antiviral drugs currently being tested or used in treatment regimens work by inhibiting the action of reverse transcriptase or by inhibiting an enzyme (protease) needed at a later stage of the HIV's course when maturation of new infectious viruses takes place (Volberding et al., 2003). To date, there are two forms of HIV: HIV-1 and HIV-2. HIV-1 is the major cause of AIDS in America and Europe. HIV-2, found primarily in Central Africa, has also been found to cause AIDS but seems

less virulent, less transmissible, and creates lower proportions of infected cells (Gould, 2002). The course of HIV/AIDS is illustrated in Figure 25–7.

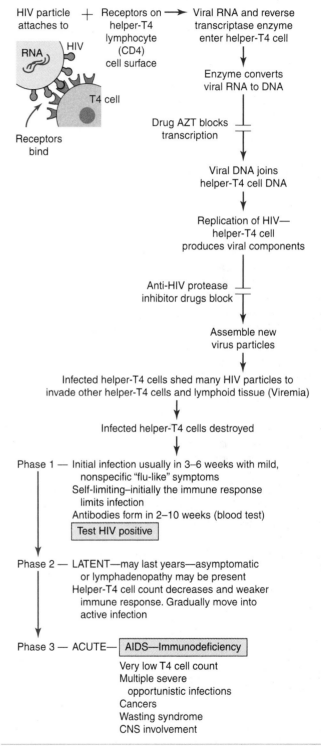

Figure 25–7 ■ HIV–AIDS (*Reprinted from Gould, B.E. (2002). Pathophysiology for the health professions (2nd ed., p. 54). Copyright 2002, with permission from Elsevier.*)

Phases of HIV Infection

The phases of HIV disease in adults are usually based either on the grouping of disease manifestations or on CD4$^+$ T cell levels, both of which reflect disease progression. Table 25–4 provides a summary of the phases of HIV infection, including primary infection, chronic asymptomatic (latency), symptomatic HIV infection, and overt AIDS.

TABLE 25–4   Phases of HIV/AIDS

PHASE	DESCRIPTION
Primary infection	Onset: 2 to 4 weeks following exposure
	Duration: Up to 2 weeks following onset of symptoms
	Clinical manifestations: Flu- or mononucleosis-like symptoms (e.g., sore throat, fever, myalgias, malaise, gastrointestinal problems, headache)
	Viral activities: Rapid HIV replication causing high viral load; within about 2 weeks, immune system musters attack and serum viral load is reduced dramatically
Chronic asymptomatic (latency)	Duration: Mean of 10 years
	Clinical manifestations: May be asymptomatic; lymphadenopathy may be evident
	Viral activities: HIV replication is occurring but is isolated in lymph nodes with very little in circulating blood; person is infectious
Symptomatic HIV infection	Onset: When clinical manifestations appear
	Duration: Until clinically meets criteria for AIDS
	Clinical manifestations: Vary, may include lymphadenopathy, mouth lesions, anemia or thrombocytopenia, neurological symptoms; no AIDS-defining illness present
	Viral activities: CD4$^+$ T cell levels are greater than 200 but less than normal; slow decline in CD4$^+$ T cell counts accompanied by increasing HIV viral load as immune defense against HIV deteriorates
Overt AIDS	Onset: When person clinically meets criteria for AIDS
	• CD4$^+$ T cell count less than 200 cells/mL **OR**
	• Presence of at least one "AIDS-defining" illness
	(most common in United States: PCP, candidiasis, CMV, and MAC^a)
	Clinical Manifestations: Wasting syndrome, dementia, malignancies, & other opportunistic infections/conditions
	Duration: Until death, usually within 2 to 3 years (without anti-viral drug therapy)
	Viral Activities: Continued drop in CD4$^+$ T cell levels and increasing HIV viral load

^{a}PCP: *Pneumocystis carinii* pneumonia; CMV: Cytomegalovirus; MAC: *Mycobacterium avium-intracellulare* complex
Data partially taken from Sweeney, K. A., & Llamoso, C. (2002). Acquired immunodeficiency syndrome. In C. M. Porth, Pathophysiology: Concepts of altered states (6th ed., pp. 379–395). Philadelphia: Lippincott Williams & Wilkins.

HIV Screening

The antibody to HIV has been identified and can be used for screening purposes. However, the latency period for HIV is longer than with many other infectious organisms. Latency period refers to the time the body takes to recognize nonself and program antibodies to the virus. The point at which serum antibodies are present in the blood is called *seroconversion*. Seroconversion usually occurs within 3 months of exposure but may not occur for up to 6 months (Sweeney & Llamoso, 2002). The prolonged latency period effectively reduces the accuracy and immediacy of host identification. One of the theories concerning this prolonged latency period is that HIV invades T cells and, in effect, sequesters itself from view of the body's surveillance system, meanwhile multiplying anomalous T cells that are ineffective for purposes of immunity. Another theory is that HIV mutates rapidly and B cells may not recognize variations effectively to produce antibodies efficiently.

Screening for the antibody is helpful to the extent that individuals can be identified who have been exposed to HIV; however, not all of these individuals actually carry the virus, nor will all of them show signs of illness. Several types of human–HIV relationships are possible.

- **Exposure.** An individual may be exposed to the virus but neither carry it nor contract the disease.
- **Carrier.** The individual may carry the virus with the capability of infecting others but without accompanying signs and symptoms.
- **Terminal disease.** The individual may be infectious, symptomatic, and terminal. It is only after signs of opportunistic infections begin to develop that an individual is actually determined to have the disease.

Laboratory testing to diagnose HIV infection relies predominantly on the presence of the antibody to p24, a major protein found in HIV. The p24 protein is an antigen that is capable of triggering a detectable immune system response to HIV. Antibodies to the p24 antigen can be detected in the blood using several testing methods, such as p24 antigen capture methods or the polymerase chain reaction (PCR); however, both of these tests are prohibitively expensive as primary screening tools for adults. They can, however, be useful in detecting the virus prior to antibody formation, which is called the window period, or in cases in which antibody tests are not conclusive. PCR is generally used only as a first-line diagnostic tool in infants.

The enzyme-linked immunosorbent assay (ELISA) is 95 to 99 percent accurate in identifying the presence of an antibody. A false-positive ELISA result could occur as a result of cross-reactive antibodies to HLA antigens, hepatic disease, gamma globulin injections, and some malignancies. A positive ELISA must be confirmed with another antibody-reliant test known as the Western blot test. Two positive ELISAs and a positive Western blot test confirm the diagnosis of HIV infection. Indeterminate tests are usually repeated at 3- and 6-month intervals. If tests continue to be negative, the result is seronegative; if the tests are questionable at this time, p24 or PCR tests may be conducted. A newer, noninvasive HIV antibody test uses the Western blot but is collected through oral mucosa transudate. This oral test is thought to be as reliable as blood tests using the regular Western blot.

The incubation period for HIV, that is, from infection to clinical symptoms, is estimated to be from 3 months to 10 years. Carriers of the virus who test positive for the antibody can remain as carriers for years with the virus in a dormant state. Although approximately one third of those who now test positive for the disease eventually will begin to show clinical manifestations, some investigators believe that the percentage of those who go on to develop the disease will eventually approach 95 percent. To diagnose AIDS, a clinician needs to know the T helper cell ($CD4^+$) lymphocyte count and if there are AIDS-defining illnesses (e.g., opportunistic infections) present.

Clinical Manifestations

Defining characteristics of AIDS were established in 1981 by the Centers For Disease Control and Prevention (CDC). Based on continued research, the AIDS case definition was revised in 1985, 1989, and 1993 for adolescents and adults, and includes 26 or more associated diseases. The 1993 revision defines AIDS as HIV infection (seropositive) with

- A $CD4^+$ count less than 200 cells/mcL OR
- The presence of at least one of 25 AIDS-defining illnesses (CDC, 1992).

Clinical manifestations of HIV infection generally are related to opportunistic infections preying on an impaired immune system. Common diseases include Kaposi's sarcoma, *P. carinii* pneumonia, tuberculosis, and others. The AIDS patient experiences increasing debilitation, fevers, wasting syndrome, severe fatigue, and pain. Death often results from uncontrollable infection (Gould, 2002). Lymphadenopathy, pharyngitis, rash, pulmonary infiltrates, and neurologic abnormalities, such as dementia, tremors, and encephalitis, contribute to the debilitated state. HIV is usually not susceptible to circulating antibodies because HIV travels from cell to cell rather than through the bloodstream and because it readily mutates. To date, there is no predictable course of curative treatment, and the mortality rate continues to be approximately 95 percent for symptomatic individuals. Two variables that predict outcomes (i.e., time to AIDS or time to death) include viral load and $CD4^+$ count. A viral load of 36,000 copies/mL is associated with a 62 percent risk of progression to clinical AIDS in 5 years and a viral load of 10,000 copies/mL has a risk of 8 percent in 5 years (Liebman et al., 2001).

Women with AIDS

Women infected with HIV may transmit the virus to the fetus; however, administration of azidothymidine (AZT) has decreased the risk of the fetus being infected with HIV during pregnancy. Some infants carry the mother's antibodies for awhile and then convert to test negative for HIV (Gould, 2002). Women with AIDS have a higher incidence of severe vaginal infections, pelvic inflammatory disease, cervical cancer, and opportunistic infections, such as oral candida and herpes infections. The occurrence of Kaposi's sarcoma is much rarer in women than in men with AIDS.

AIDS in Children

Pediatric patients with AIDS differ significantly from adults in several ways, including means of transmission, onset, trajectory, and symptom manifestation. HIV/AIDS is transmitted to infants and preschool children either through infected blood, such as during blood transfusions; through vertical transmission from mother to fetus; through breast-feeding; or, more rarely, through sexual practices such as incest and sexual abuse.

Although infected blood has been responsible for transmission of the HIV virus in many children over the past decade, blood supply screening has significantly reduced this mode of transmission. The more common transmission is now maternal–fetal or vertical transmission. Early estimates of the risk of maternal vertical transmission vary from 25 to 40 percent; the variability of potential risk rests with the infectious state and viral load of the mother. For example, the mother is most likely to transmit the virus when she is newly infected with an initial infection, with a new reinfection, or when she is symptomatic of overt AIDS. It is thought that the virus is more actively reproducing and less constrained by the mother's immune system during these times. In 1994, however, experimental studies of HIV-positive pregnant women revealed that the risk of vertical transmission dropped significantly (to 8 percent) when taking AZT. Infants infected in utero tend to have a more virulent and progressive form of HIV than infants who tested negative at birth but were likely infected during the birth process or from breast-feeding; therefore, antiretroviral therapy is now recommended for seropositive HIV pregnant women (Fowler et al., 2004).

Treatment Approaches

Various approaches to treatment have been theorized and tested. Restoration of immune function has been attempted by bone marrow transplant, transfusions of white blood cells, and interferon treatments. Unfortunately, the newest healthy cells are quickly infected by the virus. The HIV is so variable (much like the variations of flu virus) that a medication formulated against one genetic mutation of the virus may not provide protection against other strains. Pharmacological approaches using combination antiretroviral therapy rather than monotherapy (one drug) and using some of the newer protease inhibitors have been successful in maintaining viral load suppression and in treating AIDS as a long-term chronic disease in adults (Liebman et al., 2001). Antiviral drugs can reduce the viral replication process but cannot kill the virus (Gould, 2002). Antiretroviral combination therapy with reverse transcriptase inhibitors, such as zidovudine (ZBV) and lamivudine (3TC); and protease inhibitors, such as indinavir (Crixivan), has been most successful to date. Such therapy is known as *highly active antiretroviral therapy*. Combinations of three to five drugs in a "cocktail" are used to prolong the asymptomatic or latent phase as well as to reduce the viral load in the overt AIDS phase (Gould, 2002). Antiretroviral therapy for children, however, has differed in that some agree that monotherapy with reverse transcriptase inhibitors is the treatment of choice. Research continues toward the most effective antiretroviral therapy for infants and children.

$CD4^+$ T cell counts are evaluated to determine degree of immune deficiency. Viral load testing reflects viral activity and disease progression. Viral suppression is considered effective when it is less than 400 to 500 copies/mL. Rising viral load indicates disease progression (5,000 to 10,000 copies/mL) as does falling $CD4^+$ levels (less than 500 cells/mcL) (Kee, 2002).

Antiretroviral drug resistance is one of the most difficult challenges in HIV management. Incomplete HIV suppression can result in HIV resistance to treatment; therefore, long-term, uninterrupted antiviral therapy is required for HIV inhibition. Unfortunately, antiretroviral drugs can have significant side effects, which may negatively affect patient compliance. To date there are relatively few effective drugs available; and if drug resistance develops, the patient is at risk for rapid decline (Liebman et al., 2001).

Drug prophylaxis protocols for opportunistic infections of HIV/AIDS have shown promise in delaying or avoiding symptomatic infections. The goal of primary prophylaxis is to avoid or delay the onset of disease symptoms, and secondary prophylaxis seeks to prevent or delay recurrent symptomatic infection. Other treatment approaches are symptomatic, and still others continue to be under experimental investigation. The relatively recent development of highly reactive antiretroviral therapies (HAART) has significantly increased the ability to treat and prevent opportunistic infections in the AIDS patient (CDC, 2002).

The most common infectious manifestation of the immunosuppressed HIV patient is *pneumocystis carinii* pneumonia (PCP) and its recurrence. This disease was one of the first opportunistic infections to be identified as an AIDS-defining illness. Since its prevalence in the AIDS population has been followed, it continues to be the most life-threatening opportunistic infection to both adult and pediatric AIDS patients. Although the PCP organism is not considered particularly pathogenic in the immunocompetent individual, its virulence increases as the T4 cell count falls below 200 cells/mcL in the adult and 1,500 cells/mcL in the child. The infected patient presents with fever, fatigue, and weight loss months before actual respiratory symptoms develop. Coughing, shortness of breath, hypoxemia, and abnormal pulmonary function studies contribute to the clinical picture of progressive illness. Prophylaxis therapy is indicated when the $CD4^+$ cell count falls below 200 to 300 cells/mcL in the adult HIV-1 patient. Typical preventive and treatment therapy for PCP includes trimethoprim-sulfamethoxazole (TMP-SMX, Bactrim, Septra) or an aerosol of pentamidine.

Prevention of other opportunistic infections such as toxoplasmosis, tuberculosis, *Mycobacterium avium* complex (MAC), cytomegalovirus (CMV), and fungi is crucial. High-priority vaccine recommendations include pneumonia and influenza. Other vaccines, such as measles, mumps, and rubella (MMR) and chicken pox (varicella zoster), may be contraindicated because of their imposed risk as live viruses. Immune globulins can be given before or after exposures to measles, chicken pox, or hepatitis A (Liebman et al., 2001). Neupogen, a granulocyte stimulant, may be given to counteract the neutropenia related to antiretroviral therapy or to the HIV itself.

Finally, although relatively few health care professionals are at risk for HIV, treatment approaches for occupational exposure to needle sticks, blood and body fluids, or contaminated instruments have been developed. Postexposure prophylaxis protocols include determining the source and severity of the exposure, determining HIV status of the source, and recommendations for treatment. A basic postexposure prophylactic (PEP) regimen begins within 2 hours of exposure and includes 4 weeks of zidovudine (ZDV) and lamivudine (3TC) (CDC, 2001). Other protocols recommend triple combination therapy for needle-stick exposure, which includes protease inhibitors (Liebman et al., 2001).

In summary, the basic concepts of HIV transmission, cellular transformation, epidemiology, treatment, and outcome have been discussed. Great strides have been made in the past few years in an attempt to understand this disease and to begin to research its detection, treatment, and cure. It is impossible to cover all aspects of this immune deficiency disease adequately in such a brief space and to approach currency in information. The learner is encouraged to seek out current information as it becomes available while building on the basic concepts presented in this section.

SECTION EIGHT REVIEW

1. Immunodeficiency originating from embryonic anomaly, genetic predisposition, or congenital failure is categorized as
   A. primary
   B. secondary
   C. acute
   D. chronic

2. Which statement best characterizes HIV disease?
   A. symptoms result from opportunistic pathology
   B. HIV invades cells primarily through the bloodstream
   C. clinical manifestations are in a characteristic and predictable sequence
   D. people testing positive for HIV are carriers and contagious
3. Fluids known to be modes of transmission for HIV include
   A. tears
   B. perspiration
   C. plasma
   D. saliva

4. AIDS-defining illnesses include (choose all that apply)
   1. PCP
   2. Kaposi's sarcoma
   3. tuberculosis
   4. rubella (measles)
   A. 2, 3, and 4
   B. 1, 3, and 4
   C. 2 and 3
   D. 1, 2, and 3

Answers: 1. A, 2. A, 3. C, 4. D

SECTION NINE: Care of the Immunocompromised Patient

Upon completion of this section, the learner will be able to discuss nursing considerations pertinent to the assessment and care of the immunocompromised patient.

Focused Assessment

The physical examination for level of immunocompetence primarily reflects the patient's nutritional status because the proper functioning of the immune system depends on nutritional status. Consequently, if the patient is malnourished, the immune status will be negatively affected. Physical assessment techniques and critical thinking must be focused on seeking evidence of infection, either acute or chronic. This includes assessing for skin lesions, open wounds, the presence of adventitious breath sounds and abnormal sputum, enlarged liver or spleen, or palpable lymph nodes or masses.

Nursing History

The patient history gives important clues to possible altered immunocompetence. Carpenito-Moyet (2004) suggests obtaining the following historical data:

- Complaints of fever, fatigue, weakness, swollen glands, light-headedness, visual disturbances
- Loss of appetite and weight loss
- Slow wound healing history
- Unexplained rashes, mouth sores, or oral patches
- Presence of increased levels of stress, infection, malignancy, or autoimmune disease
- History of exposure to infectious diseases

- Changes in menstrual patterns, unusual bleeding or bruising (reflective of platelet dysfunction)
- Recent use of immunosuppressant drugs
- Allergy history
- Burn injury
- Exposure to work environment chemicals
- At-risk factors for development of AIDS:
    Homosexual orientation or sexual partner of homosexual
    Transfusion of blood or blood products
    IV illegal drug users or sexual partner of drug user
    Child born of mother with AIDS
- Family history of autoimmune disorders or cancer

Evidence-Based Practice

- *A review of studies assessing the effectiveness of specific nursing interventions regarding infection prevention in neutropenic patients with cancer revealed that very few studies successfully demonstrated that interventions (e.g., protective environments/clothing, and low microbial water and food) reduced infection rates in this patient population. The reviewers concluded that there are major gaps in empirical evidence in the area of protective interventions in neutropenic patients with cancer (Larson, 2004).*

- *In a 10-year retrospective study, investigators found that admission diagnoses of patients with HIV who required intensive care have changed over this time, presumably related to improved drug management of HIV. Whereas respiratory failure (particularly PCP related) used to be the major cause for admission, there has been an increasing trend of ICU admissions for non-HIV related disorders, particularly complications of HCV (hepatitis C). In addition, investigators found a significant decrease in death from acute respiratory failure over time in this population (Narasimhan et al., 2004).*

- *In a large multihospital retrospective study, investigators looked at patients with HIV. Specifically, they focused on the relationship of patient's age to admission diagnosis, severity of illness, therapeutic drug interventions, and other factors. They found that older patients were admitted with pneumonia (PCP or community acquired pneumonia [CAP]) more often than younger patients. Older patients with HIV were significantly more ill and required ICU care and mechanical ventilation more often than younger patients with HIV. In addition, although both groups received drug therapy for CAP early on, older patients had a lower rate of receiving anti-PCP therapy. The investigators called for increased awareness of the possibility that older patients have HIV and that anti-PCP prophylaxis should be considered earlier (Sureka et al., 2004).*

Immunocompetence in the High-Acuity Patient

The high-acuity patient is at high risk for development of immunocompetence problems secondary to prolonged stress, severe infections, malnutrition, diabetes, and other problems. The nurse must monitor the patient for critical cues of an underlying immunocompetence problem. Some of these major critical cues include the presence of

- Fever
- Poor wound healing
- Joint pain
- White oral patches
- Level of consciousness and mental status changes
- Abnormal complete blood count (CBC) with differential
- Abnormal coagulation studies
- Recurrent, prolonged, or severe infections
- Secondary infections
- Immunosuppressive drug therapy, such as corticosteroids or cytotoxic drugs
- Other at-risk factors, such as splenectomy, diabetes mellitus, chronic alcohol abuse, malnutrition, or renal failure

Laboratory Findings

Laboratory testing is the major diagnostic tool for establishing immune status. Tests may include common ones, such as the WBC with differential and total lymphocyte count (TLC), as well as tests establishing nutritional status, such as serum albumin or prealbumin. These tests are relatively inexpensive and easy to perform and are used as screening tests for general immune status. The nurse should be able to monitor these levels for abnormal trends. WBC with differential is presented in detail in Module 24, "Acute Hematologic Dysfunction," and will not be discussed here.

A variety of cell-specific and disorder-specific laboratory tests are available if further evaluation of immunocompetence is necessary. Many of these tests, however, are both time consuming and expensive. Immunoglobulins, T cells, and B cells can be measured both quantitatively and functionally. Skin testing may be ordered to evaluate cellular immunocompetence. Protein and immunoglobulin levels through electrophoresis can help detect diseases associated with excess or deficient immune function. The ELISA can show exposure to HIV, to rheumatoid factor, and to lupus cells (Kee, 2002).

Nursing Management

General Goals

The goals for care of the immunocompromised patient include the goals appropriate to the malnourished patient. Additional goals include reestablishing immunocompetence and preventing and treating complications.

Collaborative Interventions

1. **Laboratory testing.** Various tests may be ordered to evaluate immune status, as discussed previously. Because many of the cell-specific blood tests are not commonly performed and are both expensive and time consuming to obtain or measure, the nurse should clarify nursing responsibilities and expectations regarding the tests before drawing samples or having them drawn to prevent nursing error.
2. **Drug therapy.** Two types of drugs have a direct impact on the immune system: immunosuppressive therapy agents and agents that enhance immunity. Immunosuppressants decrease immune function. Uses include control of chronic inflammatory problems, prevention of organ transplant rejection, and others. Examples of immunosuppressant drugs are steroids and cyclosporin A. Drugs that enhance immune function in some way include immunotherapy agents, primarily used in cancer therapy; monoclonal antibodies, antibodies that act against specific antigens; and interleukin, a lymphokine used to enhance immune responses. Drug therapy is presented in more detail in Module 26, "Organ Transplantation."
3. **Environmental protection.** Severe leukopenia places the patient at high risk for infection. The severely immunocompromised patient is placed in a controlled environment. Hospitals have protocols establishing the exact nature of the environmental protection. A private room is ordered. Some hospitals have special positive airflow rooms that diminish airflow of possibly contaminated air into the protected patient's room.

Independent Nursing Interventions

When caring for the immunocompromised patient, the nurse's role centers around monitoring and preventing infection, regaining or maintaining adequate nutrition, and meeting the psychosocial needs of the patient and family. Patient and family teaching to prevent and recognize infection is essential. Monitoring for infection should focus on the mucous membranes, skin, and lungs, which are the most common sites of infection in this patient population. Two nursing diagnoses are appropriate in meeting the first two goals.

- *High risk for infection:* related to deficient immune protection
- *Alteration nutrition:* in less than body requirements

High Risk for Infection Related to Deficient Immune Protection, Neutropenia. Desired patient outcome: The patient will show no evidence of infection.

I. Monitor patient every 2 to 4 hours for signs and symptoms of infection
   A. Fever in the immunosuppressed patient; a persistent fever of 100.5°F (38 °C) or higher for more than 1 hour may be the only sign of infection
   B. Signs and symptoms of inflammation, such as pain, redness, heat, or swelling (some or all of these may be absent if neutrophils are too low)
   C. Skin or mucous membrane lesions
      1. Check all skin folds, mouth, and perianal area
      2. Check wounds and areas noted in 1 for yeast invasion (white patches)
   D. Gastrointestinal lesions
      1. Check all stools for occult blood
      2. Monitor for diarrhea or constipation
   E. Genitourinary problems
      1. Check urine for color, odor
      2. Monitor patient for pain or fever
   F. Respiratory: Monitor for adventitious breath sounds, cough, dyspnea, pain; early in the course of a pulmonary infection, the patient may only develop dyspnea, tachypnea, and fever
   G. Invasive line/tube sites: Observe all sites closely for signs or symptoms of actual or potential infection
   The severely neutropenic patient will not be able to muster a normal immune response, which significantly alters the clinical findings. The inability to form pus (a by-product of normal neutrophil activity) can significantly reduce common infection findings, such as

   ■ Cloudy urine
   ■ Purulent sputum and adventitious breath sounds
   ■ Purulent wound drainage

II. Institute measures to protect the patient environmentally
   A. Place in private room; keep door closed
   B. Screen all persons coming into contact with patient for signs and symptoms of infection. Apply mask if respiratory infection is suspected or confirmed
   C. Excellent hand washing before contact (gloves recommended)
   D. Maintain strict aseptic technique for all sterile procedures
   E. Minimize foods and objects brought into the room from outside environment: Fresh fruits and vegetables may need to be washed or peeled before being taken into the room; flowers and vases with standing water may be restricted
   F. Special daily room cleaning with disinfectants is recommended

III. Provide ongoing protection against development of infection
   A. Monitor hydration status every shift
   B. Turn every 1 to 2 hours
   C. Skin care
      1. Thorough bathing every day
      2. Keep skin clean and lubricated at all times
   D. Keep linens clean and wrinkle free
   E. Pulmonary exercises every 4 hours
      1. Incentive spirometry, deep breathing
      2. As ordered: percussion, postural drainage, vibration (percussion is contraindicated if coagulopathy exists)
   F. Minimize invasive procedures: no rectal temperatures or enemas and no injections
   G. Protect patient against injury by instructing patient as follows:
      1. No straining
      2. No sharp objects: Use electric razor
      3. Report any infection signs and symptoms
      4. Brush teeth with very soft bristle brush or toothette at least every 4 hours
   H. Meticulous central line care (if present)
IV. Institute measures that foster drug regimen compliance
   A. Clarify critical importance of regimen to prevent development of drug resistance
   B. Tailor medication regimen to patient lifestyle
   C. Direct observation, as needed
   D. Help patient and family plan ahead for changes in routine

Alteration in Nutrition: Less Than Body Requirements. The nutritional needs of the high-acuity patient are presented in detail in Module 23. Immunocompromised patients often develop stomatitis, which can interfere with consumption of food.

I. Perform actions to minimize stomatitis problems
   A. Mouth care before mealtime
   B. Offer lidocaine viscous immediately before mealtime if mouth pain is an issue during eating
   C. Provide a soft food diet with frequent small meals

Many other nursing diagnoses might apply to the immunosuppressed patient based on individual physiologic and psychosocial needs. Some of the more common ones include the following:

■ High risk for injury
■ Anxiety
■ Coping, ineffective individual
■ Pain
■ Knowledge deficit
■ Powerlessness
■ Activity intolerance
■ Social isolation
■ Self-care deficit

SECTION NINE REVIEW

1. Common patient complaints associated with altered immunocompetence include (choose all that apply)
   1. abnormal bleeding
   2. pain
   3. swollen glands
   4. fatigue
   A. 1, 2, and 3
   B. 1, 3, and 4
   C. 2, 3, and 4
   D. 1 and 2
2. A severely immunocompromised hospitalized patient should receive environmental protection, including
   A. screening visitors for infection
   B. using bedding brought from home
   C. wearing clean gloves for dressing changes
   D. placement in semiprivate room with door closed
3. Nursing actions that provide ongoing protection against development of infection in a patient with neutropenia include
   A. restricting patient's fluid intake
   B. turning patient every 1 to 2 hours
   C. bathing patient every third day
   D. encouraging patient's use of incentive spirometer once per shift

Answers: 1. B, 2. A, 3. B

POSTTEST

1. In defending the body, the immune system is activated after which defense is unsuccessful?
   A. inflammatory response
   B. skin integrity
   C. phagocytosis
   D. interferons
2. Which cells or tissue is/are primarily responsible for production of B cells?
   A. bursa equivalent
   B. thymus
   C. stem cells
   D. spleen
3. Passive immunity is acquired through
   A. exposure to live antigens through inoculation
   B. vaccination with antiserum, such as tetanus toxoid
   C. genetic determination
   D. exposure to IgA antibodies
4. The best definition of antibody titer is the
   A. amount of a specific antibody in a serum
   B. presentation of processed T lymphocytes
   C. synthesis of circulating immunoglobulins
   D. molecular weight of an antigenic determinant
5. Specific immunity is best described as
   A. an antigen–antibody response
   B. foreign material filtration
   C. phagocytosis
   D. interferon antiviral activity
6. Matching of HLA antigens is particularly critical before
   A. blood transfusions
   B. factor VIII replacement
   C. organ transplantation
   D. in vitro fertilization
7. Which type of cell is responsible for the synthesis of circulating immunoglobulins?
   A. suppressor T cells
   B. B cells
   C. macrophages
   D. memory cells
8. The macrophage is primarily responsible for antigen destruction by
   A. lysis
   B. neutralization
   C. differentiation
   D. phagocytosis
9. Cell-mediated immunity is best characterized by
   A. specific recognition and memory of antigen
   B. primary and secondary response patterns
   C. subsets of IgG, IgA, IgE, IgM, and IgD
   D. direct attack on invading antigens
10. Which immunoglobulin is found in large quantities in secretory body fluids?
    A. IgA
    B. IgE
    C. IgG
    D. IgM

11. IgG comprises several types of antibodies and
    A. provides local antibody protection in the mucosa
    B. crosses the placental barrier
    C. can be administered as active acquired immunity
    D. functions with mast cells in hypersensitivity responses
12. The best definition of the complement system is
    A. a nonspecific immune response of engulfing and ingesting foreign antigens by neutrophils
    B. the body's first line of defense against viruses
    C. the body's surveillance system for malignant cells
    D. a progressive, sequential immune response activated by IgG and IgM
13. An example of a type IV hypersensitivity reaction is
    A. blood transfusion reaction
    B. host transplant rejection
    C. allergic asthma
    D. Arthus reaction
14. Which of the following is commonly thought of as being an autoimmune phenomenon?
    A. transplant rejection
    B. polio
    C. *Pneumocystis carinii*
    D. ulcerative colitis
15. How do increased levels of cortisol released during stress affect the immune system?
    A. it increases the production of glycogen
    B. stimulation of T cell production is enhanced by cortisol
    C. cortisol inhibits the production of interleukin-1 and -2
    D. higher levels of cortisol cause accelerated production of immunoglobulins by B cells
16. Zinc plays a major role in B cell and T cell production. For what reasons might an acutely ill adult have a zinc deficiency?
    A. prolonged periods of IV potassium replacement
    B. malabsorption syndromes accompanied by severe diarrhea
    C. third-space fluid deficit
    D. hyperosmolar dehydration
17. In what ways is the immune system compromised in the patient with extensive burns?
    A. zinc levels may become dangerously high, with extensive epidermal loss
    B. the patient's serum contains substances that suppress all immune responses

    C. T cells are suppressed, but B cell activity and antibody production generally are unaffected
    D. dehydration creates an imbalance between humoral and cell-mediated immunity
18. For which reason has HIV treatment been largely disappointing?
    A. treatment against one genetic strain may not provide protection against other evolving strains
    B. the virus does not attach to immunoglobulin antigenic sites as other antigens do
    C. the HIV blocks the complement system
    D. HIV invades B cells and sequesters itself from view of the body's immune system
19. Why are individuals who receive specific blood components more at risk for acquiring HIV than the average person who receives whole blood or packed cell transfusion?
    A. the screening procedures lack the sophistication of whole blood testing
    B. the risk increases with the large numbers of donors required to produce therapeutic amounts
    C. HIV is more difficult to detect in blood components than in whole blood or packed cells
    D. the virus attaches to large amounts of factor VIII and platelets
20. The nurse should suspect an infection in an immunosuppressed patient if the patient's temperature is above _____ for more than 1 hour.
    A. 100°F (37.8°C)
    B. 100.5°F (38°C)
    C. 101°F (38.3°C)
    D. 101.5°F (38.6°C)
21. A patient experiencing significant immunosuppression may develop which symptoms EARLY in the course of a pulmonary infection? (choose all that apply)
    1. dyspnea
    2. tachypnea
    3. adventitious breath sounds
    4. fever
    A. 1, 3, and 4
    B. 2, 3, and 4
    C. 1, 2, and 4
    D. 1 and 3

POSTTEST ANSWERS

Question	Answer	Section	Question	Answer	Section
1	B	Introduction	12	D	Five
2	A	One	13	B	Six
3	B	Two	14	D	Six
4	A	Two	15	C	Seven
5	A	Three	16	B	Seven
6	C	Three	17	A	Seven
7	B	Four	18	A	Eight
8	D	Four	19	B	Eight
9	D	Five	20	B	Nine
10	A	Five	21	C	Nine
11	B	Five			

REFERENCES

Carpenito-Moyet, L. J. (2004). *Nursing diagnosis: Application to clinical practice.* Philadelphia: Lippincott Williams & Wilkins.

Centers for Disease Control and Prevention (CDC). (1992). Revised classification system for HIV infection and expanded surveillance case definitions for AIDS among adolescents and adults. *MMWR, 41,* RR 17–19.

Centers for Disease Control and Prevention (CDC). (2001). Updated U.S. Public Health Service guidelines for the management of occupational exposures to HBV, HCV, and HIV and recommendations for postexposure prophylaxis. *MMWR,* 2001; 50(No. RR-11), 23–33.

Centers for Disease Control and Prevention (CDC). (2002). Guidelines for preventing opportunistic infections among HIV-infected persons. *MMWR, 52,* RR 08 1–46.

Fowler M. G., Garcia P., Hanson C., & Sansom S. (2004). Progress in preventing perinatal HIV transmission in the United States. Emerging Infectious Diseases. Available: *http://www.cdc.gov/ncidod/EID/vol10no11/04–0622_02.htm* Accessed 11 March 2005.

Gould, B. E. (2002). Immunity and abnormal responses. In B. E. Gould, *Pathophysiology for the health professions* (2nd ed., pp. 35–59). Philadelphia: W. B. Saunders.

Guyton, A., & Hall, J. (1997). *Human physiology and mechanisms of disease* (6th ed.) Philadelphia: W.B. Saunders.

Kee, J. L. (2002). *Laboratory and diagnostic tests with nursing implications* (6th ed.). Upper Saddle River, NJ: Prentice Hall.

Larson, E. (2004). Evidence-based nursing practice to prevent infection in hospitalized neutropenic patients with cancer. *Oncology Nursing Forum, 31*(4), 717–723.

Liebman, H. A., Cooley, T. P., & Levine. (2001). The acquired immunodeficiency syndrome. In E. Beutler, M. A. Lichtman, B .S. Coller, T. J. Kipps, & U. Seligsohn (Eds.), *Williams hematology* (6th ed., pp. 985–1010). New York: McGraw Hill.

Lydyard, P. M., & Grossi, C. E. (2001). Cells, tissue and organs of the immune system. In I. Roitt, J. Brostoff, & D. Male (Eds.), *Immunology* (6th ed., pp. 15–42). Edinburgh: Mosby.

Male, D. (2001). Introduction to the immune system. In I. Roitt, J. Brostoff, & D. Male (Eds.), *Immunology* (6th ed., pp. 1–12). Edinburgh: Mosby.

Narasimhan, M., Posner, A. J., DePalo, V. A., et al. (2004). Intensive care in patients with HIV infection in the era of highly active antiretroviral therapy. *CHEST, 125*(5), 1800–1804.

Platts-Mills, T. (2001). Hypersensitivity type 1. In I. Roitt, J. Brostoff, & D. Male (Eds.), *Immunology* (6th ed., pp. 324–341). Edinburgh: Mosby.

Porth, C. M. (2002). Alterations in the immune system. In C. M. Porth (Ed.), *Pathophysiology: Concepts of altered states* (6th ed., pp. 357–378). Philadelphia: Lippincott Williams & Wilkins.

Puyana, J., Pellegrini, J., De, A., et al. (1998). Both T-helper-1 and T-helper-2 type lymphokines are depressed in posttrauma anergy. *Journal of Trauma Injury, Infection, and Critical Care, 44*(6), 1037–1045.

Sullivan, K. A., & Kipps, T .J. (2001). Human leukocyte platelet antigens. In E. Beutler, M. A. Lichtman, B. S. Coller. T. J. Kipps, & U. Seligsohn (Eds.), *Williams hematology* (6th ed., pp. 1859–1877). New York: McGraw Hill.

Sureka, A., Parada, J., Deloria-Knoll, M., Chmiel, J., et al. (2004). HIV-related pneumonia care in older patients hospitalized in the early HAART era. *AIDS Patient Care & STDs, 18*(2), pp. 99–108.

Sweeney K. A. & Llamoso, C. (2002). Acquired immunodeficiency syndrome. In C. M. Porth, *Pathophysiology: Concepts of altered states* (6th ed., pp. 379–395) Philadelphia: Lippincott Williams & Wilkins.

Volberding, P. A., Baker, K. R., & Levine, A. M. (2003). Human immunodeficiency virus hematology. In V. Broudy, N. Berliner., et al. (Eds.), *Hematology: American society of hematology education program book* (pp. 294–313). Washington, DC: American Society of Hematology.

Organ Transplantation

Diana Thacker, Connie Taylor, Kathleen Dorman Wagner

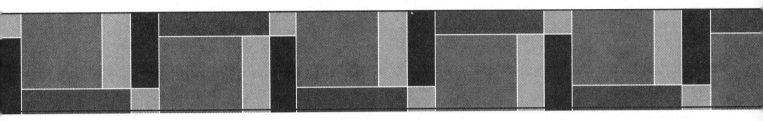

OBJECTIVES   Following completion of this module, the learner will be able to

1. Discuss the history of organ transplantation.
2. Describe types of grafts and donors.
3. Explain the general organ procurement process.
4. Discuss donor and organ management.
5. Explain the immunologic considerations of organ transplantation.
6. Describe the determination of transplant need.
7. Discuss the major complications associated with organ transplantation.
8. Describe immunosuppressant therapy.
9. Discuss the general concepts related to transplantation of selected organs, including postprocedure management implications.

This self-study module provides the learner with a broad picture of solid organ transplantation. The module is organized into two parts. As an introduction, Section One presents a brief history of solid organ transplantation.

Part I, which is composed of Sections Two through Four, focuses on the donor. Section Two differentiates between the various types of grafts and donors. It also includes a brief summary of some of the major laws intended to protect the donor and establish procurement protocols. Section Three explains organ procurement and includes discussions of establishing brain death, suitability for organ donation, obtaining consent, and working with the family to obtain consent. It concludes with the typical sequence of events involved in the procurement process. Section Four discusses management of the donor prior to organ removal and organ preservation.

Part II focuses on the organ recipient. Sections Five through Eight present specific recipient topics. Section Five explains immunologic considerations, such as histocompatibility and donor–recipient compatibility testing. Section Six describes how the need for an organ transplant is determined. Key concepts include determination of need and transplant recipient evaluation. Section Seven discusses posttransplantation complications, dividing them into three categories: technical, organ rejection, and immunosuppressant related. Section Eight describes some of the major immunosuppressants currently in use. Section Nine paints a broad picture of selected organ transplants, including kidney, heart, heart–lung, liver, pancreas, pancreas–kidney, and small bowel. The discussion of each type of organ transplant includes major indications for transplantation, preparation of the recipient, postoperative management, and evaluation of organ function. Each section includes a set of review questions to help the learner evaluate his or her understanding of the section's content before moving on to the next section. All Section Reviews and the module Pretest and Posttest include answers. It is suggested that the learner review those concepts answered incorrectly in the review questions before proceeding to the next section.

PRETEST

1. The early focal point of interest for organ transplantation was the
   A. lung
   B. kidney
   C. heart
   D. liver

2. Skin grafts were first experimented with as a treatment for
   A. leg ulcers
   B. traumatic injury
   C. skin cancer
   D. burn injury

3. The specific term referring to transplantation between identical twins is
   A. isograft
   B. autograft
   C. heterograft
   D. allograft

4. Segmental (partial) live-organ donations are usually between
   A. identical twins
   B. husband and wife
   C. parent and child
   D. human and ape

5. Under what circumstance should the nurse refer a patient to the organ procurement coordinator when death is imminent?
   A. after the patient's heart stops
   B. after the patient is pronounced brain dead
   C. when the patient is admitted to the hospital
   D. when the Glasgow Coma Score is 6 or less

6. The major advantage of early notification of the organ procurement coordinator when a potential donor has been identified is that _____ can be initiated.
   A. family counseling
   B. life-support measures
   C. signing of the consent form
   D. preliminary evaluation for suitability

7. Major management goals for caring for the donor patient include which of the following? (choose all that apply)
   1. maintaining stable hemodynamic status
   2. maintaining infections at minimum level
   3. maintaining fluid and electrolyte balance
   4. maintaining optimal oxygenation status
   A. 1 and 4
   B. 1, 3, and 4
   C. 2 and 3
   D. 1, 2, and 3

8. The most common underlying cause of hypotension in the donor is
   A. dehydration
   B. cardiac failure
   C. fluid overload
   D. increased systemic vascular resistance

9. Histocompatibility antigens are also known as
   A. monocytes
   B. macrophages
   C. human leukocyte antigens
   D. polymorphonuclear lymphocytes

10. Human leukocyte antigens (HLAs) are important because they
    A. are the source of donor organ rejection
    B. indicate the degree of organ failure
    C. are identical only within the same species
    D. reflect the need for transplantation

11. General guidelines for determination of organ transplant need include which of the following? (Choose the appropriate combination)
    1. severe functional disability
    2. end-stage organ failure
    3. psychological readiness
    4. additional serious health problems
    A. 1, 3, and 4
    B. 2 and 3
    C. 2, 3, and 4
    D. 1, 2, and 3

12. The decision as to whether a person is placed on the organ transplant waiting list as a potential recipient is usually made by
    A. the patient/family
    B. a multidisciplinary committee
    C. the organ procurement team
    D. the potential recipient's physician

13. Which of the following are examples of technical complications of organ transplantation? (choose all that apply)
    1. bleeding
    2. infection
    3. anastomosis leakage
    4. vascular thrombosis
    A. 2, 3, and 4
    B. 1, 3, and 4
    C. 1 and 3
    D. 2 and 4

14. Organ rejection that takes place within minutes to hours following transplantation and results from the presence of preformed graft-specific cytotoxic antibodies is called _____ rejection.
    A. subacute
    B. acute
    C. hyperacute
    D. chronic

15. The immunosuppressant that selectively acts against the helper T cells without affecting other types of immune cells is
    A. corticosteroids
    B. azathioprine
    C. cyclosporine
    D. OKT3

16. Long-term posttransplantation steroid therapy is particularly associated with potentially severe _____ disorders.
    A. bone
    B. heart
    C. liver
    D. blood

17. The major indication for kidney transplantation is end-stage renal disease, which most commonly results from which of the following? (choose all that apply)
    1. diabetes mellitus
    2. hypertension
    3. glomerular nephritis
    4. nephrotoxicity
    A. 2, 3, and 4
    B. 1, 3, and 4
    C. 1 and 2
    D. 1, 2, and 3

18. Dysfunction of a renal graft is most commonly associated with the
    A. preoperative condition of the donor
    B. preoperative condition of the recipient
    C. length of time the organ was preserved
    D. length of time required to perform the transplant

19. Major conditions that are associated with the need for heart transplantation include (choose all that apply)
    1. myocardial infarction
    2. congenital malformations
    3. ventricular aneurysm
    4. cardiomyopathy
    A. 2, 3, and 4
    B. 1, 2, and 3
    C. 1, 3, and 4
    D. 2 and 4

20. Major indications for liver transplantation include (choose all that apply)

    1. fulminant hepatic failure
    2. acute hepatotoxicity
    3. malignant hepatic tumors
    4. irreversible chronic liver disease
    A. 1, 2, and 3
    B. 1, 3, and 4
    C. 1 and 3
    D. 2, 3, and 4

21. Liver transplant patients are at particularly high risk for development of which early complication?
    A. hemorrhage
    B. rejection
    C. infection
    D. obstruction

22. The most common complications in the immediate postoperative period of the pancreas transplant include (choose all that apply)
    1. dehydration
    2. metabolic acidosis
    3. hyperinsulinemia
    4. infection
    A. 1, 3, and 4
    B. 2 and 4
    C. 2, 3, and 4
    D. 1, 2, and 3

23. The gold standard for diagnosing acute rejection in the intestinal transplant is a(n)
    A. significant increase in stomal output
    B. ileus
    C. endoscopic mucosal biopsy
    D. change in stomal color

Pretest Answers: 1. B, 2. D, 3. A, 4. C, 5. A, 6. D, 7. B, 8. A, 9. C, 10. A, 11. D, 12. B, 13. B, 14. C, 15. C, 16. A, 17. D, 18. C, 19. A, 20. B, 21. A, 22. D, 23. C

GLOSSARY

acute rejection   A cell-mediated immune response in which the T lymphocytes and macrophages of the host suddenly attack and destroy the graft tissue; it occurs within days, months, or even years following the transplant.

allograft   Tissue that is transplanted between members of the same species.

anastomosis   Site at which a graft is sutured into a recipient.

antigens   Substances that are capable of eliciting the immune response.

autograft   Transplantation of tissue from one part of a person's body to another part.

cadaver donor   A donor from whom tissue or an organ is recovered after death.

chronic rejection   A humoral immune response in which antibodies slowly attack and destroy the graft.

cytokine-release syndrome (CRS)   A group of clinical manifestations associated with the initial dose of monoclonal antibody therapy.

cytotoxic agents   Drugs that have the capability of destroying target cells.

donor   One who donates an organ or tissue.

graft   The transfer of tissue or organ from one part of the body to a different part, or from another donor source.

heterograft   Transplantation of tissue between two different species.

histocompatibility   The ability of cells and tissues to live without interference from the immune system.

HLA antigens   Human leukocyte antigens—proteins found on the sixth chromosome (also called histocompatibility antigens).

hyperacute rejection   A humoral immune response in which the B lymphocytes are activated to produce antibodies against the donor organ; it occurs within minutes to hours following transplantation.

immunosuppressant   A drug that suppresses the immune response.

isograft   Transplantation of tissues between identical twins.

monoclonal antibodies (mAb)   Antibodies that are pure clones of specific B lymphocytes.

polyclonal antibodies   Antibodies produced by immunizing animals with human lymphocytes.

recipient   One who receives an organ or tissue.

rejection   The activation of the immune response against a transplanted tissue or organ.

syngraft   See isograft.

tissue typing   Identification of the HLA antigens of both the donor and the recipient.

vascular thrombosis   A blood clot in the vasculature of the graft.

xenograft   See heterograft.

ABBREVIATIONS

ALG	Antilymphocyte globulin	**HIV**	Human immunodeficiency virus
Alk Phos	Alkaline Phosphatase (ALP)	**HLA**	Human leukocyte antigen
ALT	Alanine aminotransferase (SGPT)	**KODA**	Kentucky Organ Donor Affiliates
AST	Aspartate aminotransferase (SGOT)	**mAb**	Monoclonal antibody
ATG	Antithymocyte globulin	**O$_2$**	Oxygen
BUN	Blood urea nitrogen	**OPO**	Organ procurement organization
CMV	Cytomegalovirus	**OPTN**	National Organ Procurement and Transplantation Network
CRS	Cytokine-release syndrome		
CyA or CsA	Cyclosporine	**PEEP**	Positive end-expiratory pressure
ESRD	End-stage renal disease	**UAGA**	Uniform Anatomical Gift Act
GCS	Glasgow coma scale	**UNOS**	United Network for Organ Sharing
Hct	Hematocrit	**WBC**	White blood cell count
Hgb	Hemoglobin		

SECTION ONE: Brief History of Organ Transplantation

At the completion of this section, the learner will be able to discuss the history of organ transplantation. Organ transplantation is not a new concept. For centuries there have been attempts to replace various body tissues. It was not until the dawn of the twentieth century, however, that surgical skills and knowledge of immunology and immunosuppression became advanced enough to facilitate tissue survival following transplantation. This section highlights strategic events in the development of modern organ transplantation as described by Dr. Joseph Murray, a pioneer in transplantation (Murray, 1991).

1910 to 1930: The Beginnings

The kidney was the early focal point of interest for organ transplantation. Surgeons had struggled with young patients who, while otherwise healthy, were dying of end-stage renal failure. Prior to 1912, although there was interest in performing such transplants, surgeons had not yet developed a successful method of reconnecting the organ vasculature to make transplantation a feasible option. It was in 1912 that the Nobel Prize winner Dr. A. Carrel developed a landmark method of successfully suturing and transplanting blood vessels and organs. It was also during this period that animal research began exploring tissue survival following autografts and allografts.

1930 to 1950: In Search of Long-Term Success

In the early 1930s, experimentation in skin grafting as a treatment for burns contributed greatly to the advancement of transplantation knowledge. It was noted that, although no skin grafts survived for long, skin grafts from family members survived longer than those from nonfamily members. In 1937, it was discovered that skin grafting between identical twins could provide permanent graft survival. This discovery rekindled interest in organ and tissue replacement, although the reasons for tissue acceptance or rejection were still unknown.

It was in the late 1940s that renal transplantation programs began to develop in earnest. Following World War II, research began to focus on allograft rejection. A common antigen was discovered between kidney and skin allografts that would cause sensitization of a recipient for subsequent graftings. Scientists knew that if renal transplantation was to be a feasible option they must find a way to get around the immunologic problems experienced thus far. By the end of the 1940s, transplanted kidneys were surviving for up to 6 months. Long-term organ transplant survival remained just out of reach.

1950 to 1960: The Isograft and Immunosuppressant Discovery Years

In 1954, the first renal transplants between identical human twins took place. Tissue matching was performed by cross skin grafting between two twin brothers. The success of the isograft demonstrated that identical twins provided a method of bypassing the tissue incompatibility problem.

Research continued toward solving the problem of tissue incompatibility. Total body x-ray was performed experimentally, as a means to depress the immune system. After the x-ray treatments were completed, bone marrow infusions were performed and the renal allograft transplant was completed. This method, however, had only marginal success in the short term and little success in the long term.

During this decade, research also focused on pharmacologic immunosuppression. In 1959, animal experimentation began using 6-mercaptopurine, an antimetabolite, with encouraging success. It was during the next year that azathioprine (Imuran) was introduced. Early use of azathioprine was associated with patient death from high-dose–related complications. Once the correct dose was established, however, azathioprine was very successful during human clinical trials, and it continues to be a major form of immunosuppression therapy. Not long after initiating the use of azathioprine, corticosteroids were introduced as adjunctive therapy.

1961 to the Present

The 1960s saw a rapid increase in transplant knowledge. Renal transplant survival rates increased dramatically. New forms of immunosuppressive therapy were discovered. Organ procurement programs were initiated both regionally and nationally. There was great enthusiasm to take what was learned from the renal transplantation programs and expand it to transplantation of other organs.

In the late 1960s, liver and pancreas transplantation was initiated, followed by heart transplantation. Early attempts at heart transplantation were not very successful. The poor success rate associated with heart transplantation "between 1968 and 1970 was undoubtedly transplantation's darkest hour" (Murray, 1991, p. 123). Today, however, cardiac transplantation is successful, in part because of improved immunosuppressant therapy, particularly cyclosporine. Following the attainment of a successful cardiac transplant program, surgeons turned to perfecting the heart–lung, single-lung, and double-lung transplants.

In summary, the history of organ transplantation is relatively short. Most dysfunctional organs can now be replaced by healthy ones. The problems associated with histocompatibility and organ rejection required years of research to overcome. This section presented an overview of events that led to present-day organ transplant programs.

SECTION ONE REVIEW

1. The early focal point of interest for organ transplantation was the
   A. kidney
   B. lungs
   C. heart
   D. liver
2. Skin grafts were first experimented with as a treatment for
   A. leg ulcers
   B. traumatic injury
   C. skin cancer
   D. burn injury
3. One of the earliest immunosuppressants to be successfully used on transplant patients was
   A. cyclosporine
   B. azathioprine
   C. corticosteroids
   D. 6-mercaptopurine

Answers: 1. A, 2. D, 3. B

The Organ Donor

SECTION TWO: The Graft and Donor

At the completion of this section, the learner will be able to describe types of grafts and donors. The term **graft** refers to the transfer of tissue from one part of the body to a different part, or from another donor source. There are three major types of grafts: the autograft, the heterograft, and the allograft.

The Autograft

The **autograft** is the transplantation of tissue from one part of a person's body to another part. It is the ideal situation for tissue compatibility and graft survival. A common example of autografting is the skin graft. For example, when a person receives severe burns, healthy tissue can be removed from an undamaged body area and transplanted over the burned area to promote healing and recovery. Autografting is not used for organ transplantation and thus will not be discussed further in this section. (See Module 35 for more information.)

The Heterograft

The **heterograft,** also called a **xenograft,** refers to transplantation of tissue between two different species. Examples of heterografts are porcine skin grafts and experimental baboon heart transplants. At this time, heterografts are primarily used as temporary transplantations until a permanent allograft becomes available. Tissue rejection occurs rapidly because of the dissimilarities of tissues between species.

The Allograft

The **allograft** (homograft) refers to tissue that is transplanted between members of the same species. One form of allograft, the **isograft** (**syngraft**), refers to transplantation between identical twins. The allograft is the most common type of organ transplantation. Allografts, with the exception of isografts, trigger an immune reaction that will cause rejection of the graft. Allografts are obtained either from live or cadaver donors.

The Live Donor

The kidney is the primary solid organ that is recovered, en total, from a live **donor.** Ideally, the live donor is related to the recipient as part of the immediate family (e.g., parents, siblings). When a related donor is not available, a nonrelated live donor is used. Related donors are preferred because of increased histocompatibility and, therefore, longer graft life. If an isograft is used, no rejection is expected because the two tissues are completely histocompatible. Segmental (partial) organ donation, such as one lobe of a liver or lung, or part of the pancreas, may be performed using a live donor. Segmental organ donation is usually provided by the parents of a recipient child.

The Cadaver Donor

The **cadaver donor** is one who has organs or tissue recovered after death. Cadaver donors are most commonly healthy individuals who die as the result of a traumatic event or a sudden death. Cadaver donors comprise the majority of solid organ donors. Potential cadaver donors are initially evaluated for suitability. There are two types of potential cadaver donors: those who die of cardiac death and those who die of brain death.

Donors Who Die of Cardiac Death. Cardiac death refers to death by termination of cardiac and respiratory function. Transplantable tissues may be limited to heart valves, corneas, eyes, saphenous veins, skin, and bones. These tissues are to be recovered within 12 to 24 hours postdeclaration of death. On occasion, organs may be recovered following cardiac death. This must be initiated within minutes of cardiac arrest with the appropriate personnel available to complete the organ recovery.

Donors Who Die of Brain Death. Brain death refers to the cessation of the entire brain and brainstem function. Loss of brain stem function destroys the vital centers for blood pressure, temperature, and respiratory control, making cardiopulmonary death imminent. Organ donations resulting from brain death comprise the majority of cadaver organs. Transplantable tissues from this group of donors include tissues as well as solid organs, such as the kidneys, lungs, heart, liver, pancreas, and small bowel. Strict laws and formal procurement protocols have been established to protect the potential donor's rights.

Legal Aspects of Donation and Transplantation

Many laws are in place at both the national and state levels to protect the potential organ donor and to organize and facilitate organ procurement and distribution. The following are examples of some of this legislation in the United States.

Uniform Anatomical Gift Act

The Uniform Anatomical Gift Act (UAGA) authorizes the donation of all or part of the human body following death for a variety of uses (research, transplantation, and education). The act also includes guidelines regarding who can donate, how donation is to be carried out, and who can receive the organ donation. The act provides for the donor card as a means for individuals to convey their desire to be donors. The act also includes liability protection for health care providers. All states have passed the UAGA.

Required-Request Legislation

A section of the UAGA, called the "Routine Inquiry and Required Request; Search and Notification," stipulates hospital responsibilities toward identifying potential donors and providing donor information to families to make them aware of their opportunities to donate. Hospitals that do not comply with the required-request stipulations may be open to penalties or administrative actions.

National Organ Transplant Act

The National Organ Transplant Act set up the National Organ Procurement and Transplantation Network (OPTN). The OPTN establishes national registries to track potential recipients and posttransplantation organ recipients. It also provides for a national system to match organs and potential recipients. In addition, the act prohibits selling of human organs and tissues. This act has been adopted in all 50 states.

Uniform Determination of Death Act

The Uniform Determination of Death Act has been enacted as a guideline for states to establish a legal definition of death. Most states have adopted some form of this act. For example, in Kentucky, KRS 446.400: Determination of death; minimal conditions to be met, states

> For all legal purposes, the occurrence of human death shall be determined in accordance with the usual and customary standards of medical practice, provided that death shall not be determined to have occurred unless the following minimal conditions have been met: (1) When respiration and circulation are not artificially maintained, and there is a total and irreversible cessation of spontaneous respiration and circulation; or (2) When respiration and circulation are artificially maintained, and there is a total and irreversible cessation of all brain function, including the brain stem and that such determination is made by two licensed physicians.

Medicare Conditions of Participation

Enacted in 1998, these conditions must be followed by hospitals for Medicare reimbursement. The guidelines specifically indicate the responsibilities of hospitals toward notifying and working with their organ procurement organization (OPO). Specifically, hospitals must report all deaths and imminent deaths to the OPO in a timely manner. If the OPO finds a patient meets criteria for organ donation, the hospital should ensure the family is offered donation. Those who communicate with the family about donation must be employed by the OPO or have received training from the OPO on best practices for donation communication. Care must be provided to the donor to allow for donation to occur while testing and placement of organs and tissues take place. Death record reviews should be completed by the OPO, and the OPO should provide education to the hospital as needed. In addition, if the hospital performs organ transplants, data must be submitted to the Secretary of Health and Human Services when requested.

In summary, there are three major types of grafts, including the autograft, the heterograft, and the allograft. One type of allograft, the isograft, is a graft between identical twins. Allografts comprise the majority of grafts. Allografts can be obtained from live or cadaver donors. The majority of grafts are of cadaver origin. Cadaver organs and tissues come from two sources: donors who die of cardiac death and those who die of brain death. Strict laws and formal procurement protocols protect the potential donor's rights. Examples of some of the major laws include the Uniform Anatomical Gift Act, required-request legislation, the National Organ Transplant Act, the Uniform Determination of Death Act, and Medicare's conditions of participation.

SECTION TWO REVIEW

1. Tissue that is transplanted between members of the same species is the definition of
   A. autograft
   B. heterograft
   C. xenograft
   D. allograft
2. The specific term referring to transplantation between identical twins is
   A. isograft
   B. autograft
   C. heterograft
   D. allograft
3. Segmental (partial) live-organ donations are usually between
   A. identical twins
   B. husband and wife
   C. parent and child
   D. human and ape
4. The major legislation that authorizes the donation of all or part of the human body following death is called the
   A. National Organ Transplant Act
   B. Uniform Anatomical Gift Act
   C. Uniform Determination of Death Act
   D. Omnibus Reconciliation Act

Answers: 1. D, 2. A, 3. C, 4. B

SECTION THREE: Organ Procurement

At the completion of this section, the learner will be able to explain the general organ procurement process. The specific procedures used to procure and distribute organs differ among transplant programs and organizations. This section will provide information regarding the procurement process in general.

Evidence-Based Practice

- *An Internet site targeting heart recipients and their caregivers was developed as an intervention for improving several psychosocial outcomes (quality of life, medical regimen compliance, and mental health). The site provided workshops focusing on medical regimen and stress management, a discussion forum, and electronic access to transplant professionals. Preliminary results suggested that the Web-based intervention might positively affect psychosocial outcomes (Dew et al., 2004).*

- *A study of beliefs and attitudes regarding brain death and organ procurement found that the public is misinformed, unaware of, or holds beliefs that are incongruent with the definition of brain death. The investigators suggest the need for improved public education regarding brain death and organ donation (Siminoff et al., 2004).*

- *Cystic fibrosis (CF) patients with or without lung transplantation have an increased risk for digestive tract cancer. This study found that the risk of developing cancer was higher in the lung transplantation group than the nontransplantation group (Maisonneuve et al., 2003).*

Establishing Death

The Uniform Determination of Death Act defines how death is determined. Death can either be pronounced by cardiac standstill criteria or brain death criteria. Each state legislates specific criteria to be met for a death pronouncement. An example is Kentucky's legislation (KRS 446.440):

> When artificial respiration and circulation are not maintained and there is irreversible cessation of spontaneous respiration and circulation (Cardiac Standstill Death).

> When respiration and circulation are artificially maintained and there is total and irreversible cessation of all brain and brain stem function (Brain Death). Two licensed physicians must determine brain death.

When cardiac standstill occurs tissue donation is possible. Tissues that can be recovered include corneas, eyes, skin from anterior and posterior torso, buttocks and thighs, bone from the upper and lower extremities, leg veins, heart for valves, and mandible. Tissues must be recovered within 12 to 24 hours of cardiac standstill.

When brain death occurs, both organs and tissues can be donated. Organ recovery can include heart, lungs, liver, pancreas, small bowel, and kidneys. Organ perfusion and oxygenation must be maintained to allow for organ donation. The brain dead patient continues to have a beating heart and is maintained on a ventilator, sometimes requiring medications to promote adequate blood pressure and hemodynamic stability. This artificial supportive care must continue through the organ recovery to prevent ischemia and cellular death within the organs. Brain death most often occurs within a few diagnostic categories, including traumatic brain injury, bleeding in the brain, anoxia, and cerebral tumors and infections.

In 1968, the Ad Hoc Committee on Brain Death of Harvard Medical School published the report *A Definition of Irreversible Coma*. In this report, the criteria for brain death included apneic coma and an absence of elicited responses for a period of 24 hours using electroencephalogram (EEG) recordings. Its exclusions for brain death included hypothermia and drug intoxication. In 1981, the President's Commission for the Study of Ethical Problems submitted a report defining death to the president and congress. The Commission's final report was published as the *Guidelines for the Determination of Death*, which has become the guidelines for legislation in all states with regard to brain death. This document includes an exclusion for hypotension.

There are several conditions that can make a patient appear brain dead when he or she is not; therefore, when brain death is suspected, three factors must be known before brain death testing is initiated. These three factors are as follows:

- Cause of unresponsiveness must be known
- Absence of metabolic central nervous system (CNS) depression
- Absence of toxic CNS depression

Determining the cause of unresponsiveness is necessary to rule out a condition that might be reversible. Metabolic CNS depression can occur if the patient is hypotensive, hypothermic, or has severe acid–base imbalances. The president's commission has recommended that the patient must have an adequate blood pressure related to the patient's age and size (adults should have a systolic blood pressure of at least 90 mm Hg), a PaO_2 greater than 60 mm Hg, and a temperature greater than 32.2°C (90.0°F). If these parameters are not met, they must be corrected before brain death testing begins. Toxic CNS depression can occur from sedatives, alcohol, or neuromuscular blockades, which depress cranial nerve responses as well as cerebral electrical activity. In cases where any of these substances are present, there are two options available. First, the health care team can wait until the substances are eliminated from the body and then proceed with clinical or EEG testing. Second, cerebral blood flow studies can be used to determine brain death immediately.

Brain death testing determination can be done by a clinical exam, cerebral blood perfusion study, or EEG. The type of testing used is determined by the physician with consideration of the patient's injuries, his or her hemodynamic stability, and whether toxic or metabolic CNS depression is present.

Clinical Examination

Clinical examination is probably the most cost-effective testing that can be used to determine brain death and can be completed at the bedside. This test cannot be used if the patient has toxic or metabolic CNS depression. Clinical exams should not be used if the patient has an inability to initiate respiration as a result of other injuries or pathology. Examples of this include the patient with C1–C2 quadriplegia or advanced life support (ALS) requiring ventilator assistance. Each hospital should have policies in place outlining how many clinical tests are required, and how often to test for brain death (e.g., two clinical exams 12 hours apart, with continued observation between the two exams). The following criteria must be observed with all of the reflexes being absent.

- No response to any painful or verbal stimuli. The patient's Glasgow Coma Score is 3.
- No pupillary response to light.
- No eye movement (doll's eyes reflex) with head rotation.
- No eye movement to iced water calorics.
- No blink response to cornea irritation.
- No cough response to deep suctioning.
- No gag response to oral-pharyngeal stimulation.
- Apnea.

Apnea testing is typically performed once, at the time of the final clinical exam. This testing should be approached with caution and close monitoring. When performed, the patient is removed from the ventilator and observed for any respiratory movement while allowing a rise in the $PaCO_2$. The $PaCO_2$ should be raised to a level sufficient to stimulate the respiratory drive center. Prior to starting the apnea test the patient is preoxygenated on FIO_2 of 0.1 (100 percent O_2 concentration). When the patient is disconnected from the ventilator, passive oxygen must be delivered. If, during the test, the patient begins having cardiac dysrhythmias, hypotension, or the oxygen saturation falls below 70 percent, an arterial blood gas is immediately drawn and the patient is reconnected to the ventilator. In situations where the patient requires reconnection to the ventilator before apnea testing is complete and the patient's $PaCO_2$ is less than 60 mm Hg at the time of ventilator reconnection, another type of testing may be considered or the apnea test is repeated after the patient is stabilized. If the $PaCO_2$ is above 60 mm Hg and no respiratory movement is noted, the patient is considered apneic. If respiratory movement is noted during the testing, the patient is reconnected to the ventilator and the patient is not considered apneic.

Cerebral Blood Flow

Brain death can be determined if cerebral blood flow is absent. A cerebral angiogram, cerebral nuclear flow study, or transcranial doppler can be used. The patient must have an adequate blood pressure to allow cerebral blood flow. If cerebral blood flow is absent, no further testing or observation is required. Use of this test can be expensive, but it provides immediate results.

Brain blood flow is considered the gold standard of brain death determination.

Electroencephalogram

The EEG measures electrical activity of the cerebrum. Publicly, it is the most recognized test used to determine brain death. Electrodes placed on the patient's head monitor for electrical activity while the patient receives different levels of stimulation. Hospital policies vary regarding how EEGs can be used in determining brain death. Many policies require that multiple EEGs be performed over a specific period of time (e.g., two EEGs over a 48-hour interval). Electrocerebral silence or a "flat" EEG and a clinical exam with no brainstem activity are adequate for brain death determination.

Referral to the OPO

The Medicare conditions of participation state all imminent death should be referred to the OPO. Imminent death refers to the potential brain dead patient. Although the Department of Health and Human Services (DHHS) defines imminent death as that of a severely brain-injured patient with a Glasgow Coma Score of 6 or less, DHHS allows the criteria of referral to be an agreed-on value by the hospital and the OPO. After the referral, the OPO will then make a determination of suitability for organ donation and develop a plan of care with the medical staff regarding patient and family care. Should the patient become brain dead, the early notification and evaluation facilitates a timely communication with the family and OPO.

It is often the emergency room or critical care nurse who first identifies the patient as a potential organ donor because the nature of the illnesses that precedes rapid deterioration requires medical management in the emergency or critical care environment. To facilitate the referral process there are certain data the nurse can have available to help the OPO begin the evaluation process. (See Table 26–1.)

TABLE 26–1   Donor Referral Initial Nursing Database

Patient's name

Age, sex, race

Cause of brain injury

Height and weight

Current Glasgow Coma Score (GCS)

Past medical and social history

Laboratory data (if available)
    Serum electrolytes, BUN, creatinine, AST, ALT, alk phos, WBC, Hgb, Hct

Hemodynamic status (blood pressure, heart rate, O_2 saturation)

Urine output (mL/hr)

Current inotropic support (drug name and dose)

Plan of care (brain death testing scheduled, DNR status)

Determination of Patient's Suitability for Organ Donation

Several factors must be considered in determining if a patient is a candidate for donation. Some of these factors include the patient's medical and social history, compliance to medical treatments, and current hemodynamic stability and instability. Past medical and social history considers the patient's illnesses, and behaviors that affect the body's function and influence the transmission of diseases. This information is important for the transplant surgeon to consider in order to determine the risks posed to a potential organ recipient. Factors that can prevent donation from occurring include human immunodeficiency virus (HIV), acquired immune deficiency syndrome (AIDS), or active hepatitis B (HbSaG). Certain other factors, although not necessarily precluding donation, are important to take into consideration, including sepsis and any high-risk behaviors for disease transmission (e.g., IV drug abuse; male-to-male sex; extended jail; hemophilia; blood contact with a person who has HIV, AIDS, or HbSaG). Having cancer does not necessarily eliminate a person as a potential donor, particularly if the cancer is in remission, localized, and not blood borne. If the extent of the potential donor's history is unknown, he or she should still be considered a potential organ donor.

Hemodynamic status is also assessed on each potential donor patient. Some degree of hemodynamic instability usually develops related to a sequelae of physiologic events that occur with brain death. These include diabetes insipidus, initial hypertension followed by hypotension, inability to regulate body temperature, and neurogenic pulmonary edema. Although most patients go through periods of hemodynamic instability as brain death occurs, it is often sufficiently correctable to maintain adequate perfusion of the organs. The goals of management are to maintain the potential donor within the normal hemodynamic parameters (Table 26–2). However, failing to meet those criteria does not mean donation cannot occur. The OPO reviews the hemodynamics and makes a determination if the instability is significant.

TABLE 26–2   Hemodynamic Parameters of the Adult Potential Organ Donor

Blood pressure	Greater than 100 mm Hg (systolic) or MAP greater than 75 mm Hg
Heart rate	80–110/min
Sao$_2$	Greater than 95 percent
CVP	8–12 mm Hg
PCWP	10–12 mm Hg
SVR	800–1,200 dynes/sec/cm^5
Cardiac index	Greater than 2.0 L/m/m^2

MAP-mean arterial pressure; Sao$_2$-oxygen saturation; CVP-central venous pressure; PCWP-pulmonary capillary wedge pressure; SVR-systemic vascular resistance

Obtaining Consent

The Uniform Anatomical Gift Act defines the order of priority of those who give consent for donation. First is the spouse, followed by adult children, either parent, adult sibling(s), or a guardian. Some states have legislation allowing the patient priority if a signed and appropriately witnessed organ donor card, donor registry, or driver's license specifying such are available.

The Medicare Conditions of Participation states that only persons employed by the OPO or those who have received training from the OPO in best practices in the consent process should discuss donation. OPO staff will provide support to the family after receiving the patient referral. The OPO staff's initial interactions focus heavily on facilitating the family's understanding of the patient's brain injury, poor prognosis, and imminent death. A significant amount of time is devoted to helping the family understand the concept of brain death and understanding that death has occurred although the patient will sustain a heartbeat for a period of time. Only after the family develops the understanding that brain death is true death should conversations about donation begin. This process is called *decoupling*. Decoupling is the separation of conversations about brain death and its understanding by the next of kin before donation is mentioned. In a study conducted by Kentucky Organ Donor Affiliates (KODA, 1994), it was determined that if a family's acceptance of brain death did not occur before donation was mentioned, consent rates for donation were 18 percent. However, if the family understood and accepted brain death as actual death and subsequently donation was mentioned, the consent rate rose to 65 percent.

Donor Testing

After consent is obtained, care of the donor is transferred to the OPO and an OPO coordinator will initiate orders. A thorough organ evaluation is initiated as each organ is evaluated to ensure suitability for transplant. Serologic testing is performed to determine the absence or presence of transmittable diseases. Blood type and human leukocyte antigen (HLA) typing is determined. Once these tests are completed, the information is entered into the United Network for Organ Sharing (UNOS) system to identify matching recipients.

The heart evaluation includes any cardiac history and injury. An electrocardiogram (ECG), chest x-ray, and echocardiogram may be done to determine the current cardiac function and measurements. If the patient is more than 45 years of age or has a medical history consistent with the development of coronary artery disease, a cardiac catheterization may be done. If no cardiac dysfunction is present, matching a heart recipient is initiated.

The lung evaluation includes any pulmonary history including smoking or injury. An arterial blood gas, chest x-ray, and sputum gram stain are obtained. Assuming the results of these tests are adequate, a bronchoscopy is completed. If no pulmonary dysfunction is noted, matching a lung recipient(s) search is initiated.

Liver function is evaluated through investigation of any positive hepatic history, including alcohol and drug use, to evaluate whether any hepatic injury has occurred. Electrolyte and liver function tests will be initiated. If hepatic function is adequate, matching a liver recipient search is initiated.

The pancreas is evaluated by history, including diabetes and any pancreatic injury. The serum glucose, amylase, and lipase are monitored. If the patient is 10 to 50 years of age and pancreatic function is adequate, pancreas matching is initiated.

Evaluation of the kidneys includes medical history, injuries, and laboratory findings, such as blood urea nitrogen (BUN) and serum creatinine. Once HLA typing is completed and the evaluation confirms adequate kidney function, recipients are searched for.

A specific algorithm matches each organ to a recipient. In general, priority is given to recipients within the donor's local area. A significant factor for survival of a transplanted organ is a decreased cold ischemic time, the time when circulation to the organ is stopped in the donor and restored in the recipient. If a matching recipient is not found within the local area, the search continues in the region followed by a national search. Exceptions to this are "perfect matches" for a kidney or pancreas recipient. For liver patients, priority may be given to a "status 1" patient with 7 days or less to live without a transplant.

It is routine for the OPO coordinator to find recipients for the organs prior to the donor organ recovery. If the donor patient becomes hemodynamically unstable and stability cannot be established, organ placement will occur during and after the recovery completion. If the donor's hemodynamic instability is too great to expedite the organ recovery, it is unlikely that the heart or lungs can be recovered because of ischemia to these two organs. The liver and kidney can tolerate hemodynamic instability far greater than the cardiothoracic organs and often can be transplanted without compromise to the recipient. As the organ recovery occurs, the surgeon observes the organ for its functioning in the donor and assures that anatomically, all is well. Should the recovery process begin and a terminal disease process be found (such as cancer), the donation will be halted.

In the operating room (OR) the OPO coordinator continues to coordinate the recovery. An abdominal team and thoracic team of surgeons may be used. As the organ recipients are located, each surgeon has the option of being present in the operating room to recover the organ. The heart and lung surgeons often complete their own recoveries because observing the organ in the donor is often desired. The liver, pancreas, and kidney surgeons often ask a local transplant surgeon to complete the abdominal recovery. Prior to the recovery, cannulas are placed in the aorta and cold preservation fluids flush the blood from the organ to maintain a low metabolic state until transplanted. Each organ is triple bagged to maintain sterility and transported on ice to the recipient's hospital. The transplant begins immediately on arrival. Each organ must be transplanted into the recipient within a certain time frame to facilitate adequate function.

Non–Heart-Beating Organ Donation

When organ donation was first being attempted, artificial respiratory support by mechanical ventilators was unknown. It was not until the 1980s that brain death was recognized as a type of death. With the advent of brain death, there was a shift in the transplant community to pursue organ donation only in the brain-dead patient because organ perfusion could be maintained until the time of recovery. As the waiting list has continued to increase at a rate of 20 to 30 percent each year, and organ donation has remained constant, there is an increasing gap between the supply and demand of organs. Because of this widening gap, there has been a recent resurgence in pursuing non–heart-beating organ donation. For non–heart-beating organ donation to occur, an organ procurement coordinator or a trained hospital designee must be present when cardiac cessation occurs. The organs must undergo in situ cooling soon after cardiac death is pronounced, and organ recovery should occur in a short time period. Patient criteria vary in each institution and OPO regarding non–heart-beating organ donation.

In summary, organ procurement requires a carefully executed series of events. Identification of the potential brain-death patient and notification of the organ procurement agency is a crucial first step. This is followed by establishing the diagnosis of brain death in the potential donor. There are accepted medical standards for brain death, which are specific to each institutional policy and state law. Consent for organ donation is sought from the next of kin. The manner in which the family is approached in seeking permission is very important.

SECTION THREE REVIEW

1. A major advantage of early notification of the organ procurement coordinator when a potential donor has been identified is that _____ can be initiated.
   A. family counseling
   B. life-support measures
   C. signing of the consent form
   D. preliminary evaluation for suitability

2. The topic of organ donation should not be initiated with the family until the
   A. patient has died
   B. family signs the consent form
   C. family acknowledges the patient's death
   D. family asks about possible donation

SECTION FOUR: Donor Management and Organ Preservation

At the completion of this section, the learner will be able to discuss donor management and organ preservation.

Donor Management

Donor management focuses on maintaining organ function when brain death occurs. Close monitoring and evaluation of the patient's body system functions is crucial for maintaining organ viability for eventual transplantation. This section is organized by major body and organ functions that must be stabilized to adequately oxygenate and perfuse the organs to retain organ viability. Table 26–3 provides a summary of organ donor management.

Hemodynamic Instability

As brain death ensues, organ functions begin to deteriorate, which results in hemodynamic instability. Hemodynamic dysfunction, when recognized and treated early, can usually be controlled and hemodynamic stability restored and maintained. Many patients with brain injury come to the hospital in a normal hemodynamic state. Initially, the body attempts to repair the injured area of brain by increasing cerebral blood flow (CBF) and oxygen to the area of injury. The increased CBF increases cerebral edema. As cerebral edema increases, CBF eventually becomes compromised. The body responds by releasing catecholamines that increase heart rate and blood pressure in an attempt to increase cerebral blood supply. Catecholamine-induced tachycardia and hypertension continue until the body depletes its supply of catecholamines, resulting in the onset of hypotension. The hypotensive state persists unless catecholamine stores are replaced intravenously. Intropin (Dopamine) is the most common catecholamine used for this purpose, gen-

TABLE 26–3 Summary of Organ Donor Management

Functional Instability	Management
Hemodynamic	Problem: Hypotension
	Goal: Systolic blood pressure greater than 100 mm Hg is desired (Systolic blood pressure greater than 90 mm Hg may be acceptable)
	Therapy: IV catecholamine therapy—Intropin (Dopamine) most common choice; norepinephrine, neosynephrine, or epinephrine drip may be used if Intropin therapy is inadequate
Thermoregulatory	Problem: Hypothermia (occasionally hyperthermia)
	Goal: Maintain body temperature at 96°F to 100°F (35.6°C to 37.8°C)
	Therapy: Warming blanket (hypothermia); cooling blanket (hyperthermia)
Fluid and electrolyte	Problem: Dehydration and electrolyte imbalances from diabetes insipidus (DI)
	Goal: Urine output maintained at 1 to 2 ml/kg per hour; maintain adequate electrolyte balance
	Therapy: Replace ADH if necessary (DDAVP or vasopressin); IV fluids: salt-poor IV fluids and avoid hypo-osmotic fluids; placement of central line or pulmonary artery catheter; close monitoring and replacement of fluid and electrolytes
Pulmonary	Problem: Neurogenic pulmonary edema
	Goal: Maintain Pao$_2$ above 100 mm Hg
	Therapy: Mechanical ventilation; positive end-expiratory pressure (PEEP); bronchodilator (if bronchospasm is present)
Hematopoietic	Problem: Coagulopathy
	Goal: Maintain adequate hematopoietic status
	Therapy: Monitor Hgb/Hct; PT, PTT and INR; replace blood as necessary
Endocrine	Problem: Loss of thyroid hormone and cortisol production; decreased insulin production
	Goal: Maintain adequate hormone levels
	Therapy: Replace hormones as necessary—thyroid protocol: IV bolus of levothyroxine (T4), solumedrol, insulin, and 50 percent dextrose followed by continuous T4 intravenous infusion

erally correcting the patient's hypotension. However, if intropin therapy is not successful in achieving an acceptable arterial blood pressure, initiation of norepinephrine, neosynephrine, or epinephrine may be necessary. In an adult, a systolic blood pressure of 100 mm Hg is desired, although 90 mm Hg is acceptable. If the hypotension is not successfully treated, cardiac standstill is imminent, which compromises organ donation. The development of hypotension after a period of hypertension is a late sign in the brain death sequence of events and is referred to as the *herniation picture*, usually indicating brain death.

Loss of Thermoregulation

As brain death progresses the hypothalamus is destroyed and the patient can no longer regulate body temperature. Hypothermia is seen most often and warming must be initiated. If left untreated, hypothermia can cause cardiac dysrhythmias and cardiac standstill. Occasionally, hyperthermia develops and cooling blankets must be employed. Hyperthermia results in vasodilatation and worsening hypotension if untreated. The temperature should be maintained at 96°F to 100°F (35.6°C to 37.8°C).

Fluid and Electrolyte Instability

As the pituitary gland ceases functioning, antidiuretic hormone (ADH) is no longer secreted. The absence of ADH results in diabetes insipidus (DI). Symptoms of DI include urine outputs greater than 4 mL/kg/hr, urine specific gravity of less than 1.005, and urine osmolality of less than 300 mOsm/kg. Placing a central line or pulmonary artery catheter can be helpful in the measurement and treatment of adequate fluid replacement. Replacement of ADH may be necessary to manage an appropriate fluid balance. Desmopressin acetate (DDAVP) or vasopressin is the usual drug of choice in treating DI. Urine output should be maintained at 1 to 2 mL/kg/hr.

When DI is present, choosing the correct IV fluid can be challenging. IV fluids need to be salt poor. If large amounts of dextrose-containing IV fluids are used, a hyperosmolar diuresis can develop; therefore, serum glucose levels must be closely monitored and treated appropriately. Care should be taken to avoid hypo-osmotic fluids, such as sterile water, because administration of large volumes of this type of fluid can result in rhabdomyolysis (renal damage caused by myoglobin). The rapid loss of urine from diabetes insipidus can result in significant electrolyte and acid–base imbalances. Potassium, calcium, phosphorus, and magnesium are lost, whereas sodium is retained. Unresolved hypernatremia eventually causes liver dysfunction, which may result in primary liver nonfunction if transplanted. Serum electrolytes need to be closely monitored and replaced as necessary to maintain optimal cell and organ function.

Pulmonary Dysfunction

Occasionally, brain death may precipitate neurogenic pulmonary edema. This is characterized by rhonchi, pink frothy secretions, a decreasing PaO_2, and a normal to low central venous pressure (CVP). The chest x-ray shows "whited out" lungs. Judicious treatment with ventilator support is required, maximizing the FIO_2 and positive end-expiratory pressure (PEEP) to maintain the PaO_2 above 100 mm Hg. In addition, low tidal volumes are used to minimize alveolar damage. Bronchospasms are likely to occur in the acute burn patient who developed smoke-inhalation–related anoxia. In such cases, a bronchodilator may be indicated.

If symptoms of pulmonary edema are present but the CVP is high, the pulmonary edema is likely from fluid overload. To treat this problem, restricting fluids, administering diuretics, and discontinuing vasopressin may be necessary, which can cause pulmonary vasoconstriction.

Hematopoietic Dysfunction

Coagulopathies are common in the patient with a traumatic brain death. As brain death occurs, large amounts of tissue plasminogen activator, a thrombolytic enzyme, are released. Longterm hypothermia increases the likelihood of coagulopathy. Hemograms, prothrombin time (PT), partial thromboplastin time (PTT) and international normalized ratio (INR) should be monitored. Blood replacement should occur if needed.

Loss of Endocrine Function

Progressing brain death results in a loss of thyroid hormone production. In addition, cortisol production ceases and insulin production decreases. A combination of these processes causes a shift from aerobic to anaerobic metabolism. The myocardial cells become oxygen depleted and cellular death begins. OPOs now use a thyroid protocol to reverse this process. Levothyroxine (T4), solumedrol, insulin, and 50 percent dextrose are given in a bolus. A T4 drip is started and continued throughout the organ recovery process.

Preservation of Organs

A single donor may provide one or multiple organs and tissues. At a prearranged time agreed on by all the transplant teams involved, the donor is taken to the operating room and prepared for surgery. When the donor is brought to the OR, the chart must have the correct documentation present: date and time of the death declaration and the signed or recorded consent form. In addition, the hospital may require a signed death certificate or other documentation. The procedures followed in the OR are similar to any other surgery. The anesthesiologist monitors and maintains the donor's cardiopulmonary and renal status and the fluid and electrolyte balance throughout the organ recovery period. There may be more than one organ recovery team in the OR, with each team being responsible for recovering a particular organ or organ set. The donor's attending physician cannot be part of the recovery teams.

During the organ recovery surgery, the transplant surgeon(s) makes one incision from the suprasternal notch to the symphysis pubis. The surgeon inspects the donor for the presence of any unexpected disease, such as an undiagnosed cancer, and then begins the process of dissecting each organ from its surrounding anatomical structures. Once all of the organs are ready to be removed, cannulas are placed in the thoracic aorta, pulmonary artery, portal vein, and abdominal aorta. A clamp is placed on the aorta and perfusion of the organs begins with a cold preservation solution. The solution runs through each organ, removing the blood from the organ. This procedure slows the organ's metabolic rate and preserves it until the organ is transplanted. Once removed from the donor, the organ is packaged in the preservative solution and sterile triple bagged. It is then placed on ice and transported to the recipient's hospital. Table 26–4 lists the allowed cold ischemic times for each organ.

In summary, management of the donor prior to organ recovery focuses on maintenance of a stable hemodynamic status, optimal oxygenation state, normothermia, fluid and electrolyte balance, and prevention of infection. An organ donor may donate one or multiple organs. Organ recovery is performed by surgical teams in an operating room. Organs require careful handling and special preservation techniques, and they are cooled to decrease metabolic processes.

TABLE 26–4   Organ Preservation and Transplantation Time Frames

ORGAN	TRANSPLANTATION TIME FRAME (HRS)
Heart	4–6
Lungs	4–6
Liver	12–24
Pancreas	12–24
Kidneys	24–48
Small bowel	12–24

SECTION FOUR REVIEW

1. Major management goals in caring for the donor patient include (choose all that apply)
   1. maintaining a stable hemodynamic status
   2. maintaining infections at a minimum level
   3. maintaining fluid and electrolyte balance
   4. maintaining optimal oxygenation status
   A. 1 and 4
   B. 1, 3, and 4
   C. 2 and 3
   D. 1, 2, and 3
2. The most common underlying cause of hypotension in the donor is
   A. dehydration
   B. cardiac failure
   C. fluid overload
   D. increased systemic vascular resistance
3. Which of the following statements best reflects procedures related to organ recovery in the operating room?
   A. an anesthesiologist is not necessary
   B. the recipient's physician must be part of the recovery team
   C. only one organ recovery team can be present in the operating room
   D. the donor's physician is not part of the recovery team
4. The organ preservation method that is common to all organs is
   A. hypothermia
   B. concentration of electrolytes
   C. type of diuretic
   D. preservation formula

Answers: 1. B, 2. A, 3. D, 4. A

The Organ Recipient

SECTION FIVE: Immunologic Considerations

At the completion of this section, the learner will be able to explain the immunologic considerations of organ transplantation.

Histocompatibility

The term **histocompatibility** comes from the Greek word *histos*, meaning tissue, and the Latin word *compati*, meaning to sympathize with. Histocompatibility, then, refers to the ability of cells and tissues to live without interference from the immune system. In Section One, it was noted that, historically, histocompatibility problems lead to rapid tissue or organ rejection, thereby limiting successful long-term transplant results to those performed between identical twins. Why is histocompatibility so important in transplantation?

Sommer (2002) explains that major histocompatibility complexes (MHC) are special key molecules that allow the body to be able to distinguish self from nonself. In humans, MHC molecules are known as human leukocyte antigens (HLA). **Antigens** are defined as substances that are capable of eliciting the immune response. Antigens can be composed of foreign materials or they can exist as normal cellular components (such as MHC). **HLA antigens** are proteins found on chromosome six. They exist in pairs (called haplotypes) on the surface of cells and are genetically determined. MHC molecules that are involved in intracellular communication for self-recognition are classified into two groups: MHC I (or class I) antigens and MCH II (or class II) antigens.

MHC I (Class I) Antigens

The MHC I proteins have been labeled HLA-A, HLA-B, and HLA-C. They are found on the surface of essentially all nucleated cells (Sommer, 2002).

MHC (Class II) Antigens

The MHC II proteins have been labeled HLA-DR, HLA-DP, and HLA-DQ. They are primarily found on the cell surfaces of macrophages and B lymphocytes (Sommer, 2002).

The HLA antigens in the MHC I and II classes help the immune system distinguish self from nonself, functioning somewhat like "fingerprints" that are unique to the individual. Normally, the immune system is able to recognize its own HLA "fingerprint" as self, and the immune response is not triggered. HLA antigens are inherited; thus, each full sibling in a family will have some combination of HLA inherited from both biological parents. The closer the HLA antigen combination matches between two people, the more the "fingerprint" is recognized as self.

A multitude of combinations of pairings can occur; thus, complete HLA matching is virtually impossible with the exception of identical twins. Because full siblings share the same biological parents, they often have some degree of HLA matching. In contrast, cadaver organs are completely unmatched when chosen randomly for a **recipient.** For this reason, immediate family members most often make the best kidney transplant donors because they are more likely to have a better matched tissue type. Identical twins, however, have the same histocompatibility pairings and are, therefore, perfect HLA matches. In the case of identical twins, a transplanted tissue or organ is recognized as having a self-HLA fingerprint and is accepted into the recipient without an immune assault.

Donor–Recipient Compatibility Testing

Three common tests used to evaluate the compatibility of the donor's tissues to the recipient's are tissue typing, crossmatching, and ABO typing.

Tissue Typing

Tissue typing refers to the identification of the HLA (histocompatibility) antigens of both the donor and the recipient. It evaluates the degree to which the two sets of tissues are HLA matched. The closer the HLA match is between the donor and the recipient, the better chance for long-term transplant success. The opposite is true, as well.

Crossmatching

Crossmatching tests the potential recipient for antidonor (preformed) antibodies. When such preformed antibodies are present, the patient is referred to as presensitized. Histocompatibility can be tested by evaluating the degree of reactivity of the immune response to crossmatch testing of donor and recipient cells and serum. When a serum crossmatching is performed, a sample of the recipient's serum is subjected to the serum of a sample of the prospective donor's blood. The serum is analyzed for the formation of preformed antibodies (PRA). The normal value is 0 percent. A prospective crossmatch is performed immediately prior to the transplant on those patients with a PRA of 10 percent or higher. In order to suppress the preformed antibodies, the patient awaiting a transplant may undergo one or more treatment modalities with plasmapheresis, intravenous immunoglobulin (IVIg), cyclophosphamide, mycophenolate mofetil, calcineurin inhibitors, and/or steroids (Ohler, 2002). A recipient can become sensitized to foreign HLA antigens through prior organ transplantation, blood transfusion, pregnancy, connective tissue disease, or mechanical assist devices used as a bridge to cardiac transplantation (Cupples et al., 2002). In such cases, the reintroduction of a new organ containing the sensitized HLA antigens can cause rapid organ rejection and possibly death.

ABO Typing

ABO typing identifies the blood group of the donor and the recipient. ABO compatibility is an initial criterion for transplantation. The rules for blood type matching are the same as for transfusions: Unmatched protein types will cause a rapid immune reaction. The type O allograft is considered the universal transplant donor type because it can be transplanted safely into a recipient with any blood type. Type AB is considered to be the universal organ recipient because it can receive an allograft from all blood types. Types A and B can only receive an allograft from their own blood type or type O donors. Table 26–5 summarizes ABO compatibility.

TABLE 26–5   Organ Donor and Recipient ABO Compatibility

COMPATIBLE POTENTIAL	
RECIPIENT'S BLOOD TYPE	DONOR'S BLOOD TYPE
A	A or O
B	B or O
AB (universal recipient)	A, B, or O
O	O only

In summary, histocompatibility is the ability of cells and tissues to live without interference from the immune system. HLA antigens are histocompatibility antigens found on the sixth chromosome. There are two classes of HLA antigens that are involved in self-recognition and, therefore, of interest to organ transplantation. HLA antigens are inherited, with a multitude of possible pairing combinations. Identical twins have the same HLA pairings; thus, they can donate and receive each other's organs without rejection problems. To ensure the best histocompatible match, donor–recipient compatibility testing is performed. Three tests are usually performed, including tissue typing, crossmatching, and ABO typing.

SECTION FIVE REVIEW

1. Histocompatibility antigens are also known as
   A. monocytes
   B. macrophages
   C. human leukocyte antigens
   D. polymorphonuclear lymphocytes
2. HLA antigens are located on (in) the cell
   A. surfaces
   B. nucleus
   C. cytoplasm
   D. mitochondria
3. The best histocompatibility matching is found between
   A. siblings
   B. identical twins
   C. parent and child
   D. fraternal twins
4. The identification of the histocompatibility antigens of both the donor and the recipient is called
   A. crossmatching

B. ABO typing
C. antigen classifying
D. tissue typing

5. A recipient can become sensitized to foreign HLA antigens through which of the following ways? (choose all that apply)
   1. pregnancy
   2. donating blood
   3. prior organ transplantation
   4. receiving blood transfusions

   A. 2, 3, and 4
   B. 1, 3, and 4
   C. 1 and 3
   D. 3 and 4

Answers: 1. C, 2. A, 3. B, 4. D, 5. B

SECTION SIX: Determination of Transplant Need

At the completion of this section, the learner will be able to describe the determination of transplant need. Scarcity of organ resources and the physical and financial costs involved make determination of transplant need a major issue. In March of 2005, there were 87,679 patients on the waiting list for transplants (UNOS, 2005). Depending on the type, transplant surgery can cost between $60,000 and $300,000 or more. The cost of antirejection drugs can exceed $12,000 per year (Hauboldt & Ortner, 2002).

The choice of who will receive an organ is not a simple one. Hundreds or possibly thousands of patients are on the national waiting list for the same organ at any one time. Organs are allocated to recipients based on a point system established by UNOS.

Determination of Need

The criteria used for determination of need are multifaceted. Specific guidelines vary among transplant programs, but the general guidelines are fairly consistent and include end-stage organ failure, short life expectancy, severe functional disability, no additional serious health problems, and psychological readiness.

End-stage organ disease is the primary indicator for transplantation need and is established by evaluation of organ function. The short life expectancy criterion is generally considered 6 to 12 months. Measurement of functional disability evaluates the potential recipient's ability to lead a reasonable lifestyle (e.g., ability to work or perform activities of daily living). This can be evaluated by interviewing the patient and family, observation, and cardiopulmonary exercise testing. Psychological readiness is established through interviewing, assessing known history, and possible psychological testing. Because of the highly stressful nature of transplantation, the presence of additional serious medical problems increases the risk of postoperative complications and is associated with a higher mortality rate.

Transplant Recipient Evaluation

The patient is considered as a potential transplant candidate only after maximum medical therapy has become ineffective, leaving transplantation as the final option. Evaluation of the potential recipient is an extensive process. Many factors must be thoroughly evaluated prior to placing the patient on the UNOS national patient waiting list for organ transplantation. These factors usually include the potential recipient's clinical, nutritional, psychological, and financial status.

Clinical Status

Organ-specific diagnostic studies and laboratory testing are conducted; preexisting or concurrent medical problems (risk factors for transplantation) are closely scrutinized and discussed with the patient and family. Table 26–6 summarizes the common major studies and tests for organ transplantation preparation.

Nutritional Status

Malnourished patients awaiting an organ transplant are at high risk for perioperative complications such as wound infection, graft failure, cytomegalovirus (CMV) infection, and bacterial infection. Nutritional intervention is crucial in the pretransplant stage and may even require enteral or parenteral feedings. Assessments should include regular physical assessments, weights, anthropometric measurements, and laboratory tests. The

TABLE 26–6 Common Organ Evaluation Studies and Tests

ORGAN	STUDIES/TESTS
All organs	**Immune specific**
	ABO, HLA tissue typing, presensitization, crossmatching, HIV profile
	General
	Complete blood count with differential, blood chemistries, coagulation studies, urinalysis
	Cardiovascular
	ECG, echocardiogram, cardiac catheterization (if risk for heart disease)
	Radiographic
	Chest x-ray
	Other
	Blood typing and crossmatching, examination and testing for infection (e.g., culturing of blood, urine, etc.), viral titers, tuberculin skin tests, colonoscopy, gender specific tests (PSA, mammogram, PAP smear)
Kidneys	**Radiographic**
	Gastrointestinal x-rays, abdominal ultrasound, voiding cystourethrogram
Heart, heart–lung, and lung	**Cardiovascular**
	Endomyocardial biopsy (to rule out myocarditis and sarcoidosis), echocardiogram, cardiac catheterization
	Pulmonary
	Arterial blood gas, chest x-ray, pulmonary function testing, ventilation/perfusion scan, computed tomographic (CT) scan of chest, exercise testing
	Other
	Doppler study, legs duplex scan
Liver	**Laboratory Tests**
	Liver function tests, drug and alcohol screening tests
	Other
	Portal vein sonogram and doppler, abdominal CT scan, liver biopsy, endoscopic retrograde cholangiopancreatography (ERCP)
Pancreas	**Laboratory Tests**
	Pancreatic enzymes, hemoglobin A1c
	Other
	Nerve conduction studies, gastric emptying scan, ophthalmology exam
Small Bowel	**Laboratory Tests**
	Iron studies, lipid profile
	Radiographic
	Gastrointenstinal contrast studies, abdominal ultrasound
	Other
	Nutritional and metabolic assessments

severely malnourished and the severely obese patients represent the highest risk for perioperative complications (Hasse, 2002).

Psychological Status

Chronic illness and its treatment are known to have profound long-term psychological effects on the patient and family. These psychological effects may have an impact on the long-term success of the transplant. In addition, the stresses associated with organ transplantation can further strain the coping abilities of this population. For these reasons, the potential organ recipient, and possibly the family, will undergo a psychological evaluation. If problems are assessed, appropriate counseling is initiated.

Financial Status

The total cost of organ transplantation varies with the organ being grafted. Costs that are factored in include pretransplantation evaluation, interim transplantation, and posttransplantation care. Medicare, state medical programs, and private health insurance coverage vary widely. Coverage is often differentiated by the type of organ being transplanted. If financial resources are questionable, financial options are explored. In addition, the patient may be required to relocate close to the transplant center for a designated time period both pre- and posttransplant, adding an additional financial strain.

Once the decision is made to accept a patient as a suitable recipient, the patient's name and vital information are entered into the computer bank at the United Network for Organ Sharing. This organization is charged with distributing organs in an equitable and nondiscriminatory manner. The potential recipient remains on the UNOS organ waiting list until an organ becomes available.

In summary, scarcity of donor organs and the transplantation costs make determination of transplantation need a crucial issue. General guidelines to establish need include end-stage organ failure, short life expectancy, and functional disability. A person is considered for organ transplantation only after receiving maximum medical therapy. A potential recipient is evaluated in regard to clinical, nutritional, psychological, and financial status. Once need and eligibility have been established, the potential recipient's vital information is entered onto the UNOS national organ transplant waiting list.

SECTION SIX REVIEW

1. General guidelines for determination of organ transplant need include (choose all that apply)
    1. severe functional disability
    2. end-stage organ failure
    3. psychological readiness
    4. additional serious health problems
    A. 2, 3, and 4
    B. 1, 2, and 4
    C. 1 and 2
    D. 1, 2, and 3
2. The decision as to whether a person is placed on the organ transplant waiting list as a potential recipient is usually made by
    A. the patient/family
    B. a multidisciplinary committee
    C. the organ procurement team
    D. the potential recipient's physician

3. The determination of end-stage organ failure is primarily based on which of the following criteria?
    A. tissue biopsy
    B. patient history
    C. functional disability
    D. age/gender
4. A potential transplant recipient has his or her psychological status thoroughly assessed because
    A. there is a risk of posttransplant psychosis
    B. a depressed state is a major contraindication for transplantation
    C. there is a higher mortality associated with psychological distress
    D. stress associated with transplantation strains coping abilities

Answers: 1. D, 2. B, 3. A, 4. D

SECTION SEVEN: Posttransplantation Complications

At the completion of this section, the learner will be able to discuss the major complications associated with organ transplantation.

Although each type of organ transplant has many unique features, they also have commonalities; this is true also of organ transplant complications. Three major types of complications are associated with transplantation:

- Technical complications
- Graft rejection
- Immunosuppressant-related problems

Technical Complications

The technical procedures involved in performing the transplantation are not without risks. Three major groups of technical complications are associated with the surgical procedure: vascular thrombosis, bleeding, and anastomosis leakage.

Vascular Thrombosis

Vascular thrombosis is a fairly rare complication that usually develops during the early postoperative period. It refers to the development of a blood clot in the vascular system. As a complication of organ transplantation, it refers to a blood clot in the vasculature of the graft, often the major artery. The presence of a thrombosis may not be detected initially because the patient is frequently asymptomatic. Diagnostic tests may be performed soon after surgery (e.g., duplex ultrasonography) to assure arterial patency. Early detection and immediate thrombectomy are essential if the graft is to survive. Even then, the graft is at high risk for failure. Any delay in detection of thrombosis frequently leads to loss of the graft.

Bleeding

Postoperative transplantation bleeding is managed in a fashion similar to other postsurgery patients, with the exception of liver transplants. In the liver transplant patient, it is often difficult to differentiate bleeding that is secondary to coagulopathy associated with a dysfunctional liver from bleeding that has resulted from a surgical (technical) problem. Postoperatively, a transplanted liver may have some degree of coagulopathy present, which makes control of otherwise normal postoperative bleeding extremely difficult. The decision must be made as to whether to allow bleeding to continue until the coagulopathy resolves as liver function returns or whether to take the patient for exploratory surgery immediately under the assumption that the cause is surgical.

Anastomosis Leakage

The term **anastomosis** refers to the site at which the graft is sutured into the recipient. Problems at the anastomosis site usually occur 1 to 3 weeks following transplantation. The problem may be failure of the anastomosis to seal completely, usually at the epithelial layer, which results in leakage of fluids (e.g., urine following a postrenal graft, or air as in bronchial dehiscence). An anastomosis leak usually results from inadequate healing, possibly as a result of a deficient blood supply or steroid therapy. Anastomosis leaks usually require surgical exploration and repair.

Graft Rejection

Graft rejection refers to the activation of the immune response against a transplanted tissue or organ. It is the result of the body recognizing the new tissue as nonself, which then triggers an autoimmune system attack to eliminate the invader. Graft rejection is primarily the result of T lymphocyte and B lymphocyte activities. The three types of graft rejection are based on the time and speed of onset and are called hyperacute, acute, and chronic.

Hyperacute Rejection

Hyperacute rejection is a type III (Arthus) hypersensitivity response; that is, it is a humoral response in which the B lymphocytes are activated to produce antibodies. It occurs within minutes to hours following transplantation and results from the presence of preformed graft-specific cytotoxic antibodies. Because the antibodies are already formed, as soon as the graft is placed, the immune system recognizes the foreign tissue and increases graft-specific antibody production. In turn, the antibodies accumulate rapidly and trigger agglutination of platelets, activation of the complement system, and phagocytic activities. Fortunately, hyperacute rejection is now rare because of improved donor–recipient screening and matching procedures.

Acute Rejection

Acute rejection is characterized by sudden onset and usually occurs within days or months following the transplant. Acute rejection begins as a type IV hypersensitivity response; that is, it is a cell-mediated immune response in which the T lymphocytes and macrophages of the host attack and destroy the graft tissue. The graft's HLA antigens are recognized as foreign (nonself), thereby triggering T lymphocyte proliferation and attack. As the acute rejection continues, graft-specific cytotoxic antibodies are produced, which further aggravates the acute rejection process.

Chronic Rejection

Chronic rejection is a humoral immune response in which antibodies slowly attack the graft. Chronic rejection may begin at any time following transplantation and may take years to render the graft nonfunctional. The antibodies trigger the same immune response as seen with hyperacute rejection but at a very low level. In time, the organ becomes ischemic and dies.

Immunosuppressant-Related Problems

Immunosuppressants are the cornerstone to successful long-term transplantation. This group of drugs, however, is associated with side effects that can cause serious problems, such as infection, organ dysfunction, malignancy, and steroid-induced problems such as hyperglycemia.

Infection

Infection is a leading cause of death in posttransplantation patients, with specific infections occurring at different time intervals (Fig. 26–1). Common sources of infection include invasive tubes (e.g., indwelling catheters), pneumonia, abscesses, and

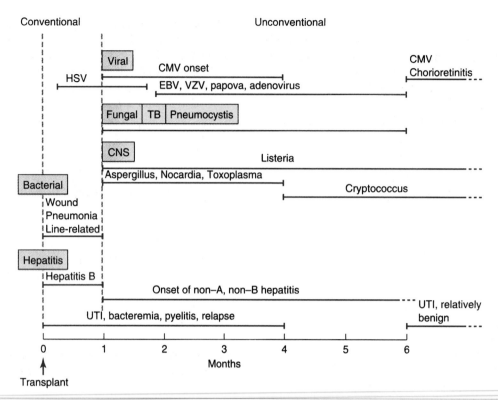

Figure 26–1 ■ Common temporal sequence of post transplantation infection. *(From Andreoli, T. E. (Ed.). (2001). Cecil essentials of medicine, (5th ed.) Philadelphia: W. B. Saunders, p. 299. With permission.)*

wound infections. Treatment of the infections with repeated runs of antibiotics may precipitate a superinfection (e.g., *Clostridium difficile* or *Candida*) or development of a resistant strain of bacteria such as ganciclovir-resistant CMV, methicillin-resistant *S. aureus* (MRSA), or vancomycin-resistant *enterococcus* (VRE) (Stitt, 2003). There is a particular risk for development of CMV infection. The CMV may have already been present in the recipient or it may have been introduced in conjunction with the transplant. CMV-seropositive patients may develop reactivation of the virus as a result of their immunosuppressed state. CMV infections may be mild or severe. A severe CMV infection can potentially cause dysfunction of multiple organs. This is especially a problem in seronegative recipients who received a seropositive organ or CMV-positive blood products. These patients receive CMV negative, leukocyte-filtered blood products (Cupples & Lucey, 2002). In addition, the recipient is at increased risk for development of opportunistic infections such as fungus (e.g., *Aspergillus*).

Infection is a major posttransplantation problem because immunosuppressant therapy compromises the immune system in some way. The immunosuppressed patient is unable to muster the same response to acute infection as a person who is immunocompetent; therefore, infection presents itself in more subtle ways. The primary symptom of infection in this population is the presence of a fever that is often low grade (about 100.5°F [38°C]). Other assessments may include tachypnea, fatigue, tachycardia, and pain. Development of a fever requires a

rapid but thorough search for the source of the infection and aggressive treatment. The lungs and urinary tract are the most common sources of nosocomial infection.

Organ Dysfunction

Almost all solid organ transplant patients receive a similar regimen of immunosuppressant therapy. Immunosuppressants are associated with multiple side effects, many of which target specific organs. Some degree of graft dysfunction is common immediately following organ transplantation. Development of nephrotoxicity and hepatotoxicity can occur with any organ transplant but are considered especially serious in kidney and liver transplants, respectively. The combination of the adverse effects of the drug and postgraft dysfunction may precipitate a severe graft crisis. Immunosuppressant therapy is discussed in Section Eight.

Malignancy

Patients on long-term immunosuppressant therapy are at increased risk for development of some form of malignancy. Malignancies that have been associated with organ transplantation include non-Hodgkin and other lymphomas, Kaposi's sarcoma, hepatobiliary and renal malignancies, skin tumors, and others. About 5 percent of renal transplant patients develop a malignant disease, which is about 100 times higher than is found in the general population (Bartucci, 1999).

Steroid-Induced Problems

Long-term steroid therapy carries with it multiple potentially serious side effects. Steroid-induced hyperglycemia, significant weight gain, and metabolic bone disease are common problems especially in the first year. Steroid therapy is discussed further in Section Eight.

In summary, three general types of complications are associated with solid organ transplantation: technical complications, graft rejection, and immunosuppressant-related problems. Technical complications include vascular thrombosis, bleeding, and anastomosis leakage. Graft rejection is due to T and B lymphocyte activities acting against the graft. There are three types of rejection: hyperacute, acute, and chronic. Immunosuppressant-related problems include infection, organ dysfunction, malignancy, and steroid-induced problems. Certain immunosuppressive agents have the potential of exacerbating organ dysfunction.

SECTION SEVEN REVIEW

1. Which of the following are examples of technical complications of organ transplantation?
   1. bleeding
   2. infection
   3. anastomosis leakage
   4. vascular thrombosis
   A. 2, 3, and 4
   B. 1, 3, and 4
   C. 1 and 3
   D. 2 and 4
2. Organ rejection that takes place within minutes to hours following transplantation and results from the presence of preformed graft-specific cytotoxic antibodies is called _____ rejection.
   A. subacute
   B. acute
   C. hyperacute
   D. chronic

3. Posttransplantation patients are at particular risk for developing a(n) _____ infection either from being seropositive prior to the transplant or by receiving a seropositive organ or blood transfusion.
   A. hepatitis A
   B. pneumonia
   C. cytomegalovirus
   D. wound
4. Posttransplant patients are at increased risk for development of malignancies secondary to

   _____.
   A. organ toxicity
   B. preexisting conditions
   C. underlying tissue incompatibility
   D. prolonged immunosuppressant therapy

Answers: 1. B, 2. C, 3. C, 4. D

SECTION EIGHT: Immunosuppressant Therapy

At the completion of this section, the learner will be able to describe immunosuppressant therapy. The long-term success of organ transplantation has been made possible by use of immunosuppressant therapy. Prior to the discovery and refinement of immunosuppressant therapy, tissue transplantation was considered only a very short-term therapy with the exception of identical twin grafts. This section presents an overview of some of the major drugs or drug groups that are administered for their ability to alter immune function.

Immunosuppressant drug therapy is carefully monitored by one of two methods to maintain therapeutic serum levels and prevent rejection while at the same time avoiding toxicity and infection. Cyclosporine and tacrolimus are concentration-controlled drugs, meaning dosage varies based on serum drug levels (Gelone & Lake, 2002; Humar & Matas, 2001; Smith, 2002). Mycophenolate mofetil (MMF) and azathioprine are dose-controlled drugs with a standard dose being delivered on a routine basis; however, dosage may be changed if the patient experiences significant changes in routine laboratory tests or clinical condition (Gelone & Lake, 2002; Humar & Matas, 2001; Smith, 2002). Sirolimus dosage is based on both the standard dosing and the serum drug level. Significant drug interactions can also develop, necessitating changes in immunosuppressant drug dosage. Other factors that can affect the dosing regimen include the organ type, the transplant center, rejection status, and the transplant date.

Cyclosporine

Cyclosporine (CyA or CsA), a unique drug of fungal origin, is the major immunosuppressant agent for prevention of allograft rejection. Cyclosporine's powerful immunosuppressant activities are directed against the helper T cells without affecting other types of immune cells, such as macrophages, B cells, granulocytes, and suppressor T cells. The high degree of specificity of cyclosporine allows the immune system to maintain some degree of protection from infection, especially bacterial infections. Cyclosporine may be used as sole or combination therapy in prevention of rejection (Barbuto et al., 1999). It is also an effective agent in treating graft-versus-host syndrome. Cyclosporine acts, in part, by blocking the production of interleukin-2 and interluekin-3 (IL-2, IL-3). It is associated with multiple serious side effects, including hepatotoxicity, nephrotoxicity, neurotoxicity, hyperglycemia, hirsutism, and gingival hyperplasia, among others. Three formulations of cyclosporine are Sandimmune, Neoral, and Gengraf.

Corticosteroids

Corticosteroids are steroid hormones. Prednisone is a synthetic corticosteroid that is commonly used as adjunct immunosuppressant therapy following organ transplantation. Corticosteroids have both anti-inflammatory and immunosuppressant capabilities. In the posttransplant patient, corticosteroids are administered primarily for their immunosuppressant activities. They significantly decrease the number of lymphocytes, particularly T lymphocytes, by interfering with the production and secretion of interleukin-2. In addition, large doses of corticosteroids suppress B lymphocyte production, particularly immunoglobulin G (IgG) and IgA, and significantly impair monocyte–macrophage function. Steroid therapy is useful for prevention of rejection and is used in rescue therapy for organ rejection; however, long-term use is associated with severe bone disorders, diabetes mellitus, and cataracts. Steroid therapy, when used postoperatively to prevent rejection, has been associated with certain complications, such as decreased wound healing and increased risk of dehiscence, or tearing of the anastomosis.

Antimetabolites

Antimetabolites, or **cytotoxic agents,** are drugs that have the capability of destroying target cells. Certain drugs target immunocompetent cells and thus are of use as immunosuppressants. Two commonly used cell cycle-specific cytotoxic agents are azathioprine and mycophenolate.

Azathioprine

Before the introduction of cyclosporine, azathioprine (AZA) was the drug of choice for prevention of graft rejection. Now it mainly has been replaced by MMF or sirolimus as part of combination immunosuppressant therapy. Azathioprine is a derivative of 6-mercaptopurine. It inhibits DNA and RNA synthesis, which ultimately causes suppression of cell-mediated immunity. Azathioprine primarily targets T lymphocytes but has some effect on B cells and, therefore, exerts a degree of inhibition on the humoral immune response. Its action is not specific to lymphocytes and can also inhibit proliferation of all blood cell lines; therefore, the patient can develop anemia and thrombocytopenia, as well as leukopenia. A common product name for azathioprine is Imuran.

Mycophenolate Mofetil

A newer drug than azathioprine, mycophenolate (MMF) is a less toxic alternative to AZA therapy. According to Bush (1999), MMF is produced from penicillin mold. It interferes with cell proliferation by inhibiting deoxyribonucleic acid (DNA) and ribonucleic acid (RNA) synthesis. B and T cell lymphocytes are targeted. MMF has been shown to be more effective than azathioprine in preventing acute rejection and is effective in rejection rescue therapy. The primary side effects of MMF are gastrointestinal, such as nausea and diarrhea. It also causes inhibition of all blood cell lines, causing anemia, thrombocytopenia, and leukopenia. A common product name for mycophenolate is CellCept.

Antibodies

Several preparations have been produced specifically as anti-lymphocyte antibodies. There are two major antibody preparations: monoclonal and polyclonal antibodies. Both types of antibodies are formed from foreign proteins that may cause recipient antibodies to form against them, resulting in sensitization of the patient and possible development of serum sickness or anaphylactic reactions (Barbuto et al., 1999). Monoclonal and polyclonal antibodies should be used as repeated therapy in sensitive individuals.

Monoclonal Antibodies

Monoclonal antibodies (mAb) were developed, in part, to increase the specificity of attack by targeting the lymphocyte subsets responsible for the immune rejection reaction. Ideally, this would allow the majority of the immune system to remain intact. Muromonab-CD3 (OKT3), a murine antihuman-CD3 monoclonal antibody, is the primary agent currently in use, although two new induction agents have recently been added to the immunosuppressant drug arsenal. OKT3 specifically targets a surface antigen (T3) located on mature T lymphocytes and forms antibody–antigen complexes, which render the T3 nonfunctioning. It can be used as rescue therapy during acute rejection or as a prophylactic antirejection agent during the early posttransplantation period (Bush, 1999; Smith, 2002).

Basiliximab (Simulect) and Daclizumab (Zenapax) are the latest monoclonal antibodies available and are currently used for induction therapy. The IL-2 receptor antagonists are modified monoclonal antibodies with most of the murine portion replaced with human antibody component (Gelone & Lake, 2002; Smith, 2002). Both bind to and block the interleukin-2 receptor alpha subunit on the surface of activated T cell lymphocytes (Gelone & Lake, 2002; Pirsch et al., 2003; Smith, 2002). Unlike OKT3 the IL-2 receptor antagonists do not trigger the cytokine-release syndrome (CRS), have relatively mild side effects, and exhibit no drug interactions (Gelone & Lake, 2002; Humar & Matas, 2001).

Cytokine-release syndrome (CRS) is a reaction that is associated with initiation of monoclonal antibody therapy, particularly OKT3. When first described, it was called "first-dose response" because it typically develops within the first hour following the initial dose of OKT3. CRS is caused by the release of cytokines following an initial activation of T lymphocytes (Bush, 1999; Smith, 2002). Cytokines are cell mediators that are responsible for cell function and growth regulation. CRS can be mild or life threatening. Severe flulike symptoms are the most common, such as chills, fever, and headache. Additional symptoms may include nausea, vomiting, and diarrhea. CRS symptoms usually diminish with each day of treatment. Severe symptoms are rare and may include pulmonary edema, hypotension, neurotoxicity, nephrotoxicity, and thrombosis. Premedication with diphenhydramine, methylprednisolone, and acetaminophen is usually given 30 minutes prior to OKT3 administration. Symptoms typically disappear after 2 to 3 days of therapy.

Polyclonal Antibodies

Polyclonal antibodies, such as antithymocyte globulin (ATG) or antilymphocyte globulin (ALG), are usually produced by immunizing animals with human lymphocytes or thymocytes. If cells from the thymus gland are used, the resulting preparation is called "antithymocyte serum," which is used to produce ATG. If cells from human lymphocytes are used, the resulting serum preparation is called "antilymphocyte serum" and the antibody is ALG. Polyclonal antibodies particularly target T lymphocytes and are used primarily for treatment of graft rejection, but can be used prophylactically in the immediate posttransplant period. Atgam and Thymoglobulin are the only preparations available.

Macrolide Antibiotics

Macrolides are a class of antibiotics like erythromycin and clarithromycin that bind to cell membranes and cause changes in protein function leading to bacteria cell death. The two immunosuppressant drugs in this class, Tacrolimus and Sirolimus, inhibit T cell proliferation suppressing the immune response.

Tacrolimus (FK 506, Prograf)

Tacrolimus is an immunosuppressive antibiotic that was originally derived from a soil fungus. Although it is unrelated to cyclosporine, it acts in a similar fashion in its attack on helper T lymphocytes. Tacrolimus was first approved for prevention of liver transplant rejection and is now also being used in renal transplantation. Tacrolimus therapy has been associated with new onset diabetes mellitus that may be reversible once therapy has been ended.

Sirolimus (Rapamune)

Sirolimus, approved in 1999, is a macrolide antibiotic originally developed as a potential antifungal drug. Similar to tacrolimus it blocks T and B cell cytokine proliferation. This drug rarely causes nephrotoxicity, neurotoxicity, or hyperglycemia. Hyperlipidemia is the most notable side effect, especially when paired with CsA and prednisone. Concomitant use with CsA potentiates the nephrotoxicity effect of CsA leading the manufacturer to recommend that Sirolimus be given 4 hours after CsA.

In summary, immunosuppressant therapy is the major reason for long-term graft success. Immunosuppressants may inhibit T cell or B cell function, or both. A newer group of drugs, monoclonal antibodies, exerts their immunosuppressant attack very specifically, thus leaving more of the immune system intact. Currently, monoclonal antibodies are used for short-term therapy. CRS is a potentially serious phenomenon associated with monoclonal antibody therapy, particularly OKT3. Symptoms usually disappear within several days of initiation of therapy. Fairly new to the immunosuppressive agent arsenal are tacrolimus and sirolimus, classified as immunosuppressive antibiotics.

SECTION EIGHT REVIEW

1. The immunosuppressant that selectively acts against the helper T cells without affecting other types of immune cells is
   A. corticosteroids   C. cyclosporine
   B. azathioprine   D. OKT3
2. Long-term posttransplantation steroid therapy is particularly associated with potentially severe _____ disorders.
   A. heart   C. liver
   B. bone   D. blood
3. The major gastrointestinal side effect common to almost all immunosuppressant drugs is
   A. nausea and vomiting
   B. heartburn
   C. abdominal cramping
   D. constipation
4. Monoclonal antibodies are unique in that they target
   A. B cells
   B. helper T lymphocytes
   C. suppressor T lymphocytes
   D. specific lymphocyte subsets
5. The MOST common symptoms associated with CRS include which of the following?
   A. chills   C. diarrhea
   B. vomiting   D. hypotension

Answers: 1. C, 2. B, 3. A, 4. D, 5. A

SECTION NINE: Overview of Selected Organ Transplantation

At the completion of this section, the learner will be able to discuss the general concepts related to transplantation of selected organs, including postprocedure management implications.

This section presents a brief overview of selected solid organ transplants, including kidney, heart, heart–lung, lung, liver, pancreas, pancreas–kidney, and small intestine. Postprocedure management and evaluation of organ function are also discussed.

Kidney Transplantation

Kidney transplants have been in the literature since the early 1930s, when a kidney was transplanted into the thigh of a young woman in Russia. Today, kidney transplants are a highly successful mode of therapy. A diagnosis of end-stage renal disease (ESRD) does not necessitate renal transplantation because dialysis can be used as an alternative therapy for ESRD. A patient who is being considered for transplantation is carefully screened to determine whether the probability of a successful transplant is sufficient to warrant transplantation rather than continuing use of dialysis. When a renal transplant is successful, it is significantly less costly than long-term dialysis therapy.

Major Indications for Transplantation

ESRD is the primary indicator for a renal transplant. ESRD can result from many problems, the three most common causes being hypertension, diabetes mellitus, and glomerulonephritis. These three conditions comprise more than half of all causes of ESRD. As of March 2005, there were more than 65,000 patients on the national waiting list for renal transplants (UNOS, 2005).

Preparation of the Recipient

When a kidney becomes available, the recipient is admitted to the hospital and pretransplant orders are initiated. Admission may be the day before a scheduled surgery if there is a living donor. If a cadaver donor is made available, preparatory time is much shorter. On notification, the patient is admitted to the transplant center, with surgery rapidly following the admission. Preoperative hemodialysis is often performed to normalize fluid and electrolyte balance. Before the patient goes to surgery, cross-matching is performed. If the results are negative, an initial dose of an immunosuppressant and prophylactic antibiotics are administered either before or after the patient is transferred to the operating room. Figure 26–2 provides an illustration of a renal transplant.

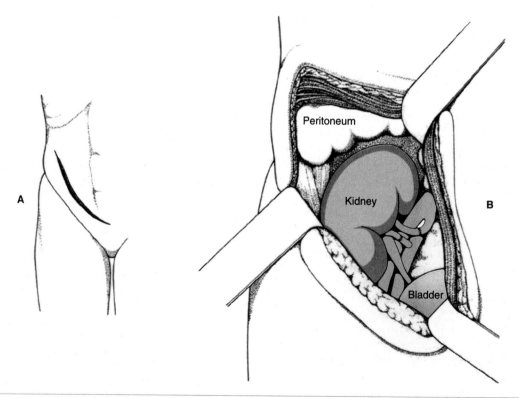

Figure 26–2 ■ Placement of the renal graft into iliac fossa. *A.* The incision is depicted for the right side of the abdomen, representing graft implantation in the right iliac fossa. *B.* The iliac vessels exposed. *(From Smith, S. L. (1990). Tissue and organ transplantation: Implications for professional nursing practice [p. 190]. St. Louis: Mosby Year Book.)*

Postoperative Management

Following transplantation, the patient is monitored closely for the first 24 hours, often in an intensive care setting. Medical and nursing priorities depend on the level of graft function and development of any complications. Typical postoperative orders for the first 24 hours include the following:

- IV fluids at a rate sufficient to keep urine output greater than 100 mL/hr; rate may also be titrated based on hourly urine outputs
- Diuretic therapy
- Daily weights
- Vital signs and central venous pressure readings
- Prophylactic antibiotic therapy
- Close monitoring of:
  - laboratory values: serum creatinine trends, electrolytes (particularly potassium, sodium, bicarbonate, calcium, and phosphorous), hemoglobin and hematocrit, serum glucose, blood urea nitrogen (BUN), arterial blood gases (ABGs), and white blood cell (WBC) count
  - intake and output balance with hourly urine output
  - blood clots, which can obstruct the urinary catheter
  - signs and symptoms of fluid volume excess
  - signs and symptoms of acute infection
- blood levels of immunosuppressant drugs (e.g., CsA, tacrolimus, and sirolimus)

Graft dysfunction is more commonly noted in cadaver grafts than in live ones. In the cadaver transplant, organ ischemia is more likely a result of the increased length of time the organ was preserved. Renal ischemia may lead to acute tubular necrosis, which causes oliguria or anuria. If the dysfunction lasts more than 48 hours, hemodialysis may be necessary until the graft begins functioning sufficiently. Recovery of the graft takes approximately 2 weeks.

Hypertension is a common problem in the kidney transplant patient. This condition can be exacerbated during the postoperative recovery period because of fluid volume imbalances precipitated by the high volume of IV fluids used to maintain a high urine flow. Antihypertensive agents may be ordered preoperatively and postoperatively to maintain the blood pressure within an acceptable range for the patient.

Evaluation of Renal Function

In addition to laboratory tests, several other procedures can be performed to evaluate function of the renal graft. A needle biopsy using ultrasound is performed to examine renal tissue. This is considered the most valuable indicator of renal function. Ultrasound of the kidney may be ordered to look for hydronephrosis, obstruction, or collections of fluid. A renal scan using radioactive isotopes also evaluates renal function.

Postrenal Transplant Complications

General complications associated with organ transplantation are presented in Section Seven. The 1-year graft survival rate for cadaver renal transplants is about 88 percent, and for living-donor transplants the graft survival rate is about 95 percent (UNOS, 2005). The most common long-term complication of renal transplantation is graft rejection.

Heart, Heart–Lung, and Lung Transplantation

Dr. Christiaan Barnard performed the first heart transplant in 1967 in South Africa (Augustine & Masiello-Miller, 1995). The first single-lung transplant was performed by Hardy in 1963, and the first successful heart–lung transplant was performed at Stanford University in 1981 (Owens & Wallop, 1995). The early history of heart, lung, and heart–lung transplants was one of poor graft success rates. Organ rejection, inadequate healing, and infection were major obstacles to success. It was not until the late 1970s (heart) and early 1980s (lung and heart–lung) that technical and immunosuppressant therapy improvements made these transplants a successful surgical option. The introduction of the immunosuppressant cyclosporine played a major role in the eventual success of these transplants.

Major Indications for Transplantation

General criteria for determination of transplant need were presented in Section Six. Specific major conditions that are associated with heart, lung, or heart–lung transplantation are listed in Table 26–7. As of March 2005, there were about 3,200 patients on the heart transplant waiting list, about 3,800 patients on the lung transplant waiting list, and about 170 on the heart–lung waiting list (UNOS, 2005).

TABLE 26–7   Major Conditions Associated with Organ Transplantation

ORGAN	MAJOR CONDITIONS
Heart	Cardiomyopathy, valvular heart disease, ventricular aneurysm, viral myocarditis, congenital malformations, arteriosclerotic coronary artery disease
Lung	*Single lung:* End-stage pulmonary fibrosis, chronic obstructive pulmonary disease, pulmonary hypertension secondary to Eisenmenger's syndrome, primary pulmonary hypertension *Double lung:* Cystic fibrosis, bronchiectasis, primary pulmonary hypertension
Heart–lung	Primary pulmonary hypertension (no known cause), congenital heart disease, Eisenmenger's syndrome
Pancreas	Type 1 diabetes mellitus (end-stage pancreatic disease) with severe metabolic complications
Small bowel	Short gut syndrome (SGS) in Crohn's disease, trauma, mesenteric thrombosis, familial adenomatous polyposis (FAP), radiation enteritis, volvulus, gastroschisis, necrotizing enterocolitis (NEC), Hirschsprung's disease

Preparation of the Recipient

Once the patient has been found suitable for organ transplantation and he or she has been placed on the transplant waiting list, the major management focus becomes maintaining the patient's cardiac and/or lung status. If the patient lives any distance from the transplant center, he or she may be asked to find lodging close to the transplant center to be readily available. In some cases, the patient may carry a portable communication device to facilitate quick communication and availability.

During the waiting period, the patient may require multiple admissions into the hospital to control cardiac or respiratory failure problems. Health maintenance is promoted through rest; control of cardiac arrhythmias, heart failure, and sodium and fluid intake; and monitoring of drug therapy for therapeutic effects. Lung transplant candidates will have pulmonary function closely monitored and controlled through bronchodilators; IV diuretics; oxygen supplementation; steroid therapy; and pulmonary vasodilator therapy, such as prostacyclin to control pulmonary hypertension. Some heart patients may require more aggressive therapy, such as IV inotropic drugs; a pacemaker-cardioverter-defibrillator; or mechanical circulatory assistance, such as the intra-aortic balloon pump (IABP) or a left ventricular assist device (LVAD) as a bridge to transplantation. Unfortunately, some patients die before they can receive a transplant because of rapid worsening of heart or lung failure, or scarcity of organ resources.

When a donor organ is available, the recipient is immediately brought to the hospital and initially prepared with appropriate laboratory tests and a chest x-ray. Preoperative teaching is performed and the patient may receive an initial dose of immunosuppressant therapy and prophylactic antibiotics. Blood is drawn for a retrospective HLA crossmatch with the donor.

As part of the transplant teaching, the patient and family are informed that the surgery will not be performed until the donor organs have been examined and have been determined to be suitable for transplantation. More specifically, the patient is taken to the operating room and intubated but the incision is not made until the procurement team has visualized the organs to be transplanted and they have given the "go-ahead." If the donor organs are determined to be not suitable, the recipient surgery is canceled. Figure 26–3 provides an illustration of a cardiac transplant.

Postoperative Management

Postoperative management of the heart and heart–lung transplant patient is similar to that of all open-heart surgery patients with the exception of denervation of the transplanted heart. Loss of cardiac autonomic innervation alters the heart's ability to respond to hypovolemia, hypotension, exercise, and certain drugs (e.g., atropine) (Cooper, 2001; Kobashigawa, 2001). In addition, a resting tachycardia is usually present because of the lack of vagal innervation. These patients generally do not experience chest pain with cardiac ischemia and infarction. Typical postoperative management includes the following:

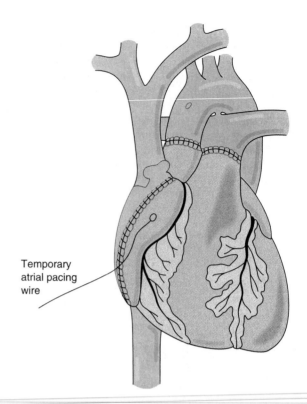

Temporary atrial pacing wire

Figure 26–3 ■ Cardiac transplantation. Suture lines connect donor and recipient atria, and then the great vessels are connected. *(From Copeland, J. G. [1984]. Modern techniques in surgery—cardiac thoracic surgery [pp. 66–75]. New York: Futura Publishing.)*

1. Maintaining or correcting problems associated with cardiac function and denervation, including
   - Hemodynamic and cardiac monitoring for cardiac failure, cardiac dysrhythmias, perioperative myocardial infarction, cardiac tamponade, and hemorrhage
   - Pharmacologic therapy based on cardiac status, possibly including diuretics, vasodilators, inotropic agents, and cardiac dysrhythmic agents
2. Maintaining or correcting problems with fluid and electrolyte balance, including
   - Monitoring intake and output balance and electrolyte trends
   - Intravenous fluid therapy titrated to fluid balance status and cardiac function status
   - Electrolyte replacement as indicated
3. Maintaining and correcting problems with renal function, including
   - Monitoring patient's urine output and renal laboratory value trends

The heart–lung and lung transplant patient is at risk for development of problems associated with pulmonary dysfunction. Denervation of the transplanted lung leads to impaired cough and mucociliary clearance resulting in infections, retained secretions, and mucous plugs (Schulman, 2001). Bronchoscopic exams, called "surveillance bronchoscopies," are often performed in the immediate postoperative period to remove retained secretions and mucous plugs, and visually assess the anastomotic site for possible dehiscence, necrosis, or stenosis. The following are management considerations related to the lungs and maintaining pulmonary function:

1. Monitor for signs and symptoms of respiratory insufficiency
   - Administer diuretic therapy
   - Fluid restriction
   - Early weaning from mechanical ventilator with reintubation, if required
   - Monitor fluid balance: intake and output, daily weights
   - Monitor ABGs, pulse oximetry, and Svo_2
   - Bronchodilator therapy, as required
   - Early ambulation
   - Incentive spirometry
2. Preventing infection
   - Strict aseptic suctioning technique
   - Aggressive postextubation pulmonary toilet
   - Cough and deep-breathing exercises
   - Incentive spirometry
   - Percussion and postural drainage
   - Early removal of invasive lines and tubes
   - Close monitoring of trends in temperature, chest x-ray, and peak expiratory flow. Although the white blood cell count will be monitored, it is anticipated that it will increase significantly for several days postop secondary to drug therapy

Evaluation of Organ Function

Postoperative organ function will be evaluated in a variety of ways, including laboratory tests, electrocardiograms, pulmonary function testing, and tissue biopsies. Organ rejection in the heart transplant patient may present as malaise, shortness of breath, new onset of peripheral edema, weight gain, or new onset of atrial fibrillation/flutter. Rejection in the lung and heart–lung transplant may be exhibited by shortness of breath, hypoxia, decrease in spirometry, elevated WBC, or a chest x-ray infiltrate (Nathan & Ohler, 2002).

The Biopsy

Heart Biopsy. A biopsy of the right ventricular wall is obtained approximately 1 week posttransplantation. A special device called an endomyocardial bioptome is inserted into the right ventricle by way of the right jugular vein (Fig. 26–4). The procedure is generally performed in the cardiac catheterization laboratory. The biopsy results can definitively indicate whether rejection is present and to what degree. Immunosuppressant therapy can then be adjusted to halt the rejection process. Biopsies are performed periodically to continue monitoring the graft status.

Lung Biopsy. Pulmonary tissue can be obtained by biopsy during a bronchoscopy procedure. In patients who have had a heart–lung transplant, the lung is usually biopsied first because rejection occurs more frequently in the lungs.

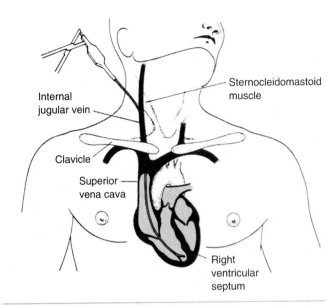

Figure 26–4 ■ Endomyocardial biopsy techniques. Transvenous biopsy approach through the right internal jugular vein. *(From Smith, S. L. [1990]. Tissue and organ transplantation: Implications for professional nursing practice [p. 219]. St. Louis: Mosby Year Book.)*

Liver Transplantation

Liver transplantation was first attempted in a human being in 1963 by Dr. Thomas Starzl. It was not until the early 1980s that the procedure became a long-term option. This change was largely because of the introduction of cyclosporine A, which rapidly increased graft survival rates to approximately 79 percent at 3 years posttransplantation (UNOS, 2005). Improvements in immunosuppressant therapy and better surgical and donor organ preservation techniques played important roles in increasing survival rates.

Major Indications for Transplantation

Three major liver problems that are referred for possible liver transplantation include patients with chronic irreversible liver disease, liver and biliary tree primary malignant tumors, and fulminant hepatic failure. Cirrhosis is the most common indicator for liver transplantation in adults. In children, indications include such disorders as biliary atresia, Alagille syndrome, and inborn errors of metabolism.

Preparation of the Recipient

As with other patients on the waiting list for organs, the waiting period is an extremely stressful period. Patients may experience anger, fear, depression, and hopelessness as their condition worsens. The patient and the family members need psychological support and possibly counseling during this period. When available, patients and their families may be encouraged to join a transplant support group at the transplant medical center.

The patient's hepatic function and nutritional status are monitored intermittently, usually including laboratory tests. The patient may require admission into the hospital for interim treatment if hepatic function decreases significantly. Preoperative teaching is often initiated during the waiting period because time is short once an organ becomes available for transplantation.

Alternative Transplant Approaches

Not all recipients receive an entire donor liver. Two alternative types of liver grafts may be used: split-liver transplants and living-related donor transplants. The split-liver transplant divides a single donor liver into two pieces to provide a graft for two recipients. Scarcity of resources and the fact that a small child recipient cannot take an entire adult donor liver triggered the original interest in split-liver transplants. The operation is extremely complex and a high morbidity and mortality rate has made this option a limited one at this time. The living-related donor transplant usually involves a donation from a parent to a small child.

Postoperative Management

Immediate postoperative management in the critical care unit focuses on prevention of complications, particularly those associated with liver dysfunction, abnormalities of fluid and electrolytes, infection, and rejection. Early management also centers on support of the other systems, such as cardiopulmonary, renal, gastrointestinal, and neurologic. The complexity of the liver transplant procedure places the recipient at risk for development of many complications. Nursing care in the intensive care unit setting requires intense multiple system monitoring and rapid analysis of abnormal assessment data.

In addition to the typical postoperative management associated with all transplant patients, the major management goal that is unique to liver transplantation is maintaining normal liver function, which includes the following assessments:

- Monitor bile drainage appearance and quantity
- Monitor laboratory tests that reflect liver function:
  - Prothrombin time (PT) and partial thromboplastin time (PTT)
  - Alanine aminotransferase (ALT) and aspartate aminotransferase (AST), alkaline phosphatase
  - Bilirubin (total and direct), ammonia levels
  - Glucose
- Monitor neurologic status

Evaluation of Organ Function

The general function of the graft is routinely monitored through laboratory testing. **Rejection** often presents itself as elevations in serum transaminases, bilirubin, alkaline phosphatase, and WBC count (Pirsch & Douglas, 2002). In addition, the patient may experience general malaise, a mild fever, disorientation, hepatomegaly, and right upper quadrant pain/tenderness. An ultrasound of the abdomen may be ordered to investigate the general condition of the liver. Liver biopsy, however, is the only means of making the definitive diagnosis of rejection.

Pancreas and Pancreas-Kidney Transplantation

William Kelly and Richard Lillehei pioneered human pancreas transplantation in 1966 at the University of Minnesota. Even though this allograft was unsuccessful, the nine combination kidney–pancreas transplants performed over the subsequent 2 years were successful. Because of the success of the dual-organ transplantation, pancreas transplantation was abandoned in favor of the kidney–pancreas transplant. The pancreas transplantation success rate has improved dramatically over the past decade because of improved donor selection and immunosuppressive therapy, advanced organ retrieval and preservation techniques, and modifications in pancreatic exocrine secretion management (Dimercurio et al., 2002; Papalois & Hakim, 2001; Pirsch & Stratta, 2001).

Major Indications and Types of Transplants

Type 1 diabetes mellitus is the leading cause of end-stage renal disease, blindness, and amputation. To date, pancreas transplantation is the single most effective physiologic method of controlling glucose metabolism, slowing the progression of end-stage organ disease and improving the quality of life in type 1 diabetes patients (Dimercurio et al., 2002; Cowan et al., 2002). The degree of nephropathy determines the type of pancreas transplant. Available options include simultaneous pancreas–kidney transplant (SPK), pancreas transplant alone (PTA), or pancreas transplant after a kidney transplant (PAK). Figure 26–5 provides an illustration of a simultaneous pancreas–kidney transplant surgery. In March 2005 there were more than 1,600 people waiting for a pancreas, more than 60,000 people waiting for a kidney, and more than 2,400 waiting for a combined kidney–pancreas (UNOS, 2005).

Preparation of the Recipient

Pretransplant care for the pancreas–kidney transplant candidate is similar to that for the patient awaiting a kidney transplant. Monitoring of common diabetic complications, such as nephropathy, retinopathy, and hyperglycemia, is followed closely by the transplant team. Depending on the degree of nephropathy present, the pretransplant patient may require renal dialysis prior to transplantation. Education is initiated during this period, focusing on the surgical procedure and method of exocrine drainage, immunosuppressant drugs, and organ rejection.

Postoperative Management

In the critical care unit, postoperative care focuses on prevention and treatment of infection, thrombosis, dehydration, meta-

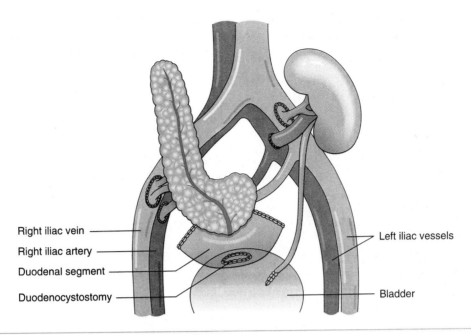

Right iliac vein
Right iliac artery
Duodenal segment
Duodenocystostomy

Left iliac vessels

Bladder

Figure 26–5 ■ Surgical technique of combined pancreas–kidney transplantation.

bolic acidosis, hyperinsulinemia, acute rejection, and graft dysfunction. In addition, management of pancreatic exocrine secretions (digestive enzymes) is essential to prevent and control enzyme-related complications. Use of the "systemic bladder" surgical technique predisposes the transplant patient to bladder infections, pyelonephritis, graft pancreatitis, and dehydration with intractable metabolic acidosis. The "portal-enteric" technique is more physiologic with normal carbohydrate and lipid metabolism. Fasting hyperinsulinemia and metabolic acidosis are avoided as are urinary tract infections, hematuria, and reflux pancreatitis. Postoperative monitoring includes

■ Serum glucose, amylase, HbA1c, C-peptide levels, CBC, and electrolytes
■ Urinary amylase levels if bladder drainage of exocrine secretions is employed
■ Hourly urine, nasogastric, and wound drainage measurements
■ Aggressive fluid volume and electrolyte replacement
■ Daily weights
■ Vital signs with central venous pressure readings
■ Observation for signs and symptoms of infection, especially urinary tract infections and pancreatitis
■ Hematuria
■ Serum drug levels to maintain therapeutic levels of immunosuppressant therapy (e.g., CsA, tacrolimus, sirolimus)

Graft dysfunction or loss may be attributed to thrombosis, pancreatitis, organ preservation, or surgical techniques. Typical signs and symptoms include pain/tenderness over the graft site, fever, elevated serum glucose and amylase levels, and decreased urinary amylase levels.

Evaluation of Organ Function

Early detection of pancreas rejection in the PAK and PTA transplant recipient remains difficult because of a lack of specific clinical markers. Signs and symptoms often mimic pancreatitis. Elevated laboratory values may be a result of drug toxicity, high dose steroids, and diuretic therapy. An elevated serum glucose occurs late in the rejection episode and is not considered a reliable indicator of rejection. The definitive diagnosis can only be made by ultrasound or CT-guided needle biopsy through a cystoscopy for bladder drained grafts or a percutaneous biopsy. In the SPK transplant a rise in the serum creatinine is an early indicator for kidney rejection and a surrogate marker for pancreas rejection because both organs reject at approximately the same time (Cowan et al., 2002; Dimercurio et al., 2002). In this case a kidney biopsy is performed to determine the grade of rejection.

Intestine Transplantation

Not until the introduction of tacrolimus in 1989 did small bowel transplantation emerge as a successful option for patients with permanent intestinal failure dependent on total parenteral nutrition (TPN). Prior to this time technical complications, sepsis from the intestinal bacterial load, and lack of effective immunosuppressive therapy against the massive lymphoid tissue prevented any long-term success. The small intestine is unique in that it is the largest immune organ in the body, is prone to infection because its contents are not sterile, and has no clinical tests to assess function of the transplanted organ (Murr & Sarr, 2001). As of March 2005 approximately 190 patients were waiting for an intestinal transplant (UNOS, 2005).

Major Indications and Types of Transplants

The major indication for intestinal transplantation is permanent and irreversible intestinal failure as a result of short gut syndrome, which is further divided into structural and functional failure. *Intestinal failure* is the inability of the gut to maintain sufficient nutrition, fluid, and electrolyte balance. *Functional failure* is associated with severe dysmotility of the gut leading to malabsorption and TPN dependency, such as chronic intestinal pseudo-obstruction syndrome (CIPS), congenital enteritis, and radiation enteritis. *Structural failure* results from trauma, bowel resection, or other abnormalities that shorten the length of the small intestine. Crohn's disease and necrotizing enterocolitis are examples of diseases that can eventually cause structural failure.

Currently, there are three types of surgical procedures performed, depending on the needs of the patient. The isolated intestinal transplant is indicated in irreversible intestinal failure accompanied by poor quality of life, failure to thrive, permanent dependence on TPN for survival, and limited central venous access for TPN therapy (Park, 2002; Williams et al., 2002). Combined intestinal and liver transplantation is necessary for patients with both irreversible intestinal failure and TPN-induced liver dysfunction/failure (Abu-Elmagd et al., 2001; Park, 2002; Williams et al., 2002). Global dysmotility of the GI tract results in the need for a multivisceral transplant (small bowel with liver, stomach, and/or pancreas).

Preparation of the Recipient

Once the patient is placed on the waiting list the focus shifts to maintaining optimum nutrition and preventing infection, especially at the vascular access site. TPN provides the needed caloric intake in addition to enteral and oral feedings, if tolerated. Blood chemistries, coagulation studies, liver function tests, and vitamin levels are assessed on a regular basis. Vascular line access for TPN therapy must remain patent and free of infection because these lines may be needed for several months posttransplant for ongoing nutritional therapy. Teaching begins with the patient and family to prepare them for prolonged daily management and care, and the change in body image associated with the ileostomy.

Postoperative Management

Postoperative management of the intestinal transplant patient presents a unique challenge to the ICU nursing staff in maintaining a balance between the appropriate level of immuno-

suppressive therapy and the predisposition to infections in the gut. In addition, denervation of the transplanted intestine has a significant effect on water and electrolyte absorption and motility function leading to diarrhea and malabsorption. Based on these issues, priorities in the immediate postoperative period include

- Strict intake and output including enteric output from the ileostomy, nasogastric tube, jejunostomy tube, and rectum
- Daily weights
- Vital signs and hemodynamic monitoring
- Assessment of postoperative ileus, which should resolve after 5 days
- Monitoring for rejection and infection
- Frequent monitoring of labs: electrolytes, vitamins, mineral and trace elements, protein, albumin, magnesium, bicarbonate, CBC, liver function tests
- Strict management of IV fluids to meet demands of stomal output
- Caloric support to meet the metabolic demands
- Maintenance of skin integrity around stomal site
- Daily monitoring of serum levels of immunosuppressive drugs (CsA, tacrolimus, sirolimus)

Evaluation of Organ Function

Unlike the kidney and liver transplants the intestinal transplant lacks a serum marker to suggest rejection. Clinically, patients may exhibit significant increase or decrease in stomal output, fever, decreased or absent bowel sounds, abdominal pain/distention, irritability, and/or change in stomal color. Surveillance endoscopy with tissue biopsy is performed as often as twice weekly through the ileostomy to diagnose rejection.

In summary, renal transplantation was the first transplant procedure to find widespread acceptance and success. The primary indication for renal transplant is end-stage renal disease. The early history of heart and lung transplantation was one of frustration and poor success rates. Graft survival rates have increased with improved technical skills and immunosuppressive therapy. Three major categories of patients undergo liver transplants: those with irreversible chronic liver disease, those with liver and biliary tree malignant tumors, and those with fulminant hepatic failure. As an alternative to transplantation of the entire liver, a partial organ transplant may be performed. Pancreas transplantation not only controls glucose metabolism and the chronic effects of diabetes mellitus but also can dramatically improve the patient's quality of life. The degree of diabetic nephropathy determines the type of transplant performed: simultaneous pancreas–kidney, pancreas only, or a pancreas transplant after a kidney transplant. Newer immunosuppressive drugs and improved surgical techniques have led to successful intestine transplantation.

1. The major indication for kidney transplantation is end-stage renal disease, which most commonly results from which problems? (choose all that apply)
    1. diabetes mellitus
    2. hypertension
    3. glomerular nephritis
    4. nephrotoxicity
    A. 2, 3, and 4
    B. 1, 3, and 4
    C. 1 and 2
    D. 1, 2, and 3

2. Dysfunction of a renal graft is most commonly associated with the
    A. preoperative condition of the donor
    B. preoperative condition of the recipient
    C. length of time the organ was preserved
    D. length of time required to perform the transplant

3. The most common cause of renal graft failure is
    A. rejection
    B. hypoperfusion
    C. hypertension
    D. nephrotoxicity

4. Major conditions that are associated with the need for heart transplantation include (choose all that apply)
    1. myocardial infarction
    2. congenital malformations
    3. ventricular aneurysm
    4. cardiomyopathy
    A. 2, 3, and 4
    B. 1, 2, and 3
    C. 1, 3, and 4
    D. 2 and 4

5. While the patient is waiting for a lung transplant, health maintenance particularly focuses on the _____ system.
    A. cardiopulmonary
    B. renal
    C. hepatobiliary
    D. neurologic

6. Postoperative management of the patient with a heart transplant includes the goal of preventing infection. Which of the following interventions most directly addresses this goal?
    A. early ambulation
    B. monitor urine output and laboratory trends
    C. monitor ABGs, pulse oximetry, SvO_2
    D. aggressive postextubation pulmonary toilet

7. Approximately 1 week following a heart transplant, a heart biopsy is performed to evaluate the recipient for
    A. anastomosis leak
    B. rejection
    C. infection
    D. ischemic tissue

8. Major indications for liver transplantation include (choose all that apply)
    1. fulminant hepatic failure
    2. acute hepatotoxicity
    3. malignant hepatic tumors
    4. irreversible chronic liver disease
    A. 1, 2, and 3
    B. 1, 3, and 4
    C. 1 and 3
    D. 2, 3, and 4

9. Liver transplant patients are at particularly high risk for development of which early complication?
    A. hemorrhage
    B. rejection
    C. infection
    D. obstruction

10. A split-liver type of transplant refers to
    A. a parent-to-small-child liver donation
    B. splitting normal from abnormal parts of liver
    C. dividing a cadaver donor liver between two recipients
    D. splitting lobes of a live donor liver between several recipients

11. Postoperative monitoring of liver function typically includes which of the following? (choose all that apply)
    1. bilirubin
    2. ammonia
    3. prothrombin time
    4. blood urea nitrogen
    A. 2, 3, and 4
    B. 1, 3, and 4
    C. 1 and 2
    D. 1, 2, and 3

12. The major indication for a pancreas transplant is
    A. type 1 diabetes mellitus
    B. end-stage renal disease
    C. diabetic retinopathy
    D. peripheral neuropathy

13. Use of the systemic bladder technique to manage the pancreatic exocrine secretions predisposes the recipient to which complications? (choose all that apply)
    1. graft pancreatitis
    2. thrombosis
    3. hematuria
    4. pyelonephritis
    A. 2 and 3
    B. 1, 3, and 4
    C. 1 and 3
    D. 1, 2, and 3

14. The most common complications in the immediate postoperative period of the pancreas transplant include (choose all that apply)
    1. hemorrhage
    2. metabolic acidosis
    3. hyperinsulinemia
    4. dehydration
    A. 2, 3, and 4
    B. 1, 2, and 3
    C. 2 and 3
    D. 1, 3, and 4

15. Clinical signs and symptoms of pancreatic graft dysfunction exhibited by the patient include which of the following? (choose all that apply)
    1. fever
    2. tenderness over graft site
    3. decreased serum amylase
    4. elevated blood sugar

A. 1 and 2
B. 2, 3, and 4
C. 1, 2, and 4
D. 1, 2, and 3

16. Irreversible intestinal failure is the primary indication for intestine transplantation. Which of the following conditions can result in intestinal failure?
    1. Crohn's disease
    2. gastroesophageal reflux disease
    3. radiation enteritis
    4. trauma to the intestine
    A. 1 and 3
    B. 1, 3, and 4
    C. 2 and 3
    D. 1, 2, and 3

17. Denervation of the transplanted small bowel results in
    A. malabsorption
    B. decreased caloric requirements
    C. constipation
    D. elevated serum sodium

18. The gold standard for diagnosing acute rejection in the intestinal transplant is
    A. a significant increase in the stomal output
    B. an ileus
    C. an endoscopic mucosal biopsy
    D. a change in stomal color

Answers: 1. D, 2. C, 3. A, 4. A, 5. A, 6. D, 7. B, 8. B, 9. A, 10. C, 11. D, 12. A, 13. B, 14. A, 15. C, 16. B, 17. A, 18. C.

 POSTTEST

The following Posttest is constructed in a case study format. A patient is presented. Questions are asked based on available data. New data are presented as the case study progresses.

Kathy S is a critically ill 23-year-old college student who recently sustained multiple trauma in a motor vehicle crash. The health care team is currently initiating evaluation of Kathy for establishing brain death.

1. If it is decided that Kathy may be a potential organ donor, she must be evaluated for suitability as a donor. Common criteria used to determine suitability include which of the following? (choose all that apply)
    1. presence of infection
    2. cardiac arrest resuscitation
    3. preexisting metastatic disease
    4. head trauma

A. 2, 3, and 4
B. 1 and 2
C. 1, 3, and 4
D. 1, 2, and 3

2. Potential donors such as Kathy are protected by law. The legislation that gives specific guidelines regarding how donation is to be carried out is the
    A. National Organ Transplant Act
    B. Uniform Anatomical Gift Act
    C. Uniform Determination of Death Act
    D. required-request legislation

3. Brain-death testing at the bedside is performed on Kathy. Required brain-death criteria include which of the following? (choose all that apply)
    1. Glasgow Coma Scale of 5
    2. negative ice calorics

    3. no doll's eye reflex

    4. no CNS depressants

  A. 2, 3, and 4

  B. 1 and 3

  C. 1, 2, and 3

  D. 2 and 3

4. The manner in which Kathy's family is approached about organ donation is important. It is suggested that her family not be approached until

  A. Kathy has been declared legally dead

  B. they have asked the physician about possible donation

  C. they have acknowledged that Kathy is brain dead

  D. it is determined whether Kathy has signed a uniform donor card

5. Prior to discussing donation with Kathy's family, she may have a preliminary evaluation performed by the donor procurement coordinator/team. Initial evaluation is performed primarily to

  A. save time

  B. evaluate for unsuitability

  C. guarantee suitability

  D. meet legal requirements

Kathy has been found suitable as a potential organ donor. Although her family has been in close contact with the physician and nurses, they are unable to be at Kathy's bedside for the next several days. They have expressed an interest in organ donation, but consent has not been given.

6. Kathy meets all of the criteria for brain death. The health care team is anxious to obtain consent to initiate donor supportive measures. Which of the following statements is correct regarding obtaining consent?

  A. any member of Kathy's family can come in to sign a consent form

  B. consent is not mandatory if the family is not available

  C. consent could be obtained over the telephone

  D. because Kathy has signed a uniform donor card, the family does not have to give consent

Kathy is now legally established as a donor.

7. As a donor, maintaining Kathy's fluid and electrolyte balance is a priority. Nursing interventions to accomplish this goal may include (choose all that apply)

    1. maintaining urine output at 20 to 25 mL/hr

    2. mL/mL replacement of urine output with IV fluid

    3. monitoring for therapeutic effects of Pitressin

    4. maintaining blood pressure above 90 mm Hg systolic

  A. 2, 3, and 4

  B. 1, 3, and 4

  C. 1, 2, and 3

  D. 2 and 4

Kathy is taken to the operating room for organ recovery to be performed.

8. Operating room procedures for donor organ recovery may include (choose all that apply)

    1. several recovery teams in the operating room

    2. Kathy's physician not in the operating room

    3. aseptic procedures not required

    4. the anesthesiologist performing functions

  A. 1, 3, and 4

  B. 2 and 3

  C. 1, 2, and 4

  D. 2, 3, and 4

Juan C, 46 years old, has a long history of chronic renal problems. He has been receiving hemodialysis for the past 5 years. Mr. C, his family, and his physician have been discussing the possibility of renal transplantation.

9. Mr. C has no siblings. Assuming that he eventually does undergo a renal transplant, he will most likely receive a(n) _____.

  A. autograft

  B. allograft

  C. isograft

  D. heterograft

10. Mr. C and his son (a possible kidney donor) have tissue typing done. Their HLA matching is likely to be

  A. partially matched

  B. identical

  C. totally unmatched

  D. unpredictable

11. Kathy's kidney is being considered for transplantation into Mr. C. He will have a sample of his blood subjected to a sample of Kathy's blood to check for preformed antibodies. This test is called

  A. antigen testing

  B. ABO typing

  C. tissue typing

  D. crossmatching

12. Mr. C has type A blood and Kathy's blood type is O. This combination of donor and recipient blood types is a(n)

  A. unacceptable match

  B. questionable match

  C. acceptable match

  D. ideal match

13. If Mr. C develops a technical type of complication associated with his kidney transplantation, it could include which of the following problems? (choose all that apply)

    1. urine leakage at the anastomosis site

    2. vascular thrombosis of the renal artery

    3. perioperative or postoperative bleeding

    4. type III hypersensitivity response

  A. 1, 3, and 4

  B. 1 and 3

  C. 2, 3, and 4

  D. 1, 2, and 3

14. If Mr. C develops a cytomegalovirus infection following the surgery, he would most likely develop it through
    A. incorrect suctioning procedures
    B. reactivation of preexisting CMV
    C. infiltration in wound infections
    D. contamination via invasive tubes
15. Mr. C is currently receiving cyclosporine (CyA). The major advantage of using this drug is that it
    A. affects only helper T cells
    B. directs its action against B cells
    C. is a cell cycle–specific cytotoxic agent
    D. has anti-inflammatory and immunosuppressant capabilities
16. If Mr. C is started on monoclonal antibody therapy, the nurse will need to monitor him closely for the first 48 hours for _____, in addition to the usual assessments.
    A. infection
    B. renal failure
    C. nausea and vomiting
    D. cytokine-release syndrome

Additional history on Mr. C: History of type 1 diabetes mellitus since age 5. Several episodes of staphylococcal pneumonia as a child. He is 5 foot 10 and weighs 150 pounds (68.2 kg). Several months ago, he was treated for a severe infection with gentamicin. He has a history of hypertension that has been well controlled with antihypertensive therapy.

17. Mr. C's end-stage renal disease most likely resulted from
    A. hypertension
    B. type 1 diabetes mellitus
    C. complications of staphylococcal pneumonia
    D. recent antibiotic therapy
18. If Mr. C develops failure of his transplanted kidney, it is most likely going to be because of
    A. nephrotoxicity
    B. hypertension
    C. hypoperfusion
    D. rejection

POSTTEST ANSWERS

Question	Answer	Section	Question	Answer	Section
1	D	Two	10	A	Five
2	B	Two	11	D	Five
3	A	Three	12	C	Five
4	C	Three	13	D	Seven
5	B	Three	14	B	Seven
6	C	Three	15	A	Eight
7	A	Four	16	D	Eight
8	C	Four	17	B	Nine
9	B	Two	18	D	Nine

REFERENCES

Abu-Elmagd, K., Reyes, J., & Fung, J. J. (2001). Clinical intestinal transplantation: Recent advances and future consideration. In D. J. Norman & L. A. Turka (Eds.), *Primer on transplantation* (pp. 610–625). Mt. Laurel, NJ: American Society of Transplantation.

Augustine, S. M., & Masiello-Miller, M. (1995). Heart transplantation. In M. T. Nolan & S. M. Augustine (Eds.), *Transplantation nursing: Acute and long-term management* (pp. 109–140). Norwalk, CT: Appleton & Lange.

Barbuto, J. A., Akporiaye, E. T., & Hersh, E. M. (1999). Immuno-pharmacology. In B. G. Katzung (Ed.), *Basic and clinical pharmacology* (7th ed., pp. 916–944). Norwalk, CT: Appleton & Lange.

Bartucci, M. R. (1999). Kidney transplantation: State of the art. *AACN Clinical Issues, 10*(2), 153–163.

Bush, W. W. (1999). Overview of transplantation immunology and the pharmacotherapy of adult solid organ transplant recipients: Focus on immuno-suppression. *AACN Clinical Issues, 10*(2), 253–269.

Cooper, D. K. C. (2001). Heart transplantation. In N. S. Hakim & G. M. Danovitch (Eds.), *Transplantation surgery* (pp. 91–121). London: Springer-Verlag.

Cowan, P. A., Wicks, M. N., Rutland, T. C., Ammons, J., & Hathaway, D. K. (2002). Pancreas transplantation. In S. L. Smith, *Organ transplantation: Concepts, issues, practice, and outcomes.* Medscape Transplantation, 2002.

Cupples, S. A., Boyce, S. W., & Stamou, S. C. (2002). Heart transplantation. In S. A. Cupples & L. Ohler (Eds.), *Solid organ transplantation: A handbook for primary health care providers* (pp. 146–188). New York: Springer-Verlag.

Cupples, S. A., & Lucey, D. R. (2002). Infectious diseases in transplant recipients. In S. A. Cupples & L. Ohler (Eds.), *Solid organ transplantation: A handbook for primary health care providers* (pp. 16–63). New York: Springer-Verlag.

Dew, M. A., Goycoolea, J. M., Harris, R. C., et al. (2004). An Internet-based intervention to improve psychosocial outcomes in heart transplant recipients and family caregivers: Development and evaluation. *Journal of Heart & Lung Transplantation, 23*(6), 745–759.

Dimercurio, B., Henry, L., & Kirk, A. D. (2002). Simultaneous kidney-pancreas transplantation. In S. A. Cupples & L. Ohler (Eds.), *Solid organ transplantation: A handbook for primary health care providers* (pp. 223–239). New York: Springer-Verlag.

Gelone, D. K., & Lake, K. D. (2002). Transplantation pharmacotherapy. In S. A. Cupples & L. Ohler (Eds.), *Solid organ transplantation: A handbook for primary health care providers* (pp. 88–130). New York: Springer-Verlag.

Hasse, J. (2002). Nutritional issues in adult organ transplantation. In S. A. Cupples & L. Ohler (Eds.), *Solid organ transplantation: A handbook for primary health care providers* (pp. 64–87). New York: Springer-Verlag.

Hauboldt, R. H., & Ortner, N. J. (2002). 2002 organ and tissue transplant costs and discussion. In *Milliman USA Research Report* (p. 23). Available at http://www.milliman.com/health/publications/research_reports/hrr_07-2002.pdf. Accessed December 15, 2003.

Humar, A., & Matas, A. J. (2001). Immunosuppressive drugs. In N. S. Hakim & G. M. Danovitch (Eds.), *Transplantation surgery* (pp. 373–393). London: Springer-Verlag.

Kobashigawa, J. A. (2001). Physiology of the transplanted heart. In D. J. Norman & L. A. Turka (Eds.), *Primer on transplantation* (2nd ed., pp. 358–362). Mt. Laurel, NJ: American Society of Transplantation.

KODA. (1994). Materials provided by Kentucky Organ Donor Affiliates (KODA). Lexington, KY: Author.

Maisonneuve, P., FitzSimmons, S. C., Neglia, J. P., et al. (2003). Cancer risk in nontransplanted and transplanted cystic fibrosis patients: A 10-year study. *Journal of the National Cancer Institute, 95*(5), 381–388.

Murr, M. M., & Sarr, M. G. (2001). Small bowel transplantation: The new frontier in organ transplantation. In N. S. Hakim & G. M. Danovitch (Eds.), *Transplantation surgery* (pp. 235–248). London: Springer-Verlag.

Murray, J. E. (1991). Nobel Prize lecture: The first successful organ transplants in man. In P. I. Terasaki (Ed.), *History of transplantation: Thirty-five recollections* (pp. 123–138). Los Angeles: UCLA Tissue Typing Laboratory.

Nathan, S., & Ohler, L. (2002). Lung and heart-lung transplantation. In S. A. Cupples & L. Ohler (Eds.), *Solid organ transplantation: A handbook for primary health care providers* (pp. 240–260). New York: Springer-Verlag.

Ohler, L. (2002). Appendix: Review of transplant immunology for community health care providers. In S. A. Cupples & L. Ohler (Eds.), *Solid organ transplantation: A handbook for primary health care providers* (pp. 394–400). New York: Springer-Varlag.

Owens, S. G., & Wallop, J. M. (1995). Heart–lung and lung transplantation. In M. T. Nolan & S. M. Augustine (Eds.), *Transplantation nursing: Acute and long-term management* (pp. 141–163). Norwalk, CT: Appleton & Lange.

Papalois, V. E., & Hakim, N. S. (2001). Pancreas and islet transplantation. In N. S. Hakim & G. M. Danovitch (Eds.), *Transplantation surgery* (pp. 211–233). London: Springer-Verlag.

Park, B. K. (2002). Intestine transplantation. In S. L. Smith, *Organ transplantation: Concepts, issues, practice, and outcomes*. Medscape Transplantation, 2002. Available at: http://www.medscape.com/viewarticle/436543. Accessed October 1, 2003.

Pirsch, J., Simmons, W. D., & Sollinger, H. (2003). Working guide to immunosuppression. In J. Pirsch, W. D. Simmons, & H. Sollinger (Eds.), *Transplantation drug manual* (4th ed., pp. 1–24). Georgetown, TX: Landes Bioscience.

Pirsch, J. D., & Douglas, M. J. (2002). Liver transplantation. In S. A. Cupples & L. Ohler (Eds.), *Solid organ transplantation: A handbook for primary health care providers* (pp. 261–291). New York: Springer-Verlag.

Pirsch, J. D., & Stratta, R. J. (2001). Pancreas and simultaneous kidney–pancreas transplantation. In D. J. Norman & L. A. Turka (Eds.), *Primer on transplantation* (2nd ed., pp. 501–511). Mt. Laurel, NJ: American Society of Transplantation.

Schulman, L. L. (2001). Physiology of the transplanted lung. In D. J. Norman & L. A. Turka (Eds.), *Primer on transplantation* (2nd ed., pp. 674–680). Mt. Laurel, NJ: American Society of Transplantation.

Siminoff, L. A., Burant C., & Youngner, S. J. (2004). Death and organ procurement: Public beliefs and attitudes. *Social Science & Medicine, 59*(11), 2325–2335.

Smith, S. L. (2002). Immunosuppressive therapies in organ transplantation. In S. L. Smith, *Organ transplantation: Concepts, issues, practice, and outcomes*. Medscape Transplantation, 2002.

Sommer, C. (2002). Immunity and inflammation. In C. M. Porth (Ed.), *Pathophysiology: Concepts of altered health states* (6th ed., pp. 331–355). Philadelphia: J. B. Lippincott.

Stitt, N. L. (2003). Infection in the transplant recipient. In S. L. Smith, *Organ transplantation: Concepts, issues, practice, and outcomes*. Medscape Transplantation, 2003.

UNOS [United Network for Organ Sharing]. (1993). Patients waiting for transplants. Richmond, VA: Author.

UNOS [United Network for Organ Sharing]. (2005). Critical data. United Network for Organ Sharing. Available at: http://www.unos.org/. Accessed March 13, 2005.

Williams, L., Horslen, S. P., & Langnas, A. N. (2002). Intestinal transplantation. In S. A. Cupples & L. Ohler (Eds.), *Solid organ transplantation: A handbook for primary health care providers* (pp. 292–333). New York: Springer-Verlag.

MODULE

27 Altered Glucose Metabolism

Diane Orr Chlebowy, Kathleen Dorman Wagner

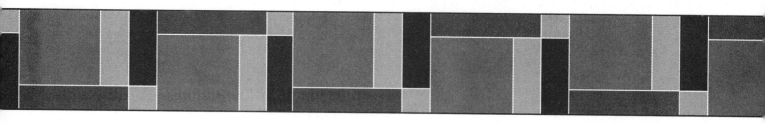

OBJECTIVES Following completion of this module, the learner will be able to

1. Discuss normal glucose metabolism.

2. Describe the effects of insulin on metabolism.

3. Explain the effects of insulin deficit.

4. Differentiate the two major types of diabetes mellitus.

5. Discuss the pathophysiology, clinical manifestations, and nursing care management of therapy-induced hypoglycemia.

6. Discuss the pathophysiology, clinical manifestations, and nursing care management of diabetic ketoacidosis.

7. Discuss the pathophysiology, clinical manifestations, and nursing care management of hyperglycemic hyperosmolar state.

8. Explain the use of exogenous insulin in the management of the client with diabetes mellitus.

9. Discuss the acute care nursing implications of chronic diabetic complications.

This self-study module focuses on physiologic processes involved in normal glucose metabolism, as well as the pathophysiologic basis of altered glucose metabolism. The three major diabetic crises are presented. Each is described in terms of pathophysiology, clinical presentation, and management. The module is composed of nine sections. Sections One and Two discuss normal glucose metabolism and the effects of insulin on metabolism. The focus then shifts to abnormal glucose metabolism. Section Three describes the impact of insulin deficit on metabolism. Section Four defines and then differentiates the two major types of diabetes mellitus (type 1 and type 2). Sections Five through Seven discuss the three acute life-threaten-

ing consequences of diabetes: therapy-induced hypoglycemia, diabetic ketoacidosis, and hyperglycemic hyperosmolar state. Section Eight reviews exogenous insulin therapy, focusing on types of insulin therapy used during acute illness. Finally, Section Nine presents an overview of chronic diabetic complications and their effects on the nursing management of the acutely ill patient. Each section includes a set of review questions to help the learner evaluate his or her understanding of the section's content before moving on to the next section. All Section Reviews and the module Pretest and Posttest include answers. It is suggested that the learner review those concepts answered incorrectly in the review questions before proceeding to the next section.

 PRETEST

1. Insulin promotes use of glucose by
   A. breaking down glucose
   B. assisting glucose into the cells
   C. converting glucose to glycogen
   D. transporting glucose in the blood

2. Which of the following is true regarding the effect of insulin on fat metabolism? It inhibits
   A. synthesis of fatty acids
   B. glucose use by tissues
   C. release of fatty acids
   D. transport of glucose into fat cells

3. When an insulin deficiency exists, the liver responds by converting
   A. fatty acids to glucose
   B. glycogen to glucose
   C. glucagon to glucose
   D. amino acids to glucose

4. Insulin-dependent cells use which of the following nutritional substances FIRST when insulin is not available?
   A. fatty acids
   B. glycogen
   C. glucagon
   D. amino acids

5. The etiology of type 1 diabetes is believed to be
   A. obesity
   B. an autoimmune reaction
   C. a bacterial infection
   D. general pancreatic dysfunction

6. A client experiencing rapid onset hypoglycemia is most likely to have predominantly _____ symptoms.
   A. cell dysfunction
   B. gastrointestinal
   C. stimulated sympathetic nervous system
   D. stimulated parasympathetic nervous system

7. Central nervous system symptoms associated with hypoglycemia are caused by lack of _____ rather than insulin deficit.
   A. glucose
   B. amino acids
   C. fatty acids
   D. glucagon

8. Clinical manifestations of severe hypoglycemia include
   A. bradycardia
   B. fruity odor of the breath
   C. mental confusion
   D. ketonuria

9. Clinical manifestations of diabetic ketoacidosis include
   A. weight gain
   B. fluid overload
   C. electrolyte depletion
   D. hypoventilation

10. Which of the following statements is correct regarding hyperglycemic hyperosmolar state?
    A. it has a higher mortality rate than diabetic ketoacidosis
    B. it is most common in young clients with type 1 diabetes
    C. it causes severe fluid volume overload
    D. significant ketosis is present

11. Exogenous insulin is
    A. used only in the treatment of type 1 diabetes
    B. often used in management of type 2 diabetes during periods of stress
    C. most often derived from animal sources
    D. seldom used in the treatment of hyperglycemic hyperosmolar state

12. Diabetic retinopathy causes blindness as a result of
    A. glucose deposits on the retina
    B. thickening of the retina
    C. destruction of the optic nerve
    D. infarction of retinal tissue

13. Diabetic nephropathy damages the nephrons by causing
    A. glomerulosclerosis
    B. glomerulonephritis
    C. chronic nephritis
    D. renal hypertension

Pretest Answers: 1. B, 2. C, 3. B, 4. A, 5. B, 6. C, 7. A, 8. C, 9. C, 10. A, 11. B, 12. D, 13. A

GLOSSARY

acetoacetic acid   Produced by fat catabolism, it is one component of ketone bodies.

acetone (dimethyl ketone)   Produced by fat catabolism, it is a component of ketone bodies.

acetyl-CoA (acetylcoenzyme A)   A product of the reaction between acetic acid and coenzyme A.

aminoacidemia   Amino acids in the blood.

anion gap   A measurement of excessive unmeasurable anions.

atherosclerosis   A form of arteriosclerosis characterized by plaque deposits.

β-hydroxybutyric acid   One component of ketone bodies.

carbohydrates   Nutritional substances composed of complex and simple sugars.

catabolism   Breakdown of a substance.

diabetes mellitus   A complex metabolic disorder in which the person has either an absolute or a relative insulin deficiency; this insulin deficiency results in impaired carbohydrate, protein, and fat metabolism.

diabetic ketoacidosis (DKA)   A potentially devastating form of metabolic acidosis, characterized by a clinical syndrome of symptoms associated with elevated blood glucose and blood ketone levels and metabolic acidosis.

glucagon   A hormone produced by the alpha cells of the islets of Langerhans of the pancreas.

gluconeogenesis   Formation of glycogen in the liver from a noncarbohydrate substance.

glycogen   The stored form of carbohydrate for conversion into glucose.

glycogenolysis   Conversion of glycogen to glucose.

glycosuria   Excretion of glucose in the urine.

glycosylated hemoglobin (Hb A$_1$c)   Hemoglobin with glucose attached to it.

hormone-sensitive lipase   A fat-splitting enzyme.

hyalinization   A degenerative cell process affecting the basement membrane of arteries and arterioles; hyalinized cells take on a glassy appearance.

hyperglycemia   Abnormally high level of glucose in the blood

hyperglycemic hyperosmolar state (HHS)   A hyperglycemic complication of diabetes mellitus that results from insulin deficiency or insulin resistance; previously referred to as hyperglycemic hyperosmolar nonketotic syndrome (HHNS).

hypoglycemia   Abnormally low level of glucose in the blood.

infarction   Death of tissue.

insulin   An anabolic hormone produced by the beta cells of the islets of Langerhans of the pancreas.

insulin-dependent cells   Cells that require insulin to facilitate diffusion of glucose through the cell membrane.

ketonuria   The presence of ketones in the urine.

ketosis   The presence of ketones in the blood.

lipogenesis   Formation of fat.

lipolysis   Breakdown or splitting of fat.

macroangiopathy   Disease of the large and medium-sized blood vessels; essentially atherosclerosis.

metabolic acidosis   An alteration in acid–base balance characterized by an arterial blood gas pH of less than 7.35 (normal is 7.35 to 7.45) with a bicarbonate level of less than 22 mEq/L (normal is 22 to 28 mEq/L).

microangiopathy   Small blood vessel disease.

microvascular disease   Disease of the capillaries.

osmotic diuresis   Excessive urinary excretion caused by osmotic shifting of fluids.

polydipsia   Excessive thirst.

polyuria   Excessive urination.

Somogyi effect   A nocturnal hypoglycemia rebound phenomenon characterized by wide swings in serum glucose levels.

synthesis   Formation of a substance.

uptake   To take a substance into a cell.

ABBREVIATIONS

CO	Cardiac output	**HHS**	Hyperglycemic hyperosmolar state (previously referred to as HHNS, hyperglycemic hyperosmolar nonketotic syndrome)
BUN	Blood urea nitrogen		
DKA	Diabetic ketoacidosis		
FFA	Free fatty acid	**HLA DR**	Human leukocyte antigen genotype
Hb (Hgb)	Hemoglobin	**ICA**	Islet cell antibodies
Hb A	Hemoglobin A	**MOsm/L**	Milliosmoles per liter
Hb A$_1$c	Glycosylated hemoglobin	**PC**	Potential complications
HCO$_3$	Bicarbonate	**PCO$_2$**	Partial pressure of carbon dioxide

SECTION ONE: Normal Glucose Metabolism

At the completion of this section, the learner will be able to discuss normal glucose metabolism.

Glucose is used by most body cells as an energy source. Some cells (e.g., brain cells) can use only glucose for energy. Glucose, however, does not cross muscle and fat cell membranes using the same mechanisms, as do most other molecules. It requires a protein carrier, facilitated by insulin, to transport it into these cells. Fat and muscle cells are, therefore, sometimes referred to as **insulin-dependent cells.** After combining with the protein carrier in the cell membrane, glucose is able to diffuse across the membrane into the cell, where the carrier releases it. Supplying the cells with glucose is a complex physiologic task based on important feedback mechanisms for regulating blood glucose levels. This mechanism is primarily controlled by two hormones, insulin and glucagon, with important support by three other hormones, epinephrine, growth hormone, and cortisol. The normal fasting plasma glucose level is 70 to 110 mg/dL (fasting) (Kee, 2002).

Insulin

Insulin is a polypeptide (small protein) produced by the beta cells of the islets of Langerhans in the pancreas. Its underlying role is to lower the blood glucose level, and it sometimes is referred to as the hypoglycemic factor. Insulin plays a crucial part in regulating carbohydrate, fat, and protein metabolism.

Insulin must bind to special insulin receptor proteins in the cell membrane to carry out its functions. Once it is attached to a receptor site, insulin combines with the carrier protein in the cell membrane. The carrier protein, with help from insulin, promotes glucose diffusion across the cell membrane. Insulin's exact role is to enhance the function of the carrier protein.

Glucagon

Glucagon, a small protein, is secreted by alpha cells in the islets of Langerhans in the pancreas. It is the major hormone responsible for raising serum glucose levels and sometimes is referred to as the hyperglycemic factor. Glucagon's effects are in opposition to those of insulin. The stimulus for glucagon release is a decrease in the serum glucose level to a hypoglycemic level (Guvan et al., 2004). Glucagon counterbalances the effects of insulin by converting hepatic **glycogen** (via **glycogenolysis**) into glucose. Once converted, hepatic glucose rapidly moves into the circulation, increasing blood glucose levels. The reciprocal relationship between insulin and glucagon assists in maintaining homeostatic blood glucose levels.

Epinephrine, Growth Hormone, and Cortisol

When serum glucose drops below normal ranges, the sympathetic nervous system is stimulated. Consequently, the adrenal glands secrete epinephrine. Epinephrine increases serum glucose levels in a manner similar to glucagon but to a lesser extent.

Pituitary growth hormone and cortisol both respond to prolonged periods of hypoglycemia. They help reestablish a more normal glucose level by decreasing the rate of glucose use by the cells. Growth hormone decreases the body's ability to use carbohydrates, which spares them as an energy source. It facilitates the transport of amino acids into the cells. Oversecretion of growth hormone can lead to glucose intolerance and the development of diabetes (Guvan et al., 2004).

In summary, glucose is the body's main source of fuel. Its control and use depend primarily on two hormones, insulin and glucagon. Three other hormones also contribute to regulating serum glucose levels. Epinephrine elevates glucose in response to a hypoglycemic state in a similar manner to glucagon. Growth hormone and cortisol decrease cellular use of glucose, promoting hyperglycemia.

SECTION ONE REVIEW

1. Insulin is produced in the
   A. kidneys
   B. pituitary gland
   C. liver
   D. pancreas
2. Insulin promotes use of glucose by
   A. breaking down glucose
   B. assisting glucose into the cells
   C. converting glucose to glycogen
   D. transporting glucose in the blood
3. Glucagon promotes
   A. decreased use of glucose
   B. conversion of hepatic glycogen
   C. protein synthesis and transport
   D. transport of glucose into the cells

4. Which of the following is true regarding growth hormone?
   A. it decreases cellular use of glucose
   B. it promotes storage of fat
   C. it decreases blood glucose levels
   D. it increases breakdown of glycogen
5. Release of cortisol
   A. increases mobilization of fats
   B. decreases use of glucose
   C. decreases secretion of insulin
   D. increases breakdown of muscle glycogen

Answers: 1. D, 2. B, 3. B, 4. A, 5. B

SECTION TWO: The Effects of Insulin on Metabolism

At the completion of this section, the learner will be able to describe the effects of insulin on metabolism.

Insulin and Carbohydrate Metabolism

The body depends on adequate levels of glucose to provide energy for normal functioning. **Carbohydrates,** nutritional substances composed of complex and simple sugars, normally provide most of the body's glucose needs. Directly after consumption of carbohydrates, the serum glucose level increases, triggering a rapid increase in insulin secretion. Under the influence of insulin, glucose is moved into cells (cellular **uptake**) for immediate use or stored for later use. The liver plays a major role in glucose storage, and, to a lesser extent, fat and muscle tissues also provide glucose storage.

Insulin and the Liver in Glucose Metabolism

Directly after a meal, glucose that is not used immediately by the cells is stored rapidly in the liver as glycogen. With the help of insulin, glucose is converted into glycogen, diffusing into the liver cells where it becomes trapped until the serum glucose level becomes low. Insulin levels alter in direct response to glucose levels. Consequently, as serum glucose levels drop (as happens between meals), insulin is no longer needed and, thus, its level rapidly declines. The lack of insulin triggers a reversal of the process, breaking down the liver glycogen into glucose phosphate and releasing it from the liver cells to move back into the circulation. Thus, glucose may be stored as glycogen or released into the circulation (Guvan et al., 2004).

Insulin and Muscle Tissue in Glucose Metabolism

During normal daily activity, muscle tissue uses fatty acids, not glucose, as its major source of energy. This is because the resting membrane of the muscle does not allow glucose into the cell without the presence of insulin. Insulin levels, however, are very low between meals, thereby requiring use of energy sources other than glucose.

Muscle cells use glucose under two circumstances. First, during heavy exercise, muscle cell membranes become highly permeable to glucose. Second, for several hours after meals, the high level of insulin in the serum enhances transport of glucose into the muscle cells. Muscle cells store available glucose as muscle glycogen for their own use. They are, however, unable to convert it back into glucose or transport it back out of the muscle tissue into the general circulation. Muscle tissue, therefore, does not contribute to counteracting the effects of insulin.

Insulin and Fat Metabolism

Insulin also has important effects on fat metabolism. Normal levels of insulin help regulate fat metabolism by

■ Facilitating glucose use by most tissues, thereby sparing fat as the major energy source
■ Promoting synthesis of fatty acids primarily in the liver; fatty acids are then transported to adipose tissue for storage

■ Inhibiting fatty acid release into the circulation
■ Facilitating transport of glucose into fat cells for fatty acid synthesis

The blood glucose level is the major determining factor as to whether the cells will use carbohydrates or fats for energy. Once the decision is made, the switch from one energy source to the other is done rapidly. When there is a lack of insulin (such as between meals), cells must rely on fat as the primary energy source in insulin-dependent tissues. When insulin is again made available in sufficient quantities, glucose resumes its function as the major energy source. The use of fats as an energy source is as important as the use of carbohydrates (Porth, 2004).

Insulin and Protein Metabolism

Insulin plays an important part in the storage of protein following ingestion of nutrients. Insulin helps regulate protein metabolism by

■ Facilitating transport of amino acids across the cell membrane
■ Promoting protein **synthesis**
■ Decreasing protein **catabolism**

In addition to glucose, amino acids also act as triggers for insulin secretion. Thus, when amino acid levels increase after ingestion of nutrients, insulin is secreted to facilitate cellular uptake, synthesis, and storage of proteins.

In summary, the effects of normal levels of insulin on carbohydrate, fat, and protein metabolism are profound. Insulin helps regulate glucose metabolism in fat and muscle (insulin-dependent) tissues. It plays an important part in the cellular uptake, synthesis, and storage of both amino acids and fatty acids. Blood glucose and amino acid levels are the major triggers of insulin secretion. Blood glucose levels are the decisive factor in the type of food (carbohydrate or fat) used as the energy source for the insulin-dependent cells.

SECTION TWO REVIEW

1. Which of the following substances supplies the primary source of cell energy?
   A. fat
   B. protein
   C. carbohydrate
   D. glucagon

2. Cells requiring insulin to facilitate diffusion of glucose into them are called
   A. insulin-dependent
   B. glucose-dependent
   C. glycogen-dependent
   D. carbohydrate-dependent

3. Excess glucose is stored in the
   A. pancreas
   B. muscle tissues
   C. adipose tissues
   D. liver
4. During normal daily activities, muscle cells use which of the following as their major energy source?
   A. glucose
   B. fatty acids
   C. amino acids
   D. glucagon

5. Which of the following is true regarding the effect of insulin on fat metabolism? It inhibits
   A. synthesis of fatty acids
   B. glucose use by tissues
   C. release of fatty acids
   D. transport of glucose into fat cells

Answers: 1. C, 2. A, 3. D, 4. B, 5. C

SECTION THREE: The Effects of Insulin Deficit

At the completion of this section, the learner will be able to explain the impact of insulin deficit on metabolism.

Insulin deficiency results in disordered carbohydrate, protein, and fat metabolism. If carbohydrates are unable to be the major glucose energy source, the liver initiates conversion of glycogen to glucose. The principal metabolic alterations associated with insulin deficiency include (1) impaired cellular uptake and use of glucose, (2) increased extracellular (serum) glucose, (3) increased mobilization of fats, and (4) tissue depletion of protein (Fig. 27–1).

Movement of glucose into insulin-dependent cells occurs in direct proportion to the amount of insulin available. When insulin-dependent tissues are deprived of glucose as a result of either insulin deficiency or insulin resistance, their functional capacities become restricted. Table 27–1 summarizes the effects of insulin deficiency on insulin-dependent tissues.

TABLE 27–1   Effects of Insulin Deficit on Insulin-Dependent Tissues

TISSUES	EFFECTS
Glucose Transport Problems	
Skeletal muscle	Fatigue; decreased strength
Cardiac muscle	Weaker contractions; decreased cardiac output; decreased peripheral circulation
Smooth muscle	Poor bowel tone; decreased vascular tone
Leukocytes	Depressed leukocyte function; impaired inflammatory response
Crystalline lens of eye	Opacity/cataracts
Fibroblasts	Impaired healing
Pituitary gland	Retarded growth; impaired regeneration of tissue; other endocrine problems
Insulin Resistance Problem	
Adipose tissue	Lipolysis; lipidemia; elevated serum ketone levels

Insulin Deficit and Carbohydrate Metabolism

Insulin deficit dramatically alters carbohydrate metabolism. Carbohydrates are the major supplier of simple and complex sugars, producing glucose as the primary energy source. Insulin deficit causes cessation in glucose uptake by insulin-dependent cells and a decrease in glucose use by the cells. The combination of decreased glucose uptake and decreased glucose use causes a rapid buildup of serum glucose, **hyperglycemia.**

In an insulin-poor environment, insulin-dependent cells are actually starving. Though abundant potential energy is available in the form of glucose, it is of no use to the cells. Other sources of energy are used, including fatty acids (the primary backup energy source) and amino acids, once fat reserves are depleted. Clinically, dysfunctional carbohydrate metabolism is evidenced as hyperglycemia, and, if it is not controlled, ketosis and aminoacidemia may result, each with its own set of complications.

Insulin Deficit and Fat Metabolism

Insulin deficit alters fat metabolism by increasing **lipolysis** (fat breakdown) and decreasing **lipogenesis** (fat formation). The decreased availability of intracellular glucose results in increased breakdown of stored triglycerides by **hormone-sensitive lipase,** causing lipolysis. Free fatty acids become the major energy source for the tissues, with the major exception of the brain. Clinically, this is evidenced as increased blood levels of free fatty acids and glycerol. The liver also converts some of the excess fatty acids into cholesterol and phospholipids. Excess fatty acid breakdown causes increased levels of **acetyl-CoA (acetylcoenzyme A),** which is used by the liver for energy. The excess is converted into **acetoacetic acid.** Some of the acetoacetic acid is further converted into **β-hydroxybutyric acid** and **acetone (dimethyl ketone).** These three substances (acetoacetic acid, β-hydroxybutyric acid, and acetone) move into the circulation as ketone bodies (see Fig. 27–1).

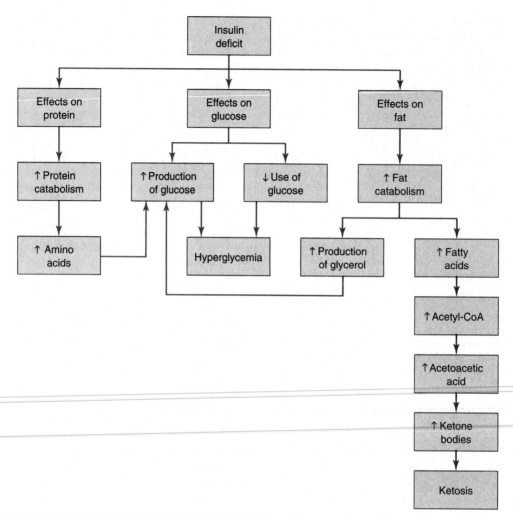

Figure 27–1 ■ Consequences of insulin deficit.

Clinically, this sequence of events has both acute and chronic consequences. Acutely, the increased levels of ketone bodies result in **ketosis** and **ketonuria.** When ketosis is extreme, severe **metabolic acidosis** and coma result (e.g., diabetic ketoacidosis). The use of fat as energy is evidenced as a significant increase in plasma lipoproteins (as much as three times normal). In the long term, high levels of lipoproteins are associated with the rapid onset of atherosclerosis, especially when high cholesterol levels are present. Many of the complications of diabetes mellitus are secondary to atherosclerotic changes.

Insulin Deficit and Protein Metabolism

Without insulin, the body is unable to store protein. There is an increase in protein catabolism and cessation of protein synthesis. Protein catabolism causes large quantities of amino acids to move into the circulation. The amino acids are then used either directly as an energy source or as part of the **gluconeogenesis** process.

Clinically, protein catabolism is evidenced by muscle wasting, multiple organ dysfunction, **aminoacidemia,** and increased urine nitrogen. If nitrogenous wastes accumulate in the body faster than they can be excreted in the urine, the patient will exhibit an altered level of consciousness and mentation. In addition, as gluconeogenesis is initiated, hyperglycemia is further aggravated.

Insulin Deficit and Fluid and Electrolyte Balance

When an insulin deficit exists, the serum glucose level increases, which causes plasma osmotic pressure to increase. The resulting change in pressure produces a shifting of body fluids from the tissues into the intravascular compartment. This shifting of fluids leads to intracellular dehydration.

As the level of hyperglycemia increases beyond the kidney's ability to reabsorb the extra glucose, **glycosuria** (excretion of glucose in the urine) develops. Urinary excretion of glucose produces an **osmotic diuresis** evidenced as **polyuria** (excessive urination). Osmotic diuresis results in excessive loss of water, potassium, sodium, chloride, and phosphate ions. Loss of these ions further increases both extracellular and intracellular dehydration. Deficits in potassium and sodium are manifested by weakness, fatigue, and other signs and symptoms associated with the specific electrolyte imbalances. As fluid is lost, serum osmolality increases. Dehydration stimulates the hypothalamic thirst center, causing excessive thirst (**polydipsia**). Dehydration also produces hemoconcentration as fluid from the vascular space is lost, which causes decreased cardiac output (CO). If the dehydration is allowed to progress, the CO may become critically low, ultimately leading to circulatory failure.

Circulatory failure has two major consequences. First, it causes poor tissue perfusion and tissue hypoxia. Decreased perfusion to the brain results in cerebral hypoxia and symptoms related to altered cerebral tissue perfusion. Second, it causes severe hypotension, which is responsible for decreased renal perfusion and may eventually result in acute renal failure. Circulatory failure is fatal if an adequate CO is not reestablished in a timely manner.

In summary, insulin deficiency severely alters metabolism of carbohydrates, proteins, and fats. When glucose is unable to move into insulin-dependent cells, cell function rapidly becomes impaired. Fluid and electrolyte balance becomes impaired as plasma osmotic pressure changes as a result of glycosuria. As fluids shift, the cells become dehydrated and electrolytes become deranged. Osmotic diuresis, if prolonged, causes hypovolemia and decreased CO, eventually leading to circulatory failure.

SECTION THREE REVIEW

1. When an insulin deficiency exists, the liver responds by converting
   - A. fatty acids to glucose
   - B. glycogen to glucose
   - C. glucagon to glucose
   - D. amino acids to glucose
2. Insulin-dependent cells use which of the following nutritional substances FIRST when insulin is not available?
   - A. fatty acids
   - B. glycogen
   - C. glucagon
   - D. amino acids
3. Insulin deficit alters fat metabolism by
   - A. increasing lipogenesis
   - B. synthesizing triglycerides
   - C. increasing lipolysis
   - D. synthesizing glycerol
4. When acetoacetic acid converts to acetone and β-hydroxybutyric acid, _____ is/are formed.
   - A. amino acids
   - B. acetyl-coA
   - C. glycerol
   - D. ketone bodies
5. Protein catabolism is evidenced by
   - A. muscle wasting
   - B. hyperexcitability
   - C. decreased urine urea nitrogen
   - D. increased triglyceride levels

Answers: 1. B, 2. A, 3. C, 4. D, 5. A

SECTION FOUR: Types of Diabetes Mellitus

At the completion of this section, the learner will be able to differentiate the two major types of diabetes mellitus.

Diabetes mellitus (diabetes) is a complex metabolic disorder in which the person has either an absolute or relative insulin deficit. It is divided into two major types: type 1 and type 2 diabetes.

Type 1 Diabetes Mellitus

Type 1 diabetes occurs when there is an absolute lack of endogenous insulin caused by autoimmune beta cell destruction. It can develop at any age but most commonly occurs before the age of 30. The human leukocyte antigen (HLA) genotype, HLA DR-3 or DR-4, is strongly associated with the occurrence of type 1 diabetes among certain racial groups. Viral and chemical agents are also proposed to be triggers for the development of type 1 diabetes. Regardless of the triggering event, it is believed that an autoimmune reaction destroys the beta cells (Ratner, 2001).

Type 2 Diabetes Mellitus

Approximately 90 percent of individuals in the United States with diabetes have type 2 diabetes. Type 2 diabetes is usually diagnosed after the age of 30 years but may also occur in children and adolescents. It is associated with a relative insulin deficiency (less insulin secretion) or insulin resistance rather than a total deficit. The major etiology of type 2 diabetes is

TABLE 27–2 Comparison of the Two Types of Diabetes Mellitus

CHARACTERISTIC	TYPE 1	TYPE 2
Usual age of onset	Younger than 30 years of age	Older than 30 years of age
Rate of onset	Rapid	Slow
Weight status	Not associated with obesity	Commonly associated with obesity
Insulin secretion (beta cell status)	Total loss of beta cells within 1 year of diagnosis; no insulin secretion	Decrease in size and number of beta cells; decreased insulin secretion
Glucagon secretion (alpha cell status)	Abnormal alpha cell function, but relative excess of glucagon in relation to insulin	Decrease in size and number of alpha cells; glucagon and insulin secretion decreased but often balanced
Ketone status	Ketone prone; high risk for ketoacidosis	Not ketone prone unless under stress; low risk for ketoacidosis
Insulin resistance	Usually only present with elevated glucose levels	Usually present
Insulin supplement status	Insulin dependent	Usually not insulin dependent
Diabetic crises associated with disorder(s)	Diabetic ketoacidosis (DKA); hypoglycemic coma	Hyperglycemic hyperosmolar state (HHS); hypoglycemic coma

progressive pancreatic dysfunction secondary to **hyalinization** of the islets of Langerhans. Over the course of the disease, both the pancreas and the liver develop fatty deposits as a result of high serum lipid levels. They also undergo tissue atrophy, associated with a decrease in size and number of functioning pancreatic and liver cells. Obesity in the presence of hereditary tendencies is considered a major risk factor for development of type 2 diabetes. Table 27–2 presents a comparison of type 1 and type 2 diabetes.

Diabetic Crises

Diabetes mellitus is associated with many clinical manifestations that are multisystemic in nature. Three acute complications, diabetic ketoacidosis (DKA), hyperglycemic hyperosmolar state (HHS), and therapy-induced hypoglycemic coma, may occur with diabetes. DKA and HHS are produced by an abnormally high blood glucose level, hyperglycemia. In contrast, hypoglycemic coma is produced by an abnormally low blood glucose level. Many clients with diabetes are admitted to the hospital for a diagnosis other than their chronic diabetic state. However, the physiologic stress caused by the acute problem may precipitate a diabetic crisis, which further complicates the client's prognosis.

The Focused History

When a diabetic crisis is suspected, specific parts of the nursing history should be obtained immediately.

- Preexisting history of type 1 or type 2 diabetes
- Self-maintenance activities
- Special diet, including adherence with diet
- Insulin or oral antidiabetes agents (type, dosage, adherence to regimen)
- Glucose testing history (blood glucose monitoring, urine testing)
- Exercise and weight loss
- Usual pattern of glucose control (stable versus occasional-to-frequent loss of glucose control)
- Possible precipitating factors (e.g., infection, presence of other physiologic or psychologic stressors, failure to follow diet or drug therapy)
- Preexisting neurologic or vascular complications of diabetes (e.g., decreased kidney function, peripheral or cardiovascular disease)
- Unexplained weight loss of 10 percent or greater.

Sections Five, Six, and Seven present the three acute complications, including assessment and management.

In summary, diabetes mellitus is a complex metabolic disorder associated with an absolute or relative insulin deficit or insulin resistance. There are two major types of diabetes mellitus: type 1 and type 2. Type 1 is associated with autoimmune destruction of the beta cells in the pancreas. Type 2 is associated with heredity, obesity, insulin resistance, or general dysfunction of the pancreas and the liver. There are many differences between these two types of diabetes. However, both cause progressive deterioration of multiple body systems.

SECTION FOUR REVIEW

1. The etiology of type 1 diabetes is believed to be
   A. obesity
   B. an autoimmune reaction
   C. a bacterial infection
   D. general pancreatic dysfunction
2. By 1 year after diagnosis of type 1 diabetes, there is
   _____ percent of functioning beta cells
   remaining in the pancreas.
   A. 0
   B. 10
   C. 30
   D. 50
3. Type 2 diabetes is associated with which of the
   following major risk factors?
   A. smoking
   B. viral infection
   C. obesity
   D. autoimmune reaction

4. In what way is pancreatic function altered in the
   patient with type 2 diabetes?
   A. beta cells become hyalinized
   B. beta cells become overactive
   C. alpha cell activity predominates
   D. alpha cells break down insulin
5. Which of the following statements is true regarding
   type 2 diabetes? Type 2 diabetes _____ than
   type 1 diabetes.
   A. is less common
   B. has a slower rate of onset
   C. usually occurs at a younger age
   D. is more commonly associated with ketones

Answers: 1. B, 2. A, 3. C, 4. A, 5. B

SECTION FIVE: Hypoglycemic Coma

At the completion of this section, the learner will be able to discuss the diabetic complication, hypoglycemic coma.

Hypoglycemia—an abnormally low blood glucose level—is the most common diabetic complication. It may occur with any type of diabetes. Hypoglycemia is triggered by imbalances among exercise, diet, and medication. Onset of symptoms is usually rapid, and, if it is prolonged, seizures and coma may result.

Clinical Presentation

Hypoglycemia can be defined clinically as a blood glucose level of less than 70 mg/dL or 3.9 mmol/L (Gonder-Frederick, 2001). Some clients, however, develop symptoms of hypoglycemia even with a serum glucose of greater than 70 mg/dL, or if the drop in glucose is very rapid. Hypoglycemia becomes symptomatic when there is insufficient glucose available to meet the energy needs of the central nervous system. Common precipitating conditions for development of hypoglycemia include

- Excessive administration of insulin or oral antidiabetes agents
- Consumption of too little food
- High activity levels
- Certain medications (e.g., propranolol) and alcohol, which potentiate the effects of the pharmacologic regimen
- Hormonal changes

Patients receiving oral antidiabetes agents (e.g., sulfonylureas) are at highest risk for severe and prolonged symptoms of hypoglycemia because of the extended half-life of these agents.

A patient's clinical presentation is primarily related to central nervous system (CNS) effects and catecholamine effects.

Central Nervous System Effects

The CNS depends on available glucose for its energy source and is sensitive to insufficient levels of glucose. CNS effects reflect the inability of brain cells to function normally without an adequate energy source. Progressive symptoms include

- Decreased ability to reason and remember (slow thinking)
- Changing mental status
- Emotional lability
- Headache, dizziness
- Thickened, slurred speech
- Loss of coordination
- Loss of proprioception
- Numbness
- Drowsiness
- Convulsions
- Coma

Catecholamine Effects

The lack of circulating glucose triggers the secretion of stress hormones, subsequently causing production of glucose from alternate body sources, such as hepatic gluconeogenesis. The presence of increased levels of the hormone epinephrine, a catecholamine, triggers a sympathetic response. This stress response accounts for many of the symptoms of hypoglycemia such as

- Anxiety
- Tremors, nervousness
- Cold, clammy skin
- Tachycardia, palpitations
- Hyperventilation
- Tingling in extremities
- Nausea and vomiting
- Hunger
- Diaphoresis

The rate of onset and the patient's age influence the type of symptoms that predominate.

Rapid Onset. When the onset of hypoglycemia is rapid, sympathetic nervous system symptoms often predominate. A significant, rapid drop of blood glucose level stimulates the sympathetic nervous system, which initiates secretion of epinephrine. Epinephrine causes gluconeogenesis in the liver, thereby increasing the serum glucose level. Concurrently, growth hormone and cortisol also are secreted to assist in increasing glucose levels by decreasing glucose use by the cells.

Slow Onset. When the onset of hypoglycemia is slow, the symptoms of CNS dysfunction may predominate. Over a period of time, the body is able to adapt to a slow decline in blood glucose. Brain cells are not insulin dependent and take in glucose directly. Central nervous system symptoms, therefore, are caused by lack of available glucose rather than an insulin deficit. The brain is a high-energy tissue, requiring large amounts of glucose to maintain normal functioning. Without glucose, particularly over a prolonged period, the brain can sustain permanent damage that may be either minor or severe (irreversible coma).

The Influence of Age. The age of the patient has an impact on the clinical presentation of hypoglycemia. The elderly tend to have more severe symptoms and may become symptomatic at higher serum glucose levels. CNS symptoms, particularly those relating to altered levels of consciousness, may be misdiagnosed in chronically ill elderly if the onset is very slow. In the elderly, the hypoglycemic symptoms may be masked as worsening dementia.

Medical Interventions. The major goal of interventions is rapid restoration of normal serum glucose levels. The specific type of intervention is based partially on the patient's level of consciousness.

The Conscious Hypoglycemic Patient. Reversal of hypoglycemia in the conscious patient is relatively simple to accomplish. Patients with blood glucose levels less than 70 mg/dL should eat or drink 10 to 15 g of glucose-or carbohydrate-containing foods or beverages. If blood glucose levels are less than 50 mg/dL, 20 to 30 g of glucose or carbohydrate may be needed. Blood glucose levels should be tested 15 to 20 minutes after initiating treatment. If the blood glucose levels remain low, the treatment should be repeated (Gonder-Frederick, 2001)

The Unconscious Hypoglycemic Patient. If a hospitalized adult patient with diabetes becomes hypoglycemic, exhibiting confusion or coma, the following regimen is suggested (Barnett, 2001):

1. If possible, draw a stat blood sample prior to initiating therapy.
2. Administer a 50 mL intravenous (IV) bolus of 50 percent glucose.
3. If 50 percent glucose is not available, administer glucagon 1 mg (subcutaneous (SQ), intramuscular (IM), or IV).
4. Follow the glucose bolus with a continuous IV glucose infusion (5 to 10 percent) to maintain the plasma glucose at a level greater than 100 mg/dL.

In summary, hypoglycemia is a condition in which there is insufficient glucose to meet cellular energy needs. It may be a result of excessive administration of insulin or antidiabetes agents, too little food, high-activity levels, certain medications and foods, or hormones. Hypoglycemia triggers the sympathetic response, causing secretion of epinephrine, which initiates the conversion of glycogen to glucose. The clinical presentation of hypoglycemia is the result of sympathetic nervous system stimulation and starvation of neural cells. The primary goal of treatment is restoration of blood glucose levels to as close to normal as possible.

SECTION FIVE REVIEW

1. Which of the following statements is TRUE regarding hypoglycemia?
   A. it is defined only in terms of blood glucose levels
   B. it is defined only in terms of clinical presentation
   C. it becomes symptomatic only when excessive insulin is present
   D. it becomes symptomatic at different blood glucose levels

2. Conditions that increase the risk of hypoglycemia include
   A. dietary fasting
   B. high-fat diet
   C. little exercise
   D. too little insulin

3. Of the following, the clinical presentation of hypoglycemia partially reflects
   A. lack of glucose within the cells
   B. excessive glucose within the cells
   C. stimulation of parasympathetic nervous system
   D. excessive circulating insulin
4. A patient experiencing rapid onset hypoglycemia is most likely to have predominantly _____ symptoms.
   A. cell dysfunction
   B. gastrointestinal
   C. stimulated sympathetic nervous system
   D. stimulated parasympathetic nervous system
5. Central nervous system symptoms associated with

hypoglycemia are caused by lack of _____ rather than insulin deficit.
   A. glucose
   B. amino acids
   C. fatty acids
   D. glucagon
6. In the unconscious hypoglycemic patient with a venous access, the treatment of choice is
   A. 50 percent glucose (IV)
   B. 0.5 to 2 mg glucagon (IM)
   C. 10 percent dextrose and water (IV)
   D. 8 ounces of orange juice (orally)

Answers: 1. D, 2. A, 3. A, 4. C, 5. A, 6. A

SECTION SIX: Diabetic Ketoacidosis

At the completion of this section, the learner will be able to describe the diabetic complication, diabetic ketoacidosis.

Diabetic ketoacidosis (DKA) results from an absolute or relative deficiency in insulin. It is a potentially severe, sometimes life-threatening complication characterized by ketosis, acidosis, hyperglycemia, dehydration, and electrolyte imbalances (Davidson & Schwartz, 2001).

Focused Assessment

A rapid assessment of the severity and state of compensation of DKA helps establish management priorities. The signs and symptoms of DKA are multisystemic in nature; thus, a systematic assessment is necessary. Not every patient exhibits all the clinical manifestations of DKA, and confirmation is made by evaluation of appropriate laboratory tests. Table 27–3 summarizes the major cardinal signs and their specific associated signs and symptoms. A brief description of the pathophysiologic basis of the cardinal signs of diabetic ketoacidosis follows.

Pathophysiologic Basis of DKA Symptomatology

Hyperglycemia. The origin of **hyperglycemia** is an absolute or relative deficit in insulin, which causes the inability of glucose to move into cells, thus increasing serum glucose levels. Fat from adipose tissue is converted into free fatty acids (FFAs). The FFAs, in turn, are converted to glucose by gluconeogenesis in the liver. The liver also causes glycogenolysis, which converts glycogen to glucose. All these factors contribute to worsening hyperglycemia (see Fig. 27–1).

TABLE 27–3 Cardinal Signs and Specific Signs and Symptoms of Diabetic Ketoacidosis

CARDINAL SIGNS	SPECIFIC SIGNS AND SYMPTOMS
Hyperglycemia	Elevated serum glucose (greater than 250 mg/dL)
	Elevated urine glucose
Metabolic acidosis	Elevated serum and urine ketones
	Acidotic serum pH (less than 7.30)
	Acidotic serum HCO_3 (less than 15 mEq/L)
	Positive high anion gap (greater than 17 mEq/L)
	Alkalotic serum Pco_2 (less than 35 mm Hg)
	Elevated respiratory rate and depth (Kussmaul breathing)
	Fruity odor to breath
Osmotic diuresis	Polyuria
	Polydipsia
	Dehydration
	Hypotension
	Hemoconcentration
	Electrolyte abnormalities
	Azotemia (elevated BUN and creatinine)
	Elevated serum osmolarity (but less than 350 mg/dL)
Compensation	Decreased urine output
	Increased serum sodium levels
	Increased blood pressure, pulse, respirations
	Peripheral vasoconstriction

Metabolic Acidosis. Free fatty acids are broken down by the CNS into ketone bodies for energy faster than they can be converted to glucose. Because of the lack of insulin, muscle cells cannot oxidize the ketone bodies sufficiently, causing a buildup of ketone bodies. Increased levels of circulating ketone bodies decreases the pH, and as the pH falls below 7.20, the respiratory center is stimulated to excrete carbonic acid via the lungs in the form of carbon dioxide and water (Kussmaul breathing). Acetone, which is contained in ketone bodies, is excreted through the lungs (ketone breath) and the kidneys (ketonuria). Bicarbonate reserves become overwhelmed and then exhausted by the severity and prolonged state of the acidosis, which causes a drop in serum bicarbonate levels.

Osmotic Diuresis. Elevated serum glucose levels increase intravascular osmotic pressure. The increased pressure draws extravascular fluids into the intravascular compartment. As the levels of glucose and intravascular volume increase, the kidneys respond by dramatically increasing excretion of glucose and urine. This is associated with increased loss of electrolytes, hemoconcentration, and increasing dehydration. Gastrointestinal symptoms associated with DKA may be related to abnormally low electrolyte levels.

Compensatory Mechanisms. The renin–angiotensin–aldosterone system is activated to increase sodium and water reabsorption. Antidiuretic hormone (ADH) is secreted by the posterior pituitary to cause retention of water and sodium. Urine output also is controlled by compensatory vasoconstriction, which limits renal blood flow. The autonomic nervous system is stimulated to secrete catecholamines and glucocorticoids, which results in vasoconstriction; thus increasing the blood pressure and decreasing urine output. Blood pressure, pulse, and respirations are all increased as a result.

Decompensation. The client with severe DKA can eventually develop failure of compensatory mechanisms. Decompensation represents exhaustion of compensatory mechanisms, which rapidly leads to cardiovascular collapse. The level of consciousness deteriorates and blood pressure and pulse can no longer maintain adequate organ perfusion. The supply of catecholamines becomes exhausted, causing loss of the body's ability to maintain peripheral vasoconstriction. Urine output decreases and ceases as hypoperfusion to the kidneys causes them to fail.

Anion Gap. DKA is only one cause of metabolic acidosis. Measuring **anion gap** is one way to help isolate DKA from some other acidotic conditions. Gaining a basic understanding of the concept of anion gap may facilitate early diagnosis and treatment of DKA.

Metabolic acidosis exists either as normal anion gap acidosis (from loss of bicarbonate ions) or as high anion gap acidosis (from an accumulation of fixed acids in the serum).

Anions are negatively charged particles (e.g., CO_2^-, HCO_3^-, and Cl^-). They are the opposite of cations, or positively charged particles (e.g., Na^+ and K^+). Normally, cations and anions are in balance with each other. Anion gap represents the level of unmeasurable anion excess that exists in the body. Measurement of

the anion gap is helpful in differentiating the type of metabolic acidosis present. It is expressed as

$$\text{Anion gap} = (Na^+ + K^+) - (Cl^- + HCO_3^-)$$

Anion gap has a normal range of 10 to 17 mEq/L (Kee, 2002). This normal range is a function of such unmeasured serum anions as phosphates, sulfates, ketones, and lactic acid.

High Anion Gap Acidosis. An anion gap of greater than 17 mEq/L indicates an accumulation of these unmeasured anions and warrants immediate attention. When metabolic acidosis is caused by elevations in organic acids, the anion gap increases. Such states as starvation, lactic acidosis, and DKA cause a high anion gap.

Normal Anion Gap Acidosis. When metabolic acidosis is caused by a loss of bicarbonate (buffer) anions, the anion gap remains normal. This occurs in such states as high chloride intake, renal failure, and diarrhea.

A person admitted with a potential or actual DKA may have an anion gap determination performed. Although anion gap alone is inconclusive for DKA, it is used as adjunctive data in clustering critical cues for differential diagnosis.

Causes of Diabetic Ketoacidosis

DKA is caused by extreme insulin deficiency. Infection is the primary precipitating factor for development of DKA (American Diabetes Association, 2003). Illness and infection increase the production of glucocorticoids by the adrenal gland supporting the production of new glucose by the liver (gluconeogenesis). Epinephrine and norepinephrine levels are also increased causing further breakdown of glycogen into glucose (glycogenolysis). Diabetic ketoacidosis is seen most commonly in type 1 diabetics.

Any condition or situation that increases the insulin deficit can precipitate DKA, for example, infection, stroke, myocardial infarction, trauma, alcohol abuse, and drugs (American Diabetes Association, 2003). In addition, new-onset type 1 diabetes and omission of exogenous insulin in diagnosed type 1 individuals commonly leads to DKA (American Diabetes Association, 2003). In about 20 percent of cases, no specific precipitating event is found (Johnson, 1998).

Stress as a Major Precipitating Factor

An increased level of stress causes further production of stress hormones (e.g., epinephrine, growth hormone, and cortisol). As discussed in Section One, when secreted, these hormones increase blood glucose levels by either increasing conversion of glycogen to glucose or decreasing cellular use of glucose. When the stress is severe, as in a severe acute infection or illness, the increase in glucose can be substantial, thus precipitating an imbalance in the glucose/insulin relationship.

Severe infection with systemic involvement also is typically accompanied by hyperthermia (fever). Hyperthermia increases the metabolic rate, thus greatly increasing cellular need for insulin. Therefore, in the presence of infection, there is both an increased supply and an increased demand for glucose. In such a situation, it would seem that a balance in glucose would exist. This is not the case, however, with type 1 diabetes. A balance can be maintained or regained only when sufficient insulin is present to meet the increased glucose needs of the cells. DKA is precipitated by a relative insulin deficiency in this situation. If insulin dosage is not increased in response, there is insufficient insulin to meet the increased glucose supply as well as the increased metabolic demand.

A similar situation can occur with a patient with type 2 diabetes whose condition normally is controlled by diet, antidiabetes agents, or both. In situations of high stress (infection, trauma, surgery), the level of insulin secretion in the pancreas often is insufficient to meet the increased supply of and demand for glucose; thus, this type of patient clinically exhibits hyperglycemia, which often requires temporary exogenous insulin therapy. Sliding scale insulin is then administered until the level of physiologic stress is sufficiently reduced and balance is regained between the glucose level and the endogenous insulin supply.

Management of Diabetic Ketoacidosis

The DKA-related treatment goals include

- Correcting fluid and electrolyte imbalances
- Decreasing serum glucose
- Correcting acidosis
- Preventing further complications
- Providing client education (Davidson & Schwartz, 2001).

Nursing interventions are based on activities that help the patient meet expected outcomes. They consist of collaborative interventions: (1) activities ordered by the physician or advanced nurse practitioner but requiring some actions by the nurse and (2) activities that are within the nursing scope of practice (independent nursing orders).

Collaborative Interventions

The American Diabetes Association (2003) has established guidelines for the management of diabetic ketoacidosis (see Fig. 27–2 for the ADA protocol). These guidelines include

1. **IV therapy.** The patient's initial management requires rapid rehydration. Osmotic diuresis precipitated by elevated glucose levels severely depletes body fluids. Initial fluid replacement will be with one-half normal (0.45 percent) or normal (0.9 percent) saline. As soon as the serum glucose level is decreased to approximately 250 mg/dL, dextrose (5 percent) may be added to the intravenous fluids.

The patient will receive nothing by mouth until the crisis state is resolved.

2. **Insulin therapy.** Correction of the hyperglycemic state depends on careful use of insulin. During the crisis state, only short-acting insulins are used because of their fast results in reducing glucose levels, which facilitate better control. Insulin management generally is via continuous, low-dose intravenous infusion with regular insulin. Regular insulin is the only insulin that can be given intravenously. The patient's glucose levels should be monitored hourly while receiving insulin IV.

3. **Sodium bicarbonate therapy.** Sodium bicarbonate ($NaHCO_3$) is the drug of choice for rapid correction of most metabolic acidosis problems. However, with DKA, treatment with sodium bicarbonate is controversial and not recommended by the majority of endocrinologists. Sodium bicarbonate may be recommended with severe cases of metabolic acidosis if the arterial pH is 7.0 or less or if the serum bicarbonate level is less than 5 mEq/L. When ketoacidosis is corrected too rapidly, it can precipitate cerebrospinal fluid (CSF) acidosis, causing potentially severe neurologic complications. Cerebrospinal fluid acidosis is difficult to correct because sodium bicarbonate does not cross the blood–brain barrier. Diabetic ketoacidosis often corrects itself with the use of insulin, electrolyte therapy, and IV fluid replacement.

4. **Electrolyte replacement.** Potassium, sodium, and phosphate are three of the major electrolytes requiring replacement during a DKA episode. Sodium is replaced primarily during the initial rehydration phase of treatment using 0.9 percent and 0.45 percent normal saline IV solutions. Particular care is taken in managing potassium replacement because serum levels decrease as the acidotic state is corrected and normal urine output is regained. In cases of severe hypokalemia, insulin treatment should be delayed until potassium levels are greater than 3.3 mEq/L to prevent cardiac dysrhythmias or cardiac arrest as shown in Figure 27–2. Phosphate, a buffer, may become depleted during periods of acidosis, particularly if the acidosis is prolonged. Adequate levels of phosphate are important in managing the acidosis. When replacement is warranted, it is generally administered IV in the form of potassium phosphate.

5. **Correction of underlying problems.** A key to successful management of a hyperglycemic crisis is finding and aggressively treating the underlying cause. If an infection is the underlying problem, antibiotic therapy is initiated, and if a wound is present (such as an open ulcer), it may be debrided. The pathophysiologic effects of diabetes prevent the patient from healing well, increasing the risk of further infectious complications.

6. **Laboratory and other tests.** The patient's status will be closely monitored throughout the DKA period. Initially, close monitoring of serum pH, glucose, ketones, osmolality,

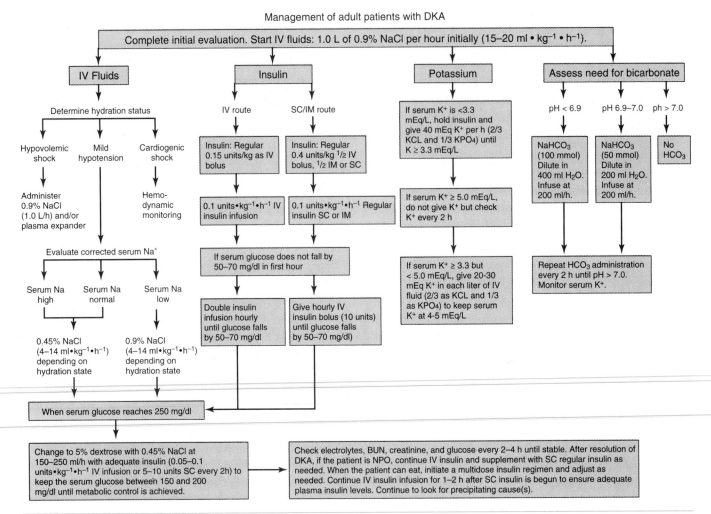

Figure 27–2 ■ Management of adult patients with DKA. *(From American Diabetes Association [ADA]. (2003). Hyperglycemic crises in patients with diabetes mellitus. Diabetes Care, 26, S111. With permission.)*

and electrolytes is necessary. The patient may have an electrocardiogram (ECG) and cardiac monitoring ordered to monitor serum potassium effects on the heart. A culture and Gram stain of potentially infected secretions or fluids confirm the type of organism so that IV antibiotic therapy can be most effective.

Independent Nursing Interventions

Fluid Volume Deficit

1. Assess for signs and symptoms of fluid volume deficit; report abnormals.
2. Monitor hemodynamics as available; report worsening trends: pulmonary artery pressure, pulmonary artery wedge pressure, and central venous pressure.
3. Monitor laboratory and other test results; report abnormals: blood urea nitrogen (BUN) and creatinine, electrolytes, hemoglobin, and hematocrit.

4. Monitor for therapeutic and nontherapeutic effects of fluid replacement therapy; report abnormals.
5. When taking oral fluids, force fluids if underlying problems permit.

Altered Nutrition: Less Than Body Requirements

1. Monitor for therapeutic and nontherapeutic effects of insulin therapy; report abnormals.
2. Monitor laboratory and other test results; report abnormals: serum glucose, ketones, albumin, transferrin, CBC with differential.
3. Monitor and document dietary intake.
4. Encourage intake of prescribed diet.
   A. Avoid painful procedures immediately before meals or feedings.
   B. Administer pain medications before meals, when needed; assess effectiveness of PRN medications.
5. Implement measures to reduce energy requirements.

Potential Complication (PC): Electrolyte Imbalances; Metabolic Acidosis

1. Assess for signs and symptoms of electrolyte imbalances; report abnormals (specify imbalances based on specific disorder).
2. Assess for signs and symptoms of metabolic acidosis; report abnormals.
3. Monitor laboratory (e.g., serum electrolytes) and other test results; report abnormals
4. Monitor for therapeutic and nontherapeutic effects of electrolyte and acidosis drug therapy; report abnormals.
5. Monitor ECG for changes consistent with electrolyte imbalance, such as dysrhythmias, *T* wave changes, *ST* segment changes.

6. Encourage intake of appropriate nutrients.
7. Restrict intake of undesirable nutrients based on electrolyte levels.
8. Encourage intake of fluids if fluid volume deficit exists.

In summary, DKA is an acute life-threatening consequence of diabetes mellitus, which can be prevented by thorough rapid intervention, client education, and medical management. It is a type of high anion gap metabolic acidosis caused by accumulation of ketone bodies. Anion gap is one method of differentiating DKA from several other types of acidosis. DKA may be precipitated by any event that increases the insulin deficit. Physiologic stress and acute infection are two major precipitating conditions.

SECTION SIX REVIEW

1. Which of the following set of laboratory results best reflects diabetic ketoacidosis?
   A. pH 7.28, HCO_3 34 mEq/L, blood glucose 260 mg/dL
   B. pH 7.18, HCO_3 13 mEq/L, blood glucose 120 mg/dL
   C. pH 7.26, HCO_3 14 mEq/L, blood glucose 450 mg/dL
   D. pH 7.38, HCO_3 24 mEq/L, blood glucose 620 mg/dL
2. Typical clinical manifestations of diabetic ketoacidosis include
   A. absence of ketonuria
   B. fluid overload
   C. electrolytes within normal range
   D. progressive dehydration
3. Ketosis results from mobilization of
   A. amino acids
   B. glucagon

   C. glucose
   D. fatty acids
4. A high anion gap acidosis is consistent with which of the following problems?
   A. diarrhea
   B. high intake of chloride
   C. starvation
   D. high intake of sodium
5. A common precipitating factor for development of diabetic ketoacidosis is
   A. a stress-free lifestyle
   B. decreased exercise
   C. infection
   D. food/insulin balance

Answers: 1. C, 2. D, 3. D, 4. C, 5. C

SECTION SEVEN: Hyperglycemic Hyperosmolar State

At the completion of this section, the learner will be able to discuss the diabetic complication, hyperglycemic hyperosmolar state.

Hyperglycemic hyperosmolar state (HHS) is a hyperglycemic complication of diabetes mellitus that results from insulin deficiency or insulin resistance. It is sometimes overlooked and primarily occurs in elderly patients, particularly sick elderly, with type 2 diabetes. HHS has a higher mortality rate than DKA because of its severe metabolic changes and the delay in diagnosis. The major precipitating factor for development of HHS is infection (American Diabetes Association, 2003). Other precipitating factors include severe diarrhea, severe burns, peritoneal

dialysis, myocardial infarction, thiazide usage, and hypertonic feeding (Davidson & Schwartz, 2001).

Pathophysiologic Basis of HHS

The patient with type 2 diabetes produces moderate levels of insulin. In the presence of a precipitating event, the type 2 diabetic's relative lack of insulin can trigger hyperglycemia by way of acceleration of hepatic gluconeogenesis and decreased peripheral glucose utilization. The result of these events is extreme hyperglycemia (may be in excess of 2,000 mg/dL) while avoiding significant ketoacidosis. Failure to develop significant ketoacidosis is attributed to the type 2 diabetic's ability to produce sufficient insulin to prevent or minimize lipolysis and ketogenesis.

The excess glucose accumulates in the extracellular spaces because it cannot be transported into the cells or metabolized normally, resulting in a progressive increase in osmolality. As extracellular osmolality increases, water is pulled from the intracellular spaces into the extracellular spaces. As the level of hyperglycemia increases and exceeds the renal threshold, osmotic diuresis significantly increases, precipitating progressive dehydration of intracellular and extracellular spaces. Severe dehydration of the intracellular and extracellular spaces results in hyperosmolar coma if the serum osmolality increases to 320 mOsm/L or higher (Davidson & Schwartz, 2001).

Clinical Presentation

DKA and HHS have many similarities; both are associated with

- An absolute or relative insulin deficit
- Hyperosmolality secondary to hyperglycemia and water loss
- Depletion of volume secondary to osmotic diuresis
- Electrolyte abnormalities secondary to the osmotic diuresis
- Altered mental status

There are also many major differences between DKA and HHS that assist the clinician in differentiating the two disorders. Some of the major differences include

- DKA is associated with rapid onset, whereas HHS develops more slowly and insidiously.
- Hyperglycemia is more severe with HHS.
- Hyperosmolality is more severe in HHS, causing profound dehydration.
- Water loss associated with HHS is significantly greater than with DKA.

- HHS is associated with severe neurologic signs (e.g., coma, seizures); in addition, mental status changes may occur over a period of days with HHS.

The clinical features commonly associated with HHS include hyperglycemia, dehydration, absence of significant ketosis, and neurological signs. Table 27–4 presents a comparison of diagnostic criteria for DKA and HHS.

Medical Interventions

Medical goals for management of the patient with HHS are essentially the same as for the patient with DKA. In management of HHS, the first priority is rehydration and restoration of normal electrolyte levels. Other goals include correction of the precipitating event (if possible) and prevention of complications. Fluid replacement needs in the HHS patient are greater than in the DKA patient because of the more profound state of dehydration. Careful monitoring is necessary to prevent complications associated with too rapid rehydration, though complications associated with fluid volume overload during fluid resuscitation of the HHS patient is rare. Because the individual with type 2 diabetes may be sensitive to exogenous insulin, insulin generally is administered in lower doses in treatment of the HHS patient than in the DKA patient. Figure 27–3 provides a protocol for management of HHS in adult clients.

In summary, hyperglycemic hyperosmolar state (HHS) is a type of hyperglycemic diabetic crisis associated with type 2 diabetes mellitus. The hallmark of HHS is a hyperglycemic hyperosmolar state without significant ketosis. The degree of hyperglycemia and dehydration is more severe in HHS than in DKA. Treatment of DKA and HHS is similar, although HHS requires higher volumes of fluids and lower doses of insulin.

TABLE 27–4   Diabetic Ketoacidosis (DKA) and Hyperglycemic Hyperosmolar State (HHS): Comparison of Major Salient Features

	CONDITIONS	
FEATURE	**DKA**	**HHS**
Age of patient	Usually less than 40 years old	Usually less than 60 years old
Duration of symptoms	Usually less than 2 days	Usually greater than 5 days
Plasma glucose level	Usually less than 600 mg/dL (less than 33.3.mmol/L)	Usually greater than 600 mg/dL (33.3 mmol/L)
Sodium concentration	More likely to be normal or low	High, normal, or low
Potassium concentration	High, normal, or low	High, normal, or low
Bicarbonate concentration	Low	Normal
Ketone bodies	At least 4+ in 1:1 dilution	Less than 2+ in 1:1 dilution
Arterial pH	Low	Normal
Serum osmolality	Often less than 320 mOsm/kg (less than 320 mmol/kg)	Usually greater than 320 mOsm/kg (greater than 320 mmol/kg)
Cerebral edema	Often subclinical; occasionally clinical	Subclinical has not been evaluated; rarely clinical
Prognosis	3 to 10 percent mortality	10 to 20 percent mortality
Subsequent course	Insulin therapy required in virtually all cases	Insulin therapy not required in many cases

From Davidson, M. B. (1998). Diabetic ketoacidosis and hyperosmolar nonketotic coma (pp. 159–194). In M. B. Davidson (Ed.). Diabetes mellitus: Diagnosis and treatment, *(4th ed.). Philadelphia: W. B. Saunders. Copyright 1998, with permission from Elsevier.*

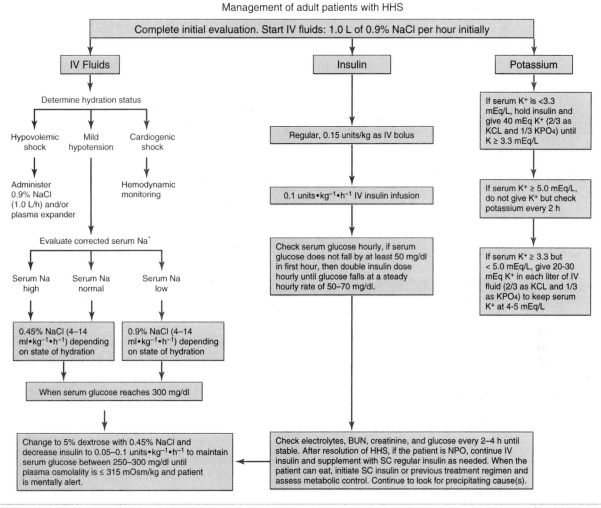

Figure 27–3 ■ Management of adult patients with HHS. *(From American Diabetes Association [ADA]. (2003). Hyperglycemic crises in patients with diabetes mellitus. Diabetes Care, 26[1], S112. With permission.)*

SECTION SEVEN REVIEW

1. Which of the following statements is correct regarding HHS?
   A. it has a high mortality rate
   B. it is most common in type 1 diabetes
   C. it causes severe fluid volume overload
   D. death occurs from severe metabolic acidosis

2. Common precipitating events causing HHS include which of the following?
   A. hemodialysis
   B. infection
   C. chronic infection
   D. high fat diet

3. HHS does not cause ketosis because
   A. lipolysis does not occur
   B. protein catabolism is occurring
   C. high glucagon levels prevent it
   D. hyperglycemia is not sufficiently severe

4. Which of the following statements regarding the differences between DKA and HHS is correct?
   A. the onset of HHS is faster
   B. dehydration is less severe in HHS
   C. hyperosmolality is more severe in HHS
   D. mental status changes more rapidly in HHS

5. Which of the following statements is correct regarding insulin management of the patient with HHS?
   A. insulin management is contraindicated
   B. the patient usually requires low-dose insulin management
   C. the type 2 diabetic is resistant to exogenous insulin
   D. the type 1 diabetic is resistant to exogenous insulin

Answers: 1. A, 2. B, 3. A, 4. C, 5. B

SECTION EIGHT: Exogenous Insulin Therapy

At the completion of this section, the learner will be able to explain the use of exogenous insulin in the management of the client with diabetes mellitus.

Individuals with type 1 diabetes require exogenous insulin replacement. Type 2 diabetics do not always require exogenous insulin. However, during a period of stress (e.g., illness or surgery), the type 2 diabetic may experience hyperglycemia, requiring temporary insulin therapy until the condition is resolved and glucose levels return to normal. Type 2 diabetics may require exogenous insulin later in their therapy when oral antidiabetes agents and lifestyle modifications are ineffective for control.

Sources of Exogenous Insulin

Insulin is derived from the pancreases of animals or synthesized in a laboratory. Insulin produced from animal pancreases is further divided into two types: beef (bovine) and pork (porcine). Of all types of exogenous insulin, bovine insulin differs most from human insulin and, therefore, generally is not used as commonly as other forms. Bovine insulin is not available in the United States (White et al., 2001). Porcine insulin is structurally similar to human insulin and usually is well accepted by the body.

Synthetic insulin is rapidly replacing animal-based insulins and is used almost exclusively in the United States. Synthetic insulin is developed in a laboratory setting and involves structural conversion of a substance into the amino acid chains identical to human insulin. Various substances, such as *Escherichia coli* or saccharomyces cerevisiae, are used to manufacture biosynthetic human insulin using recombinant DNA technology.

Certain factors dictate which type of insulin is best suited to a specific person. Some of these factors include the presence of the following:

- Insulin allergy
- Insulin resistance
- Adipose tissue atrophy at injection sites
- Religious restriction against pork
- Cost of insulin

The final choice of insulin often is based on trial and error in finding which product best meets the individual needs of the person. Insulins are not interchangeable because they have differing efficacy levels and possible allergy implications. For this reason, it is important for the nurse to be aware of the type of insulin ordered and to take precautions that the same type of insulin is administered. For example, the patient who normally receives synthetic insulin should not be given porcine or bovine insulin without specific orders to do so.

Factors That Influence Insulin

Many factors have an impact on insulin dosage or effectiveness. Table 27–5 lists some of the major factors and how they influence insulin dosages.

Types of Insulin

Insulin is divided into four major categories according to its duration of action. The four categories include rapid acting, short acting, intermediate acting, and long acting. There are also several insulins that are categorized as premixed. These

TABLE 27–5 Factors Affecting Insulin Dosage

FACTOR	EFFECT
Drug Interactions	
Thiazide diuretics, glucocorticoids, thyroid preparations, nicotine, rifampin	May increase glucose levels and insulin requirements
MAO inhibitors, oral antidiabetes agents, anabolic steroids, salicylates	May reduce glucose levels and insulin requirements
Beta-adrenergic blocking agents	May mask hypoglycemic symptoms
Other	
Exercise	May reduce glucose levels and insulin requirements
Acute illness	Increases blood glucose levels and insulin requirements; often requires sliding-scale insulin administration
Nutritional support	Increases blood glucose levels and insulin requirements; often requires sliding scale insulin administration

TABLE 27–6 Insulins Available in the United States

CLASSIFICATION	HUMAN RECOMBINANT INSULINS	PURIFIED PORK INSULINS
Rapid-acting insulin	Lispro (Humalog)	
	Aspart (Novolog)	
Short-acting insulin	Regular (Humulin R)	Regular Iletin II
	Regular (Novolin R)	
	Regular (Velosulin BR)	
Intermediate-acting insulin	NPH (Humulin N)	NPH Iletin II
	NPH (Novolin N)	Lente Iletin II
	Lente (Humulin L)	
	Lente (Novolin L)	
Long-acting insulin	Ultralente (Humulin U)	
	Glargine (Lantus)	
Combination therapy (premixed)	NPH/regular 70/30 (Humulin 70/30)	
	NPH/regular 70/30 (Novolin 70/30)	
	NPH/regular 50/50 (Humulin 50/50)	
	NPH/lispro 75/25 (Humalog Mix 75/25)	

insulins combine neutral protamine Hagedorn (NPH) with regular insulins. Lispro insulin (Humalog), a synthetic insulin, has an altered in structure that results in a shortened action time. This rapid-acting insulin has a peak of 30 to 90 minutes and duration of 6 to 8 hours. It has become the preferred meal coverage insulin for many diabetics (Semb, 2004). Table 27–6 differentiates the various insulins according to these categories. Figure 27–4 differentiates between the categories based on the extent and duration of action of the various insulins.

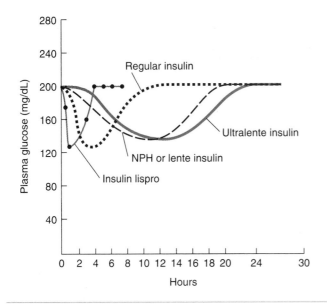

Figure 27–4 ■ Extent and duration of action of various types of insulin (in a fasting diabetic). *(From Katzung, B. G. [2004]. Basic and clinical pharmacology, (8th ed., p. 716). New York: McGraw-Hill. Reproduced with permission of the McGraw-Hill Companies.)*

Side Effects of Insulin

Administration of too much insulin causes hypoglycemia. The patient is at greatest risk for hypoglycemia during peak action time. It is crucial to be aware of the type of insulin administered (e.g., rapid acting), when the dose was administered, and what type of nutrition has been consumed after administration. A person receiving a short-acting insulin, such as regular insulin, at 8:00 A.M. would have peak within 2 to 4 hours after subcutaneous administration. This would mean that the risk for hypoglycemia is greatest between the hours of 10:00 A.M. and 12:00 noon.

A patient receiving an intermediate-acting insulin (such as NPH) at 8:00 A.M. would peak about 6 to 12 hours later, placing him or her at greatest risk for hypoglycemia between the hours of 2:00 P.M. and 8:00 P.M. Many acutely ill patients require supplemental rapid-acting insulin (regular insulin) as well as their usual intermediate- or long-acting insulin. Mixing types of insulin gives the patient multiple insulin peak periods throughout a 24-hour period. Other factors commonly seen in acutely ill patients, such as prolonged NPO status and nutritional support, all have an impact on glucose levels and insulin needs.

Continuous Low-Dose Intravenous Insulin Infusion

Fleckman (1993) stated that, historically, treatment of DKA in its early stages consisted of large doses of insulin (hundreds of units). Over time, clinicians found that continuous low-dose IV insulin made regulation easier and provided better control of glucose levels. Other advantages include fewer complications associated with hypokalemia and hypoglycemia, and rapid rate of insulin dissipation.

During a hyperglycemic crisis, a continuous infusion of regular insulin may be ordered to provide better control of serum insulin levels. When preparing to administer IV insulin, it is important to remember that

- Only regular insulin is administered IV.
- Insulin binds to polyvinylchloride in IV bags and tubing, lowering the insulin concentration in the fluid. One form of insulin, Velosulin, has been buffered with phosphate, which prevents the insulin from binding to plastic tubing.
- Blood glucose levels must be monitored frequently to avoid hypoglycemia.

Sliding-Scale Insulin Administration

During periods of physiologic stress, glucose levels may be very unstable, requiring supplemental insulin in addition to the patient's usual insulin coverage. Consequently, insulin dosage must reflect current blood glucose levels. Orders may be written to titrate the insulin dose to specific glucose levels. This type of insulin regimen is called *sliding-scale insulin* coverage. Table 27–7 gives an example of a sliding-scale insulin order.

It is recommended that sliding-scale insulin administration be carried out based on blood glucose rather than urine glucose measurements. Urine glucose does not reflect hour-by-hour changes in glucose levels. Thus, its value for tight glucose control is diminished.

Intensive Insulin Therapy

Traditionally, moderate levels of hyperglycemia were expected and accepted in high acuity patients at the time of admission, and often, the hyperglycemia was not treated unless the blood glucose level rose to 200 mg/dL or higher (Montori et al., 2002). In the 1990s, however, it became apparent that even moderate levels of hyperglycemia could have deleterious effects on highly stressed body systems during acute illness. Stress hyperglycemia in the critically ill patient has been associated with a higher incidence of complications and decreased long-term survival

(Capes, et al., 2000; Lewis et al., 2004; Malmberg et al., 1999; Van den Berghe, et al., 2001). *Stress hyperglycemia* refers to elevated blood glucose levels that develop because of the stress response. During times of crisis, the stress response triggers an outflow of stress hormones, particularly cortisol, which significantly increase blood glucose levels.

Malmberg et al. (1999) studied adult diabetic patients with acute myocardial infarctions (AMI). They concluded that the severity of a diabetic patient's admission glycometabolic state (measured as Hb A_1c and blood glucose levels) was a significant predictor of mortality, and that intensive insulin therapy (defined by them as continuous intravenous insulin therapy followed by subcutaneous insulin injections for a minimum of three months after the AMI) reduced long-term mortality. Capes et al. (2000) further concluded that stress hyperglycemia was harmful to high acuity nondiabetic patients, as well those with diabetes. In 2000, Van den Berghe et al. (2001) initiated their landmark investigation involving diabetic and nondiabetic critically ill adult patients. They recommended maintaining tight control of blood glucose levels to 110 mg/dL or less to reduce mortality and morbidity in critically ill patients regardless of whether or not they are diabetics. Several years later, Van den Berghe et al. (2003) further recommended use of an insulin titration algorithm to optimally control hyperglycemia in the critically ill patient population. Currently there is no universally accepted titration algorithm and intensive insulin therapy protocols vary widely. Table 27–8 provides an example of an insulin titration algorithm.

Nursing care of the patient receiving intensive insulin therapy includes frequent monitoring of blood glucose levels, titrating the insulin infusion according to the protocol, closely monitoring the patient for development of hypoglycemia as glucose levels approach normal, and intervening rapidly if hypoglycemia occurs to return the patient to a normoglycemic state without complications. Maintaining the blood glucose levels within the normal range is often challenging, particularly if the patient's condition is complex and unstable.

The Somogyi Effect: An Insulin Dosage Problem

Some patients, particularly those who are acutely ill, have wide swings in serum glucose levels from early morning to postprandial testings caused by an excessive insulin dosage. One explanation of this phenomenon is the **Somogyi effect**. The effect is triggered by nocturnal hypoglycemia. Hypoglycemia causes release of stress hormones, ultimately increasing serum glucose, which, in turn, creates a state of hyperglycemia. Morning urine ketones may be noted as well as an elevated serum glucose caused by catabolic processes. The resulting hyperglycemia, if accompanied by increased insulin dosage, precipitates another episode of hypoglycemia that may be worse than the preceding episode (Fig. 27–5).

TABLE 27–7   Example of Sliding-Scale Insulin Regimen

BLOOD GLUCOSE LEVEL (MG/DL)	REGULAR INSULIN DOSE (SUBCUTANEOUSLY)
200–250	5 units
251–300	10 units
301–350	12 units
351–400	15 units
Greater than 400	Call physician

TABLE 27–8 Example of Insulin Titration Algorithm

BLOOD GLUCOSE LEVEL (MG/DL)	INSULIN RATE (UNITS PER HOUR)	ACTIONS AND FOLLOW-UP PROCEDURES
Admission:		
If > 220	Initiate at 4	Initiate insulin infusion
If > 110	Initiate at 2	Check blood glucose level every hour
Maintenance:		
Rapid reduction of glucose > 5% change	Reduce insulin dose to half	Check blood glucose every 30 min.
> 140	Increase to 2	
110–140	Increase to 1	
Approaching normal	Adjust dose up or down by 0.1 to 0.5 units/hr	
Within normal limits	Maintain current dose	
60–80	Reduce dose adequately (some algorithms stop insulin infusion at this glucose level)	Rate of insulin decrease depends on previous blood glucose level Check blood glucose every 30 min.
40–60	Stop insulin infusion	Assure baseline glucose intake Check blood glucose level every 30 min.
< 40	Stop insulin infusion	Assure baseline glucose intake Give 25 mL dextrose 50% water ($D_{50}W$) Check blood glucose level every 30 min.

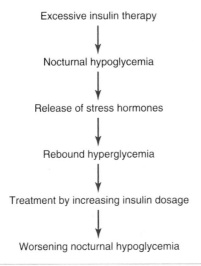

Figure 27–5 ■ The Somogyi effect.

Recognition of the presence of the Somogyi effect has important treatment implications. The administration of more insulin worsens the level of nocturnal hypoglycemia, further aggravating the problem. When the Somogyi effect is suspected, the insulin dosage actually may need to be decreased, or a bedtime snack of protein may be added to the diet to slow down the rebound cycle.

In summary, exogenous insulin therapy is a necessity for the client with type 1 diabetes. The type 2 diabetic may require it, particularly during periods of physiologic stress. Exogenous insulin is available from either animal or synthetic sources. Animal sources of insulin are similar but not identical to human insulin, making them potentially less acceptable to the body. Synthetic insulin is a laboratory duplication of human insulin. Choice of type of insulin based on source usually is decided by trial and error.

SECTION EIGHT REVIEW

1. Which of the following situations would be MOST likely to necessitate exogenous insulin use in the type 2 diabetic client?
   A. a localized toe infection
   B. a mild common cold
   C. a high carbohydrate meal
   D. an abdominal hysterectomy
2. Which of the following are sources of insulin? (choose all that apply)

   1. pork
   2. beef
   3. Staphylococcus aureus
   4. Escherichia coli
   A. 1, 2, and 3
   B. 1 and 2
   C. 1, 2, and 4
   D. 2

3. Exogenous insulin is
   A. seldom used in the treatment of HHS
   B. most often derived from animal sources
   C. used only in the treatment of type 1 diabetes
   D. often required in management of type 2 diabetes during stress periods
4. Which of the following are factors that dictate the type of insulin that is best suited for a specific person? (choose all that apply)
   1. a patient's weight
   2. insulin resistance
   3. a patient's allergies
   4. adipose tissue condition

A. 2, 3, and 4
B. 2 and 3
C. 1, 2, and 3
D. 3 and 4

5. Which of the following factors would MOST likely decrease insulin need?
   A. acute illness
   B. steroid therapy
   C. nutritional support
   D. oral antidiabetic agents

Answers: 1. A, 2. C, 3. D, 4. A, 5. D

SECTION NINE: Acute Care Implications of Chronic Complications

At the completion of this section, the learner will be able to discuss the acute care implications of chronic diabetic complications.

Glucose Control and Complications

There are many factors that influence acutely ill patient outcomes, such as preexisting chronic diseases. Diabetes is a chronic disease that profoundly affects patient outcomes because of the many acute and chronic complications that can result from it. Though diabetes mellitus is caused by dysfunction of one organ—the pancreas—it causes dysfunction of virtually all organs. Maintaining long-term glucose control is essential in the prevention or reduction of diabetes-related complications.

Overall glucose control can be monitored using the **glycosylated hemoglobin (Hb A$_1$c)** test. According to Kee (2002), the predominant type of hemoglobin is hemoglobin A (Hb A). Normally, about 4 to 8 percent of hemoglobin A has glucose attached to it and is referred to as glycosylated hemoglobin (Hb A$_1$). Hb A$_1$ forms slowly throughout the 120-day life span of hemoglobin. Hb A$_1$ is made up of three different molecules, one of which is Hb A$_1$c. This particular molecule is about 70 percent glycosylated. The amount of glycosylated hemoglobin depends on the amount of glucose in the blood and is a good indicator of the average serum glucose level over a 120-day period. The normal range of glycosylated hemoglobin (Hb A$_1$c) is 4.5 to 7.5 percent of the total hemoglobin (Kee, 2002). Uncontrolled diabetes mellitus is present if a glycosylated hemoglobin level is more than 15 percent of the total hemoglobin.

Chronic Complications

Chronic complications can be divided into three types: peripheral neuropathy, microvascular, and macrovascular. The remainder of this section will present an overview of major long-term complications associated with diabetes mellitus.

Diabetic Peripheral Neuropathies

Peripheral neuropathies are the most common complications of diabetes mellitus. They begin early in the course of the disease, affecting both type 1 and type 2 diabetics. Peripheral neuropathies primarily alter sensory perception. The underlying cause of neuropathies is poorly understood. They may result from thickening of vessel walls that supply peripheral nerves, thus impairing nutrition to the nerves. They may result from a segmental demyelinization that results in slowed or disrupted conduction. There is also some evidence that sorbitol may accumulate in the nerve cells, impairing conduction. Whatever the cause, the result is an alteration in sensory perception.

Neuropathies initially may cause pain or abnormal sensations or both. As nerve degeneration progresses, the patient may experience loss of the ability to discriminate fine touch, a decrease in proprioception, and local anesthesia.

The autonomic nervous system also may be affected. As the myelin sheath undergoes degenerative changes, functions governed by the autonomic nerves are affected adversely. The patient may experience an increase in gut motility and diarrhea, postural hypotension, or other autonomic nervous system–related complications.

The neuropathies experienced by diabetics vary in type, severity, and clinical manifestations. Because of this diversity, it is not possible to predict which neuropathy any individual will develop.

Acute Care Implications. When feasible, patients with diabetes should be assessed for the presence and degree of peripheral neuropathy. The presence of a diminished sense of touch and pain may mask injury or infection. The client must be protected from injury at all times to prevent damage to affected tissues. The diabetic patient must also be protected from hyperthermic burns. Excessive heat may not be sensed, which increases the risk of burns by heating pads, hyperthermia blankets, and bathing. Some neuropathies are associated with progressive, permanent damage to the neurons. However, others are reversible when good glucose control is maintained.

Microvascular Disease

Microvascular disease is associated with capillary membrane thickening, which causes **microangiopathy** (small blood vessel disease). As the capillary membrane thickens, the tissues become increasingly hypoperfused, and organs become hypoxic and ischemic. Prolonged ischemia eventually causes **infarction** (death of tissue). The degree of microvascular disease may be influenced most by the duration of diabetes rather than the level of glucose control. Two organs are at particular risk for microvascular disease secondary to diabetes mellitus: the retina of the eyes (retinopathy) and the kidneys (nephropathy).

Retinopathy. Diabetic retinopathy is responsible for a significant portion of newly diagnosed blindness in the United States. It is caused by an underlying microangiopathy of the retina, leading to retina microvascular occlusion. Once occlusion exists, the retina undergoes increasing areas of ischemia and infarction, eventually leading to blindness. Damage occurs in two complex stages. Stage I is associated with increased capillary permeability, aneurysm formation, and hemorrhage. Stage II is associated with increasing retinal ischemia and eventual infarction, causing blindness. Diabetic retinopathy is associated with both type 1 and type 2 diabetes.

Acute Care Implications. The acutely ill diabetic patient may have moderate to severe visual impairment. Early assessment of visual status is important, either by questioning the patient directly or by interviewing the family. Medical and nursing management and teaching must be altered to meet the needs of a visually impaired patient. In the high-acuity patient, blindness affects pupillary changes and must be taken into consideration when performing a neurologic assessment. A visually impaired patient in a critical care environment may have more difficulty making sense of distracting noises and equipment surrounding the bedside. Frequent explanation and reorientation may be necessary.

Nephropathy. Diabetic nephropathy is a disease of the glomeruli. The glomerular basement membrane becomes thickened, resulting in intracapillary glomerulosclerosis (hardening

and thickening of the glomeruli). Glomeruli become enlarged and eventually are destroyed, ultimately resulting in renal failure. As the degree of renal failure increases, the patient may require a decreased insulin dosage to prevent hypoglycemia. Reduced renal function decreases the ability of the kidneys to metabolize insulin. Insulin not metabolized remains available to facilitate glucose metabolism.

Acute Care Implications. The acutely ill patient with some degree of preexisting renal impairment is at risk for further impairment from hypotensive episodes, nephrotoxic drug therapy, or the multisystemic complications associated with many acute illnesses. Kidney function must be carefully monitored at regular intervals. Drug therapy may need to be altered based on kidney function. Kidney failure, as a disease entity, has its own set of actual and potential complications.

Macrovascular Disease

Macrovascular disease (**macroangiopathy**) refers to atherosclerosis. **Atherosclerosis** is a form of arteriosclerosis (thickening and hardening of arterial walls), characterized by plaque deposits of lipids, fibrous connective tissue, calcium, and other blood substances. Atherosclerosis, by definition, affects only large arteries (excluding arterioles). The cause of rapid development of atherosclerosis in the diabetic patient is described in Section Three.

Macrovascular disease is associated with the development of coronary artery disease, peripheral vascular disease, brain attack (stroke), and increased risk of infection. Type 2 diabetes is more closely associated with macrovascular diseases than type 1 diabetes. Peripheral vascular disease and increased risk of infection have important implications in the care of the acutely ill patient.

Peripheral Vascular Disease. Progressive atherosclerotic changes in peripheral arterial circulation lead to decreasing arterial blood flow to peripheral tissues. As the disease progresses, small arteries become occluded, precipitating a tissue ischemia/infarction sequence of events. In the type 2 diabetic, this is typically noted as small isolated patches of gangrene, particularly on the feet and toes. As circulation becomes increasingly compromised, areas of gangrene become larger, and amputation may be required.

Acute Care Implications. The client with peripheral vascular disease is at increased risk for complications secondary to poor tissue perfusion and loss of skin integrity. Of particular concern in the acutely ill patient is the development of decubitus ulcers and infection. Development of either of these two problems could potentially lead to gangrene and possible amputation. Careful limb positioning, excellent skin hygiene, and close monitoring of skin integrity are extremely important.

Increased Risk of Infection. The diabetic client is at high risk for development of infection for a variety of reasons.

1. **Diminished early warning system.** Impaired vision and peripheral neuropathy contribute to the decreased ability of the diabetic patient to perform self-monitoring. Breaks in skin integrity may not be seen or felt because of the underlying disease process.
2. **Tissue hypoxia.** Vascular disease causes tissue hypoxia. When skin integrity is broken, there is a decreased ability to heal, secondary to lack of oxygen. Glycosylated hemoglobin in RBCs decreases release of oxygen to the tissues, thus contributing to hypoxia.
3. **Rapid proliferation of pathogens.** Once inside the body, pathogens rapidly multiply because of increased glucose in body fluids, which acts as an energy source for the pathogens.
4. **Impaired white blood cells.** Diabetes is associated with the development of abnormal white blood cells, particularly phagocytes, and also alters chemotaxis (movement of WBCs to the site of infection).
5. **Impaired circulation.** A diminished blood supply decreases the ability of WBCs to move into the infected area.

Acute Care Implications. The acutely ill diabetic patient is at increased risk for the development of severe, difficult-to-treat infections. Any infection, no matter how minor it begins, may become life-threatening in this population. Close monitoring for infection and rapid, aggressive intervention are needed. Decreased kidney function may be a complicating factor in aggressive antibiotic therapy.

Wound healing also is impaired in the diabetic for several reasons. Impaired tissue perfusion, especially in the distal extremities, interferes with healing in those areas because of lack of circulation and tissue hypoxia. Hyperglycemic states adversely affect wound healing by interfering with collagen concentrations in a wound. Good control of blood glucose significantly facilitates wound healing.

In summary, the multisystemic nature of the chronic complications of diabetes strongly influences patient outcomes in acute illness. There are three major categories of complications: (1) peripheral neuropathies; (2) microvascular complications, including retinopathy and nephropathy; and (3) macrovascular complications, including coronary artery disease, brain attack (stroke), peripheral vascular disease, and increased risk of infection.

SECTION NINE REVIEW

1. Peripheral neuropathies primarily affect
   A. motor functions
   B. sensory functions
   C. optic functions
   D. vascular functions
2. Microvascular diseases are associated with
   A. deposits of lipoproteins
   B. deposits of calcium products
   C. large blood vessel disease
   D. small blood vessel disease
3. Diabetic retinopathy causes blindness as a result of
   A. glucose deposits on the retina
   B. thickening of the retina
   C. destruction of the optic nerve
   D. infarction of retinal tissue
4. Diabetic nephropathy damages the nephrons by causing
   A. glomerulosclerosis
   B. glomerulonephritis
   C. chronic nephritis
   D. renal hypertension

5. Diabetes-induced atherosclerosis is associated with which of the following complications? (choose all that apply)
   1. peripheral vascular disease
   2. brain attack (stroke)
   3. gastrointestinal ulcers
   4. coronary artery disease
   A. 1, 2, and 3
   B. 2, 3, and 4
   C. 1, 2, and 4
   D. 1 and 3
6. Diabetes increases a patient's chance of infection as a result of which of the following?
   A. abnormal white blood cells
   B. abnormal platelet function
   C. slow proliferation of pathogens
   D. decreased body fluid glucose levels

Answers: 1. B, 2. D, 3. D, 4. A, 5. C, 6. A

POSTTEST

The following Posttest is constructed in a case study format. A patient is presented. Questions are asked based on available data. New data are presented as the case study progresses.

Connie D is a 44-year-old housewife with a history of diabetes mellitus. She has been admitted to the hospital for reevaluation of insulin dosage. She has been having periods of drowsiness and confusion at home.

1. Connie's brain cells
   A. do not require glucose for energy
   B. require fatty acids as their major energy source
   C. do not require insulin for cellular uptake of glucose
   D. require high levels of insulin for cellular uptake of glucose

2. When Connie's blood glucose drops below normal, the sympathetic nervous system stimulates secretion of
   A. epinephrine
   B. cortisol
   C. glucagon
   D. growth hormone

3. Which statement best reflects the effect of insulin on glucose metabolism in Connie's liver? Insulin facilitates conversion of _____.
   A. excess amino acids into glucose
   B. excess fatty acids into glycogen
   C. excess glycogen into glucose
   D. excess glucose into glycogen

4. When Connie's blood amino acid levels increase, insulin
   A. facilitates storage of proteins
   B. inhibits synthesis of protein
   C. facilitates protein catabolism
   D. inhibits transport of amino acids into cell

Connie has an absolute insulin deficit.

5. An absolute insulin deficit would affect her carbohydrate metabolism in which of the following ways?
   A. brain cells rapidly become glucose starved
   B. insulin-dependent cells become glucose starved
   C. brain cells convert glycogen to glucose directly
   D. insulin-dependent cells take in glucose directly

6. In which way does insulin deficit affect Connie's protein metabolism?
   A. protein synthesis is increased
   B. protein catabolism is halted
   C. protein cannot be stored without insulin
   D. protein cannot be used as energy without insulin

Connie's diabetes is characterized by the following. Her mother also had diabetes. Connie was diagnosed with diabetes at the age of 32. She is 5 feet 5 inches (16.5 meters) tall and weighs 173 pounds (78.6 kg). She requires insulin on a daily basis.

7. Which of the preceding data is most suggestive of type 1 diabetes?
   A. her mother also had diabetes
   B. she was diagnosed at the age of 32
   C. she is 5 feet 5 inches (16.5 m) tall and weighs 173 pounds (78.6 kg)
   D. she requires insulin on a daily basis

8. If Connie had type 2 diabetes, the most common etiologic factors include
   A. viral infection and obesity
   B. obesity and genetic predisposition
   C. immune reaction and viral infection
   D. obesity and autoimmune reaction

During her hospitalization, Connie was kept NPO for 8 hours for a particular set of blood tests. She, however, did receive her usual morning insulin dosage. Consequently, Connie experiences symptoms typical of a hypoglycemic episode.

9. Typical clinical manifestations of Connie's hypoglycemia would include which of the following? (choose all that apply)
   1. bradycardia
   2. tremor
   3. diaphoresis
   4. vomiting
   A. 2, 3, and 4
   B. 1, 3, and 4
   C. 1, 2, and 3
   D. 1 and 3

10. Common causes of hypoglycemic episodes include
    A. lack of dietary intake
    B. heavy carbohydrate meal
    C. insufficient insulin dose
    D. decreased exercise level

Connie has developed an infection from an ingrown toenail. She currently has a temperature of 100°F (37.8°C) (oral). A rapid assessment reveals the following: opens eyes and groans to mild shaking but closes them immediately after stimulation.

11. What other clinical manifestations would help confirm a diagnosis of diabetic ketoacidosis at this time?
    A. polydipsia
    B. hand tremors
    C. fruity breath odor
    D. shallow respirations

12. Which laboratory result would be most diagnostic of diabetic ketoacidosis?
    A. pH 7.34
    B. anion gap 18 mEq/L
    C. HCO_3 17 mEq/L
    D. Pa_{CO_2} 28 mm Hg

It has been decided that Connie's diabetic ketoacidosis was precipitated by her foot infection.

13. Infection can precipitate a diabetic ketoacidosis episode as a result of
    A. stress response
    B. increased insulin resistance
    C. increased glucagon levels
    D. diminished cortisol activity
14. Connie's diabetic ketoacidosis can be differentiated best from hyperglycemic hyperosmolar state (HHS) by measuring
    A. pH
    B. ketones
    C. bicarbonate
    D. blood glucose

Connie is experiencing large swings in her glucose levels throughout the day. The physician orders a larger insulin dose to better control the hyperglycemia. The next day, her hyperglycemia is worse. It is decided that she may be experiencing the Somogyi effect. Connie is confused but conscious.

15. The Somogyi effect is characterized by a rebound phenomenon caused by release of
    A. glucagon
    B. amino acids
    C. fatty acids
    D. stress hormones
16. Considering her status, which of the following interventions would be most appropriate?
    A. 5 units of regular insulin
    B. glucagon 1.5 mg (IM)
    C. bed time snack
    D. 50 percent dextrose (IV)

During her diabetic ketoacidosis episode, Connie receives a continuous drip of IV insulin.

17. Important rules to remember in infusing IV insulin include which of the following? (choose all that apply)
    1. only regular insulin is used IV
    2. insulin binds to plastic bags and tubing
    3. obtain urine glucose every hour
    4. IV doses usually are small
    A. 1, 2, and 3
    B. 2, 3, and 4
    C. 1, 2, and 4
    D. 1 and 2

On Connie's history, you note that she has a long history of peripheral neuropathy, poor vision, and peripheral vascular disease.

18. Connie's peripheral neuropathy is best controlled by
    A. steroid therapy
    B. good glucose control
    C. vitamin supplementation
    D. nothing; there is no slowing the process
19. Connie's vision has become progressively impaired over the duration of her diabetes. Diabetic retinopathy is a result of
    A. glucose deposits on retina
    B. macrovascular occlusion
    C. fatty deposits on retina
    D. microvascular occlusion
20. Connie's peripheral vascular disease may lead to further complications because it causes
    A. tissue ischemia
    B. acute infection
    C. peripheral edema
    D. coronary artery disease

POSTTEST ANSWERS

Number	Answer	Section
1	C	One
2	A	One
3	D	Two
4	A	Two
5	B	Three
6	C	Three
7	D	Four
8	B	Four
9	A	Five
10	A	Five

Number	Answer	Section
11	C	Six
12	B	Six
13	A	Six
14	B	Seven
15	D	Eight
16	C	Eight
17	C	Eight
18	B	Nine
19	D	Nine
20	A	Nine

REFERENCES

American Diabetes Association. (2003). Hyperglycemic crises in patients with diabetes mellitus. *Diabetes Care, 26*(1), S109–S117.

Barnett, P. (2001). Hypoglycemia. In T. E. Andreoli, C. C. Carpenter, R. C. Griggs, & J. Loscalzo (Eds.), *Cecil's essentials of medicine* (5th ed., pp. 599–604). Philadelphia: W. B. Saunders.

Capes, S. E., Hunt, D., Malmberg, K., & Gerstein, H. C. (2000). Stress hyperglycemia and increased risk of death after myocardial infarction in patients with and without diabetes: a systematic overview. *The Lancet, 355,* 773–778.

Davidson, M. B., & Schwartz, S. (2001). Hyperglycemia. In M. J. Frantz (Ed.), *A core curriculum for diabetes education: Diabetes and complications:* (4th ed., pp. 19–42). Chicago: American Association of Diabetes Educators.

Fleckman, A. M. (1993). Diabetic ketoacidosis. *Endocrinology Metabolic Clinics of America, 22*(2), 181–206.

Furnary, A., Gao, G., Grunkemeir, G., Wu, Y., Zerr, K., et al. (2003). Continuous insulin infusion reduces mortality in patients with diabetes undergoing coronary artery bypass grafting. *Journal of Thoracic and Cardiovascular Surgery, 125*(5), 1007–1021.

Gonder-Frederick, L. A. (2001). Hypoglycemia. In M. J. Frantz (Ed.), *A core curriculum for diabetes education: Diabetes management therapies:* (4th ed., pp. 229–260). Chicago: American Association of Diabetes Educators.

Guvan, S., Kuenzi, J. A., & Matfin, G. (2004). Diabetes mellitus. In C. M. Porth (Ed.), *Essentials of pathophysiology* (pp. 560–579). Philadelphia: Lippincott Williams & Wilkins.

Johnson, D. (1998). Endocrine disorders. In M. R. Kinney et al. (Eds.), *AACN's clinical reference for critical-care nursing* (4th ed., pp. 849–872). St. Louis: C. V. Mosby.

Kee, J. L. (2002). *Laboratory and diagnostic tests with nursing implications* (6th ed.). Upper Saddle River, NJ: Prentice Hall.

Lewis, K., Kane-Gill, S., Bobek, M., & Dasta, J. (2004). Intensive insulin therapy for critically ill patients. *The Annals of Pharmacotherapy, 38,* 1243–1251.

Malmberg, K., Norhammar, A., Wedel, H., & Ryden, L. (1999). Glycometabolic state at admission: Important risk marker of mortality in conventionally treated patients with diabetes mellitus and acute myocardial infarction. *Circulation, 99,* 2626–2632.

Montori, V. M., Bistrian, B. R., & McMahon, M. M. (2002). Hyperglycemia in acutely ill patients. *JAMA, 288*(17), pp. 2167–2169.

Porth, C. M. (2004). *Pathophysiology: Concepts of altered health states* (7th ed.). Philadelphia: Lippincott, Williams & Wilkins.

Ratner, R. E. (2001). Pathophysiology of the diabetes disease state. In M. J. Frantz (Ed.), *A core curriculum for diabetes education: Diabetes and complications* (4th ed., pp. 1–18). Chicago: American Association of Diabetes Educators.

Semb, S. (2004). Nursing management: Diabetes mellitus. In S. M. Lewis, M. M. Heitkemper, & S. R. Dirksen (Eds.), *Medical-surgical nursing: Assessment and management of clinical problems* (6th ed., pp. 1268–1302). St. Louis: C. V. Mosby.

Van den Berghe, G., Wouters, P., Bouillon, R., Weekers, F., Verwaest, C, et al. (2003). Outcome benefit of intensive insulin therapy in the critically ill: Insulin dose versus glycemic control. *Critical Care Medicine, 31*(2), 359–366.

Van den Berghe, G., Wouters, P., Weekers, F., Verwaest, C., Bruyninckx, F., et al. (2001). Intensive insulin therapy in critically ill patients. *New England Journal of Medicine, 324*(19), 1359–1367.

White, J. R., Campbell, R. K., & Yarborough, P. C. (2001). Pharmacologic therapies. In M. J. Frantz (Ed.), *A core curriculum for diabetes education: Diabetes management therapies* (4th ed., pp. 89–105). Chicago: American Association of Diabetes Educators.

28 Acute Renal Dysfunction

Kathleen Dorman Wagner

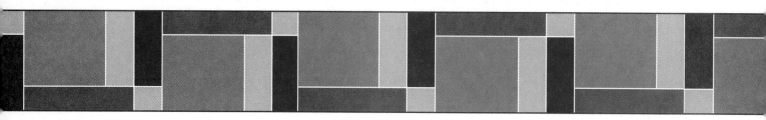

OBJECTIVES Following completion of this module, the learner will be able to

1. Briefly explain normal kidney function.
2. Discuss the influences of selected body systems on renal function.
3. Identify the categories of acute renal failure as prerenal, interstitial, or postrenal.
4. Describe the phases of acute renal failure.
5. Describe the effects of acute renal dysfunction on fluid and electrolyte balance.
6. Discuss assessment and diagnosis of renal failure.
7. Provide a brief overview of the collaborative management of the patient with acute renal failure.
8. Discuss dialysis as a treatment modality for acute renal failure.
9. Discuss the implications of caring for a high-acuity patient who has chronic renal failure.

This self-study module focuses on the physiologic as well as pathophysiologic processes involved in acute renal failure. It is composed of nine sections. Sections One and Two discuss normal renal function. The module then shifts its focus to abnormal kidney function, specifically acute renal failure. Sections Three and Four present categories and phases of acute renal failure. Section Five describes the effects of acute renal failure on fluid and electrolyte balance. Section Six presents assessment and diagnosis of renal failure, including the nursing history and assessment, and laboratory tests and procedures used for diagnosing acute renal failure. Section Seven provides an overview of collaborative management of acute renal failure.

Section Eight presents an overview of renal dialysis, including hemodialysis, peritoneal dialysis, and continuous renal replacement therapy (CRRT). Finally, in Section Nine the focus shifts from acute renal failure to chronic renal failure, with an overview of the implications for care for the high-acuity patient who has chronic renal failure. Each section includes a set of review questions to help the learner evaluate his or her understanding of the section's content before moving on to the next section. All Section Reviews and the module Pretest and Posttest include answers. It is suggested that the learner review those concepts answered incorrectly in the review questions before proceeding to the next section.

 ## PRETEST

1. The functional unit of the kidney is the
   A. nephron
   B. glomerulus
   C. renal tubule
   D. Bowman's capsule

2. Fluid and solutes are moved from the vascular system into the tubular system of the nephron by
   A. tubular reabsorption
   B. glomerular filtration
   C. vascular resistance
   D. tubular secretion

3. A receptor that increases the blood pressure by increasing production of antidiuretic hormone (ADH) is a(n)
   A. baroreceptor
   B. chemoreceptor
   C. osmoreceptor
   D. stretch receptor

4. The influence of aldosterone on the maintenance of body fluid levels is based on which principle?
   A. sodium follows water
   B. potassium follows sodium
   C. water follows sodium
   D. sodium follows potassium

5. Approximately _____ percent of patients treated early in the course of acute renal failure have little to no residual loss of renal function.
   A. 10
   B. 25
   C. 50
   D. 75

6. Acute tubular necrosis (ATN) is caused primarily by which of the following two factors?
   A. myoglobin and nephrotoxic drugs
   B. hypoperfusion and myoglobin
   C. myoglobin and hemoglobin
   D. nephrotoxic drugs and hypoperfusion

7. Renal ischemia has which effect on renal blood flow?
   A. vasospasm
   B. vasodilation
   C. vasoconstriction
   D. decreased vascular resistance

8. The maintenance phase of acute renal failure ends when the blood urea nitrogen (BUN) and creatinine
   A. cease decreasing
   B. begin to decrease
   C. slow their increase
   D. return to normal

9. Which laboratory value can be used to differentiate acute tubular necrosis from prerenal hypoperfusion?
   A. BUN and chloride
   B. calcium and chloride
   C. sodium and potassium
   D. specific gravity and urine osmolality

10. Renal biopsy would most likely be used to further investigate
    A. prerenal failure
    B. intrinsic renal failure
    C. renal thrombosis
    D. renal calculi obstruction

11. Which imbalances most commonly occur secondary to acute renal failure?
    A. hyperkalemia, hyperphosphatemia, metabolic acidosis
    B. hypokalemia, hyponatremia, hypercalcemia
    C. hyperkalemia, hypocalcemia, metabolic alkalosis
    D. hypernatremia, hypermagnesemia, hypercalcemia

12. Potassium imbalance secondary to acute renal dysfunction is associated with which factors? (choose all that apply)
    1. increased excretion
    2. metabolic acidosis
    3. decreased excretion
    4. increased tissue breakdown
    A. 1, 3, and 4
    B. 2 and 3
    C. 2, 3, and 4
    D. 3 and 4

13. Which statement is correct regarding how acute renal failure affects the cardiovascular system?
    A. it causes hypotension
    B. it causes congestive heart failure
    C. it causes atherosclerosis
    D. it causes increased renal blood flow

14. Acute renal failure can precipitate gastrointestinal bleeding as a result of increased levels of
    A. uric acid
    B. creatinine
    C. urea
    D. ammonia

15. Common rapid access sites for short-term hemodialysis are
    A. subclavian and femoral veins
    B. femoral and brachial arteries
    C. radial and femoral arteries
    D. internal jugular and subclavian veins

16. Which statement is correct regarding diffusion?
    A. it occurs up a concentration gradient
    B. it moves particles (solute) across a membrane
    C. it occurs down a concentration gradient
    D. it disperses solute within a solution with no membrane

17. Catabolic processes that are present in patients with acute renal failure make restriction of _____ necessary.
    A. carbohydrates
    B. fats
    C. protein
    D. essential amino acids

18. The major cause of death from acute renal failure is
    A. hyperkalemia
    B. metabolic acidosis
    C. fluid excess
    D. infection

Pretest Answers: 1. A, 2. B, 3. A, 4. C, 5. C, 6. D, 7. C, 8. B, 9. D, 10. B, 11. A, 12. C, 13. B, 14. D, 15. A, 16. C, 17. C, 18. D

GLOSSARY

acid–base balance   A stable concentration of hydrogen ions in body fluids.

acidosis   An increased hydrogen ion concentration in the blood or a pH less than 7.35.

active transport   Movement of substances across a membrane without a pressure gradient, using the expenditure of energy.

acute renal failure   A syndrome of multiple etiologies that is characterized by a sudden onset and rapid decline of renal function.

acute tubular necrosis (ATN)   A destructive process of the renal tubules.

aldolase   An enzyme present in large quantities in cardiac and skeletal muscles.

aldosterone   A hormone produced by the adrenal cortex, responsible for excretion of potassium and absorption of sodium in the renal tubules, leading to reabsorption of water into the blood volume.

anions   Electrons with a negative charge.

antidiuretic hormone (ADH)   A hormone produced by the hypothalamus and secreted by the posterior pituitary.

anuria   Cessation of urine production.

autoregulation   A compensatory mechanism that maintains renal blood flow even when there is a great variance in perfusion pressure.

azotemia   The accumulation of uremic toxins (urea, uric acid, and creatinine) in the blood.

Bowman's capsule   The initial structure of the tubular system of the nephron.

cardiac output   The amount of blood the heart pumps in 1 minute.

cations   Electrons with a positive charge.

chronic renal failure (CRF)   The slow, progressive, and irreversible destruction of the kidneys.

dialysis   A process of diffusion by which dissolved particles can be transported across a semipermeable membrane from one fluid compartment to another.

diuretic   Medication that reduces the reabsorption of sodium and water in the kidneys, resulting in an increase in urine excretion.

electrolytes   Elements or compounds that when dissolved in a fluid dissociate into ions and can carry an electrical current.

glomerular filtration   The process by which fluid and solutes are moved from the vascular system into the tubular system of the nephron.

glomerular filtration rate (GFR)   Measurement of the plasma volume that can be cleared of any given substance within a certain time frame.

glomerulus   A cluster of capillaries located in the nephron; its primary function is to filter solutes.

homeostasis   The normal state of chemical balance within the body.

hyperkalemia   A greater than normal amount of potassium in the blood.

hypertension   Abnormally elevated blood pressure persistently exceeding 150/90 mm Hg.

hypervolemia   Increase in the amount of fluid in the circulating blood volume.

hypotension   Abnormally low blood pressure, inadequate for normal tissue perfusion and oxygenation.

Intrinsic renal failure   Kidney dysfunction caused by direct damage to the renal parenchyma.

myoglobin   An oxygen-binding protein with a structure similar to hemoglobin that is found primarily in skeletal and cardiac muscle.

nephron   The functional unit of the kidney.

oliguria   Excretion or formation of an abnormally small amount of urine.

passive transport (diffusion)   Movement of molecules from an area of higher concentration to an area of lower concentration; does not require the expenditure of energy.

permeability   The capability of spreading or flowing through small holes or gaps.

postrenal failure   Kidney dysfunction caused by bilateral obstruction of urine flow distal to the kidney parenchyma.

prerenal failure   Kidney dysfunction caused by inadequate renal blood flow.

rhabdomyolysis   A syndrome characterized by excessive skeletal muscle breakdown that causes release of muscle cell contents, including myoglobin.

tubular secretion   The process by which substances are secreted into the tubules to be excreted in the final stage of urine formation.

uremia   Clinical symptoms of azotemia.

ABBREVIATIONS

ADH	Antidiuretic hormone	**CRRT**	Continuous renal replacement therapy
ATN	Acute tubular necrosis	**CVP**	Central venous pressure
BUN	Blood urea nitrogen	**CVVH**	Continuous venovenous hemofiltration
CAVH	Continuous arteriovenous hemofiltration	**CVVH-D**	Continuous venovenous hemofiltration–dialysis
CAVH-D	Continuous arteriovenous hemofiltration–dialysis	**GFR**	Glomerular filtration rate
CRF	Chronic renal failure		

SECTION ONE: Normal Kidney Function

At the completion of this section, the learner will be able to briefly explain normal kidney function.

The Urinary System

The urinary system, with all of its structures intact, includes two kidneys, two ureters, a urinary bladder, and a urethra (Fig. 28–1). This system maintains **homeostasis** by removing waste products and by either conserving or excreting fluid and electrolytes. An individual requires only one functioning kidney to maintain normal regulatory mechanisms. The kidneys are the only means by which urine is transported and excreted.

The Kidney

A cross-section view of the kidney reveals the cortex, medulla, and pelvis (Fig. 28–2). The cortex and medulla are called the renal parenchyma. The medulla contains the renal pyramids, or collecting ducts. The cortex and medulla house all of the nephrons, which are composed primarily of tubular structures and blood vessels surrounding the nephrons. The nephrons produce urine, which then drains to the papilla, located at the base of the pyramid. The papilla acts as a collecting area, funneling urine to the renal pelvis, where it flows out of the kidney via the ureter. Renal blood supply to the kidney is from the renal artery,

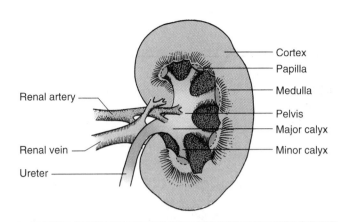

Figure 28–2 ■ Gross anatomy of the kidney. *(From Ulrich, B. T. [1989]. Nephrology nursing: Concepts and strategies [p. 3]. Norwalk, CT: Appleton & Lange.)*

a direct branch of the abdominal aorta. The renal artery subdivides further, with some branches nourishing the kidney and others taking part in the filtration process. Almost all of the blood being filtered returns to the normal circulation via the renal vein.

Nephron

The **nephron** is the functional unit of the kidney. Each nephron is composed of three major structures: a glomerulus, tubular apparatus, and collecting duct (Fig. 28–3). There are approximately 1 million nephrons in each kidney composed of vascular (blood flow) and tubular (urine flow) systems that promote the formation of urine. The vascular system of a nephron includes the glomerulus and vasa recta. The **glomerulus** is composed of a tight cluster of capillaries, and the afferent and efferent loops. The afferent loop becomes the glomerulus, and the efferent loop continues distal to the glomerulus to become the vasa recta, encircling the convoluted tubules and the loops of Henle.

Surrounding each glomerulus is a **Bowman's capsule,** the initial structure of the tubular system. Connected to the Bowman's capsule is the proximal convoluted tubule, which then becomes the loop of Henle. The loop of Henle is a hairpin-shaped section of the tubule. At the distal end of the loop of Henle is the distal convoluted tubule. This section is continuous with a system of collecting ducts that becomes progressively larger, eventually dumping urine into the renal pelvis.

The primary function of the nephron unit is to filter waste products from the blood as it flows through the kidneys. Approximately 1,200 mL of blood (about 21 percent of the resting cardiac output) passes through the kidneys every minute (Guyton & Hall, 1997). This large amount of blood is needed to produce the volume of filtrate necessary for glomerular filtration to occur. Urine formation is made possible by glomerular filtration and tubular reabsorption and secretion. Figure 28–4 shows nephron transport of substances, as well as their fate in the filtration process.

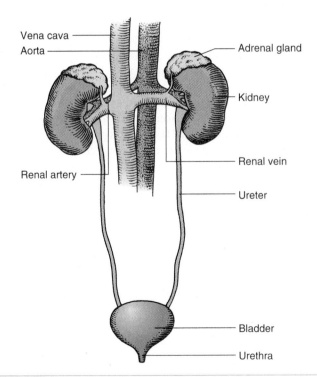

Figure 28–1 ■ Gross anatomy of the renal system. *(From Ulrich, B. T. [1989]. Nephrology nursing: Concepts and strategies [p. 2]. Norwalk, CT: Appleton & Lange.)*

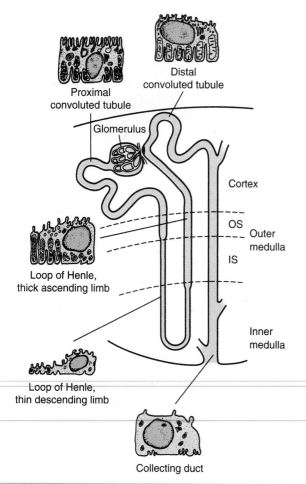

Proximal convoluted tubule

Distal convoluted tubule

Glomerulus

Cortex

OS
Outer medulla
IS

Loop of Henle, thick ascending limb

Inner medulla

Loop of Henle, thin descending limb

Collecting duct

Figure 28–3 ■ The nephron. *(From Ganong, W. F. [1985]. Review of medical physiology, (13th ed., p. 581). East Norwalk, CT: Appleton & Lange.)*

Glomerular Filtration. **Glomerular filtration** is the process by which fluid and solutes are moved from the vascular system into the tubular system of the nephron, from an area of relatively high pressure to an area of low pressure. The glomerulus is a high-pressure, semipermeable capillary bed. For filtration to occur, there must be adequate blood volume in the intravascular space, and adequate hydrostatic pressure from the cardiac output and vascular resistance. Glomerular filtrate is composed of

- Water (H_2O), hydrogen ions (H^+)
- Electrolytes: sodium (Na^+), potassium (K^+), calcium (Ca^{++}), magnesium (Mg^+), chloride (Cl^-), bicarbonate ($\mathbf{HCO_3^-}$), phosphate ($\mathbf{PO_4^-}$)
- Waste products: urea, creatinine, uric acid
- Metabolic substrates: glucose and amino acids

The **glomerular filtration rate (GFR)** measures the plasma volume that can be cleared of any given substance within a certain time frame. In a person with normal renal function, the GFR is about 180 L per day. The GFR can be used as an indicator of the adequacy of renal function. The rate of glomerular filtration is altered by any disease condition that changes plasma flow through the glomeruli or the **permeability** of the cell membrane.

Tubular Reabsorption.   Not all filtrate is excreted. Some is reabsorbed and returned to the blood through tubular reabsorption. Tubular reabsorption is accomplished in the proximal convoluted tubules of the kidneys. Reabsorption occurs as a result of two transport systems:

1. **Active transport.** Movement of substances across a membrane without a pressure gradient, using the expenditure of energy. Potassium, sodium, calcium, phosphates, glucose, and amino acids all require active transport.
2. **Passive transport (diffusion).** Movement of molecules from an area of higher concentration to an area of lower concentration. Passive transport does not require an expenditure of energy. Water, chloride, urea, and some phosphate and bicarbonate are reabsorbed by passive transport.

Tubular Secretion. **Tubular secretion** is the process by which substances, such as potassium, hydrogen, and antibiotics, are secreted into the tubules to be excreted in the final stage of urine formation. The final concentration or dilution of urine occurs in the distal tubules and collecting ducts that lead to the bladder. The volume of urine excreted is about 1,500 mL per day.

Effects of Aging on Renal Function

Under normal circumstances renal function remains adequate throughout life. The renal cortex loses mass with normal aging, with a 30 to 50 percent reduction in functional glomeruli (Pikna, 2002). As the glomerular filtration rate decreases with aging, so does muscle mass, which results in a reduction in creatinine production. This helps explain why serum creatinine levels do not significantly increase as GFR decreases. As with other organs, however, the aging kidneys are subject to decreased reserve capacity, which increases the risk for development of renal insufficiency or failure if the kidneys come under stress. Decreased renal function increases the risk for renal-based fluid and electrolyte imbalances during illness. Aging causes a decrease in urine concentration capacity and response to antidiuretic hormone (ADH). The aging patient is also more prone to dehydration as a result of development of an impaired thirst mechanism (Pikna, 2002).

In summary, the kidneys are the primary organs responsible for excretion of body wastes and excess fluid, electrolytes, and metabolites. The nephron is the functioning unit of the kidneys and is composed of a glomerulus, Bowman's capsule, and the tubular system. Glomerular filtration is the process by which fluid and substances are moved across the nephron vascular cell membrane into the tubular system for either reabsorption or eventual excretion. Glomerular filtration occurs by either an active or a passive transport system. Although there are many age-related renal changes, under normal circumstances, renal function remains adequate throughout life. When placed under stress, however, the decreased renal reserve capacity places the aging patient at increased risk for development of impaired renal function and acute renal failure.

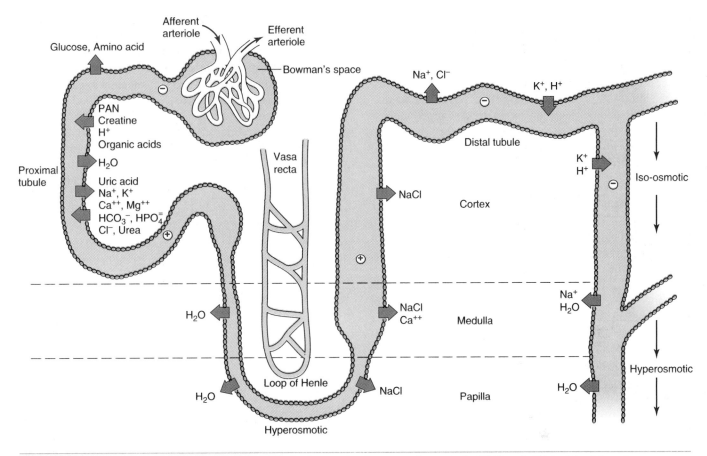

Figure 28–4 ■ Nephron transport. *(From Ulrich, B. T. [1989].* Nephrology nursing: Concepts and strategies *[p. 15]. Norwalk, CT: Appleton & Lange.)*

SECTION ONE REVIEW

1. The functional unit of the kidney is the
   - A. nephron
   - B. ureter
   - C. medulla
   - D. glomerulus
2. The term *renal parenchyma* refers to
   - A. renal pelvis
   - B. renal tubules
   - C. renal cortex and medulla
   - D. renal blood supply
3. Fluid and solutes are moved from the vascular system into the tubular system of the nephron by
   - A. tubular reabsorption
   - B. glomerular filtration
   - C. vascular resistance
   - D. tubular secretion

4. The movement of substances across a membrane without a pressure gradient using energy is called
   - A. active transport
   - B. tubular secretion
   - C. passive transport
   - D. tubular reabsorption
5. Normal aging has what effect on the number of functioning glomeruli?
   - A. no change
   - B. reduction by 10 to 20 percent
   - C. reduction by 30 to 50 percent
   - D. reduction by 50 to 75 percent

Answers: 1. A, 2. C, 3. B, 4. A, 5. C

SECTION TWO: Influences of Body Systems on Renal Function

At the completion of this section, the learner will be able to discuss the influences of selected body systems on renal function.

Renal function depends on the interrelated functioning of the cardiovascular, nervous, and endocrine systems. This section provides a brief overview of the influences of various body systems on renal function.

Cardiovascular System

The heart and blood vessels provide the kidneys with sufficient plasma to permit regulation of water and electrolytes in the body fluids. The cardiovascular system delivers blood to be filtered, maintains the blood pressure necessary for organ perfusion and glomerular filtration and provides the nephron vascular system. The kidneys receive 1 to 1.5 L of blood per minute, which is 20 to 25 percent of the cardiac output. This high blood flow state is required to adequately filter waste products from the blood and for regulation of fluid and electrolytes. The glomerular filtration rate is about 125 mL per minute but it can vary widely from almost zero to 200 mL per minute.

Nervous System

The nervous system helps regulate blood pressure through the sympathetic nervous system. Several types of receptors located in the large arteries of the neck and chest help maintain normal arterial blood pressure. *Baroreceptors* are sensitive to blood pressure changes, activating the hypothalamus when stimulated to alter antidiuretic hormone (ADH) production appropriately. *Chemoreceptors* in the carotid and aortic bodies send messages to the vasomotor center to increase blood flow when hydrogen ions and carbon dioxide content is high and oxygen levels are low. In addition, hypothalamic *osmoreceptors* are sensitive to changes in water osmolality. As water osmolality changes, the osmoreceptors communicate these changes to the hypothalamus, which results in altered ADH production.

The nervous system influences fluid balance by regulating the thirst mechanism. The thirst center is located in the brain's hypothalamus and is highly sensitive to fluid osmolality. In circumstances such as cellular dehydration, the hypothalamus sends impulses to stimulate thirst. Conversely, the drive to drink is diminished when overhydration is present.

Endocrine System

The endocrine system affects renal function directly through secretion of two hormones, antidiuretic hormone and aldosterone. **Antidiuretic hormone (ADH)** is produced by the hypothalamus and secreted by the posterior pituitary. It is responsible for the ability of water to follow sodium as it is excreted or reabsorbed. ADH secretion is stimulated by baroreceptors, which are sensitive to changes in arterial blood pressure, and by osmoreceptors, which are sensitive to changes in serum osmolality. It increases the permeability of the nephron cell membranes to water, allowing more water to be reabsorbed. Urinary output declines in response to the action of ADH.

Aldosterone, produced by the adrenal cortex, is influenced by serum levels of sodium and potassium. Aldosterone causes the kidney tubules to excrete potassium and absorb sodium, leading to reabsorption of water into the intravascular space. Fluid deficit stimulates production of this hormone. Angiotensin is a major controller of aldosterone secretion; thus, it is crucial in control of sodium levels. It also is an important part of the renin–angiotensin system, which strongly influences arterial blood pressure, as well as water and sodium regulation.

Compensatory Mechanisms

Compensatory mechanisms for maintaining renal perfusion and prevention of ischemic damage are the renin–angiotensin mechanism and autoregulation.

Renin–Angiotensin System. The renin–angiotensin system is important in the control of blood pressure. Renin is an enzyme secreted by the juxtaglomerular apparatus of the kidneys. It is theorized that a decreased blood pressure (**hypotension**), low intratubular sodium, or possibly catecholamines may stimulate renin production. Once produced, renin combines with angiotensin I, which originates in the liver, and is converted to angiotensin II in the lungs. Angiotensin II causes peripheral vasoconstriction and stimulates aldosterone release. Aldosterone stimulates the expansion of the circulatory volume through the reabsorption of sodium and water in the distal tubules. Figure 28–5 shows the sequence of events involved in the renin–angiotensin system.

Autoregulation. **Autoregulation** maintains a constant renal blood flow by regulating resistance of blood flow even when there are great variances in perfusion pressure. Through autoregulatory feedback mechanisms, the GFR and renal blood flow remain normal as long as the perfusion pressure remains between 75 and 160 mm Hg (Guyton & Hall, 1997); and it assures that renal metabolic needs are met. Autoregulation requires that resistance to renal blood flow must vary in direct proportion to arterial blood pressure (Porth, 2002a). When autoregulation is intact, if blood pressure drops below normal, the GFR decreases as blood flow through the glomeruli diminishes and less sodium and water are passed into the filtrate. The resulting conservation of sodium and water increases fluid volume in the intravascular space and blood pressure increases. The mechanism of autoregulation is unknown. It is theorized that it may result from renal vasoconstriction or vasodilation in response to decreases or increases in blood pressure.

In summary, renal function depends on multiple body systems. The cardiovascular system provides blood to the kidneys for filtering and sufficient blood pressure for perfusion and au-

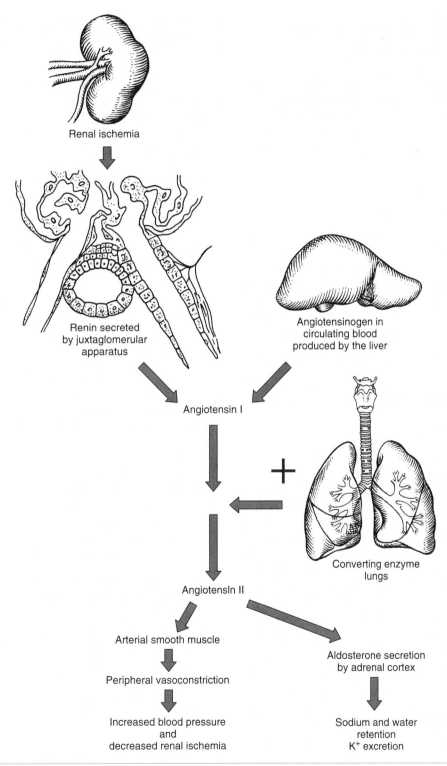

Figure 28–5 ■ The renin–angiotensin system. *(From Ulrich, B. T. [1989].* Nephrology nursing: Concepts and strategies *[p. 22]. Norwalk, CT: Appleton & Lange.)*

toregulation. The nervous system provides special receptors to help control blood pressure and fluid balance. Receptors stimulate the hypothalamus to alter production of ADH to either stimulate or inhibit production. The hypothalamus is also responsible for regulation of thirst in response to the level of hy-

dration. The endocrine system in conjunction with the nervous system is responsible for secretion of ADH and aldosterone. ADH alters water reabsorption, and aldosterone alters sodium and potassium serum levels, influencing water balance and arterial blood pressure.

SECTION TWO REVIEW

1. About _____ percent of the cardiac output comprises the total renal blood flow.
   A. 10
   B. 20
   C. 30
   D. 40
2. A receptor that increases the blood pressure by increasing production of ADH is
   A. baroreceptor
   B. chemoreceptor
   C. osmoreceptor
   D. ADH receptor
3. The influence of aldosterone on the maintenance of body fluid levels is based on which principle?
   A. sodium follows water
   B. potassium follows sodium
   C. water follows sodium
   D. sodium follows potassium
4. The thirst center in the hypothalamus is sensitive to
   A. blood pressure
   B. fluid osmolality

C. potassium level
D. sodium level

5. The renin–angiotensin system is important in the control of
   A. blood pressure
   B. autoregulation
   C. potassium excretion
   D. ADH production
6. Aldosterone causes the kidneys to
   A. vasodilate
   B. absorb potassium
   C. excrete water
   D. absorb sodium
7. True or False: For renal autoregulation to work, blood flow resistance must vary in direct proportion to the arterial blood pressure.

Answers: 1. B, 2. A, 3. C, 4. B, 5. A, 6. D, 7. True

SECTION THREE: Categories of Acute Renal Failure

At the completion of this section, the learner will be able to identify the categories of acute renal failure as prerenal, intrinsic, or postrenal.

It is estimated that about 15 percent of critically ill patients develop acute renal failure (ARF) with a mortality rate that may run as high as 60 to 70 percent (Ferrone, 2003). About 30 percent of patients with acute renal failure require renal dialysis (Albright, 2001), which increases the mortality rate even higher (as high as 80 percent) (Agraharkar, 2002; Esson & Schrier, 2002). The mortality rate is particularly high when multiple organ dysfunction syndrome (MODS) is present.

A single definition of acute renal failure has not been agreed on, however, the terms *syndrome, rapid onset,* and *rapid decline of function* are typically noted in the myriad definitions. For the purposes of this module, **acute renal failure** is defined as a syndrome with multiple etiologies that is characterized by a sudden onset and rapid decline of renal function. It may develop suddenly, within hours, or over a period of days. Acute renal failure is often reversible if diagnosed and treated early; however, if left unrecognized or if inadequately treated, it can cause permanent damage to the renal parenchyma.

Acute renal failure is categorized based on the location of the insult, being designated as prerenal, intrinsic, or postrenal. Table 28–1 provides a list of common causes of acute renal failure.

Prerenal Failure

Prerenal failure stems from problems that alter renal blood flow, causing renal hypoperfusion. Prerenal problems are the most common causes of renal failure overall but they are the second most common causes of hospital acquired renal failure (Ferrone, 2003). Underlying conditions that can precipitate prerenal failure include decreased cardiac output, vascular obstruction, and drug-induced altered glomerular hemodynamics.

Decreased Cardiac Output

Any problem that significantly diminishes **cardiac output (CO)** can cause prerenal failure (see Table 28–1). When cardiac output decreases, the kidneys rapidly respond through renal capillary vasoconstriction, which shunts blood away from the kidneys and increases blood supply to other, more critical core organs. In the short term, this is a benign, adaptive response; however, if the low renal blood flow state becomes prolonged, renal tissue ischemia and possibly necrosis results.

The kidneys are able to tolerate a wide variation in blood flow without causing tissue damage; however, as blood flow falls, so does the glomerular filtration rate. Porth (2002a) explains that as renal blood flow approaches zero, renal oxygen consumption approximates that required to keep renal tubular cells viable. This occurs when blood flow falls to about 20 percent of normal and results in onset of ischemic renal changes.

TABLE 28–1   Common Causes of Acute Renal Failure

Prerenal	Intrinsic (Intrarenal)
Excessive fluid loss	*Ischemia*
■ Vascular: Hemorrhage	■ Secondary to prerenal failure
■ Skin: Severe burns	*Nephrotoxicity*
■ Gastrointestinal: Vomiting, diarrhea	■ Drugs
■ Renal: Polyuria	■ Aminoglycosides, contrast dyes, ethylene glycol, NSAIDS, others
Decreased renal perfusion	■ Rhabdomyolysis
■ Decreased cardiac output	■ Causes: Severe crush injuries, severe burns, compartment syndrome, severe exertion or seizure activity, adverse effect of certain drugs (e.g., statins, agents for cholesterol lowering, paramethoxyamphetamine [ecstasy]), other
■ Congestive heart failure	
■ Myocardial infarction	*Intratubular obstruction*
■ Third spacing of fluids	■ Cellular debris, myoglobin casts, uric acid crystals
■ Increased vascular capacity	
■ Shock	
■ Sepsis	
■ Vascular obstruction	
■ Embolus	
■ Dissecting aortic aneurysm	
■ Tumor	
Drug-related altered glomerular hemodynamics	**Postrenal**
■ Selected drugs known to either inhibit vasodilation or cause vasoconstriction of glomerular arterioles include	*Mechanical causes*
■ ACE-inhibitors	■ Blood clots, calculi, tumors, prostatic hypertrophy, urethral strictures
■ Amphotericin B	*Functional causes*
■ Angiotensin receptor blockers	■ Diabetic neuropathy, neurogenic bladder, certain drugs (e.g., ganglionic blockers)
■ Cocaine	
■ Cyclosporine	
■ NSAIDs	
■ Tacrolimus	

The tubules are the most vulnerable to low-flow states because of their high metabolic rate; thus, ischemic tubular epithelial damage occurs first. If the low blood flow state is prolonged (more that 20 to 30 minutes), tubular epithelial cell necrosis sets in.

Clinically, the nurse monitors the mean arterial blood pressure and urine output as indicators of adequate renal blood flow. It is important to maintain a mean arterial pressure of at least 70 mm Hg (ideally greater than 75 mm Hg) to adequately perfuse the kidneys. Adequate urine output, as an indicator of GFR, should be maintained above 25 to 30 mL per hour.

Vascular Obstruction

Whereas decreased cardiac output is a systemic cause of acute renal failure, vascular obstruction is a localized cause. When the vessels serving the kidneys suddenly lose their patency, perfusion distal to the obstruction becomes compromised and can precipitate acute renal failure.

Drug-Induced Altered Glomerular Hemodynamics

Usually, in a discussion of renal failure, drugs are implicated as being major culprits in nephrotoxic intrinsic damage to the kidneys. Certain drugs, however, can alter the hemodynamics of the glomeruli. Ferrone (2003) uses nonsteroidal anti-inflammatory drugs (NSAIDs) as the exemplar drugs associated with this phenomenon. NSAIDs effectively inhibit synthesis of prostaglandins and prostaglandins are mediators of glomerular afferent arteriole vasodilation; thus, NSAIDs can ultimately decrease glomerular capillary pressure. This phenomenon becomes more significant if the patient has coexisting renal injury risk factors present.

Intrinsic Failure

Intrinsic renal failure is caused by problems involving the renal parenchyma (renal tissue) and is categorized by the primary injury site (e.g., acute tubular necrosis and acute interstitial nephritis). Intrinsic failure accounts for the majority (up to 60 percent) of hospital acquired acute renal failure cases (Ferrone, 2003). Acute tubular necrosis is the most common intrinsic renal disorder. Other causes include renal vascular disease (e.g., renal artery stenosis, diabetic sclerosis, and renal vein thrombosis), glomerulonephritis, and acute interstitial nephritis (e.g., pyelonephritis, hypercalcemia).

Acute Tubular Necrosis

Acute tubular necrosis (ATN) refers to necrosis (death) of renal tubule tissue. It accounts for about 85 percent of intrinsic renal failure cases (Ferrone, 2003). Acute tubular necrosis can result from ischemia, nephrotoxic agents, tubular obstruction, or severe infection (e.g., sepsis). ATN is associated with tissue destruction; thus, the incidence of permanent renal damage is high.

Renal Tubular Ischemia. Recall that tissue ischemia develops when the mean arterial blood pressure falls below 60 to 70 mm Hg for a prolonged length of time. Renal ischemic damage usually occurs in patches of individual cells or in small clusters of cells in the kidneys (Agraharkar, 2002). Tubular damage is primarily in the proximal tubules but damage to the distal nephrons may also be noted. Damage may be mild and reversible if the duration of the ischemia is 25 minutes or less; however, prolonged ischemia (more than 60 minutes) usually causes severe, permanent renal damage.

Nephrotoxicity. Nephrotoxicity can develop from exogenous or endogenous agents. Common exogenous agents include radiographic contrast dye, aminoglycoside antibiotics, NSAIDs, and others. Risk for nephrotoxicity caused by many of these agents can be reduced by keeping the patient well hydrated and maintaining an adequate hemodynamic status. Not all agents harm the kidneys equally. Ferrone (2003) explains that although aminoglycosides are nephrotoxic agents, they cause mild tubular epithelial sloughing that is usually reversible if the drug is withdrawn promptly. Ethylene glycol (found commonly in antifreeze), however, destroys the entire nephron, causing severe, irreversible damage. Two major problems associated with endogenous nephrotoxicity include rhabdomyolysis and hepatorenal syndrome (described in Module 31 "Acute Hepatic Dysfunction").

Rhabdomyolysis is a syndrome characterized by excessive muscle breakdown that causes release of muscle cell contents (including electrolytes and myoglobin) in large quantities. In the high-acuity setting, the most common cause is severe crush injury, such as is seen in multiple trauma. It is the increased serum myoglobin aspect of rhabdomyolysis that is of interest to acute tubular necrosis. Kee (2002) describes **myoglobin** as an oxygen-binding protein that is found primarily in cardiac and skeletal muscle. It is a ferrous (iron) compound that is similar to hemoglobin in composition. Myoglobin is both directly and indirectly toxic to renal tubular cell epithelium. Normally, there is little free myoglobin circulating in the blood and none found in the urine. When skeletal or cardiac muscle is destroyed, myoglobin escapes and increased levels can be found in the serum within 2 to 6 hours following injury and in the urine (myoglobinuria) within 3 hours of injury. While a small amount of myoglobin is readily filtered through the glomerular system because of its small size, large quantities are toxic and cause acute tubular necrosis.

Clinically, the nurse should be aware of any risk factors a patient has for development of rhabdomyolysis. Myoglobin may be noted in the urine, making it appear tea or cola colored. It is easily measured in the serum, with the normal adult value range of 12 to 90 ng/mL (Kee, 2002). Other tests that may help in diagnosing rhabdomyolysis include a urine dipstick that is positive for heme but negative for red blood cells (Kaplan, 2002). Serum creatine kinase (CK) levels are elevated as is **aldolase** (an enzyme present in large quantities in cardiac and skeletal muscle), which has a normal adult serum value of less than 6 units per liter.

Intratubular Obstruction. The glomerular tubules can become obstructed when cellular debris, myoglobin or hemoglobin casts, or uric acid crystals become trapped in the filtration system.

Postrenal Failure

Postrenal failure refers to renal dysfunction caused by an obstruction to the outflow of urine from the kidneys. To precipitate renal failure, the obstruction must block urine outflow bilaterally, or unilaterally when there is only one functioning kidney. Renal failure results from backup pressure caused by the increasing volume of urine proximal to the obstruction. Postrenal failure can be caused by obstruction of the bladder, ureters, or urethra, which may be of mechanical or functional origin (see Table 28–1 for examples of both causes).

In summary, there are three categories of acute renal failure: prerenal, which stems from decreased renal perfusion; intrinsic (usually acute tubular necrosis), caused by problems involving the renal tissue; and postrenal, which results from obstruction of urine flow. Acute tubular necrosis accounts for the majority of intrinsic renal failure cases. It can result from renal tubule ischemia or nephrotoxicity. Rhabdomyolysis in the high-acuity setting most commonly results from crush injury. The release of large quantities of myoglobin into the blood can cause obstruction in the glomeruli as well as toxic damage. Should acute renal failure be left unrecognized or inadequately treated, increased kidney tissue damage will result and lead to permanent damage, regardless of the cause.

SECTION THREE REVIEW

1. Congestive heart failure, hemorrhage, and shock are examples of possible etiologic factors for development of which type(s) of renal failure?
   A. prerenal
   B. intrinsic
   C. postrenal
   D. prerenal and postrenal

2. Approximately what percentage of critically ill patients develop acute renal failure?
   A. 5
   B. 10
   C. 15
   D. 20

3. Acute tubular necrosis is caused primarily by which of the following two factors?
   A. myoglobin and nephrotoxic agents
   B. hypoperfusion and myoglobin
   C. myoglobin and hemoglobin
   D. nephrotoxic agents and hypoperfusion

4. Renal tissue ischemia occurs when the mean arterial blood pressure drops to below _____ mm Hg.
   A. 50 to 60
   B. 60 to 70
   C. 70 to 80
   D. 80 to 90

5. Agents that are considered highly nephrotoxic include (choose all that apply)
   1. radiographic contrast dyes
   2. aminoglycosides
   3. cardiac glycosides
   4. NSAIDs
   A. 1, 2, and 4
   B. 1 and 2
   C. 2, 3, and 4
   D. 2 and 4

6. Which statement reflects the relationship between renal blood flow and glomerular filtration rate (GFR)?
   A. as blood flow decreases, GFR increases
   B. as blood flow decreases, GFR decreases
   C. as blood flow increases, GFR decreases
   D. there is no direct relationship

7. In the presence of renal hypoperfusion, what renal cells are injured first? (fill in the blank)

   _____

8. Rhabdomyolysis results from which type of tissue breakdown?
   A. smooth muscle
   B. immunoglobin
   C. blood cell
   D. skeletal muscle

Answers: 1. A, 2. C, 3. D, 4. B, 5. A, 6. B, 7. Tubular epithelium, 8. D

SECTION FOUR: The Phases of Acute Renal Failure

At the completion of this section, the learner will be able to explain the phases of acute renal failure.

Changes in renal function can be considered on a continuum that ranges from mild renal impairment to complete renal failure. Renal impairment begins when the kidneys are not able to meet the demands of dietary or metabolic stress. It may not be discovered until as much as 80 percent of the nephrons have lost normal functioning. Hypertrophy and hyperplasia of the remaining nephrons permit an increase in their workload and in their ability to maintain function. The progressive course of acute renal failure is fairly predictable and can be reflected in three phases: onset, maintenance, and recovery. Table 28–2 provides a summary of the three phases.

Onset (Initiating) Phase

The onset phase begins at the time of the precipitating event and has a short duration (hours to days). It ends when the renal tubules become injured. There are no clinical manifestations associated with this phase because renal injury has not yet been established. Clinically, the nurse should be aware of which patients are at high risk for development of acute renal failure because of the presence of risk factors for such an event. Interventions should be taken to assure that the patient's mean arterial pressure remains above 70 mm Hg and that the patient's hydration and oxygenation status are optimal. These steps can help prevent further insult to the kidneys.

TABLE 28–2 Phases of Acute Renal Failure

PHASE	ONSET	CHARACTERISTICS
Onset	Precipitating event	■ Renal damage has not yet occurred ■ No renal-specific signs and symptoms
Maintenance	When manifestations appear (often within 48 hours of event)	■ Renal tubules are damaged causing reduction in GFR 　■ Fluid excess: Edema, congestive heart failure (CHF), water intoxication, if prolonged, hypertension may develop 　■ Azotemia: Elevated BUN, creatinine, uric acid 　■ Hyperkalemia ■ Severity: May be mild or severe
Recovery	When urine output begins to increase and azotemia begins to decrease	■ Period of tissue repair ■ As GFR increases 　■ Increased urine output (UO) with initial concentration problems 　■ Decreasing BUN, creatinine, potassium

Maintenance Phase

The maintenance phase is heralded in with a sudden drop in the glomerular filtration rate, reflecting acute injury to the renal tubules. It generally begins about 48 hours after the precipitating event and may last for several weeks. The patient rapidly develops **azotemia,** hyperkalemia, and fluid volume overload. Urine output falls to its lowest point during this phase, and may drop to less than 400 mL per 24 hours (**oliguria**) or less than 50 mL per 24 hours (**anuria**). In the past, this phase was called oliguric/anuric because urine output usually fell to those levels. With the advent of improved forms of therapy, however, patients may no longer have such dramatic decreases in urine output. This more mild (nonoliguric) form of renal failure reflects the presence of higher numbers of functional renal tubules; thus, these patients have less severe elevations in metabolic wastes, moderate fluid overload problems, and fewer complications (Porth, 2002b).

In severe acute renal failure, the longer the patient remains in an oliguric/anuric state, the higher the risk of irreversible renal damage and chronic renal failure.

Recovery (Convalescent) Phase

Eventually, the kidneys begin the slow process of tissue repair. When the tubules are sufficiently healthy, urine output will slowly increase and metabolic waste levels will begin to decrease in the serum. Increasing urine output is an early sign of recovery; however, urine concentration problems may continue as repair progresses. Clinically, this may be seen as urine output recovery that is more rapid than the restoration of normal serum creatinine and blood urea nitrogen (BUN) levels. The recovery phase may be prolonged, lasting 6 months to a year. The kidneys are extremely vulnerable during this phase; thus, it is important to avoid use of nephrotoxic agents or further hypoperfusion episodes. The patient requires close monitoring and management of fluid and electrolyte levels and evaluation of the degree of permanent renal damage.

In summary, there are three phases of acute renal failure, including onset, maintenance, and recovery. These phases occur in the same progressive order, with varying degrees of reduced urine output. If urine output decreases to less than 400 mL per day, it is called oliguria and if it falls to less than 50 mL per day, it is called anuria. Fluid and electrolytes must be monitored carefully and controlled during each phase. Early diagnosis and treatment are crucial to prevent or minimize permanent renal damage.

SECTION FOUR REVIEW

1. As many as _____ percent of the nephrons may be lost before significant renal dysfunction is noted.
   A. 40
   B. 60
   C. 80
   D. 100

2. When urine output falls to below _____ mL per 24 hours, the renal term *oliguria* is appropriate.
   A. 50
   B. 100
   C. 200
   D. 400

3. Renal ischemia has which effect on renal blood flow?
   A. vasospasm
   B. vasodilation
   C. vasoconstriction
   D. decreased vascular resistance
4. The maintenance phase ends when the BUN and creatinine
   A. cease to decrease
   B. begin to decrease
   C. slow their increase
   D. return to normal
5. The onset phase of acute renal failure is associated with which manifestation?
   A. slow increase in BUN
   B. rapid increase in creatinine

   C. slow decrease in urine output
   D. no manifestations
6. To prevent or minimize renal damage, the mean arterial pressure should ideally be maintained above _____ mm Hg.
   A. 60
   B. 70
   C. 80
   D. 90
7. True or False: During the recovery phase, the serum creatinine levels return to normal more rapidly than the urine output. Usually, urine volume returns to normal before metabolic wastes.

Answers: 1. C, 2. D, 3. C, 4. B, 5. D, 6. B, 7. False, usually the urine volume recovers before metabolic wastes.

SECTION FIVE: The Effects of Renal Dysfunction on Fluid and Electrolyte Balance

At the completion of this section, the learner will be able to describe the effects of acute renal failure on fluid and electrolyte balance.

When a patient develops renal failure, the kidneys are no longer able to function normally, losing the ability to regulate reabsorption and excretion of fluids and electrolytes. The body's fluids (primarily composed of water and electrolytes) are found in essentially every organ system. Therefore, because renal failure profoundly alters fluid and electrolyte balance, it also has negative influences on all body systems.

Fluid Balance

The importance of fluid regulation is apparent, considering that 60 to 70 percent of the body's composition consists of water. Body water is divided into two compartments: intracellular (fluid within the cells) and extracellular (fluid outside the cells). The extracellular fluid compartment can be further divided into intravascular fluid within the blood vessels (plasma) and interstitial water in the tissue spaces.

Failure of the kidneys to excrete water unbalances the normal homeostasis of the body, causing serious consequences. Fluid imbalance triggers one of two problems: hypervolemia, an increase in circulatory and body water, or hypovolemia, an inadequate amount of circulating fluid volume. Acute renal failure (during the maintenance phase) is associated with development of an accumulation of fluids (**hypervolemia**) produced by failure of the kidneys to perfuse and filter fluids properly. Hypervolemia is associated with many complications, including congestive heart failure, pulmonary edema, and hypertension.

Electrolyte Balance

In addition to the regulatory mechanisms of the endocrine system, the kidneys control the balance of electrolytes within the body fluid. **Electrolytes** help maintain fluid osmolality. The major **cations** regulated by the kidneys are potassium, sodium, calcium, and magnesium. Major **anions** under renal regulation include chloride and bicarbonate. Renal failure can cause any of the following electrolyte imbalances: hyperkalemia, hypernatremia, hyponatremia, hypocalcemia, hyperphosphatemia, hypermagnesemia, and metabolic acidosis.

Potassium Imbalance

Hyperkalemia is a major concern in renal failure. **Hyperkalemia** is caused by decreased excretion of potassium by the kidneys and increased cellular release of potassium through tissue breakdown and acidosis. Hyperkalemic changes manifest most frequently in cardiac and neuromuscular changes. Although serum potassium may not elevate significantly, under certain circumstances, such as gastrointestinal (GI) bleeding, severe tissue trauma, or hypercatabolic state, it may rise to a life-threatening level.

Occasionally, hypokalemia has been implicated in acute renal failure as a possible causative factor. Hypokalemia can alter the interstitium of the renal medulla, impairing renal function and precipitating acute renal failure.

Sodium Imbalance

Acute renal failure generally causes increased serum sodium; however, this is not always true. Hypernatremia occurs when the GFR is decreased and sodium is unable to be excreted in sufficient amounts. Because sodium conservation occurs mainly in the renal medulla, any deterioration of this area of the kidney may cause excessive sodium loss (hyponatremia). For these reasons, sodium levels are variable in acute renal failure.

Calcium and Phosphate Imbalances

Calcium follows a similar reabsorption pathway as sodium. Serum calcium is reduced in acute renal failure as a result of decreased absorption from the gastrointestinal tract caused by an inability of the kidneys to produce the active component of vitamin D (1,25–dihydroxycholecalciferol). Loss of this active component results in diminished use of calcium and hypocalcemia. Calcium maintains an inverse relationship with phosphate (PO_4^{++}); therefore, as calcium levels decrease, phosphate levels increase, causing hyperphosphatemia.

Magnesium Imbalance

Acute renal failure is a major cause of hypermagnesemia. Hypermagnesemia occurs because, like potassium, magnesium is excreted primarily by the kidneys. When the kidneys lose their ability to excrete magnesium, serum levels increase. Hypermagnesemia may also result from use of magnesium-containing drugs, such as antacids.

Metabolic Acidosis

The kidneys play an important role in maintaining normal pH by urinary excretion of excess hydrogen ions. Metabolic **acidosis** can result from two problems: First, it develops as the result of the kidneys' inability to excrete hydrogen ions; as hydrogen ions accumulate, the pH falls and an acidotic state develops. Second, renal failure also can cause metabolic acidosis by loss of renal bicarbonate buffering capabilities. In addition, acidosis potentiates the effects of potassium on the heart, which increases the risk of life-threatening dysrhythmias (Shah, 2001).

In summary, acute renal failure has a profound impact on fluid and electrolyte balance. Hypervolemia is caused by an inability of the kidneys to excrete adequate volumes of body fluids, which leads to fluid volume excess. Renal failure causes electrolyte imbalances primarily through loss of the ability to excrete adequate amounts of electrolytes, such as potassium and sodium. This, in turn, interferes with vitamin D production, precipitating hypocalcemia and hyperphosphatemia. The loss of the kidneys' ability to excrete sufficient amounts of hydrogen ions results in metabolic acidosis.

SECTION FIVE REVIEW

1. Interstitial fluid is located
   A. inside the cells
   B. inside the blood vessels
   C. within the tissue spaces
   D. within the intracellular compartment
2. Which set of imbalances most commonly occur secondary to acute renal failure?
   A. hyperkalemia, hyperphosphatemia, metabolic acidosis
   B. hypokalemia, hyponatremia, hypercalcemia
   C. hyperkalemia, hypocalcemia, metabolic alkalosis
   D. hypernatremia, hypermagnesemia, hypercalcemia
3. Potassium imbalance secondary to acute renal failure is associated with which factors? (choose all that apply)
   1. increased excretion
   2. metabolic acidosis
   3. decreased excretion
   4. increased tissue breakdown

A. 1, 3, and 4
B. 2 and 3
C. 2, 3, and 4
D. 3 and 4
4. An inability of the kidneys to produce 1,25 dihydroxycholecalciferol, the active component of vitamin D, lowers the serum levels of which electrolyte?
   A. sodium
   B. magnesium
   C. phosphate
   D. calcium
5. Metabolic acidosis is closely associated with acute renal failure because of the kidneys' inability to
   A. retain sodium ions
   B. excrete hydrogen ions
   C. retain bicarbonate ions
   D. excrete potassium ions

Answers: 1. C, 2. A, 3. C, 4. D, 5. B

SECTION SIX: Assessment and Diagnosis of Renal Failure

This section presents nursing assessment of the patient with renal failure and highlights major diagnostic tests. At the completion of this section, the learner will be able to discuss assessment and diagnosis of renal failure.

Renal Success or Renal Failure?

Assessment of a rapid decrease in urine output to abnormally low levels over several successive hours should make the nurse suspicious that some significant event is occurring. The difficulty in this situation is often not in recognizing a potential problem but rather it is in determining whether the kidneys have sustained damage (acute renal failure) or whether they are performing normal fluid conservation activities.

When a patient initially develops renal hypoperfusion, the renal tubules conserve sodium and water to increase intravascular fluid volume and increase perfusion. This activity is considered organ protective rather than pathologic. In such cases, if perfusion is reestablished quickly, urine output will rapidly return to normal—hence the name, renal "success." In an earlier section, we learned that there is a window of about 20 to 30 minutes following a renal hypoperfusion event to correct the problem and prevent serious renal tubule ischemic damage. It is imperative, then, that the nurse first recognize the situation and then follow up with the physician or advanced practitioner immediately. Rapid assessment and effective interventions can prevent, or at least minimize, renal damage, thereby making the difference between renal success and renal failure.

The Focused Renal Assessment

In the acutely ill patient, renal dysfunction often has an insidious onset. It initially may be suspected when urine output stays below normal despite attempts to increase it. It also may be initially detected first when electrolyte (particularly serum potassium $[K^+]$) or BUN values develop abnormal trends. As renal failure progresses, the resulting signs and symptoms reflect the progressive loss of normal kidney functions, such as excretion of waste products, and loss of fluid, electrolyte, and acid–base regulation.

Nursing History

Important recent history data to be aware of include the following:

- Previous history of renal problems
- Recent use of nephrotoxic substances (e.g., contrast dyes, nephrotoxic antibiotics, especially aminoglycosides), particularly in the presence of dehydration
- Recent exposure to heavy metals or organic solvents
- Recent hypotensive episode of 25 minutes or greater
- Presence of tumor or multiple clots that might cause renovascular or urine outflow obstruction bilaterally
- Presence of infection

At times, it may be important to differentiate between acute renal failure and chronic renal failure. History that suggests chronic renal failure includes chronic weight loss and fatigue, nocturia, anorexia, and pruritus (Agraharkar, 2002) and azotemia. Other data that favor chronic renal failure include anemia and abnormally small kidneys (Shah, 2001).

Physical Assessment

Assessment of the patient with renal failure requires particular attention to the cardiopulmonary and renal systems to evaluate fluid and hemodynamic status. In addition, the nurse should focus the assessment on monitoring for any manifestations of uremia. Although **uremia** is a clinical syndrome that develops in end-stage renal disease (chronic renal failure), the patient with severe acute renal failure is likely to develop some of the manifestations of uremia (Young, 2003). Figure 28–6 provides an illustration of the multisystem effects of uremia. A brief overview of the multisystem effects of prolonged renal failure on body systems and related clinical manifestations follows.

Neurologic Effects

Accumulation of nitrogenous waste products from impaired renal excretion and metabolic acidosis contributes to a decrease in mental functioning. As uremic toxins build up in the brain tissue, uremic encephalopathy develops. Accumulation of toxins can slow peripheral nerve conduction, producing peripheral neuropathy. In addition, fluid volume excess, caused by renal failure, can precipitate cerebral edema, which may increase intracranial pressure and alter level of consciousness.

Cardiovascular and Pulmonary Effects

Hypertension is a common manifestation of renal failure. It is caused by systemic and central fluid volume excess and increased renin production. In the presence of renal ischemia, the renin–angiotensin system is triggered, which results in increased blood pressure and increased renal blood flow (see Section Two). Fluid volume excess and electrolyte imbalances are the basis of most cardiovascular symptoms. The presence of fluid volume excess may cause congestive heart failure accompanied by peripheral and pulmonary edema. The inability of the kidneys to excrete hydrogen ions and electrolytes adequately causes them to accumulate in the body. The resulting electrolyte imbalance can precipitate cardiac arrhythmias, metabolic acidosis, and other complications.

Patients with acute renal failure require close monitoring for signs and symptoms of pneumonia. These patients are at increased risk for developing this complication as a result of decreased level of consciousness, weakness, thick secretions, decreased cough reflex, and decreased pulmonary macrophage activity.

Gastrointestinal Effects

Electrolyte imbalances and increasing levels of uremic toxins are the primary contributors to gastrointestinal (GI) manifestations. As urea decomposes in the GI tract, it releases ammonia. Ammonia in the GI tract increases capillary fragility and GI mucosal irritation. As the ammonia levels increase, small mucosal ulcerations may develop, causing GI bleeding. Acute renal failure alters GI motility largely as a result of electrolyte imbalances. The patient may develop constipation or diarrhea, depending on the GI motility status.

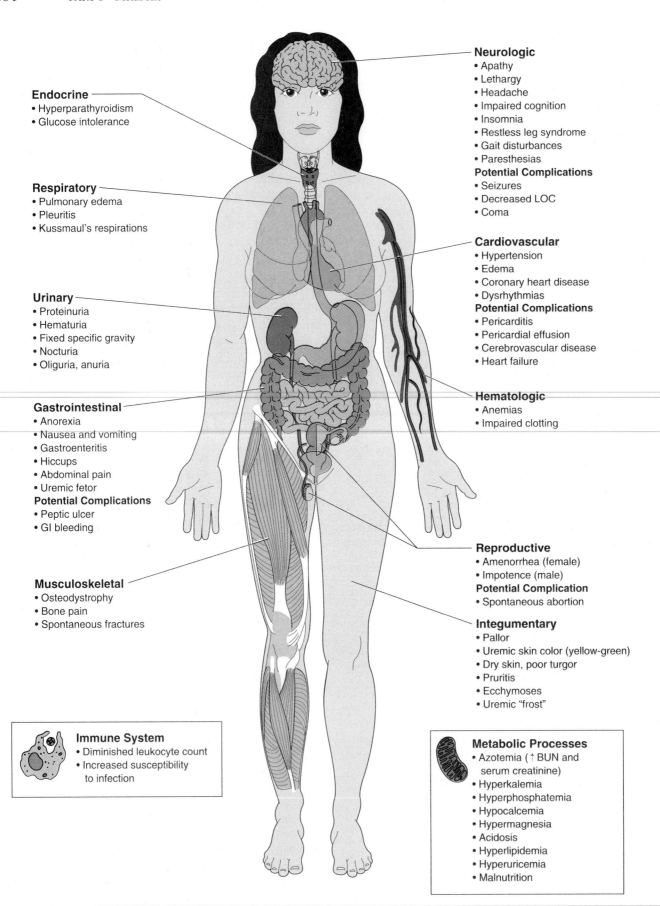

Neurologic
• Apathy
• Lethargy
• Headache
• Impaired cognition
• Insomnia
• Restless leg syndrome
• Gait disturbances
• Paresthesias
Potential Complications
• Seizures
• Decreased LOC
• Coma

Endocrine
• Hyperparathyroidism
• Glucose intolerance

Respiratory
• Pulmonary edema
• Pleuritis
• Kussmaul's respirations

Cardiovascular
• Hypertension
• Edema
• Coronary heart disease
• Dysrhythmias
Potential Complications
• Pericarditis
• Pericardial effusion
• Cerebrovascular disease
• Heart failure

Urinary
• Proteinuria
• Hematuria
• Fixed specific gravity
• Nocturia
• Oliguria, anuria

Hematologic
• Anemias
• Impaired clotting

Gastrointestinal
• Anorexia
• Nausea and vomiting
• Gastroenteritis
• Hiccups
• Abdominal pain
• Uremic fetor
Potential Complications
• Peptic ulcer
• GI bleeding

Reproductive
• Amenorrhea (female)
• Impotence (male)
Potential Complication
• Spontaneous abortion

Musculoskeletal
• Osteodystrophy
• Bone pain
• Spontaneous fractures

Integumentary
• Pallor
• Uremic skin color (yellow-green)
• Dry skin, poor turgor
• Pruritis
• Ecchymoses
• Uremic "frost"

Immune System
• Diminished leukocyte count
• Increased susceptibility
  to infection

Metabolic Processes
• Azotemia (↑ BUN and
  serum creatinine)
• Hyperkalemia
• Hyperphosphatemia
• Hypocalcemia
• Hypermagnesia
• Acidosis
• Hyperlipidemia
• Hyperuricemia
• Malnutrition

Figure 28–6 ■ The multisystem effects of uremia.

Hematologic Effects

The kidneys produce erythropoietin, which is necessary for normal red blood cell (RBC) production. When kidney function fails, red blood cell production becomes compromised and the life span of existing RBCs may decrease. Platelet function is also impaired by the presence of uremic toxins, which increases the risk of bleeding problems. The combination of hematopoietic factors, GI irritation, and blood loss from hemodialysis all contribute to the development of anemia.

Integumentary Effects

Because the uremic toxins cannot be excreted via the kidneys, they may accumulate on the skin surface causing pruritus and dry skin. The patient's skin appears pale and may develop a yellow cast. The yellow skin coloring is different from the jaundice associated with liver disease. The color is duller and does not affect the sclera of the eyes. Bruising is frequently noted as a result of dysfunctional platelets. The development of uremic frost, a late-stage phenomenon of renal failure, has become less common in the acute care setting because of earlier, more effective management. The term *uremic frost* refers to a fine, white layer of urate crystals that develops on the skin. In addition, protein wasting may cause thin hair and brittle, thin nails.

Skeletal Effects

Under normal circumstances, about seven eighths of ingested calcium is excreted in the feces without being absorbed. The remaining eighth is absorbed by the intestines and is eventually excreted by the kidneys (Guyton & Hall, 1997). Because of the limited ability of the kidneys to metabolize vitamin D in acute renal failure, absorption of calcium in the intestines is further impaired. In long-term renal failure, skeletal disorders occur related to decreased calcium absorption.

Laboratory Tests

Blood Urea Nitrogen and Creatinine

The diagnosis and management of renal failure largely depend on laboratory tests measuring uremic toxins and renal excretion. Blood urea nitrogen (BUN) and creatinine are the two most important laboratory measurements of renal status.

Urea is the major nonprotein end-product of protein breakdown and it is eliminated from the body via the kidneys. Urea nitrogen levels are influenced by a person's hydration status, catabolic processes, protein intake, and gastrointestinal bleeding. The presence of any of these factors must be considered when evaluating BUN levels. BUN is small in size and has the ability to be reabsorbed back into the blood if given sufficient time. This becomes evident when GFR falls significantly and BUN levels rise rapidly.

Creatinine is the end product of muscle metabolism and is created by the breakdown of creatinine phosphate in the mus-

TABLE 28–3 Major Laboratory Values Measuring Kidney Function

LABORATORY TEST	NORMAL VALUES	ABNORMAL TREND
Serum		
Blood urea nitrogen	5–25 mg/dL	Increased
Creatinine	0.5–1.5 mg/dL	Increased
Uric acid		
Male	3.5–8.0 mg/dL	Increased
Female	2.8–6.8 mg/dL	Increased
Potassium	3.5–5.3 mEq/L	Increased
Calcium	9–11 mg/dL	Decreased
Chloride	95–105 mEq/L	Increased
Phosphorus	2.5–4.5 mg/dL	Increased
Albumin	3.5–5.0 g/dL	Decreased
Urine		
Protein	0–5 mg/dL/24 hr	Increased
Creatinine clearance	85–135 mL/min	Decreased
Urea clearance	64–100 mL/min	Decreased

Normal serum values are from Kee, J. L. (2002). Laboratory and diagnostic tests with nursing implications, *(6th ed.). Upper Saddle River, NJ: Prentice Hall.*

cles. Creatinine is produced at a relatively steady rate that depends on an individual's muscle mass. Creatinine is larger in size, does not reabsorb back into the blood, and will be eliminated to the degree that remaining renal function will allow.

The reabsorption ability of BUN but not creatinine helps explain the reason that the BUN level increases more rapidly than creatinine. Under normal circumstances, BUN and creatinine maintain a ratio of about 10:1 to 15:1. This ratio, however, becomes altered (favoring BUN) in the presence of renal failure. Clinically, a BUN-to-creatinine ratio of 20:1 or higher is considered suspicious of renal failure (Agraharkar, 2002).

Table 28–3 summarizes major laboratory values measuring kidney function. Note that serum and urine values have an inverse relationship.

Osmolality

The relationship of urine and blood osmolality is monitored as an indicator of adequate renal function. When renal function is normal, the urine and blood (plasma) osmolality maintain a direct relationship (i.e., as one rises, the other also rises). If renal perfusion becomes diminished, the urine osmolality becomes more elevated than the blood osmolality, and urine specific gravity increases.

Assessment of Electrolyte Imbalances

Assessment of serum and urine electrolytes provides important information regarding renal status and alerts the health care professional to potential complications based on abnormal values. Electrolyte imbalances cause a wide range of functional problems, particularly in the neurologic, musculoskeletal, cardiovascular, and gastrointestinal systems. The signs and symptoms of imbalances often reflect either hyperactive or hypoactive system function, depending on the nature of the imbalance. Module 3, "Fluid and Electrolyte Balance in the High-Acuity Patient," describes the effects of the various electrolyte imbalances.

Special Procedures

Occasionally, the acutely ill patient requires radiographic testing or invasive procedures to help verify the exact etiology of acute renal failure. Following are brief descriptions of some of the more common tests performed to help make a differential diagnosis.

Renal Biopsy

Renal biopsy is an invasive procedure performed by needle aspiration of renal tissue. Once it is obtained, the tissue is examined microscopically. Renal biopsy may be used when the exact nature of intrinsic acute renal failure is unknown.

Intravenous Pyelogram

Intravenous pyelogram (IVP) uses a flat plate film of the abdomen before and after injection of a contrast medium into the kidneys via the bloodstream. The IVP is able to outline the kidneys, showing size, shape, and the ability to concentrate and excrete the dye. The nurse should be aware that contrast dyes can be nephrotoxic and can potentially precipitate intrinsic renal damage.

Renal Ultrasound

Renal ultrasound uses high-frequency sound waves directed at the kidneys to measure various densities. Ultrasound can distinguish tumors, fluid masses, and obstructions. Major advantages of renal ultrasound are that it is noninvasive and can be performed at the bedside with minimal discomfort to the acutely ill patient.

Computed Tomography Scan

The computed tomography (CT) scan uses a three-dimensional concept of radiography by taking x-ray slices of an organ. The CT scan provides information regarding the size and shape of the kidneys and the presence of lesions, cysts, calculi, and congenital anomalies. Masses are detected easily with this method.

Renal Arteriogram

The renal arteriogram requires injection of a contrast dye into the renal artery via the femoral artery. The arteriogram visualizes blood flow through the renal vessels. Prerenal obstruction can be diagnosed using this method. Because renal arteriogram uses contrast dye, nephrotoxicity is a possibility.

In summary, early diagnosis of acute renal failure generally is made based on urine and blood chemistry alterations. Certain tests help differentiate the exact nature of the acute renal failure. The acutely ill patient may require a combination of blood, urine, radiographic, or other tests to help differentiate the etiology.

SECTION SIX REVIEW

1. When a patient experiences diminished renal perfusion, how will the urine/plasma osmolality relationship change?
   A. plasma osmolality decreases more than urine osmolality
   B. urine osmolality decreases more than plasma osmolality
   C. plasma osmolality increases more than urine osmolality
   D. urine osmolality increases more than plasma osmolality
2. Which laboratory value can be used to differentiate acute tubular necrosis from prerenal hypoperfusion?
   A. BUN and chloride
   B. calcium and chloride
   C. sodium and potassium
   D. specific gravity and osmolality
3. Renal biopsy would most likely be used to further investigate which renal disorder?
   A. prerenal failure
   B. intrinsic failure
   C. renal thrombosis
   D. renal calculi obstruction
4. Which test would most likely be performed to diagnose a prerenal vascular obstruction?
   A. CT scan
   B. intravenous pyelogram
   C. renal biopsy
   D. renal arteriogram
5. A renal diagnostic procedure requiring contrast dye is
   A. arteriogram
   B. biopsy
   C. ultrasound
   D. CT scan

6. Alterations in mental function secondary to acute renal failure are caused primarily by
   A. uremic toxins
   B. magnesium imbalance
   C. hypoglycemia
   D. fluid overload

7. Peripheral neuropathy can manifest in which way? (choose all that apply)
   1. seizures
   2. tingling
   3. numbness
   4. itching
   A. 1, 2, and 3
   B. 2 and 3
   C. 1 and 4
   D. 2, 3, and 4

8. Which statement is correct regarding how acute renal failure affects the cardiovascular system?
   A. it causes hypotension
   B. it causes congestive heart failure
   C. it causes atherosclerosis
   D. it causes increased renal blood flow

9. Acute renal failure can precipitate gastrointestinal bleeding as a result of increased levels of
   A. uric acid
   B. creatinine
   C. urea
   D. ammonia

10. Which of the following best reflects the effects of acute renal failure on the integumentary system?
    A. thickened hair follicles
    B. excessively oily skin
    C. excessive bruising
    D. thickened nailbeds

11. The BUN-to-creatinine ratio is considered a good indicator of probable acute renal failure when it rises to _____ or higher.
    A. 10:1
    B. 15:1
    C. 20:1
    D. 25:1

Answers: 1. D, 2. D, 3. B, 4. D, 5. A, 6. A, 7. D, 8. B, 9. D, 10. C, 11. C

SECTION SEVEN: Collaborative Management of the Patient in Acute Renal Failure

At the completion of this section, the learner will be able to provide a brief overview of the collaborative management of the patient with acute renal failure.

Management of the patient in acute renal failure is primarily collaborative. Initial interventions focus on correction of the precipitating event (e.g., a hypotensive episode, an obstruction), support of the body systems until kidney function stabilizes, and prevention or treatment of complications. Nursing care is complex because renal failure patients are extremely sick and unstable during the early stages of the disorder.

Acute renal failure is a physiologic complication that has the capacity to cause dysfunction of multiple other body systems. A major part of the management of patients with acute renal failure is prevention and treatment of complications. Four major potential complications are routinely addressed:

- Fluid overload
- Catabolic processes
- Electrolyte/acid–base imbalance
- Infection

Fluid Overload

Fluid overload is the result of two mechanisms: retention of sodium and water, and the renin–angiotensin–aldosterone system. Fluid overload can result in development of congestive heart failure (CHF) and pulmonary edema. Interventions focus on preventing fluid excess or, if it is present, regaining fluid balance. There are a variety of ways that these goals are accomplished, including fluid restriction, diuretic therapy, and dialysis.

Fluid Restriction

Fluid replacement may be restricted to urine output plus insensible water loss (about 800 mL to 1 L per day). Accurate measurement of output (e.g., urine, nasogastric tube or fistula drainage, diarrhea, etc.) is crucial to be able to replace fluid on a one-to-one basis. The free water can be distributed evenly over the 24-hour day or it can be divided into shifts to provide the patient with fluid to drink with meals or to take with oral medications. The free water also can be used for tube feeding flushes. Uremic patients may experience extreme thirst; thus, oral fluids in small quantities often increase patient comfort.

Diuretic Therapy and Dialysis

If the kidneys have maintained some level of function, **diuretic** therapy may decrease fluid excess to varying degrees. Dialysis is an invasive but effective means of controlling fluid excess. Because it is an invasive procedure, it places the patient at increased risk for multiple complications. Dialysis is presented in Section Eight.

Nursing Diagnoses. Nursing diagnoses that readily apply to fluid overload issues include

■ Excess fluid volume
■ Decreased cardiac output

Desired Outcomes. The client will attain

1. Reduced or absence of edema
2. Clear or improved lung sounds
3. Absence of shortness of breath
4. Weight trend toward baseline
5. Improved blood pressure toward baseline

Nursing Interventions. Nursing interventions focus on monitoring the patient for fluid volume excess and heart failure, following through on physician's orders related to fluid overload, monitoring for therapeutic and nontherapeutic effects of therapy, and evaluating patient outcomes.

Catabolic Processes

The high-acuity patient in acute renal failure generally is undergoing accelerated catabolic processes as a result of hypermetabolism triggered by high stress levels, infection, trauma, or other acute problems. Hypermetabolism significantly increases nutritional requirements, particularly protein; thus, it increases formation of nitrogen waste products. The injured kidneys, however, cannot rid the body of nitrogen waste and the uremic toxins. They accumulate rapidly and produce azotemia. Elevated concentrations of nitrogenous waste products impair the functions of multiple body systems (refer to Section Six). The brain (renal encephalopathy) and the gastrointestinal tract (GI bleeding) are at particular risk for serious complications.

Nursing Diagnoses. Nursing diagnoses that apply to the problem of catabolic processes include

■ Altered nutrition: Less than body requirements
■ Altered thought processes
■ Altered bowel elimination: Diarrhea
■ Altered bowel elimination: Constipation
■ Potential complication: GI bleeding

Desired Outcomes (for nursing diagnoses). The client will attain

1. Weight trend toward baseline
2. Serum protein (e.g., albumin, prealbumin) trends toward normal ranges

3. Nitrogen balance
4. Usual mental status
5. Stools of soft formed consistency and usual frequency

Nursing Implications. To combat the accelerated catabolic processes, the patient requires nutritional support. The nurse should consider an early nutrition consult to establish estimated nutritional support needs for the patient. The diet should be restricted in protein, sodium, potassium, and fluids; and high in carbohydrates, fats, and essential amino acids. Nutrition given orally or via feeding tube routes is preferable to the IV route in order to minimize the risk of infection. If dietary restrictions are insufficient in maintaining acceptable nitrogenous waste levels (e.g., BUN and creatinine), dialysis may be initiated.

Weight should be monitored daily, with the understanding that rapid weight shifts are probably secondary to fluid excess problems. Serum protein levels should be monitored regularly to evaluate whether the patient's nutritional status is worsening or improving. The patient's mental status needs to be monitored at least every shift to observe for onset of renal encephalopathy. Stool consistency and frequency is monitored and orders are obtained as needed to attain/maintain adequate bowel evacuation patterns. Refer to Module 23, "Metabolic Responses to Stress," for more information on meeting nutritional needs.

Electrolyte/Acid–Base Imbalance

Electrolyte imbalances are a frequent complication associated with acute renal failure. Two major electrolytes that require close monitoring and management are potassium and sodium.

Potassium

Hyperkalemia is an ongoing, potentially lethal complication of acute renal failure. Treatment may include drug therapy or dialysis. Drug therapy may consist of several options. Cation exchange resins may be used either rectally or orally to physically remove the potassium from the body. Sodium bicarbonate, insulin, or hypertonic glucose may be ordered to attempt to drive potassium back into the cells. Dialysis may be ordered to control potassium, particularly when the hyperkalemia is accompanied by excess fluid volume.

Sodium

Sodium levels vary in the acute renal failure patient and management depends on whether levels are normal, high, or low. The close relationship between sodium and water make it important to control; therefore, values are monitored closely. Sodium is restricted in the diet and in IV fluids to control fluid excess and prevent dilutional hyponatremia. Maintaining a balance of intake and output helps prevent or control hypernatremia. If renal function is sufficient, diuretic therapy may be ordered to lower sodium levels.

Metabolic Acidosis

Metabolic acidosis can become severe in acute renal failure, creating disruption of normal cellular functions.

Nursing Diagnoses. Collaborative problems that apply to electrolyte and **acid–base balance** include

- Potential complication: Metabolic acidosis
- Potential complication: Electrolyte imbalance
- Fluid volume excess

Desired Patient Outcomes. The patient will attain/maintain

1. pH within normal limits (7.35 to 7.45)
2. Serum electrolytes within normal limits

Nursing Implications. The nurse monitors the patient for the clinical manifestations of electrolyte imbalances, particularly potassium, sodium, calcium, phosphate, and magnesium. The patient's arterial blood gas values are closely monitored to evaluate acid–base status. Sodium bicarbonate may be ordered sparingly, to minimize the hypernatremic effects. Dialysis may also be initiated to help control acidosis.

Infection

Infection is a major cause of death from acute renal failure because of an immunocompromised status.

Nursing Diagnoses. The nursing diagnosis that applies to the patient with a potential infection is

- High risk for infection

Desired Patient Outcomes. The patient will be free of infection as evidenced by

1. WBC count within acceptable limits
2. Absence of fever
3. Cultures are negative

Nursing Implications. The nurse focuses care on monitoring the patient for signs and symptoms of infection. Scrupulous hygienic maintenance is necessary to minimize the risk of infection. Major sources of infection in the acute renal failure patient include urinary tract infection, pneumonia, septicemia, and skin/wound infections. Minimal use of invasive lines and tubes is crucial. If the patient becomes symptomatic of infection, potential sources should be cultured and antibiotic therapy initiated. Antibiotic therapy requires dose adjustments based on the severity of renal impairment. If antibiotics are ordered, the nurse monitors for the therapeutic and nontherapeutic effects of therapy.

Related Nursing Diagnoses

In addition to the nursing diagnoses previously listed, the patient in acute renal failure frequently meets the critical criteria for the following:

- Activity intolerance
- High risk for injury
- High risk for altered mucous membranes
- High risk for altered skin integrity
- Altered renal tissue perfusion
- Pain
- Anxiety
- Knowledge deficit

In summary, a general overview of collaborative management of the high-acuity patient in acute renal failure has been presented. Because acute renal failure is a complication that results in further complications, it requires a strong collaborative effort between physicians and nurses. The nurse performs frequent assessments to evaluate the function of multiple body systems, implements and evaluates actions based on physician's orders, and performs independent nursing actions based on the individual needs of the patient. Four major potential complications are routinely addressed: fluid overload, catabolic processes, electrolyte/acid–base imbalance, and infection.

SECTION SEVEN REVIEW

1. Major complications that are routinely addressed in the patient with acute renal failure include (choose all that apply)
   1. fluid overload
   2. acid–base imbalance
   3. anabolic processes
   4. infection
   A. 2, 3, and 4
   B. 2 and 3
   C. 1, 2, and 4
   D. 1, 2, and 3

2. To restrict fluid intake of the patient with acute renal failure, a common method is to
   A. maintain strict nothing-by-mouth status
   B. match the intake to the output
   C. restrict intake to less than 50 mL per hour
   D. infuse IV fluid at 400 mL per 24 hours

3. Catabolic processes that are present in patients with acute renal failure make restriction of _____ necessary.
   A. carbohydrates
   B. fats

C. proteins
D. essential amino acids
4. Hyperkalemia is frequently treated with what pharmacologic agent?
A. cation exchange resin
B. sodium bicarbonate
C. calcium chloride
D. phosphate

5. The major cause of death from acute renal failure is
A. hyperkalemia
B. metabolic acidosis
C. fluid excess
D. infection

Answers: 1. C, 2. B, 3. C, 4. A, 5. D

SECTION EIGHT: Dialysis—An Acute Renal Failure Treatment Modality

At the completion of this section, the learner will be able to discuss dialysis as a treatment modality for acute renal failure.

A major portion of the management of acute renal failure focuses on maintaining fluid, electrolytes, and azotemia within acceptable limits. During the maintenance phase, severe kidney dysfunction can cause life-threatening abnormalities in fluid, electrolyte, and uremic toxin levels. Medical management of acute renal failure varies with the type of failure (prerenal, intrinsic, or postrenal). This section focuses on dialysis as one distinct feature in the management of acute renal failure.

Early in the course of the disorder, tests may be performed to define the type of renal failure (e.g., diminished renal function secondary to a postshock state [prerenal] versus parenchymal tubular damage [intrinsic]). To differentiate between these two etiologies, a diuretic challenge may be given, using either mannitol (an osmotic diuretic) or furosemide (a loop diuretic). If the kidneys are able to respond to the diuretic by increasing urinary output, fluid replacement and additional diuretics are given to treat a prerenal type of problem. If, however, there is no response from the diuretic challenge, acute tubular necrosis is considered seriously, and dialysis may become a viable treatment option. Patients who experience the oliguria for more than 4 to 5 days generally require dialysis. Dialysis has significantly improved the prognosis of patients experiencing ATN.

TABLE 28–4 Comparison of Acute Renal Failure Treatment Modalities

FACTORS	HEMODIALYSIS	CRRT	PERITONEAL DIALYSIS
Indications for use	Acute poisoning Acute/chronic renal failure Transfusion reaction Hepatic coma	Multiple organ dysfunction syndrome Sepsis Acute renal failure Inability to tolerate hemodialysis or peritoneal dialysis	Hemodynamic instability Severe cardiovascular disease Hemodialysis not available Less rapid treatment is appropriate Inadequate vascular access
Disadvantages	Requires vascular access and heparin Restricts activity level	Requires vascular access Slow process Restricts activity level Risk of contamination	Slower than hemodialysis Abdominal discomfort Decreased mobility Risk of peritonitis
Contraindications	Coagulopathy Age extremes Hemodynamic instability	Acute poisoning Hematocrit greater than 45 percent Inability to anticoagulate Low mean arterial pressure Congestive heart failure	Adhesions of peritoneum or abdomen Peritonitis Recent abdominal surgery
Complications	Infection Decreased cardiac output Cardiac arrhythmias Disequilibrium syndrome[a] Air embolism Disconnection hemorrhage	Infection Bleeding Infiltration Air embolism	Infection Decreased cardiac output Fluid overload Hyperglycemia Metabolic alkalosis Respiratory insufficiency Abdominal pain

[a]Symptoms of disequilibrium syndrome include disorientation, seizures, headache, agitation, and nausea and vomiting.

Dialysis

Dialysis is a process of diffusion by which dissolved particles are transported across a semipermeable membrane from one fluid compartment to another. Dialysis does not correct renal dysfunction. It only corrects metabolic waste, fluid, electrolyte, and acid–base imbalances. Return of normal renal function depends on treatment of the underlying problem and the ability of the body to heal the damaged tubules. Hemodialysis, continuous renal replacement therapy, and peritoneal dialysis are three types of treatment for acute renal failure. Table 28–4 provides a comparison of the three treatment modalities.

Hemodialysis

Hemodialysis requires a direct access into the vascular compartment. For short-term use, as is seen frequently in the high-acuity patient, a temporary access site may be used. The two most common sites are the subclavian and femoral veins, using a relatively simple percutaneous venous access, which is effective for hemodialysis on a temporary basis. For long-term use, an internal arteriovenous fistula, shunt, or graft may be formed surgically, usually in the lower arm. Figure 28–7 illustrates three types of venous access.

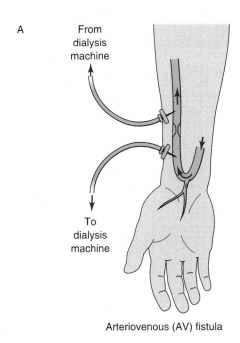

Arteriovenous (AV) fistula

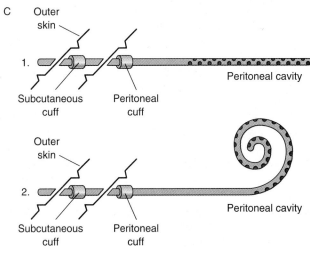

Temporary venous access

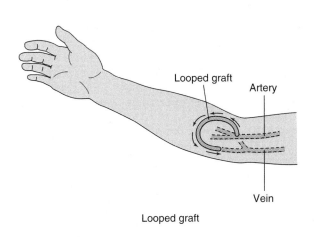

Looped graft

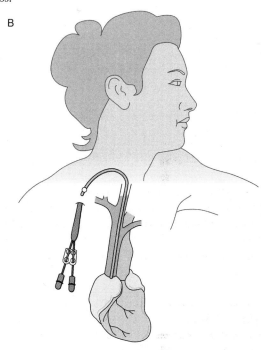

Two double-cuff Tenckhoff peritoneal catheters:
1. Standard; 2. Curled

Figure 28–7 ■ Types of renal dialysis access. *A.* The arteriovenous (AV) fistula and graft are used for long-term hemodialysis. *B.* A temporary venous access can be placed centrally or into the femoral vein for use in treating acute renal failure. *C.* The Tenckhoff catheter is used for peritoneal dialysis and is inserted through the lower abdominal wall. *From National Kidney and Urologic Diseases Information Clearinghouse [NKUDIC]. [2004]. National Institute of Diabetes and Digestive and Kidney Diseases [NIDDK], NIH. Available at:* http://kidney.niddk.nih.gov/kudiseases. *Accessed July 1, 2004.*

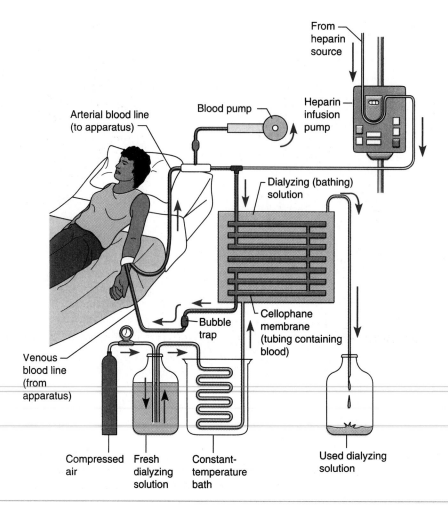

Figure 28–8 ■ Hemodialysis system.

Hemodialysis cleans the blood by pumping it out of the patient via a venous access. The blood then passes through a dialyzer, which removes fluid and solutes, returning the filtered blood back to the patient. The semipermeable membrane necessary for diffusion in hemodialysis is penetrable, thin cellophane. The blood comprises the first fluid compartment, and the dialysate is the second one. The semipermeable membrane pores are large enough to allow small substances to pass across (e.g., creatinine, urea and uric acid, and water molecules) but too small to allow larger particles to diffuse (e.g., proteins, blood cells, and bacteria). Figure 28–8 illustrates hemodialysis.

Diffusion occurs down a concentration gradient because the blood has a higher solute concentration than the dialysate has. This causes the flow of urea, creatinine, and other relatively concentrated solutes to move across the semipermeable membrane (the cellophane) into the dialysate solution.

Continuous Renal Replacement Therapy

Continuous renal replacement therapy (CRRT) is a relatively new type of dialysis that is used when hemodialysis is not feasible (e.g., hemodynamic instability or intolerance to peritoneal dialysis). At this time, CRRT is primarily seen in the critical care setting because frequent assessments and ongoing monitoring are essential.

CRRT, a continuous form of therapy (8 hours or more), is used primarily to remove fluid and, if necessary, waste products and excess electrolytes. The two most commonly used forms of CRRT are continuous arteriovenous hemofiltration (CAVH) and continuous venovenous hemofiltration (CVVH). When continuous dialysis is added to CAVH or CVVH, it is referred to as CAVH-D and CVVH-D, respectively.

Continuous Arteriovenous Hemofiltration (CAVH). Blood enters the CAVH circuit using the patient's own arterial blood pressure. Therefore, both an arterial and a venous access are necessary. The most common access site is the femoral artery and vein because of easy access and large vessel size. The volume within the extracorporeal circuit at any one time is small, making it less hemodynamically traumatic than conventional hemodialysis.

Blood in the circuit flows past a hemofilter, which maintains a lower pressure than the blood circulating past it. This pressure difference facilitates movement of solutes and water across its semipermeable membrane. The resulting ultrafiltrate

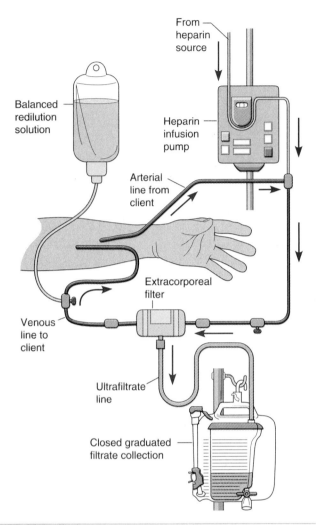

Figure 28–9 ■ Configuration of continuous arteriovenous hemofiltration.

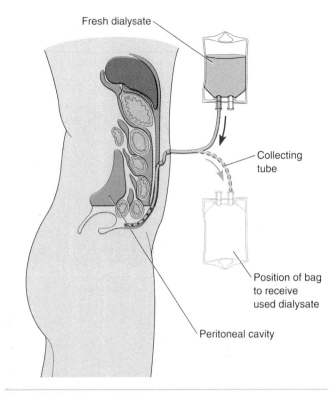

Figure 28–10 ■ Peritoneal dialysis.

drains into a collection apparatus. The level at which the collection device is hung determines the ultrafiltration rate. The ultrafiltration rate can also be adjusted by several other means, such as clamping the ultrafiltrate line or using an infusion control device. Once the blood passes the hemofilter, it is diluted again with a predetermined bath of electrolytes, water, and nutrients, based on the patient's fluid, electrolyte, and nutritional status. Figure 28–9 provides an illustration of CAVH.

Continuous Arteriovenous Hemofiltration–Dialysis (CAVH-D). CAVH-D is the addition of continuous dialysis to CAVH. CAVH-D uses a dialysate solution that infuses into the hemofilter at the venous end. The dialysate solution flows in the opposite direction of the blood, which creates a continual diffusion gradient throughout the hemofilter; thus, the removal of waste products and excess electrolytes is facilitated.

Continuous Venovenous Hemofiltration (CVVH). CVVH uses only a double-lumen catheter placed in a vein, which eliminates the need for an arterial catheter with its potential complications. CVVH uses a small pump to propel the blood from one

lumen of the catheter through the hemofilter and back into the vein through the second lumen of the catheter. The pump serves to control the blood flow and fluid removal rate.

Continuous Venovenous Hemofiltration–Dialysis (CVVH-D). CVVH-D is the addition of continuous dialysis to the process of CVVH. The dialysate solution is infused through the hemofilter in the same manner as in CAVH-D.

Peritoneal Dialysis

Peritoneal dialysis uses the patient's own peritoneal lining to serve as the semipermeable membrane through which diffusion, osmosis, and filtration occur (Fig. 28–10). The desired outcome of peritoneal dialysis is the same as other forms of dialysis—to remove metabolic wastes and correct fluid and electrolyte imbalances. It can be performed either manually or by use of automatic cycling machines. Dialyzing fluid is introduced into the peritoneal cavity via a peritoneal catheter (such as the Tenckhoff), which is secured in place (see Fig. 28–7, c). Once in the abdominal cavity, it is held there for a specified period of time, allowing adequate time for the transfer of fluid and solutes across the peritoneal lining. Once the dialyzing pass time is completed, the dialyzing fluid, with its additional fluid and solutes, is drained out of the abdomen.

Automatic Peritoneal Dialysis Cyclers.   In the high-acuity setting, automatic cyclers are frequently used when peritoneal dialysis is ordered. The major advantage of the automatic cycler is

Cycle Description

GENERAL DESCRIPTION

The cycler is a simple two-system dialysis unit. The **inflow system** consists of the dialysate *solution supply*, a *last bag*, a *heater bag*, a pump, connecting tubing, and a peritoneal dialysis catheter that is inserted into the peritoneal cavity (e.g., Tenckhoff catheter). The pump only activates when fluid must flow against gravity (e.g., pushing new dialysate up into the heater bag). At other times, simple gravity flow is used to move fluid. A *last bag* may be ordered when cycling is intermittent. The last bag is the final bag of dialysate to be used during a particular dialysis cycle. It may have a different composition from the regular dialysate in the solution supply. The **outflow system** consists of the peritoneal catheter, connection tubing, *weigh bag*, pump, and *disposal container*. The cycler machine also has an alarm system that activates if a problem in the inflow or outflow system occurs.

CYCLES

A. Patient Fill

Prior to the first patient fill, the dialysate is pumped from the *Solution Supply* into the *Heater Bag*, where it is warmed to body temperature. The warmed dialysate flows from the heater bag into the peritoneal cavity by gravity flow.

B. Dwell

The dwell time is the prescribed time in which the dialysate remains in the peritoneum. During the patient dwell period, the cycler system is closed to the patient. The cycler performs two activities during dwell time: 1) it pumps the next round of dialysate from the solution supply (or last bag) into the heater bag; and 2) it pumps any used dialysate from the *Weigh Bag* into the *Disposal Container* bag.

C. Patient Drain

Directly following the dwell period, the system opens up between the patient and the weigh bag. Used dialysate exits the peritoneal cavity by gravity force and flows into the weigh bag where it is weighed and measured and then pumped into the *disposal container* for eventual discard. Weighing the used dialysate helps evaluate the amount of fluid being removed from the body during the dialysis process.

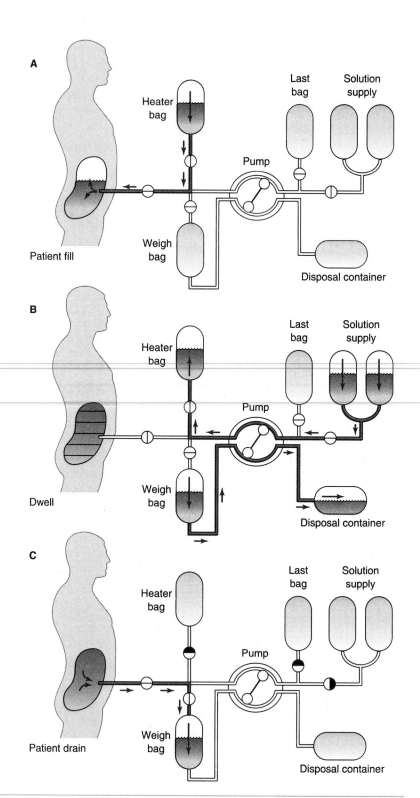

Figure 28–11 ■ Common components of a cycler-assisted peritoneal dialysis. *(Illustration from National Kidney and Urologic Diseases Information Clearinghouse [NKUDIC]. National Institute of Diabetes and Digestive and Kidney Diseases [NIDDK], NIH. Available at:* http://kidney.niddk.nih.gov/kudiseases. *Accessed July 1, 2004.*

that it can be programmed to deliver a set volume on a schedule. Cycler systems include solution storage, a pump, heater bag, weigh bag, disposal container, and alarms (NKUDIC, 2001). Figure 28–11 illustrates and describes a typical dialysis cycler system.

Nursing management of the patient undergoing dialysis or hemofiltration focuses on activities that maintain catheter or venous access patency and prevent complications. Many nursing interventions apply to all treatment modalities. Table 28–5 summarizes nursing activities based on type of treatment modality.

Dialysate Solutions

The exact nature of the dialysate is based on the fluid and electrolyte status of the patient. It consists of a combination of water and variable concentrations of electrolytes. Electrolytes common to dialysate solutions include potassium, sodium, chloride, magnesium, and calcium. Electrolyte concentrations are manipulated carefully depending on whether the serum level of each electrolyte is high, low, or within normal range. Acute renal failure usually is associated with higher-than-normal levels of potassium, sodium, magnesium, and phosphate. For this reason, the electrolyte levels in the dialysate solution will be either within normal range or below normal to pull excess electrolytes out of the blood and into the dialysate solution (down the concentration gradient).

Glucose is commonly added to the solution to increase filtration of the fluid and a buffer is included, either bicarbonate or acetate. Buffers help stabilize any existing metabolic acidosis and keep electrolytes in solution form. Table 28–6 shows one example of the composition of hemodialysis dialysate, including normal serum levels of each component.

TABLE 28–6 Composition of Dialysate

COMPONENT	DIALYSATE LEVEL	NORMAL SERUM LEVELS
Sodium	133–142 mEq/L	135–145 mEq/L
Potassium	0.0–4.0 mEq/L	3.5–5.3 mEq/L
Chloride	103–105 mEq/L	95–105 mEq/L
Calcium	2.5–3.5 mEq/L	2.2–2.5 mEq/L
Magnesium	1.0–1.5 mEq/L	1.5–2.5 mEq/L
Glucose	0.0–200 mg/100 mL	70–110 mg/dL
Acetate	33–38 mEq/L	—
Bicarbonate	As ordered	24–28 mEq/L

Data from Ulrich, G. T. (1989). Nephrology nursing: Concepts and strategies (p. 130). Norwalk, CT: Appleton & Lange. Normal serum levels from Kee, J. L. (2002). Laboratory and diagnostic tests with nursing implications (6th ed.). Upper Saddle River, NJ: Prentice Hall.

Drug Therapy and Dialysis

Administration of drugs requires special consideration when the patient is receiving dialysis. First, between intermittent dialysis treatments, drugs that do not break down fully in the body continue to circulate in active form because they cannot be excreted via the kidneys. Continuing to deliver the usual normal doses in such a patient can lead to severe toxic effects. Second, during dialysis many drugs cross the semipermeable membrane and are removed from the blood, which creates postdialysis subtherapeutic drug levels of those particular pharmacologic agents. This capability makes dialysis a useful

TABLE 28–5 Nursing Considerations During Dialysis Treatment

	HEMODIALYSIS	CRRT	PERITONEAL DIALYSIS
Goals	Maintain shunt, fistula, or catheter patency	Maintain catheter patency	Maintain catheter patency
	Prevent complications	Prevent complications	Maintain balanced intake and output
			Prevent complications
Nursing Care	Monitor vital signs and hemodynamic status	Monitor vital signs and hemodynamic status	Monitor vital signs and hemodynamic status
	Weigh before and after dialysis	Weighs daily	Weigh daily
	Monitor for signs and symptoms of complications	Monitor for signs and symptoms of complications	Monitor for signs and symptoms of complications
	Monitor laboratory values for therapeutic levels	Monitor laboratory values for therapeutic levels	Monitor laboratory values for therapeutic levels
	Daily sterile shunt site care	Daily catheter care	Daily catheter care
	Daily fistula care until site is healed	Monitor hourly intake and output	Precise documentation of intake and output
	No blood pressure cuff, injection, IV insertions, or tourniquets on limb with shunt or fistula	Observe color if ultrafiltrate is used with every exchange	Obtain intermittent cultures of drainage dialysate and catheter tip (if removed)
	Keep clamps at bedside at all times	Assess for patency (presence of palpable thrill on both tubings)	Turn side to side to facilitate drainage
			Observe color of drainage dialysate

option for rapid removal of intentional or accidental over-doses of dialyzable drugs.

The nurse caring for the patient receiving dialysis should be aware of which drugs are dialyzable. Many hospitals have a listing of drugs that will be dialyzed out. These drugs should be scheduled appropriately to avoid undesired dialysis. Table 28–7 is a partial listing of the dialyzability of some commonly ordered drugs.

In summary, when the kidneys are no longer able to adequately cleanse the blood of excess waste products, fluid, and electrolytes, artificial means often are required to correct the imbalances. Three methods were described: hemodialysis, CRRT, and peritoneal dialysis. Each modality carries with it indications, contraindications, and disadvantages. The nurse must be aware of the effect of hemodialysis on drug therapy. Problems of either toxic or subtherapeutic drug levels are associated with acute renal failure and dialysis.

TABLE 28–7   Dialyzability of Common Drugs

DRUGS DIALYZED OUT OF BLOOD	DRUGS NOT SIGNIFICANTLY DIALYZED OUT OF BLOOD[a]
Acetaminophen	Albumin
Aspirin	Diazepam
Captopril	Digoxin
Mannitol	Furosemide
Methyldopa	Heparin
Metoclopramide (partially)	Hydralazine
Protamine sulfate	Iron products
Pyridoxine	Levothyroxine
Theophylline	Nifedipine
General[b]:	Prazosin HCl
Beta blockers	Prochlorperazine
Penicillin drugs	Propranolol HCl
Aminoglycosides	Quinidine
Cephalosporins	Verapamil

[a]Drugs that are protein bound or have large molecules that are not removed during dialysis.

[b]Many specific agents in these groups dialyze out and may require additional dosing.

SECTION EIGHT REVIEW

1. If the patient responds to a diuretic challenge by increasing urine output, the nurse would anticipate which type of follow-up intervention?
   A. hemodialysis
   B. peritoneal dialysis
   C. large doses of diuretics
   D. fluid replacement and diuretics

2. The major purpose of using dialysis is to
   A. remove proteins from the blood
   B. correct imbalances of fluid and electrolytes
   C. remove drugs from the blood
   D. correct renal dysfunction

3. Common rapid access sites for short-term hemodialysis are
   A. subclavian and femoral veins
   B. femoral and brachial arteries
   C. radial and femoral arteries
   D. internal jugular and subclavian veins

4. Which statement is correct regarding diffusion?
   A. it occurs up a concentration gradient
   B. it moves particles (solute) across a membrane
   C. it occurs down a concentration gradient
   D. it disperses out within a solution with no membrane

5. CRRT would most likely be used on which patient?
   A. a 6-year-old patient diagnosed with prerenal failure
   B. a hemodynamically stable, 7-year-old cardiac patient
   C. a 2-year-old patient diagnosed with postrenal failure
   D. a hemodynamically unstable 4-year-old trauma patient

6. When peritoneal dialysis is performed, the semipermeable membrane is the
   A. peritoneal lining
   B. hemofilter
   C. cellophane membrane
   D. renal lining

7. Assuming that a patient's electrolytes have undergone the typical imbalances associated with acute renal failure, the dialysate solution will contain low levels of which electrolyte?
   A. calcium
   B. chloride
   C. potassium
   D. bicarbonate

Answers: 1. D, 2. B, 3. A, 4. C, 5. D, 6. A, 7. C

SECTION NINE: The High-Acuity Patient with Chronic Renal Failure

At the completion of this section, the learner will be able to discuss the implications of caring for a high-acuity patient who has chronic renal failure.

Evidence-Based Practice

- *Chronic renal failure patients who presented at an emergency department with complaints of chest pain were found to have a higher percentage of heart failure and myocardial infarction within 30 days of being seen than non-CRF patients with the same complaint (McCullough et al., 2003).*

- *End-stage renal failure was found to significantly increase complications and mortality following coronary angioplasty (Reinecke et al., 2003).*

- *Post-myocardial infarction patients with severe renal disease had a higher incidence of death while still in the hospital and following discharge (Wright et al., 2003).*

- *In patients with end-stage renal disease who were receiving hemodialysis, an elevated fibrinogen level was a risk factor for death from a cardiovascular event—the higher the fibrinogen level, the higher the risk of dying (Zoccali et al., 2003).*

Chronic renal failure (CRF) refers to the slow, progressive, and irreversible destruction of the kidneys (Porth, 2002b). It is characterized by progressive renal mass destruction with loss of nephrons over months or years (Verrelli, 2004). Chronic renal failure can result from a primary renal disorder (e.g., glomerulonephritis or polycystic kidney disease) or as a secondary disorder (e.g., as a complication of diabetes mellitus or hypertension). The most common causes of chronic renal failure are diabetes, hypertension, and glomerulonephritis. CRF is fairly common, with more than 375,000 people in the United States diagnosed as having end-stage renal disease (ESRD). In patients with CRF who require dialysis, the 5-year survival rate in the United States is about 35 percent, and if the patient is also a diabetic, it drops to about 20 percent (Verrelli, 2004). These statistics change if renal transplantation is performed and the patient no longer requires dialysis. Table 28–8 summarizes statistics on renal failure for the year 2000.

Until the early 1970s, people with chronic renal failure progressed in their disease process and died of its complications. Today, however, advances in medical science and technology have significantly increased the number of living persons with end-stage renal disease, thus increasing the number of patients with chronic renal failure who may require high-acuity care for treatment of severe illnesses that may or may not relate directly to their CRF.

TABLE 28–8 Chronic Renal Failure Statistics (2000)

Gender: Males more than females (about 10 percent)

Age: 75 percent older than 45 years of age

Race: White: about 60 percent, African American: about 32 percent

Associated disorders (by frequency)

    Diabetes: 35 percent

    Hypertension: 23 percent

    Glomerulonephritis: 16 percent

More than 275,000 on dialysis and 100,000 with functioning renal transplants

About 67 deaths per year, secondary to kidney failure

Data from National Kidney Foundation (NKF). (2004). Fact sheets: End-stage renal disease in the United States. Available at: www.kidney.org/. Accessed June 28, 2004.

Stages of Chronic Renal Failure

Chronic renal failure is commonly staged by the percentage of normal GFR remaining. There are usually four stages in the disease process beginning with diminished renal reserve and ending with end-stage renal disease. Table 28–9 lists the stages and highlights the clinical findings associated with each stage.

Diminished Renal Reserve

The first stage of CRF is diminished renal reserve, which lasts until the GFR drops to about 50 percent of normal (Porth, 2002b). During this period, nephrons are being destroyed but adequate compensatory mechanisms are in place to maintain normal renal function. One such mechanism is hypertrophy of the remaining normal nephrons, which increases their filtration capacity. The person is clinically unaware of this stage because of the lack of clinical manifestations. Should the kidneys become further stressed, however, they can progress to the next stage. Nephrotoxins, such as aminoglycoside antibiotics, NSAIDs, and IV contrast dye, may cause further renal insult. A person with 50 percent renal reserve would be free of clinical manifestations during this first stage, especially considering the fact that many people lead completely normal lives with only one kidney (Porth, 2002b).

Renal Insufficiency

The second stage, renal insufficiency, begins when the GFR has dropped to 20 to 50 percent of normal (Porth, 2002b). It is often heralded in by development of a particular type of polyuria called "isothenuria." This form of polyuria has a tonicity that is similar to that of plasma because of loss of sodium and water, which results from loss of the kidneys' capacity for regulating sodium and water balance. Clinical manifestations appear

TABLE 28–9 Stages of Chronic Renal Failure

STAGE	GFR (% OF NORMAL)	ASSOCIATED CLINICAL MANIFESTATIONS
Diminished renal reserve	About 50	*General:* Asymptomatic; at increased risk for nephrotoxicity from drugs and toxins *Renal function laboratory tests:* Normal
Renal insufficiency	20–50	*General:* Onset of hypertension and anemia, development of polyuria ("isosthenuria") *Renal function laboratory tests:* Onset of azotemia
Renal failure	Less than 20	*General:* Onset of renal failure manifestations *Renal function laboratory tests:* Continue to deteriorate
End-stage renal disease	Less than 5	*General:* Worsening of manifestations *Renal function laboratory tests:* Reflect total loss of renal function

Data from Porth, C. M. (Ed.). (2002). Pathophysiology: Concepts of altered health states, (6th ed.). Philadelphia: Lippincott Williams & Wilkins

during this stage that reflect the initial loss of the kidney's compensatory mechanisms. As the renal insufficiency stage progresses, any additional stress placed on the remaining functional nephrons can result in rapid progression to renal failure (Porth, 2002b).

Renal Failure

The third stage, renal failure, begins when the GFR has dropped below 20 percent of normal (Porth, 2002b). Volume and solute regulation is lost and the person develops metabolic acidosis, hyperkalemia, and edema. It is at this point that the person may develop signs and symptoms of uremia, which are multisystem in nature. Uremia is discussed further with end-stage renal disease.

End-Stage Renal Disease

The final stage, end-stage renal disease (ESRD), occurs when GFR is almost totally lost (less than 5 percent of normal). Structurally, the nephrons are scarred, with loss of capillaries and tubular fibrosis and atrophy. The kidneys are grossly abnormal, shriveled in appearance, and nonfunctional. If the person is to survive, dialysis or renal transplantation is required. Uremia is the primary characteristic of this stage (Porth, 2002b). Uremia is differentiated from azotemia, azotemia only refers to the abnormally elevated levels of nitrogenous wastes, whereas uremia refers to the numerous multisystem signs and symptoms associated with ESRD.

The effects of uremia reflect the failure of crucial kidney functions, including elimination of body wastes, regulation of fluid and electrolytes, acid–base balance, and the release of several hormones, such as erythropoietin (RBC production), renin (blood pressure regulation), and the active form of vitamin D (important in maintenance of calcium in bones and chemical balance). Refer to Figure 28–6 for the multisystem effects of uremia.

Nursing Considerations

The high-acuity patient with chronic renal failure enters the hospital setting with significant, preexisting health problems that potentially have altered the majority of body functions because of the multisystem nature of uremic syndrome. Minimally, the nurse can anticipate the following:

■ Dialysis will be required. The patient will require continued dialysis, which may or may not be on the same schedule and of the same type as ordered prior to hospitalization.

■ Hypertension is likely to be present. Hypertension is usually present related to excess extracellular fluid (ECF), particularly if the patient is admitted before routine dialysis has been performed.

■ Some degree of hypoxia may be present. The patient is likely to be chronically anemic because of loss of erythropoietin. If the patient develops a fever or other hypermetabolic process, hypoxia will worsen. It is recommended that the hemoglobin level be targeted at 11 to 12 g/dL (Gregory, 2003). Maintaining adequate hemoglobin and hematocrit levels will increase tissue oxygenation.

■ Increased risk for infection is present. Chronic renal failure patients are prone to infection for several reasons: First, they frequently are admitted with preexisting protein-calorie malnutrition as a result of protein catabolism and lack of protein dietary intake, and impaired glucose metabolism related to impaired insulin secretion (Wells, 2003). Second, the patient is likely to be immunodepressed (via malnutrition and altered immune response related to elevated metabolic wastes) or immunosuppressed (via steroid therapy or immunosuppressant drug therapy).

In addition, there are myriad health issues and complications associated with chronic renal failure that increase morbidity and mortality. The presence of chronic renal failure in a high-acuity patient has significant implications in prognosis and recovery from a severe acute illness. This fact can be readily understood by examining the deleterious effects of uremic syndrome on the entire body. Chronic renal failure patients are particularly at risk for problems associated with cardiovascular disease, which is the major cause of death in this patient population (Uyeharra et al., 2002).

Care of the high-acuity patient with chronic renal failure then requires monitoring of all major body systems, rapid recognition of development of complications, and timely interventions. The nursing diagnoses that might apply to this patient population are numerous. Following are some common diagnoses that apply to the chronic renal failure patient (Ulrich & Canale, 2001).

- Altered fluid and electrolyte balance
- Altered nutrition: Less than body requirements
- Activity intolerance
- Risk for infection
- Risk for constipation (p. 533)

In addition, the following potential complications (PC) apply:

- PC: Uremic syndrome
- PC: Hypertension

The potential complication *uremic syndrome* is specific to the renal failure patient. Some of the major nursing interventions that are suggested for this problem include

1. Assess for clinical manifestations of uremia (refer to Fig. 28–6)
2. Assess for and report abnormal changes in serum, electrolytes, creatinine clearance, BUN and creatinine, and platelets
3. Implement measures for reduction of nitrogenous wastes: Control intake of proteins, prevent/reverse catabolic processes

In summary, this section provided a brief overview of chronic renal failure and implications for care in high-acuity situations. Four stages of chronic renal failure were identified as diminished renal reserve, renal insufficiency, renal failure, and ESRD. It is at the final stage that a person must either be started on dialysis or receive a renal transplant to survive. The primary cause of death in the CRF patient is cardiovascular disease. Major problems that can be anticipated when a patient with CRF is to be admitted were listed, as were common nursing diagnoses and potential complications. Finally, a brief set of nursing interventions relevant to the potential complication, uremic syndrome, was provided.

SECTION NINE REVIEW

1. List the three major causes of chronic renal failure.

   _____

   _____

   _____

2. Chronic renal failure is staged based on what criteria?
   A. etiology of failure
   B. number of symptoms present
   C. urinary output and creatinine levels
   D. percentage of normal GFR remaining
3. During the diminished reserve stage, the kidneys compensate in which way?
   A. dying nephrons are rapidly replaced
   B. nephrons conserve energy
   C. remaining normal nephrons hypertrophy
   D. renal vessels vasodilate
4. Isosthenuria (a form of polyuria) develops during which stage of chronic renal failure?
   A. diminished renal reserve
   B. renal insufficiency
   C. renal failure
   D. end-stage renal disease
5. The renal failure stage of chronic renal failure begins when the GFR has dropped to _____ percent of normal.
   A. less than 5
   B. less than 20

C. 20 to 50
D. 50

6. The renal failure stage of chronic renal failure is characterized by the development of which problems? (choose all that apply)
   1. edema
   2. hypocalcemia
   3. hypercalcemia
   4. metabolic alkalosis
   5. metabolic acidosis
   A. 1, 3, and 5
   B. 3 and 4
   C. 1, 2, and 5
   D. 3 and 5
7. The appearance of the kidneys during the end-stage renal disease stage is best described as
   A. small and shriveled
   B. necrotic and sloughing
   C. large and bloated
   D. inflamed & edematous
8. True or False: Azotemia differs from uremia because azotemia only refers to elevated nitrogenous waste levels, whereas uremia is a multisystem syndrome.

9. Patients with chronic renal failure are at increased risk for some degree of hypoxia because of
  A. pulmonary complications
  B. malnutrition
  C. electrolyte imbalances
  D. chronic anemia
10. Give two reasons the patient with chronic renal failure is at increased risk for development of infection.
  _____
  _____

11. Managing nitrogenous wastes in the chronic renal failure patient requires close control of which nutrient?
  A. proteins
  B. fats
  C. carbohydrates
  D. vitamins and minerals

Answers: 1. diabetes, hypertension, glomerulonephritis; 2. D, 3. C, 4. B, 5. B, 6. A, 7. A, 8. True, 9. D, 10. impaired immune response, protein-calorie malnutrition; 11. A

POSTTEST

The following Posttest is constructed in a case study format. A patient is presented. Questions are posed based on available data. New data are presented as the case study progresses.

Maria G, a 32-year-old teacher, has been admitted through the emergency department after sustaining multiple injuries in a motor vehicle crash (MVC). The emergency medical team relates that when she was found at the scene of the event, she was noted to have an arterial blood pressure of 76/42. It was believed that the ambulance had arrived 20 minutes after the crash. In the emergency department, she was found to have a ruptured spleen and she was prepared immediately for surgery. She has no known history. It has been almost 48 hours since the event. You note that Maria's urine output has been approximately 25 mL for 2 successive hours.

1. For glomerular filtration to take place, it is important that Maria maintain
  A. a low hydrostatic pressure
  B. an adequate cardiac output
  C. a low renal blood volume
  D. a high renal vascular resistance
2. Certain ions, such as potassium and hydrogen, undergo renal tubular "secretion." This term refers to the process by which substances are moved
  A. into the tubules for excretion
  B. back into the vascular system
  C. into the interstitial compartment
  D. back into the glomerulus from Bowman's capsule
3. Assuming Maria's nervous system is intact, how would it respond to her low blood pressure?
  A. osmoreceptors would inhibit antidiuretic hormone production
  B. stretch receptors would vasoconstrict peripheral arterioles

  C. chemoreceptors would stimulate production of aldosterone
  D. baroreceptors would stimulate antidiuretic hormone production
4. The renin–angiotensin system assists in increasing Maria's arterial blood pressure by
  A. causing vasoconstriction
  B. decreasing circulatory volume
  C. increasing hydrogen ion concentration
  D. inhibiting reabsorption of sodium

The following data are now available. It is believed that Maria's blood pressure remained low for at least 30 minutes directly after the crash. The emergency team had difficulty obtaining a vascular access with which to administer fluids. Her daughter has informed you that Maria has no known chronic conditions except for mild arthritis, which she controls with aspirin on a daily basis.

5. Considering Maria's recent history, the origin of her renal problem is most likely?
  A. postrenal
  B. prerenal
  C. intrinsic
  D. perirenal

Five days have passed since the crash. Maria's urine output has fallen to 350 mL over the past 24 hours. She has just received a diuretic challenge, to which she had no response. Her blood pressure is now 165/94.

6. Considering the latest changes, what specifically is Maria most likely developing?
  A. prerenal failure
  B. acute tubular necrosis
  C. postrenal failure
  D. perirenal failure

7. Maria is at high risk for developing renal failure because ischemia occurs when the mean arterial blood pressure drops to below _____ mm Hg for more than 30 minutes.
   A. 50 to 60
   B. 60 to 70
   C. 70 to 80
   D. 80 to 90

Maria is now in acute renal failure secondary to acute tubular necrosis. Her urine output has been approximately 350 mL over the past 24 hours, and her BUN is now 100 mg/dL. She is confused and drowsy.

8. According to the latest data, Maria is experiencing the _____ stage of acute renal failure.
   A. onset
   B. maintenance (oliguric)
   C. maintenance (anuric)
   D. recovery

It has been 18 days since the onset of Maria's acute renal failure. Her urine output is now 500 mL over the past 24 hours, and her BUN and creatinine have both leveled off.

9. According to the latest available data, Maria is in which of the following stages of acute renal failure?
   A. recovery
   B. maintenance (oliguric)
   C. onset
   D. maintenance (nonoliguric)

Maria's laboratory values are as follows:

48 Hours Postinjury:	5 Days Postinjury:
BUN/creatinine ratio 24:1	BUN/creatinine ratio 13:1
Urine sodium 38 mEq/L	Urine sodium 52 mEq/L
Specific gravity 1.028	Specific gravity 1.008
Serum osmolality 650 mOsm/L	Serum osmolality 285 mOsm/L

10. Maria's pattern of renal laboratory findings are consistent with an initial _____ failure which became a(n) _____ failure.
    A. postrenal, intrinsic
    B. prerenal, postrenal
    C. prerenal, intrinsic
    D. intrinsic, acute tubular necrosis
11. A renal ultrasound is ordered. Which statement is correct regarding ultrasound?
    A. it is an invasive procedure
    B. it requires use of a contrast dye
    C. it can be performed at the bedside
    D. it requires a local anesthetic

Maria experienced some of the clinical manifestations of uremic syndrome. She was complaining of tingling and numbness of her feet.

12. Maria's symptoms of tingling and numbness were most likely caused by
    A. hyperkalemia
    B. hypocalcemia
    C. stimulated stretch receptors
    D. peripheral neuropathy
13. Skin bruising in acute renal failure is secondary to the effects of
    A. increased erythropoietin
    B. decreased ammonia levels
    C. severe hypocalcemia
    D. excessive uremic toxins
14. Maria's serum phosphate is elevated. Which of the following reasons is most likely the cause?
    A. hypermagnesemia
    B. hypocalcemia
    C. hypomagnesemia
    D. hypercalcemia
15. She is at risk for developing metabolic acidosis primarily as a result of
    A. decreased excretion of potassium
    B. increased excretion of hydrogen ions
    C. increased excretion of potassium
    D. decreased excretion of hydrogen ions

Maria had the following hourly urine outputs recorded:

3:00: 32 mL
4:00: 41 mL
5:00: 43 mL

16. Based on common fluid restriction practice, and assuming that she has no other output during this period, you would anticipate giving Maria _____ mL of fluid between 5:00 and 6:00.
    A. 41
    B. 43
    C. 84
    D. 116
17. Maria is to begin receiving nutritional support. The nurse would anticipate that the preferred route to be used is
    A. oral/GI tract
    B. Hickman catheter
    C. peripheral parenteral nutrition
    D. central venous IV line
18. Maria's nutritional plan will require restriction of
    A. minerals
    B. fats
    C. protein
    D. carbohydrates

It has been decided that Maria needs dialysis. Her present status is as follows. She is hemodynamically stable, and she is 8 days postabdominal surgery. She has generalized edema and severe electrolyte abnormalities.

19. Based only on the available data, which type of dialysis is most likely to be ordered for Maria?
    A. hemodialysis
    B. peritoneal dialysis
    C. continuous ultrafiltration
    D. combination of hemodialysis and peritoneal dialysis
20. She is receiving a drug that is highly protein bound while in circulation. What would be the significance of

drug protein binding and hemodialysis if this treatment were ordered?
    A. protein-bound drugs will be released during dialysis
    B. protein-bound drugs break down rapidly in the blood
    C. protein-bound molecules are too large to dialyze out
    D. protein-bound drugs in tissues move into circulation during dialysis

POSTTEST ANSWERS

Question	Answer	Section
1	B	One
2	A	One
3	D	Two
4	A	Two
5	B	Three
6	B	Three
7	B	Three
8	B	Four
9	A	Four
10	C	Five

Question	Answer	Section
11	C	Five
12	D	Five
13	D	Five
14	B	Six
15	D	Six
16	B	Seven
17	A	Seven
18	C	Seven
19	A	Eight
20	C	Eight

REFERENCES

Agraharkar, M. (2002). Acute renal failure. Available at: *www.emedicine. com/MED/topic1595.htm.* Accessed March 9, 2004.

Albright, R. C. (2001). Acute renal failure: A practical update. *Mayo Clinic Proceedings, 76,* 67–74.

Esson, M. L., & Schrier, R. W. (2002). Diagnosis and treatment of acute tubular necrosis. *Annals of Internal Medicine, 137,* 744–752.

Ferrone, M. (2003). Pharmaceutical interventions in acute renal failure. *U.S. Pharmacist, 28*(10).

Gregory, N. (2003). Effect of higher hemoglobin levels on health-related quality of life parameters. *Nephrology Nursing Journal, 30*(1), 75–78.

Guyton, A. C., & Hall, J. E. (1997). *Human physiology and mechanisms of disease* (6th ed.). Philadelphia: W. B. Saunders.

Kaplan, A. A. (2002). Renal failure. In F. S. Bongard & D. Y. Sue (Eds.), *Current critical care: Diagnosis and treatment* (2nd ed., pp. 342–375). New York: Lange Medical Books/McGraw Hill.

Kee, J. L. (2002). *Laboratory and diagnostic tests with nursing implications* (6th ed.). Upper Saddle River, NJ: Prentice Hall.

McCullough, P. A., Nowak, R. M., & Foreback, C. (2003). Chronic renal disease is a marker for outcomes in emergency department patients presenting with chest pain. *Kidney, 12*(3), 114–115.

NKUDIC. (2001). NIH Publication No. 01-4688. Available at: *http://kidney. niddk.nih.gov/kudiseases/pbs/peritoneal/.* Accessed May 4, 2004.

Pikna, J. K. (2002). Concepts of altered health in older adults. In C. M. Porth (Ed.), *Pathophysiology: Concepts of altered health states* (6th ed., pp. 43–60). Philadelphia: Lippincott Williams & Wilkins.

Porth, C. M. (2002a). Control of renal function. In C. M. Porth (Ed.), *Pathophysiology: Concepts of altered health states* (6th ed., pp. 673–691). Philadelphia: Lippincott Williams & Wilkins.

Porth, C. M. (2002b). Renal failure. In C. M. Porth (Ed.), *Pathophysiology: Concepts of altered health states* (6th ed., pp. 777–793). Philadelphia: Lippincott Williams & Wilkins.

Reinecke, H., Regetmeier, A., Matzkies, F., et al. (2003). Even moderate chronic failure is associated with impaired acute and long-term outcome after coronary angioplasty. *Nephrology, 8*(3), 110–116.

Shah, S. V. (2001). Acute renal failure. In T. E. Andreoli (Ed.), *Cecil essentials of medicine* (5th ed., pp. 283–290). Philadelphia: W. B. Saunders.

Ulrich, S. P., & Canale, S. W. (2001). *Nursing care planning guides* (5th ed.). Philadelphia: W. B. Saunders.

Uyeharra, G., Young, L., Miller, M., Takvorian, L., & Vogel, S. (2002). Cardiac disease, infectious disease, and chronic renal failure. *Nephrology nursing Journal, 29*(2), 199–201.

Verrelli, M. (2004). Chronic renal failure. Available at: *www.emedicine. com/med/topic374.htm.* Accessed March 9, 2004.

Wells, C. (2003). Optimizing nutrition in patients with chronic kidney disease. *Nephrology Nursing Journal, 30*(6), 637–648.

Wright, R. S., Reeder, G. S., & Herzog, C. A. (2003). Renal failure patients at increased risk of death after acute myocardial infarction. *Kidney, 12*(3), 118 [abstract].

Young, B. A. (2003). Uremia. *E-medicine.* Available at: *http://www.emedicine. com/med/topic2341.htm.* Accessed July 4, 2004.

Zoccali, C., Mallamaci, F., Tripepi, G., Cutrupi, S., et al. (2003). Fibrinogen, mortality and incident cardiovascular complications in end-stage renal failure. *Journal of Internal Medicine, 254*(2), 132–139 [abstract].

Nursing Care of the Patient with Altered Metabolic Function

Kathleen Dorman Wagner

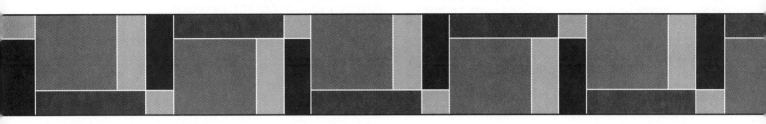

OBJECTIVES   Following completion of this module, given a specific clinical situation, the learner will be able to

1. Interpret the significance of laboratory data.
2. Interpret the significance of assessment data.
3. Develop appropriate desired patient outcomes.

4. Apply knowledge of the patient with altered nutrition/ metabolism to develop a plan of nursing interventions.
5. Describe the nursing management of the patient with altered nutrition/metabolism status.

This module is designed to integrate the major points discussed in Part VI, "Metabolic." This module summarizes relationships among key concepts and assists the learner in clustering information to facilitate clinical application. The module applies content in an interactive learning style using a case study format. The learner is encouraged to cluster data and derive as well as prioritize nursing diagnoses. The module ends with a brief summary of major points. All normal ranges for laboratory values are taken from Kee (2002).

Developing a Plan of Care

Assessment

Each module in Part VI, "Metabolic," presented material on assessments appropriate to the module's specific topic. Once data collection is complete, the nurse clusters the critical cues based on the presence of abnormal data or missing normal data, collects any necessary additional data, and develops a list of nursing diagnoses.

Nursing Diagnoses

Nursing diagnoses are based on frequently recurring functional problems rather than body systems, which is characteristic of medical diagnoses. Therefore, the disorders presented in Part VI, "Metabolic," have many nursing diagnoses in common even though the disorders cause dysfunctions in different body systems. Although the etiologic factors associated with each nursing diagnosis may differ based on the underlying patho-physiologic problem, the desired patient outcomes and nursing management remain essentially the same. This nursing care–oriented module presents some of the major nursing diagnoses and desired patient outcomes (evaluative criteria) commonly associated with problems of nutrition and metabolism.

Problems of Nutrition

Three North American Nursing Diagnosis Association (NANDA)–approved nursing diagnoses directly reflect nutrition:

- Imbalanced nutrition: Less than body requirements *
- Imbalanced nutrition: More than body requirements
- Risk for more than body requirements.

Problems of Metabolism

Many metabolic alterations, such as starvation, renal failure, and diabetes, are associated with shifts in body fluid and electrolytes, placing the high-acuity patient at risk for developing problems in these areas.

Fluid Imbalance

Problems of metabolism often affect fluid balance, though in different ways. Three NANDA-approved nursing diagnoses focus on fluid balance:

- Fluid volume deficit
- Fluid volume excess
- Risk for fluid volume imbalance

Fluid volume excess is presented in Part I, "Special Topics," and Part III, "Perfusion," and will not be discussed here.

Electrolyte Imbalances

Electrolyte imbalances are not addressed directly in any NANDA-approved nursing diagnosis. They are physiologic complications that are collaborative problems. Collaborative problems are based on physiologic complications. The nurse focuses on monitoring the patient for clinical manifestations that indicate onset of the complication, as well as monitoring the patient for changes in clinical status.

Collaborative problems require a combination of physician-ordered and nurse-ordered interventions to treat the complication effectively. Using a collaborative problem model, electrolyte imbalance can be addressed in a plan of care as follows:

- Potential complication (PC): Electrolyte imbalances

---

* The disorders presented in Part VI, "Metabolic," are associated primarily with nutritional deficits rather than excesses.

Ulrich and Canale (2001) suggest an alternative nursing/collaborative diagnosis that combines fluid and electrolyte problems. They recommend the following:

- Altered fluid and electrolyte balance

Altered Immunocompetence

Metabolic problems frequently alter immune function. Infection, therefore, is a relatively common complication. The following NANDA-approved nursing diagnosis addresses infection:

- Risk for infection

Carpenito-Moyet (2004) and Ulrich and Canale (2001) suggest the following additional collaborative problems related to immunocompetence (PC = potential complication):

- PC: Opportunistic infections
- PC: Sepsis
- PC: Allergic reaction
- PC: Donor tissue rejection
- PC: Immunodeficiency

An additional nursing diagnosis, *Hyperthermia*, may be included in the plan of care if the nurse views fever as a distinctly separate problem.

Additional Nursing Diagnoses

Many other nursing diagnoses potentially could be included in the plan of care for the patient with a disorder affecting nutrition and metabolism. Some of these include

- Activity intolerance (risk for or actual)
- Impaired oral mucous membranes
- Altered respiratory function
- Disturbed thought processes
- Ineffective tissue perfusion (specify)
- Anxiety
- Fatigue
- Impaired skin integrity (high risk for or actual)
- Impaired tissue integrity
- Knowledge deficit
- Pain (specify acute or chronic)
- Self-care deficit (specify type)

Desired Patient Outcomes

The desired outcomes (evaluative criteria) presented here are standard ones as suggested by Ulrich and Canale (2001). On an actual plan of care, each outcome would need to be written more specifically, reflecting outcomes that are realistic for the individual needs and capabilities of the patient.

Imbalanced Nutrition: Less than Body Requirements

Desired outcomes: The patient will maintain adequate nutrition, as evidenced by

1. Serum glucose, albumin, prealbumin, transferrin, hemoglobin, hematocrit, lymphocyte, blood urea nitrogen (BUN), and creatinine within acceptable ranges
2. Weight trends moving toward normal for patient
3. Mucous membranes healthy
4. Strength and activity tolerance usual or improved

Fluid Volume Deficit Related to (Applicable Etiologies)

Desired outcomes: The patient will regain fluid and electrolyte balance as evidenced by

1. Stable weight
2. Normal skin turgor
3. Normal mental status for patient
4. Blood pressure and pulse within normal range for patient
5. Serum osmolality within normal range
6. Serum BUN, creatinine, glucose, hemoglobin, and hematocrit within acceptable ranges
7. Urine output greater than 30 mL per hour
8. Moist mucous membranes
9. Intake approximately equal to output
10. Capillary refill less than 3 to 5 seconds
11. Urine specific gravity within normal range

PC: Electrolyte Imbalances

Desired outcomes: The patient will maintain/regain electrolyte balance, as evidenced by

1. Electrolyte levels within normal ranges
2. Absence of cardiac dysrhythmias

3. Normal neurologic status for patient
4. Normal muscle strength and tone for patient
5. Normal neuromuscular status for patient
6. Normal blood pressure, pulse, and respirations for patient
7. Absence of abdominal pain, nausea, or vomiting

The desired outcomes presented here are generic. If the patient is experiencing several specific significant electrolyte abnormalities, the plan can separate each abnormality. When split up, each specific abnormality would include its own list of desired patient outcomes and interventions.

Risk for Infection

Desired outcomes: The patient will be free of infection as evidenced by

1. Pulse and temperature within normal range
2. Absence of lesions with redness, swelling, heat, or drainage
3. Absence of chills
4. Negative cultures
5. Skin integrity intact
6. Absence of adventitious breath sounds
7. White blood cell differential counts within acceptable ranges
8. Urine clear
9. Voiding asymptomatic

Interventions

Collaborative and independent nursing interventions are presented in each module. In addition, interventions are applied in the upcoming case study.

Case Study

BEATRICE J, A PATIENT WITH COMPLEX METABOLIC DYSFUNCTION

Beatrice J, a 53-year-old woman, was brought into the emergency department by her husband, who simply stated that his wife "just looks real bad."

Initial Appraisal

On approaching Beatrice's stretcher, you make the following rapid assessment.

GENERAL APPEARANCE. Beatrice is a moderately obese Caucasian female. Her hair is gray and unkempt, and she is wearing a soiled nightgown.

SIGNS OF DISTRESS. Beatrice's breathing is even but deep. No facial grimacing is noted, and her limbs are outstretched in a relaxed fashion. She is mumbling in a confused manner. She appears drowsy.

OTHER. You note that her left foot is swollen, with a makeshift bandage on the heel. The wound has a foul odor emanating from it. She does not have any tubes or intravenous lines attached at this time. A man who states that he is Beatrice's husband, George, is standing beside the stretcher.

Recent History

George gives you the following brief history. Beatrice has a 15-year history of type 1 diabetes. About 3 weeks ago, she had a left heel spur removed in an outpatient surgery. Four days before this admission, Beatrice began experiencing abdominal pain and nausea, with intermittent vomiting. Her husband relates that for the past 2 days, his wife had omitted her insulin because "she didn't need it because she hadn't been able to eat anything." Although she was complaining of her foot hurting, she adamantly refused to have her husband call the doctor. Over the past week, her foot had become increasingly swollen and red, with a bad odor. For the past 3 days, she required frequent assistance into the bathroom to urinate, but she had not urinated in the past 8 hours. George adds that Beatrice has become increasingly confused and disoriented. Because of these developments, he felt the need to bring her into the hospital.

QUESTION

Based on these preliminary data, you would focus your assessment first on her _____ status.

- **A.** renal
- **B.** diabetes
- **C.** nutrition
- **D.** immunocompetence

ANSWER

The correct answer is B. During the initial appraisal, a critical cue was noted: no insulin in 2 days. Based on this single cue, the nurse can quickly cluster other similar critical cues, including history of type 1 diabetes, recent and acute physiologic stressors (surgery, probable wound infection), abdominal pain, nausea and vomiting, change in level of consciousness, failure to take insulin, no food consumption for several days, and a pattern of polyuria changing to diminished urine output. The exact nature of the diabetic crisis remains uncertain until laboratory results are evaluated. While waiting for laboratory results, if available, the nurse can obtain a capillary glucose specimen or urine sample for sugar and acetone.

The Focused Diabetic Assessment

Beatrice's initial appraisal, brief recent history, and data clustering are suggestive of a diabetic crisis. Immediate attention should be focused on obtaining more data to test this hypothesis. The results are as follows. Beatrice is drowsy and responds rapidly to light shaking. Her respirations are deep and even at 28/min (Kussmaul type). When bending down to examine her eyes, a fruity odor is noted on her breath. Her blood pressure is now 82/48, pulse 115/min (cardiac monitor shows sinus tachycardia), and temperature 102°F (38.9°C). Her skin is flushed, hot, and dry. Her mucous membranes

also are dry. You note that her jugular veins are collapsed when she is lying in a flat position.

Stat laboratory samples are drawn, and the results come back as follows:

Arterial Blood Gas (ABG)

pH:	7.20	
P_{CO_2}:	28 mm Hg	
P_{O_2}:	88 mm Hg	
HCO_3:	14 mEq/L	
Anion Gap:	30 mEq/L	(normal, 10 to 17 mEq/L)
Serum Glucose:	400 mg/dL	(normal, 70 to 110 mg/dL)
Hemoglobin A_1c (Hgb A_1c):	6.2 percent	(normal 4.5 to 7.5 percent)
Serum Ketones:	Positive	(normal, negative)
Serum BUN and creatinine:	28 and 1.5	(normal, BUN: 5 to 25 mg/dL and creatinine: 0.5-1.5)

Serum Electrolytes

Sodium (Na) = 152 mEq/L	(normal, 135 to 145 mEq/L)
Chloride (Cl) = 108 mEq/L	(normal, 95 to 105 mEq/L)
Potassium (K) = 5.8 mEq/L	(normal, 3.5 to 5.3 mEq/L)
Calcium (Ca) = 8.3 mg/dL	(normal, 9 to 11 mg/dL)
Hgb = 15.4 g/dL	(normal for females, 12 to 15 g/dL)
Hct = 48.2 percent	(normal for females, 36 to 46 percent)

QUESTION

Based on the data collected thus far, you hypothesize that Beatrice's clinical presentation is most consistent with which type of crisis?

- **A.** hypoglycemia
- **B.** Somogyi effect
- **C.** diabetic ketoacidosis (DKA)
- **D.** hyperosmolar hyperglycemic state (HHS)

ANSWER

The correct answer is C. Beatrice's history, clinical presentation, and laboratory data are consistent with diabetic ketoacidosis. Her ABG, anion gap, ketones, and serum glucose all suggest DKA rather than HHS.

Question: How would her history, presentation, and labs differ if she had HHS?

Review of Beatrice's lab values:

1. ABG results: Her low pH, low P_{CO_2}, and low bicarbonate levels inform us that she is in metabolic acidosis, as does her high anion gap.
2. Serum glucose, ketones, and HgbA$_1$c: Beatrice's elevated serum glucose and ketones confirm that she is in diabetic ketoacidosis. Note that her HgbA$_1$c, although on the high side of normal, is not abnormally high, which suggests that her hyperglycemia is due to her acute condition rather than being long term.
3. BUN and creatinine: The BUN is elevated but it is difficult to interpret it because BUN values elevate with hemoconcentration. (This will be investigated further.)
4. Serum electrolytes: Her electrolytes suggest hemoconcentration, which we would expect in the presence of dehydration.
5. Hemoglobin and hematocrit: Her Hgb and Hct suggest hemoconcentration, secondary to dehydration.

QUESTION

Examine her admission vital signs. What concerns do you have, if any? (short answer)

ANSWER

Beatrice's tachycardia is probably compensatory, secondary to her fever and hypotension. Her fever is likely related to her infection and state of dehydration. Her deep, rapid respirations are compensatory to blow off CO_2 and bring the pH back toward alkaline. Our major concern, however, is Beatrice's admission blood pressure of 82/48! Her mean arterial pressure (MAP) is 59 mm Hg. This should raise a red flag that she is at risk for complications of hypoperfusion organ ischemia. We should be concerned that her kidneys are at risk, as are her other organs.

The Systematic Bedside Assessment

Beatrice has a large-bore intravenous (IV) catheter inserted, and appropriate medical interventions for DKA are initiated based on her blood pressure and laboratory results. Interventions include fluid replacement and IV insulin drip. She is then moved from the emergency department to a critical care unit.

On arrival in the critical care unit, Beatrice is transferred to a bed. An updated report from the emergency department nurse is given, and a systematic bedside assessment is performed.

HEAD AND NECK. Beatrice's face appears flushed, and her lips are dry and cracked. She now moans and opens her eyes when moderately shaken. Her pupils are equal and react briskly to light. Her neck veins are flat. No abnormalities are noted.

CHEST. *Pulmonary status.* Breath sounds are present and equal bilaterally. No adventitious breath sounds are auscultated. Rate and quality are the same as previously noted.

Cardiac Status. S1 and S2 with no murmur is auscultated. The cardiac monitor shows sinus tachycardia at 120 beats per minute. Rhythm is regular.

ABDOMEN. The abdomen is slightly distended. Hypoactive bowel sounds are auscultated in all quadrants. The abdomen is soft to palpation.

PELVIS. A urinary catheter is in place. The urine output over the past 2 hours is 25 mL. The urine is clear, dark amber, with a specific gravity of 1.045.

EXTREMITIES. There is poor skin turgor. The skin is hot and dry. No peripheral edema is noted. The nailbeds are pale. Peripheral pulses are present in all four extremities but weak. The left foot is hot and edematous. You note a 15-cm open wound on the left heel, with a moderate amount of green purulent drainage. Touching the foot causes Beatrice to moan and grimace.

POSTERIOR. No skin breakdown is noted and no sacral edema. Posterior breath sounds are clear.

Developing the Plan of Care

Beatrice's DKA is brought under control through appropriate medical management. The nurse writes the following initial list of nursing diagnoses based on Beatrice's current status.

- Imbalanced nutrition: less than body requirements
- Decreased cardiac output
- Pain
- Altered tissue perfusion: peripheral
- Fluid volume deficit
- Self-care deficit
- PC: Infection

QUESTION

Which of the preceding diagnoses would be considered top priority during the first 4 hours after admission?

A. PC: infection
B. Fluid volume deficit
C. Altered tissue perfusion: peripheral
D. Altered nutrition: less than body requirements

ANSWER

The correct answer is B. A second cluster of critical cues is as follows: blood pressure 82/48 mm Hg, pulse 115 beats per minute. Lips and mucous membranes are dry. There is poor skin turgor. Neck veins are collapsed when lying flat. A history is given of an elimination pattern change from polyuria to oliguria over the past few days. At this time, we do not know whether the kidney function is failing or if they are compensating for the dehydration. These critical cues are very suggestive of fluid volume deficit. Correction of the fluid volume deficit is a priority if complications of hypovolemic shock are to be avoided. Correcting the fluid volume deficit also should increase Beatrice's cardiac output, assuming her cardiovascular system remains intact. **Immediate fluid resuscitation is required as a priority collaborative intervention to elevate her MAP to at least 70 mm Hg.**

Nursing implications: The nurse is responsible for hanging the appropriate fluids, running them at the prescribed rate, and monitoring Beatrice for the therapeutic effects (e.g., increased blood pressure and MAP, increased urine output, and CVP within normal limits) and for any nontherapeutic effects, particularly congestive heart failure (e.g., jugular vein distention, dependent edema, pulmonary crackles, elevated CVP).

The presence of a large-bore IV catheter is necessary to allow rapid IV infusion rates. Central venous pressure line placement early in the course of treatment will facilitate appropriate management of fluid rates to meet her needs. If closer monitoring of fluid and cardiac status is considered desirable, a flow-directed pulmonary artery catheter may be inserted.

QUESTION

Fluid resuscitation has been initiated on Beatrice. The nurse can anticipate that the second set of priority interventions will focus on initiating

A. electrolyte replacement
B. sodium bicarbonate
C. antibiotic therapy
D. insulin therapy

ANSWER

The correct answer is D. Beatrice's hyperglycemia must be addressed as soon as there is IV access and fluid replacement has been initiated. These two collaborative interventions will be performed in rapid succession. Electrolyte levels will be monitored carefully until her condition stabilizes. Her serum potassium is currently high; however, it will drop rapidly when her insulin therapy begins to drive potassium back into the cells. Potassium therapy is often held initially unless it is low at admission. In addition, her phosphate level should be obtained and monitored carefully. Because phosphate is a buffer, her acidotic state may have depleted it. If replacement therapy is necessary, it may be administered in the form of potassium phosphate (K-Phos).

EXERCISE

The nurse is developing a list of desired patient outcomes that are appropriate for the nursing diagnosis, *fluid volume deficit.* List at least six evaluative criteria that would be appropriate for this nursing diagnosis.

1.
2.
3.
4.
5.
6.

ANSWER

1. Weight stable
2. Normal skin turgor
3. Blood pressure and pulse within normal range for patient
4. Serum osmolality within normal range
5. Serum BUN, creatinine, glucose, hemoglobin, and hematocrit within acceptable ranges
6. Urine output greater than 30 mL per hour
7. Normal mental status for patient
8. Capillary refill less than 3 to 5 seconds
9. Urine specific gravity within normal range
10. Moist mucous membranes

QUESTION

What is the relationship between Beatrice's acute infection and the onset of her DKA? (short answer)

ANSWER

Development of a serious infection is a leading cause of DKA. The presence of a serious infection triggers increased secretion of stress hormones, which in turn prompt the release of an increased glucose load into the bloodstream to meet increased metabolic demands created by the infection. In the nondiabetic, increased insulin would be released to match the increased glucose load. In the patient with diabetes, however, the elevated serum glucose circulates in the absence of increased levels of insulin, creating hyperglycemia. Without adequate insulin coverage, glucose cannot meet the hypermetabolic demands of the body; subsequently, the body turns to fatty acids for energy and diabetic ketoacidosis develops. Acutely ill diabetic patients, whether type 1 or type 2, develop some degree of hyperglycemia when faced with situations that significantly stress the body. Increased insulin dosage is usually required until the stress is relieved. When working with a type 2 diabetic patient who requires temporary insulin therapy, it is important for the nurse to explain the reason for this therapy during acute illness to allay fears of worsening diabetes.

Beatrice's infection will require aggressive antibiotic therapy to destroy the infection. Until the infection is gone, her glucose levels will remain high and probably difficult to control.

Case Study Update: Seven Days Postadmission

Beatrice remains in the critical care unit. Although her DKA was resolved within the first 48 hours, her glucose levels remain elevated. An updated systematic assessment shows the following:

HEAD AND NECK. Neurologically, Beatrice is confused and drowsy, oriented to name only. A Salem sump tube is in place in her right nostril, and correct gastric placement is confirmed. Mucous membranes are pink and moist. Positive jugular vein distention (JVD) is noted at a 45-degree angle.

CHEST. *Cardiovascular status.* S1, S2, and S3 are present, with no murmurs. Rhythm is regular with a sinus tachycardia at 110 to 115 beats per minute. *T* waves are peaked on the electrocardiogram (ECG). Blood pressure is 174/92.

Respiratory status. Breath sounds are heard in all lung fields. Bases are diminished, with crackles to midfields bilaterally. Occasional nonproductive cough is noted.

ABDOMEN. A nasogastric tube is connected to intermittent low wall suction. Nasogastric drainage is dark green and negative for blood. Bowel sounds are hypoactive in all four quadrants. The abdomen is moderately distended and tight.

PELVIS AND GENITOURINARY TRACT. Urinary catheter remains in place. Urine output for the past 24 hours has been a total of 425 mL.

EXTREMITIES. Edema (4+) is noted in all extremities. The skin is dry and flaky. Pulses are difficult to palpate secondary to edema.

LEFT FOOT WOUND STATUS. The wound remains open and draining. It appears pale, with large areas of blackened tissue and patches of white. No healthy tissue is evident.

POSTERIOR. The coccyx is reddened, although the skin is still intact. With Beatrice positioned on her right side, crackles are auscultated over the posterior fields (right more than left).

OTHER. Temperature is 100°F to 102°F (37.8°C to 38.9°C). A 5-pound (2.3 kg) weight gain is noted over the past 48 hours. Beatrice continues to receive 5 percent dextrose in normal saline at 125 mL per hour. She is receiving total parenteral nutrition (TPN) at 75 mL per hour.

Current Drug Therapy

Current drug therapy includes regular and NPH Humulin insulin (SQ), gentamicin (IV), heparin (SQ), and ranitidine (IV).

QUESTION

Of the following, which assessment is most suggestive of the presence of an underlying nutritional problem?

- A. edema
- B. flaky, dry skin
- C. hypoactive bowel sounds
- D. absence of wound healing

ANSWER

The correct answer is D. Following Beatrice's wound debridement and antibiotic therapy, some degree of wound healing would be expected; however, her wound is again deteriorating according to the latest assessment data. Beatrice's ability to heal is further complicated by her long-standing diabetes, as well as possible renal failure, because both of these conditions suppress healing.

QUESTION

Besides Beatrice's prolonged hypotensive episode as a major risk factor for development of acute renal failure, which drug is particularly associated with nephrotoxicity?

- A. gentamicin
- B. insulin
- C. heparin
- D. ranitidine

ANSWER

The correct answer is A. Aminoglycosides, such as gentamicin, are nephrotoxic. Gentamicin peak and trough levels should be drawn routinely to monitor for toxic blood levels. To monitor renal function for development of nephrotoxicity, serum BUN and creatinine also are measured routinely.

Current Serum Laboratory Results
(Abnormal Values Only)

Glucose: 320 mg/dL
Albumin: 2.2 g/dL   (normal, 3.5 to 5.0 g/dL)
Transferrin: 112 mg/dL   (normal, 200 to 430 mg/dL)
White Blood Cell Count: 4,300/mL   (normal, 5,000 to 10,000/mL)

WBC Differential

Neutrophils = 75 percent   (normal, 50 to 70 percent)
Bands = 15 percent   (normal, 0 to 5 percent)
Lymphocytes = 20 percent   (normal, 25 to 35 percent)
BUN and creatinine: 80 mg/dL   (normal, 5 to 25 mg/dL) and
Creatinine 3.2 mg/dL   (normal, 0.5 to 1.5 mg/dL)

Electrolytes

Sodium (Na) = 162 mEq/L
Chloride (Cl) = 115 mEq/L
Potassium (K) = 6.0 mEq/L
Calcium (Ca) = 11.2 mEq/L

QUESTION

Which statement best reflects the reason that Beatrice's serum creatinine is elevated?

- A. controlled diabetes causes increased breakdown of protein
- B. malnutrition causes increased excretion of creatinine
- C. gluconeogenesis increases the amount of serum creatinine
- D. nephrons are unable to cleanse the waste products from the blood

ANSWER

The correct answer is D. Creatinine is a waste product of muscle metabolism. When the kidneys go into failure, they can no longer perform their normal functions, and creatinine remains in the blood rather than being excreted. While Beatrice is in acute renal failure, you would anticipate that although her serum creatinine and BUN increase, creatinine and urea nitrogen clearance in the urine would decrease. Keep in mind that in acute renal failure, the BUN elevates more rapidly than creatinine. Calculating a BUN-to-creatinine ratio can be helpful in determining whether a person is likely in acute renal failure (ARF). A BUN-to-creatinine ratio of greater than 20:1 is considered suspicious for ARF. Beatrice's ratio is 25:1.

QUESTION

What type of acute renal failure is Beatrice most likely experiencing? (short answer)

ANSWER

Acute tubular necrosis (ATN). Acute tubular necrosis is the most common interstitial form of acute renal failure and is usually of prerenal origin (secondary to a prolonged hypotensive/hyperfusion episode). Her clinical presentation is consistent with development of ATN.

QUESTION

Beatrice has become drowsy and confused. Reexamine her updated data. What is probably the source of her altered level of consciousness? (short answer)

ANSWER

Elevated BUN and creatinine. Elevated levels of nitrogenous waste products readily cross the blood–brain barrier and are toxic to the brain cells. Their buildup in the brain can result in uremic encephalopathy. Characteristics of uremic encephalopathy include twitching, asterixis, agitation, seizures, confusion, stupor, coma, and others. Although Beatrice has not had a liver profile drawn, we cannot discount the possibility that in addition to compromising her kidneys, her hypotension episode may have also caused liver damage. Evaluating her liver enzymes and serum ammonia should be done. Ammonia is toxic to the brain and can cause hepatic encephalopathy, which clinically presents with some of the same features as uremic encephalopathy.

QUESTION

Beatrice's leukopenia is most likely caused by which combination of physiologic insults?

- **A.** hyperglycemic crisis and hypotension
- **B.** malnutrition and overwhelming infection
- **C.** acute renal failure and hyperglycemia
- **D.** hypotension and malnutrition

ANSWER

The correct answer is B. Beatrice's malnutrition is a major factor in failure of the immune system. This has been complicated by a severe infection of prolonged duration that may well have exhausted available neutrophils and lymphocytes.

QUESTION

A *disadvantage* of using serum albumin as an indicator of malnutrition is that it

- **A.** reflects muscle protein
- **B.** has a short half-life
- **C.** reflects plasma protein
- **D.** has a long half-life

ANSWER

The correct answer is D. Although considered a good indicator of nutritional status, the long half-life of serum albumin make the laboratory values misleading as to current status. Serum prealbumin, another indicator, is better at reflecting current status because of its short half-life.

Beatrice's malnourished state is severely hindering her recovery. Goals for managing this problem include

1. Halt the state of catabolism
2. Regain positive nitrogen balance
3. Prevent and treat complications

Collaborative Interventions

1. **Laboratory testing.** High-acuity patients need to have blood drawn for intermittent laboratory tests that measure various aspects of nutritional status. These tests include CBC with differential, serum albumin (and/or transferrin), prealbumin, and BUN and creatinine. Urine clearance testing of urea and creatinine may be ordered. Clearance testing helps determine the extent of damage to the nephrons, the effectiveness of renal disease treatment, and the baseline function of the kidneys before initiating treatment.

2. **Dietary orders.** Beatrice's deteriorating nutritional status requires consultation with the nutritional support team, as well as the medical team. Although total parenteral nutrition may be adequate for a brief period, it does not meet all of the nutritional needs of a patient for an extended period. The more physiologically compromised the patient is, the more complex the nutritional needs become. It is essential that Beatrice's nutritional needs be met to facilitate healing and to build up her immune system, which is dangerously compromised. Beatrice's acute renal failure complicates the team's ability to supply her with the protein necessary for regaining immunocompetence and healing. As

discussed in the acute renal dysfunction module, protein breaks down into nitrogenous wastes, which cannot be eliminated from the body when the kidneys are not functioning adequately.

3. **Nutritional supplementation.** Various supplements consisting of vitamins and minerals may be ordered to meet Beatrice's current nutritional needs, which are important in healing and blood cell formation. These supplements may include vitamins, iron, zinc, and folic acid. Nutritional support is presented in depth in Module 23, "Metabolic Responses to Stress."

Independent Nursing Interventions

Imbalanced nutrition: less than body requirements is the primary nursing diagnosis that is included on Beatrice's plan of care to address her state of malnutrition. Other significant nursing diagnoses pertinent to care of the malnourished patient include the following.

- Risk for infection
- Activity intolerance
- Self-care deficit
- Pain
- PC: Electrolyte imbalance or *altered fluid and electrolyte balance*

Case Update

Though her DKA has been resolved, Beatrice's general condition has not significantly improved over the past week. Her renal function has stabilized over the past 24 hours, however, with her more recent BUN being 69 mg/dL and a creatinine of 3.3 mg/dL. Today, the nurse has noted progressive mental changes in Beatrice. The latest neurologic assessment resulted in the following data:

> Over the past 24 hours, her Glasgow Coma Scale has dropped from 15 to 11. She is disoriented to place and time, and her speech pattern has become slurred and confused. She is drowsy and lethargic, requiring mild shaking before she opens her eyes. She has been vomiting. Her temperature is 100°F (37.8°C), blood pressure is 164/95 mm Hg, pulse is 106 beats per minute, and respirations are rapid at 30 breaths per minute; light crackles are auscultated in her bilateral lung bases. Her skin is diaphoretic and hand tremors are noted.

EXERCISE

Based on the available data, what problems could Beatrice be developing? List at least three potential problems.

1.
2.
3.

ANSWER

Beatrice's current assessment could have several possible sources. Based on her history of diabetes, vital signs, changes in clinical presentation, and recent development of acute renal failure, potential sources of her new signs and symptoms include hypoglycemia, a gas exchange problem, electrolyte imbalances, worsening of her acute renal failure with developing uremic encephalopathy, or she possibly could be developing hepatic encephalopathy. To make matters more difficult, her recent changes may be a combination of problems as a result of multiple organ dysfunction.

QUESTION

Is there sufficient data to develop nursing diagnoses? If YES, list the diagnoses. If NO, what further data do you need to obtain to write a nursing diagnosis (or diagnoses)?

ANSWER

No. Through clustering existing data, it has been hypothesized that Beatrice may be having a problem with hypoglycemia, gas exchange, electrolyte imbalances, uremic encephalopathy, or hepatic encephalopathy (all physiologic complications). Currently, however, there is insufficient data to write a complete diagnostic statement because the potential origins of the problem have not been investigated. Because physiologic complications are collaborative problems that require laboratory or other tests to diagnose, it is most expedient for the nurse to contact the physician to discuss the status change and receive orders. Prior to contacting the physician, however, the nurse may want to obtain additional critical data that will help differentiate the diagnosis, including a fingerstick glucose level, Spo_2 by pulse oximetry, and rapid focused assessment of nailbeds and mucous membranes—the fingerstick glucose level and Spo_2 can be obtained rapidly, cheaply, and often as independent nursing functions.

The change in Beatrice's status is communicated to the physician, who orders diagnostic laboratory tests, including arterial blood gas, serum glucose, BUN and creatinine, serum electrolytes, and liver function profile (LFP). The laboratory test results are as follows:

ABGs

pH:	7.48
Pco_2:	32 mm Hg
Po_2:	88 mm Hg
HCO_3:	31 mEq/L
Sao_2:	97 percent
Serum Glucose:	65 mg/dL

Serum Electrolytes

Sodium (Na) = 130 mEq/L
Potassium (K) = 5.2 mEq/L

Renal Function Profile

BUN = 68 mg/dL
Creatinine = 3.2 mg/dL

Liver Function Profile (LFP)

ALT = 1,200 U/mL	(normal, 5 to 35 U/mL)
AST = 1,500 U/L	(normal, 0 to 35 U/L)
ALP (alk phos) = 120 U/L	(normal, 20 to 90 U/L)

QUESTION

Based on the laboratory results, which hypotheses can be discarded? Circle your decision.

Hypoglycemia	Discard/Do not discard
Gas exchange problem	Discard/Do not discard
Electrolyte imbalances	Discard/Do not discard
Renal encephalopathy	Discard/Do not discard
Hepatic encephalopathy	Discard/Do not discard

ANSWER

Based on the available data, the ABGs are not sufficiently abnormal to cause Beatrice's new clinical signs and symptoms—discard gas exchange. Her renal function labs, while abnormal, continue to be stable and would probably not account for the acute status change—discard renal encephalopathy as the most probable source of the change in status. Her electrolyte imbalances are not consistent with her acute status changes—discard. Her serum glucose as well as some of her acute changes are consistent with hypoglycemia—do not discard. Her clinical presentation is suspicious of hepatic encephalopathy and her LFP is consistent with liver dysfunction—do not discard. Her hypoglycemia problem may be caused by the hepatic dysfunction.

Based on Beatrice's clinical manifestations and current laboratory data, the physician makes a tentative diagnosis of acute hepatic failure. Acute hepatic dysfunction is presented in Module 31.

Since Beatrice has had a series of nutrition/metabolic problems, her care plan already contains most of the nursing diagnoses associated with hepatic dysfunction. The nurse can anticipate adding the following nursing diagnoses to Beatrice's plan of care:

- Altered respiratory function
- Nausea
- Acute Pain: upper abdominal
- PC: Bleeding

EXERCISE

List three desired outcomes that would be appropriate for the following collaborative problem: PC: Bleeding

1.
2.
3.

ANSWER

PC: Bleeding
1. Blood pressure and pulse within normal range
2. No blood in urine, stool, or vomitus
3. No purpura, petechiae, ecchymoses of skin or mucous membranes
4. Improved or stable hemoglobin and hematocrit
5. Stable abdominal girth

The nurse is developing nursing interventions that will help protect Beatrice from developing bleeding problems. Ulrich and Canale (2001) suggest the following interventions:

1. Injection and venous access sites: Use small-gauge needles; apply prolonged, gentle pressure to site after removal of needle/catheter
2. Blood pressures: Avoid overinflation of cuff and inflate cuff only as needed
3. Place pads on side rails if restless or confused
4. Avoid trauma to gums: No stiff toothbrush or floss
5. Avoid rectal trauma (no rectal temps, no rectal tubes, no straining during bowel movement)
6. As ordered, administer and monitor for therapeutic effects of
   A. Vitamin K
   B. Fresh plasma (or blood)
   C. Platelets

7. If bleeding occurs, take immediate steps to control it:
   A. Apply firm pressure over site, when appropriate
   B. For epistaxis:
      1. Position in high-Fowler's position
      2. Apply pressure, apply ice pack
   C. For gastric or esophageal bleeding:
      1. Position on side
      2. Administer vasopressin, as ordered
      3. Assist with esophageal-gastric balloon insertion, as ordered
      4. Administer vitamin K and blood products, as ordered
   D. Monitor for signs and symptoms of hypovolemic shock
   E. Provide patient and family with emotional support

Evaluation and Revision of the Plan of Care

Evaluation of the effectiveness of Beatrice's plan of care is based on how well she meets the desired outcomes within each nursing diagnosis. The care plan is a working document subject to frequent changes. Interventions that have not been effective must be scrutinized to pinpoint why they are ineffective. Revision of the plan is then made, removing ineffective actions and adding alternative ones.

Beatrice's problems are complex and require aggressive interventions, both collaborative and independent, if she is to regain her prehospitalization state of health.

Ultimately, following failure of her left heel wound to heal and subsequent development of sepsis, Beatrice required amputation of her left leg to below the knee. On removal of this major physiologic stressor, she rapidly recovered and was eventually able to be discharged home.

In summary, this module has provided the learner with the opportunity to apply the concepts learned in the metabolic section of the book to a complex patient situation. In addition, the case study has attempted to show how one type of metabolic disorder can precipitate an imbalance in other body systems. This case study presented a sequence of events that in reality does occur, profoundly affecting the patient's prognosis. Although each disorder had a different etiology, they shared many of the same nursing diagnoses.

REFERENCES

Carpenito-Moyet, L. J. (2004). *Handbook of nursing diagnosis* (10th ed.). Philadelphia: Lippincott Williams & Wilkins.

Kee, J. L. (2002). *Laboratory and diagnostic tests with nursing implications* (6th ed.). Upper Saddle River, NJ: Prentice Hall.

Ulrich, S. P., & Canale, S. W. (2001). *Medical–surgical nursing care planning guides* (5th ed.). Philadelphia: W. B. Saunders.

PART

7

Gastrointestinal

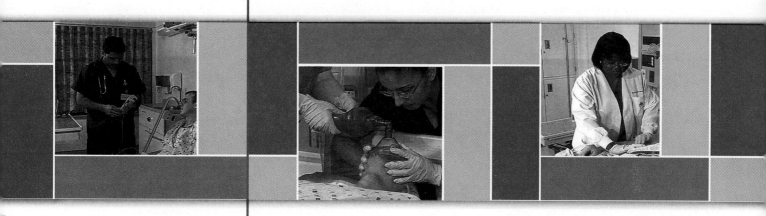

MODULE 30 Acute Gastrointestinal Dysfunction

MODULE 31 Acute Hepatic Dysfunction

MODULE 32 Acute Pancreatic Dysfunction

MODULE 33 Nursing Care of the Patient with Altered Gastrointestinal Function

30 Acute Gastrointestinal Dysfunction

Melanie Hardin–Pierce

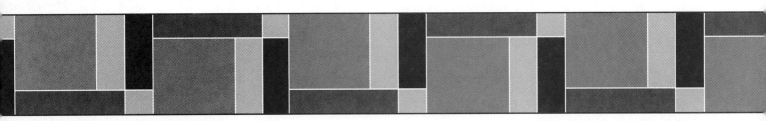

OBJECTIVES   Following completion of this module, the learner will be able to

1. Identify the anatomic structures of the GI tract.
2. Discuss the functions of the GI tract.
3. Discuss factors influencing circulation to the GI tract.
4. Describe the neurologic control of the GI tract.
5. Describe the mechanisms that exist to protect the integrity of the GI tract.
6. Describe the evaluation of GI function using laboratory and diagnostic tests.
7. Describe the incidence and clinical manifestations associated with acute GI bleeding.
8. Describe the etiology and pathophysiology of acute upper GI bleeding.
9. Describe the etiology and pathophysiology of acute lower GI bleeding.
10. Describe an overview of the management of acute GI bleeding.
11. Describe the etiology, pathophysiology, and management of acute intestinal obstruction and paralytic ileus.
12. Describe the nursing diagnosis and management of acute GI bleeding and bowel obstruction.

This self-study module presents the physiologic and pathophysiologic processes involved in acute gastrointestinal (GI) dysfunction and management of the patient with acute GI bleeding, problems in motility, and intestinal ischemia. The module is composed of 11 sections. Section One presents an overview of the anatomy and physiology of the GI system, including organs and functions. Section Two explains the GI blood supply and nervous system innervation. Section Three explains the defense mechanisms of the GI tract, including lymphatic and immune function. Section Four describes the various laboratory and diagnostic tests used to evaluate GI function. Section Five describes the incidence and clinical manifestations of acute GI bleeding. Section Six describes the etiology and pathophysiology of acute upper GI bleeding. Section Seven describes the etiology and pathophysiology of acute lower GI

bleeding. Section Eight provides an overview of the collaborative management of acute GI bleeding including pharmacotherapy and therapeutic and surgical interventions. Section Nine explains the etiology, pathophysiology, and management of acute intestinal obstruction and paralytic ileus. Section Ten introduces the concept of intra-abdominal hypertension and abdominal compartment syndrome. Finally, Section Eleven describes the nursing diagnosis and management of acute GI bleeding and paralytic ileus. Each section includes a set of review questions to help the learner evaluate her or his understanding of the section's content before moving on to the next section. All Section Reviews and the module Pretest and Posttest include answers. It is suggested that the learner review those concepts answered incorrectly in the review questions before proceeding to the next section.

 ## PRETEST

1. The primary function of the GI tract is to
   A. metabolize toxic agents
   B. produce clotting factors
   C. provide nutrients needed for metabolism
   D. eliminate carbon dioxide

2. The outermost layer of the GI tract is the
   A. peritoneum
   B. submucosa
   C. mucosa
   D. serosa

3. Blood flow through the gut, spleen, pancreas, and liver comprise the
   A. portal circulation
   B. mesenteric circulation
   C. splanchnic circulation
   D. extrinsic circulation

4. The arterial blood supply to the mesentery and intestines is known as the _____ circulation.
   A. mesenteric
   B. portocaval
   C. visceral
   D. aortic

5. Gut-associated lymphoid tissue (GALT) includes
   A. thyroid, duodenum, gastric mucosa
   B. tonsils, appendix, Peyer's patches
   C. adrenal glands, cecum, stomach
   D. goblet cells, salivary glands, parietal cells

6. The main aerobic bacteria within the GI tract is
   A. *Escherichia coli*
   B. *Bacteroides fragilis*
   C. *Staphylococcus aureus*
   D. beta-hemolytic *streptococcus*

7. Which laboratory measures are important in evaluating the need for clotting factor replacement?
   A. hemoglobin and hematocrit
   B. platelet count and hematocrit
   C. thrombin time and mean corpuscular volume
   D. prothrombin time and partial thromboplastin time

8. Elevations in the white blood cell (WBC) count suggests a(n)
   A. inflammatory or infectious process
   B. immunocompromised host
   C. normal nonimmunologic gut defense response
   D. hemoconcentration as a result of fluid volume deficit

9. The appearance of melena is described as
   A. bright red in color from a lower GI tract source
   B. black and tarry in color from an upper GI source
   C. light brown in color from an upper GI source
   D. "coffee ground" in appearance from the colon

10. A patient passes a large amount of loose, maroon-colored stool. When documenting this event, the correct term that applies to this description is
    A. melena
    B. diarrhea
    C. hematochezia
    D. hematemesis

11. Infections associated with peptic ulcer disease include
    A. *Escherichia coli* infection
    B. *Helicobacter pylori*
    C. beta-hemolytic *streptococcus*
    D. *Staphylococcus aureus*

12. Drugs known to disrupt the mucosal barrier are
    A. nonsteroidal anti-inflammatory drugs (NSAIDs)
    B. angiotensin-converting enzyme (ACE) inhibitors

    C. cephalosporins
    D. histamine receptor antagonists

13. The elderly are at increased risk of developing ischemic bowel complications. What is another risk factor for the development of bowel ischemia in this population?
    A. atrial fibrillation
    B. hypertension
    C. immobility
    D. obesity

14. Twenty-five percent of all bleeding from ischemic bowel disease is associated with
    A. recreational drug use
    B. severe malnutrition
    C. anticoagulant use
    D. traumatic injury

15. A good measure of perfusion for the nurse to monitor is
    A. arterial blood gas (ABG)
    B. complete blood count (CBC)
    C. urine output
    D. skin temperature

16. Complications of vasopressin include
    A. hypoglycemia
    B. hypernatremia
    C. decreased coronary blood flow
    D. increased portal pressures

17. Acute paralytic ileus (adynamic ileus) is associated with
    A. adhesions following abdominal surgery
    B. a loss of intestinal peristalsis
    C. volvulus of the intestines
    D. hyperperistalsis of the intestines

18. Medications that are known to contribute to the development of acute paralytic ileus include
    A. ACE inhibitors
    B. aminoglycosides
    C. opioids
    D. beta blockers

19. The _____ system inhibits GI motility.
    A. sympathetic
    B. parasympathetic
    C. intrinsic
    D. enteric

20. Colonoscopy allows inspection of the
    A. duodenal bulb
    B. large intestine
    C. gastric mucosa
    D. small intestine

21. Prophylactic measures to prevent the development of peptic ulcers in acutely ill patients include
    A. early enteral feeding and histamine receptor antagonists
    B. surgical resection of all affected mucosa and antacids
    C. total parenteral nutrition and proton pump inhibitors
    D. sclerotherapy and sucralfate

22. Impaired gut perfusion is a risk factor in which of the following conditions?
    A. hypernatremia
    B. diabetes mellitus
    C. hypertension
    D. hypotension

GLOSSARY

abdominal compartment syndrome (ACS)   Occurs when the intra-abdominal pressure increases to a point where vascular tissue is compromised with subsequent loss of tissue viability and function.

brush border   Consists of villi and microvilli; necessary for absorption to take place.

cardiac glands   Gastric glands that secrete mucous.

chief cells   A fundic gland that secretes pepsinogen for protein digestion.

cholecystokinin (CCK)   Hormone that stimulates pancreatic enzymes, increases contractility of the gallbladder, and inhibits gastric motility.

chyme   A mixture of partly digested food and digestive secretions within the stomach and small intestine.

fundic glands   Gastric glands that consist of chief and parietal cells.

gastric inhibitory peptide (GIP)   Hormone that helps digest carbohydrates and fats.

gastric tonometry   A technique to assess gut perfusion by using a gastric balloon to measure the mucosal CO_2 level.

gastrin   A hormonal regulator produced by cells located in the pyloric region of the stomach; stimulates gastric glands to produce hydrochloric acid and pepsinogen.

gut   Refers to the bowel or intestine.

hematemesis   Vomiting of bright red blood or blood that resembles "coffee grounds."

hematochezia   Bright red blood or maroon stool secondary to bleeding.

hydrochloric acid   Secreted by the parietal cells to lower gastrointestinal pH and to regulate bacterial growth.

intestinal strangulation   Intestine twists to such an extent that circulation to the twisted area is impaired.

intrinsic factor   Secreted by the parietal cells; necessary for vitamin B_{12} absorption.

melena   Black, tarry, foul-smelling stools containing blood.

mesenteric circulation   Blood flow to the intestines.

mesentery   Part of the peritoneum that suspends the small intestine to the abdominal wall.

microvilli   Fingerlike projections covering the villi.

mucosa   Innermost layer of the GI wall.

muscularis   Muscular layer of the GI wall.

parietal cells   A fundic gland that secretes hydrochloric acid for pH regulation and intrinsic factor for vitamin B_{12} absorption.

pepsinogen   An enzyme secreted by chief cells; converts to its active form of pepsin for protein digestion.

peritoneum   Serous membrane that lines the abdominal cavity and abdominal organs.

Peyer's patches   Lymph tissue on the outer wall of the intestine.

secretin   Hormone that stimulates release of pancreatic bicarbonate and water.

serosa   Outermost layer of the GI wall.

severe abdominal compartment syndrome   IAP greater than 25 mm Hg.

splanchnic circulation   Blood flow through the gut, spleen, pancreas, and liver.

submucosa   Layer of the GI wall that contains blood and lymphatic vessels.

villi   Fingerlike projections covering intestinal folds.

ABBREVIATIONS

ACS	Abdominal compartment syndrome
AVM	Arteriovenous malformation
BUN	Blood urea nitrogen
CO	Cardiac output
CO_2	Carbon dioxide
EGD	Esophagogastroduodenoscopy
GALT	Gut-associated lymphoid tissue
GI	Gastrointestinal
IAH	Intra-abdominal hypertension
IAP	Intra-abdominal pressure
ICU	Intensive care unit
NSAIDs	Nonsteroidal anti-inflammatory drugs
$Prco_2$	Partial pressure of carbon dioxide, reflects CO_2 level in the stomach mucosa
$Prco_2$–$Paco_2$ Gap	The difference between the gastric and arterial carbon dioxide levels
PUD	Peptic ulcer disease

SECTION ONE: Anatomy and Physiology of the Gastrointestinal Tract

At the completion of this section, the learner will be able to identify the anatomic structures and functions of the gastrointestinal (GI) tract.

The primary function of the GI system is to provide the necessary nutrients needed by cells to sustain function and growth. The GI tract provides the mechanisms for the digestion and absorption of those nutrients through the processes of ingestion, digestion, and absorption. The anatomic structures of the GI tract are the mouth, pharynx, and esophagus in the upper GI tract, and the stomach and small and large intestines in the lower GI tract (Fig. 30–1).

Gastrointestinal Wall

The gastrointestinal wall is comprised of four major layers. These layers, from the inside out, are the mucosa, submucosa, muscularis, and serosa (Fig. 30–2). The outermost layer is called the **serosa.** The serosa is derived from the visceral peritoneum, as it adheres to the visceral organs of the abdomen. The serosa secretes mucus, which prevents friction between the abdominal organs. The **muscularis** is a muscular layer, providing the rhythmic contraction needed to mechanically break down food, mix it with enzymes, and propel it through the GI tract. The next layer, the **submucosa,** contains loose, connective tissue and elastic fibers, blood vessels, and lymphatic vessels. The submucosa also contains one plexus of the enteric nervous system (Meissner's nerve plexus), a part of the

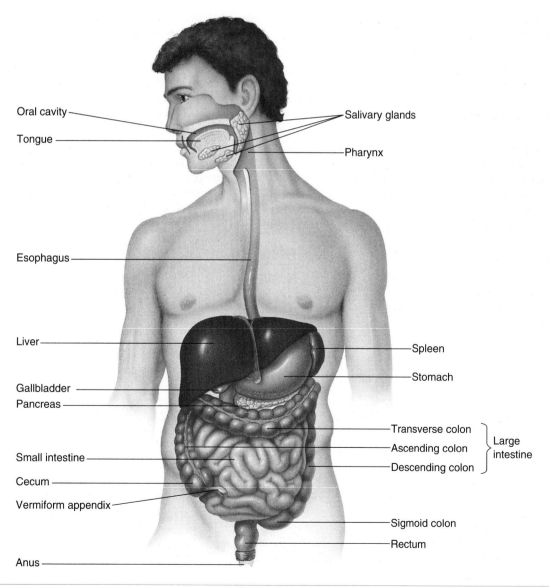

Figure 30–1 ■ The gastrointestinal tract.

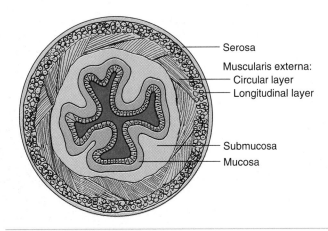

Serosa

Muscularis externa:
Circular layer
Longitudinal layer

Submucosa
Mucosa

Figure 30–2 ■ Cross-section of the gut wall.

autonomic nervous system (Andreoli et al., 2000; Lingappa, 2003; Tucker, 2000).

The **mucosa,** the innermost layer, absorbs both nutrients and fluids and receives the majority of the blood supply. The mucosa contains specialized cells throughout the GI tract whose function varies depending on the anatomic location. These cells mostly secrete mucus or digestive enzymes to aid in the passage or digestion of food (Gray, 1995; Lingappa, 2003). In critical illness, the integrity of the mucosa can break down as a result of trauma, hypoperfusion, stress, medications, or surgery. The result of impaired mucosal integrity can be inflammation, bleeding, and infection.

The **peritoneum,** the largest serous membrane in the body, consists of a visceral and a parietal layer. The parietal peritoneum lines the wall of the abdominal cavity. The visceral peritoneum covers most of the abdominal organs and constitutes their serosa. The peritoneum contains large folds that weave in and out between the organs. These folds function to bind the organs to each other and contain the blood vessels, lymph tissue, and the nerves that supply the abdominal organs. The potential space between the visceral and parietal layers of the peritoneum is called the *peritoneal space.* Inflammation of the peritoneum is called *peritonitis.* One of the most important functions of the peritoneum is to prevent friction between contiguous organs.

The **mesentery** is the large outward fold of peritoneum that suspends the small intestine to the abdominal wall. It functions to bind the small intestine to the abdominal wall and facilitates intestinal motility while supporting blood vessels, nerves, and lymphatics. Impaired blood flow through the mesentery can result in intestinal ischemia. This can occur as a result of shock in critically ill patients (Bongard, 2002; Markey, 1999).

Gastric Enzymes

The primary function of the GI tract is digestion of food and absorption of nutrients. The cardiac (proximal) and pyloric (distal) sphincters of the stomach control the rate of food passage through the GI tract. Secretion of gastric enzymes is necessary

for digestion. Enzymes are secreted by the cardiac and fundic glands, which are located in the stomach. The **cardiac glands** secrete mucus, which acts as a lubricant and mucosal barrier from acids. The **fundic glands** consist of the chief cells and the parietal cells. The **chief cells** secrete **pepsinogen,** which converts to pepsin (its active form) in an acid environment. Pepsin is necessary for protein digestion. **Parietal cells** secrete (1) **hydrochloric acid,** which lowers pH and kills bacteria, and (2) **intrinsic factor,** which is necessary for vitamin B_{12} absorption. **Gastrin,** a hormonal regulator produced by cells located in the pyloric region of the stomach, stimulates the gastric glands to produce the hydrochloric acid and pepsinogen (Del Valle, 2001; Lingappa, 2003; Tucker, 2000).

Small Intestine

The small intestine extends from the pylorus to the ileocecal valve and consists of the duodenum, the jejunum, and the ileum (see Fig. 30–1). Its primary function is absorption of nutrients and water. The mucosa and submucosal layers of the small intestine are arranged in folds, which actually project out into the lumen of the intestine. These folds function to slow the passage of **chyme** through the small intestine in order to allow more time for digestion and absorption to occur. Fingerlike projections covering the intestinal folds are called **villi.** Each individual villus is covered with tiny absorptive fingerlike projections called **microvilli.** The villi and the microvilli collectively make up the **brush border** of the small intestine. The folds, villi, and microvilli greatly increase the absorptive surface of the small intestine. The villi contain two cell types: (1) goblet cells, which produce mucus, and (2) absorptive cells (microvilli), which are responsible for absorption of nutrients. The villi also produce digestive enzymes along the brush border, which complete the process of digestion as absorption takes place (Fig. 30–3). Diseases of the small intestine that cause atrophy and flattening of the brush border greatly reduce the surface area for absorption, resulting in malabsorption (Del Valle, 2001; Lingappa, 2003; Tucker, 2000).

The small intestine secretes hormones that have both stimulatory and inhibitory effects necessary in the regulation of intestinal digestion. Recall that the gastric pH is acidic. When acidic chyme comes into contact with the duodenal mucosa, hormones are secreted that regulate the digestive process. These hormones include cholecystokinin, secretin, and gastric inhibitory peptide. **Cholecystokinin (CCK)** is secreted in response to the presence of fat, protein, and an acidic pH. The role of cholecystokinin is to (1) stimulate the release of pancreatic digestive enzymes necessary for the digestion of protein and fat, (2) increase the contractility of the gallbladder so that bile is released into the duodenum to aid in the absorption of fats, and (3) inhibit gastric motility in order to slow things down a little so that digestion and absorption can take place. Gastric acid in contact with the intestinal mucosa causes the release of another hormone, secretin. **Secretin** stimulates the release of pancreatic

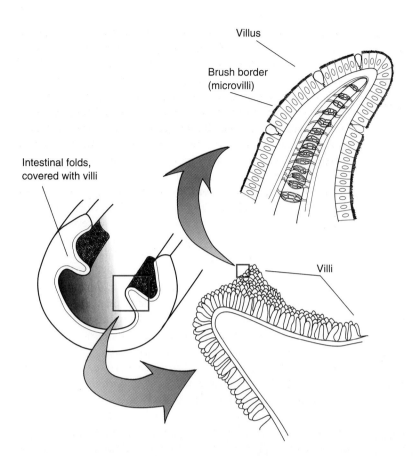

Villus

Brush border
(microvilli)

Intestinal folds,
covered with villi

Villi

Figure 30–3 ■ Cross-section of small intestine. This cross-section of the intestinal wall shows an intestinal fold covered with villi from three different magnifications.

bicarbonate and water ("pancreatic juice"). Pancreatic juice is alkaline and, therefore, functions to increase the pH of the chyme within the duodenum. Pancreatic digestive enzymes are active only in an alkaline environment. **Gastric inhibitory peptide (GIP)** is another hormone secreted by the small intestine to facilitate the digestion of carbohydrates and fats. GIP is secreted in response to the presence of carbohydrates and fats within the small intestine. GIP inhibits motility and the secretion of gastric acid. Furthermore, GIP stimulates insulin secretion. The inhibition of gastric acid is to maintain a basic pH environment necessary for the pancreatic proteolytic enzymes to metabolize proteins and fats. The inhibition of gastric motility aids absorption by decreasing transit time (Lingappa, 2003; Tucker, 2000). Table 30–1 provides a summary of intestinal hormones.

Large Intestine

The large intestine is a hollow, muscular tube, extending from the terminal ileum at the ileocecal valve to the anus (approximately 5 feet [15.2 m] in length). The main functions of the large intestine are the completion of water and nutrient absorption, the manufacture of certain vitamins, the formation of feces, and the expulsion of feces from the body. The large intestine is divided into the cecum, colon, and rectum (see Fig. 30–1). The cecum lies below the ileocecal valve, which controls the flow of chyme from the ileum of the small intestine into the cecum. This

TABLE 30–1   Intestinal Hormones

HORMONE	ACTION
Secretin—secreted in response to acidic chyme and alcohol entering the duodenum	Stimulates release of pancreatic bicarbonate and water Stimulates release of bile Potentiates the action of CCK
Cholecystokinin (CCK)—secreted in response to the presence of fat, protein, and acidic chyme	Stimulates release of pancreatic digestive enzymes Increases contractility of gallbladder Inhibits gastric motility
Gastric inhibitory peptide (GIP)— secreted in response to carbohydrates and fat	Inhibits gastric acid secretion and motility Stimulates insulin secretion

From: Lindseth, G. L. (2003). Disorders of the small intestine . In S. L. Price & L. M. Wilson (Eds.). Pathophysiology: Clinical concepts of disease processes. *(6th ed., p.328). St. Louis: C.V. Mosby.*

valve also prevents backflow of fecal material from the large intestine into the small intestine. The opposite end of the cecum joins with the colon. The colon is divided into four portions: ascending, transverse, descending, and sigmoid. The absorption of water and electrolytes is largely completed in the ascending colon. In fact, the colon absorbs approximately 1,000 mL per day of water and electrolytes (Lingappa, 2003). The last portion of the large intestine is the rectum. The rectum extends from the sigmoid colon to the anus, which is the opening to the outside of the body. The internal and external muscles regulate the anal sphincter.

The wall of the large intestine differs from the wall of the small intestines. The mucosal layer of the large intestine is thicker and contains no villi or folds. The mucosa of the large intestine contains more mucus-producing goblet cells than does the mucosa of the small intestine. The mucus facilitates the passage of fecal contents through the colon by lubricating and protecting the mucosa (Guyton, 2000).

The digestion that does occur in the large intestine results from bacterial rather than enzymatic action. The normal flora bacteria that reside within the large intestine break down dietary cellulose and synthesize folic acid, vitamin K, riboflavin, and nicotinic acid.

The movements of the large intestine are called haustral churning. These movements are slow and cause the intestinal contents to move back and forth in a kneading action, thus allowing time for absorption to occur. As the rectal wall becomes full of stool and distends, the defecation reflex is initiated.

In summary, the GI tract, through the processes of ingestion, digestion and absorption, provides the body with the nutrients required for function and growth. The gastrointestinal wall is composed of the mucosa, submucosa, muscularis, and serosa; each plays a crucial role in digestive and absorptive processes. The mucosa contains the majority of the GI blood supply and is in charge of absorption of nutrients and fluids. It also contains special cells that secrete mucus and digestive enzymes. The submucosa provides structure to the GI tract and contains blood and lymphatic vessels as well as the Meissner's nerve plexus. The muscularis layer, composed of muscle, mechanically breaks down food and moves food through the GI tract. Finally, the serosa has a protective function, decreasing friction between the abdominal organs through secretion of mucus. The stomach acts as a holding and processing tank for ingested food and fluid. The stomach produces several important gastric enzymes. Gastric enzymes, which are secreted by the chief and parietal cells, are necessary for digestion. The chief cells secrete pepsinogen, which converts to pepsin to digest proteins. The parietal cells secrete hydrochloric acid (which reduces pH and destroys bacteria) and intrinsic factor (required for vitamin B_{12} absorption). Gastrin stimulates production of hydrochloric acid and pepsinogen. The small intestine consists of the duodenum, the jejunum, and the ileum. Its major functions are nutrient and water absorption. The large intestine is responsible for final water and nutrient absorption, vitamin formation, and formation/excretion of feces.

SECTION ONE REVIEW

1. The innermost layer of the GI tract which is responsible for secretion of mucus and enzymes is the
   A. submucosa
   B. muscularis
   C. mucosa
   D. mesentery
2. The _____ line(s) the wall of the abdominal cavity.
   A. peritoneum
   B. mucosa
   C. microvilli
   D. brush border
3. Parietal cells secrete
   A. gastrin
   B. pepsinogen
   C. hydrochloric acid
   D. mucus
4. CCK is secreted in response to
   A. fats, acidic pH, and protein
   B. alkaline pH, secretin, and protein
   C. fats, carbohydrates, and alkaline pH
   D. acidic pH, secretin, and carbohydrates
5. Absorption of water and electrolytes takes place in the
   A. transverse colon
   B. descending colon
   C. sigmoid colon
   D. ascending colon

Answers: 1. C, 2. A, 3. C, 4. A, 5. D

SECTION TWO: Blood Supply and Nervous System Innervation of the GI Tract

At the completion of this section, the learner will be able to discuss factors influencing circulation to the GI tract and describe the neurologic control of the GI tract.

The GI system receives about one fourth of the resting cardiac output, more than any other organ system (Podolsky & Isselbacher, 2001). The organs of the abdomen are known as *viscera*. The term *splanchnic* refers to the viscera. The combination of the portal and mesenteric circulatory systems is called the **splanchnic circulation.** The splanchnic circulatory system includes blood flow through the **gut,** spleen, pancreas, and liver (Guyton, 2000) (Fig. 30–4).

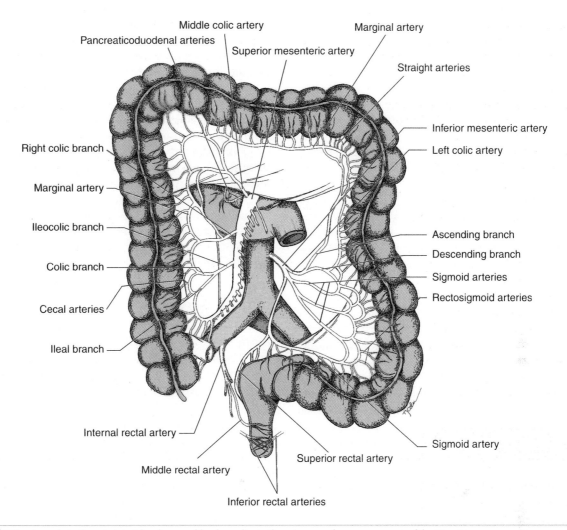

Figure 30–4 ■ Blood supply to the gut. Arterial and venous blood supplies to the primary and accessory organs of the GI system.

Arterial Blood Supply to the Intestines

The arterial blood supply to the mesentery and the intestines is called the **mesenteric circulation,** and it is a part of the extensive splanchnic circulation. The mesenteric circulation begins at the aorta, flowing through the aortic arch to the celiac artery and the superior and inferior mesenteric arteries. Arteries that branch off of the larger celiac artery supply blood to the stomach, esophagus, duodenum, gallbladder, pancreas, and spleen. The superior mesenteric artery supplies arterial blood to the small intestine, the ascending colon, and part of the transverse colon. The inferior mesenteric artery supplies the remainder of the transverse colon, the descending colon, sigmoid colon, and the rectum (Guyton, 2000; Tucker, 2000; Lingappa, 2003). Table 30–2 summarizes the arterial blood supply to the gut via the branches of the celiac artery and the superior and inferior mesenterics.

TABLE 30–2   Arterial Blood Supply

ARTERY (BRANCH OF CELIAC)	AREA SUPPLIED WITH BLOOD
Left gastric	Stomach and esophagus
Hepatic to right gastric	Stomach
Gastroduodenal	Duodenum, gallbladder, stomach
Cystic	Gallbladder
Splenic	Stomach, spleen, pancreas
Superior mesenteric	Ascending colon, cecum, ileum, jejunum, transverse colon
Inferior mesenteric	Rectum, sigmoid colon, transverse colon

From Krumberger, J. M. (1998). Gastrointestinal clinical physiology. In M.R. Kinney, S. B. Dunbar, J. A. Brooks–Brunn, N. Molter, & J. M. Vitello–Cicciu (Eds.), AACN's clinical reference for critical care nursing. (4th ed., p. 328) St. Louis: C. V. Mosby; Lindseth, G. L. (2003). Disorders of the stomach and duodenum. In S. L. Price & L. M. Wilson (Eds.). Pathophysiology: Clinical concepts of disease processes, *(6th ed., p. 985) St. Louis: C. V. Mosby.*

TABLE 30–3 Portal Vein Branches and their Drainage Sites

PORTAL VEIN BRANCH	DRAINAGE SITE
Gastric	Esophagus, stomach
Splenic	Duodenum, esophagus, gallbladder, stomach, pancreas
Superior mesenteric	Ascending and transverse colon, small intestine
Inferior mesenteric	Descending and sigmoid colon, rectum

From Krumberger, J. M. (1998). Gastrointestinal clinical physiology. In M. R. Kinney, S. B. Dunbar, J. A. Brooks–Brunn, N. Molter, & J. M. Vitello–Cicciu (Eds.), AACN's clinical reference for critical care nursing, (4th ed., p. 985). St. Louis: C. V. Mosby; Lindseth, G. L. (2003). Disorders of the stomach and duodenum. In S. L. Price & L. M. Wilson (Eds.), Pathophysiology: Clinical concepts of disease processes, (6th ed.). St. Louis: C.V. Mosby.

Venous Drainage

Venous drainage from the GI tract and the liver passes through the portal vein system. Venous drainage passes through the inferior vena cava and the external iliac vein. Table 30–3 summarizes the veins that branch off from the portal vein and the specific sites from which they drain (Del Valle, 2001; Guyton, 2000; Markey, 1999; Tucker, 2000;).

Sympathetic stimulation directly affects the splanchnic circulation by causing vasoconstriction of the arterioles within the gut wall, resulting in a decrease in blood flow. Prolonged vasoconstriction, as occurs in shock states or with high doses of vasopressor drugs, can lead to ischemia and ulceration of the gut mucosal lining. The breakdown in the integrity of the intestinal walls results in an inability to serve as a barrier against bacteria and foreign toxins. Gram-negative bacteria from within the intestines can translocate through the damaged mucosal lining to the general circulation, resulting in sepsis. Ulceration of the mucosal barrier can lead to ulcers and GI bleeding (Croghan, 2004; Guyton, 2000; Markey, 1999).

Innervation of the GI Tract

The stomach receives its nerve supply from the autonomic nervous system, which can be further divided into the extrinsic and intrinsic nervous systems.

Extrinsic Nervous System

The extrinsic nervous system consists of the parasympathetic and sympathetic systems. Parasympathetic fibers arise from the medulla and spinal segments (vagus nerves). This parasympathetic system (1) enhances GI functions by secretion of the neurotransmitter acetylcholine, (2) increases glandular secretion and muscle tone, and (3) decreases sphincter tone. The net result of parasympathetic stimulation is increased propulsion of contents through the GI tract. The sympathetic motor and sensory fibers arise from the thoracic and lumbar segments of the spinal cord with distribution via the sympathetic ganglia (celiac plexus). Sympathetic fibers run alongside the blood vessels secreting the neurotransmitter norepinephrine.

Stimulation of the sympathetic nervous system inhibits activity in the GI tract, causing effects essentially opposite to those of the parasympathetic stimulation (inhibiting peristalsis and increasing sphincter tone). The net result of sympathetic stimulation is greatly slowed propulsion of contents through the GI tract (Del Valle, 2001; Guyton, 2000; Tucker, 2000). Figure 30–5 compares the sympathetic and parasympathetic nervous systems.

Intrinsic Nervous System

The GI tract also has an intrinsic nervous system, known as the *enteric nervous system,* which coordinates GI motility and secretion. The enteric nervous system is considered the third component of the autonomic nervous system. It consists of two networks located within the wall of the GI tract: the myenteric (Auerbach's) plexus and the submucosal (Meissner's) plexus (Fig. 30–6). The myenteric plexus influences muscle tone, contractions, velocity, and excitation of the stomach. The submucosal plexus influences secretions of the stomach (Del Valle, 2001; Guyton, 2000; Smith, 1998; Tucker, 2000).

In summary, blood flow to the gut, spleen, pancreas, and liver is supplied by the splanchnic circulatory system, which comprises about one fourth of the resting cardiac output. The mesenteric circulation, a part of the splanchnic circulation, supplies blood to the mesentery and the intestines. The portal vein system drains venous blood from the GI tract and liver. Vasoconstriction of the arterioles within the gut wall occurs due to GI tract sympathetic nervous system stimulation. When this sympathetic stimulation is prolonged, vasoconstriction can cause bleeding, ischemia, and ulceration of the gut wall. Mucosal integrity allows gram-negative bacteria and toxins from within the intestines to translocate through the impaired mucosal barrier to the general circulation, resulting in sepsis. The extrinsic nervous system consisting of the parasympathetic and sympathetic systems is part of the autonomic nervous system that innervates the stomach. Parasympathetic stimulation results in the secretion of acetylcholine, increases glandular secretion and muscle tone, and decreases sphincter tone so that propulsion of GI contents or peristalsis occurs. Sympathetic stimulation inhibits peristalsis and increases sphincter tone so that the propulsion of GI contents is slowed. The intrinsic nervous system, also known as the enteric nervous system, coordinates GI motility and secretion.

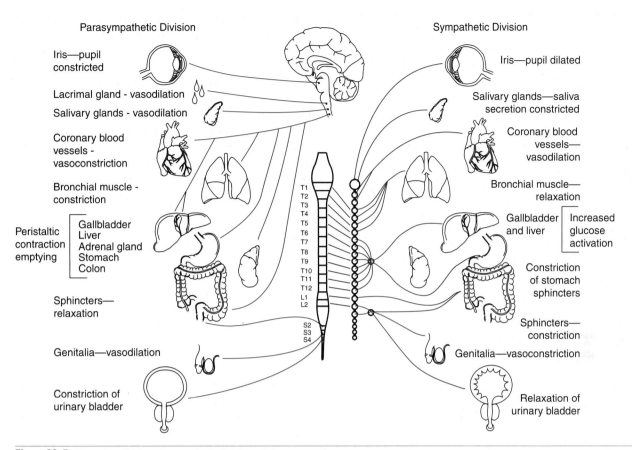

Parasympathetic Division

Iris—pupil constricted

Lacrimal gland - vasodilation

Salivary glands - vasodilation

Coronary blood vessels - vasoconstriction

Bronchial muscle - constriction

Peristaltic contraction emptying { Gallbladder Liver Adrenal gland Stomach Colon

Sphincters— relaxation

Genitalia—vasodilation

Constriction of urinary bladder

Sympathetic Division

Iris—pupil dilated

Salivary glands—saliva secretion constricted

Coronary blood vessels— vasodilation

Bronchial muscle— relaxation

Gallbladder and liver } Increased glucose activation

Constriction of stomach sphincters

Sphincters— constriction

Genitalia—vasoconstriction

Relaxation of urinary bladder

T1 T2 T3 T4 T5 T6 T7 T8 T9 T10 T11 T12 L1 L2

S2 S3 S4

Figure 30–5 ■ Parasympathetic and sympathetic divisions of the autonomic nervous system.

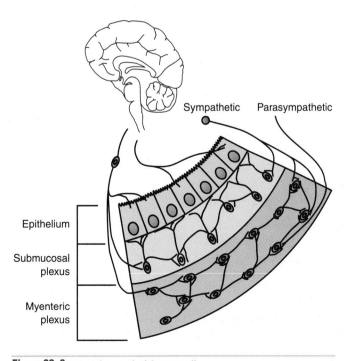

Sympathetic   Parasympathetic

Epithelium

Submucosal plexus

Myenteric plexus

Figure 30–6 ■ Neural control of the gut wall.

SECTION TWO REVIEW

1. The mesenteric circulation begins its flow at the
   A. celiac artery
   B. hepatic artery
   C. aorta
   D. superior vena cava
2. The portal venous system drains the GI tract and the
   A. spleen
   B. liver
   C. pancreas
   D. kidneys
3. Sympathetic stimulation of the splanchnic circulation results in
   A. vasoconstriction of the arterioles within the gut wall
   B. vasodilation of the arterioles within the gut wall
   C. translocation of bacteria across the gut wall
   D. ulceration of the gut wall mucosa
4. The portal venous system includes the
   A. superior vena cava and the external iliac vein
   B. inferior vena cava and the external portal vein
   C. superior vena cava and the inferior celiac vein
   D. inferior vena cava and the external iliac vein
5. The Meissner's (submucosal) plexus influences
   A. muscle tone
   B. stomach secretions
   C. muscle contractions
   D. stomach excitation

Answers: 1. C, 2. B, 3. A, 4. D, 5. B

SECTION THREE: Gut Defenses

At the completion of this section, the learner will be able to describe the mechanisms that exist within the GI tract to protect the integrity of the gut.

When food is ingested, so are foreign antigens and microorganisms. Simply licking the lips or placing the fingers into the mouth allows a multitude of bacteria to enter the GI tract. Because of its easy accessibility to potentially pathologic organisms, the GI system must play a major role in the body's defense against bacteria, parasites, and other toxic pathogens. The GI system has two major mechanisms of defense: nonimmunologic and immunologic.

Nonimmunologic Defense Mechanisms

Nonimmunologic defense mechanisms are those provided by salivary secretions, gastric acid, peristalsis, mucous coat, and commensal bacteria.

Salivary Secretions

Food enters the mouth, where it comes into contact with saliva. Saliva contains substances that are active against foreign antigens and bacteria ingested with the food.

Gastric Acid

Pathogenic microorganisms surviving the mouth pass along to the stomach, where the effects of the gastric acidity (pH less than 4.0) create an environment that is unfavorable to pathogen growth. The acid environment inhibits bacteria from entering the small intestine, where the pH must remain basic (pH of 7.0 or greater) in order for the pancreatic proteolytic enzymes to become active and participate in the digestive process. Offending organisms that survive the gastric acidic environment have difficulty adhering to the epithelial surface of the GI tract in order to colonize and invade the gut wall. This difficulty in attachment to the epithelial surface is partly because of the tight junctions that exist between the epithelial mucosal cells, preventing colonization and invasion.

Peristalsis

Peristaltic motility further inhibits pathogen attachment to the gut mucosa by pushing contents along, decreasing contact time needed by the pathogens to colonize. Continuous peristalsis movement prevents stagnation of chyme and reflux of duodenal contents back up into the stomach (Braunwald, 2001; Guyton, 2000; Markey, 1999).

Mucous Coat

Further mechanical resistance to offending pathogenic invaders is provided by the overlying mucous coat covering the epithelial surface. Goblet cells within the submucosa of the GI tract secrete mucus which covers the intestinal surface, providing a physical barrier to the passage of potential pathogens. The mucous coat may actually facilitate the removal of these microorganisms by allowing them to slide through the GI tract.

Commensal Bacteria

Commensal or indigenous bacteria are the normal flora existing within the ileum and large intestine that limit proliferation and adherence of potentially pathologic bacteria. *Bacteroides fragilis* is the main anaerobic bacteria, and *Escherichia coli* is the main aerobic bacteria that prevent overgrowth of other gram-negative and gram-positive bacteria. These normal flora are stable and protective in healthy persons. They break down cellulose and synthesize vitamin K, folic acid, riboflavin, and nicotinic acid. They limit pathologic infections by competing with nutrients and adhesion sites, and by producing inhibitory fatty acids within the epithelium (Lingappa, 2003; Markey, 1999). The stomach, duodenum, and jejunum are sterile.

Immunologic Defense Mechanisms

The immunologic defense is provided by the gut-associated lymphoid tissue (GALT). The GI tract is a major immune organ, with 70 to 80 percent of all immunologic-secreting cells being located within the intestinal wall, and about 25 percent of the intestinal mucosa being composed of lymphoid tissue (Markey, 1999). GALT includes the tonsils, lymph tissue within the intestinal wall, and appendix. The tonsils are strategically located to intercept airborne and ingested pathogens. **Peyer's patches** are nodules of lymph tissue located on the outer wall of the intestines. The appendix is a blind tube about the size of the little finger located in the ileocecal region of the small intestine. These tissues include T helper cells (of the CD4 type), B cells, plasma cells, mucosal mast cells (goblet cells), and macrophages that respond to gastrointestinal pathogens. Immunoglobulins produced by GALT migrate to the GI tract, tear ducts, and salivary glands to defend against pathogen penetration of epithelial surfaces (Guyton, 2000; Lindseth, 2003b).

Mechanisms That Maintain Mucosal Integrity

Superficial epithelial cells secrete mucus and bicarbonate, which aid in maintaining a pH gradient between the lumen and the mucosa to protect the underlying epithelial tissues from damage by gastric acid and pepsin. Mucosal blood flow is also believed to be an important mechanism to maintain mucosal integrity (Fig. 30–7) (Andreoli et al., 2000; Guyton, 2000; Lindseth, 2003a).

Trauma, shock, intestinal obstruction, protein malnutrition, and parenteral nutritional therapy can all cause disruption of the intestinal mucosal integrity. When patients are treated with total parenteral nutrition (TPN), it has been observed that the lack of enteral stimulation results in mucosal atrophy and bacterial overgrowth. Impaired gut barrier function facilitates bacterial translocation of bacteria across the mucosal barrier and into the lymphatic vessels and portal circulation. This potentially pathologic bacterium may enter the systemic

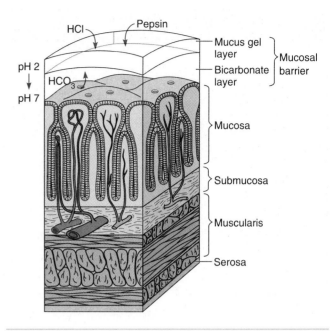

Figure 30–7 ■ Mechanisms for maintaining mucosal integrity. Superficial epithelial cells secrete mucus and bicarbonate, which aid in maintaining a pH gradient between the lumen and mucosa, and protect the underlying epithelial cells from damage by acid and pepsin. Mucosal blood flow is also believed to be a mechanism important in maintaining mucosal integrity.

circulation and cause sepsis. Intestinal bacteria have been observed to cause systemic disease in immunodeficient patients, such as the critically ill (Andreoli et al., 2000; Guyton, 2000; Urden et al., 2001).

In summary, the nonimmunologic and immunologic defense mechanisms protect against potentially pathological bacteria, parasites, and other toxins that can enter through ingestion or through translocation into the general circulation directly from the gut through damaged mucosa. Saliva, along with the acid environment in the stomach, the mucous coat, the presence of commensal bacteria or normal flora in the intestines, and peristalsis inhibit bacterial colonization and growth in the GI tract. The lymphatic tissue within the intestinal wall makes up the largest immune-secreting tissue in the body. These tissues provide T helper cells, B cells, plasma cells, mucosal mast cells, and macrophages that respond defensively to GI pathogens. Mucous and bicarbonate, which are secreted by the superficial epithelial cells, coat the mucosa and protect it from being damaged by the gastric acid and pepsin. Risk factors for disruption of mucosal integrity and the subsequent migration of gut bacteria into the systemic circulation include trauma, shock, intestinal obstruction, protein malnutrition, the use of parenteral nutritional therapy, and prolonged sympathetic stimulation.

SECTION THREE REVIEW

1. Commensal bacteria are a part of the gut's
   A. enteric defense mechanism
   B. nonimmunologic defense mechanism
   C. gut-associated lymphatic tissue
   D. immunologic defense mechanism
2. Peristalsis promotes gastrointestinal health by
   A. pushing intestinal contents along the GI tract and preventing reflux
   B. creating an acid environment that is unfavorable to pathogen growth
   C. secreting substances that are active against foreign antigens
   D. covering the epithelial surface with mucus
3. The mucous coat
   A. maintains an acid environment
   B. activates protective digestive enzymes

   C. provides a physical barrier against invasion by pathogens
   D. interferes with bacterial replication
4. Goblet cells secrete
   A. gastrin
   B. hydrochloric acid
   C. secretin
   D. mucus
5. The initial nonimmunologic defense mechanism that is active against antigens is provided by
   A. salivary secretions
   B. intestinal peristalsis
   C. *Escherichia coli* bacteria
   D. Peyer's patches

Answers: 1. B, 2. A, 3. C, 4. D, 5. A

SECTION FOUR: Laboratory and Diagnostic Studies

At the completion of this section, the learner will be able to describe the laboratory findings and diagnostic tests used in the management of acute GI problems.

Laboratory Findings

Laboratory tests used to make a differential diagnosis in GI bleeding and acute abdominal pain include electrolytes, end products of metabolism, enzymes, hematology, and arterial blood gases (ABGs). They are summarized in Table 30–4.

Electrolytes

Electrolyte levels that should be monitored with GI dysfunction include calcium, chloride, magnesium, potassium, and sodium. These electrolytes are primarily absorbed by the small intestine and may be lost, depleted, or increased with gastrointestinal disorders (e.g., potassium loss occurs with diarrhea and vomiting).

Blood Urea Nitrogen (BUN)

Elevated BUN (greater than 40 mg/dL) in the absence of underlying renal disease, as evidenced by a normal serum creatinine, may indicate significant blood loss (loss of 2 or more units). Furthermore, an elevated BUN-to-creatinine ratio may occur in upper GI bleeding and volume depletion as a result of hemo-

concentration from a fluid volume deficit. Following a GI bleed, old blood may be within the intestines and is digested as it passes through the GI tract, resulting in the production of urea nitrogen as a by-product of metabolism, thus elevating the BUN (Andreoli et al., 2000; Arnell, 2002; Haist & Robbins, 2002; Nicoll et al., 2004; Stamos, 2002; Urden et al., 2001;). Bowel obstruction can cause azotemia because stasis of intestinal contents within the intestines allows more digestion to take place, which produces more by-products of protein metabolism.

Enzymes

Aspartate aminotransferase (AST) and lactic dehydrogenase (LDH) may be elevated in liver disease. Elevated AST and LDH levels may be significant in the presence of GI bleeding because liver dysfunction may contribute to GI bleeding (see Module 31). Alkaline phosphatase elevations occur with intestinal, liver, and bone tissue injury. Serum amylase elevations occur with pancreatitis, peptic ulcer disease (PUD), small bowel obstruction, and ischemic bowel.

Hematologic Levels

Serum hematocrit (Hct) and hemoglobin (Hgb) may be abnormal in gastrointestinal bleeding; thus, serial measures are most helpful. During acute hemorrhage, however, the hematocrit may not reflect the volume of blood loss. Prior to fluid resuscitation, the Hct may be higher than expected as a result of hemoconcentration from volume loss. The hematocrit may fall precipitously after aggressive fluid resuscitation because of hemodilution effects. It takes 24 to 72 hours for the Hct to equilibrate with the

TABLE 30–4 Laboratory Tests

TEST	NORMAL VALUES	COMMENTS
Electrolytes		
Calcium	Total, 4.5–5.5 mEq/L Ionized, 4.4–5.0 mg/dL	Absorbed by the small intestine and may be lost, depleted, or increased with GI disorders
Chloride	95–105 mEq/L	
Magnesium	1.5–2.5 mEq/L	
Potassium	3.5–5.3 mEq/L	
Sodium	135–145 mEq/L	
Chemistry		
Blood urea nitrogen	5–25 mg/dL	Bowel obstruction can cause azotemia; lactic acid is elevated in bowel infarction and metabolic acidosis
Lactic acid	Arterial: 0.5–2.0 mEq/L Venous: 0.5–2.0 mEq/L	
Enzymes		
Alkaline phosphatase	20–90 U/L	Found in bone, intestine, and liver, and released with destruction of those tissues
Amylase	25–125 U/L	Elevated in peptic ulcer disease, intestinal obstruction, mesenteric thrombosis, and after abdominal surgery
Hematologic		
Complete blood count with differential		
Hemoglobin	M: 14–18 g/dL F: 12–16 g/dL	Hct, Hgb are decreased with GI bleeding and with malabsorption; with acute blood loss, Hct may not decrease for several hours
Hematocrit	M: 40–54 percent F: 37–47 percent	
White blood cells	4,500–10,000/mm^3	White blood cell count elevated with infection, and inflammation
Arterial blood gases		
pH	7.35–7.45	Metabolic acidosis may result from ischemic bowel
Paco$_2$	35–45 mm Hg	
Pao$_2$	80–100 mm Hg	
Sao$_2$	> 95 percent	
HCO$_3$	22–26 mEq/L	
BE	+2 to -2 mEq/L	
Helicobacter antibodies	Negative	Used to detect *Helicobacter pylori* infection in peptic ulcer disease

Data from Westfall, U. E. (1999). Gastrointestinal laboratory and diagnostic tests. In L. Bucher & S. Melander (Eds.). Critical care nursing. *Philadelphia: W. B. Saunders; Urden, L., Stacy, K., & Lough, M. (2001).* Thelan's critical care nursing: Diagnosis and management, *(4th ed.). St. Louis: C. V. Mosby.*

extravascular fluid following administration of large amounts of fluids or blood products (Haist & Robbins, 2002; Lefor et al., 2002). Platelets may be increased or decreased with GI bleeding. A prolonged prothrombin time (PT) and partial thromboplastin time (PTT) can make stabilization of the patient with a GI bleed very challenging. Platelets and clotting factors are also lost with rapid bleeding. It is important to evaluate PT and PTT levels in order to determine requirements for replacement of clotting factors. A decreased mean corpuscular volume (MCV) suggests the possibility of iron-deficiency anemia secondary to chronic GI blood loss. White blood cell (WBC) count elevations suggest an inflammatory or infectious process. This can occur with peptic ulcer with perforation, and with ischemic bowel.

Arterial Blood Gases (ABGs)

ABG measures are useful in evaluation of respiratory status and pH deviations. Hypoxemia is an early sign of sepsis. Metabolic acidosis may result from sepsis, ischemic bowel, or peptic ulcer perforation. Decreased oxygen-carrying capacity as a result of blood loss is a common complication from severe upper GI hemorrhage.

Antibodies

Helicobacter antibodies may be detected in the serum of persons with *H. pylori* infection. *H. pylori* infection is associated with PUD and will be discussed further in another section of this module.

Diagnostic Studies

Diagnosing GI disorders can be challenging because the complex disease status of the high acuity patient may mask the development of gastrointestinal complications. GI symptoms often are vague initially and may have an insidious onset; thus, early GI manifestations may be overlooked in the presence of other high priority health concerns. Diagnostic studies, either invasive or noninvasive, are often required to definitively diagnose an acute GI problem. The remainder of this section provides a brief overview of some of the major studies used in diagnosing GI disorders. Both noninvasive and invasive tests are used to diagnose GI disorders.

X-ray exam or flat plate of the abdomen is helpful in diagnosing intra-abdominal problems such as intestinal obstruction, rupture, masses, abnormal fluid or air levels, and foreign bodies. An upper GI series with contrast medium is another type of x-ray exam; it allows visualization of the GI tract in order to diagnose tumors, masses, hernias, obstructions, ulcers, fistulas, or diverticular disease. The patient must ingest a contrast material, usually barium, prior to the actual x-ray. The contrast medium allows visualization of any abnormalities. It is important to ask about the client's allergy history prior to administration of the contrast medium in order to prevent serious allergic reactions. Furthermore, it is important to assist the patient in expelling the contrast (barium).

Computed tomography (CT) is another test allowing visualization of the abdomen, retroperitoneal structures, masses, abscesses, and abnormal fluid or air levels, which might be visible if perforation has occurred. This exam requires the person to ingest a barium contrast solution prior to the exam.

Ultrasound sonography allows visualization of abdominal and retroperitoneal soft tissue structures to diagnose fluid or air pockets, abscesses, masses, and to observe movement. This procedure may be done at the bedside. Transducing gel is applied to the skin, and mild pressure is applied with a transducer. Adipose tissue, air, and barium may diminish ultrasound wave transmission.

Magnetic resonance imaging (MRI) is useful to assess abdominal and retroperitoneal structures for masses, abscesses, and fluid or air pockets. All external metal objects and dental appliances must be removed. Internal metal objects or foreign bodies are a contraindication to MRI. It is very important that the patient lie still for this test; therefore, he or she must be able to cooperate.

A *nuclear scan* allows visualization of organs, gastrointestinal motility, and bleeding. An intravenous contrast medium is administered, making allergic reactions a risk with this test; therefore, an allergy history should be obtained. Nuclear scan is contraindicated in pregnancy, breast-feeding, or recent nuclear exposure. All metal must be removed from these patients also. Nonuniform radioactive uptake in tissues often indicates disease.

Angiography allows visualization of blood flow in selected vascular beds. Bleeding vessels can be identified with this test. A contrast medium is administered intravenously; therefore, allergy history is important (Urden et al., 2001; Westfall, 1999).

Endoscopy allows inspection of internal surfaces of organs. It includes a series of diagnostic tests for the GI system using fiber-optic light and a lens system. Removal of tissue for testing (biopsy), as well as some treatments, such as sclerotherapy, suction, and cauterization of bleeding vessels, may be performed during endoscopy of the upper or lower GI tract. An endoscopic exam of the upper GI tract, known as esophagogastroduodenoscopy (EGD), can include inspection of structures from the mouth to the ligament of Treitz (the junction of the duodenum and jejunum) to diagnose the source of bleeding or ulceration of the GI tract mucosa. Colonoscopy allows inspection of the large intestine to identify a lower GI bleeding source or other disease (Arnell, 2002; Urden et al., 2001; Westfall, 1999). Common endoscopic tests are summarized in Table 30–5.

Gastric Tonometry is an invasive monitoring technique that allows the assessment of gut perfusion. This technique uses a gastric balloon to measure the carbon dioxide (CO_2) level of the gastric mucosa, which rises when the GI tract is underperfused. Tonometry provides an early warning of reduced gastric perfusion, which can occur when a patient is hypovolemic or in shock. During a period of hypoperfusion, the GI tract is one of the first organ systems to suffer reduced blood flow. A decrease in the delivery of oxygen rich blood to the gut mucosa results in anaerobic metabolism. Tonometry measures the changes in the pH and CO_2 levels of the gut that is indicative of GI tract perfusion; specifically, tonometry measures the balance of CO_2 removal (dependent on perfusion) and CO_2 production (dependent on metabolism) (Ackerman & Ashe, 2000; Schulman, 2002).

Tonometry can be measured using a gas permeable balloon attached to the end of a nasogastric tube (Fig. 30–8). This special nasogastric tube contains an additional lumen that attaches the tonometer balloon to a monitor. After a calibration procedure, the monitor fills the balloon with air. Carbon dioxide that is produced by the gastric mucosa diffuses through the gas permeable balloon wall and equilibrates with the air inside of the balloon. The monitor calculates the level of CO_2 in the balloon, known as the $PrCO_2$ (partial pressure of carbon dioxide). The $PrCO_2$ level is measured and displayed on the monitor every 10 minutes. Changes in the $PrCO_2$ level reflect changes in anaerobic and aerobic metabolism, thus perfusion of the GI tract.

Normal $PrCO_2$ is less than 50 mm Hg, which reflects the CO_2 level in the gastric mucosa. A normal **$PrCO_2$–$PaCO_2$ gap,** which is the difference between arterial and gastric CO_2 levels, is less than 10 mmHg. As perfusion to the gut decreases, the $PrCO_2$ increases and the $PrCO_2$–$PaCO_2$ gap level becomes larger (Ackerman & Ashe, 2000; Schulman, 2002). Table 30–6 provides an interpretation of gastric tonometry values.

Nursing Considerations

The identification of GI hypoperfusion via gastric tonometry can help clinicians prevent or avoid organ damage in hemodynamically unstable patients. Measures to improve gut perfusion are warranted when the $PrCO_2$ and the $PrCO_2$–$PaCO_2$ gap rises.

TABLE 30–5   Endoscopies of the Gastrointestinal System

TEST	INDICATIONS	CONTRAINDICATIONS
Esophagogastroduodenoscopy (EGD)	Visualization of upper GI tract for diagnosis or treatment; locate upper GI bleeding source	Cardiovascular and/or respiratory instability
Colonoscopy	Visualization of the large intestine for diagnosis or treatment; locate lower GI bleeding source	Perforation, peritonitis, recent bowel surgery, cardiovascular and/or respiratory compromise, inability of the patient to tolerate bowel prep
Proctoscopy, sigmoidoscopy, proctosigmoidoscopy, anoscopy	Visualization of sigmoid colon and rectal/anal mucosa for diagnosis or treatment; locate source of sigmoid, rectal, or anal bleeding	Perforation, infection, peritonitis, surgery, cardiovascular and/or respiratory compromise

From Westfall, U. E. (1999). Gastrointestinal laboratory and diagnostic tests. In L. Bucher & S. Melander (Eds.), Critical care nursing. *Philadelphia: W.B. Saunders; Urden, L., Stacy, K., & Lough, M. (2001).* Thelan's critical care nursing: Diagnosis and management, *(4th ed.). St. Louis: C.V. Mosby; Arnell, T. (2002). Gastrointestinal bleeding. In F. S. Bongard & D. Y. Sue (Eds.),* Current critical care diagnosis and treatment, *(2nd ed., p. 756). New York: Lange.*

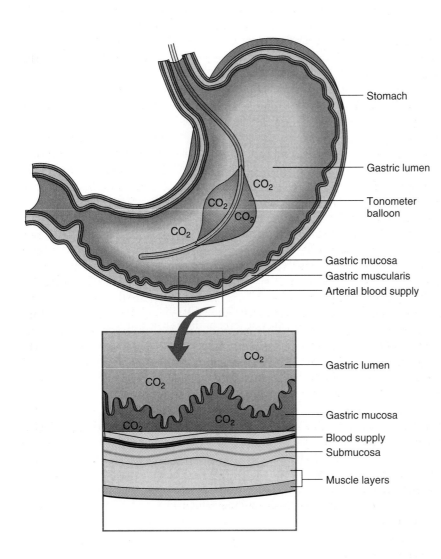

Figure 30–8 ■ Gastric tonometry. A special gastric tube with a balloon on the distal end is inserted into the stomach to measure the CO_2 level of the gastric mucosa. Gastric CO_2 ($PrCO_2$) rises when the mucosa is hypoperfused.

Such measures might include oxygen administration to maintain an oxygen saturation of 92 percent or greater. It is also beneficial to reduce oxygen consumption by managing tachycardia, tachypnea, shivering, fever, pain, or agitation. The patient's cardiac output, hemoglobin, and oxygenation levels should be optimized with the use of crystalloids, colloids, and inotropic and vasopressor medications (Ackerman & Ashe, 2000; Schulman, 2002). When measuring gastric $PrCO_2$ levels, enteral feeding is stopped for 30 minutes before taking the measurement (Schulman, 2002).

TABLE 30–6 Interpretation of Gastric Tonometry Values

Prco$_2$	Prco$_2$–Paco$_2$	Interpretation
Greater or equal to 61 mm Hg	Greater or equal to 16 mm Hg	Persistent elevations in these values are indicative of compromised gut perfusion Aggressive measures to restore perfusion are warranted
51–60 mm Hg	11–15 mm Hg	The patient's gut perfusion should be closely monitored; hemodynamic status should be evaluated
Less than 50 mm Hg	Less than 10 mm Hg	These values are normal; no interventions are warranted based on these values

From Ackerman, M. H., & Ashe, T. R. (2000). *The latest in gastrointestinal care: Find out how gut perfusion monitoring can help you identify warnings of shock.* Nursing 2000, 30(5 suppl), 36–38.

Sublingual capnometry is a simple, noninvasive technology that provides immediate and continuous measures of partial pressure of arterial carbon dioxide ($PaCO_2$). Recent studies have shown that this test is an accurate indicator of splanchnic perfusion. A special CO_2 probe is placed beneath the tongue. Unfortunately, patients often need to be sedated to tolerate both the probe and the endotracheal tube. The presence of orogastric or nasogastric tubes does not appear to affect the accuracy of the results. With sublingual capnometry, enteral feedings do not need to be stopped to obtain measures. Additional studies in human subjects are necessary, however, before this technology will be available for bedside use (Weil, 1999; Schulman, 2002).

In summary, multiple laboratory and diagnostic tests are indicated in gastrointestinal dysfunction. Blood urea nitrogen (BUN) as well as electrolytes, such as calcium, chloride, magnesium, potassium, and sodium, should be closely monitored in patients with acute GI dysfunction, GI bleeding, or acute abdominal pain. Laboratory enzyme tests that are useful when determining the etiology of acute GI dysfunction include AST, LDH, alkaline phosphatase, and serum amylase. Elevations in these enzymes can suggest liver disease, pancreatitis, PUD, small bowel obstruction, and ischemic bowel. Gastrointestinal bleeding requires the evaluation and monitoring of the serum hematocrit; hemoglobin; platelets, which can be decreased; as well as studies of coagulation (prothrombin time and partial thrombo-

plastin time), which can be prolonged. Elevations in the WBC count suggest possible infection or inflammation as a result of bowel perforation or ischemia. Respiratory status and arterial blood gases should be monitored for pH deviations and hypoxia. If PUD is diagnosed, detection of serum *Helicobacter* antibodies should be included in the plan of care. There are multiple diagnostic studies, both noninvasive and invasive, used to diagnose GI disorders. Abdominal x-ray or flat plate, upper GI series with contrast medium allows for the detection or visualization of intestinal obstruction, rupture, masses, ulcers, fistulas, diverticular disease, or abnormal collections of air or fluid. CT scans with and without contrast, ultrasound sonography, and magnetic resonance imaging (MRI) allow visualization of abdominal and retroperitoneal structures, masses, abscesses, and abnormal fluid or air levels. The nuclear scan with contrast allows visualization of organs, GI motility problems, and bleeding. An angiography with IV contrast allows visualization of bleeding vessels. Endoscopic procedures allow inspection of the internal surfaces of the GI tract and allow for the removal of tissue for biopsy. Gastric tonometry is a technique that allows the assessment of gut perfusion through continuous monitoring of the carbon dioxide level of the gastric mucosa. Sublingual capnometry is the noninvasive technology that provides continuous measures of the $PaCO_2$, an accurate indicator of splanchnic perfusion.

SECTION FOUR REVIEW

1. BUN is commonly elevated following a GI bleeding event. Which of the following best explains why this abnormal laboratory measure occurs?
   A. acute renal failure
   B. fluid volume overload
   C. metabolic acidosis
   D. hemoconcentration of the blood
2. BUN elevation (greater than 40 mg/dL), in the absence of underlying renal disease, may suggest

A. loss of 2 or more units of blood
B. impaired circulation to renal tissues
C. significant fluid volume overload
D. onset of acute renal failure
3. Bowel obstruction can cause a(n)
   A. elevated AST
   B. elevated BUN
   C. decreased LDH
   D. decreased MCV

4. *H. pylori* infection is associated with
   A. upper GI bleeding
   B. chronic lower GI bleeding
   C. liver disease
   D. PUD
5. _____ may contribute to GI bleeding.
   A. Pulmonary disease
   B. Hepatic dysfunction
   C. Autoimmune complications
   D. Connective tissue disease
6. Gastric tonometry measures the
   A. $PrCO_2$ and $PrCO_2$–$PaCO_2$ gap
   B. $PaCO_2$ and PaO_2–FIO_2 ratio

   C. gastric pH and $PaCO_2$
   D. gastric hemoglobin levels
7. Persistent elevations in the $PrCO_2$ and the $PrCO_2$–$PaCO_2$ gap levels include
   A. impaired gas exchange
   B. hypoperfusion of GI tract
   C. acid hypersecretory state
   D. normal gut wall metabolism

Answers: 1. D, 2. A, 3. B, 4. D, 5. B, 6. A, 7. B

SECTION FIVE: Incidence and Clinical Manifestations of Acute GI Bleeding

Following the completion of this section, the learner will be able to describe the incidence of and clinical manifestations of acute GI bleeding.

Incidence

GI bleeding is a common clinical problem. The incidence per year of upper GI bleeding is 150 per 100,000 people (Farrell & Friedman, 2001; Lingenfelser & Ell, 2001), with a mortality of 5 to 10 percent. GI bleeding can range in severity from a very slow occult blood loss to a sudden, massive hemorrhage. About 80 percent of acute GI bleeding stops without intervention, but some recurrent bleeding can become a life-threatening emergency (Andreoli et al., 2000). Upper GI bleeding, from vessels proximal to the ligament of Treitz, is more likely to produce arterial hemorrhage because of the large arterial blood supply needed for digestion, whereas lower GI bleeding is more commonly of venous origin. In persons with acute upper GI hemorrhage, comorbid or concurrent disease is the cause of death approximately 70 percent of the time. Patients with acute lower GI bleeding tend to be older than those with upper GI bleeding, have more concomitant medical problems, and experience increased morbidity. The mortality rate for acute lower GI bleeding is the same as for acute upper GI bleeding (Farrell & Friedman, 2001; Lingenfelser & Ell, 2001).

Clinical Manifestations

Gastrointestinal blood loss may be (1) acute (sudden or massive with hypovolemia) or (2) chronic (slow and often unnoticed by the patient). Blood that is present in the GI tract but not really visible is called *occult blood*. Occult bleeding is often detected by chemical testing of a stool or nasogastric specimen. This process is known as *hemoccult* or *guaiac testing*. Acute GI bleeding may present in one of several ways:

1. **Hematemesis**—vomiting of bright red blood or blood that looks like coffee grounds. This bleeding is often brisk and is usually from an upper GI arterial source.
2. **Melena**—black, tarry, foul-smelling stools passed after a bleed of 100 to 500 mL of blood, usually from an upper GI source. However, a small intestine or right colon bleeding source may also be the cause.
3. **Hematochezia**—bright red blood or maroon stool from the rectum, usually the result of lower GI bleeding or massive upper GI bleeding.

Clients with chronic GI bleeding often present with fatigue, dyspnea, syncope, angina, a positive fecal occult blood test, or iron-deficiency anemia (Andreoli et al., 2000; Haist & Robbins, 2002; Podolsky & Isselbacher, 2001; Urden et al., 2001).

In summary, GI bleeding is a common clinical problem. In persons with acute upper GI bleeding, comorbid or concurrent disease is commonly the cause of death. Patients with lower GI bleeding tend to be older than those with upper GI bleeding, and have more concomitant medical problems, and experience increased morbidity. The mortality rates for either type of GI bleeding are similar. Clinical manifestations of acute GI bleeding can include blood loss, fatigue, dyspnea, syncope, angina, and iron-deficiency anemia. The blood loss can be acute, chronic, or occult in nature, presenting as hematemesis, melena, or hematochezia.

SECTION FIVE REVIEW

1. The section of the GI tract that is involved in an upper GI hemorrhage is
   A. proximal to the ligament of Treitz
   B. proximal to the ileocecal valve
   C. distal to the pyloric sphincter
   D. distal to the duodenal bulb
2. The mortality rate for acute lower GI bleeding is
   A. twice as high as the mortality rate for acute upper GI bleeding
   B. less than the mortality rate for acute upper GI bleeding
   C. the same as the mortality rate for acute upper GI bleeding
   D. slightly higher than the mortality rate for acute upper GI bleeding
3. Characteristics of acute lower GI bleeding include
   A. bleeding commonly of arterial origin
   B. bleeding commonly of venous origin
   C. bleeding massive 80 percent of the time
   D. bleeding always occult
4. A client presents to the emergency department after vomiting bright red blood. The client becomes hypotensive soon after and is admitted into the hospital with GI bleeding. The presentation of this episode of bleeding is
   A. occult
   B. chronic
   C. subacute
   D. acute
5. Clients with occult GI bleeding often present with
   A. nausea and vomiting
   B. mental status changes
   C. headache and abdominal pain
   D. fatigue and syncope

Answers: 1. A, 2. C, 3. B, 4. D, 5. D

SECTION SIX: Acute Upper GI Bleeding

At the completion of this section, the learner will be able to describe the etiology and pathophysiology of acute upper GI bleeding.

Etiology

More than 90 percent of upper GI bleeding cases are caused by peptic ulcer, erosive gastritis, Mallory–Weiss tears, or esophagogastric varices (Arnell, 2002). Other etiologies of upper GI bleeding include tumors, arteriovenous malformations, and stress ulcers. Table 30–7 summarizes the causes of upper GI bleeding.

The amount and degree of upper GI bleeding varies. When an ulcer erodes through an artery, the bleeding is profuse. Therefore, the manifestations of GI bleeding depend on the source, the rate of bleeding, and comorbid disease. Severe GI bleeding may seriously aggravate coronary artery disease, hypertension, diabetes mellitus, pulmonary disease, and renal failure, and it often presents as shock. Lesser degrees of bleeding may present as orthostatic changes in pulse (a change of greater than 10 beats per minute) or blood pressure (a drop of 10 mm Hg or greater) secondary to compensatory mechanisms (Arnell, 2002; Beers & Berkhow, 1999; Prakash, 2000a, 2001).

TABLE 30–7 Causes of Upper GI Bleeding

ETIOLOGY	OCCURRENCE (PERCENTAGE OF TOTAL UPPER GI BLEED CASES)
Peptic ulcers	45
Gastric	23
Duodenal	22
Gastritis	20–30
Varices	15–20
Esophagitis	13
Mallory–Weiss tear	5–10
Arteriovenous malformation	Less than 5

From Beers, M. H., & Berkhow, R. (Eds.). (1999). The Merck manual of diagnosis and therapy, (17th ed.). Whitehouse Station, NJ: Merck Research Laboratories; Arnell, T. (2002). Gastrointestinal bleeding. In F. S. Bongard & D. Y. Sue (Eds.), Current critical care diagnosis and treatment, (2nd ed., p. 756). New York: Lange.

Studies have found that the most common cause of death in GI hemorrhage is the result of exacerbation of the underlying disease rather than intractable hypovolemic shock (Andreoli et al., 2000; Farrell & Friedman, 2001). However, GI hemorrhage, if unrecognized or treated too late, can lead to hypovolemic shock and ultimately death.

Peptic Ulcer Disease

PUD is the most common cause of upper GI bleeding. Ulcers range in size from several millimeters to several centimeters and are characterized by a break in the mucosa extending through the muscularis mucosae. Peptic ulcers occur in the portion of the GI tract exposed to acid–pepsin secretion, which includes the stomach and the duodenum (Figs. 30–9 and 30–10).

Traditional theories on the cause of peptic ulcer disease have been focused on acid hypersecretion or the inability of the mucosa to secrete mucus for protection. It is now known that acid hypersecretion is not the primary mechanism by which ulceration occurs. It appears that certain associated factors, namely infection with *H. pylori* bacteria and the use of nonsteroidal anti-inflammatory drugs (NSAIDs), disrupt the mucosal defense barrier, making it susceptible to the damaging effects of acid. Cigarette smoking has been linked to an increased incidence of ulcer disease, slower healing rates, and higher rates of ulcer recurrence (Elliot, 2002; Isenkery et al., 1995). Other risk factors include a family history of ulcer disease and the use of aspirin (Urden et al., 2001). Mortality, as a result of peptic ulcer disease is quite low; however, patients suffer substantial pain as a result of the chronic nature of this disease. Interestingly, peptic ulcer disease is the most common cause of upper GI bleeding in critically ill patients. Peptic ulcer disease accounts for approximately 40 percent of patients admitted to an intensive care unit (ICU) specifically for bleeding and 50 percent of patients admitted for some other reason who develop upper GI hemorrhage during their stay (Arnell, 2002).

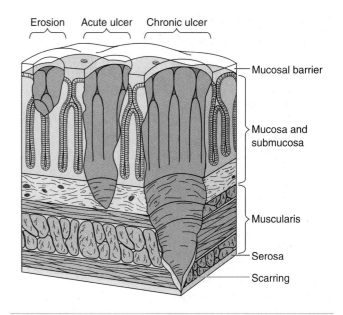

Figure 30–10 ■ Erosion and ulcerations of the upper gastrointestinal tract. Acute and chronic ulcers may penetrate the entire wall of the stomach.

H. pylori can be cultured from the stomachs of approximately 70 to 90 percent of patients with gastric ulcers, and 80 to 95 percent of patients with duodenal ulcers (Falk, 2001). *H. pylori* is able to secrete its own protective covering, which protects it from gastric acid, allowing it to thrive in a high-acid environment. The mechanism by which *H. pylori* impairs mucosal integrity is poorly understood. The organism is responsible for the production of ammonia, cytotoxins, and mucolytic enzymes that erode the mucous barrier, making the mucosa more susceptible to acid damage. NSAIDs inhibit prostaglandin production and action. Inhibition of prostaglandins is believed to be the most important causative factor to the development of ulcers. Prostaglandins function to increase mucous secretion, bicarbonate secretion, and mucosal blood flow as well as to inhibit gastric acid secretion. Because NSAIDs interfere with the normal prostaglandin actions, they contribute to the formation of peptic ulcers (Fig. 30–11).

Peptic ulcer disease can be subdivided into duodenal ulcers and gastric ulcers. Duodenal ulcers constitute approximately 80 percent of peptic ulcers (Lingappa, 2003; Smith, 1998). The most frequent sites for duodenal ulcers are the gastric pylorus and the first portion of the duodenum. Duodenal ulcers can occur at any age but are most common among young adults, especially in persons with type A blood, who smoke, abuse alcohol, and who report a positive family history of peptic ulcers. Duodenal ulcer pain tends to be consistent. The pain is absent on awakening but returns around midmorning. It is relieved by food but recurs 2 to 3 hours after eating. Antacids provide some temporary relief. Intense pain that awakens the patient from sleep at night is common with duodenal ulcer.

Gastric ulcer symptoms usually do not follow a consistent pattern. For example, eating often causes pain. Gastric ulcers

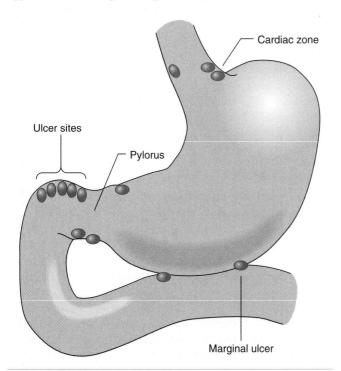

Figure 30–9 ■ Common sites of peptic ulcers. Causes of peptic ulcers: (1) high acid and pepsin content, (2) irritation, (3) poor blood supply, (4) poor secretion of mucus, and (5) infection.

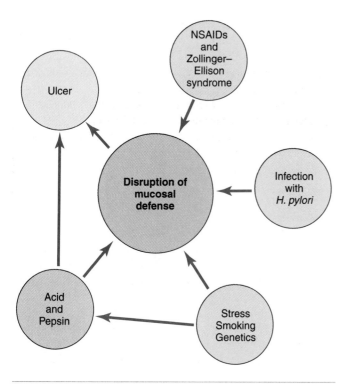

Figure 30–11 ■ Etiological factors in ulcer development. Acid and pepsin activity overpowers mucosal defense to produce ulcers most commonly when mucosal defense is impaired. Two factors, nonsteroidal anti-inflammatory drugs and *H. pylori* infection, appear to be linked to the impairment of mucosal defense.

affect older adults and are associated with malignancy. Gastric ulcers tend to be chronic, usually involving branches of the left gastric artery, and can produce severe hemorrhage if erosion into the arterial wall occurs. If the gastric ulcer is located in the pyloric canal (the narrow region of the stomach that opens through the pylorus into the duodenum), the symptoms are often associated with obstruction (e.g., bloating, nausea, vomiting) (Beers & Berkhow, 1999; Prakash, 2001).

Diagnosis and Treatment

Diagnosis of peptic ulcer disease is largely suggested by history and is confirmed by visualization with fiber-optic endoscopy, the diagnostic tool of choice. Conversely, approximately 10 percent (Beers & Berkhow, 1999; Podolsky & Isselbacher, 2001) of duodenal ulcers may be missed using endoscopy. For this reason, a follow up barium x-ray exam may be ordered if clinical suspicion for peptic ulcer is high. Determination of a duodenal or gastric ulcer by upper endoscopy or radiographic study should be followed by confirmation of *H. pylori* infection. *H. pylori* infection can be definitively diagnosed using endoscopy. Diagnostic tests for the presence of *H. pylori* vary and include serologic testing, carbon-labeled urea breath tests, rapid urease assay (Clotest), and culture or histologic analysis of endoscopic biopsies (Lindseth, 2003b; Prakash, 2000a, 2001).

Treatment of peptic ulcer disease involves antibiotics (for eradication of *H. pylori*), histamine (H_2) receptor antagonist agents (as an antisecretory), proton pump inhibitors (for acid secretion inhibition), prostaglandins (to inhibit acid secretion and enhance mucosal barrier), sucralfate (to promote mucosal barrier), and antacids (to give symptomatic relief and raise gastric pH). Many high-acuity patients have nasogastric as well as small-bore enteric feeding tubes. The appropriate route of administration for sucralfate and antacids is through the nasogastric tube to allow for direct contact with the gastric mucosa. If the nasogastric tube is attached to suction, it must be interrupted for 30 to 60 minutes. Eliminating foods that cause distress is helpful. Surgery is indicated only to manage severe bleeding and perforation complications of peptic ulcers (Altman, 2001; Deglin & Vallerand, 2001; van Lanschot et al., 2002). The pharmacologic interventions will be discussed further in upcoming sections of this module.

Acute Erosive or Hemorrhagic Gastritis

Acute erosive or hemorrhagic gastritis involves severe inflammation of the gastric mucosa. The most common clinical manifestation of erosive gastritis is upper GI bleeding, which presents as hematemesis, "coffee ground" emesis, or bloody aspirate in a patient receiving nasogastric suction, or as melena. Because erosive gastritis involves superficial lesions, bleeding is not as rapid as with a lesion that extends deeper into the mucosa and may erode into a blood vessel. The slow loss of blood can be noted in continuously decreasing hemoglobin and hematocrit levels. Causes of erosive gastritis include NSAIDs, alcohol, and acute stress. Uncommon causes of gastric mucosal erosion include radiation, viral infections, caustic ingestion, and direct trauma (e.g., nasogastric tubes). Gastritis is often asymptomatic but may cause epigastric pain, nausea, vomiting, and bleeding. GI bleeding as a result of gastritis is usually not severe, except in the critically ill. Diagnosis of gastritis is accomplished by direct visualization with endoscopy (Arnell, 2002; McQuaid, 1999).

NSAID Gastritis

Thirty percent of patients receiving long-term NSAID therapy have gastritis at one time or another. NSAID-induced ulcers are more common in persons 55 years of age or older (Forsmark et al., 2000). Other factors that may increase the risk of NSAID-induced ulcers include previous history of peptic ulcer disease, corticosteroid use, high doses of NSAIDs, and recent use of NSAIDs. Also, the incidence is slightly higher in females (Arnell, 2002; Lingappa, 2003). NSAIDs compete with prostaglandin receptor sites in the gastric mucosa. Prostaglandins, particularly prostaglandin E, have been linked to mucosal repair and maintenance of mucosal integrity (Lindseth, 2003b). When these prostaglandin defense mechanisms are inhibited by the action of NSAIDs, severe inflammation and erosive injury can occur to the gastric mucosa. The incidence of NSAID gastritis may decrease with greater use of Cox 2 inhibitors. These new NSAIDs do not produce GI side effects because they do not inhibit prostaglandin E.

Alcoholic Gastritis

Chronic alcohol ingestion can result in inflammation of the gastric mucosa. The inflammation can progress to erosions and hemorrhage. Episodes of upper GI bleeding as a result of gastritis are usually mild and respond to withdrawal of alcohol and to pharmacologic therapy (2 to 3 weeks of H_2 receptor antagonists or sucralfate therapy) (Tucker, 2000).

Stress Gastritis

Bleeding associated with stress-related gastritis comes from diffuse, superficial lesions or erosions in the gastric mucosa. Decreased blood flow to the gut during times of severe stress may contribute to the breakdown in normal mucosal defenses (Flannery & Tucker, 2002; Lindseth, 2003b). Risk factors for stress gastritis include severe burns, sepsis, central nervous system trauma, shock, respiratory failure with mechanical ventilation, hepatic and renal failure, multiorgan dysfunction, and high doses of vasopressor agents (dopamine or Levophed). Increased length of stay in an ICU and increased length of time the patient has gone without enteral nutrition are associated with higher risk of developing stress-related gastritis. Endoscopic studies have shown that stress-related mucosal damage occurs in 52 to 100 percent of patients within 18 to 24 hours of admission to an ICU (Flannery & Tucker, 2002; Tucker, 2000). Diagnosis of gastritis is confirmed by direct endoscopic visualization.

Prevention and Treatment

Once significant GI bleeding from gastritis occurs (in about 2 percent of ICU patients), the mortality rate is more than 60 percent (Arnell, 2002; Beers & Berkhow, 1999; Prakash, 2001). Severe bleeding from a localized lesion may be treated with endoscopic sclerotherapy to cauterize the bleeding lesion. Diffusely bleeding lesions may respond to vasopressin administered intravenously or intra-arterially into a bleeding vessel. Vasopressin (also known as antidiuretic hormone) is a potent stimulator of smooth muscle, particularly those of capillaries and arterioles. It exerts its therapeutic effect in the management of GI bleeding by vasoconstriction of the splanchnic vessels, which reduces blood flow through the bleeding vessel. Vasopressin exerts its vasoconstricting effects systemically; therefore, untoward side effects of abdominal cramping, angina, hypertension, arrhythmias, and headache may occur. Concomitant use of nitroglycerin may reduce vasopressin effects on the coronary arteries, especially in persons with coronary artery disease (Prakash, 2000a, 2001). Surgical resection of the involved portions of the stomach is indicated if bleeding does not respond to more conservative treatment.

The incidence of stress-related gastritis can usually be decreased or prevented if the gastric pH is maintained above 4.0. This can be accomplished with the prophylactic administration of histamine receptor antagonists or oral antacids to all at-risk patients to raise the gastric pH above 4.0 (Beers & Berkhow, 1999; Lindseth, 2003b; McQuaid, 1999; Prakash, 2000b, 2001). Sucralfate, a mucosal binding agent that forms a protective barrier over the erosion, given orally is also effective in reducing stress-related bleeding. Early enteral feeding has been advocated as a means of lowering the incidence of bleeding in acutely ill persons.

Conservative treatment for NSAID-induced gastritis includes discontinuation of the drug, reduction to the lowest effective dose, or administration with meals. Patients with persistent gastritis or who are at increased risk of developing gastric mucosal injury should be treated with sucralfate, histamine receptor antagonists, or with a proton pump inhibitor (omeprazole). Misoprostol can be administered along with NSAID therapy to prevent ulcer formation. Misoprostol is a synthetic prostaglandin E analog that replaces the protective prostaglandins consumed with prostaglandin-inhibiting therapies (e.g., NSAIDs). Misoprostol is reserved for use with long-term NSAID therapy in high-risk persons (Prakash, 2000a). If the patient has adequate renal function, switching the patient to a Cox 2 inhibitor NSAID may prevent NSAID-induced gastritis.

Esophageal and Gastric Varices

Upper GI bleeding from esophageal or gastric varices is associated with cirrhosis, portal hypertension, and portal or splenic vein thrombosis. Bleeding from esophagogastric varices is usually massive and occurs without warning. Portal hypertension causes the development of collateral venous pathways, called *varices,* which are located in the esophagus and stomach. Hepatic cirrhosis as a result of alcohol abuse is the most common cause of variceal bleeding in the United States. (See Module 31, "Acute Hepatic Dysfunction," for an overview of the etiology, pathophysiology, and treatment of bleeding esophageal or gastric varices.)

Mallory–Weiss Tears

A Mallory–Weiss tear is a small laceration in the mucosa at the gastroesophageal junction. Fifty percent of these patients give a history of vomiting that precedes the hematemesis (Andreoli et al., 2000; Forsmark et al., 2000; Prakash, 2001). High-risk patients are those with a history of alcohol abuse. Bleeding as a result of a Mallory–Weiss tear often presents with mild to massive hematemesis. Most tears stop bleeding spontaneously, and rebleeding is infrequent. Diagnosis is confirmed by upper GI endoscopy, and treatment consists of histamine receptor antagonists, antacids, and embolization or selective infusion of vasopressin into the bleeding vessel (Forsmark et al., 2000).

Arteriovenous Malformation

An arteriovenous malformation (AVM), sometimes referred to as an *angiodysplasia*, is a small, abnormal mucosal or submucosal blood vessel that has a tendency to bleed. Arteriovenous malformations can occur in both the upper GI and the lower GI tracts, but they are most commonly located in the cecal region of the lower GI tract. The cause of arteriovenous malformations is unknown but appears to be genetic. Once GI bleeding from an arteriovenous malformation occurs, recurrent GI bleeding, chronic anemia, or severe acute GI bleeding is the usual clinical course (Beers & Berkhow, 1999; Flannery & Tucker, 2002). Gastrointestinal arteriovenous malformations are common in the elderly with other comorbid illness, such as valvular heart disease, chronic renal failure, liver disease, and collagen vascular disease, and those undergoing radiotherapy. Upper GI bleeding as a result of an arteriovenous malformation is most commonly diagnosed by upper GI endoscopy. Definitive treatment of the underlying or concomitant conditions (e.g., valvuloplasty or kidney transplantation) can cure bleeding arteriovenous malformations. Endoscopic sclerotherapy is used palliatively because new arteriovenous malformations can continue to develop in high-risk patients (Farrell & Friedman, 2001).

In summary, peptic ulcer disease (PUD) accounts for the most common cause of upper GI bleeding and is frequently associated with *H. pylori* bacterial infection. Peptic ulcer disease erodes the gastric mucosa making it susceptible to the damaging effects of acid. Peptic ulcers can be classified as duodenal or gastric, with duodenal ulcers being the most common type. Another etiology of upper GI bleeding is acute erosive or hemorrhagic gastritis, which involves severe inflammation and erosion of the gastric mucosa. The most common clinical manifestation of erosive gastritis is upper GI bleeding. Causes of erosive or hemorrhagic gastritis include use of NSAIDs, alcohol, and acute physiological stress. Prevention of stress-related gastritis can be accomplished by maintaining the gastric pH above 4.0 with the administration of histamine receptor antagonists or oral antacids to all at-risk patients. Early enteral feeding can lower the incidence of gastritis in acutely ill persons. Esophageal and gastric varices are further etiologies of upper GI bleeding, and are associated with cirrhosis, portal hypertension, and portal or splenic vein thrombosis. Mallory–Weiss tears are also responsible for upper GI bleeding in patients with a history of alcohol abuse, and a history of vomiting that precedes the hematemesis. Arteriovenous malformation occurs in both the upper and lower GI tracts, and has a tendency to bleed. The cause of arteriovenous malformation is unknown but is more common in the elderly with comorbid illness.

SECTION SIX REVIEW

1. Which of the following is a cause of acute upper GI bleeding?
   A. Mallory–Weiss tear
   B. diverticula
   C. ischemic bowel disease
   D. ulcerative colitis
2. _____ is the most common cause of upper GI bleeding.
   A. Esophageal varices
   B. Peptic ulcer disease
   C. Arteriovenous malformation
   D. Stress gastritis
3. Peptic ulcers occur in the
   A. stomach and ileum
   B. duodenum and colon
   C. stomach and peritoneum
   D. stomach and duodenum
4. A 35-year-old male is diagnosed with PUD. His father had a gastric ulcer. He smokes one pack of cigarettes per day, takes a diuretic to treat his hypertension, and is obese (310 pounds at 6 feet tall). He takes aspirin every day for his "arthritis." How many risk factors for PUD does this person have?

A. two
B. three
C. four
D. five
5. Peptic ulcers are caused by
   A. colonization of bacteria within the GI tract
   B. hypersecretion of pancreatic enzymes
   C. underproduction of bicarbonate
   D. disruption of the mucosal barrier
6. Gastric ulcer symptoms
   A. are relieved by eating
   B. are aggravated by eating
   C. are not affected by eating
   D. follow a consistent pattern
7. Stress-related mucosal damage occurs in 52 to 100 percent of patients within _____ hours of admission to an ICU.
   A. 24 to 48
   B. 8 to 16
   C. 18 to 24
   D. 48 to 72

8. Which drug is often prescribed along with long-term NSAID therapy in high-risk patients to prevent the development of ulcers?
   A. neomycin
   B. misoprostol
   C. sucralfate
   D. antacids

9. GI bleeding as a result of a Mallory–Weiss tear often presents with
   A. hematemesis
   B. hematochezia
   C. melena
   D. pain

Answers: 1. A, 2. B, 3. D, 4. B, 5. D, 6. B, 7. C, 8. B, 9. A

SECTION SEVEN: Acute Lower GI Bleeding

At the completion of this section, the learner will be able to describe the etiology and pathophysiology of acute lower GI bleeding.

The two most common causes of acute lower GI bleeding are diverticulosis and AVM. Other common causes of chronic lower GI bleeding are internal hemorrhoids and neoplasms. Table 30–8 summarizes the causes and characteristics of lower GI bleeding. Bleeding stops spontaneously in 80 to 90 percent of patients, with a risk of recurrence in 25 percent of the patients. Unlike upper GI bleeding, the majority of lower GI bleeds are slow and intermittent and do not require hospitalization. Less frequent causes of lower GI bleeding include ischemic bowel disease and inflammatory bowel disease. Lower GI bleeding is included in this module because 10 to 20 percent of the acute lower GI bleeding cases do not resolve spontaneously and, therefore, require high-acuity nursing (Arnell, 2002).

TABLE 30–8 Causes and Characteristics of Lower GI Bleeding

CAUSE	CHARACTERISTICS
Diverticula	Sustained, dark, occasionally massive bleeding throughout the colon
Arteriovenous malformation	Intermittent, both dark and bright red bleeding, clots, coming from cecal area
Internal hemorrhoids	Bright red blood per rectum, intermittent with bowel movements
Ischemic bowel disease	Intermittent, mostly dark blood; abdominal tenderness, fever, leukocytosis
Carcinoma	Occult bleeding with intermittent melena, right colon tumors
Inflammatory bowel disease	Intermittent bleeding, mixed with frequent bowel movement

Data from Krumberger, J. M., & Hammer, B. (1998). Gastrointestinal disorders. In M. R. Kinney, S. B. Dunbar, J. A. Brooks-Brunn, N. Molter, & J. M. Vitello-Cicciu (Eds.). AACN's clinical reference for critical care nursing, (4th ed.). St. Louis: C. V. Mosby; Driscoll, C. J. (1999). Acute gastrointestinal bleed. In L. Bucher & S. Melander (Eds.). Critical care nursing. Philadelphia: W. B. Saunders; Arnell, T. (2002). Gastrointestinal bleeding. In F. S. Bongard & D. Y. Sue (Eds.), Current critical care diagnosis and treatment, (2nd ed., p.762). New York: Lange.

Diverticular Bleeding

Diverticular bleeding can be massive and life threatening but occurs in only 3 percent of patients with diverticulosis. It is the most common etiology of major lower GI bleeding. Bleeding from a diverticulum occurs when an artery penetrates and ruptures into the sac of the diverticulum, a result of pressure erosion (Arnell, 2002). Bleeding stops spontaneously in 80 percent of patients, with no further intervention necessary. However, 25 percent of these cases rebleed requiring surgical intervention or angiography with intra-arterial infusion of vasopressin (Beers & Berkhow, 1999).

Arteriovenous Malformations

Bleeding from an arteriovenous malformation is usually slow, chronic, and can be occult. Patients usually present with weakness, fatigue, dyspnea on exertion, and guaiac-positive stools. Bleeding from an arteriovenous malformation is rarely massive. A typical bleeding episode requires less than 2 to 4 units of blood and is not associated with hypotension. The elderly have increased risk of severe blood loss from this type of GI bleed. Arteriovenous malformations are angiodysplastic lesions that are usually small, superficial, multiple, and located in the colon and cecum. The cause of an arteriovenous malformation is not clear, but they appear to be associated with cardiac disease, low-flow states, and the aging process. Bleeding occurs from weakened, friable vessel wall lesions caused by chronic tension and dilation of blood vessels most commonly located in the cecal area of the intestine. In cases in which the bleeding does not stop spontaneously, arterial embolization and surgery may be necessary (Arnell, 2002; Stamos, 2002).

Ischemic Bowel Disease

Ischemic bowel disease can be defined as inflammation of the colon resulting from an interruption of the colonic blood supply (Arnell, 2002; Beers & Berkhow, 1999). It may result from occlusion of a major artery, small-vessel disease, venous obstruction, low-flow states (e.g., cardiogenic shock), or intestinal obstruction. Intestinal ischemia can develop postoperatively following vascular bypass or colon resection with anastomosis. In the elderly, risk factors for developing ischemic bowel disease include atherosclerosis, atrial fibrillation, and hypotension. Older patients are most commonly affected, although younger patients with diabetes, pancreatitis, heart disease, sickle cell disease, or systemic lupus erythematosus are also at risk.

Bleeding from ischemic bowel disease is often associated with anticoagulant use (25 percent of all bleeding cases) (Arnell, 2002; Beers & Berkhow, 1999; Braunwald, 2001; Stamos, 2002). The bleeding is usually intermittent, with mixed dark and bright red blood and clots visible from the rectum. Fever and abdominal pain are usually present. Lower GI endoscopy reveals purple discoloration of the bowel, often in the presence of erosion and ulceration. Radiographic x-rays are nonspecific but may reveal abnormal air pockets if perforation is present. Barium contrast studies reveal characteristic "thumbprints," suggesting a necrotic process. Arterial or venous occlusion of the mesenteric vasculature should be suspected and ruled out when ischemia of the bowel is included in the differential diagnosis. Treatment of ischemic bowel disease involves restoration of blood circulation to the intestines and might include fluid resuscitation, optimization of cardiac output, and treatment of any underlying disease. Antibiotics may be required for infections. Resection of the affected bowel may be necessary for fulminant disease or severe bleeding. Patients with ischemic bowel disease often have other medical problems, including multiple organ failure, and, therefore, have a mortality rate of about 50 percent (Beers & Berkhow, 1999; Crittormson & Burbick, 1989).

Inflammatory Bowel Disease

Bloody diarrhea is the most common symptom of inflammatory bowel disease. The degree of bleeding is usually light to moderate but it can be massive. In very rare instances, life-threatening bleeding can result when the underlying inflammation ulcerates into adjacent arteries (Arnell, 2002). The treatment of bleeding associated with inflammatory bowel disease is management of the underlying disorder with corticosteroids (Arnell, 2002; Flannery & Tucker, 2002). If the bleeding is uncontrollable by medical means, then surgical resection of the affected portion of the bowel is necessary.

Neoplasms

Benign and malignant tumors and polyps are common among the elderly, with 10 to 20 percent of these patients developing bleeding lesions (Lingenfelser & Ell, 2001). Bleeding from neoplasms is usually slow, chronic, and self-limiting. Only rarely is there acute blood loss of significant proportions from a neoplasm. In these cases, bowel resection and tumor excision are indicated.

In summary, the two most common causes of acute lower GI bleeding are diverticulosis and arteriovenous malformation. Other causes include internal hemorrhoids and neoplasms. Lower GI bleeding is slow and intermittent and does not require hospitalization. However, 10 to 20 percent of patients with acute lower GI bleeding require hospitalization to stop the bleeding. Diverticular bleeding can be massive and life threatening and is the most common etiology of significant lower GI bleeding. Treatment with surgical resection and/or angiography with intra-arterial infusion of vasopressin are indicated in cases with recurrent and significant bleeding. Bleeding from arteriovenous malformations is usually slow, chronic, and can be occult associated with weakness, fatigue, dyspnea on exertion, and occult blood in the stools. In cases in which the bleeding does not stop spontaneously, arterial embolization and surgery may be necessary. Lower GI bleeding from ischemic bowel disease is the result of inflammation of the colon from an interruption of the colonic blood supply. Bleeding from ischemic bowel disease is often associated with anticoagulant use and is often intermittent. Lower GI endoscopy allows visualization of the affected bowel. Treatment involves restoration of blood circulation to the intestines and may include fluid resuscitation, optimization of cardiac output, and treatment of any underlying disease. Resection of the affected bowel may be necessary for fulminant disease or severe bleeding. Bloody diarrhea from inflammatory bowel disease is usually light to moderate. In rare instances, life-threatening bleeding can result when the underlying inflammation ulcerates into adjacent arteries. Treatment involves management of the underlying disorder with corticosteroids. Benign and malignant tumors and polyps are common among the elderly. Bleeding from neoplasm is usually slow, chronic, and self-limiting, rarely involving significant blood loss. Bowel resection and tumor excision are indicated in cases where bleeding is significant.

SECTION SEVEN REVIEW

1. Diverticula are found throughout the
   A. stomach
   B. small intestine
   C. colon
   D. GI tract

2. Sustained, dark red lower GI bleeding from the large intestine is a characteristic of a bleeding
   A. diverticula
   B. hemorrhoid
   C. tumor
   D. angiodysplasia

3. Angiodysplasia (arteriovenous malformation) of the lower GI tract is associated with
  A. renal disease
  B. cardiac disease
  C. a high-fat diet
  D. an inflammatory process

4. Ischemic bowel disease is defined as a(n)
  A. malignant process
  B. infectious process

  C. chronic stress process
  D. inflammatory process

5. Treatment of ischemic bowel disease involves
  A. steroid administration
  B. high-dose narcotics
  C. fluid resuscitation
  D. enemas until clear

Answers: 1. C, 2. A, 3. B, 4. D, 5. C

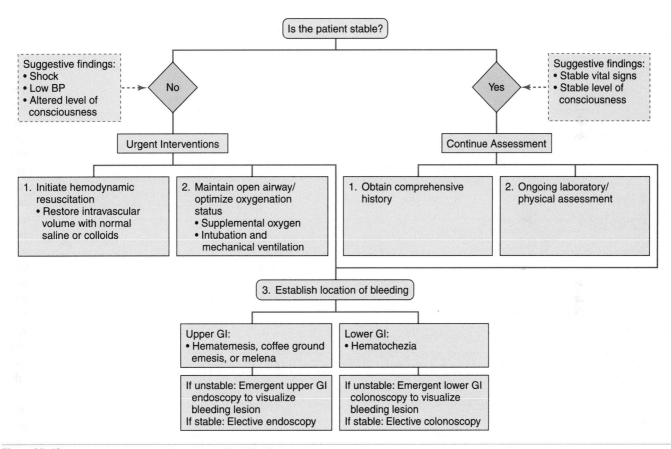

Figure 30–12 ■ Diagnostic approach to the patient with GI bleeding.

SECTION EIGHT: Management of Acute Gastrointestinal Bleeding

At the completion of this section, the learner will be able to describe the management of acute GI bleeding.

Patients who are experiencing acute GI bleeding must be approached in a systematic manner (Fig. 30–12). This approach should be collaborative and include (1) initial assessment, (2) resuscitation, (3) definitive diagnosis, and (4) treatment.

Caring for the patient with acute GI bleeding is a collaborative endeavor. The nurse's role includes the following (in collaboration with the physician):

■ Assess the severity of blood loss.
■ Replace a sufficient amount of fluids and blood products to counteract shock.
■ Assist in the diagnosis of the cause of the bleeding.
■ Plan and implement treatment.
■ Manage the ongoing plan of care and monitor progress.

■ Provide supportive care and education to the patient and significant others because any bleeding experience is potentially life threatening.

Initial Assessment

To assess severity of blood loss, the nurse must determine hemodynamic stability. Evidence of instability includes decreased blood pressure or orthostatic hypotension, decreased or altered level of consciousness, and decreased urine output (which is suggestive of fluid volume deficit). Evidence of hemodynamic instability in the presence of hematemesis, hematochezia, or melena should be considered an emergency until proven otherwise, and admission to an ICU is recommended. The following are guidelines for admission to an ICU:

1. Clearly documented frank hematemesis
2. Coffee-ground emesis and either melena or hematochezia
3. Hemodynamic instability (hypotension, tachycardia, or orthostatic hypotension)
4. A drop in hematocrit of 5 points after fluid resuscitation
5. A significant unexplained increase in the BUN when GI bleeding is suspected (increased BUN suggests fluid volume deficit or metabolism of blood within the GI tract)

Resuscitation

Resuscitation is the primary goal of early management in the hemodynamically unstable patient and mandates the maintenance of intravascular volume and tissue oxygenation. Blood specimens for type and crossmatching, CBC, PT/PTT, and chemistries should be obtained. Nasal oxygen and pulse oximetry are useful, especially in the elderly or in patients with a history of cardiac or pulmonary disease. Close nursing assessment of the patient's level of consciousness and oxygenation status is important in the acute phase. Endotracheal intubation should be considered for decreased level of consciousness, shock, or massive bleeding, and the nurse should have emergency intubation and oxygen equipment ready if needed. Vital signs, orthostatic blood pressure changes, and urine output are valuable clinical indicators of perfusion and blood volume. An indwelling catheter should be placed to monitor urine output because this is a good measure of perfusion. Central venous pressures or pulmonary capillary wedge pressures are also helpful to monitor volume status.

Volume resuscitation is accomplished with crystalloid (normal saline or lactated Ringer's) at a rate to maintain a systolic blood pressure of higher than 90 mm Hg through at least two large-bore IV lines. If, after 2 to 3 liters of crystalloid infusion, the patient remains unstable, an infusion of blood products (packed red cells or whole blood) should be considered. Vasoconstricting drugs (vasopressors) are generally not indicated because hypovolemia is usually the cause of the hypo-

tension. Packed red cells are transfused for massive bleeding to keep the hematocrit higher than 28 to 30 percent. Patients with cardiac or pulmonary disease may require transfusion to a higher hematocrit (higher than 30 percent). Transfusions of whole blood may be considered in massively bleeding patients because they provide increased colloid osmotic pressure, thus decreasing the patient's total fluid requirements. O-negative blood can be used until the patient's blood has been cross-matched. A blood warmer should be considered for rapid fluid or blood administration to prevent hypothermia. Each unit of blood should elevate the hematocrit by 3 points. Fresh frozen plasma is considered for patients who have a coagulopathy (increased PT or PTT) or who have been on Coumadin therapy. If the patient has thrombocytopenia, platelet transfusion should be considered to maintain the platelet count above 50,000/mm^3 (Andreoli et al., 2000; Beers & Berkhow, 1999; Haist & Robbins, 2002; Lefor et al., 2002; Prakash, 2000a, 2001). An early surgical consult is essential and should be obtained within the first few hours of the onset of bleeding.

For patients with persistent bleeding, some type of therapeutic intervention is necessary. This intervention can be pharmacotherapy, mechanical (balloon) tamponade (Sengstaken–Blakemore tube), endoscopic therapy (sclerotherapy), or surgery. Once blood volume is restored, the patient is monitored for evidence of further bleeding (e.g., tachycardia, decreased blood pressure, hematemesis, bloody or tarry stools). Specific therapy depends on the bleeding site (refer to previously discussed etiologies of GI bleeding for specific treatments). Tables 30–9 through 30–11 summarize therapeutic pharmacologic and interventional therapies in the setting of acute GI bleeding. Definitive diagnosis of the source of the GI bleeding should be undertaken as soon as the patient is stable. Table 30–12 summarizes the various endoscopies of the GI system.

Arterial Angiotherapy Interventions in Persistent GI Hemorrhage

Selective arterial infusion of vasopressin is used to control massive bleeding in patients who have peptic ulcer disease, stress ulcers, erosive gastritis, Mallory–Weiss tear, and arteriovenous malformation. Selective catheterization of the bleeding artery is required for infusion of vasopressin. Arterial embolization is an alternative to arterial vasopressin where the bleeding vessel is selectively catheterized and a coagulant is placed in the vessel (Beers & Berkhow, 1999; Prakash, 2001).

Therapy for Specific Lesions

Bleeding peptic ulcers can often be diagnosed and treated with endoscopy. Surgery is considered for severe hemorrhage or recurrent bleeding. Arterial angiography can be used to control massive bleeding from peptic ulcers in patients who are considered to be poor surgical risks.

TABLE 30–9 Therapeutic Pharmacologic Interventions in Acute GI Bleeding

INTERVENTION	EFFECTS	COMMENTS
Antacids	Neutralize gastric acidity	Therapy for peptic ulcer disease and gastritis
		Must act in the stomach, in direct contact with the gastric mucosa
Histamine receptor antagonists (H₂ blockers)	Block histamine stimulation of acid-secreting cells; reduce acid secretion	Therapy for peptic ulcer disease and gastritis
Sucralfate	Forms a protective barrier, allowing ulcer healing	Therapy for peptic ulcer disease and gastritis
		Must act in the stomach, in direct contact with the gastric mucosa
Proton pump inhibitors	Inhibits acid secretory pump (H⁺, K⁺-ATPase)	Therapy for peptic ulcer disease and gastritis
Prostaglandins (misoprostol)	Inhibits gastric secretion, and stimulates mucosal defense mechanisms	Adjunct prophylactic therapy to prevent development of ulcers with chronic nonsteroidal anti-inflammatory drug use

Data from McQuaid, K. R. (1999). Alimentary tract. In L. M. Tierney, S. J. McPhee, & M. A. Papadakis (Eds.), Current medical diagnosis and treatment, *(38th ed.). Norwalk, CT: Appleton & Lange; Deglin, J., & Vallerand, A. (2001).* Davis's drug guide for nurses, *(8th ed.). Philadelphia: F. A. Davis.*

TABLE 30–10 Interventions for Severe GI Hemorrhage (Evidence of Hemodynamic Instability and/or Persistent Bleeding)

INTERVENTION	EFFECTS	COMMENTS
Vasopressin	Decreases portal pressure by vasoconstricting splanchnic arteries. Untoward effects include decreased coronary blood flow, increased blood pressure	Treatment of severe hemorrhage as a result of upper GI variceal bleeding, erosive gastritis, arteriovenous malformations, and Mallory–Weiss tears
Somatostatin	Decreases portal pressure by vasoconstriction of splanchnic circulation	See above
Octreotide	A synthetic analog of somatostatin; has same action as somatostatin	See above
Mechanical tamponade	Provides tamponade to actively bleeding gastric/esophageal varices	Treatment of bleeding esophageal and gastric varices

Data from McQuaid, K. R. (1999). Alimentary tract. In L. M. Tierney, S. J. McPhee, & M. A. Papadakis (Eds.), Current medical diagnosis and treatment, *(38th ed.). Norwalk, CT: Appleton & Lange; Deglin, J., & Vallerand, A. (2001).* Davis's drug guide for nurses, *(8th ed.). Philadelphia: F. A. Davis.*

TABLE 30–11 Arterial Angiotherapy Interventions in GI Hemorrhage

INTERVENTION	DESCRIPTION	COMMENTS
Selective arterial infusion of vasopressin	Requires selective catheterization of the bleeding artery for infusion of vasopressin.	Used to control massive bleeding in those patients who have peptic ulcer disease, stress ulcers, erosive gastritis, and Mallory–Weiss tear
Arterial embolization	An alternative to arterial vasopressin where the bleeding vessel is selectively catheterized, and a coagulant is placed in the vessel	

From Beers, M. H., & Berkhow, R. (Eds.). (1999). The Merck manual of diagnosis and therapy, (17th ed.). Whitehouse Station, NJ: Merck Research Laboratories; Del Valle, J. (2001). Peptic ulcer disease and related conditions. In E. Braunwald, A. Fauci, D. Kasper, S. Hauser, D. Longo, & J. L. Jameson (Eds.), Harrison's principles of internal medicine, (15th ed.). New York: McGraw Hill; Prakash, C. (2001). Gastrointestinal diseases: Gastrointestinal bleeding. In S. N. Ahya, K. Flood, & S. Paranjothi (Eds.), The Washington manual of medical therapeutics, (3rd ed., p. 349). Philadelphia: J. B. Lippincott.

Bleeding from esophageal or gastric varices requires ICU admission. These patients will need endotracheal intubation and early endoscopy. Sclerotherapy should be performed as soon as a diagnosis of variceal bleeding is confirmed. Rebleeding occurs in 50 percent of cases following sclerotherapy (Prakash, 2001). Intravenous vasopressin or octreotide (somatostatin analog) may be used as an alternative to sclerotherapy (or concomitantly) to reduce portal pressures (see Module 31). Balloon tamponade therapy is an effective temporary method to stop variceal bleeding while awaiting more definitive therapy. Shunt surgery or transjugular intrahepatic portosystemic shunt (TIPS) should be considered if the risk is high for recurrent variceal bleeding (see Module 31).

TABLE 30–12 Endoscopic Interventions in GI Hemorrhage

INTERVENTION	DESCRIPTION	COMMENTS
Endoscopic injection sclerotherapy	Sclerosing agent is injected into bleeding vessel	Treatment bleeding from varices, Mallory–Weiss tears, arteriovenous malformations, ulcers
Endoscopic electrocoagulation	Direct electric current is applied to bleeding lesion = fibrosis	See above
Endoscopic laser therapy	Direct application of heat to coagulate bleeding lesion	See above
Endoscopic heater probe	Direct electric current is applied to coagulate bleeding lesion	See above

Data from McQuaid, K. R. (1999). Alimentary tract. In L. M. Tierney, S. J. McPhee, & M. A. Papadakis (Eds.), Current medical diagnosis and treatment, (38th ed.). Norwalk, CT: Appleton & Lange; Laine, L. (2001). Gastrointestinal bleeding. In E. Braunwald, A. Fauci. D. Kasper, S. Hauser, D. Longo, & J. L. Jameson (Eds.), Harrison's principles of internal medicine, (15th ed.). New York: McGraw Hill.

Bleeding Mallory–Weiss tears that do not stop spontaneously require therapeutic endoscopy or selective arterial angiotherapy, whereas bleeding AVMs of the colon can be treated with arterial angiotherapy or therapeutic endoscopic procedures. In diverticular bleeding, selective arterial vasopressin is often effective in stopping the bleeding. Selective arterial therapy requires catheterization of the bleeding vessel for infusion of vasopressin. Surgery is needed when the bleeding is severe (Beers & Berkhow, 1999; Forsmark et al., 2000; Laine, 2001; McQuaid, 1999; Prakash, 2001).

In summary, patients who are experiencing acute GI bleeding must be managed in a systematic, collaborative approach, which includes initial assessment, resuscitation, definitive diagnosis, and treatment. Initial assessment of the severity of blood loss must include an assessment of the patient's hemodynamic stability. Patients are evaluated for admission to an ICU using evidence-based criteria, which includes frank hematemesis, melena, or hematochezia; hemodynamic instability; reduction in serum hematocrit of 5 points after fluid resuscitation; and significant, unexplained increase in the BUN. Resuscitation is the primary goal of early management in the hemodynamically unstable bleeding patient and mandates the maintenance of intravascular volume and tissue oxygenation. This management might involve blood collection for type and cross matching, CBC, PT/PTT, and chemistries; oxygen administration or endotracheal intubation; frequent nursing assessment of level of consciousness, hemodynamics, vital signs, urine output, and volume status. Volume resuscitation is accomplished with crystalloid or blood product infusion.

SECTION EIGHT REVIEW

1. The first step in the collaborative treatment of a patient who is experiencing an acute GI bleed is
   A. assessment
   B. resuscitation
   C. diagnosis
   D. treatment

2. To assess the severity of blood loss, the nurse should determine
   A. respiratory status
   B. hemodynamic status
   C. level of consciousness
   D. the degree of impairment

3. Signs and symptoms that provide supporting evidence of a fluid volume deficit are
   A. abdominal distention
   B. unchanged level of consciousness
   C. orthostatic hypotension
   D. increased urine output

4. In a patient who has had a GI bleed, an increased BUN suggests fluid volume deficit or
   A. onset of acute renal failure
   B. development of systemic inflammatory response
   C. an acute infectious process
   D. metabolism of blood in the gut

5. Laboratory tests needed in the management of a patient with an acute GI hemorrhage include
   A. hourly ABG measurements
   B. blood and urine cultures
   C. type and crossmatch blood for possible transfusion
   D. stool culture for occult blood

6. Volume resuscitation is usually accomplished with
   A. intravenous crystalloid infusion
   B. vasoconstricting drugs
   C. blood transfusion
   D. normal saline via a nasogastric tube

Answers: 1. A, 2. B, 3. C, 4. D, 5. C, 6. A

SECTION NINE: Acute Intestinal Obstruction and Paralytic Ileus

At the completion of this section, the learner will be able to describe the etiology, pathophysiology, and management of acute intestinal obstruction and paralytic ileus.

Acute Small-Bowel Obstruction

Obstruction of the small intestine is a common surgical complication, often as a result of the development of adhesions following abdominal surgery. Other causes of obstruction are hernias, volvulus, Crohn's disease, and tumors. Most obstructions result from actual occlusion of the intestinal lumen (mechanical or physical), resulting in distention and gas and fluid accumulation above the obstruction. When the small bowel is obstructed, distention with gas and fluid occurs proximal to the obstruction. Swallowed air is the major cause of the distention. Bacterial fermentation within the lumen of the intestine produces other gases (methane). Inflammation leads to transudation of fluid from the extracellular space into the intestinal lumen and peritoneal cavity. Fluid and electrolytes become trapped within the obstructed bowel and may leak out into the peritoneum, further disturbing electrolyte and fluid balance. The inflammatory process causes large amounts of fluid and sodium to accumulate within the intestine (mass effect). Fluid losses may be so severe that hypotension results, which can result in cardiovascular collapse unless the condition is recognized and treated. In severe cases, perforation of the intestinal wall can occur, with spillage of the bowel contents into the peritoneal cavity (Krumberger, 1998; Podolsky & Isselbacher, 2001; Prakash, 2001; Stamos, 2002; Urden et al., 2001).

In severe cases of bowel obstruction, the intestine can become strangulated. **Intestinal strangulation** occurs when the intestine "twists" itself to such an extent that circulation is interrupted. Strangulation can result in necrosis, perforation, and sepsis. Corrective surgery is generally the treatment of choice to prevent ischemic bowel problems. Appropriately treated, simple obstruction has a low mortality rate (less than 2 percent), whereas strangulation is associated with a high mortality rate (up to 25 percent if surgery is delayed). When the obstruction is located in the colon, it usually stems from a malignant tumor (McQuaid, 1999; Podolsky & Isselbacher, 2001; Stamos, 2002).

Acute Paralytic Ileus

Paralytic ileus (adynamic ileus) involves bowel obstruction as a result of a loss of intestinal peristalsis in the absence of any mechanical (physical) obstruction commonly seen in hospitalized patients. It can occur anywhere along the GI tract as a complication from trauma, handling of the bowel during surgery, electrolyte disturbances (hypokalemia, hypocalcemia, and hy-

pomagnesemia), intestinal ischemia, peritonitis, and sepsis. In addition, there are multiple medications that reduce gastric motility (e.g., opioids, anticholinergics, and phenothiazines), thus contributing to the development of paralytic ileus (Podolsky & Isselbacher, 2001).

Ogilvie's syndrome involves paralytic ileus of the colon. This is a severe form of ileus that often arises in bedridden patients who have serious systemic illnesses. The abdomen is usually silent, and abdominal cramping is not present, but tenderness may be noted. Abdominal x-rays show a dilated colon. Dehydration is usually present as a consequence of fluid translocation into distended loops of intestine (Lindseth, 2003a; Prakash, 2001; Prakash & Clouse, 2000).

Clinical Manifestations

Laboratory and radiologic examinations, along with history and physical findings, aid in diagnosing intestinal obstruction. The hallmark clinical manifestation of intestinal obstruction is abdominal distention. Small-bowel obstruction is characterized by cramping and periumbilical pain that occurs in waves, with periods of relative comfort in between the waves of pain. Vomiting, possibly profuse, soon follows the onset of pain and is usually bilious with a large quantity of mucus. Electrolyte imbalances and intraluminal loss of fluids occur, with dehydration soon following. Visible peristaltic waves may be observed on the abdomen, and high-pitched tinkles are auscultated during the painful spasms. The abdomen may be tender to palpation. If rebound tenderness develops, the nurse should observe for signs and symptoms of shock as a result of perforation. Symptoms of colonic paralytic ileus (Ogilvie's syndrome) include abdominal distention and diminished bowel sounds without pain (Stamos, 2002).

Laboratory Findings

Hematology, electrolyte, and chemistry studies will reflect inflammation, fluid, and electrolyte imbalances. Mild leukocytosis (greater than 15,000) is common, whereas WBC elevations from 15,000 to 25,000 may occur with strangulation and perforation (Silen, 2001; Urden et al., 2001). Serum BUN, creatinine, sodium, and osmolality levels become elevated as fluid and electrolytes leak out of the obstructed bowel and third spacing (translocation of electrolytes and fluid into the intestinal lumen) occurs. Increases in serum amylase levels are common.

Radiologic Findings

Radiology films are taken with the patient in upright, flat, and side-lying positions. Distended bowel loops will reveal air–fluid levels in a "ladderlike" pattern. Distention is more pronounced within the colon in patients with paralytic ileus. Direct visualization and barium studies may help to confirm the diagnosis (McQuaid, 1999; Silen, 2001; Stamos, 2002).

Treatment

It is imperative to identify those patients at risk for developing a bowel obstruction or motility problem. Patients at risk for developing bowel obstruction are the elderly, postoperative, bedridden, and those with dysfunction of multiple body systems. Initial therapy is directed toward fluid resuscitation and stabilization of the patient. Oral food and fluids are withheld, and a nasogastric tube (Salem-sump) is inserted and attached to low, intermittent suction to relieve vomiting and to decompress abdominal distention. Colonoscopy with decompression is sometimes useful in Ogilvie's syndrome. Isotonic intravenous fluid administration should be used to treat dehydration. Electrolyte losses should be replaced and continually monitored by the nurse. The extent of fluid resuscitation is best guided by the urine output, though in the elderly or those with cardiopulmonary disease, a pulmonary artery catheter (Swan–Ganz) is the best means of determining fluid volume needs. The nurse should closely monitor the patient's urine output using an indwelling urinary drainage catheter. (Refer to Module 9 for an explanation of pulmonary artery catheters.) If the patient demonstrates peritoneal signs (boardlike abdominal distention with severe pain) and strangulation is suspected, broad-spectrum antibiotics should be considered to provide anaerobic and gram-negative coverage. Early surgical consult is advised in high-risk patients. All cases of complete obstruction require surgical resection of the affected bowel (Beers & Berkhow, 1999; McQuaid, 1999; Prakash, 2001; Prakash & Clouse, 2000; Silen, 2001; Stamos, 2002).

In summary, acute intestinal obstruction and paralytic ileus are common surgical complications. Acute intestinal obstruction is often a result of the development of adhesions following abdominal surgery. Hernias, volvulus, Crohn's disease, and tumors are other causes of obstruction. Acute small-bowel obstruction is associated with distention as a result of fluid and gas accumulation above the point of obstruction, which results in inflammation. The inflammation is associated with transudation of fluid and electrolytes with fluid losses that can be severe resulting in homodynamic instability and perforation of the intestinal wall. Corrective surgery is often indicated to prevent ischemic bowel complications. If the patient exhibits peritoneal signs, intestinal strangulation should be suspected, and broad-spectrum antibiotics should be administered. Early surgical consult for resection of affected bowel is advised in high-risk patients. Paralytic ileus involves bowel obstruction as a result of a loss of intestinal peristalsis in the absence of any mechanical obstruction anywhere along the GI tract as a complication of prolonged immobility, surgery, trauma, electrolyte disturbances, intestinal ischemia, peritonitis, and sepsis. Medications that can reduce gastric motility include opioids, anticholinergics, and phenothiazines. Clinical manifestation of intestinal obstruction includes abdominal distention, cramping, vomiting, electrolyte imbalances, dehydration, and loss of bowel sounds. Laboratory findings consistent with intestinal obstruction include leukocytosis, and elevated serum BUN, creatinine, sodium, amylase, and osmolality levels as fluid and electrolytes leak out of the obstructed bowel occurs. Direct visualization and barium studies may help to confirm the diagnosis of bowel obstruction. Treatment involves fluid resuscitation, decompression of abdominal distention, and electrolyte replacements.

SECTION NINE REVIEW

1. Common mechanical causes of small-bowel obstruction are
   A. adhesions
   B. myocardial infarction
   C. closed-head injury
   D. inflammatory bowel disease

2. If a patient with a small-bowel obstruction develops rebound tenderness with "boardlike" distention, the nurse should suspect
   A. constipation
   B. perforation
   C. Ogilvie's syndrome
   D. retroperitoneal bleeding

3. _____ accumulates in the bowel proximal to the actual bowel obstruction, resulting in distention.
   A. Fluid
   B. Blood
   C. Stool
   D. Pus

4. Bowel that "twists" itself to such an extent that circulation is interrupted is known as
   A. peritonitis
   B. perforation
   C. strangulation
   D. peristalsis

5. Strangulation is associated with a mortality rate of
   A. less than 2 percent
   B. 50 percent or less
   C. 80 percent or less
   D. 25 percent or less

Answers: 1. A, 2. B, 3. A, 4. C, 5. D

SECTION TEN: Intra-abdominal Hypertension and Abdominal Compartment Syndrome

At the completion of this section, the learner will be able to describe the etiology, pathophysiology, assessment, and management of intra-abdominal hypertension and abdominal compartment syndrome.

Abdominal compartment syndrome (ACS) is a rare but life-threatening condition resulting from an acute expansion of abdominal contents. Increased abdominal pressure (IAP) causes intra-abdominal hypertension (IAH) which impairs blood flow to multiple organs, causing tissue ischemia and organ failure. It is important to recognize patients who are at risk for abdominal compartment syndrome and identify early signs of trouble so that appropriate treatment can be initiated.

IAH/ACS Continuum

The terms *intra-abdominal hypertension* and *abdominal compartment syndrome* are sometimes used interchangeably, but it is generally accepted that the two represent a continuum of pathophysiologic changes. The critical pressure level varies between patients, but intra-abdominal hypertension is present when increased abdominal pressure reaches 10 to 15 mm Hg, whereas abdominal compartment syndrome is defined as intra-abdominal hypertension greater than 20 mm Hg, causing end-organ dysfunction that is improved by abdominal decompression (Malbrain, 2001).

Etiology

Intra-abdominal hypertension can occur because of a variety of chronic and acute causes, including the accumulation of fluid, pregnancy, blood clots, or third-spacing fluid losses. Sudden elevations of increased abdominal pressure are usually associated with abdominal surgery or trauma (Table 30–13). Patients who are at the most risk for developing intra-abdominal hypertension and abdominal compartment syndrome include those with abdominal trauma who are postop for repair of the injuries. Because the abdomen functions as a single compartment, an increase in its contents, for example, from fluids, may cause an elevation in intra-abdominal pressure, leading to intra-abdominal hypertension. Other conditions that place patients at increased risk for developing IAH/ACS include ruptured abdominal aortic aneurysm, bowel obstruction, hemorrhagic pancreatitis, ascites, and intra-abdominal neoplasm. Therapies, such as intra-abdominal packing during surgery, pneumatic antishock garments, and gas insufflation of the abdominal cavity during laparoscopic procedures, are also associated with abdominal compartment syndrome (Bailey & Shapiro, 2000; Gallagher, 2000; Tiwari et al., 2002; Webber & Mills, 2002). In nonsurgical patients the most common cause of IAH/ACS is bowel edema and distention. Factors predisposing an individual to development of bowel edema include hypothermia (less than 93.2°F [34°C]), acidosis (pH less than 7.2), massive transfusion or fluid resuscitation, coagulopathy or disseminated intravascular coagulation (DIC), and septic shock with capillary leak (Malbrain, 2001; Webber & Mills, 2002).

TABLE 30–13 Risk Factors for Development of IAH and ACS

Abdominal aortic aneurysm rupture
Abdominal trauma
Acute pancreatitis
Hepatic transplantation
Ileus
Intestinal obstruction
Intra-abdominal or retroperitoneal hemorrhage
Massive volume resuscitation
Pregnancy
Severe ascites
Shock states

Multisystem Effects of IAH

Multiple organ systems are affected by intra-abdominal hypertension (Table 30–14). The gastrointestinal tract is affected first by rising increased abdominal pressure, which compromises perfusion to the intestinal mucosa. The intestinal mucosa becomes ischemic, allowing bacteria to translocate into the bloodstream, predisposing the patient to systemic inflammatory response syndrome and sepsis. Gastrointestinal signs and symptoms of abdominal compartment syndrome include increased gastric carbon dioxide level (as measured by gastric tonometry, see Section Four), decreased arterial pH, and elevated serum lactic acid. These abnormalities may indicate intestinal ischemia (Bailey & Shapiro, 2000; Gallagher, 2000; Tiwari et al., 2002; Webber & Mills, 2002).

Cardiovascular System

The cardiovascular system is most affected by increased IAH/ACS. The most prevalent sign of abdominal compartment syndrome is hemodynamic change. As intra-abdominal hypertension elevates the diaphragm, intrathoracic pressure rises, causing an increase in ventricular wall tension that is evidenced by an increase in systemic vascular resistance. The increased pressure in the abdomen causes femoral venous pressure to rise, which in turn raises both central venous and right atrium pressures. Venous return (preload) decreases, resulting in reductions in cardiac volume and filling pressures. Tachycardia is a common symptom as the heart tries to maintain cardiac output and

TABLE 30–14   System Effects of IAH/ACS

BODY SYSTEM	EFFECTS OF INCREASED INTRA-ABDOMINAL PRESSURE	POTENTIAL OUTCOMES
Cardiovascular	Increased thoracic pressure because of increased pressure on diaphragm	Hemodynamic changes Elevated SVR, CVP, and RAP Tachycardia (compensatory) Decreased CO Hypotension (late sign)
Pulmonary	Decreased lung excursion and expansion because of increased diaphragmatic pressure	Decreased lung compliance Hypercapnia Hypoxemia Elevated PIP
Renal	Decreased renal blood flow because of elevated IAP and decreased CO, which decreases GFR and renal ischemia.	Oliguria Azotemia Prerenal failure
Neurologic	Decreased cerebral perfusion pressure (CPP) because of elevated ICP, which results from decreased venous drainage from the head	Increased ICP Altered level of consciousness
Gastrointestinal	Decreased blood flow to abdominal organs which results in tissue hypoxia, conversion to anaerobic metabolism, and generation of free radicals, and lactic acidosis	Small bowel ischemia Translocation of bacteria from gut Sepsis Further increase in intra-abdominal pressure Multiple organ dysfunction

SVR: systemic vascular resistance; CVP: central venous pressure; RAP: right atrial pressure; CO: cardiac output; PIP: peak inspiratory pressure; IAP: intra-abdominal pressure; GFR: glomerular filtration rate; ICP: intracranial pressure

compensate for decreased stroke volume. If this deterioration is not halted, left ventricular failure, increased afterload, and a further reduction in cardiac output and stroke volume occur, which eventually can result in hypotension and shock. Hypotension is a late and ominous sign because blood pressure remains essentially normal early in the shock process because of compensatory mechanisms (Bailey & Shapiro, 2000; Gallagher, 2000; Tiwari et al., 2002; Webber & Mills, 2002). Additionally, IAH impairs venous return from the legs. The resulting venous stasis, in combination with other risk factors such as immobility and coagulation defects, places the patient at increased risk for developing deep-vein thrombosis (Gallagher, 2000).

Pulmonary System

The pulmonary system is affected by IAH/ACS. Increased pressure on the patient's diaphragm prevents normal excursion and lung expansion. Complications include hypercapnia and hypoxemia because alveolar ventilation and oxygenation are impaired. Lung compliance is reduced, resulting in elevations in peak inspiratory pressures (Bailey & Shapiro, 2000).

Renal System

Renal system impairments from IAH/ACS occur early as a result of renal ischemia. Urine output and glomerular filtration rate decrease. Oliguria and eventually anuria develop, along with late elevations in serum BUN and creatinine (Bailey & Shapiro, 2000).

Neurologic System

Neurologic system complications are also caused by abdominal compartment syndrome. These include increased intracranial pressure and altered level of consciousness because of decreased cerebral perfusion pressure (Bailey & Shapiro, 2000).

Measurement of Intra-Abdominal Pressure

If the patient develops signs of organ system dysfunction and is at risk for the development of IAH/ACS, it is important to consider abdominal compartment syndrome as a complication. The sequelae of abdominal compartment syndrome are often life threatening, and many clinicians advocate using routine, noninvasive abdominal pressure monitoring for all critically ill patients at risk for developing IAH/ACS. Although the most accurate and direct technique for measuring increased abdominal pressure would be to insert a catheter directly into the peritoneal cavity, this invasive procedure requires tube placement in the abdomen, increasing the risk of bowel injury or peritoneal contamination. However, it has been validated that transurethral bladder pressure reflects the increased abdominal pressure indirectly (Iberti et al., 1989; Kron et al., 1984).

Alterations in intra-abdominal pressure are indirectly reflected by changes in bladder pressure (Kron et al., 1984). When the bladder is filled with approximately 50 to 100 mL of fluid, there is virtually no pressure exerted on the bladder wall, enabling it to act as a passive diaphragm capable of transmitting

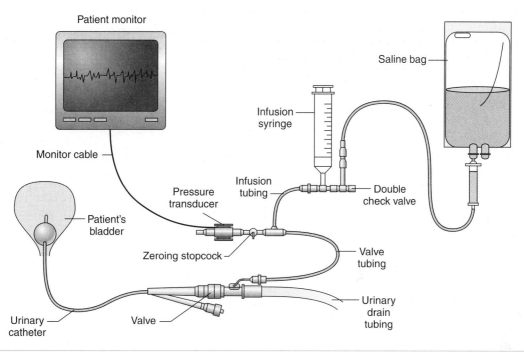

Figure 30–13 ■ Measurement of bladder pressure.

abdominal pressure without imparting additional pressure from its own musculature. Two methods of measuring intra-abdominal pressure using a urinary bladder catheter are the transducer and fluid manometer methods. It is important to ensure that the urinary catheter is draining freely and the bladder is empty for either method. The transducer method uses a conventional cardiac transducer monitoring system, which is connected to the patient's urinary catheter drainage system. Using this method, 60 to 100 mL of saline is injected through a catheter port. The pressure transducer is then connected to the urinary catheter using a 16-gauge needle inserted into the aspiration port at the level of the patient's pubis. The resulting bladder pressure waveform can be viewed on a monitor screen. The fluid manometer method uses the urinary catheter as a manometer. To use this method, 60 to 100 mL of normal saline is instilled into the urinary catheter's aspiration port. The catheter is held at a 90 degree angle to the patient's pelvis, and the height of the fluid in the tubing above the pelvis is measured to determine the pressure reading (Gallagher, 2000) (Fig. 30–13).

Normal bladder pressure is 0 mm Hg. After abdominal surgery, bladder pressures between 0 and 15 mm Hg are not uncommon. Higher pressures indicate the onset of intra-abdominal hypertension (the precursor to abdominal compartment syndrome) and may be associated with early organ system pathophysiology (Gallagher, 2000).

Treatment

Treatment of abdominal compartment syndrome focuses on decompression and preserving cardiopulmonary and renal function. Interventions vary with the severity of the intra-abdominal pressure elevation.

Mild ACS

For mild abdominal compartment syndrome (IAP of 15 to 20 mm Hg), elevating the head of the bed helps to minimize pressure on the diaphragm, allowing maximum lung expansion. Additionally, assisting the patient to turn, cough, breathe deeply, and use an incentive spirometer will help to improve alveolar ventilation, reduce the risk of atelectasis, and prevent ventilation–perfusion mismatch (shunt) (King, 2001; Webber & Mills, 2002).

Moderate ACS

If moderate abdominal compartment syndrome (IAP of 20 to 25 mm Hg) develops, the patient should be transferred to an intensive care unit for closer monitoring. Sedation or neuromuscular blockade to chemically paralyze and sedate the patient may be indicated (Ivatury et al., 2001). If the patient is hemodynamically unstable, demonstrating, for example, low cardiac output or hypotension, surgical decompression of the abdomen may be indicated. It is important to ensure that a surgical service is consulted early in the course of treatment in case surgical decompression using a laparotomy procedure is required. It should be noted that there have been no randomized clinical trials to support the use of routine abdominal decompression through midline laparotomy for treatment of abdominal compartment syndrome (De Waele et al., 2003). A major concern with surgical intervention is that the morbidity of a midline laparotomy in a critically ill patient is considerable (Barker et al., 2000).

Severe ACS

Severe abdominal compartment syndrome (IAP greater than 25 mm Hg) requires urgent surgical decompression of the abdominal cavity or removal of excess fluid, blood, packing, or blood clots. In cases of trauma, the abdomen is sometimes left open after exploratory laparotomy to prevent ACS; however, even with this preventive measure, abdominal pressure may still rise to a dangerous level (Gallagher, 2000; Ivatury et al., 2001; Stamos, 2002; Tiwari et al., 2002; Webber & Mills, 2002).

Surgical decompression of the abdomen, if necessary for severe ACS, involves a risk for hypotension once the abdomen is opened. This hypotension may be caused by reperfusion, and researchers recommend volume resuscitation with fluids containing mannitol and sodium bicarbonate immediately before and during decompression surgery, which may prevent unstable arrhythmias (Bailey & Shapiro, 2000; Gallagher, 2000; Ivatury et al., 2001; Tiwari et al., 2002; Webber & Mills, 2002).

Complications of ACS

Complications of abdominal compartment syndrome may include reperfusion asystole, which occurs when by-products from ischemic areas circulate to the heart, causing acidosis-related impairments of electrical activity. Resuscitation equipment and emergency medications should be available in the event asystole occurs. The physician may order an intravenous infusion of sodium bicarbonate and mannitol to prevent this phenomenon.

Pulmonary embolism can occur if thrombi break loose from leg veins. This is also considered a complication that is associated with reperfusion. The nurse should monitor for signs and symptoms of pulmonary embolism, such as dyspnea, pleuritic chest pain, and signs of shock. Oxygen administration, evaluation for and administration of thrombolytic drugs, and anticoagulants may be required if pulmonary embolism occurs.

Nursing Implications

Unless complications occur, abdominal decompression usually improves the patient's condition. If the ACS treatment is effective, end points of therapy will include decreased ventilation pressures, increased oxygenation, and improved cardiovascular and renal function. After surgery, nursing care will consist of maintaining the patient's oxygenation and hemodynamic stability; caring for the abdominal wound; monitoring for infection; and measuring fluid intake and output, including wound drainage, to determine the patient's fluid requirements. The patient may require mechanical ventilation, aggressive volume resuscitation, and vasopressor and inotropic drugs. Management of the patient with ACS is a challenge. It is critical for the nurse to recognize the signs of ACS early, so that prompt treatment can be initiated to avoid organ failure and death.

In summary, IAH and (ACS) are potentially life-threatening complications resulting from an acute expansion of abdominal contents and increased abdominal pressure, which impairs blood flow to organs, causing tissue ischemia and organ failure. The critical pressure level for abdominal compartment syndrome varies between patients, but IAH is present when increased abdominal pressure reaches 10 to 15 mm Hg, whereas moderate ACS is defined as intra-abdominal hypertension greater than 20 mm Hg, causing end-organ dysfunction that is improved by abdominal decompression. Patients who are at the highest risk for developing ACS are those with abdominal trauma who are postop for repair of the injuries. As intra-abdominal hypertension increases and abdominal compartment syndrome develops, a continuum of decompensation signs develop. The most prevalent sign of abdominal compartment syndrome is hemodynamic change consistent with decreased preload, tachycardia, and reductions in cardiac output and stroke volume. If impaired abdominal perfusion continues, left ventricular failure, increased afterload, hypotension, and shock results. The sequelae of ACS are often life threatening, and routine pressure monitoring for all critically ill patients at risk for developing IAH/ACS are indicated, such as transurethral bladder pressure monitoring. Nursing interventions focus on maximizing the patient's oxygenation and keeping him or her hemodynamically stable. Unless complications such as reperfusion asystole and pulmonary embolism occur, abdominal decompression usually improves the patient's condition.

SECTION TEN REVIEW

1. Which patient represents the population with the highest risk of developing abdominal compartment syndrome?
   A. a patient with chronic obstructive pulmonary disease
   B. a patient who is status postmyocardial infarction
   C. a patient who is postoperative for repair of a liver laceration
   D. a patient who is status posthip replacement
2. Renal effects of increasing intra-abdominal hypertension include
   A. increased urine output
   B. increased sodium and water concentration

C. decreased glomerular filtration rate
D. decreased renal tubular acidosis
3. Which statement correctly reflects the effects of ACS on preload and cardiac output?
A. preload and cardiac output are decreased
B. preload and cardiac output are increased

C. preload and cardiac output are normal
D. preload is increased; cardiac output is decreased
4. True or False: Decreased blood pressure is an early sign of ACS.

Answers: 1. C, 2. C, 3. A, 4. False

SECTION ELEVEN: Gastrointestinal Nursing Diagnoses and Management

At the completion of this section, the learner will be able to describe the nursing diagnosis and management of acute GI bleeding and paralytic ileus.

The care of patients with acute GI bleeding is complex and requires close assessment and monitoring of the patient's condition and progress. Collaborative management of physiological problems as well as concern for the patient's psychosocial response to the acute illness are priorities for the nurse. Because fear and anxiety often accompany acute GI bleeding, patients and their significant others need information and support during this time. Nurses coordinate plans for the patient's ongoing care based on accurate and ongoing nursing assessment. Nursing diagnoses that are appropriate for patients diagnosed with GI bleeding, paralytic ileus, and acute intestinal ischemia are listed in Table 30–15.

TABLE 30–15 Nursing Diagnoses

PROBLEM STATEMENT	ETIOLOGIC FACTORS
Gastrointestinal Bleeding	
Fluid volume deficit, risk for	Hypovolemia secondary to blood loss; NPO; vomiting; diarrhea
Tissue perfusion, altered: cerebral, cardiac, respiratory, renal, peripheral, mesenteric	Hypovolemia and decreased oxygenation secondary to anemia, hypotension, shock
Gas exchange, impaired	Hypovolemia, anemia
Anxiety	Fear of bleeding, threat of death
Aspiration, risk for	Hematemesis and potential changes in level of consciousness
Nutrition, less than body requirements, altered	Decreased appetite secondary to bowel irritability; NPO
Pain	Bleeding and discomfort
Diarrhea	Decrease in intestinal transit time secondary to cathartic effects of blood in GI tract
Thought processes, altered	Hypoxia secondary to anemia
Infection, risk for	Immune suppression; intestinal ischemia/infarction secondary to hypotension and shock
Fatigue	Anemia, decreased oxygenation
Knowledge deficit	Precipitating factors; therapeutic procedures/interventions; discharge information
Paralytic Ileus	
Ineffective breathing pattern	Abdominal distention
Fluid volume deficit, actual	Vomiting, distention, electrolyte imbalance, hypovolemia (loss of fluid/electrolytes due to stasis of bowel contents)
Tissue perfusion, risk for, bowel	Decreased oxygenation to tissues secondary to bowel strangulation, perforation, and/or shock
Infection, risk for	Perforation, strangulation, bowel ischemia → infarction → necrosis → sepsis
Bowel elimination, altered	Absent bowel sounds; NPO; electrolyte loss; constipation
Pain/discomfort, actual	Distention; intestinal angina; perforation
Knowledge deficit, actual	Illness, treatments, procedures, and outcome
Intestinal Ischemia	
Pain/comfort, actual	Intestinal angina; distention; infarction; peritonitis
Infection, risk for	Infarction → necrosis → sepsis
Fluid volume deficit, risk for	Electrolyte imbalance; NPO; vomiting; diarrhea; third spacing; shock if perforation occurs
Knowledge deficit, actual	Illness, treatments, procedures, and outcome

Data from Krumberger, J. M., & Hammer, B. (1998). Gastrointestinal disorders. In M. R. Kinney, J. B. Dunbar, J. A. Brooks-Brun, N. Molter, & J. M. Vitello_Cicciu (Eds.), AACN's clinical reference for critical care nursing, *(4th ed.). St. Louis: C.V. Mosby; Urden, L., Stacy, K., & Lough, M. (2001)* Thelan's critical care nursing: Diagnosis and management, *(4th ed.). St. Louis: C.V. Mosby; Carpenito-Moyet, L. J. (2003).* Nursing diagnosis: Application to clinical practice, *(10th ed.). Philadelphia: J. B. Lippincott.*

A life-threatening complication of acute GI bleeding and bowel infarction is shock (hypovolemic or septic shock). Key nursing goals for the patient with hypovolemic or septic shock include maintenance of adequate tissue perfusion/oxygenation, prevention of fluid volume deficit related to blood loss and third spacing of fluids, and optimization of hemodynamic status. Regardless of what has caused the shock (GI hemorrhage or sepsis), the nurse must first see that venous access is achieved so that fluid and blood resuscitation therapy can begin. Tables 30–9 through 30–11 list common interventions used to stop the hemorrhage. Ensuring adequacy of intravenous infusions remains a nursing priority for the duration of the treatment of shock. In order to maintain adequate gas exchange and tissue perfusion, the nurse should

1. Ensure an open airway and administer supplementary oxygen
2. Initiate continuous monitoring for cardiac dysrhythmias
3. Prepare for insertion of a pulmonary artery catheter and record and monitor cardiac filling pressures once placement has been achieved
4. Prepare the patient for emergent surgical intervention to control bleeding or resect necrotic bowel (Krumberger, 1998; Schulman, 2002; Urden et al., 2001)

Table 30–16 summarizes some nursing interventions specific to the care of the patient at risk for hypovolemia as a result of GI bleeding. These interventions also apply to the patient who is in shock secondary to sepsis.

In summary, the nursing care of patients with acute GI bleeding is complex and requires collaboration with other disciplines for close assessment and monitoring of the patient's condition and progress. Additionally, the nurse is concerned with the psychosocial response of the patient and significant others to the acute, often critical, illness. There are a number of nursing diagnoses that are appropriate for patients diagnosed with GI bleeding, paralytic ileus, and acute intestinal ischemia. Key nurs-

TABLE 30–16 Clinical Application: Nursing Interventions for Patients at Risk for Hypovolemia Due to GI Bleeding

- Assess for signs and symptoms of shock; vital signs, urine output, hemodynamic measures (PAP, PCWP, CI, CO, SVR, CVP), Sao$_2$ (oxygen saturation), diminished peripheral pulses, restlessness, agitation, cool, pale, or moist skin
- Assess fluid status; intake and output (urine output, gastric drainage)
- Assess electrolyte levels (may become altered from fluid loss or fluid shifts)
- Assess hemoglobin, hematocrit, RBC, coagulation studies (PT, PTT), renal function (BUN, serum creatinine)
- Test gastric drainage, emesis, or stools for occult blood
- Assess gastric pH; consult with physician/practitioner about specific pH range and antacid administration
- Consult with physician/practitioner about replacing fluid losses based on assessment findings
- Administer replacement fluids and blood products as directed
- Assess for adverse reaction to blood products

PAP, pulmonary artery pressure; PCWP, pulmonary capillary wedge pressure; CI, cardiac index; CO, cardiac output; SVR, systemic vascular resistance; CVP, central venous pressure; RBC, red blood count; PT, prothrombin time; PTT, partial thromboplastin time; BUN, blood urea nitrogen.

Data from Carpenito-Moyet, L. (2003). Nursing diagnosis: Application to clinical practice, *(10th ed.). Philadelphia: J. B. Lippincott; Schulman, C. (2002). End point of resuscitation. Choosing the right parameters to monitor.* Dimensions of Critical Care, 21*(1), 2–14.*

ing goals for patients with hemodynamic compromise from acute GI dysfunction include maintenance of adequate tissue perfusion/oxygenation, prevention of fluid volume deficit related to blood and fluid loss, and resuscitation and optimization of hemodynamic status. Nursing interventions specific to the care of the patient at risk for hypovolemia as a result of GI bleeding and shock are summarized.

SECTION ELEVEN REVIEW

1. A life-threatening complication of acute GI bleeding and bowel infarction is
   A. renal failure
   B. abdominal aorta aneurysm
   C. shock
   D. pancreatitis

2. When providing nursing care for a patient experiencing GI bleeding or paralytic ileus/necrotic bowel, the nurse should prepare the patient for
   A. surgery
   B. placement of a urinary catheter
   C. endotracheal intubation
   D. obtaining blood cultures

Answers: 1. C, 2. A

POSTTEST

1. The normal flora that reside within the large intestine break down cellulose and synthesize
   A. hydrochloric acid, vitamin C, calcium, and carbolic acid
   B. vitamin E, phosphorous, creatine, and folic acid
   C. vitamin K, carbon dioxide, methane, and riboflavin
   D. vitamin K, folic acid, riboflavin, and nicotinic acid

2. The ileocecal valve
   A. prevents backflow of feces from large to small intestine
   B. prevents backflow of chyme from the duodenum to the stomach
   C. allows stomach contents to move into the small intestine
   D. allows passage of feces through the rectum

3. The stomach receives its nerve supply from the
   A. autonomic nervous system
   B. gastrointestinal nervous system
   C. mesenteric nervous system
   D. splanchnic nervous system

4. The enteric nervous system coordinates
   A. sphincter tone and glandular secretion
   B. splanchnic blood supply and sensation
   C. GI motility and secretion activities
   D. absorption of fluid and electrolytes

5. Chronic total parenteral nutritional therapy without enteral stimulation may result in
   A. regeneration of intestinal mucosa cells
   B. enhanced immunologic defense mechanisms
   C. mucosal atrophy and bacterial overgrowth
   D. enhanced production of mucus by goblet cells

6. Intact gut barrier function inhibits
   A. bacterial translocation across mucosal barriers
   B. GALT defense mechanisms
   C. rapid response of macrophages to pathogens
   D. immunoglobulin production by GALT

7. _____ may contribute to gastrointestinal bleeding.
   A. Pulmonary disease
   B. Hepatic dysfunction
   C. Autoimmune complications
   D. Cardiac disease

8. In the case of GI bleeding, angiography allows visualization of
   A. vascular beds and flow
   B. GI motility
   C. abscesses
   D. masses

9. All external metal objects must be removed in order for a(n) _____ to be performed.
   A. ultrasound sonography
   B. angiography
   C. CT scan
   D. MRI

10. Occult bleeding is usually
    A. unnoticed by the patient
    B. massive in its presentation
    C. acute in its presentation
    D. bright red in appearance

11. NSAIDs interrupt mucosal integrity by
    A. inhibiting gastric acid production
    B. increasing mucus production
    C. inhibiting prostaglandin function
    D. decreasing bicarbonate secretion

12. Upper GI bleeding from esophageal or gastric varices is associated with
    A. acute renal failure
    B. gastric acid hypersecretion
    C. chronic renal failure
    D. portal hypertension

13. Gastrointestinal arteriovenous malformations are most common in
    A. the young, healthy adult population
    B. the elderly with chronic disease
    C. females with diabetes mellitus
    D. males with human immunodeficiency virus (HIV)

14. Duodenal ulcer pain is characteristically
    A. consistent
    B. sporadic
    C. worse on awakening
    D. aggravated by food

15. The mortality rate for patients with ischemic bowel disease is
    A. 20 percent
    B. 30 percent
    C. 40 percent
    D. 50 percent

16. _____ is the most common symptom of inflammatory bowel disease.
    A. Nausea and vomiting
    B. Bloody diarrhea
    C. Constipation
    D. Abdominal distention

17. A patient requires a blood transfusion. The blood bank has not typed and crossmatched the patient's blood; therefore, packed red cells cannot be transfused because of the risk of allergic reaction. The patient needs blood now, and the decision is made to transfuse whole blood that does not require type and crossmatch. Which type of whole blood can be used in this situation?
    A. type A
    B. type AB
    C. type B
    D. type O

18. The nurse notes that the patient's heart rate is 125 beats per minute (increased from 85). The patient's blood pressure is decreased to 88/40 from 126/62, and the patient is suddenly anxious. These assessment findings can indicate
   A. rebleeding
   B. pain
   C. hypervolemia
   D. hyperglycemia

19. Ogilvie's syndrome involves paralytic ileus of the
   A. colon
   B. ileum
   C. jejunum
   D. duodenum

20. Complete bowel obstruction requires
   A. rapid initiation of enteral feeding
   B. stat soapsuds enema
   C. surgical resection of bowel
   D. evacuation by colonoscopy

21. When gut perfusion is compromised, which of the following occurs?
   A. gastric CO_2 level increases
   B. gastric $PrCO_2$ decreases
   C. the $PrCO_2$–$PaCO_2$ gap decreases
   D. GI tract metabolism is anaerobic

22. Interventions that directly improve gut perfusion include
   A. optimizing cardiac output
   B. optimizing hemoglobin levels
   C. administering supplemental oxygen
   D. all of the above

23. An intravenous infusion of _____ before surgical decompression may decrease the occurrence of reperfusion asystole.
   A. epinephrine and furosemide
   B. vasopressin and nitroglycerine
   C. octreotide and calcium chloride
   D. sodium bicarbonate and mannitol

POSTTEST ANSWERS

Question	Answer	Section
1	D	One
2	A	One
3	A	Two
4	C	Two
5	C	Three
6	A	Three
7	B	Four
8	A	Four
9	D	Four
10	A	Five
11	C	Six
12	D	Six

Question	Answer	Section
13	B	Six
14	A	Six
15	D	Seven
16	B	Seven
17	D	Eight
18	A	Eight
19	A	Nine
20	C	Nine
21	A	Four
22	A	Four
23	D	Ten

REFERENCES

Ackerman, M. H., & Ashe, T. R. (2000). The latest in gastrointestinal care: Find out how gut perfusion monitoring can help you identify warning signs of shock. *Nursing, 2000, 30*(5 suppl), 36–38.

Altman, D. (2001). Drugs used in gastrointestinal diseases. In B. G. Katzung (ed.). *Basic & clinical pharmacology* (8th ed.). New York: Lange.

Andreoli, T. E., Bennett, J. C., Carpenter, C. C., & Plum, F. (2000). *Cecil's essentials of medicine* (5th ed.). Philadelphia: W. B. Saunders.

Arnell, T. (2002). Gastrointestinal bleeding. In F. S. Bongard & D. Y. Sue (Eds.), *Current critical care diagnosis and treatment* (2nd ed., p. 756). New York: Lange.

Bailey, J., & Shapiro, M. (2000). Review: Abdominal compartment syndrome. *Critical Care Forum, 4*(1), 23–29.

Barker, D., Kaufman, H., Smith, L., Ciraulo, D., Richart, C., & Burns, R. (2000). Vacuum pack technique of temporary abdominal closure: A 7-year experience with 112 patients. *Journal of Trauma, 48,* 201–206.

Beers, M. H., & Berkhow, R. (Eds.). (1999). *The Merck manual of diagnosis and therapy* (17th ed.). Whitehouse Station, NJ: Merck Research Laboratories.

Bongard, F. S. (2002). Shock and resuscitation. In F. S. Bongard & D. Y. Sue (Eds.), *Current critical care diagnosis and treatment* (2nd ed., pp. 242–258). New York: Lange.

Braunwald, E. (2001). *Harrison's principles of internal medicine* (15th ed.). New York: McGraw Hill.

Carpenito-Moyet, L. (2003). *Nursing diagnosis: Application to clinical practice* (10th ed.). Philadelphia: J. B. Lippincott.

Crittormson, W. L., & Burbick, M. P. (1989). Mortality from ischemic colitis. *Diseases of Colon Rectum, 32,* 469–472.

Croghan, A. (2004). Nursing assessment of the gastrointestinal system. In S. M. Lewis, M. M. Heitkemper, & S. R. Dirksen (Eds.), *Medical-surgical nursing* (6th ed., p. 946). St. Louis: C. V. Mosby.

Deglin, J., & Vallerand, A. (2001). *Davis's drug guide for nurses* (8th ed.). Philadelphia: F. A. Davis.

Del Valle, J. (2001). Peptic ulcer disease and related conditions. In E. Braunwald, A. Fauci, D. Kasper, S. Hauser, D. Longo, & J. L. Jameson (Eds.), *Harrison's principles of internal medicine* (15th ed.). *CD-ROM version 1.0.* New York: McGraw Hill.

De Waele, J., Benoit, D., Hoste, E., & Colardyn, F. (2003). A role for muscle relaxation in patients with abdominal compartment syndrome? *Intensive Care Medicine, 29,* 332.

Elliot, D. (2002). The treatment of peptic ulcers. *Nursing Standard, 13*(22), 37–42.

Falk, G. W. (2001). Diseases of the stomach and duodenum. In T. E. Andreoli, C. Carpenter, R. C. Griggs, & J. Loscalzo (Eds.), *Cecil essentials of medicine* (5th ed., pp. 332–343). Philadelphia: W. B. Saunders.

Farrell, J., & Friedman, L. (2001). Gastrointestinal bleeding in the elderly. *Gastroenterol Clinic North America, 30*(2), 377–407.

Flannery, J., & Tucker, D. (2002). Pharmacologic prophylaxis and treatment of stress ulcers in critically ill patients. *Critical Care Clinics of North America, 14*(1), 39–51.

Forsmark, C., Rockey, D., & Van Dam, J. (2000). Current management of upper GI tract bleeding. *Patient Care* (January), 20–42.

Gallagher, J. (2000). What you should know about abdominal compartment syndrome. *Critical Care Choices, 44,* 46–48.

Gray, H. (1995). *Gray's anatomy: The anatomical basis of medicine and surgery* (38th ed.). New York: Churchill.

Guyton, A. (2000). *Textbook of medical physiology* (10th ed.). Philadelphia: W. B. Saunders.

Haist, S., & Robbins, J. (2002). *Internal medicine on call* (3rd ed.). New York: Lange.

Iberti, T., Lieber, C., & Benjamin, E. (1989). Determination of intra-abdominal pressure using a transurethral bladder catheter clinical validation technique. *Anesthesiology, 70*(1), 47–50.

Isenkery, J. I., McQuaid, K. R., Laine, I., et al. (1995). Acid peptic disorders. In T. Yamada (Ed.), *Textbook of gastroenterology.* Philadelphia: J. B. Lippincott.

Ivatury, R., Sugerman, H., & Peitzman, A. (2001). Abdominal compartment syndrome: Recognition and management. *Advances in Surgery, 35,* 251–269.

King, J. (2001). Blunt abdominal trauma. In S. D. Melander (Ed.), *Case studies in critical care nursing: A guide for application and review* (2nd ed.). Philadelphia: W. B. Saunders.

Kron, I., Harman, P., & Nolan, S. (1984). The measurement of intra-abdominal pressure as a criterion for abdominal re-exploration. *Annals of Surgery, 199,* 28–30.

Krumberger, J. M. (1998). Gastrointestinal clinical physiology. In M. R. Kinney, S. B. Dunbar, J. A. Brooks-Brunn, N. Molter, & J. M. Vitello-Cicciu (Eds.), *AACN's clinical reference for critical care nursinig* (4th ed.). St Louis: C. V. Mosby.

Laine, L. (2001). Gastrointestinal bleeding. In E. Braunwald, A. Fauci, D. Kasper, S. Hauser, D. Longo, & J. L. Jameson (Eds.), *Harrison's principles of internal medicine* (15th ed.). CD-ROM Version 1.0. New York: McGraw Hill.

Lefor, A., Bogdonoff, D., Geehan, D., & Maldonado, L. (2002). *Critical care on call.* New York: Lange.

Lindseth, G. L. (2003a). Disorders of the small intestine. In S. L. Price & L. M. Wilson (Eds.), *Pathophysiology: Clinical concepts of disease processes* (6th ed., p. 341). St. Louis: C. V. Mosby.

Lindseth, G. L. (2003b). Disorders of the stomach and duodenum. In S. L. Price & L. M. Wilson (Eds.), *Pathophysiology: Clinical concepts of disease processes* (6th ed., p. 328). St. Louis: C. V. Mosby.

Lingappa, V. R. (2003). Gastrointestinal disease. In S. J. McPhee, V. R. Lingappa, & W. F. Ganong (Eds.), *Pathophysiology of disease: An introduction to clinical medicine* (pp. 340–356). New York: Lange.

Lingenfelser, T., & Ell, C. (2001). Gastrointestinal bleeding in the elderly. *Best Practices Clinical Gastroenterology, 15*(6), 963–982.

Malbrain, M. (2001). Intra-abdominal pressure on the intensive care unit: Clinical tool or toy? In J. L. Vincent (Ed.), *2001 year book of intensive care and emergency medicine* (pp. 547–585). New York: Springer-Verlag.

Markey, D. W. (1999). Gastrointestinal anatomy and physiology. In L. Bucher & S. Melander (Eds.), *Critical care nursing* (pp. 675–691). Philadelphia: W. B. Saunders.

McQuaid, K. R. (1999). Alimentary tract. In L. M. Tierney, S. J. McPhee, & M. A. Papadakis (Eds.), *Current medical diagnosis and treatment* (38th ed.). Norwalk, CT: Appleton & Lange.

Nicoll, D., McPhee, S., & Pignone, M. (2004). *Pocket guide to diagnostic tests* (4th ed.). New York: Lange.

Podolsky, D. K., & Isselbacher, K. J. (2001). Disorders of the alimentary tract. In E. Braunwald, A. Fauci, D. Kasper, S. Hauser, D. Longo, & J. L. Jameson (Eds.), *Harrison's principles of internal medicine* (15th ed.). CD-ROM Version 1.0. New York: McGraw Hill.

Prakash, C. (2000a). Gastrointestinal bleeding: Principles of diagnosis and management. In R. S. Irwin & J. M. Rippe (Eds.), *Manual of intensive care medicine* (3rd ed., p. 433). Philadelphia: Lippincott Williams & Wilkins.

Prakash, C. (2000b). Stress ulcer syndrome. In R. S. Irwin & J. M. Rippe (Eds.), *Manual of intensive care medicine* (3rd ed., p. 437). Philadelphia: Lippincott Williams & Wilkins.

Prakash, C. (2001). Gastrointestinal diseases: Gastrointestinal bleeding. In S. N. Ahya, K. Flood, & S. Paranjothi (Eds.), *The Washington manual of medical therapeutics* (30th ed., p. 349). Philadelphia: Lippincott Williams & Wilkins.

Prakash, C., & Clouse, R. (2000). Intestinal pseudoobstruction (ileus). In R. S. Irwin & J. M. Rippe (Eds.), *Manual of intensive care medicine* (3rd ed., p. 445). Philadelphia: Lippincott Williams & Wilkins.

Schulman, C. (2002). End point of resuscitation: Choosing the right parameters to monitor. *Dimensions of Critical Care, 21*(1), 2–14.

Silen, W. (2001). Acute intestinal obstruction. In E. Braunwald, A. Fauci, D. Kasper, S. Hauser, D. Longo, & J. L. Jameson (Eds.), *Harrison's principles of internal medicine* (15th ed.). CD-ROM Version 1.0. New York: McGraw Hill.

Smith, S. L. (1998). The gastrointestinal system. In J. G. Alspach (Ed.), *AACN's core curriculum for critical care nursing* (5th ed.). Philadelphia: W. B. Saunders.

Stamos, M. (2002). Acute abdomen. In F. S. Bongard & D. Y. Sue (Eds.), *Current critical care diagnosis and treatment* (2nd ed., p. 748). New York: Lange.

Tiwari, A., Haq, A. I., Myint, F., & Hamilton, G. (2002). Acute compartment syndromes. *British Journal of Surgery, 89,* 397–412.

Tucker, D. A. (2000). Normal and altered function of the gastrointestinal system. In B. Bullock & R. Henze (Eds.), *Focus on pathophysiology* (pp. 721–728). Philadelphia: J. B. Lippincott.

Urden, L., Stacy, K., & Lough, M. (2001). *Thelan's critical care nursing: Diagnosis and management* (4th ed). St. Louis: C. V. Mosby.

van Lanschot, J., van Leerdam, M., Delden, O., & Fockens, P. (2002). Management of bleeding gastroduodenal ulcers. *Digestive Surgery, 19,* 99–104.

Webber, S. J., & Mills, G. H. (2002). The abdominal compartment syndrome: Ban under-recognized and inadequately treated condition? *Care of the Critically Ill, 18*(4), 115–117.

Weil, M. H. (1999). Sublingual capnometry: A new noninvasive measurement for diagnosis and quantification of severity of circulatory shock. *Critical Care Medicine, 27*(7), 1225–1229.

Westfall, U. E. (1999). Gastrointestinal laboratory and diagnostic tests. In L. Bucher & S. Melander (Eds.), *Critical care nursing.* Philadelphia: W. B. Saunders.

31 Acute Hepatic Dysfunction

Allison Steele, Melanie Hardin-Pierce

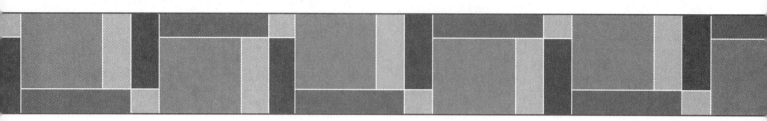

OBJECTIVES Following completion of this module, the learner will be able to

1. Identify the anatomic structures of the liver.
2. Discuss the functions of the liver.
3. Discuss liver function through evaluation of laboratory test results.
4. Describe the etiology and clinical manifestations associated with acute hepatitis.
5. Describe the etiology and clinical manifestations associated with acute hepatic dysfunction and failure.
6. Describe the complications of acute hepatic dysfunction.
7. Describe an overview of the medical management of the patient with acute hepatic dysfunction.
8. Describe the nursing implications appropriate to management of the patient experiencing acute hepatic dysfunction.

This module presents the physiologic and pathophysiologic processes involved in acute hepatic dysfunction and management of the patient with acute hepatic failure. The module is composed of eight sections. Sections One through Three present a review of the anatomy and physiology of the liver, including liver functions and evaluation of liver function through laboratory testing. Section Four provides an overview of acute hepatitis. Section Five describes acute hepatic failure based on causative factors. It then describes the clinical manifestations of acute hepatic failure. Section Six explains the multisystem complications of hepatic dysfunction. Sections Seven and Eight complete the module, with an overview of medical management, therapeutic goals, nursing assessment, and frequently occurring nursing diagnoses. Each section includes a set of review questions to help the learner evaluate his or her understanding of the section's content before moving on to the next section. All Section Reviews and the module Pretest and Posttest include answers. It is suggested that the learner review those concepts answered incorrectly in the review questions before proceeding to the next section.

 PRETEST

1. The functional unit of the liver is called the
   A. hepatocyte
   B. lobule
   C. canaliculi
   D. capsule
2. Bile is secreted by the
   A. terminal bile ducts
   B. quadrate lobe
   C. canaliculi
   D. hepatocytes
3. The primary substance in bile is
   A. bile salts
   B. bilirubin
   C. cholesterol
   D. electrolytes

4. The major function of bile salts is to assist with
   A. absorption of fat products
   B. blood clotting
   C. conversion of vitamin D
   D. protein synthesis

5. The majority of iron is located in
   A. the liver
   B. bone
   C. fat
   D. hemoglobin

6. The major by-product of amino acid deamination is
   A. bilirubin
   B. ammonia
   C. fatty acids
   D. glucose

7. Serum enzyme levels are obtained to measure
   A. clotting factors
   B. organ function
   C. cellular injury
   D. tissue oxygenation

8. Serum isoenzyme levels often provide better data than parent enzyme levels because they are
   A. faster to obtain
   B. more tissue specific
   C. more plentiful
   D. easier to measure

9. Which combination of lactic dehydrogenase (LDH) isoenzymes best reflects hepatic injury?
   A. LDH1 and LDH2
   B. LDH2 and LDH3
   C. LDH3 and LDH4
   D. LDH4 and LDH5

10. Acute hepatitis is most commonly caused by
    A. bacterial invasion
    B. viral invasion
    C. yeast invasion
    D. an autoimmune reaction

11. The major cause of acute and chronic hepatitis and cirrhosis is
    A. cytomegalovirus
    B. hepatitis C virus
    C. Epstein–Barr virus
    D. hepatitis B virus

12. Classic hepatitis is characterized by
    A. localized necrosis
    B. a greatly enlarged liver
    C. the development of fibrosis
    D. the development of fulminant hepatic failure

13. Which statement is correct regarding fulminant hepatic failure?
    A. it causes necrosis of liver tissue
    B. it has a mortality of less than 50 percent
    C. it is characterized by stage I to II encephalopathy
    D. it has a slow, insidious onset

14. A major hepatotoxin that is known to cause fulminant hepatic failure is
    A. acetaminophen
    B. gentamicin
    C. aspirin
    D. cephalosporin

15. In the United States cirrhosis of the liver is most commonly caused by
    A. hepatitis A virus
    B. alcohol abuse
    C. hepatitis B virus
    D. Epstein–Barr virus

16. A major cause of ascites is
    A. hyperalbuminemia
    B. low colloid osmotic pressure
    C. hepatorenal syndrome
    D. fluid volume overload

17. A major factor contributing to the onset of acute renal failure as a complication of hepatic failure is
    A. hepatotoxins
    B. a hypotensive episode
    C. high ammonia levels
    D. portal vein shunting

18. The onset of type 2 hepatorenal syndrome usually occurs in the presence of
    A. hepatotoxins
    B. a hypotensive episode
    C. high ammonia levels
    D. severe ascites

19. Dietary management of the patient with acute viral hepatitis would include
    A. high protein, low fat
    B. low fat, high carbohydrate
    C. low carbohydrate, low fat
    D. low protein, high fat

20. A patient with acute viral hepatitis will most likely be admitted to the hospital if he or she is experiencing
    A. severe fatigue
    B. occasional nausea
    C. elevated bilirubin
    D. hepatic encephalopathy

21. The patient with fulminant hepatic failure will require strict nutritional control of
    A. protein
    B. fat
    C. carbohydrate
    D. fiber

Pretest Answers: 1. B, 2. D, 3. A, 4. A, 5. D, 6. B, 7. C, 8. B, 9. D, 10. B, 11. D, 12. A, 13. A, 14. A, 15. B, 16. B, 17. B, 18. D, 19. B, 20. D, 21. A

GLOSSARY

acute hepatitis   An inflammatory liver disease, usually of viral origin, that results in liver injury and necrosis.

alanine aminotransferase (ALT, SGPT)   An enzyme primarily found in the cells of the liver, kidneys, heart, and skeletal muscles.

alkaline phosphatase (Alk Phos, ALP)   An enzyme primarily found in the cells of the liver and kidneys.

anicteric hepatitis   Hepatitis with no jaundice present.

ascites   An abnormal collection of fluid in the abdominal cavity.

aspartate aminotransferase (AST, SGOT)   An enzyme primarily found in the cells of the liver, kidneys, heart, pancreas, and brain.

bile   A substance produced by the hepatocytes that is essential to normal digestion, particularly for fats.

bilirubin   The end product of hemoglobin degradation.

cholestatic hepatitis   Hepatitis with retention of bile as a result of biliary obstruction.

conjugated bilirubin   Bilirubin that has been joined with glucuronic acid to make it water soluble.

enzymes   Catalyst substances found in cells that assist in cellular activities.

fulminant hepatic failure (FHF)   A rapidly developing (less than 8 weeks) acute failure of the liver, characterized by severe encephalopathy (stage III or IV), that develops in a person with no preexisting liver dysfunction.

hepatic encephalopathy   An altered neurologic status that is caused by a buildup of circulating toxins of hepatic origin.

hepatic failure   The inability of the liver to perform its normal functions.

hepatorenal syndrome (HRS)   Acute renal failure associated with advanced liver dysfunction.

isoenzymes   A subgrouping of parent enzymes that are more specific to a particular cell type.

jaundice   A yellow cast of the skin, sclera, and mucous membranes caused by elevated bilirubin, a yellow pigment.

Kupffer's cells   Fixed tissue macrophages found in the liver.

lobule   The functional unit of the liver.

partial thromboplastin time (PTT)   Measures the intrinsic coagulation pathway.

portal hypertension   Elevated portal vein pressure that is sustained at above-normal levels.

prothrombin time (PT)   Measures the coagulation extrinsic pathway.

splanchnic circulation   The combination of the portal venous and arterial circulatory systems of the viscera.

unconjugated bilirubin   Fat-soluble bilirubin that has not yet joined with glucuronic acid.

urea   A nitrogen substance produced by the liver from ammonia.

urobilinogen   Bilirubin in the urine.

varices   Dilated veins. Singular form is varix.

ABBREVIATIONS

AHF	Acute hepatic failure
Alk Phos	Alkaline phosphatase (ALP)
ALT	Alanine aminotransferase (SGPT)
AST	Aspartate aminotransferase (SGOT)
BUN	Blood urea nitrogen
FHF	Fulminant hepatic failure
GFR	Glomerular filtration rate
GGT	Gamma glutamyl transferase
GI	Gastrointestinal
HAV	Hepatitis A virus
HBsAg	Hepatitis B surface antigen
HBV	Hepatitis B virus
HCV	Hepatitis C virus
HDV	Hepatitis D virus
HEV	Hepatitis E virus
HIV	Human immunodeficiency virus
HRS	Hepatorenal syndrome
INR	International normalized ratio
LDH	Lactic dehydrogenase
mcg	Micrograms
OCT	Ornithine carbamoyl transferase
PT	Prothrombin time
PTT	Partial thromboplastin time
SGOT	Serum glutamic oxaloacetic transaminase (AST)
SGPT	Serum glutamic pyruvic transaminase (ALT)
SIRS	Systemic inflammatory response syndrome
STD	Sexually transmitted disease
5'-N	5'-nucleotidase

SECTION ONE: Anatomy of the Liver

At the completion of this section, the learner will be able to identify the anatomic structures of the liver.

Located in the right upper quadrant of the abdominal cavity, the liver lies directly underneath the diaphragm. The liver has two major lobes, the right and the left. The right lobe can be further differentiated into the caudate and quadrate lobes, located on the posterior and inferior liver surfaces, respectively (Fig. 31–1). It is enclosed in visceral peritoneum and covered with Glisson's capsule, a connective tissue structure that provides support to the liver. The capsule subdivides into branches, called septa, that extend into the liver parenchyma to form individual liver lobules.

The **lobule** is the functional unit of the liver (Fig. 31–2). It is a cylindrically shaped unit that surrounds a central vein in a spokelike fashion. Each lobule is composed of hepatic cellular plates that radiate out from the central vein. The hepatic cells (hepatocytes) secrete bile, which flows into the bile canaliculi, a small space separating the hepatic cellular plates. From the canaliculi, bile flows into terminal bile ducts located in the septa, or spaces, lying between adjoining lobules. The septa contain the portal venules, which provide blood flow from the portal veins. The portal venules supply the blood that flows by the hepatic cellular plates, and ultimately flows into the central vein of the lobule. The physiologic structure of the lobule allows continuous exposure of blood to the hepatic cells.

Bile is composed primarily of bile salts. It also contains bilirubin, cholesterol, electrolytes, and other substances. Bile

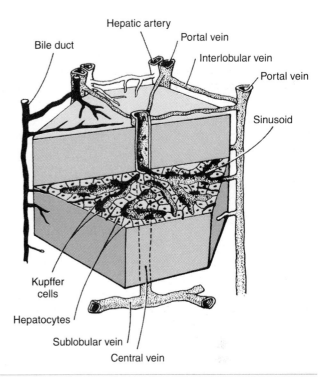

Figure 31–2 ■ Microscopic structure of hepatic function unit (liver lobule). *(From Wilson, L. M., & Lester, L. B. [1992]. Liver, biliary tract, and pancreas. In S. A. Price & L. M. Wilson [Eds].* Pathophysiology: Clinical concepts of disease processes, *(4th ed., p. 338). St. Louis: Mosby Year Book.)*

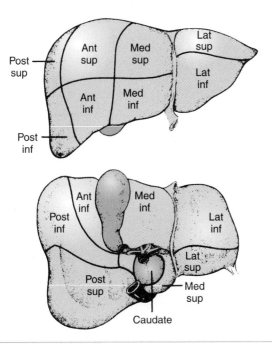

Figure 31–1 ■ Segmental anatomy of the liver. The major lobar fissure, separating the right and left lobes, passes from the inferior vena cava through the gallbladder bed. *(Reproduced with permission from Way, L. W. [1985].* Current surgical diagnosis and treatment, *(7th ed., p. 398). Norwalk, CT: Appleton & Lange.)*

flows through the bile duct system, which ultimately dumps bile into either the gallbladder or the duodenum. Approximately 0.5 to 1.0 L of bile is formed each day; the capacity of the gallbladder is only about 50 mL. Once in the gallbladder, the bile's water and inorganic salt content is absorbed by blood vessels and lymphatics, increasing the bile concentration by about 10 times. Bile is intermittently emptied from the gallbladder via contraction, which is stimulated by the presence of chyme in the duodenum. Foods with high fat content provide the strongest contraction stimulus (Guyton & Hall, 2000).

Splanchnic Circulation

The term *splanchnic* refers to the viscera (the abdominal organs). The combination of the portal venous and arterial circulatory systems of the viscera is called the **splanchnic circulation** (Fig. 31–3). Approximately 10 to 15 percent of the cardiac output (about 1.5 L per minute) flows through the liver (Bass & Yao, 2002). The volume of blood flowing into the liver is primarily determined by the volume of blood flow through the spleen and gastrointestinal (GI) tract, both of which are parts of the splanchnic circulation. The liver is richly supplied with both arterial and venous blood (Fig. 31–4). The arterial blood supply is the hepatic artery, a branch of the aorta. The portal vein brings in blood from the spleen, intestines, pancreas, and stomach. The hepatic veins drain blood away from the liver to the inferior vena cava.

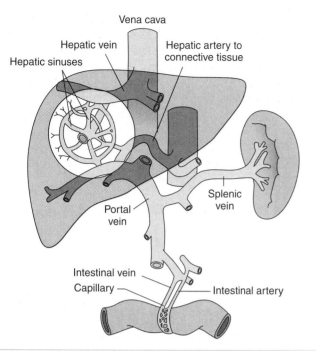

Figure 31–3 ■ The splanchnic circulation. *(Reproduced with permission from Guyton, A. C. [1992]. Human physiology and mechanisms of disease. (5th ed., p. 485). Philadelphia: W. B. Saunders.)*

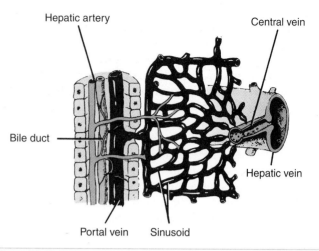

Figure 31–4 ■ Vascular anatomy of liver lobule. *(Reproduced with permission from Way, L. W. [1985]. Current surgical diagnosis and treatment, (7th ed., p. 404). Norwalk, CT: Appleton & Lange.)*

In summary, the liver is located in the right upper quadrant of the abdominal cavity. The lobule is the functional unit and consists of hepatic cellular plates. Hepatocytes secrete bile, which is stored in the gallbladder in a highly concentrated state until it is needed. Splanchnic circulation accounts for a significant portion of the cardiac output. Both the spleen and GI tract are important in determining the volume of hepatic blood flow.

SECTION ONE REVIEW

1. The functional unit of the liver is called the
   - A. hepatocyte
   - B. lobule
   - C. canaliculi
   - D. capsule
2. Bile is secreted by
   - A. terminal bile ducts
   - B. the quadrate lobe
   - C. canaliculi
   - D. hepatocytes
3. The primary substance in bile is
   - A. bile salts
   - B. bilirubin
   - C. cholesterol
   - D. electrolytes
4. The blood volume flowing through the liver represents what percentage of cardiac output?
   - A. 10 percent
   - B. 20 percent
   - C. 30 percent
   - D. 40 percent

5. The portal vein brings in blood from which organs? (choose all that apply)
   1. kidneys
   2. spleen
   3. intestines
   4. pancreas
   - A. 2, 3, and 4
   - B. 1, 2, and 3
   - C. 3 and 4
   - D. 1, 3, and 4

Answers: 1. B, 2. D, 3. A, 4. A, 5. A

SECTION TWO: The Functions of the Liver

At the completion of this section, the learner will be able to discuss the functions of the liver. The liver provides multiple functions that are essential to life, including metabolism, blood filtration, blood clotting, and acting as a blood volume reservoir.

Metabolic Functions

The liver plays a crucial role in fat, carbohydrate, and protein metabolism because of its ability to synthesize, convert, degrade, or store these nutritional substances. In addition, the liver is important in maintaining normal levels of fat-soluble vitamins and iron in the body.

Fat Metabolism

The liver is responsible for the synthesis of phospholipids and cholesterol. Through oxidation of fatty acids, the liver can supply the body with massive amounts of energy. A major function of the liver is the production and excretion of bile. A major component of bile—bile salts—are necessary for normal digestion. In the intestines, bile salts assist in absorption of fat products, such as fatty acids, cholesterol, and fat-soluble vitamins. Bile salts also assist in the breakdown of fat molecules through a detergentlike action. A second major component of bile is bilirubin, a bile pigment (discussed in Section Three).

Carbohydrate Metabolism

The liver plays a major role in maintaining normal blood glucose levels. Glucose is stored in the liver as glycogen, which is converted back into glucose as needed by the body through the process of glycogenolysis. The liver is also able to convert amino acids to glucose through the process of gluconeogenesis.

Protein Metabolism

Protein metabolism is essential to life. The liver is responsible not only for synthesis of the majority of the body's proteins but it also degrades amino acids for energy use through the process of deamination. The major by-product of deamination is ammonia, which is toxic to tissues. The liver is responsible for converting ammonia into **urea,** a nontoxic substance. Urea diffuses from the liver into the circulation for urinary excretion. When liver failure occurs, ammonia cannot be converted to urea and levels rapidly build in the blood.

Vitamin- and Mineral-Related Functions

Adequate levels of bile are needed for absorption of the fat-soluble vitamins A, D, E, and K. Should the production of bile be deficient, fat absorption decreases and the levels of these vitamins become significantly reduced. The liver requires vitamin K for production of clotting factors. If the level of vitamin K is low, clotting factor production will be reduced, possibly causing coagulation deficit complications. The liver also plays a crucial role in the early steps of the conversion of vitamin D into its active product 1,25-dihydroxycholecalciferol, which helps control the concentration of calcium.

The liver is the major storage center for iron. Ten percent of iron is bound to ferritin within hepatocytes and is released into the body as iron levels become depleted (Stolz, 2002). Iron is an important part of hemoglobin synthesis; more than half the body's iron is located in hemoglobin. Liver damage (e.g., cirrhosis) can decrease the hepatocytes' ability to store iron. If iron stores become depleted, iron-deficiency anemia can develop.

Blood Volume Reservoir

The liver serves as a reservoir for blood. Its massive vascular bed and its ability to expand and compress provide a large potential overflow receptacle. During periods of high fluid volume states in the right heart, the liver is able to accept approximately 1 L of the excess volume by distending, which decreases circulating fluid volume. In periods of fluid volume deficit, the liver is able to compress, shifting blood into the intravascular space, thereby increasing circulating fluid volume.

Blood Filter

Blood flowing through the intestines becomes contaminated with a variety of pathogens. Special fixed macrophages in the liver called **Kupffer's cells** efficiently and rapidly engulf and destroy bacteria, viruses, and other pathogens before the blood moves back into general circulation. The Kupffer's cells, which are located in the sinusoids on endothelial cells, are part of the tissue macrophage system (also called the reticuloendothelial system). The tissue macrophage system consists of mobile macrophages that are able to move freely through the tissues, and fixed macrophages that are attached to tissues. Fixed macrophages, such as the Kupffer's cells, are able to detach from their tissue when stimulated in order to carry out their phagocytic activities. The Kupffer's cells also filter out foreign particles and old cells.

Blood Clotting Factors

The liver is responsible for the formation of most blood clotting factors. Normal formation of clotting factors requires synthesis of vitamin K by the intestines. When vitamin K synthesis is hindered, the formation of clotting factors is inhibited, leading to bleeding tendencies. The liver also produces fibrinogen, a protein that forms fibrin threads and blood clots when acted on by thrombin.

Drug Metabolism and Detoxification

The liver plays a major role in the metabolism of fat-soluble drugs. Through biotransformation, it changes potentially harmful drugs into harmless substances that are then excreted by the kidneys. The liver also has the ability to detoxify harmful endogenous substances.

In summary, the liver lobule is the functional unit of the liver. It plays a crucial role in many body functions. Table 31–1 lists the major functions of the liver.

TABLE 31–1 Major Functions of the Liver

GENERAL FUNCTION	COMMENTS
Metabolic	Fat metabolism—massive energy source; produces bile
	Carbohydrate metabolism—maintains normal blood glucose
	Protein metabolism—synthesis of proteins and deamination of amino acids; converts ammonia to urea
	Vitamin and minerals—major role in absorption of fat-soluble vitamins (A, D, E, and K); major storage area for iron
Blood volume reservoir	Able to distend and compress to alter circulating blood volume
Blood filter	Tissue macrophages, Kupffer's cells, purify the blood of bacteria
Blood clotting factors	Produces clotting factors including prothrombin and fibrinogen
Drug metabolism and detoxification	Responsible for metabolism of drugs; is able to deactivate potentially harmful substances and ready them for excretion in a harmless form

SECTION TWO REVIEW

1. The major function of bile salts is to assist with
   A. absorption of fat products
   B. blood clotting
   C. conversion of vitamin D
   D. protein synthesis
2. The majority of iron is located in
   A. the liver
   B. bone
   C. fat
   D. hemoglobin
3. The major by-product of amino acid deamination is
   A. bilirubin
   B. ammonia
   C. fatty acids
   D. glucose
4. The blood filtering capabilities of the liver are primarily the result of the presence of
   A. Kupffer's cells
   B. immunoglobulins
   C. ammonia
   D. bile

Answers: 1. A, 2. D, 3. B, 4. A

SECTION THREE: Evaluation of Liver Function Through Laboratory Tests

At the completion of this section, the learner will be able to discuss liver function through evaluation of laboratory test results. A variety of common laboratory tests are available to evaluate the liver's ability to carry out its major metabolic and blood clotting activities.

Serum Enzyme Studies

Many cell activities require **enzymes** acting as catalysts to carry out their normal functions. Under normal circumstances, intracellular enzymes remain within their cell confines. When cell walls are damaged, these enzymes are released and can be found in surrounding tissues and in the serum. Most enzymes are found in two or more types of cells. For example, alanine aminotransferase is most highly concentrated in the liver, but it is also found in the kidneys, heart, and skeletal muscles. For this reason, a diagnosis of hepatic dysfunction is made based on clinical presentation and serum tests.

Hepatic Enzymes

The liver's multiple metabolic functions require the assistance of a variety of enzymes. Three of the most common are

- **Alanine aminotransferase (ALT, SGPT)**
- **Aspartate aminotransferase (AST, SGOT)**
- **Alkaline phosphatase (Alk Phos, ALP)**

Table 31–2 summarizes information on the three major liver enzymes.

Although they are of great value, enzyme levels cannot be used as definitive tests for hepatic dysfunction because they are nonspecific to the liver. If the patient's clinical presentation and initial enzyme levels do not give a clear diagnostic picture, the physician may order isoenzyme levels.

Isoenzymes

Isoenzymes are subgroups of the parent enzymes and are more specific to a particular type of cell. Several alkaline phosphatase isoenzymes found in the liver include 5'-nucleotidase (5'-N), gamma glutamyl transferase (GGT), and ornithine carbamoyl transferase (OCT). Two isoenzymes of lactic dehydrogenase (LDH) also predominate in the liver. These are LDH isoenzymes 4 and 5 (LDH4 and LDH5). Table 31–3 summarizes information concerning these isoenzymes.

Bilirubin

Bilirubin is the end product of hemoglobin degradation, which occurs in the liver. It is the pigmented portion of heme. Through the oxidation process, heme is turned into bilirubin and then is released into the bloodstream. There are two types of bilirubin: fat soluble and water soluble. Fat-soluble bilirubin has not yet passed through the liver (prehepatic). Prior to undergoing a

TABLE 31–2 Enzyme Studies Measuring Liver Function

ENZYME	NORMAL RANGE	TREND IN LIVER DISEASE	COMMENTS
Alanine aminotransferase (ALT, SGPT)	5–35 U/mL	Increased up to 20 times normal	False elevations noted with various drugs and alcohol; more specific to liver than to other organs. The ratio of AST/ALT usually is greater than 1 in alcoholic cirrhosis and liver congestion and less than 1 in acute hepatitis.
Aspartate aminotransferase (AST, SGOT)	0–35 U/L (female values slightly lower)	Increased	False elevations noted with various drugs; rises with damage to kidneys, heart, pancreas, and brain as well as liver
Alkaline phosphatase (Alk Phos)	20–90 U/L	Increased; levels will elevate two to three times normal when bile duct obstruction is present	False high or low values occur with a variety of drugs; rises with damage/disease of kidneys and bone as well as liver; a sensitive measure of biliary tract obstruction

Normal ranges from Kee, J. (2002). Laboratory and diagnostic tests with nursing implications, (6th ed.). Upper Saddle River, NJ: Prentice Hall. Comments from Kee, J. (2002) and Krumberger, J. M. (1998). Gastrointestinal patient assessment. In M. R. Kinney et al. (Eds.), AACN's clinical reference for critical care nurses, (4th ed., pp. 1011–1012). St. Louis: C. V. Mosby.

TABLE 31–3 Isoenzymes for Evaluation of Liver Function

ISOENZYME	NORMAL RANGE	TREND IN DYSFUNCTION	COMMENTS
LDH isoenzymes (LDH4 and LDH5)	LDH4: 8–16 LDH5: 6–16	Increased	This combination of LDH isoenzymes is common only to liver and skeletal muscle injury; many drugs result in false elevations of LDH
Alk Phos isoenzymes (5'-nucleotidase [5'-N])	Less than 17 U/L	Increased	5'-N is the most hepatobiliary tissue-specific ALP isoenzyme; elevated levels suggest a hepatobiliary problem
Gamma glutamyl transferase (GGT)	0–45 U/L	Increased	GGT is fairly specific to hepatobiliary tissues; it is, however, also present in pancreatic and renal cells; elevated GGT is present in serum of alcohol abusers

All normal ranges are from Kee, J. (2002). Laboratory and diagnostic tests with nursing implications, (6th ed.). Upper Saddle River, NJ: Prentice Hall.

conversion in the liver, it is called **unconjugated bilirubin.** Once in the liver, bilirubin is first split from albumin molecules by the hepatocytes and then is conjugated (joined) with glucuronic acid. In this conjugated state, it becomes water-soluble bilirubin.

Water-soluble bilirubin is also called **conjugated,** or posthepatic, **bilirubin.** In this state, it is transported as bile from the liver into the intestines. From the intestines, most of the bilirubin is excreted through the feces. A small amount is excreted through the urine (urobilinogen). Very little conjugated bilirubin remains in the circulation to return to the liver; therefore, when bilirubin is measured, it is primarily the unconjugated (prehepatic) level that is being measured.

Testing for Bilirubin

Conjugated (or "direct") bilirubin (posthepatic, water soluble) is measured using a direct method because it requires no modifications before being measured. Unconjugated (or "indirect") **bilirubin** (prehepatic, fat soluble) is measured using an indirect method because it must be altered to a water-soluble state using a solvent before it can be measured. **Urobilinogen** is measured as a sensitive test for hepatic damage. It may increase before serum bilirubin levels increase. In early hepatitis or mild liver cell damage, the urine urobilinogen level will increase despite an unchanged serum bilirubin level. However, with severe liver failure, the urine urobilinogen level may decrease because less bile will be produced. This test might be ordered along with a urinalysis. Table 31–4 summarizes the different types of bilirubin testing. Note the very small normal serum levels.

Bilirubin is a yellow pigment that provides a yellow cast to its surroundings. For example, bilirubin provides the brown color of stool. When normal elimination of bilirubin is obstructed, the characteristic yellow color becomes noticeably absent from stool and becomes evident in body fluids, as well as on the skin, sclera, and mucous membranes. This condition is called **jaundice.** Jaundice does not usually become clinically apparent until total bilirubin exceeds 2.5 mg/dL.

Testing Coagulation

The liver has an important role in maintaining normal coagulation because it produces prothrombin, vitamin K, and other clotting factors that are essential to the coagulation cascade. If liver function becomes compromised and these substances can no longer be synthesized in adequate quantities, the patient is at increased risk for serious bleeding complications. Two common blood tests are used to measure the two coagulation pathways, prothrombin time and partial thromboplastin time.

The **prothrombin time (PT)** measures the extrinsic coagulation pathway. Prothrombin (factor II of the coagulation cascade) is produced by the liver and is dependent on vitamin K, which is also produced by the liver. Hepatocytes produce most of the clotting factors, each of which has a predictable serum half-life; thus, monitoring clotting factor levels is often used as an indirect indicator of hepatic function (Pratt & Kaplan, 2001). Prolonged prothrombin times may be seen with chronic liver disease (e.g., cirrhosis) or vitamin K deficiency. Normal prothrombin time is 10 to 13 seconds (Kee, 2002). Unfortunately, the traditional measurement of prothrombin time can vary depending on the reagent and method used. For this reason, the preferred measure of prothrombin time is the international normalized ratio (INR). The normal range of INR is 2.0 to 3.0 (Kee, 2002). INR is particularly recommended for monitoring long-term warfarin therapy although it is not to be used until the dose has been stabilized.

Partial thromboplastin time (PTT) measures the intrinsic coagulation pathway. It is a more sensitive test than PT in detecting clotting deficiencies in all factors except VII and XIII. Elevations of PTT are seen with severe liver disease or heparin therapy. Normal PTT is 60 to 70 seconds (Kee, 2002). Activated partial thromboplastin time (APTT) is a more sensitive test than PTT in the detection of defects in clotting factors, including minor defects. The APTT differs from the PTT test only in that the reagent contains an activator. Normal APTT is 20 to 35 seconds (Kee, 2002).

TABLE 31–4 Bilirubin Testing

TYPE	NORMAL VALUES	COMMENTS
Total bilirubin	0.1–1.2 mg/dL	Measures both conjugated and unconjugated bilirubin
		Elevations seen with biliary obstruction
Indirect bilirubin	0.1–1.0 mg/dL	Measures prehepatic, unconjugated bilirubin; elevations associated with viral hepatitis and other disease processes where lysis of red blood cells occur
Direct bilirubin	0.1–0.3 mg/dL	Measures posthepatic conjugated bilirubin; elevations associated with multiple intrahepatic and bile duct dysfunctions
Urobilinogen	Negative in freshly voided urine	Measures posthepatic urobilinogen in the urine; elevations associated with early or recovery phase liver cell damage
		Antibiotics may decrease levels

Normal ranges from Kee, J. (2002). Laboratory and diagnostic tests with nursing implications, (6th ed.). Upper Saddle River, NJ: Prentice Hall. Comments from Kee (2002) and Krumberger, J. M. (1998). Gastrointestinal patient assessment. In M. R. Kinney et al. (Eds.), AACN's clinical reference for critical care nurses, (4th ed., pp. 1011–1012). St. Louis: C.V. Mosby.

Serum Ammonia

Elevated levels of serum ammonia indicate that the liver is not adequately converting ammonia to urea for proper elimination in the urine. Serum ammonia levels may be drawn intermittently to evaluate trends. As levels increase, the patient will present with increasing signs of hepatic encephalopathy. Arterial ammonia levels are recommended over venous specimens because they more accurately reflect the stage of encephalopathy. The normal range for serum ammonia is 15 to 45 mcg/dL (Kee, 2002). Ammonia will be discussed in more detail in Section Five.

Serum Albumin

The liver synthesizes albumin and many other proteins; thus as liver function decreases, protein levels will also decrease. Serum albumin is a good indicator of general protein levels. The half-life of albumin is relatively long (19 to 21 days) so serum albumin levels are poor indicators of acute hepatic injury (Ghany & Hoofnagle, 2001; Green & Flamm, 2002). Serum level trends are evaluated in conjunction with other nutritional and liver function data. Reduced levels are associated with several severe illnesses. The normal range for serum albumin is 3.5 to 5.0 g/dL (Kee, 2002). Refer to Module 23 for a detailed discussion of other nutritional measurement data that reflect liver function.

Evidence-Based Practice

- *The risk of developing a complication following the TIPS procedure is high (49 percent), with a high 3-month mortality rate following the procedure (32 percent). The three most common complications found in this study included encephalopathy (49 percent), infection (19 percent), and renal failure (17 percent) (Silva et al., 2004).*

- *Serum venous ammonia levels correlated positively with the severity of hepatic encephalopathy in patients with a preestablished encephalopathy score. Venous ammonia levels were found to be an acceptable measurement when compared to measuring partial arterial or venous ammonia pressures (Ong et al., 2003).*

- *Eradication of gastric H. pylori in patients with pneumonia reduces serum and gastric ammonia levels (Demirturk et al., 2001).*

- *Patients who come into the emergency department with gross GI bleeding should be evaluated for possible colonic ischemia (Ullery et al., 2004).*

In summary, laboratory tests are a major source of diagnostic data. Although enzyme studies can give general information regarding tissue injury, isoenzymes often provide data that is more specific to liver tissue injury. Other laboratory tests that provide important data include serum bilirubin, prothrombin time, partial thromboplastin time, ammonia levels, and albumin levels. Data from these tests are used in conjunction with clinical presentations to diagnose a specific liver dysfunction and differentiate it from other disease processes. These tests are generally obtained intermittently to evaluate trends.

SECTION THREE REVIEW

1. Serum enzyme laboratory levels are obtained to measure
   - A. clotting factors
   - B. organ function
   - C. cellular injury
   - D. tissue oxygenation

2. Serum isoenzyme levels often provide better data than parent enzyme levels because they are
   - A. faster to obtain
   - B. more tissue specific
   - C. more plentiful
   - D. easier to measure

3. Which combination of LDH isoenzymes best reflects hepatic injury?
   - A. LDH1 and LDH2
   - B. LDH2 and LDH3
   - C. LDH3 and LDH4
   - D. LDH4 and LDH5

4. Bilirubin is
   - A. secreted by hepatocytes
   - B. broken down into bile salts
   - C. produced primarily in the pancreas
   - D. the end product of hemoglobin degradation

5. When a serum bilirubin is obtained, it primarily measures _____ bilirubin.
   - A. unconjugated
   - B. posthepatic
   - C. conjugated
   - D. water-soluble

Answers: 1. C, 2. B, 3. D, 4. D, 5. A

SECTION FOUR: Acute Hepatitis

At the completion of this section, the learner will be able to describe the etiology and clinical manifestations associated with acute hepatitis.

Acute hepatitis is defined as an inflammatory liver disease, usually of viral origin, that results in liver injury and necrosis. The term *acute* implies that the condition lasts less than 6 months and ends either in complete resolution of the injured hepatic tissue or in rapid deterioration to liver failure and death (Fallon et al., 2001a). Acute hepatitis affects multiple body systems.

Etiology and Epidemiology

Five common viruses are associated with acute hepatitis: hepatitis A (HAV), hepatitis B (HBV), hepatitis C (HCV), hepatitis D (HDV), and hepatitis E (HEV). Other viral sources include cytomegalovirus (CMV), and Epstein–Barr virus (EBV). Less common causes of acute hepatitis include drug toxicity (e.g., acetaminophen, erythromycin, and isoniazid) and alcohol abuse.

Hepatitis A (infectious hepatitis, HAV) is transmitted through the fecal–oral route only during acute infection and is most commonly found in children and young adults. HAV is frequently associated with epidemics and is transmitted primarily through contaminated food or water. There is a high incidence of HAV in underdeveloped countries. Eating contaminated raw shellfish is sometimes responsible for HAV. Immunity occurs following acute illness. HAV is not associated with development of chronic hepatitis. A vaccine against HAV has been approved in the United States. It is recommended for high-risk populations (e.g., health care and childcare workers, travelers to endemic areas of the world, and persons who are immunosuppressed). Immune globulin should be administered to those with close contacts with HAV as prophylaxis therapy (Deinsteig & Isselbacher, 2001).

Hepatitis B (serum hepatitis, HBV) is transmitted through contaminated blood serum or body fluids. There are 1.0 to 1.25 million people in the United States with chronic HBV infection (Berenger & Wright, 2002). The prevalence of HBV has decreased over the past 15 to 20 years because of increased safe sexual practices in view of the human immunodeficiency virus (HIV) epidemic, as well as the development and wide distribution of HBV vaccine. People who are exposed to contaminated needles or body fluids are at risk for contracting hepatitis B. The at-risk population for HBV is similar to the HIV at-risk group (Table 31–5); it is considered a significant sexually transmitted disease (STD). Hepatitis B is seen in all age groups. It occurs throughout the world and is endemic in many parts of the world, though not in the United States. It is a major cause of acute and chronic hepatitis and cirrhosis. A vaccine is available to protect at-risk populations from HBV.

Hepatitis C (HCV) is a major cause of chronic hepatitis, cirrhosis, and hepatocellular carcinoma. An estimated 3 million to

TABLE 31–5 At-Risk Population for Hepatitis B Virus (HBV)

- Illicit drug users
- Health care workers
- Male homosexuals
- People who require frequent transfusions (e.g., hemophiliacs)
- People with decreased immunocompetence
- Sexual partners of people infected with HBV
- Newborns of mothers infected with HBV

4 million people are infected with HCV in the United States (Deinsteig & Isselbacher, 2001). HCV is primarily transmitted through blood and blood products. Major risk factors for developing HCV include blood transfusions prior to 1992, injection drug use, and occupational exposure. HCV is a major indication for liver transplantation (Lauer & Walker, 2001).

Hepatitis D (HDV), also known as delta virus, is not a complete virus and requires the surface antigen of the hepatitis B virus (HBsAg) to act as its outer shell in order to be a viable virus. Patients who do not test positive for HBV need not be tested for HDV. HDV is primarily transmitted through the blood serum and in the United States is primarily found in hemophiliacs and intravenous drug users.

Hepatitis E (HEV) is similar to HAV in its transmission through a fecal–oral route. Most cases of HEV follow contamination of water supplies in endemic areas of Africa, Asia, India, and Central America. It is rarely encountered in the United States.

Pathophysiologic Basis of Acute Hepatitis

The pathologic effects of acute hepatitis are the same regardless of the causative agent. Acute hepatitis can be divided into three categories based on the severity of the disease: classic hepatitis, submassive hepatic necrosis, and massive hepatic necrosis. Acute hepatitis is generally considered a reversible disease unless complications develop.

Classic hepatitis is characterized by a liver that is normal in size and color, or by one that has mild enlargement and edema with bile staining present. Necrosis is localized but inflammation is generalized. The liver tissue structures remain intact throughout the disease process.

Submassive hepatic necrosis is characterized by more generalized necrosis, with a large number of necrotic hepatocytes. Inflammation is severe and injury leads to the collapse of hepatic tissues with subsequent loss of lobule structure. Fibrosis of hepatic tissue may develop during the healing stage.

Massive hepatic necrosis is characterized by extensive necrosis with loss of entire lobules. This type of acute hepatitis is associated with the development of fulminant hepatic failure, which is discussed further in Section Five of this module.

Clinical Manifestations of Acute Hepatitis

Viral hepatitis is generally associated with a prodromal period in which the person develops flulike symptoms. The urine may become dark several days before bilirubinemia causes jaundice to be present. Jaundice usually peaks by week 2 of onset (Ghany & Liang, 2003).

Only about 25 percent of people with acute hepatitis develop jaundice. Based on this manifestation, hepatitis can be divided into anicteric and cholestatic hepatitis. **Anicteric hepatitis** refers to hepatitis with no jaundice. Patients with anicteric hepatitis may have severely compromised liver function that is overlooked because of lack of jaundice. **Cholestatic hepatitis** refers to hepatitis with retention of bile as a result of a biliary obstruction (usually secondary to the inflammatory process). Persons with cholestatic hepatitis usually are severely jaundiced, urine is dark, and feces are clay colored. Serum bilirubin becomes greatly elevated with obstructive disease. The clinical manifestations of acute viral hepatitis are summarized in Table 31–6.

In summary, acute hepatitis is primarily of viral origin. Multiple viruses can cause acute hepatitis, including hepatitis A, B, C, D, and E; cytomegalovirus; and Epstein–Barr virus. Acute hepatitis causes hepatic injury and necrosis that is generalized throughout the organ. The severity of acute hepatitis can be divided into three categories: classic, submassive, and massive. Acute hepatitis is usually reversible. The clinical manifestations of acute hepatitis typically include a prodromal period in which the patient experiences flulike symptoms. If the patient has cholestatic hepatitis, jaundice will develop and serum bilirubin levels will significantly increase.

TABLE 31–6 Clinical Manifestations of Acute Viral Hepatitis

Prodromal period

"Flulike" symptoms: malaise, headache, anorexia, hyperpyrexia, nausea and vomiting, arthritis, myalgia, abdominal pain

Jaundice

Anicteric hepatitis—no jaundice is present

Cholestatic hepatitis—jaundice that may be severe; dark urine is present several days before jaundice appears; stool is clay colored; serum bilirubin is 20 to 30 mg/dL

SECTION FOUR REVIEW

1. Acute hepatitis is most commonly caused by
   A. bacterial invasion
   B. viral invasion
   C. yeast invasion
   D. an autoimmune reaction
2. The major cause of acute and chronic hepatitis and cirrhosis is
   A. cytomegalovirus
   B. hepatitis C virus
   C. Epstein–Barr virus
   D. hepatitis B virus
3. Classic hepatitis is characterized by
   A. localized necrosis
   B. a greatly enlarged liver
   C. development of fibrosis
   D. development of fulminant hepatic failure

4. If a patient has anicteric hepatitis, the nurse would expect to see
   A. dark urine
   B. clay-colored stool
   C. normal-colored urine
   D. black stool
5. If a patient has cholestatic hepatitis, the nurse would anticipate serum bilirubin levels to
   A. fall below normal range
   B. remain within normal range
   C. elevate slightly above normal
   D. rise significantly above normal

Answers: 1. B, 2. D, 3. A, 4. C, 5. D

SECTION FIVE: Acute Hepatic Failure

At the completion of this section, the learner will be able to describe the etiology and clinical manifestations associated with acute hepatic failure.

The term **hepatic failure** refers to the inability of the liver to perform its normal functions. Acute hepatic failure (AHF) results from one of the three following situations:

1. As a primary disease process in the absence of preexisting hepatic disease

2. As a complication of chronic liver disease
3. In association with multiple organ failure in the critically ill

Regardless of the cause of AHF, many of the clinical manifestations are the same.

Acute Hepatic Failure as a Primary Disease

Although uncommon, acute hepatic failure (AHF) can occur without preexisting liver disease. Four possible etiologies include shock, virulent viral infection, hepatotoxins, and systemic inflammatory response (see multiple organ failure, below).

Shock

The liver is extremely vulnerable to ischemic injury, as are the other splanchnic organs. A sustained hypotensive episode (shock) can result in insufficient oxygenation of liver tissue, which can precipitate ischemic hepatitis. In response to hypoxia, the delicate endothelial lining of the hepatic capillaries becomes damaged and more permeable. Increased permeability allows fluid to leak from the capillaries into the hepatic tissue. As fluid shifts out of the vasculature, microthrombi develop, partly as a result of the high concentration of particulate matter remaining in the vessels. Microthrombi can cause a blockage of blood flow with subsequent tissue ischemia and necrosis distal to the blockages. Though the liver has a large reserve, if tissue destruction exceeds this reserve, acute liver failure will result. Ischemic hepatitis may spontaneously resolve or it may degenerate into acute hepatic failure. The longer the initial hypotensive episode continues, the more severe the liver destruction will be.

Viral Infection and Hepatotoxins

A particularly severe form of acute hepatic failure is called **fulminant hepatic failure (FHF)**. Fulminant hepatic failure can result from multiple causes. Two major causes are acute viral infections and hepatotoxins. Hepatitis A and B are the most common viral causes. The most common hepatotoxin precipitating fulminant hepatic failure is acetaminophen. In some cases no cause is found, although an undetected viral etiology is generally suspected. A more extensive listing of known causes of fulminant hepatic failure is presented in Table 31–7.

Definitions of fulminant hepatic failure vary widely. For the purposes of this module, the definition of FHF is based on the following criteria: the level of encephalopathy, the preexisting liver status, and the rate of onset. Fulminant hepatic failure is defined as a form of acute hepatic failure in a patient with no preexisting history of liver disease that develops rapidly (in less than 8 weeks) accompanied by encephalopathy. FHF causes rapid, massive deterioration and destruction of liver tissue with widespread hepatocellular necrosis. The result is severe hepatic dysfunction with subsequent development of encephalopathy. FHF is a medical emergency responsible for 2,000 deaths a year in the United States (Yee & Lidofsky, 2002). Survival is 20 percent without liver transplantation.

Acute Hepatic Failure as a Complication of Chronic Liver Disease

Cirrhosis of the liver is the third leading cause of death in people between the ages of 25 and 65 (Mihas, 2001). Fallon and colleagues (2001b) define cirrhosis as "the irreversible end result of fibrous scarring and hepatocellular regeneration that constitute the major responses of the liver to a variety of longstanding inflammatory, toxic, metabolic, and congestive insults" (p. 387). The onset of cirrhosis is insidious and progressive. In the United States, the two most common causes of cirrhosis are alcohol abuse and hepatitis C. Over time, the progressive deterioration of hepatic function becomes sufficient to compromise the normal functioning of the liver.

Acute Hepatic Failure as Part of Multiple Organ Failure

A major body insult, such as sepsis, can set off a systemic inflammatory response that, in turn, leads to a series of physiologic events. This response is called the *systemic inflammatory response syndrome (SIRS)*. When SIRS develops, the normally localized inflammatory response becomes a systemic, malignant process. SIRS results in a single or multiple organ inflammatory insult. In the liver, the inflammatory response sets off a massive release and assault by the liver macrophages (Kupffer's cells), causing destruction of liver tissue. The inflammatory response also causes the endothelial lining of the vessels to become more permeable, allowing fluids to leak into the liver parenchyma and resulting in organ edema and microthrombi. The microthrombi and inflammation eventually lead to the damage of hepatocytes and the blockage of bile flow. When damage becomes severe, hepatic failure ensues. Acute hepatic failure as part of the multiple organ dysfunction syndrome is discussed in Module 16.

Clinical Manifestations of Acute Hepatic Failure

The massive tissue destruction caused by AHF produces essentially the same manifestations regardless of its etiology. The clinical manifestations of AHF reflect severe hepatic encephalopathy and multiple metabolic dysfunctions.

TABLE 31–7   Causes of Fulminant Hepatic Failure (FHF)

Viral infections: Hepatitis A, B, C, and D; cytomegalovirus (CMV); Epstein–Barr virus (EBV)

Hepatotoxins: Acetaminophen, mushroom toxins, isoniazid (INH), hydrocarbons

TABLE 31–8 Stages of Hepatic Encephalopathy

STAGE[a]	CLINICAL MANIFESTATIONS
I	Awake, apathetic, restless, sleep pattern changes, mental clouding, impaired computational ability, impaired handwriting, subtle intellectual function changes, diminished muscle coordination; electroencephalogram (EEG) shows mild-to-moderate abnormalities
II	Decreased level of consciousness, lethargy, drowsiness, disorientation to time and place, confusion, asterixis, diminished reflexes, slurring of speech; EEG shows moderate-to-severe abnormalities
III	Stupor (arousable), no spontaneous eye opening, hyperactive reflexes, seizures, rigidity, abnormal posturing: decorticate, decerebrate, extensor plantar responses; EEG shows severe abnormalities
IV	Coma (may or may not respond to painful stimuli), seizures, pupillary dilation, flaccidity; EEG shows severe abnormalities

[a]Stage 0 encephalopathy may be used to describe subclinical intellectual impairment.

Hepatic Encephalopathy

Encephalopathy is the hallmark of acute hepatic failure. **Hepatic encephalopathy,** also called hepatic coma or "portosystemic encephalopathy," is defined as an altered neurologic status caused by a buildup of circulating toxins of hepatic origin (e.g., ammonia). The encephalopathy associated with FHF is frequently associated with hypoglycemia and cerebral edema. Cerebral edema is the leading cause of death in FHF. Hepatic encephalopathy has been staged (graded) according to clinical manifestations for clarity (Table 31–8). Hepatic encephalopathy is also considered a complication of AHF and is further discussed in Section Six.

Metabolic Dysfunction

Liver failure develops when more than 60 percent of hepatocytes are injured, reflected in the organ's inability to perform its multiple metabolic functions. Liver failure results in the following metabolically related clinical manifestations:

- **Protein metabolic dysfunction.** Ascites, hypoalbuminemia, hepatic encephalopathy, evidence of impaired clotting factors (hemorrhage, epistaxis, purpura)
- **Carbohydrate metabolism dysfunction.** Hypoglycemia
- **Fat metabolism dysfunction.** Nausea and vomiting, anorexia, constipation or diarrhea, prolonged PT

These metabolic dysfunctions are expressed in alterations in body systems, as noted in Table 31–9.

In summary, acute hepatic failure can develop as a primary disease process or as a complication of chronic liver disease or multiple organ failure. The clinical manifestations of acute hepatic failure reflect encephalopathy and the loss of many liver functions. Fulminant hepatic failure is a critical illness with a high mortality rate, characterized by massive hepatic necrosis and severe encephalopathy. The presence of hepatic encephalopathy, primarily from high ammonia levels, is considered the hallmark of hepatic failure.

TABLE 31–9 Effects of Hepatic Failure on Body Systems

SYSTEM	CLINICAL MANIFESTATIONS
Neurologic	Stage I to IV encephalopathy
Cardiovascular	Pulmonary edema, hypotension
Gastrointestinal	Nausea and vomiting, constipation or diarrhea, anorexia, ascites
Hematopoietic	Impaired coagulation, prolonged PT
Pulmonary	Tachypnea, crackles (rales)

SECTION FIVE REVIEW

1. Which of the following statements is true regarding fulminant hepatic failure?
   A. it causes necrosis of liver tissue
   B. it has a mortality of less than 50 percent
   C. it is characterized by stage I and II encephalopathy
   D. it has a slow, insidious onset
2. A major hepatotoxin that is known to cause fulminant hepatic failure is
   A. acetaminophen
   B. gentamicin
   C. aspirin
   D. cephalosporin
3. In the United States, cirrhosis of the liver is most commonly caused by
   A. hepatitis A virus
   B. alcohol abuse

   C. hepatitis B virus
   D. Epstein–Barr virus
4. Stages III and IV hepatic encephalopathy are characterized by
   A. stupor, coma
   B. lethargy, asterixis
   C. restlessness, slurred speech
   D. sleep pattern changes, drowsiness
5. Hepatic encephalopathy is primarily caused by high levels of
   A. bilirubin
   B. bile
   C. ammonia
   D. blood urea nitrogen (BUN)

Answers: 1. A, 2. A, 3. B, 4. A, 5. C

SECTION SIX: Complications of Hepatic Dysfunction

At the completion of this section, the learner will be able to describe complications of hepatic dysfunction.

The inability of the liver to meet all of the demands placed on it by other systems places the patient at risk for many multisystem complications. The severity of the complications is related to the level of liver dysfunction. Table 31–10 lists the major complications of hepatic dysfunction.

Hepatic Encephalopathy

As previously discussed, hepatic encephalopathy is caused by toxic levels of circulating ammonia, which readily crosses the blood–brain barrier. Normally, the liver rapidly converts ammonia into urea, which is then excreted in the urine. When the liver is unable to convert ammonia to urea, toxicity rapidly develops.

Contributing Factors

A variety of factors contribute to increased nitrogenous waste, thus contributing to increased ammonia levels.

- **Constipation.** Nitrogenous wastes remain in the GI tract longer, providing more opportunity for conversion to ammonia
- **Blood in the GI tract.** As blood in the tract is broken down, ammonia is released
- **Azotemia.** Contributes to the build up of nitrogenous wastes
- **Dietary protein consumption.** Provides amino acids, thus more ammonia buildup
- **Certain drugs.** Tranquilizers, sedatives, and analgesics remain longer in the body

Portal Hypertension

Normal hepatic venous flow meets moderate resistance (8 to 10 mm Hg) when compared with the low resistance level (2 to 8 mm Hg) of the connecting vena cava. When hepatic tissue is in-

TABLE 31–10 Common Complications of Hepatic Failure

- Hepatic encephalopathy
- Portal hypertension
- Esophageal varices
- Ascites
- Infections: Sepsis and spontaneous bacterial peritonitis
- Acute renal failure

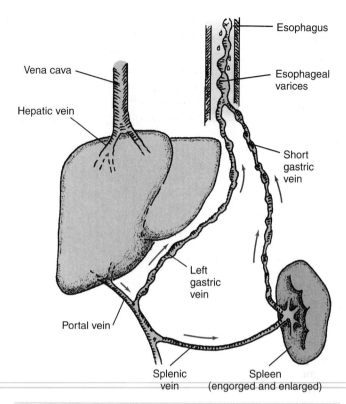

Figure 31–5 ■ Portal hypertension. Damage to liver tissue increases vascular resistance. Venous flow becomes blocked in the liver, causing portal vein pressure to increase. Blood backs up through the splenic vein into the spleen and collateral venous circulation (such as the short and left gastric veins).

jured or destroyed, blood flowing through the damaged areas requires more pressure to maintain organ blood flow. Consequently, increased hepatic capillary resistance occurs in a fashion similar to that which is created in the lungs when they sustain parenchymal damage.

Portal hypertension results from increased resistance within the portal venous system. This is usually caused by cirrhosis, which disrupts the normal lobular structure of the liver. This disruption causes resistance to blood flow into, through, and out of the liver with resultant portal hypertension. Over time, as in chronic hepatic dysfunction, the liver develops a system of collateral circulation that helps to relieve the increase in pressure. These collateral veins are called **varices** and are characterized by their dilated, tortuous appearance. In acute hepatic failure, however, collateral circulation does not have sufficient time to develop, and back flow leads to congestion of other organs in the splanchnic circulation. Figure 31–5 illustrates how circulation is affected by portal hypertension.

Esophageal Varices

Esophageal varices are a major complication of portal hypertension. Blood naturally flows through vessels with the least resistance, seeking the easiest path. This diversion of flow is called shunting. The esophageal veins (varices) in the lower portion of the esophagus provide a common collateral flow diversion. Esophageal varices dilate to accept shunted blood. A rapid increase in pressure (e.g., coughing, vomiting, straining) can cause these dilated varices to rupture, precipitating hemorrhage. Bleeding esophageal varices are considered a medical emergency. Esophageal varices develop in 50–60 percent of patients with cirrhosis (Bass & Yao, 2002).

Ascites

Ascites is defined as an abnormal collection of fluid in the abdominal cavity. Ascites develops during advanced-stage hepatic dysfunction. Two major causes of ascites are decreased colloid osmotic pressure and portal hypertension. Colloid osmotic pressure decreases as a result of a reduction in albumin. Hypoalbuminemia is caused by the inability of the liver to carry out its usual protein metabolism functions. When colloid osmotic pressure becomes too low, fluid shifts from the intravascular compartment into other body compartments (e.g., the intra-abdominal cavity). In addition, cirrhotic patients can develop extreme sodium retention by the kidneys, which leads to ascites. This phenomenon is caused by an alteration in renal sodium and water excretion related to hypoalbuminemia, hyperaldosteronism, and increased antidiuretic hormone levels (Garcia & Sanyal, 2001).

Hepatorenal Syndrome

Hepatorenal syndrome (HRS) refers to renal failure in patients with severe liver failure in the absence of renal pathology (Wong & Blendis, 2001). A diagnosis of hepatorenal syndrome should not be made until other types of acute renal failure are ruled out. Hepatorenal syndrome can be divided into two subgroups: type 1 and type 2.

Type 1 hepatorenal syndrome (type 1 HRS) is characterized by severe, rapidly progressive renal failure with a doubling of the serum creatinine to a level greater than 2.5 mg/dL or halving of the creatinine clearance to less than 20 mL per minute in less than 2 weeks (Arroyo et al., 2002; Garcia & Sanyal, 2001; Wong & Blendis, 2001). Type 1 HRS often occurs following a precipitating event that results in a hypotensive episode, such as aggressive diuresis, large volume paracentesis, spontaneous bacterial peritonitis, gastrointestinal bleeding, a major surgical procedure; or acute viral hepatitis superimposed on cirrhosis. Type 1 HRS is "the complication of cirrhosis with the poorest prognosis with a mean survival after onset of 2 weeks" (Arroyo et al., 2002, p. 1663). Type 1 HRS is associated with a 90 percent mortality without liver transplantation (Garcia & Sanyal, 2001).

Type 2 hepatorenal syndrome (type 2 HRS) has a slower, chronic, more progressive increase in the serum creatinine level to greater than 1.5 mg/dL or a creatinine clearance of less than 40 mL per minute (Arroyo et al., 2002; Wong & Blendis, 2001).

TABLE 31–11   Clinical Characteristics of Hepatorenal Syndrome

- Presence of liver failure
- Decreasing glomerular filtration rate (GFR)
- Reduced urine sodium (less than 10 mEq/24 hours)
- Presence of azotemia (elevated creatinine and blood urea nitrogen)
- Oliguria or anuria
- High BUN/creatinine ratio

Data from Fallon et al. (2002). Cirrhosis of the liver and its complications. In T. E. Andreoli, C.C. J. Carpenter, R. C. Griggs, & J. Loscalzo (Eds.). Cecil essentials of medicine, (5th ed., pp. 387–393). Philadelphia: W. B. Saunders.

Patients with type 2 HRS usually exhibit signs of liver failure and arterial hypotension to a lesser degree than patients with type 1 HRS. Most patients with type 2 HRS have severe ascites refractive to diuresis (Vargas, 2002). Those patients with type 2 HRS are predisposed to the development of type 1 HRS. HRS may be a clinical continuum and not two separate entities. The clinical characteristics of hepatorenal syndrome are presented in Table 31–11.

Infections: Sepsis and Spontaneous Bacterial Peritonitis

The Kupffer's cells play a crucial part in controlling the inflammatory response and in cleansing gram-negative intestinal bacteria from the blood. Their ability to detoxify bacteria and vasoactive substances inhibits development of a systemic inflammatory response and hemodynamic instability. In addition, the liver produces special proteins and enzymes that assist in controlling the inflammatory response. The loss of Kupffer's cells in the liver to cleanse the blood as well as loss of protein synthesis places the hepatic failure patient at risk for development of sepsis and SIRS.

The patient with acute hepatic failure is also at risk for development of spontaneous bacterial peritonitis. This form of peritonitis occurs when ascites becomes infected. Bacteria are able to translocate (migrate) into the ascites when the bowel wall loses its integrity as a result of endothelial damage secondary to tissue ischemia or infarct. Intestinal bacteria move across the injured intestinal wall and seed themselves in the ascites fluid. A hypotensive episode is the most common cause of intestinal wall injury in this patient population. The bowel is the primary source of bacteria in both sepsis and spontaneous bacterial peritonitis.

In summary, there are multiple serious complications associated with hepatic failure that can negatively impact the patient's prognosis. Complications of acute hepatic failure include hepatic encephalopathy, hepatorenal syndrome, sepsis, and spontaneous bacterial peritonitis. Portal hypertension can result in esophageal varices.

SECTION SIX REVIEW

1. Portal hypertension is caused by
   A. increased vascular resistance
   B. decreased portal vein blood flow
   C. increased hepatic artery volume
   D. decreased hepatic blood flow
2. Esophageal varices dilate in response to
   A. decreased hepatic blood flow
   B. hepatic vasoconstriction
   C. shunted splanchnic blood
   D. increased cardiac output
3. A major cause of ascites is
   A. hyperalbuminemia
   B. low colloid osmotic pressure
   C. hepatorenal syndrome
   D. fluid volume overload
4. A major factor contributing to onset of acute renal failure as a complication of hepatic failure is
   A. hepatotoxins
   B. a hypotensive episode

C. high ammonia levels
   D. portal vein shunting
5. The onset of type 2 hepatorenal syndrome usually occurs in the presence of
   A. hepatotoxins
   B. a hypotensive episode
   C. high ammonia levels
   D. severe ascites
6. The hepatic failure patient is at risk for spontaneous bacterial peritonitis as a result of
   A. translocation of intestinal bacteria
   B. increased bacterial growth in intestines
   C. secondary hepatic bacterial infection
   D. unknown causes

Answers: 1. A, 2. C, 3. B, 4. B, 5. D, 6. A

SECTION SEVEN: Medical Management

At the completion of this section, the learner will be able to describe an overview of the medical management of the patient with hepatic dysfunction. Management of the patient with acute hepatic dysfunction is primarily supportive regardless of the causative agent.

Management of Acute Viral Hepatitis

There is no specific therapy for treatment of viral hepatitis. Table 31–12 summarizes the general focuses for medical management of acute viral hepatitis. Patients with this diagnosis do not necessarily require hospitalization.

Management of Acute Hepatic Failure Complications

Failure of the liver to adequately carry out its many functions has a deleterious effect on multiple body systems. The patient will remain at high risk for complications until the liver has healed adequately to regain its functions. Management is primarily supportive and complications are addressed as they arise. When a complication is identified, management focuses on reversal, reduction, or correction to prevent permanent damage

TABLE 31–12 Supportive Medical Management for Acute Viral Hepatitis

FOCUS	GENERAL MANAGEMENT
Activity/rest	Limit activities based on level of fatigue
	Require rest based on severity of symptoms
Hydration/nutritional needs	Maintain balanced hydration status Diet: high carbohydrate, low fat; no alcohol intake
	Nausea management: metoclopramide and hydroxyzine in small doses
	Vitamin K, if needed
Hospitalization criteria	Hospitalization is indicated if severe nausea and vomiting develops, deteriorating liver function is noted (e.g., hepatic encephalopathy and/or prolonged prothrombin time)

Data from Fallon et al. (2001b). Cirrhosis of the liver and its complications. In T. E. Andreoli, C. C. J. Carpenter, R. C. Griggs, & J. Loscalzo (Eds.). Cecil essentials of medicine, (5th ed., pp. 387–393). Philadelphia: W.B. Saunders.

or death. The remainder of this section focuses on major complications that often develop during acute hepatic failure, including hepatic encephalopathy, hypoglycemia, metabolic abnormalities, gastrointestinal hemorrhage, fulminant hepatic failure, cerebral edema, and esophageal varices.

Hepatic Encephalopathy

Management of hepatic encephalopathy centers around four goals. Three of the four goals focus on control and elimination of ammonia:

- Identify and treat the precipitating factors when possible
- Reduce the amount of bacteria in the bowel
- Eliminate or reduce generation of ammonia toxins
- Prevent movement of ammonia toxins from the bowel

Identify and Treat the Precipitating Factors. Hepatic encephalopathy can be triggered or worsened by certain precipitating factors (Table 31–13). It is important to rapidly identify and aggressively treat precipitating factors to reduce the severity of the encephalopathy.

Reduce Bacteria in the Bowel. The aminoglycoside, neomycin, is frequently ordered to suppress ammonia-producing intestinal bacteria. One gram of neomycin administered orally every 6 to 8 hours can maintain long-term suppression for the treatment of hepatic encephalopathy. Neomycin is not well absorbed through the gastrointestinal tract; thus, its effects are primarily local. As with all aminoglycosides, the patient must be monitored for the potential side effects of ototoxicity and nephrotoxicity. Metronidazole (Flagyl) 250 mg administered three or four times a day is as effective as oral neomycin without the risks of ototoxicity or nephrotoxicity. Treatment with metronidazole should not exceed 2 weeks to avoid the development of peripheral neuropathy (Abou-Assi & Vlahcevic, 2001).

Gastrointestinal bleeding and constipation can precipitate hepatic encephalopathy. In the event of GI bleeding or constipation, the bowels should be cleansed of all residual blood and stool by administration of enemas. This will prevent further buildup of nitrogenous waste by speeding transit of blood through the bowel (Fitz, 2002).

Eliminate or Reduce Ammonia Toxins. Protein intake must be either eliminated or tightly controlled. There is evidence that controlling protein intake (including the type of protein) rather than eliminating it may be useful in decreasing hepatic encephalopathy. Dietary protein is often limited to 60 g per day. Vegetable proteins rather than animal proteins may have

---

TABLE 31–13 Precipitating Factors Associated with Hepatic Encephalopathy

- Infection
- Elevated protein intake
- Worsening hepatic function
- Constipation
- Azotemia (elevated blood urea nitrogen and creatinine)
- Gastrointestinal bleeding
- Hypovolemia

---

a beneficial effect because of lower rates of ammonia production (Fitz, 2002).

Prevent Movement of Ammonia Toxins. The synthetic disaccharide, lactulose, may be ordered to help prevent absorption of ammonia from the bowel. The laxative effect of lactulose moves stool through the intestines more rapidly, thus decreasing the amount of ammonia formed before the stool is eliminated. Lactulose also may facilitate trapping of ammonia ions in the intestines for unknown reasons. Lactulose breaks down into lactic acid and other organic acids that may facilitate the ammonia-trapping action. It is also theorized that lactulose may modify the intestinal flora in some manner, thereby causing a reduction in absorption of bacteria through the bowel. Typically, 15 to 30 mL of lactulose is administered four times a day (oral or enema) or adjusted as necessary to attain three to five soft stools per 24 hours (Abou-Assi & Vlahcevic, 2001; Fitz, 2002).

Hypoglycemia

Liver failure interferes with normal carbohydrate metabolism. Thus, the patient may develop hypoglycemia secondary to decreased gluconeogenesis. Management consists of frequent monitoring of serum glucose levels and close observation for the development of hypoglycemic symptoms. Treatment of hypoglycemia may consist of a continuous IV infusion of 10 percent dextrose solution. If the hypoglycemia is severe, 50 percent dextrose may be ordered as immediate treatment.

Metabolic Abnormalities

Electrolyte abnormalities, such as hyponatremia and hypokalemia, are common in patients with liver failure. Hyponatremia results from sodium loss due to diuretic therapy, the hemodilution effect, and sodium restriction. Hypokalemia is caused by diuretic therapy and elevated aldosterone levels, which result from the loss of the liver's ability to metabolize aldosterone. In addition, the renin–angiotensin–aldosterone system is activated by diminished renal blood flow.

Acid–base imbalances are also common occurrences. The acute hepatic failure patient is at risk for developing metabolic acidosis for two major reasons. First, hepatic cellular damage releases lactic acid, which results in lactic acidosis. Second, metabolic acidosis is a complication of acute renal failure, a common sequela of hepatic failure. Respiratory alkalosis may develop from hyperventilation associated with compensatory mechanisms. Treatment of acid–base imbalances consists of correcting the underlying problems and administering bicarbonate if necessary.

Gastrointestinal Hemorrhage

The acute hepatic failure patient is at risk for development of GI hemorrhage for several reasons. One is the stress associated with severe illness, which can precipitate development of stress ulcers. Another is the presence of abnormal clotting factors, which increases the risk for abnormal bleeding. The mortality rate is high for the first episode of GI bleeding and, should the patient survive the first episode, repeated bleeds are common. Therapy generally consists of prevention of stress ulcers using histamine antagonists or antacids, and controlling the coagulopathy through use of vitamin K and blood products. Table 31–14 summarizes the supportive medical management of acute hepatic failure based on common complications.

TABLE 31–14 Summary of Supportive Medical Management of Acute Hepatic Failure Complications

COMPLICATION	MANAGEMENT
Hepatic encephalopathy	Correct the precipitating cause, if possible
	No protein intake, or consider control of protein intake
	Enema if constipation or gastrointestinal bleeding
	Lactulose (PO, NG, rectal), 15–30 mL administered qid or as necessary to attain three to five soft stools per 24 hours
	Neomycin, 1–4 g (PO or enema) every 6 to 8 hrs
	Metronidazole 250 mg (PO) three to four times a day
	Intubate and mechanically ventilate
Hypoglycemia	10 percent dextrose continuous IV infusion
	50 percent dextrose IV, as required
	Monitor for low serum glucose and clinical manifestations of hypoglycemia
Metabolic abnormalities	Frequent monitoring of serum electrolytes and pH
	Correct electrolyte abnormalities
	Administer bicarbonate, as necessary
Gastrointestinal hemorrhage	Vitamin K
	Oral antacids or H$_2$ receptor antagonists (IV to keep gastric pH greater than 5
	Fresh frozen plasma, possibly platelets
Cerebral edema	Intracranial pressure monitoring
	IV mannitol
	Consider barbiturate-induced coma, if indicated
	Elevate head of bed 20 to 30 degrees
Hepatorenal syndrome	Liver transplanation
	Fluid resuscitation
	May consider transjugular intrahepatic portosystemic (TIPS) shunt
	Dopamine, 5–10 mcg/kg per minute (to increase renal blood flow)
Spontaneous bacterial peritonitis	Antibiotic therapy
	Third-generation cephalosporin, usually administered for 5 to 7 days (until ascitic fluid cell count is normal)

Data from Fallon et al. (2001b). Cirrhosis of the liver and its complications. In T. E. Andreoli, C. C. J. Carpenter, R. C. Griggs, & J. Loscalzo (Eds.). Cecil essentials of medicine, (5th ed., pp. 387–393). Philadelphia: W. B. Saunders; Arnell, T. D. (2002). Gastrointestinal bleeding. In F. S. Bongard & D. Y. Sue (Eds.). Current critical care diagnosis and treatment, (2nd ed., pp. 756–767). New York: Lange.

Fulminant Hepatic Failure

As soon as fulminant hepatic failure (FHF) is suspected, the patient should be transferred to a critical care unit. When feasible, it is also recommended that FHF patients be transferred to medical centers that specialize in FHF management because the patient's survival may often depend on rapid identification and management of multisystem complications. The causative problem of FHF is not usually treatable; therefore, the primary focus of medical management is supportive. Liver transplantation is usually required in patients who do not spontaneously recover from FHF. This requires transfer of the patient to a liver transplant center as soon as the decision is made. The survival rate of patients with fulminant hepatic failure restricted to medical management is less than 20 percent, whereas the survival rate associated with liver transplantation is greater than 60 percent (Yee & Lidofsky, 2002). Transplantation is discussed in detail in Module 26.

Cerebral Edema

Cerebral edema is an ominous complication of FHF. Its etiology is unknown yet its presence significantly reduces the patient's chances of survival. If edema cannot be adequately controlled, intracerebral herniation may result and is generally fatal.

Esophageal Varices

Portal hypertension leads to formation of venous collateral vessels between the portal and systemic circulations. These collateral vessels become dilated, tortuous veins (varices) within the submucosa of the esophagus and stomach. Esophageal varices are unpredictable; they can rupture at any time. Their close association with cirrhosis, and its specific pathologic features, places the patient at high risk for hemorrhage. Management of the patient with bleeding esophageal varices is summarized in Table 31–15.

In summary, medical management of the patient with hepatic dysfunction is primarily supportive. The person with acute viral hepatitis may be managed at home unless complications develop. Rest, control of activities, hydration, and special diet are baseline interventions. Management of acute hepatic failure complications is based on the exact complication that has developed. Hepatic encephalopathy results from high serum ammonia levels, which are toxic to the brain. Management includes identifying and treating the precipitating cause, reducing bacteria in the bowel, eliminating or reducing ammonia toxins, and preventing movement of ammonia toxins. Hypoglycemia can develop because of decreased gluconeogenesis. Treatment focuses on close monitoring of serum glucose and observing the patient for the clinical manifestations of hypoglycemia. Infusions of 10 to 50 percent dextrose may be required if hypoglycemia becomes severe. Metabolic abnormalities resulting from hepatic failure include electrolyte and acid-base abnormalities. Close monitoring of serum electrolyte and serum pH is required and the underlying causes are treated. GI hemorrhage can develop from stress ulcer formation. Bleeding is further

TABLE 31–15 Management of the Patient with Esophageal Varices

FOCUS OF TREATMENT	INTERVENTIONS
Control bleeding	**IV vasopressin** Reduces splanchnic blood flow Initial dose of 20 units followed by continuous IV infusion of 0.4–0.6 units per minute **Somatostatin** (or synthetic analog octreotide) Reduces splanchnic blood flow and portal pressure Less systemic vasoconstrictive effects than vasopressin Initial dose of 50 mcg per hour continuous IV infusion **Nitroglycerin** Given with vasopressin to decrease systemic vasoconstrictive effects (i.e., cardiac or mesenteric ischemia) **Fresh frozen plasma** A replacement of clotting factors; Platelets may be ordered, although their efficacy is controversial
Aggressive correction of bleeding varices	**Sengstaken-Blakemore** or Minnesota tube placement An inflated balloon that tamponades bleeding varices (see Fig. 31–6) **Portal systemic shunt surgery** Portocaval anastomosis Transjugular intrahepatic shunt (TIPS) (see Fig. 31–7) Distal splenorenal shunt
Preventive therapy	Therapy to reduce portal pressure: Nonselective beta blockers (i.e., propanolol, nadolol) Mononitrates (i.e., isosorbide mononitrate) Elective shunt surgery Endoscopic sclerotherapy Endoscopic variceal banding The varix is isolated and banded, which results in oblation

Data from Fallon et al. (2001b). Cirrhosis of the liver and its complications. In T. E. Andreoli, C. C. J. Carpenter, R. C. Griggs, & J. Loscalzo (Eds.). Cecil essentials of medicine, (5th ed., pp. 387–393). Philadelphia: W. B. Saunders; Arnell, T. D. (2002). Gastrointestinal bleeding. In F. S. Bongard & D. Y. Sue (Eds.), Current critical care diagnosis and treatment, (2nd ed., pp. 756–767). New York: Lange.

complicated by an impaired clotting ability, which can result in severe hemorrhage in this patient population. The development of fulminant hepatic failure (FHF) is a medical emergency, requiring aggressive supportive treatment. Liver transplantation is the treatment of choice if the patient's liver does not spontaneously recover. Cerebral edema is an ominous complication of FHF and may result in brain herniation if not corrected quickly. Esophageal varices result from portal hypertension in the presence of severe liver damage. The varices are often unstable and can rupture, causing severe upper GI hemorrhage.

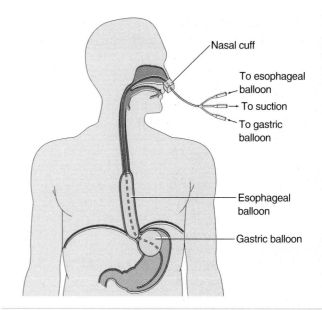

Figure 31–6 ■ Sengstaken-Blakemore tube.

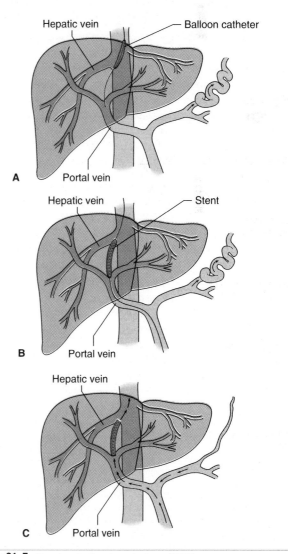

Figure 31–7 ■ Transjugular intrahepatic shunt (TIPS).

SECTION SEVEN REVIEW

1. Dietary management of the patient with acute viral hepatitis should include
   A. high protein, low fat
   B. low fat, high carbohydrate
   C. low carbohydrate, low fat
   D. low protein, high fat
2. A patient with acute viral hepatitis will most likely be admitted to the hospital if he or she experiences
   A. severe fatigue
   B. occasional nausea
   C. elevated bilirubin
   D. hepatic encephalopathy
3. The patient with acute hepatic failure will require strict nutritional control of
   A. protein
   B. fat
   C. carbohydrates
   D. fiber
4. The patient with acute hepatic failure would most likely receive which of the following continuous IV infusions based on altered glucose metabolism?
   A. lactated Ringer's
   B. 5 percent dextrose
   C. 10 percent dextrose
   D. normal saline

5. To correct bleeding in the patient with bleeding esophageal varices, the treatment of choice is
   A. sclerotherapy
   B. portosystemic shunt
   C. packed red blood cells
   D. Hespan
6. As a treatment for hepatic encephalopathy, intestinal bacteria levels are suppressed by
   A. lactulose
   B. neomycin
   C. tyrosine
   D. Histamine antagonists
7. Acute hepatic failure is associated with development of hyponatremia, which is precipitated by
   1. hemodilution
   2. diuretic therapy
   3. sodium restriction
   4. hepatic cell damage
   A. 2, 3, and 4
   B. 1, 3, and 4
   C. 1 and 2
   D. 1, 2, and 3

Answers: 1. B, 2. D, 3. A, 4. C, 5. A, 6. B, 7. D

SECTION EIGHT: Nursing Implications

At the completion of this section, the learner will be able to describe the nursing implications appropriate to managing care of the patient experiencing acute hepatic dysfunction.

General Goals

Medical management of acute hepatic dysfunction, particularly during the most active disease stages, is collaborative. Evaluation of hepatic function is performed through laboratory testing and other diagnostic procedures (noninvasive and invasive), which typically require a physician's orders and diagnostic expertise. The two goals that drive the majority of management activities are

1. To determine and correct the underlying cause
2. To support the patient until liver function returns

Collaborative interventions to support the patient center around two goals: (1) promoting stable hemodynamic and ventilatory status and (2) preventing or minimizing secondary complications.

The nurse plays a crucial role in improving patient outcomes by being responsible for bedside assessment and analysis of the patient's status on a continual basis. A major focus of the nursing assessment involves monitoring the patient for the signs and symptoms of multisystem complications. The nurse facilitates the medical diagnostic process by preparing the patient and family for procedures, assisting with procedures, and monitoring the patient's status during and after procedures. The nurse also develops nursing hypotheses and subsequent independent nursing diagnoses based on the patient's response to the illness, rather than the illness itself. This section provides a description of that part of a comprehensive nursing history and physical assessment, which focuses specifically on hepatic function.

The Focused Nursing Database

On admission, it is crucial that the nurse obtain a comprehensive nursing database. The nurse particularly focuses on data that may have a positive or negative impact on patient outcomes.

The Focused Nursing History

General historical data to collect include preexisting medical conditions; surgeries; and recent history information, such as the events leading up to the patient's admission and a description of the patient's symptoms.

Focused Health Maintenance History

When obtaining the health maintenance portion of the history, the nurse should focus on obtaining information regarding

- Diet and eating patterns
- Usual appetite prior to admission
- Weight fluctuations
- History of skin or wound healing problems

Focused Cognitive–Perceptual History

Information regarding the patient's usual mental status, ability to communicate, and presence of discomfort or pain provides important baseline data.

Focused Value–Belief History

Acute hepatic dysfunction may place the patient at significant risk. Information regarding the value–belief patterns of the patient and family can assist the nurse with planning appropriate supportive interventions.

The Focused Nursing Assessment

Assessment of the patient with acute hepatic dysfunction has two major focuses: (1) monitoring for potential complications, a collaborative effort, and (2) monitoring the progress of the independent nursing diagnoses. The following sections present some of the major assessments that may be obtained on an ongoing basis during an acute hepatic dysfunction episode to monitor the patient for potential complications.

Respiratory/Circulatory Assessment

Hepatic failure can significantly alter cardiopulmonary function, primarily through severe third spacing of fluids with subsequent intravascular fluid volume deficit. The nurse must monitor the patient for

- Signs and symptoms of fluid volume deficit
- Edema, which may be peripheral or generalized, or may be present in the form of pulmonary edema
- Diminished or adventitious breath sounds (crackles, in particular)
- Abnormal trends in blood pressure and pulse

Elimination Assessment

The adequacy of renal function is closely monitored because of the risk for development of hepatorenal syndrome. This is accomplished through observation of ordered renal function laboratory tests (e.g., blood urea nitrogen [BUN], creatinine, urine sodium) and evaluation of renal function by measuring intake and output balance and urinary output volume.

Neurologic Assessment

The patient's neurologic status requires close monitoring throughout the duration of the acute illness because hepatic failure can lead to hepatic encephalopathy and is also known to cause cerebral edema. The clinical manifestations of hepatic encephalopathy are described in Section Five and contributing factors are presented in Section Six. The neurologic assessment should minimally include the following.

Focused Cognitive–Perceptual Assessment

- **Glasgow Coma Scale (GCS).** The GCS is a useful trending tool that assesses the arousal component of consciousness. An altered level of consciousness is an early finding in hepatic encephalopathy. The GCS specifically addresses eye opening, verbal response, and motor response.

Focused Muscular–Skeletal Assessment

- **Coordination.** Coordination becomes increasingly impaired in the early stages of encephalopathy.
- **Reflexes.** Reflexes become hypoactive in the early stages of hepatic encephalopathy and hyperactive in the later stages.
- **Movement.** Asterixis (also called *liver flap* when associated with liver failure) refers to an involuntary tremor that is particularly noted in the hands but may also be seen in the feet and tongue. It becomes evident at stage II of hepatic encephalopathy.

Focused Neurosensory Assessment

- **Seizures.** Seizures may develop in the later stages of hepatic encephalopathy.

Gastrointestinal and Integumentary Assessment

Hepatic dysfunction is associated with a variety of GI and integumentary clinical manifestations. The majority of the manifestations result from the accumulation of hepatotoxins, third-spaced body fluids, coagulopathies, decreased protein levels, and complications resulting from portal hypertension. Some of the more common GI and integumentary related problems are listed as follows.

Focused GI Assessment.   The nurse should assess for

- **Nausea and vomiting, anorexia**
- **Presence of diarrhea or constipation**

- **Ascites.** Enlarging abdominal girth; shifting dullness on percussion of the abdomen; abdominal fluid wave; protruding umbilicus. In addition, the patient may develop dyspnea, diminished breath sounds, or the clinical manifestations of fluid volume deficit.
- **Bleeding esophageal varices.** The nurse does not independently evaluate the patient for the existence of varices. Instead, the nurse monitors the patient for active variceal bleeding. This is most directly accomplished by assessing nasogastric fluids for blood. If blood is present, the assessment should also include the volume and characteristics of the blood, as well as close assessment for development of the signs and symptoms of hypovolemic shock.
- **Hepatic tenderness and enlargement on palpation**

Focused Integumentary Assessment. The nurse should assess for

- Jaundice
- Pruritus
- Edema
- Dry, flaky skin
- Poor skin turgor
- Caput medusa (visible veins over the umbilical area caused by congestion and dilation of superficial abdominal wall veins associated with portal vein obstruction)

In addition, the skin can be assessed for several clinical manifestations of problems with coagulation, bleeding, and diminished proteins that usually occur with severe hepatic dysfunction, including

- Evidence of poor wound healing
- Ecchymosis or petechiae
- Bleeding gums
- Pale mucous membranes and nailbeds

The Nursing Care Plan

The nursing care plan of the patient experiencing an acute hepatic dysfunction episode usually includes both collaborative problems and independent nursing diagnoses.

Frequently Occurring Collaborative Problems

According to Carpenito-Moyet (2003) and Ulrich and colleagues (2001), the following potential complications (PCs) are commonly associated with hepatic dysfunction:

- PC: Hemorrhage (bleeding)
- PC: Metabolic disorders
- PC: Drug toxicity
- PC: Renal insufficiency

- PC: Progressive liver degeneration
- PC: Portosystemic encephalopathy

Frequently Occurring Nursing Diagnoses

On completion of the nursing database, the nurse clusters data and develops a set of nursing hypotheses based on the available data. Additional critical data that may either support or eliminate each hypothesis should also be identified and obtained. Once the hypotheses have been established, the nurse is ready to develop a list of nursing diagnoses.

For the patient with acute hepatic dysfunction, a variety of nursing diagnoses frequently occur during the crisis period. The following is a partial list of some of these frequently occurring nursing diagnoses, as suggested by Carpenito-Moyet (2003) and Ulrich and colleagues (2001):

- *Ineffective breathing pattern* related to pressure on diaphragm from ascites, weakness, pleural effusion, and thought processes impairment from ammonia toxins
- *Fluid volume deficit* related to reduced intravascular volume, variceal bleeding, and coagulopathy
- *Activity intolerance* related to decreased energy secondary to impaired liver metabolism, tissue hypoxia, and decreased nutritional intake
- *Altered nutrition: Less than body requirements* related to impairment of nutrient absorption and metabolism, decreased nutritional intake, and fat-soluble vitamin malabsorption
- *Altered comfort* related to pruritus secondary to buildup of bile salts and bilirubin pigment
- *Pain: Upper abdominal* related to ascites and enlarged liver
- *Altered thought processes* related to impaired clearance of drugs and ammonia, bleeding, and dehydration
- *High risk for infection* related to leukopenia secondary to hypoproteinemia; and splenic hyperactivity

Many of these nursing diagnoses and their interventions are addressed in other modules. Coagulopathy, which is frequently noted with hepatic dysfunction, is presented as a collaborative problem (PC: bleeding) in Module 29.

In summary, care of the patient with acute hepatic dysfunction requires both collaborative and independent nursing activities. Collaborative interventions center around the medical management goals of supporting the patient and preventing secondary complications until the liver tissue heals and function returns. Monitoring the patient for potential complications during the acute phase of illness requires ongoing and frequent multiple body system assessments. Independent nursing activities are based on the patient's responses to his or her illness rather than the disease process itself. A listing of some of the more frequently occurring nursing diagnoses is provided.

SECTION EIGHT REVIEW

1. A major underlying management goal that drives the majority of medical management activities is to
   A. promote stable hemodynamic status
   B. prevent secondary complications
   C. promote stable ventilatory status
   D. support the patient until liver function returns
2. In the later stages of hepatic encephalopathy, the reflexes typically become
   A. nonactive
   B. hypoactive
   C. normoactive
   D. hyperactive
3. The presence of asterixis indicates that _____ is/are present.
   A. involuntary tremor
   B. loss of coordination
   C. focal seizures
   D. skeletal muscle rigidity

4. The nurse notes the presence of ascites. Assessments for the presence of ascites include (choose all that apply)
   1. abdominal fluid waves
   2. retracting umbilicus
   3. shifting abdominal dullness
   4. enlarging abdominal girth
   A. 1 and 4
   B. 1, 3, and 4
   C. 2, 3, and 4
   D. 1, 2, and 3
5. Dermatologic findings commonly noted in the patient with acute hepatic dysfunction include
   A. oily skin
   B. generalized rash
   C. pruritus
   D. shiny skin

Answers: 1. D, 2. D, 3. A, 4. B, 5. C

POSTTEST

The following Posttest is constructed in a case study format. Questions are asked based on available data. New data are presented as the case study progresses.

Jerome J, 32 years old, was admitted 7 days ago with a severe drug overdose of acetaminophen. He has been in the medical intensive care unit since admission. Jerome's Glasgow Coma Scale peaked at 15 and during the past 24 hours has steadily decreased. The nurse notifies the physician of the change in neurologic status. Based on their assessment, the medical team suspects liver dysfunction.

1. Jerome's liver is extremely important. Blood flowing through the liver accounts for what percentage of his total cardiac output?
   A. 10 to 15 percent
   B. 25 to 30 percent
   C. 35 to 40 percent
   D. 45 to 50 percent
2. If Jerome's splanchnic blood flow is altered, it would directly affect which organs? (choose all that apply)
   1. intestines
   2. spleen
   3. liver
   4. kidneys
   A. 1, 3, and 4
   B. 2 and 3

   C. 2, 3, and 4
   D. 1, 2, and 3
3. If Jerome is experiencing liver dysfunction, his altered fat metabolism will cause
   A. a decrease in his energy availability
   B. an inability to convert glycogen
   C. an increase in serum ammonia
   D. a decrease in stored iron
4. If he is experiencing congestive heart failure, the liver will respond by
   A. vasoconstricting
   B. expanding in size
   C. secreting more bile
   D. secreting antidiuretic hormone

Jerome has serum enzymes ordered. The results are as follows:

ALT = 1,500 units/L

AST = 1,500 units/L

Alk Phos = 140 units/L

5. Jerome's serum enzyme levels indicate that _____ is present.
   A. hepatorenal syndrome
   B. encephalopathy
   C. severe hepatocellular injury
   D. severe cellular injury

6. The physician orders alkaline phosphatase (Alk Phos) isoenzymes for Jerome. Which Alk Phos isoenzyme is considered most hepatobiliary specific?
   A. 5'-nucleotidase
   B. gamma glutamyl transferase (GGT)
   C. ornithine carbamoyl transferase (OCT)
   D. lactic dehydrogenase (LDH) isoenzymes 4 and 5

The nurse notes that Jerome's urine has become dark amber. The quantity was 150 mL in the past hour.

7. Based on the early diagnosis of an acute hepatic dysfunction, the color of Jerome's urine suggests that the nurse can expect
   A. ammonia to decrease
   B. low serum proteins
   C. acute renal failure
   D. jaundice to develop

8. If Jerome is diagnosed as having acute hepatitis, he will most likely receive _____ therapy.
   A. antibiotic
   B. antiviral
   C. antifungal
   D. no specific

9. Which type of viral hepatitis is a major cause of chronic hepatitis, cirrhosis, and hepatocellular carcinoma?
   A. hepatitis A
   B. hepatitis B
   C. hepatitis C
   D. hepatitis D

10. If Jerome develops mild hepatic enlargement and edema, with generalized inflammation but localized necrosis, it would be classified as _____ hepatitis.
    A. classic
    B. submassive
    C. massive
    D. anicteric

11. If he has developed cholestatic hepatitis, you would anticipate assessing for
    A. the absence of jaundice
    B. the presence of gallstones
    C. severe jaundice
    D. an inflamed gallbladder

12. Typical prodromal symptoms of the patient developing acute hepatitis include (choose all that apply)
    1. hyperpyrexia
    2. increased intracranial pressure
    3. nausea and vomiting
    4. arthritis and myalgia
    A. 2, 3, and 4
    B. 1, 3, and 4
    C. 2 and 3
    D. 1, 2, and 3

13. If Jerome had developed stage III encephalopathy, you would anticipate a neurologic presentation to include
    A. restlessness, reversal of sleep rhythm
    B. lethargy, drowsiness
    C. disorientation, asterixis
    D. stupor, hyperactive reflexes

14. Based on Jerome's history, he is at risk for developing fulminant hepatic failure based on which cause?
    A. hepatotoxin ingestion
    B. hepatitis virus
    C. multiple organ failure
    D. complication of chronic failure

15. Jerome has no preexisting history of hepatic dysfunction. It is unlikely that he will develop
    A. acute renal failure
    B. esophageal varices
    C. sepsis
    D. acid–base disorders

16. If he develops spontaneous bacterial peritonitis, it is probably caused by
    A. septicemia
    B. translocation of intestinal bacteria
    C. spread of hepatic infective agent
    D. autoimmune reaction

17. Jerome's encephalopathy is worsening. The nurse notes that he has not had a bowel movement in 3 days. What physician order can the nurse anticipate?
    A. increase dietary protein
    B. neomycin 1 to 2 times per day
    C. daily milk of magnesia
    D. lactulose every hour until desired effect

18. The majority of patients experiencing fulminant hepatic failure ultimately require which intervention?
    A. liver transplantation
    B. portosystemic shunt
    C. sclerotherapy
    D. Sengstaken–Blakemore tube

19. The majority of Jerome's plan of care will focus on which underlying goal?
    A. evaluation of renal function
    B. promotion of stable hemodynamic status
    C. support for the patient until liver function resumes
    D. prevention of secondary complications

20. While assessing his integumentary status, the nurse notes visible veins over the umbilical area. In a patient with hepatic dysfunction, this finding is called
    A. asterixis
    B. ecchymosis
    C. ascites
    D. caput medusa

21. Based on the typical fluid status of the patient with acute hepatic dysfunction, the most appropriate nursing diagnosis to be added to Jerome's plan of care would be
    A. fluid volume deficit
    B. fluid volume excess
    C. cardiac output: decreased
    D. nutrition: more than body requirements

POSTTEST ANSWERS

Question	Answer	Section	Question	Answer	Section
1	A	One	12	B	Four
2	D	One	13	D	Five
3	A	Two	14	A	Five
4	B	Two	15	B	Six
5	D	Three	16	B	Six
6	A	Three	17	D	Seven
7	D	Three	18	A	Seven
8	D	Four	19	C	Eight
9	C	Four	20	D	Eight
10	A	Four	21	A	Eight
11	C	Four			

REFERENCES

Abou-Assi, S., & Vlahcevic, Z. R. (2001). Hepatic encephalopathy: Metabolic consequences of cirrhosis often is reversible. *Postgraduate Medicine, 109*(2), 52–70.

Arroyo, V., Guevara, M., & Gines, P. (2002). Hepatorenal syndrome in cirrhosis: Pathogenesis and treatment. *Gastroenterology, 122*(6), 1658–1676.

Bass, N. M., & Yao, F. Y. (2002). Portal hypertension and variceal bleeding. In M. Feldman, L. S. Friedman, M. H. Sleisenger, & B. F. Scharschmidt (Eds.), *Sleisenger and Fordtran's gastrointestinal and liver disease: Pathophysiology, diagnosis, and management* (7th ed., pp. 1487–1516). Philadelphia: W. B. Saunders.

Berenger, M., & Wright, T. L. (2002). Viral hepatitis. In M. Feldman, L. S. Friedman, M. H. Sleisenger, & B. F. Scharschmidt (Eds.), *Sleisenger and Fordtran's gastrointestinal and liver disease: Pathophysiology, diagnosis, and management* (7th ed., pp. 1278–1342). Phildelphia: W. B. Saunders.

Carpenito-Moyet, L. J. (2003). *Nursing care plans and documentation: Nursing diagnoses and collaborative problems* (4th ed.). Philadelphia: Lippincott Williams, & Wilkins.

Deinsteig, J. L., & Isselbacher, K. J. (2001). Acute viral hepatitis. In E. Braunwald, A. S. Fauci, D. L. Kasper, S. T. Hauser, D. L. Longo, & J. L. Jameson (Eds.), *Harrison's principles of internal medicine* (15th ed., pp. 1721–1737). New York: McGraw Hill.

Demirturk, L., Yazagan, Y., Izci, O., et al. (2001). The effect of *Helicobacter pylori* eradication on gastric juice and blood ammonia concentrations and on visual evoked potentials in cirrhotics. *Helicobacter, 6*(4), 325–331.

Fallon, M. B., McGuire, B. M., Abrams, G. A., & Arguedes, M. R. (2001a). Acute and chronic hepatitis. In T. E. Andreoli, C. C. J. Carpenter, R. C. Griggs, & J. Loscalzo (Eds.), *Cecil essentials of medicine* (5th ed., pp. 376–384). Philadelphia: W. B. Saunders.

Fallon, M. B., McGuire, B. M., Abrams, G. A., & Arguedes, M. R. (2001c). Cirrhosis of the liver and its complications. In T. E. Andreoli, C. C. J. Carpenter, R. C. Griggs, & J. Loscalzo (Eds.), *Cecil essentials of medicine* (5th ed., pp. 387–393). Philadelphia: W. B. Saunders.

Fallon, M. B., McGuire, B. M., Abrams, G. A., & Arguedes, M. R. (2001b) Fulminant hepatic failure. In T. E. Andreoli, C. C. J. Carpenter, R. C. Griggs, & J. Loscalzo (Eds.), *Cecil essentials of medicine* (5th ed., pp. 385–386). Philadelphia: W. B. Saunders.

Fitz, J. G. (2002). Hepatic encephalopathy, hepatopulmonary syndromes, hepatorenal syndrome, coagulopathy, and endocrine complications of liver disease. In M. Feldman, L. S. Friedman, M. H. Sleisenger, & B. F. Scharschmidt (Eds.), *Sleisenger and Fordtran's gastrointestinal and liver disease: Pathophysiology, diagnosis, and management* (7th ed., pp. 1543–1566). Philadelphia: W. B. Saunders.

Garcia, N., & Sanyal, A. J. (2001). Minimizing ascites: Complication of cirrhosis signals clinical deterioration. *Postgraduate Medicine, 109*(2), 91–102.

Ghany, M., & Hoofnagle, J. H. (2001). Approach to the patient with liver disease. In E. Braunwald, A. S. Fauci, D. L. Kasper, S. T. Hauser, D. L. Longo, & J. L. Jameson (Eds.), *Harrison's principles of internal medicine* (15th ed., pp. 1707–1711). New York: McGraw Hill.

Ghany, M. G., & Liang, J. T. (2003). Acute viral hepatitis. In T. Yamada, D. H. Alpers, L. Laine, N. Kaplowitz, C. Owyang, & Powell (Eds.), *Textbook of gastroenterology* Vol. 2. (4th ed., pp. 2276–2309). Philadelphia: Lippincott Williams & Wilkins.

Green. R. M., & Flamm. S. (2002). AGA technical review on the evaluation of liver chemistry tests. *Gastroenterology, 123*(4), 1367–1384.

Guyton, A. C., & Hall, J. E. (2000). *Textbook of medical physiology* (10th ed.). Philadelphia: W. B. Saunders.

Kee, J. L. (2002). *Laboratory and diagnostic tests with nursing implications* (6th ed.). Upper Saddle River, NJ: Prentice Hall.

Lauer, G. M., & Walker, B. D. (2001). Hepatitis C virus infection. *The New England Journal of Medicine, 345*(1), 41–52.

Mihas, A. A. (2001). Cirrhosis of the liver: A three article symposium. *Postgraduate Medicine, 109*(2), 49–50.

Ong, J. P., Aggarwal, A., Easley, K. A., et al. (2003). Correlation between ammonia levels and the severity of hepatic encephalopathy. *American Journal of Medicine, 114*(3), 188–194.

Pratt, D. S., & Kaplan. M. M. (2001). Evaluation of liver function. In E. Braunwald, A. S. Fauci, D. L. Kasper, S. T. Hauser, D. L. Longo, & J. L. Jameson (Eds.), *Harrison's principles of internal medicine* (15th ed., pp. 1711–1715). New York: McGraw Hill.

Silva, R. F., Arroyo Jr., P. C., Duca, W. J., et al. (2004). Complications following transjugular intrahepatic portosystemic shunt: A retrospective analysis. *Transplantation Proceedings, 36*(4), 926–929.

Stolz, A. (2002). Liver physiology and metabolic function. In M. Feldman, L. S. Friedman, M. H. Sleisenger, & B. F. Scharschmidt (Eds.), *Sleisenger and Fordtran's gastrointestinal and liver disease: Pathophysiology, diagnosis, and management* (7th ed., pp. 1201–1226). Philadelphia: W. B. Saunders.

Ullery, B. S., Boyko, A. T., Banet, G. A., & Lewis, L. M. (2004). Colonic ischemia: An under-recognized cause of lower gastrointestinal bleeding. *Journal of Emergency Medicine, 27*(1), 1–6.

Ulrich, S. P., Weyland, W., & Canale, S. W. (2001). *Nursing care planning guides* (5th ed.). Philadelphia: Lippincott Williams & Wilkins.

Vargas, H. I. (2002). Hepatobiliary disease. In F. S. Bongard & D. Y. Sue (Eds.), *Current critical care diagnosis and treatment* (2nd ed., pp. 768–776). New York: Lange.

Wong, F., & Blendis, L. (2001). New challenge of hepatorenal syndrome: Prevention and treatment. *Hepatology, 34*(6), 1242–1251.

Yee, H. F., & Lidofsky, S. D. (2002). Acute liver failure. In M. Feldman, L. S. Friedman, M. H. Sleisenger, & B. F. Scharschmidt (Eds.), *Sleisenger and Fordtran's gastrointestinal and liver disease: Pathophysiology, diagnosis, and management* (7th ed., pp. 1567–1576). Philadelphia: W. B. Saunders.

32 Acute Pancreatic Dysfunction

Allison Steele, Melanie Hardin-Pierce

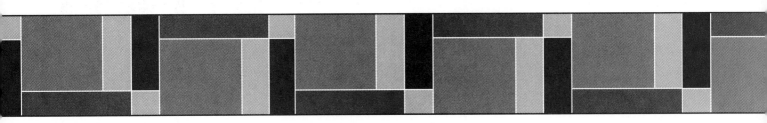

OBJECTIVES Following completion of this module, the learner will be able to

1. Describe the anatomy of the pancreas.
2. Explain the exocrine functions of the pancreas.
3. Describe the pathophysiologic basis of acute pancreatic dysfunction.
4. Describe medical data used in the diagnosis of acute pancreatic dysfunction.
5. Discuss assessment of the patient with acute pancreatic dysfunction.

6. Explain the complications of acute pancreatitis.
7. Describe the medical management of a patient with acute pancreatitis.
8. Discuss the nursing plan of care for a patient with acute pancreatic dysfunction.

This self-study module focuses on assessment and management of concepts related to the patient with a disruption of normal exocrine pancreatic function. Disruption of normal endocrine pancreatic function is presented in Module 27: "Altered Glucose Metabolism." Sections One and Two provide a brief review of basic anatomy and physiology of the exocrine pancreas, including pancreatic exocrine functions. Section Three describes the pathophysiologic basis of pancreatic dysfunction, including etiologic factors. Section Four describes laboratory tests and diagnostic procedures used to diagnose acute pancreatitis. Section Five discusses the nursing assessment of a patient with acute pancreatitis. Section Six offers a brief overview of the major complications associated with acute pancreatitis, and Section Seven describes the medical management. The module closes with Section Eight, which provides the reader with a list of independent nursing diagnoses and collaborative problems. Two nursing diagnoses, *Altered comfort: nausea and vomiting* and *Pain,* are developed, including desired patient outcomes and interventions. Each section includes a set of review questions to help the learner evaluate his or her understanding of the section's content before moving on to the next section. All Section Reviews and the module Pretest and Posttest include answers. It is suggested that the learner review those concepts answered incorrectly in the review questions before proceeding to the next section.

PRETEST

1. The functional unit of the pancreas is called the
   A. ampulla of Vater
   B. pancreatic acinus
   C. alpha cell
   D. islets of Langerhans

2. The duct of Wirsung shares the opening into the duodenum with the
   A. acinar cells
   B. common bile duct
   C. gallbladder
   D. duct of Santorini

3. The pH of pancreatic juice is
   A. highly acidic
   B. moderately acidic
   C. neutral
   D. highly alkaline

4. The pancreas is protected from autodigestion by
   A. bicarbonate and water
   B. the presence of the hormone secretin
   C. protective pancreatic cell wall coverings
   D. the production of enzymes in their inactive states

5. A common cause of acute pancreatitis is
   A. chronic alcohol abuse
   B. steroid therapy
   C. duodenal ulcers
   D. viral infections

6. Regardless of the etiology of acute pancreatitis, the primary physiologic event is
   A. hemorrhage
   B. edema
   C. autodigestion
   D. pain

7. Alcohol has which of the following effects on the pancreas?
   A. decreases enzyme secretion
   B. depresses secretion of secretin
   C. inhibits the inflammatory response
   D. causes spasm of the sphincter of Oddi

8. The primary laboratory test used to help make a diagnosis of pancreatitis is serum
   A. amylase
   B. calcium
   C. lactic dehydrogenase (LDH)
   D. elastase

9. The typical pain associated with acute pancreatitis is characterized as (choose all that apply)
   1. severe
   2. relieved by vomiting
   3. radiating to the flank
   4. continuous
   A. 1 and 3
   B. 1, 3, and 4
   C. 2, 3, and 4
   D. 1, 2, and 3

10. Shock associated with acute pancreatitis can be caused by (choose all that apply)
    1. dehydration
    2. vasodilation
    3. hemorrhage
    4. third spacing
    A. 2, 3, and 4
    B. 1, 3, and 4
    C. 3 and 4
    D. 1, 2, and 3

11. Pulmonary complications are attributed to which of the following pancreatic enzymes?
    A. trypsin
    B. elastase
    C. amylase
    D. phospholipase A

12. If a pancreatic pseudocyst were to rupture into the peritoneal cavity, the patient would most likely develop
    A. peritonitis
    B. acute renal failure
    C. paralytic ileus
    D. septicemia

13. The release of myocardial depressant factor by injured pancreatic tissue is believed to have what effect on the heart?
    A. decreases heart rate
    B. decreases cardiac output
    C. increases blood pressure
    D. increases cardiac output

14. Clinical findings consistent with "peritoneal signs" include (choose all that apply)
    1. rebound tenderness
    2. rigid abdomen
    3. hyperactive bowel sounds
    4. leukocytosis
    A. 2, 3, and 4
    B. 1 and 3
    C. 1, 2, and 4
    D. 2 and 3

15. Cullen's sign may be noted under which circumstances?
    A. acute tubular necrosis (ATN)
    B. hemorrhage
    C. hypovolemic shock
    D. respiratory failure

16. The highest priority in the management of the patient with severe acute pancreatitis is to
    A. control pain
    B. correct the underlying problem
    C. minimize pancreatic stimulation
    D. stabilize the hemodynamic status

17. The drug of choice in pain management of the patient with acute pancreatitis is
    A. morphine sulfate
    B. codeine
    C. meperidine (Demerol)
    D. ibuprofen

Pretest Answers: 1. B, 2. B, 3. D, 4. D, 5. A, 6. C, 7. D, 8. A, 9. B, 10. A, 11. D, 12. A, 13. B, 14. C, 15. B, 16. D, 17. C

GLOSSARY

acinus   The exocrine functional unit of the pancreas; composed of acinar cells that produce, store, and secrete digestive enzymes and ductal cells that secrete bicarbonate and water (plural: acini).

ampulla of Vater   Formed by the junction at the duodenum of the main pancreatic duct and the common bile duct.

amylolytic   Facilitating the breakdown of carbohydrates.

autodigestion   Breakdown of pancreatic tissues by its own enzymes.

chyme   The mixture of partially digested food and secretions of digestion found in the stomach and small bowel.

chymotrypsin   A proteolytic pancreatic enzyme.

duct of Santorini   An accessory duct of the pancreas that exists in approximately 70 percent of the population.

duct of Wirsung   The main pancreatic duct.

elastase   A proteolytic pancreatic enzyme; its proenzyme, proelastase, requires trypsin to become activated; responsible for erosion of blood vessels contributing to hemorrhage in severe acute pancreatitis.

endoscopic retrograde cholangiopancreatography (ERCP)   An invasive endoscopic test that allows cannulation and direct viewing of the ampulla of Vater, and the pancreatic and bile ducts.

kallikrein   An enzyme found in plasma, body tissues, and urine that forms kinin; it normally circulates in the plasma in its inactive state, as the proenzyme kallikreinogen; when activated by trypsin, it is an extremely potent vasodilator.

lipase   A lipolytic pancreatic enzyme; its action contributes to necrosis of fatty tissue surrounding the pancreas in the presence of pancreatitis.

lipolytic   Facilitating the breakdown of fats.

magnetic resonance cholangiopancreatography (MRCP)   A test using magnetic resonance imaging to produce images of the hepatobiliary tree.

pancreatitis   Inflammation of the pancreas; it may occur as an acute or chronic condition.

phospholipase A   A lipolytic pancreatic enzyme, activated by either bile salts or trypsin; contributes to the development of pulmonary complications (acute respiratory distress syndrome [ARDS]) by decreasing surfactant in the lungs.

proteolytic   Facilitating the breakdown of proteins.

secretin   A hormone present in the small bowel mucosa that stimulates sodium bicarbonate secretion by the pancreas and bile secretion by the liver; it decreases gastrointestinal peristalsis and motility.

sphincter of Oddi   A circular muscle that surrounds the ampulla of Vater; it helps control the rate of pancreatic enzyme and bile flow into the duodenum.

trypsin   A proteolytic pancreatic enzyme; it exists in the pancreas in its proenzyme (inactive) state as trypsinogen. Most of the other pancreatic enzymes require trypsin for activation.

ABBREVIATIONS

ATN	Acute tubular necrosis	**ERCP**	Endoscopic retrograde cholangiopancreatography
CCK	Cholecystokinin	**LDH**	Lactic dehydrogenase
DIC	Disseminated intravascular coagulation	**MDF**	Myocardial depressant factor

SECTION ONE: Anatomy of the Pancreas

At the completion of this section, the learner will be able to describe the anatomy of the pancreas.

The pancreas is a multifunctional organ, having both endocrine and exocrine functions. It is located in the upper abdominal cavity, lying in a horizontal position (Fig. 32–1). It has three divisions: the head, the body, and the tail. The head lies adjacent to the duodenum, within its curve. The pancreatic body lies directly behind the stomach, and the tail is adjacent to the spleen. This module focuses on exocrine structures. Pancreatic endocrine structures are covered in detail in Module 27, "Altered Glucose Metabolism."

Exocrine Anatomic Structure

The majority of the pancreatic tissue consists of exocrine tissues. The functional exocrine unit of the pancreas is the pancreatic **acinus** (Fig. 32–2). The acinus is composed of acinar cells that produce, store, and secrete digestive enzymes, and ductal cells that secrete bicarbonate and water (Guyton & Hall, 2000; Pandol, 2002). Acini are clustered into larger units called pancreatic lobules. The lobules are separated from each other by septa.

The digestive enzymes flow through a ductal system into the duodenum (see Fig. 32–3). Once enzymes have been released from the acinar lumina, they flow into small duct lumina and on into a connecting network of ducts, eventually terminating at the main pancreatic duct (the **duct of Wirsung**). The

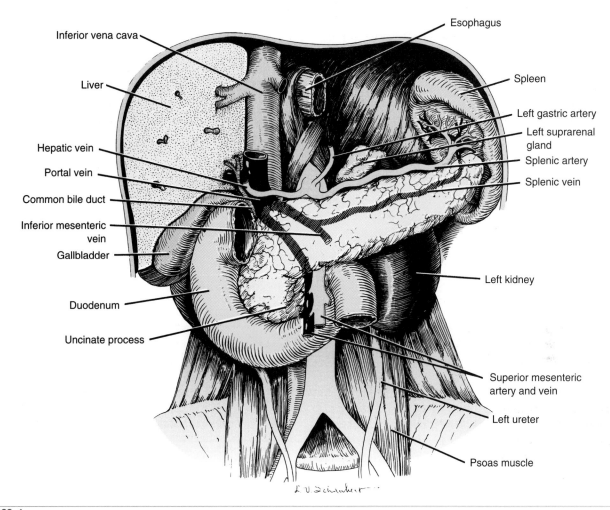

Figure 32–1 ■ The pancreas, showing relations of the major vessels, venous drainage, and adjoining structures. *(From Lindner, H. H. [1989].* Human anatomy *[p. 426]. Norwalk, CT: Appleton & Lange. Reproduced with permission of the McGraw-Hill Companies.)*

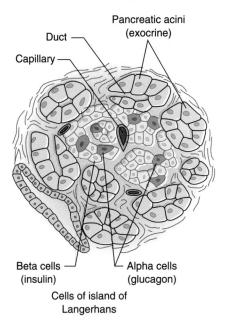

Figure 32–2 ■ Pancreatic acinar units. *(From Wilson, L. M., & Lester, L. B. [1992]. Liver, biliary tract, and pancreas. In S. A. Price & L. M. Wilson [Eds].* Pathophysiology: Clinical concepts of disease processes, *(4th ed., p. 338). St. Louis: Mosby-Year Book.)*

main pancreatic duct runs through the center of the organ from head to tail. It joins with the common bile duct, sharing the same opening into the duodenum at the **ampulla of Vater,** which is surrounded by the **sphincter of Oddi.** Located at the junction of the common bile duct and the duodenum, the sphincter of Oddi helps control the rate of pancreatic enzyme and bile flow into the duodenum. A second duct, the accessory pancreatic duct (**duct of Santorini**), exists in approximately 70 percent of people (Magee & Burdick, 2002; Simeone & Mulholland, 2003). When present, it joins the duodenum at the minor duodenal papilla, which is located proximal to the main pancreatic duct.

In summary, the pancreas has both exocrine and endocrine functions. It is located in the upper abdominal cavity. The pancreatic acinus is the functional unit of the pancreas. It secretes digestive enzymes capable of breaking down carbohydrates, proteins, and fats. Once secreted, the pancreatic juice flows through a network of duct systems and eventually passes through the ampulla of Vater and flows into the small intestines.

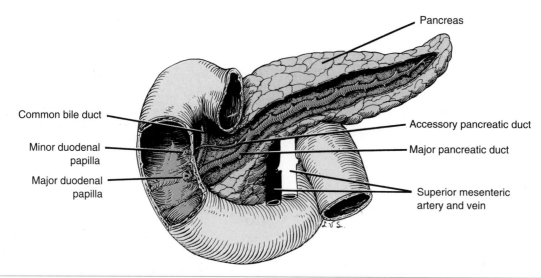

Figure 32–3 ■ The ductal system of the pancreas. *(From Lindner, H. H. [1989]. Human anatomy [p. 430]. Norwalk, CT: Appleton & Lange. Reproduced with permission of the McGraw-Hill Companies.)*

SECTION ONE REVIEW

1. The functional unit of the pancreas is called the
   A. ampulla of Vater
   B. acinus
   C. alpha cell
   D. islets of Langerhans
2. Which structures are part of the pancreatic anatomic structure? (choose all that apply)
   1. body
   2. tail
   3. arm
   4. head
   A. 2, 3, and 4
   B. 1, 2, and 3
   C. 1, 2, and 4
   D. 1 and 2

3. The sphincter of Oddi primarily serves which purpose?
   A. control of the rate of pancreatic enzyme flow into intestines
   B. control of the activation of the pancreatic enzymes
   C. regulation of the level of intestinal secretin
   D. regulation of the rate of bicarbonate secretion
4. The duct of Wirsung shares the opening into the duodenum with the
   A. acinar cells
   B. duct of Santorini
   C. gallbladder
   D. common bile duct

Answers: 1. B, 2. C, 3. A, 4. D

SECTION TWO: The Exocrine Functions of the Pancreas

At the completion of this section, the learner will be able to explain the exocrine functions of the pancreas.

Exocrine Functions

The pancreas normally secretes up to 4 L of pancreatic juice per day, with a pH of approximately 8.3. Pancreatic juice is composed of water, bicarbonate, electrolytes (particularly potassium and sodium), and digestive enzymes (Pandol, 2002). The pan-

creas is important in neutralizing the acids in the small intestines and in providing digestive enzymes.

Control of pH

Chyme is the mixture of partially digested food and intestinal secretions as it exists in the stomach and small bowel. The acidic pH of the chyme that enters the duodenum from the stomach stimulates mucosal secretion of the hormone **secretin** by the proximal end of the small intestines. Secretin is essential in the regulation of intestinal pH. Release of secretin is stimulated by a drop in pH to less than 4.5. This serves several functions. First, when intestinal pH becomes too acidic, secretin stimulates the pancreas to secrete large quantities of bicarbonate and water.

Bicarbonate raises the intestinal pH, which protects the mucosa. Second, pancreatic enzymes work best within a pH level that is neutral to slightly alkaline. The alkaline pH of the small bowel is important in the formation of pepsin, which protects the delicate intestinal mucosa and facilitates normal digestive enzyme processes.

Pancreatic Enzymes

Normal digestion depends on the digestive enzymatic activities of the pancreatic enzymes. Pancreatic digestive enzymes are responsible for the breakdown of proteins (proteolytics), fat (lipolytics), and carbohydrates (**amylolytics**). Table 32–1 summarizes the major pancreatic enzymes.

Pancreatic Secretion Regulation

Secretion of pancreatic enzymes is regulated by both hormonal and neural factors, though hormonal influences are more important. There are four major stimuli of pancreatic secretion: gastrin, cholecystokinin (CCK), secretin, and acetylcholine. Large quantities of gastrin are secreted by the stomach in response to neural stimulation. The intestinal hormones, secretin, and CCK are stimulated by stomach acids, amino acids, and fats, respectively. Gastrin, secretin, and CCK stimulate the pancreatic acinar cells and are responsible for the release of large quantities of pancreatic enzymes. Acetylcholine is secreted by parasympathetic vagal and other cholinergic nerve endings throughout the gut. Vagal influence stimulates secretion of pancreatic enzymes, which are then placed in temporary storage in the acini, await-

ing a transport mechanism to move them into the intestines (Guyton & Hall, 2000).

Pancreatic Self-Protective Properties

The **proteolytic** pancreatic enzymes (e.g., **trypsin, chymotrypsin,** and elastase) are responsible for the breakdown of proteins. Proteolytic enzymes make up about 90 percent of pancreatic digestive enzymes. The **lipolytic** pancreatic enzyme, phospholipase A, is responsible for breaking down phospholipids into fatty acids. Without some protective mechanism, these enzymes are capable of digesting the pancreatic tissues, a process called **autodigestion.** Under normal circumstances, several mechanisms exist to prevent autodigestion. First, pancreatic proteolytic enzymes (refer to Table 32–1) are produced in an inactive, precursor form, remaining inactive while in the pancreas. Second, a trypsin inhibitor (secreted by the acinar cells) maintains trypsin in its inactive (inhibited) state while it is present in the pancreatic ducts and cells (Bentrem & Joehl, 2003; Greenberger & Toskes, 2001; Guyton & Hall, 2000).

In summary, pancreatic juice, composed of water, electrolytes, pancreatic enzymes, and bicarbonate, maintains a highly alkaline pH and is used to increase the pH of chyme. Two major pancreatic exocrine functions are control of intestinal pH and secretion of digestive enzymes. Regulation of pancreatic enzyme secretion is influenced by hormonal and neural factors. Secretin plays an important role in intestinal pH regulation. Normally, the pancreas is protected from digesting itself by several protective mechanisms (Bentrem & Joehl, 2003; Greenberger & Toskes, 2001).

TABLE 32–1 Major Pancreatic Enzymes

ENZYME	TARGET	PRECURSOR NAME	COMMENTS
Trypsin	Proteins	Trypsinogen	Most abundant proteolytic enzyme; activated in intestinal mucosa by enterokinase or by preexisting trypsin
Elastase	Proteins	Proelastase	Activated by trypsin; breaks down elastic tissue; can break down blood vessel walls
Chymotrypsin	Proteins	Chymotrypsinogen	Activated by trypsin; splits (via hydrolyzing) proteins into peptones
Pancreatic amylase	Carbohydrates	—	Splits glycogen, starches, and other carbohydrates, with the exception of cellulose, into disaccharides (primarily)
Lipase	Fats	—	Requires bile salts; splits fats into monoglycerides and fatty acids
Phospholipase A	Fats	—	Activated by trypsin or bile salts; splits phospholipids into fatty acids; breaks down cell membranes and is capable of causing pancreatic and fat tissue necrosis

SECTION TWO REVIEW

1. The pH of pancreatic juice is
   A. highly acidic
   B. moderately acidic
   C. neutral
   D. highly alkaline

2. The function of secretin is to
   A. lower the pancreatic pH
   B. stimulate secretion of pancreatic enzymes
   C. directly activate pepsin production
   D. inhibit secretion of pancreatic enzymes

3. The most abundant pancreatic enzyme is
   A. chymotrypsin
   B. lipase
   C. trypsin
   D. elastase

4. The pancreas is protected from autodigestion by
   A. bicarbonate and water
   B. the presence of the hormone secretin
   C. protective pancreatic cell wall coverings
   D. the production of enzymes in their inactive states

Answers: 1. D, 2. B, 3. C, 4. D

SECTION THREE: Pathophysiologic Basis of Acute Pancreatitis

At the completion of this section, the learner will be able to describe the pathophysiologic basis of acute pancreatitis.

Pancreatitis is defined as inflammation of the pancreas. It can occur either as an acute or chronic condition. Acute pancreatitis is the sudden onset of pancreatic inflammation. It is characterized by varying degrees of abdominal pain, pancreatic tissue edema, necrosis of pancreatic tissue, and, possibly, hemorrhage. The severity of acute pancreatitis ranges from mild to severe. The majority of patients (80 to 90 percent) with acute pancreatitis have a mild form called interstitial or edematous pancreatitis (Triester & Kowdley, 2002). In mild acute pancreatitis, there are areas of fat necrosis in and around the pancreas accompanied by interstitial edema. This form of acute pancreatitis is usually mild and self-limited, resolving within 5 to 7 days (Triester & Kowdley, 2002). In the more severe form of acute pancreatitis, called necrotizing or hemorrhagic pancreatitis, there is extensive necrosis in and around the pancreas, pancreatic cellular necrosis, and hemorrhage within the pancreas. Severe pancreatitis is associated with local and systemic complications. The mortality rate associated with severe acute pancreatitis is 10 to 15 percent, which rises to 25 to 30 percent when complications are present (Beckingham & Bornman, 2001; Yousaf et al., 2003). Table 32–2 lists the characteristics of nonhemorrhagic and hemorrhagic acute pancreatitis.

TABLE 32–2 Characteristics of Nonhemorrhagic and Hemorrhagic Acute Pancreatitis

NONHEMORRHAGIC (INTERSTITIAL)	SEVERE HEMORRHAGIC (NECROTIZING)
• Short term	• Longer duration
• Pancreatic edema and swelling	• Pancreatic hemorrhage
• Little to no necrosis	• Extensive fat and tissue necrosis
• Localized inflammation	• Extrapancreatic invasion of pancreatic enzymes
• Reversible	• Irreversible damage to pancreas and surrounding tissues
• Good prognosis	• Poor prognosis—associated with sepsis and multiple organ dysfunction

Etiologies

There are multiple causes of acute pancreatitis, but in the United States gallstones and chronic alcohol abuse account for approximately 80 percent of cases (Conwell, 2001; Grendell, 2000; Topazian & Gorelick, 2003). Gallstone-induced pancreatitis is more common in women and alcohol-induced acute pancreatitis is more common in men. Gallstone-induced pancreatitis is caused by obstruction of the common bile duct by a lodged gallstone. The obstructing gallstone can either obstruct outflow of enzymes from the pancreatic duct or it can cause reflux of bile into the pancreatic duct. Either mechanism is believed to trigger activation of pancreatic enzymes in the pancreatic duct (Porth, 2005). Alcohol may induce acute pancreatitis by triggering spasms of the sphincter of Oddi, resulting in transient obstruction. Alcohol may also change the composition of pancreatic secretions, causing the formation of plugs within the pancreas, and alcohol or its metabolites may directly injure the acinar cells. An estimated 2 to 5 percent of cases of acute pancreatitis may be drug induced, perhaps through a hypersensitivity reaction or through the generation of a toxic metabolite (Dimangno & Chari, 2002; Greenberger & Toskes 2001). Hypercalcemia and hypertriglyceridemia are metabolic causes of acute pancreatitis. Idiopathic pancreatitis may develop during pregnancy, administration of total parenteral nutrition, or major surgery. Endoscopic manipulation of the ampulla of Vater or abdominal trauma may also precipitate acute pancreatitis. Table 32–3 lists the major causes of acute pancreatitis.

Pathophysiology

Most causes of acute pancreatitis involve an initial injury to the pancreatic acinar cells. Regardless of the cause, acute pancreatitis develops when pancreatic enzymes become prematurely activated within the pancreas. This premature activation results in autodigestion of the pancreas and peripancreatic tissues. The exact mechanism behind premature activation of pancreatic enzymes is not fully understood, but the initiating event is thought to be the activation of trypsinogen into its active form, trypsin, in quantities sufficient to overwhelm the normal protective mechanisms. Intrapancreatic release of trypsin promotes further release of trypsin and activation of the precursors to phospholipase A, elastase, and carboxypeptidase into active enzymes.

TABLE 32–3 Major Causes of Acute Pancreatitis

Alcohol abuse

Biliary disease: Gallstones, microlithiasis, or biliary sludge; common bile duct obstruction

Drugs: 6-Mercaptopurine, ace-inhibitors, azathioprine, estrogen, furosemide, procainamide, sulfonamides, tetracycline, thiazide diuretics, valproic acid

Hypercalcemia

Hypertriglyceridemia

Idiopathic

Infection/toxin

  Viral: Mumps, coxsackievirus, cytomegalovirus (CMV), HAV, HBV

  Bacterial: *Mycoplasma, Legionella, Salmonella*

  Fungal: *Aspergillus, Candida albicans*

  Parasitic: *Toxoplasma, Cryptosporidium*

Pancreas divisum

Trauma: Blunt or penetrating abdominal trauma; post-ERCP; surgical trauma

Activation of two pancreatic enzymes is thought to cause the most damage. These enzymes are phospholipase A and elastase. **Phospholipase A** digests phospholipids on the cell membranes, and **elastase** digests elastic tissue of vessel walls. As vessel walls sustain increasing damage, both capillary and lymphatic vessels become injured, which results in hemorrhage and edema, respectively. As the damage progresses, more acini are triggered to activate and secrete their digestive enzymes, which further increases autodigestive activities.

As a part of the inflammatory process, kallikrein is activated by the trypsin. **Kallikrein** is a basophil mediator of inflammation. It is responsible for causing bradykinin formation. Kallikrein is thought to increase local damage and precipitate systemic hypotension. It causes vasodilation and increases permeability of blood vessels, pain, and leukocyte invasion. Once kallikrein has been activated, systemic hypotension may lead to shock and multisystem dysfunction or failure (such as acute respiratory distress syndrome and acute renal failure); thus, the initial local insult of acute pancreatitis may become a complex multisystemic dysfunction disease process (Bentrem & Joehl, 2003; Cole, 2001; Dimangno & Chari, 2002; Schlapman, 2001).

In summary, pancreatitis is an inflammation of the pancreas. Acute pancreatitis may present as a mild form called interstitial or edematous pancreatitis or a more severe necrotizing or hemorrhagic pancreatitis. Most cases of pancreatitis are mild and self-limited, and are precipitated by either alcohol abuse or biliary tract disease. Other possible causes include drug toxicity and metabolic causes. The exact pathophysiologic mechanisms of injury are not yet clearly understood. The major pathophysiologic event is autodigestion of the organ, which activates an inflammatory cascade resulting in local, and in severe cases, systemic, complications.

SECTION THREE REVIEW

1. Acute necrotizing or hemorrhagic pancreatitis is characterized by (choose all that apply)
     1. severe bleeding
     2. vasoconstriction
     3. tissue necrosis
     4. extrapancreatic invasion
   A. 2, 3, and 4
   B. 1, 3, and 4
   C. 3 and 4
   D. 1, 2, and 3
2. A common cause of acute pancreatitis is
   A. chronic alcohol abuse
   B. steroid therapy
   C. duodenal ulcers
   D. viral infections
3. Regardless of the etiology of acute pancreatitis, the primary physiologic event is
   A. hemorrhage
   B. edema
   C. autodigestion
   D. pain
4. It is theorized that acute pancreatitis can be triggered by reflux of
   A. digestive juices through the sphincter of Oddi
   B. pancreatic enzymes into the common bile duct
   C. digestive juices through the common bile duct
   D. pancreatic enzymes into the duodenum
5. Premature activation of the pancreatic enzymes _____ and _____ is thought to cause the most pancreatic damage.
   A. trypsin, amylase
   B. lipase, chymotrypsin
   C. phospholipase A, elastase
   D. elastase, amylase
6. Obstruction by gallstones is most commonly seen in which patient population?
   A. persons with diabetes
   B. alcoholic men
   C. those ages 30 to 40
   D. obese women
7. Alcohol affects the pancreas by
   A. decreasing enzyme secretion
   B. depressing secretion of secretin
   C. inhibiting the inflammatory response
   D. causing spasm of sphincter of Oddi

Answers: 1. B, 2. A, 3. C, 4. A, 5. C, 6. D, 7. D

SECTION FOUR: Diagnosing Acute Pancreatitis

At the completion of this section, the learner will be able to describe medical data used in the diagnosis of acute pancreatitis.

The initial clinical presentation of the patient with acute pancreatitis is similar to that of a variety of other acute abdominal disorders. Diagnosing acute pancreatitis requires data from multiple sources, including laboratory tests and other diagnostic procedures. In addition, the patient history and physical assessment provide valuable information that will support or help rule out a diagnosis of acute pancreatitis. The nursing history and assessment are presented in Section Five.

Laboratory Assessment of Acute Pancreatitis

Laboratory testing is an important part of monitoring a patient for the development or progression of acute pancreatitis. Enzymes produced by the pancreas escape into the serum and urine when there is damage to the pancreatic parenchyma. The trends in pancreatic enzyme values are closely evaluated as an indication of disease progress. A variety of other laboratory tests may be ordered to further evaluate the pancreatitis as well as the status of any multisystem involvement. A brief description of important laboratory assessments follows.

Pancreatic Enzyme Levels

Measurement of pancreatic enzyme levels is usually obtained from the serum and urine. Cellular enzymes leak into the blood when pancreatic tissue is injured, thereby increasing serum enzyme levels. The most commonly measured pancreatic enzymes are serum amylase and **lipase.**

Serum amylase levels rise within 2 to 12 hours in the course of acute pancreatitis and return to normal within 3 to 5 days after disease onset (Smotkin & Tenner, 2002). Serum amylase can increase for a variety of reasons because the enzyme is nonspecific to the pancreas. Altered serum amylase levels, therefore, are examined in the context of other supportive clinical data. Amylase is secreted from both the salivary glands and pancreas, each with a distinct isoenzyme. Measurement of amylase isoenzyme P (P refers to pancreatic) is useful in ruling out nonpancreatic elevations in serum amylase.

Serum lipase levels rise later than amylase and remain elevated for approximately 1 to 2 weeks postonset (Smotkin & Tenner, 2002). Measuring lipase levels provides a longer period for trending values than that provided by serum amylase levels. Serum lipase levels can be elevated by use of opioids or consumption of food within 8 hours before the serum level is drawn (Kee, 2002).

An ALT greater than 150 units/L has a positive predictive value for acute gallstone pancreatitis (Smotkin & Tenner, 2002).

TABLE 32–4 Differential Laboratory Diagnosis of Acute Pancreatitis

LABORATORY TEST	NORMAL VALUES[a]	TRENDS	TREND VALUES	COMMENTS
Serum				
Amylase	30–170 U/L	↑↑	> 500 U/L	Peaks 2–12 hours post onset; may remain elevated 3–5 days; level does not correlate well with severity
Isoamylase P (pancreatic)	30–55%	↑	> 55%	
Lipase	14–280 U/L	Rapid ↑	> 280 U/L	May remain elevated after amylase returns to normal
Glucose	70–110 mg/dL	Transient ↑	> 180 mg/dL	Secondary to islet cell malfunction; criteria used in absence of preexisting history of hyperglycemia
Calcium	9–11 mg/dL	↓	< 7.5 mg/dL	Secondary to necrosis of fat causing calcium soap formation; also attributed to hypoalbuminemia (decreased availability of protein for calcium binding)
White blood cell count	4,500–10,000/mL	↑	> 15,000/mL	Secondary to inflammatory process
Blood urea nitrogen	5–25 mg/dL	↑	> 45 mg/dL	Level remains elevated following correction of fluid volume deficit
Direct bilirubin (posthepatic)	0.1–0.3 mg/dL	↑	> 0.3 mg/dL	Associated with biliary obstruction
LDH	70–250 U/L	↑	> 350 U/L	Associated with biliary obstruction and pancreatitis; LDH3 isoenzyme is found in pancreas and other organs
AST (SGOT)	5–40 U/mL	↑↑	> 250 U/mL	
Serum albumin	3.5–5.0 g/dL	↓	< 3.2 g/dL	Associated with protein deficiency
Pao$_2$	80–100 mm Hg	↓	< 60 mm Hg	Associated with pulmonary involvement
Stool				
Fat	< 6 g/24 hr	—	> 6 g/24 hr	Steatorrhea; stool is pale or gray, smells foul; caused by deficiency in pancreatic enzymes in bowel

[a] Values may vary slightly according to the laboratory performing the test

Source: All normal values are from Kee, J. L. (2002). Laboratory and diagnostic tests with nursing implications, *(6th ed.). Upper Saddle River, NJ: Prentice Hall.*

Other Laboratory Tests

A variety of laboratory tests may be helpful in evaluating acute pancreatitis and multisystem involvement, particularly the liver and gallbladder. Table 32–4 summarizes some of the major laboratory tests used in making a differential diagnosis of acute pancreatitis.

Diagnostic Tests

Diagnosis of acute pancreatitis requires data from a variety of sources. Frequently ordered major diagnostic tests include abdominal x-rays, ultrasound, computed tomography (CT) scan, endoscopic retrograde cholangiopancreatography (ERCP), magnetic resonance cholangiopancreatography (MRCP), and aspiration biopsy.

Abdominal and Chest Radiography

Radiographs of the abdomen and chest are used to exclude intestinal ileus, perforation, pericardial effusion, and pulmonary disease as causes of abdominal pain. The abdominal radiograph may be used initially as a quick means of revealing abdominal distention as well as gross abdominal abnormalities, such as an ileus. It is limited in its usefulness as a tool for diagnosing organ disorders. Chest films are valuable in revealing pulmonary complications associated with acute pancreatitis, such as atelectasis and pleural effusion.

CT Scan and Ultrasound

A CT scan confirms diagnosis and is used in determination of severity. Dynamic contrast CT helps to distinguish interstitial from necrotizing pancreatitis. The CT scan provides a noninvasive means of viewing the structure of the pancreas, the bile ducts, and the gallbladder. Damaged pancreatic tissue and lesions can be visualized. CT scan is currently considered one of the best tests for assessing pancreatic necrosis. Ultrasound uses high-frequency sound waves rather than radiation. It provides a "real-time" view of the structure being tested. In diagnostic testing for acute pancreatitis, ultrasound is particularly valuable in viewing the bile ducts and can identify gallstones more readily than the CT scan. However, abdominal ultrasound is of limited usefulness in visualization of the pancreas because of intestinal gas or obesity (Dimangno & Chari, 2002).

Cholangiopancreatography

Endoscopic retrograde cholangiopancreatography (ERCP) is an invasive endoscopic test that allows cannulation and direct viewing of the ampulla of Vater, and the pancreatic and bile ducts. It requires injection of a radiographic contrast medium followed by a series of x-rays under fluoroscopy. ERCP is particularly useful in diagnosing obstructions. In addition, the ERCP provides the opportunity for direct removal of mechanical obstructions, such as a gallstone or pancreatic stone, stent place-ment to provide drainage through a stricture, and biopsy (Banks, 1997).

Magnetic resonance cholangiopancreatography (MRCP) uses magnetic resonance imaging to produce images to evaluate the hepatobiliary tree. Because MRCP is noninvasive, and requires no contrast, MRCP has a decreased morbidity compared to ERCP. MRCP has greater than 90 percent sensitivity for bile duct stone (Topazian & Gorelick, 2003). The usefulness of MRCP is limited by the inability to intervene with stone extraction, stent insertion, and biopsy.

Aspiration Biopsy

Aspiration biopsy involves the removal of a small plug of tissue using a syringe and needle technique. It is useful in diagnosing the severity of pancreatic tissue damage, diagnosing types of lesions, and draining pseudocysts. It is also helpful in distinguishing sterile necrosis from infected necrosis (Dimangno & Chari, 2002). Aspiration biopsy can be performed during ultrasound or CT scan, to enable visualization of correct needle placement.

Predicting the Severity of an Acute Pancreatitis Episode

The Ranson criteria (Table 32–5) are commonly used to predict patient outcome, having been shown to be highly accurate (96 percent accuracy). Using these criteria, the following assumptions can be made:

- A person who has less than three criteria at the time of admission has a mortality risk of less than 1 to 2 percent
- A score of 3 or greater indicates severe acute pancreatitis (Triester & Kowdley, 2002)
- A person who is admitted with three or four criteria has a mortality risk of 15 percent
- A person who is admitted with five or six criteria present has a mortality risk of 40 percent
- A person who is admitted with seven or more criteria present has a 100 percent risk of mortality (Triester & Kowdley, 2002)
- Obesity is a risk factor independent of Ranson criteria for a poor prognosis possibly because of increased fat deposits in the peripancreatic and retroperitoneal spaces, which increase the risk for fat necrosis (Triester & Kowdley, 2002).

In summary, the diagnosis of acute pancreatitis primarily is made on the basis of laboratory findings and presenting symptoms. The hallmark of the disease is a rapid, significant increase in serum amylase and lipase levels in the presence of risk factors and complaints of severe abdominal pain. A variety of diagnostic tests can be used in differentiating the diagnosis, such as ultrasound, CT scan, ERCP, MRCP, and aspiration biopsy. Ranson criteria provide an accurate method of predicting patient mortality associated with acute pancreatitis. A differential diagnosis cannot be made on the basis of the patient history and physical assessment alone.

TABLE 32–5 Ranson Criteria for Predicting Severity of Acute Pancreatitis

RISK FACTOR	PRESENT AT TIME OF ADMISSION	RISK FACTOR	PRESENT AT TIME INITIAL 48 HOURS
Age	> 55	Hct	Decrease of > 10 percent
WBC	> 16,000 mm^3	BUN	Rise of > 5 mg/dL
Serum glucose	> 200 mg/dL	Serum calcium	< 8 mg/dL
Serum LDH	> 350 IU/L	Pao$_2$	< 60 mg/dL
Serum SGOT	> 250 U/dL	Base deficit	> 4 mEq/L
		Estimated fluid sequestration	> 6 L

Associated Mortality Based on Number of Risk Factors:[a]

# Risk Factors	Mortality (%)
< 3	0.9
3–4	15
5–6	40
≥ 7	Near 100

[a] *Additional risk factors: Respiratory failure with intubation, shock, hypocalcemia, and massive colloid administration (if ≥ 3 of these factors are present, mortality increases to near 65%)*

Adapted from Ranson, J. C. (1985). Risk factors in acute pancreatitis. Hospital Practice, 20(4), 69–73.

WBC: White blood cells. LDH: Lactic dehydrogenase. SGOT: Serum glutamic-oxaloacetic transaminase (now called AST). BUN: blood urea nitrogen, Pao$_2$: Partial pressure of oxygen.

SECTION FOUR REVIEW

1. The primary laboratory test obtained to help make a diagnosis of pancreatitis is serum
   A. amylase
   B. calcium
   C. LDH
   D. elastase

2. Severe acute pancreatitis will most likely have the following effect on serum glucose:
   A. severe hypoglycemia
   B. transient hypoglycemia
   C. no effect
   D. transient hyperglycemia

3. According to Ranson criteria for predicting the risk of mortality in acute pancreatitis patients, a patient who is admitted with five criteria would have a mortality risk of _____ percent.
   A. less than 1
   B. 40
   C. 60
   D. 100

Answers: 1. A, 2. D, 3. B

SECTION FIVE: Nursing Assessment of the Patient with Acute Pancreatitis

At the completion of this section, the learner will be able to discuss nursing assessment of the patient with acute pancreatitis.

Pain History and Assessment

Pain is the most consistent complaint associated with acute pancreatitis and is a high-priority assessment. The classic pattern of pain is described as a sudden onset of sharp, knifelike, twisting and deep, upper abdominal (epigastric) pain that frequently radiates to the flank, chest, or other parts of the abdomen. The pain may be further described as steady, sharp, and knifelike (Greenberger & Toskes, 2001). The patient may report some degree of relief by assuming a leaning forward or fetal position (Greenberger & Toskes, 2001; Schlapman, 2001), and may report an increase in pain when doing activities that increase abdominal pressure (e.g., coughing). The pain intensity varies greatly from patient to patient. The pain may be described as vague and mild, or it may be excruciating and refractory to analgesic therapy. The intensity often reflects the degree to which the disease process has extended beyond the confines of the pancreas. If localized, the pain is usually more vague and mild; however, once pancreatic functions infiltrate extrapancreatic tissues (into the peritoneum), the pain becomes well defined and sharp, and the intensity increases significantly. The pain is believed to be a result of edema and distention of the pancreatic capsule, chemical burn of the peritoneum by pancreatic enzymes, and the release of kinin peptides or biliary obstruction (Cole, 2001). Initially, the patient's complaints of pain intensity may seem out of proportion to other clinical manifestations. The pain intensity does not always correlate with the degree of pancreatic inflammation.

The Focused History and Assessment

The majority of the clinical manifestations of acute pancreatic dysfunction are of GI origin; thus, while taking the nursing history, the nurse should particularly focus on gaining information related to this system. The remainder of this section presents the major signs and symptoms associated with acute pancreatitis.

Gastrointestinal Assessment

The presence of abdominal pain is a major finding in acute pancreatitis. Additional GI clinical manifestations include

- Anorexia
- Upper abdominal tenderness without rigidity
- Abdominal distention
- Nausea and vomiting
- Diarrhea
- Peritoneal signs (noted in severe cases):
  Diminished or absent bowel sounds (ileus may develop)
  Increased pain
  Abdominal rigidity, guarding, rebound tenderness
  Other: leukocytosis, tachycardia, and fever
- Diminished breath sounds

Additional Assessments

In addition to the major GI clinical manifestations, a variety of other common or classic signs and symptoms are commonly associated with the disease process.

Integumentary

If the patient has hemorrhagic pancreatitis, two uncommon but classic signs may be observed:

1. **Cullen's sign.** A bluish discoloration around the umbilicus
2. **Grey Turner's sign.** A bluish discoloration of the flank region

Other observations that may be noted by skin inspection are jaundice and edema. If the patient develops shock, the skin will become pale, cold, and moist.

Cardiopulmonary

Cardiac signs and symptoms usually present themselves in conjunction with the complication of shock or the release of myocardial depressant factor (MDF), which is discussed in Section Six. The nurse should observe the patient for the signs and symptoms of hypovolemic shock (tachycardia, hypotension with decreased systemic vascular resistance) and MDF release (decreased cardiac output with increased systemic vascular resistance).

Respiratory signs and symptoms include those typical of

- Pleural effusion—adventitious breath sounds, particularly crackles (usually left sided) (Greenberger & Toskes, 2001; Schlapman, 2001)
- Respiratory insufficiency or failure (refer to Module 5, "Alterations in Pulmonary Gas Exchange")
- Pulmonary edema (noncardiogenic)
- Pneumonia

Neurologic

The patient with acute pancreatitis frequently develops an alteration in level of consciousness. The nurse can rapidly trend the state of arousal using the Glasgow Coma Scale (GCS). Common neurologic manifestations include confusion, restlessness, and agitation.

Renal

The patient must be closely monitored for the development of acute tubular necrosis (refer to Module 28, "Acute Renal Dysfunction"). The urine can also be observed. As increased levels of bile are excreted through the urine, it develops a brownish color and may become foamy.

Hematologic

The nurse should monitor the patient for clinical manifestations of disseminated intravascular coagulation (refer to Module 24).

Electrolyte Imbalances

Hypocalcemia may develop as a result of fat necrosis because serum calcium migrates to the extravascular space surrounding the pancreas where the fat necrosis is taking place. Two classic signs of hypocalcemia are

1. **Chvostek's sign.** The facial nerve is tapped directly in front of the ear. A positive sign is present when the facial muscles contract on the same side of the face as the tapping.
2. **Trousseau's sign.** A blood pressure cuff is inflated on the upper arm to a level directly above the patient's systolic blood pressure for 2 minutes. A positive sign is present when the hand flexes (carpopedal spasm) in response to the test.

In addition to hypocalcemia, the patient should be monitored for the hypokalemia and hypomagnesemia that may result from GI loss and insufficient intake (Cole, 2001). (Refer to

Module 3, "Fluid and Electrolyte Balance in the High-Acuity Patient," for a listing of the clinical manifestations of hypocalcemia, hypokalemia, and hypomagnesemia.)

In summary, assessment of the patient with acute pancreatitis focuses primarily on pain and the gastrointestinal system.

The severity of the signs and symptoms varies greatly and largely depends on whether the disease process is localized or has extended beyond the confines of the pancreas. Extrapancreatic invasion into the peritoneal spaces can cause chemical peritonitis, which carries with it multiple additional signs and symptoms.

SECTION FIVE REVIEW

1. The classic pattern of pain typically described by the patient with acute pancreatitis is
   A. dull, diffuse, and poorly defined
   B. sharp and confined to the epigastric area
   C. well defined, dull, localized in the flank area
   D. sharp, knifelike, often radiating to the flank
2. The intensity and description of pain associated with acute pancreatitis varies, often based on the
   A. pH of the pancreatic enzymes
   B. degree to which extrapancreatic invasion has occurred
   C. pain threshold of the individual patient
   D. degree of release of myocardial depressant factor (MDF)
3. Peritoneal signs include (choose all that apply)
   1. rebound tenderness
   2. rigid abdomen
   3. hyperactive bowel sounds
   4. leukocytosis
   A. 2, 3, and 4
   B. 1 and 3
   C. 1, 2, and 4
   D. 2 and 3

4. Cullen's sign may be noted under which circumstance?
   A. acute tubular necrosis
   B. hemorrhage
   C. hypovolemic shock
   D. respiratory failure
5. The cardiopulmonary assessment of the patient with acute pancreatitis focuses on monitoring for the development of
   A. hypercapnia
   B. hypertension
   C. cardiac arrhythmias
   D. decreased cardiac output
6. If the pancreatitis is localized, assessment of the abdomen would show (choose all that apply)
   1. tenderness
   2. rigidity
   3. distention
   4. diminished bowel sounds
   A. 1 and 2
   B. 1, 3, and 4
   C. 1, 2, and 3
   D. 2, 3, and 4

Answers: 1. D, 2. B, 3. C, 4. B, 5. D, 6. B

SECTION SIX: Complications of Acute Pancreatitis

At the completion of this section, the learner will be able to explain the complications of acute pancreatitis.

Acute pancreatitis is considered a multisystemic disease process. Complications are common and can be divided into two types: local and systemic.

Local Complications

Pancreatic abscess and pseudocyst are two local complications. Pancreatic abscess results from a localized infectious process. It generally occurs late in the course of a severe episode and may be fatal if not aggressively treated, usually with surgery and antibiotics. A pancreatic pseudocyst is composed of pancreatic enzymes, necrotic tissue, and possibly blood. Although not truly

encapsulated, the pseudocyst is enclosed either by some type of adjacent tissue or by pancreatic tissues. Some pseudocysts resolve on their own; however, while they are present, they may become infected or rupture into the peritoneal cavity, which can precipitate chemical peritonitis.

Systemic Complications

The complications of acute pancreatitis have the potential to interfere with virtually all of the body's functions.

Neurologic

A decreased level of consciousness is a common problem in severe pancreatitis and is related to several potential etiologies; including analgesia and pancreatic encephalopathy. The alleviation of pain associated with acute pancreatitis requires large doses of opioids and possibly sedation. Cerebral function is altered by either of these therapies. The pathophysiologic basis of pancreatic encephalopathy is unclear but may be attributed to pancreatic lipase activity (Dimangno & Chari, 2002).

Pulmonary

Hypoxemia is present in the majority of severe acute pancreatitis patients within the first 2 days of onset. Respiratory insufficiency and failure are common complications of acute pancreatitis. They are attributed to the release of pancreatic enzyme phospholipase A, which destroys the phospholipid, surfactant. Loss of surfactant decreases vital capacity and lung compliance and damages the pulmonary capillary endothelium (Bentrem & Joehl, 2003). The patient is at risk of developing pneumonia and/or pleural effusion and, in severe cases, acute respiratory distress syndrome (ARDS). Pleural effusions may also result from enzyme-induced inflammation of the diaphragm (Cole, 2001). Atelectasis may result from decreased diaphragmatic excursion as a result of abdominal distention or from direct injury from exposure to pancreatic enzymes (Cole, 2001; Topazian & Gorelick, 2003).

Cardiovascular

Pancreatic enzymes released into the bloodstream can have devastating effects on the cardiovascular system through two mechanisms: release of MDF and hypovolemic shock.

Myocardial Depressant Factor. MDF is a chemical mediator that is believed to originate from ischemic pancreatic tissue. When MDF is released, it depresses myocardial function, resulting in decreased cardiac output with increased systemic vascular resistance (compensatory). MDF is one of the chemical mediators implicated in the sequence of events leading to shock.

Hypovolemic Shock. Vasoactive substances are released from damaged pancreatic tissue. Trypsin activates the powerful vasodilating circulating enzyme, kallikrein, which forms two plasma kinins (kallidin and bradykinin). These two substances are responsible for vasodilation, decreased systemic vascular resistance, and increased permeability of endothelial linings of vessels. As vessels become more porous, intravascular fluids are able to shift into other compartments and into the retroperitoneal cavity, causing hypovolemia and third spacing. Fluid shifts can account for up to 6 to 10 L of fluid, which can produce hypovolemic shock (Bentrem & Joehl, 2003).

Hemorrhage is also a major cause of hypovolemic shock in hemorrhagic pancreatitis. When it is prematurely activated, the pancreatic enzyme elastase is able to break down duct and blood vessel elastic fibers, causing hemorrhage (Schlapman, 2001). Hemorrhage can also occur as a result of other complications, such as a bleeding ulcer or tissue necrosis.

Renal

Acute tubular necrosis (ATN), a type of renal failure, is a fairly common sequela in severe acute pancreatitis. It results from renal ischemia secondary to hypotension. If fluid resuscitation is timely and adequate, the kidney damage may be temporary.

Hematologic

Disseminated intravascular coagulation (DIC) is associated with severe acute pancreatitis. It may be a result of activation of the coagulation cascade by trypsin (Cole, 2001).

In summary, acute pancreatitis is capable of precipitating both local and systemic complications. Locally, the pancreas can develop abscesses and pseudocysts. The presence of a pancreatic abscess is a critical complication that may cause death if it is not treated rapidly. Systemically, most body systems can become involved. Many of the complications are multisystemic in nature and are a result of hypotension and tissue hypoxia. Table 32–6 summarizes the major systemic complications.

TABLE 32–6   Major Systemic Complications of Acute Pancreatitis

BODY SYSTEM/FUNCTION	COMPLICATIONS
Neurologic	Encephalopathy
Pulmonary	Hypoxia, respiratory failure, pneumonia, pleural effusion, atelectasis, acute respiratory distress syndrome (ARDS)
Cardiovascular	Hemorrhage, hypotension, shock, pericardial effusion, pericardial tamponade
Gastrointestinal	Bleeding
Renal	Acute renal failure
Metabolic	Metabolic acidosis, hypocalcemia, hyperglycemia
Hematologic	Vascular thrombosis, disseminated intravascular coagulation (DIC)

SECTION SIX REVIEW

1. Pancreatic pseudocyst is composed of (choose all that apply)
   1. necrotic tissue
   2. air
   3. blood
   4. pancreatic enzymes

   A. 1 and 4
   B. 1, 3, and 4
   C. 1, 2, and 3
   D. 2, 3, and 4

2. If a pseudocyst were to rupture into the peritoneal cavity the patient would most likely develop
   A. septicemia
   B. acute renal failure
   C. paralytic ileus
   D. peritonitis

3. In the acute pancreatitis patient, hypovolemic shock usually results from (choose all that apply)
   1. hemorrhage
   2. third spacing
   3. renal failure
   4. kallikrein release
   A. 1, 3, and 4
   B. 3 and 4
   C. 1, 2, and 4
   D. 2, 3, and 4

4. Pulmonary complications are attributed to which of the following pancreatic enzymes?
   A. trypsin
   B. elastase
   C. amylase
   D. phospholipase A

5. The release of MDF by injured pancreatic tissue is believed to have what effect on the heart?
   A. decreases cardiac output
   B. decreases heart rate
   C. increases blood pressure
   D. increases cardiac output

Answers: 1. B, 2. D, 3. C, 4. D, 5. A

SECTION SEVEN: Medical Management

At the completion of this section, the learner will be able to describe the medical management of the patient with acute pancreatitis.

The medical management of the patient with acute pancreatitis may be either supportive or curative but is often a combination of both. Supporting the patient's hemodynamic and oxygenation status is essential while correction of the underlying problem (mechanical obstruction) is undertaken or the underlying problem is allowed to resolve itself (alcohol induced).

Evidence-Based Practice

- *In patients with acute pancreatitis, enteral feedings should be considered the nutritional treatment of choice. Enteral nutrition is associated with a lower incidence of infections and a reduction in the need for surgical interventions for controlling the pancreatitis. Use of enteral feedings does not increase mortality or the incidence of noninfectious complications (Marik & Zaloga, 2004).*

- *In patients with severe acute pancreatitis (SAP), initiation of total enteral nutrition (TEN) within the first 48 hours following admission produced fewer complications, was less costly, and resulted in a shorter length of stay when compared to use of total parenteral nutrition (Gupta et al., 2003).*

- *Transthyretin is a sensitive biomarker of metabolic stress and protein status in patients admitted with acute and chronic pancreatitis (Lasztity et al., 2002).*

Supportive Therapy

Medical management is based on prioritized goals, including stabilizing hemodynamic status, controlling pain, minimizing pancreatic stimulation, correcting the underlying problem, and preventing or treating complications. A summary of general physician orders related to supportive management of the acute pancreatitis patient is listed in Table 32–7.

Goal 1: Stabilize the Patient's Hemodynamic Status

Hypovolemia must be identified and treated aggressively. Hemodynamic stability is accomplished primarily through two types of interventions: fluid resuscitation and inotropic therapy. Fluid resuscitation includes crystalloids, possibly colloids, and plasma expanders. It is essential to closely monitor the patient's hemodynamic status as treatment progresses. Hemodynamic status monitoring might include

- Blood pressure and pulse
- Pulmonary artery pressure
- Pulmonary artery wedge pressure
- Central venous pressure
- Cardiac output, cardiac index
- Intake and output (hourly), daily weights
- Hematocrit and serum blood urea nitrogen (BUN) levels

Goal 2: Control the Patient's Pain

Acute pancreatitis is extremely painful. Controlling the level of pain is essential for comfort and to decrease secretion of pancreatic enzymes. The drug of choice is meperidine (Demerol)

TABLE 32–7 Supportive Therapy for Acute Pancreatitis

TYPE OF SUPPORT	GENERAL PHYSICIAN ORDERS
Fluid resuscitation	May consist of up to 10–20 L of fluid during the first 24 hours, as required
	Fluids may be crystalloids or colloids
	If hypoalbuminemic, consider albumin replacement
	If hemoglobin ≤ 10 mg/dL, consider blood transfusion
	As experimental therapy to deactivate systemic proteolases, fresh frozen plasma may be ordered
Inotropic	When hypotension predominates, consider dopamine therapy
	When poor tissue perfusion predominates, consider dobutamine therapy
Respiratory	If Pao_2 is less than 60 mm Hg in the presence of high oxygen concentration, and/or respiratory rate is greater than 30/min, consider early intubation and mechanical ventilation with sedation and analgesia
Renal	In the presence of impaired renal function, consider dopamine at a low "renal" dose to increase renal perfusion; timely and adequate fluid resuscitation is essential to prevent permanent damage
Nutritional	Once hemodynamic stability has been achieved, total parenteral nutrition (TPN) or nasojejunal enteral feeding is initiated
	Monitor serum glucose closely, maintaining levels at approximately 150 mg/dL if possible
	High doses of insulin may be necessary because of severe insulin resistance

Data from Conwell, D. L. (2002). Diseases of the pancreas. In T. E. Andreoli, C. C. J. Carpenter, R. C. Griggs, & J. Loscalzo (Eds). Cecil essentials of medicine, (5th ed., pp. 356–363). Philadelphia: W. B. Saunders; Naude, G. P. (2002). Gastrointestinal failure in the ICU. In F. S. Bongard & D. Y. Sue (Eds.), Current critical care diagnosis and treatment, (2nd ed., pp. 376–390). New York: Lange.

rather than morphine sulfate. Dilaudid (hydromorphone) may also be effective in pain management. Opiates, such as morphine, can cause spasms of the sphincter of Oddi, which may further aggravate the disease process.

Goal 3: Minimize Pancreatic Stimulation

It is important to reduce the stimulation of pancreatic secretion as much as possible. Keeping the GI tract at rest facilitates pancreatic rest and reduces the amount of pancreatic juice secreted. Organ rest needs to continue until serum amylase levels have returned to normal and pain has subsided. This may take up to 7 weeks. The physician may order the following:

- Initial nothing-by-mouth (NPO) status
- Placement of a nasogastric tube to low-wall suction
- Drug therapy, such as antacids or anticholinergics (anticholinergics reduce GI motility)

Patients who are experiencing acute pancreatitis are especially hypermetabolic and hypercatabolic. They have extremely high nutritional demands but are unable to consume nutrients orally for a prolonged period. Nutritional support is essential to improving the patient's outcome.

Curative Therapy

Goal 4: Correct the Underlying Problem

Generally, medical interventions are more desirable than surgical ones. Some triggering events, such as binge alcohol abuse, may subside spontaneously if given sufficient rest time using supportive therapy. If the etiology is mechanical, however, the underlying problem can be corrected surgically. For example, if a patient has a biliary obstruction, such as a gallstone, a cholecystectomy may be performed to relieve the obstruction. Certain surgical procedures to relieve obstructions can be performed during an ERCP, as explained in Section Four.

Goal 5: Prevent or Treat Complications

It is imperative that complications be recognized early in their development and then treated aggressively. Close patient monitoring is a crucial part of meeting this goal. Medical interventions are based on correcting or supporting system dysfunctions as they develop. In addition to the various supportive physician orders listed in Table 32–7, the physician may need to order any of the following:

- Electrolyte replacement
- Insulin therapy
- Antibiotic therapy
- Arterial blood gases
- Oxygen therapy
- Pulmonary toilet (e.g., incentive spirometry)
- Radiographic studies
- Cardiac monitoring
- Pulmonary artery flow-directed catheter

Surgical debridement may be indicated if the patient develops infected pancreatic necrosis or abscess (Greenberger & Toskes, 2001). Unfortunately, surgical incisions of pancreatic tissue may lead to the development of pancreatic fistulas, which can result in the entry of pancreatic juice into other tissues, causing further damage and new complications. Pancreatic abscess is treated by percutaneous drainage (Greenberger & Toskes, 2001).

In summary, the medical management of the patient with acute pancreatitis is based on complex multisystem needs. Five major supportive treatment focuses provide the basis for the majority of medical care: fluid resuscitation; inotropic drug therapy; and respiratory, renal, and nutritional support. The major prioritized goals that help organize medical management of acute pancreatitis include stabilizing hemodynamic status, controlling pain, minimizing pancreatic stimulation, correcting the underlying cause, and preventing or treating complications. Many physician orders will be written as the patient's status changes.

SECTION SEVEN REVIEW

1. The highest priority in management of the patient with severe acute pancreatitis is to
   A. control pain
   B. stabilize hemodynamic status
   C. minimize pancreatic stimulation
   D. correct the underlying problem
2. The drug of choice in pain management of the patient with acute pancreatitis is
   A. morphine sulfate
   B. codeine
   C. meperidine
   D. ibuprofen
3. Anticholinergics may be ordered for the patient with acute pancreatitis for the primary purpose of
   A. reducing GI motility
   B. reducing pain

C. increasing pancreatic stimulation
D. increasing gastric pH

4. The effective management of complications depends on (choose all that apply)
   1. close monitoring
   2. early recognition
   3. aggressive treatment
   4. age of the patient
   A. 1, 3, and 4
   B. 2, 3, and 4
   C. 2 and 3
   D. 1, 2, and 3

Answers: 1. B, 2. C, 3. A, 4. D

SECTION EIGHT: The Nursing Care Plan

At the completion of this section, the learner will be able to discuss the nursing plan of care for a patient with acute pancreatic dysfunction. The nursing care plan for the patient experiencing an acute pancreatic dysfunction episode includes both collaborative problems and independent nursing diagnoses.

Frequently Occurring Collaborative Problems

Acute pancreatitis carries the risk of many potential complications. On a nursing plan of care, potential complications are dealt with as collaborative problems (Carpenito-Moyet, 2003). Collaborative problems require a combination of physician and nursing orders to manage the problem optimally. Potential complications (PCs) that are commonly noted in patients with acute pancreatitis include

- PC: Hyperglycemia
- PC: Hemorrhage
- PC: Peritonitis
- PC: Sepsis
- PC: Noncardiogenic pulmonary edema
- PC: Fluid and electrolyte imbalances
- PC: Pleural effusion
- PC: Hypovolemic shock

- PC: Acute tubular necrosis
- PC: Disseminated intravascular coagulation
- PC: Pancreatic abscess
- PC: Pancreatic pseudocyst

Frequently Occurring Nursing Diagnoses

On completion of the nursing database, the nurse clusters data and develops a set of nursing hypotheses based on the available data. Additional critical data that may either support or eliminate each hypothesis should also be identified and obtained. Once the hypotheses have been established, the nurse is ready to develop a list of nursing diagnoses based on the patient's response to the illness rather than on the illness itself.

In the patient with acute pancreatic dysfunction, a variety of nursing diagnoses frequently occur during the crisis period. The following is a partial list of some of these nursing diagnoses as suggested by Carpenito-Moyet (2003) and Ulrich and Canale (2001):

- *Pain: Epigastric or abdominal* related to localized peritonitis, pancreatic capsule distention, and nasogastric suction
- *Altered nutrition: Less than body requirements* related to vomiting, anorexia, and impaired digestion secondary to decreased pancreatic enzymes
- *Ineffective breathing pattern* related to abdominal pain, depressant effects of opioid therapy, and decreased lung expansion

- *Anxiety* related to unfamiliar environment; discomfort; lack of understanding of diagnosis, diagnostic tests, and interventions; and fear of death
- *Altered comfort: Nausea and vomiting* related to stimulation of the vomiting center

Many of the nursing diagnoses listed here are presented in other modules. Two nursing diagnoses—*Alteration in comfort: Nausea and vomiting,* and *Pain*—are of particular interest to this patient population.

Nausea and Vomiting

Nausea and vomiting frequently accompany and further aggravate abdominal pain in the patient with acute pancreatitis. Some patients develop dry heaves rather than actual vomiting. The following is a plan of care for managing nausea and vomiting as suggested by Ulrich and Canale (2001).

Alteration in comfort: Nausea and vomiting related to vomiting center stimulation

Desired Patient Outcomes. The patient will experience relief of nausea and vomiting as evidenced by

- No vomiting
- No dry heaves
- Patient states relief of nausea

Nursing Interventions

1. Assess patient for nausea, vomiting, and dry heaves.
2. Implement interventions to relieve nausea, vomiting, and dry heaves.
   A. Prevent/relieve gastric distention:
      Potential collaborative action: Insertion of nasogastric tube
      Related independent actions: Maintain tube patency
   B. Restrict oral intake, as ordered (NPO status is often ordered).
   C. When nauseated:
      Encourage deep, slow breathing.
      Change positions slowly.
   D. Oral hygiene every 2 hours and as necessary postvomiting.
   E. Administer antiemetic therapy as ordered: Monitor for therapeutic and nontherapeutic effects of therapy.
3. Consult with physician if current therapy fails to meet desired outcomes.

Pain

The severe pain associated with acute pancreatitis is a major nursing concern. It negatively affects patient outcomes and can be difficult to control. The following presents a partial care plan for addressing this problem, as suggested by Ulrich and Canale (2001).

Pain: Epigastric or abdominal related to localized peritonitis, pancreatic capsule distention, and nasogastric suction

Desired Patient Outcomes. The patient will experience decreased pain, as evidenced by

- Verbalization of pain relief
- Relaxed body positioning
- Relaxed facial expression
- Blood pressure, pulse, and respirations shifting toward baseline

Nursing Interventions

1. Assess patient's perception of pain experience through self-report methods.
2. Assess patient for factors that increase and decrease the pain.
3. Implement interventions to decrease pain.
   A. Nothing by mouth during acute phase.
   B. Insert nasogastric tube as ordered.
   C. Administer medications to reduce gastric acid quantity and neutralize acid.
   D. Administer analgesics as ordered; avoid use of morphine sulfate. Encourage use of patient-controlled analgesia (PCA) if ordered.
   E. Monitor for therapeutic and nontherapeutic effects of analgesic therapy.
   F. Help patient assume body positioning that reduces pain (e.g., sit/lie with knees flexed and trunk slightly flexed).
4. Consult with physician if current interventions are not adequately meeting desired outcomes.

For further information regarding acute pain management, refer to Module 2, "Acute Pain in the High-Acuity Patient."

In summary, acute pancreatic dysfunction is a potentially severe health problem that requires complex management. This section has presented collaborative problems based on potential complications and frequently occurring nursing diagnoses that may apply to the care of the patient with acute pancreatitis. Two nursing diagnoses—*Altered comfort: Nausea and vomiting,* and *Pain*—have been presented in detail.

SECTION EIGHT REVIEW

1. Which of the following potential complications (PCs) is commonly found in the patient with acute pancreatitis?
    1. PC: Hyperglycemia
    2. PC: Sepsis
    3. PC: Brain abscess
    4. PC: Acute tubular necrosis
    5. PC: Heart failure
    A. 1, 2, and 5
    B. 2, 3, and 4
    C. 1, 2, and 4
    D. 1, 4, and 5
2. In developing a plan of care for the patient with acute pancreatitis, which nursing diagnosis statement would be correct? *Pain: epigastric or abdominal* related to

A. gastric distention
B. pancreatic ischemia
C. gastric or duodenal wall erosion
D. localized peritonitis, pancreatic capsule distention

3. Nursing interventions that would directly address the nursing diagnosis *pain: epigastric or abdominal* in a patient in the acute phase of acute pancreatitis would include
    A. Nothing by mouth
    B. Encourage soft food diet
    C. Monitor for therapeutic effects of morphine
    D. Encourage patient to assume a prone position to reduce pain

Answers: 1, C. 2, D. 3, A

POSTTEST

The following Posttest is constructed in a case study format. A patient is presented. Questions are asked based on available data. New data are presented as the case study progresses.

Joan M, 63 years old, presents in the emergency department with complaints of severe abdominal pain. Because of her past history, she is admitted with a diagnosis of "rule out pancreatitis."

1. Joan's pancreas is located
    A. adjacent to the liver
    B. in front of the stomach
    C. behind the spleen
    D. within the curve of the duodenum
2. Under normal circumstances, Joan's pancreas empties into the small bowel at the
    A. ampulla of Vater
    B. duct of Wirsung
    C. acinus
    D. tail
3. Joan's pancreatic regulation of pH is accomplished by
    A. formation of pepsin
    B. release of secretin
    C. activation of enzymes
    D. secretion of cholecystokinin
4. Under normal circumstances, Joan's pancreas is protected from autodigestion because the pancreatic enzymes
    A. are inhibited by acetylcholine
    B. are activated only by an acid pH
    C. exist in precursor form in the pancreas
    D. are used immediately, with no storage capabilities

5. Joan's pancreas secretes the enzyme trypsin, which
    A. is responsible for breakdown of fats
    B. splits phospholipids into fatty acids
    C. splits carbohydrates into disaccharides
    D. is the most abundant proteolytic enzyme

Joan is 5 feet 4 inches (16.4 m) tall and weighs 161 pounds (73 kg). She gives a history of smoking about one pack per day for 40 years. She drinks a glass of wine several days a week with her evening meal. She denies a history of diabetes or heart problems but states that she has had several "gallbladder attacks" over the past several years.

6. Joan is more likely to have which type of pancreatitis?
    A. acute intersitial
    B. chronic interstitial
    C. acute hemorrhagic
    D. chronic hemorrhagic
7. Which piece of Joan's history represents the strongest etiologic factor for development of pancreatitis?
    A. smoking history
    B. gallbladder disease
    C. alcohol consumption
    D. obesity
8. If Joan is diagnosed with acute interstitial pancreatitis, it typically is characterized by
    A. a long duration
    B. fat necrosis
    C. irreversible damage
    D. localized inflammation

9. If Joan's pancreatitis has been caused by pancreatic duct obstruction, the obstruction is most likely caused by
   A. a gallstone
   B. edema
   C. a stricture
   D. severe spasms

The physician orders a battery of diagnostic tests that include, among others, serum amylase, serum lipase, and ERCP.

10. Serial serum lipase levels may be ordered in preference to serum amylase levels because serum lipase
    A. is more accurate
    B. is more specific to pancreatitis
    C. remains elevated for a longer period
    D. requires no special analysis technique

11. A major advantage of performing an ERCP is that
    A. it is a noninvasive procedure
    B. it can be performed at the bedside
    C. it provides access to the gallbladder and pancreas
    D. mechanical obstructions can be directly removed

12. If Joan's description of her pain is typical of the classic pattern associated with acute pancreatitis, it would have which characteristics?
    1. piercing
    2. slow onset
    3. epigastric
    4. sharp
    A. 2, 3, and 4
    B. 1, 3, and 4
    C. 1 and 2
    D. 1, 2, and 3

13. If Joan develops peritoneal signs as a result of extrapancreatic invasion of enzymes, the nurse would assess
    A. abdominal rigidity
    B. hyperactive bowel sounds
    C. dulling of abdominal pain
    D. onset of bradycardia

14. The nurse can assess Joan for Chvostek's sign by
    A. checking for bluish discoloration of umbilicus
    B. tapping the facial nerve in front of ear
    C. inflating arm with blood pressure cuff
    D. checking for flank bluish discoloration

15. If Joan should develop cardiovascular complications associated with her acute pancreatitis, no matter what the mechanism is, the consistent end result is
    A. increased systemic vascular resistance
    B. increased cardiac output
    C. decreased systemic vascular resistance
    D. decreased cardiac output

16. The major pulmonary complications of acute pancreatitis include (choose all that apply)
    1. cor pulmonale
    2. pleural effusion
    3. hypoxia
    4. respiratory failure
    A. 2, 3, and 4
    B. 1, 2, and 3
    C. 1, 3, and 4
    D. 2 and 3

17. If Joan develops a severe case of acute pancreatitis, the initial medical management will focus on
    A. controlling pain
    B. minimizing pancreatic stimulation
    C. stabilizing hemodynamic status
    D. correcting the underlying problem

18. Joan is complaining of severe abdominal pain. The nurse can anticipate administering which drug as the first choice?
    A. meperidine
    B. morphine
    C. hydromorphone
    D. codeine

POSTTEST ANSWERS

Question	Answer	Section
1	D	One
2	A	One
3	B	Two
4	C	Two
5	D	Two
6	A	Three
7	B	Three
8	D	Three
9	A	Three

Question	Answer	Section
10	C	Four
11	D	Four
12	B	Five
13	A	Five
14	B	Five
15	D	Six
16	A	Six
17	C	Seven
18	A	Seven

REFERENCES

Banks, P. A. (1997). Practice guidelines in acute pancreatitis. *American Journal of Gastroenterology, 92*(3), 377–386.

Beckingham, I. J., & Bornman, P. C. (2001). Acute pancreatitis. *British Medical Journal, 322*(7286), 595–598.

Bentrem, D. J., & Joehl, R. J. (2003). Pancreas: Healing response in critical illness. *Critical Care Medicine, 31*(8), S582–S589.

Carpenito-Moyet, L. J. (2003). Nursing care plans and documentation: Nursing diagnoses and collaborative problems (4th ed.) Philadelphia: Lippincott Williams & Wilkins.

Cole, L. (2001). Unraveling the mystery of acute pancreatitis. *Nursing, 31*(12), 58–64.

Conwell, D. L. (2001). Acute and chronic pancreatitis. *Practical Gastroenterology, 25*(12), 47–55.

Dimangno. E. P., & Chari, S. (2002). Acute pancreatitis. In M. Feldman, L. S. Friedman, M. H. Sleisenger, & B. F. Scharschmidt (Eds.), *Sleisenger and Fordtran's gastrointestinal and liver disease: Pathophysiology, diagnosis, and Management* (7th ed., pp. 913–937). New York: McGraw Hill.

Greenberger, N. J., & Toskes, P. P. (2001). Acute and chronic pancreatitis. In E. Braunwald, A. S. Fauci, D. L. Kasper, S. T. Hauser, D. L. Longo, & J. L. Jameson, (Eds.), *Harrison's principles of internal medicine* (15th ed., pp. 1792–1804). New York: McGraw Hill.

Grendell, J. H. (2000). Acute pancreatitis. *Clinical Perspective in Gastroenterology, 3*(6), 327–333.

Gupta, R., Patel, K., Calder, P. C., Yaqoob, P., Primrose, J. N., & Johnson, C. D. (2003). A randomized clinical trial to assess the effect of total enteral and total parenteral nutritional support on metabolic inflammatory and oxidative markers in patients with predicted severe acute pancreatitis (APACHE II > or =6). *Pancreatology, 3*(5), 406–413.

Guyton, A. C., & Hall, J. E. (2000). *Textbook of medical physiology* (10th ed.). Philadelphia: W. B. Saunders.

Kee, J. L. (2002). *Laboratory and diagnostic tests with nursing implications* (6th ed.). Upper Saddle River, NJ: Prentice Hall.

Lasztity, N., Biro, L., Nemeth, E., Pap, A., & Antal, M. (2002). Protein status in pancreatitis—Transthyretin is a sensitive biomarker of malnutrition in acute and chronic pancreatitis. *Clinical Chemistry and Laboratory Medicine: CCLM, 40*(12), 1320–1324.

Magee, D. J., & Burdick, J. S. (2002). Anatomy, histology, embryology, and developmental anomalies of the pancreas. In M. Feldman, L. S. Friedman, M. H. Sleisenger, & B. F. Scharschmidt (Eds.), *Sleisenger and Fordtran's gastrointestinal and liver disease: Pathophysiology, diagnosis, and management* (7th ed., pp. 859–870). New York: McGraw Hill.

Marik, P., & Zaloga, G. (2004). Meta-analysis of parenteral nutrition versus enteral nutrition in patients with acute pancreatitis. *British Medical Journal, 328*(7453), 1407–1410.

Pandol, S. J. (2002). Pancreatic physiology and secretory testing. In M., Feldman, L. S. Friedman, M. H. Sleisenger, & B. F. Scharschmidt (Eds.), *Sleisenger and Fordtran's gastrointestinal and liver disease: Pathophysiology, diagnosis, and management* (7th ed., pp. 871–880). New York: McGraw Hill.

Porth, C. M. (2005). Disorders of hepatobiliary and exocrine pancreas function. In C. M. Porth (Ed.), *Pathophysiology: Concepts of altered health states* (7th ed., pp. 917–948). Philadelphia: Lippincott Williams & Wilkins.

Schlapman, N. (2001). Spotting acute pancreatitis *RN, 64*(11), 54–59.

Simeone, D. M., & Mulholland, M. W. (2003). Pancreas: Anatomy, and structural anomalies. In T. Yamada, D. H. Alpers, L. Laine, N. Kaplowitz, C. Owyang, & D. W Powell (Eds.), *Textbook of gastroenterology* Vol. 2. (4th ed., pp. 2013–2026). Philadelphia: Lippincott Williams & Wilkins.

Smotkin, J., & Tenner, S. (2002). Laboratory diagnostic tests in acute pancreatitis. *Journal of Clinical Gastroenterology, 34*(4), 459–462.

Topazian, M., & Gorelick, F. S. (2003). Acute pancreatitis. In T. Yamada, D. H. Alpers, L. Laine, N. Kaplowitz, C. Owyang, & D. W. Powell (Eds.), *Textbook of gastroenterology* Vol. 2. (4th ed., pp. 2026–2061). Philadelphia: Lippincott Williams & Wilkins.

Triester, S. L., & Kowdley, K. V. (2002). Prognostic factors in acute pancreatitis. *Journal of Clinical Gastroenterology, 34*(2), 167–176.

Ulrich, S. P., & Canale, S. W. (2001). *Nursing care planning guides* (5th ed.). Philadelphia: Lippincott Williams & Wilkins.

Yousaf, M., McCallion, K., & Diamond T. (2003). Management of severe acute pancreatitis. *British Journal of Surgery, 90*(4), 407–420.

Nursing Care of the Patient with Altered Gastrointestinal Function

Melanie Hardin-Pierce

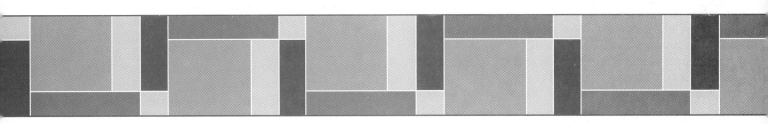

OBJECTIVES Following completion of this module, the learner will be able to

1. Describe an appropriate database for a patient with GI dysfunction.

2. Explain the assessment of a patient with GI dysfunction.

3. Discuss the development of nursing diagnoses appropriate for a patient with GI dysfunction.

4. Discuss the development of a plan of care for the patient with GI dysfunction.

This module is designed to integrate major points discussed in Modules 29 through 31. This module summarizes key relationships between concepts and assists the learner in clustering information to facilitate clinical application. Content is presented in an interactive learning style. Using a case study format, the learner is encouraged to identify nursing actions based on the assessment of a patient experiencing gastrointestinal (GI) dysfunction. The consequences of selecting a particular action are discussed. Rationale for all answers is presented.

ABBREVIATIONS

ABG	Arterial blood gas	**IV**	Intravenous
ADH	Antidiuretic hormone	**JVD**	Jugular venous distention
ALT (or SGPT)	Alanine aminotransferase	**LOC**	Level of consciousness
ARDS	Acute respiratory distress syndrome	**NG**	Nasogastric
BP	Blood pressure	**NSAID**	Nonsteroidal anti-inflammatory drug
BUN	Blood urea nitrogen	**PT**	Prothrombin time
GCS	Glasgow Coma Scale	**PTT**	Partial thromboplastin time
GGT	Gamma glutamyl transferase	**RBC**	Red blood cell
GI	Gastrointestinal	**SpO$_2$**	Peripheral arterial oxygen saturation
Hct	Hematocrit	**TPN**	Total parenteral nutrition
HR	Heart rate	**WBC**	White blood cell
ICU	Intensive care unit		

Case Study 1

UPPER GI BLEED

Mike P is a 45-year-old white male admitted to your unit with a diagnosis of acute upper GI bleeding. He was brought by car to the emergency department by two of his friends after he vomited blood earlier in the day. He was intoxicated on arrival at the hospital. His friends, who were also intoxicated, left immediately. He was transferred to the medical intensive care unit (ICU). On arrival at the ICU, the patient promptly vomited coffee-ground emesis. His medical diagnoses are (1) acute upper GI bleed and (2) hypovolemic shock.

Initial Appraisal

On approaching Mike's bed, you make the following rapid assessment.

GENERAL APPEARANCE. Mike is a thin, Caucasian male with a distended abdomen. His hair is blond and dirty, with typical male pattern baldness. He appears older than his stated age.

SIGNS OF DISTRESS. Mike's respiratory rate is approximately 24 breaths per minute, shallow and even, without apparent distress. No facial grimacing is noted, and his limbs are outstretched in a relaxed manner. He is mumbling and disoriented. He appears drowsy. His pulse is weak and thready; skin is pale and diaphoretic.

OTHER. You note the odor of alcohol on Mike's breath. He has one 18-gauge intravenous (IV) catheter in each of his arms with 0.9 percent normal saline solution infusing at 125 mL per hour. There is evidence of dried blood around the patient's mouth. His abdomen is distended, whereas his face and extremities are thin and emaciated. The nurse notes that his skin has a yellowish cast to it.

Focused Nursing History

Hospital records reveal that the patient was last hospitalized 3 months ago for decreased level of consciousness (LOC) and pneumonia. His pneumonia was treated with antibiotics, and his LOC returned to baseline. He was discharged home, where he resides with his elderly aunt. He did not show up for his scheduled follow-up appointment. His past medical history includes alcohol abuse and hypertension, for which he has been prescribed a diuretic. There is documentation of one previous episode of bleeding esophageal varices 3 years ago for which he was hospitalized. The patient is unable to provide any further history or information.

QUESTION

You note that he is ventilating without apparent distress. Based on the patient's past medical history and his history of present illness (vomiting blood), you would next focus your assessment on his _____ status.
- **A.** renal
- **B.** neurological
- **C.** fluid volume
- **D.** nutritional

ANSWER

C is the correct answer. During the initial appraisal, the nurse noted a critical cue, hematemesis (vomiting blood, dried blood around patient's mouth). Based on this single cue, the nurse can quickly cluster other similar critical cues, including a weak pulse and history of alcohol abuse, and, therefore, possible hepatic dysfunction. There are additional cues that direct the nurse to consider the possibility of hepatic dysfunction, such as distended abdomen (possible ascites); thin, emaciated extremities indicative of a poor nutritional status; and jaundice.

You scan his admission orders. An arterial blood gas (ABG); pulse oximetry; oxygen at 2 L per nasal cannula; nasogastric (NG) tube to low, intermittent suction; and urinary catheter have been ordered.

QUESTION

You decide that the NG tube and urinary catheter can wait. Which of the remaining orders would you implement first?
- **A.** pulse oximetry
- **B.** oxygen
- **C.** ABG

ANSWER

B is the correct answer. You should administer the oxygen first because you have noted the critical cues: rapid but shallow respirations, decreased LOC, confusion, and a probable upper GI bleeding event signifying blood loss. Reduced oxygen-carrying capacity accompanies active blood loss. In Mike's case, because he is symptomatic of a decreased oxygen-carrying capacity and has obviously experienced acute blood loss, oxygen should be administered first. It is also important to obtain a baseline ABG, and sometimes this should be done initially before applying oxygen in persons who are not symptomatic. In Mike's case, you should notify the laboratory regarding how much oxygen Mike is receiving and for how long he has been receiving it in order to get a true baseline ABG measurement. This intervention should be followed by a measurement of his peripheral arterial oxygenation saturation (SpO_2), which will help you to monitor Mike's response to the oxygen therapy. If you delay the oxygen administration, Mike could become hypoxic and go into respiratory failure. An NG tube is placed and Mike is lavaged with room temperature normal saline. The return aspirate consists of coffee-ground emesis.

Focused Nursing Assessment

Mike's initial appraisal, brief recent and past histories, and data clustering are suggestive of an upper GI bleeding crisis. Immediate action should be focused on obtaining more data to confirm this hypothesis. Focused neurological and respiratory assessments are indicated because Mike has a decreased LOC and he may have aspirated some of the vomitus into his lungs.

Focused Neurological Assessment

Mike is drowsy and oriented to his name only. He is mumbling inappropriate word phrases, and his Glasgow Coma Scale (GCS) score is 13 (opens eyes spontaneously, verbalizes inappropriate words, appears confused but able to obey simple commands). He moves all of his extremities on command and has a weak but equal hand grasp. Pupils are equal in size (4 mm), round, midline, and briskly reactive to light.

Focused Respiratory Assessment

Auscultation of his lungs reveals fine bibasilar crackles. Respiratory rate is 32 breaths per minute and shallow. Spo$_2$ per pulse oximetry is 86 percent on 4 L of oxygen per nasal cannula.

Focused Gastrointestinal and Fluid Volume Assessment

A focused GI and fluid volume assessment reveals 2 + pitting edema in his lower extremities. His skin and sclera are markedly icteric, and spider angiomas are noted over a grossly distended abdomen with ascites present. Palpation of the liver reveals enlargement and mild tenderness. Bowel sounds are noted on auscultation. He demonstrates significant orthostatic hypotension of greater than 10 points difference when lying and sitting (with legs dangling over the side of the bed). He complains of lightheadedness when in sitting position.

Focused Cardiovascular Assessment

A focused cardiovascular assessment reveals sinus tachycardia with a heart rate of 135, blood pressure 88/52, and absent jugular venous distention (JVD). Auscultation of his heart reveals an audible S1 and S2, without murmur or gallop.

Focused Integument and Temperature Assessment

- Skin is cool and dry to touch with palpable peripheral pulses. The nurse notes a yellowish tinge to the skin, and scleras are also yellow. Rectal temperature is 100°F.
- Mike suddenly vomits a large amount of bright red blood. Measurement of his vital signs at this time reveals the following: blood pressure 80/45, heart rate 152, with a respiratory rate of 36 breaths per minute. Pulse oximetry reveals oxygen saturation (Spo$_2$) of 85 percent. His LOC has further deteriorated.

QUESTION

How would you interpret Mike's blood pressure and pulse?
   A. they are directly related to his loss of skeletal muscle mass
   B. they are indicative of alcohol withdrawal
   C. they are directly related to his hypovolemia
   D. they are indicative of severe fluid volume overload

ANSWER

The correct answer is C. Patients with acute blood loss may become hypotensive and tachycardic as a result of hypovolemic shock. On arrival at the hospital, Mike also demonstrated orthostatic hypotension of greater than 20 points when going from a supine position to sitting up with his feet dangling. Orthostasis suggests fluid volume deficit.

Significant admission laboratory results were as follows:
   Hematocrit: 17 (normal, 40 to 54 percent [males])
   Hemoglobin: 7 (normal, 13.5 to 17 g/dL [males])
   WBC: 6,000 (normal, 5,000 to 10,000)

Coagulation Panel
   Prothrombin time (PT): 15.1 seconds (normal, 11 to 15 seconds) with an international normalized ratio (INR) of 1.9 (normal, 1.0)
   Partial thromboplastin time (PTT): 62 seconds (normal, 60 to 70 seconds)

Liver Function Tests
   Alanine aminotransferase (ALT or SGPT): 1,000 (normal, 3 to 35 units/mL)
   Gamma glutamyl transferase (GGT): 210 (normal, 4 to 23 IU/L)
   Total bilirubin: 5.0 (normal, 0.1 to 1.2 mg/dL)
   Ammonia: 62 (normal, 15 to 45 mcg/dL)

Blood Alcohol Level
   252 mg/dL (normal, zero mg/dL; indicative of alcohol intoxication, greater than 150 mg/dL; severe alcohol intoxication, 250 mg/dL; comatose, 300 mg/dL; fatal greater than 400 mg/dL)
   Blood urea nitrogen (BUN): 67 mg/dL (normal, 5 to 25 mg/dL in adults)
   Serum creatinine: 1.0 mg/dL (normal, 0.5 to 1.5 mg/dL)
   Sodium: 148 (normal, 135 to 145 mEq/L)
   Potassium: 3.1 mEq/L (normal, 3.5 to 5.3 mEq/L)
   Glucose: 78 (normal, 70 to 110 mg/dL)

Arterial Blood Gas
   pH: 7.35 (normal, 7.35 to 7.45)
   Paco$_2$: 30 (normal, 35 to 45 mm Hg)
   Pao$_2$: 82 (normal, 75 to 100 mm Hg)
   Sao$_2$: 90 percent (normal, greater than 95 percent)
Chest x-ray: Right lower lobe infiltrate

(All normal values from Kee [2002].)

QUESTION

What is the significance of the laboratory and radiographic data?

ANSWER

1. The hematocrit (Hct) is low, perhaps in response to the actual blood loss. This patient's bleeding is probably significant because the Hct is so low. Usually, the Hct value does not change substantially during the first hours after an episode of acute GI bleeding and, therefore, is not a reliable measure of the amount of blood loss (Kee, 2002). Serial measurements of Hct values are useful to evaluate continued blood loss and adequacy of red blood cell (RBC) replacement. Because the Hct value represents a percentage of RBC mass to total intravascular volume, the absolute value for the Hct must be evaluated in relation to other parameters of fluid status. The Hct value may be normal or even elevated during the hypovolemic event. Once rehydration occurs with IV fluids, significant decreases of Hct can occur without any significant change in the amount of RBCs.

2. The BUN level is also important to monitor because elevated levels may be seen with hypovolemia and renal failure. If the BUN is rising and the creatinine level remains relatively unchanged, a

decreased intravascular volume is suggested. In fact, BUN elevations of two to five times normal are associated with blood loss of greater than 1,000 mL. The BUN level also increases because of the intestinal absorption of blood proteins (George-Gay, 2001). This patient's BUN is elevated, whereas the creatinine is normal, suggesting hypovolemia.

3. This patient's hemoglobin (Hgb) is low. Decreased Hgb values are seen with severe hemorrhage, cirrhosis of the liver, and with large amounts of IV fluids as a result of hemodilution. Chronic anemia may also be an underlying problem with this patient.

4. This patient's white blood cell (WBC) count is on the low side of normal. If Mike has chronic alcohol problems, he may be malnourished. It would be beneficial to know his serum protein and WBC differential levels, to better assess his nutritional and immune status—he may not be immunocompetent secondary to chronic malnutrition related to his alcoholism. If he is not immunocompetent, it can cause complications, such as delayed healing and infection, which can negatively influence his length of hospital stay, prognosis, and mortality.

5. The coagulation panel values consisting of the PT and the PTT are normal. Liver function values (ALT or SGPT, GGT, and total bilirubin) are elevated and suggest underlying liver disease.

6. The patient's elevated liver enzymes suggest liver damage. His ammonia is elevated from the inability of the liver to convert ammonia to urea for elimination. As ammonia builds up in the body, hepatic encephalopathy develops. The serum ammonia level, however, does not necessarily directly correlate with the level of encephalopathy.

7. This patient's blood alcohol level is elevated, suggesting severe alcohol intoxication.

8. The serum sodium value is slightly elevated, suggesting hypovolemia as a result of hemoconcentration. This level should decrease following fluid resuscitation. The potassium level is decreased and will need replacement to promote optimal myocardial function.

9. The serum glucose level is normal but should be monitored closely for decreased levels.

10. This patient's ABG values are adequate on 2 L of oxygen per nasal cannula. The Spo_2 should be monitored continuously per pulse oximetry for decreased levels. Protection of the airway is critical in this patient. Endotracheal intubation should be considered by the medical team because a risk of aspiration exists (vomiting, continued decreased LOC, hypoxia). Note that he is in mild metabolic acidosis with respiratory compensation. Chronic alcoholism can result in a form of metabolic acidosis (called alcoholic ketoacidosis) related to ethanol metabolism, malnutrition, and other factors.

11. The patient's chest x-ray reveals a right lower lobe infiltrate consistent with pneumonia. Close surveillance of this patient's oxygenation status is indicated because of the high risk of aspiration pneumonia. Aspiration pneumonia is particularly problematic because it not only contaminates the lower airway but also may chemically harm the delicate lung structures, which can result in severe oxygenation problems or even acute respiratory distress syndrome.

Development of Nursing Diagnoses

You are now ready to develop the nursing diagnoses based on the available subjective and objective data. To cluster your data, look for abnormal values and findings discovered during the assessment. Mike's major symptoms at this time are bleeding, hypotension, and decreased LOC; thus, these primary symptoms can initiate your first cluster of critical cues.

CLUSTER 1

Subjective data. The patient has a decreased LOC and is unable to give you any information. His friends reported that he had vomited blood prior to arrival.

Objective data. Mike is hypotensive and vomiting bright red blood. His LOC has deteriorated from his initial GCS score of 13. His Hct is markedly decreased, whereas his BUN value is elevated. His serum creatinine is normal. Cardiac monitoring reveals sinus tachycardia.

QUESTION

Based on the preceding data, which nursing diagnosis is the priority diagnosis at this time for Mike?

A. decreased cardiac output
B. impaired gas exchange
C. fluid volume excess
D. fluid volume deficit

ANSWER

The correct answer is D. Mike is experiencing hypovolemic shock from active blood loss. The nursing diagnosis of *fluid volume deficit* related to active blood loss is supported by the data. A Foley catheter is inserted, resulting in only 35 mL of "tea"-colored urine. This finding of a decreased urine output further supports the diagnosis of fluid volume deficit.

Other nursing "diagnoses that apply to this patient include

- *Tissue perfusion, altered: cerebral, respiratory, renal, peripheral,* as evidenced by the decreased Hct and Hgb with decreased oxygen-carrying capacity, altered LOC, tachycardia, tachypnea, decreased urine output, cool skin, and weakly palpable pulses.
- *Aspiration, risk for,* related to decreased level of consciousness and vomiting.
- *Thought processes, altered,* related to alcohol intoxication, risk for alcohol withdrawal symptoms, and anemia.
- *Anxiety,* related to fear of bleeding, threat of death, and decreased oxygenation.

Collaborative Plan of Care

1. Stop the bleeding and achieve hemostasis.
2. Replace lost blood volume.
3. Correct hypovolemic shock.
4. Maintain adequacy of oxygenation status.

To deal with a presumed variceal bleed, Mike is started on intravenous vasopressin at 0.4 units per minute. Aggressive fluid resuscitation is begun. He receives 8 units of packed red blood cells to replace blood loss, 4 units of fresh frozen plasma to correct clotting factors, and 7 L of crystalloid solution (lactated Ringer's and 0.9 percent normal saline). Because of vomiting and hypotension, Mike is electively intubated to protect his airway. Diagnostic endoscopy is performed and large esophageal varices 2 to 4 centimeters above the gastroesophageal junction are found. Sclerotherapy is then performed.

QUESTION

What is the purpose of sclerotherapy?

ANSWER

Endoscopic sclerotherapy is currently the most common method of treatment in acute variceal hemorrhage. The purpose of this treatment is to sclerose (scar) the bleeding vessel, thus halting or preventing further hemorrhage. A sclerosing agent is injected into or around the bleeding vessel (George-Gay, 2001; Urden et al., 2002).

QUESTION

What nursing interventions are important in caring for a patient undergoing this procedure?

ANSWER

Nursing interventions during the procedure include
- Providing the patient and family with information concerning the procedure
- Positioning the patient
- Administering sedation if the patient is agitated

The nurse also continuously observes the patient for any signs of distress during the procedure. Postprocedure interventions include
- Assessing for further bleeding
- Monitoring for complications. Complications of sclerotherapy can include dysphagia, aspiration, esophageal perforation, mediastinitis, substernal pain, mucosal ulcerations, esophageal strictures, septicemia, fever, and pulmonary complications (Urden et al., 2002; George-Gay, 2003).

Variceal band ligation is gaining in popularity as an alternative to sclerotherapy because sclerotherapy is associated with significant complications. Transjugular intrahepatic portosystemic shunt (TIPS) is another potential intervention (see Module 31, "Acute Hepatic Dysfunction," for more information).

QUESTION

What is vasopressin? What should the nurse assess for in patients who are receiving intravenous vasopressin?

ANSWER

Vasopressin causes systemic vasoconstriction, especially of the splanchnic arteriolar system. It occurs naturally in the body as antidiuretic hormone (ADH), which is produced by the posterior pituitary. Vasopressin increases mesenteric vascular resistance, causing a reduced portal venous blood flow. These actions result in a concomitant decrease in portal venous pressure and esophageal variceal pressure, thus reducing bleeding. Unfortunately, vasopressin has some undesirable and dangerous systemic effects. These other side effects include decreased cardiac output, myocardial ischemia,

and decreased coronary blood flow. In fact, chest pain is not uncommon in patients receiving intravenous vasopressin, particularly in those who have a positive history for coronary artery disease. Nitroglycerin is often used simultaneously with a vasopressin infusion to maximize coronary blood flow and perfusion. Other complications of vasopressin for which the nurse should monitor are abdominal cramping secondary to splanchnic vasoconstriction and mesenteric ischemia, hyponatremia secondary to free water retention and antidiuretic action, hypertension secondary to systemic vasoconstriction, and bradycardia secondary to reflex responses to hypertension. Vasopressin must be weaned off slowly in order to avoid rebound effects, such as hypotension. Hypotension may also signal rebleeding. Nitroglycerin is weaned off along with the vasopressin. Diuresis may occur as the circulating ADH returns to a physiologic level, necessitating close monitoring of electrolytes, especially sodium and potassium.

Octreotide, a somatostatin analogue, has an action similar to vasopressin (splanchnic vasoconstriction/reduced portal pressure) but with fewer systemic side effects. Octreotide is administered intravenously and may offer efficacy similar to vasopressin with fewer side effects (Arnell, 2002; Zhou et al., 2002).

Therapeutic Goals and Desired Patient Outcomes

The following are critical therapeutic goals and outcomes as outlined by George-Gay (2001):

MAINTAIN HEMODYNAMIC STABILITY. The patient will attain/regain hemodynamic stability as evidenced by (AEB)

1. Systolic blood pressure (BP) greater than 90 mm Hg
2. Mean arterial pressure greater than 70 mm Hg
3. Heart rate (HR) less than 110 beats per minute
4. Hematocrit value greater than 30 percent
5. Hemoglobin value 12 to 14 g/100 mL

RESTORE TISSUE PERFUSION. The patient will have restored tissue perfusion AEB:

1. Urine output greater than 0.5 mL/kg body weight per hour
2. Capillary refill less than 3 seconds
3. Warm skin with strongly palpable peripheral pulses
4. Clear lung sounds
5. Oxygen saturation 90 percent or greater, or equal to baseline
6. Mental status returned to baseline
7. Absence of chest pain, dysrhythmia, or electrocardiographic abnormalities

ACHIEVE HEMOSTASIS/CORRECT COAGULATION DEFICITS. The patient will attain/regain hemostasis AEB:

1. No evidence of active bleeding
2. RBC, Hbg, and Hct returning to baseline
3. PT/PTT within normal limits

ACHIEVE RESPIRATORY STABILITY. The patient will achieve respiratory stability AEB:

1. Respiratory rate (RR) returned to baseline (less than 20 to 24 breaths per minute)
2. Absence of shortness of breath and crackles

3. ABG values within normal limits with baseline Spo_2 greater than 90 percent and Pao_2 75 to 100 mm Hg or within acceptable limits for patient

RESTORE NORMAL SERUM ELECTROLYTES. The patient will attain/regain electrolyte homeostasis AEB:

1. Serum sodium, potassium, calcium, glucose, and magnesium within normal limits

ACHIEVE COMFORT. The patient will be free of discomfort or will have pain and anxiety controlled at an acceptable level AEB:

1. States level of anxiety is reduced or at acceptable level
2. States pain is absent or has been reduced to acceptable level
3. Absence of nonverbal behaviors that suggest pain or anxiety
4. Vital signs (BP, HR, and RR) within acceptable ranges for patient

UNDERSTAND TREATMENT PLAN. The patient and family will understand the treatment plan AEB:

1. Patient and family verbalize understanding of and participate in treatment plan

Medical and Nursing Management and Patient Outcome

Fourteen hours after ICU admission, Mike's bleeding was stabilized. No further bleeding ensued. Fluid volume balance was maintained effectively, with urine output 50 to 100 mL per hour and electrolytes within normal limits. BUN and creatinine also were within normal limits. Mike still required sedation while on the ventilator, demonstrating agitation and thrashing about in bed as the sedation wore off. Although vital signs were stable (blood pressure 102/52; heart rate 110; respiratory rate 16), his rectal temperature rose to 100.4°F, and rhonchi were audible in both lung fields. WBC was 11,500 and ABG values were pH 7.51; Pco_2 30 mm Hg; Po_2 68 mm Hg; O_2 saturation 90 percent.

Revised Medical and Nursing Diagnoses

MEDICAL DIAGNOSES (COLLABORATIVE PROBLEMS, POTENTIAL COMPLICATIONS [PC])

- PC: Acute GI bleeding (resolving)
- PC: Pneumonia
- PC: Delirium tremens/alcohol withdrawal syndrome

NURSING DIAGNOSES

- *Impaired gas exchange* related to alveolar hypoventilation secondary to pneumonia
- *Sensory/perceptual alterations* related to alcohol withdrawal

Revised Plan of Care

Culture sputum, blood, and urine
Chest x-ray to evaluate for presence of infiltrates
Replace all invasive lines with new ones
Begin empiric antibiotic therapy

Sedation as needed
Continue respiratory ventilator support as needed
Begin aggressive pulmonary hygiene measures

Independent Nursing Interventions

The onset of acute upper GI bleeding and the resultant crisis-oriented interventions present a terrifying ordeal for the patient and family; therefore, emotional and spiritual support is needed. Additionally, the nurse should provide comfort measures. The patient needs frequent mouth care. Because of the presence of tubes (endotracheal, nasogastric, and in some cases a Sengstaken–Blakemore tube) in the nasal and oral cavities, the patient becomes a mouth breather. Hematemesis leads to the accumulation of blood in the oral cavity. The presence of tubes causes difficulty in swallowing saliva. To prevent undue discomfort from these invasive tubes, an emesis basin, tissues, and suction catheter should be kept within easy reach of the patient. The patient can be taught to suction out the mouth with a special handheld oral suction device, sometimes called a "Yankauer." To prevent undue irritation of the nares, they should be regularly cleansed and lubricated with a water-soluble substance. Epigastric discomfort can occur. Mike was kept NPO (nothing by mouth) until all evidence of bleeding was absent. Occasional ice chips or specially prepared oral lubricants per physician order may be provided to relieve mouth dryness. Humidification of supplemental oxygen is beneficial to prevent drying of delicate tissues as well as thinning pulmonary secretions so that they may be more easily expectorated.

Psychological and Family Implications

GI bleeding episodes create a crisis for the patient and the family. Not only can independent nursing interventions affect the outcome of this crisis but they can also influence the adaptation that the patient and family continue to make to the situation.

THE PATIENT. The loss of any quantity of blood may evoke panic and fear of death in the patient. The response is more complicated, with additional behavioral problems, if the patient is an alcoholic or drug abuser. Based on the idea that crisis situations have predictable outcomes, timely explanations of ongoing interventions and anticipated results help the patient cope with the overwhelming anguish and anxiety (Bucher, 2004). Decisive and supportive nursing care will help Mike to regain control of his own behavior and cooperate with the health team in therapy.

THE FAMILY. The family may display a variety of emotional reactions similar to those experienced by the patient. The need for the nurse to be keenly aware of the family and to assess the family as well as the patient should be self-evident if optimal crisis care is to be given. It is important for the patient and the family to be offered counseling following discharge to home. The family and significant others will play a critical role in the patient's eventual recovery and rehabilitation from alcohol.

Patient Outcome

The remainder of Mike's stay was uneventful. His urine culture was positive for *Escherichia coli;* blood and sputum cultures were positive for *Staphylococcus aureus.* His sputum culture was also positive for

Hemophilus influenzae. He was started on the appropriate antibiotics and was given aggressive pulmonary toilet by his nurses. Sedation was decreased, and ventilatory support was withdrawn without complications. Mike was effectively coughing up copious pulmonary secretions, his temperature had decreased to 99°F, and he was taken off all supplemental oxygen. His LOC returned to baseline (GCS score of 15). No further evidence of GI bleeding occurred, and he was discharged to home to live with his sister, who agreed to help him make his follow-up clinic appointments. Mike's nurse referred him to a local support group to help him deal with his alcohol abuse.

Case Study 2

BLEEDING PEPTIC ULCER

Mrs. H. is an 80-year-old woman with rheumatoid arthritis. She visited her local emergency department with complaints of dizziness, shortness of breath, and chest pain. Her daughter, with whom she resides, drove her to the hospital. Although she is a poor historian, her daughter relates that her mother's symptoms have been occurring with increasing frequency over the past 2 weeks.

Initial Appraisal

On approaching Mrs. H., you make the following assessment.

GENERAL APPEARANCE. Mrs. H. is a mildly obese, Caucasian female who appears her stated age. Her hair is gray and well kept. Her clothes are clean and appropriate. She is carrying a small handbag and a paper sack filled with her prescribed medications. Her daughter is appropriately attentive and concerned.

SIGNS OF DISTRESS. Mrs. H.'s breathing is rapid and even. No facial grimacing is noted, and her posture is relaxed. Her speech is clear and appropriate. She is oriented to her surroundings. Her skin is pale and cool to touch.

OTHER. Initial evaluation reveals a heart rate of 110, respiratory rate of 28 beats per minute, and Spo$_2$ of 92 percent. Continuous cardiac monitoring and 4 L of oxygen supplementation are initiated. A 12-lead electrocardiogram (ECG) is performed.

Focused Nursing History

Additional questioning reveals that Mrs. H. has smoked two packs of cigarettes a day for the past 60 years, has a history of coronary disease, and has been taking corticosteroids and nonsteroidal anti-inflammatory drugs (NSAIDs) for the management of her rheumatoid arthritis. Hospital records reveal that she was last hospitalized 3 months ago for a kidney infection. Her infection was treated with antibiotics, and she was discharged to home without further complications.

Focused Nursing Assessment

On physical examination, Mrs. H.'s lungs are clear to auscultation. Respirations are unlabored but rapid. No dysrhythmias are noted, and her ECG is normal, although her pulse is weak. Nailbeds are pale and capillary refill is sluggish. Her skin is pale, cool, and dry. Her heart sounds are audible, and no murmurs or gallops are present. She is alert and cooperative. She states that her chest pain has stopped since she has been resting. She also states that her chest pain occurs with exertion, which she describes as brisk walking and climbing stairs. Her abdomen is soft and nontender, bowel sounds are hyperactive, and rectal exam reveals tarry-colored stool that tests positive for blood. During this time, Mrs. H. tells you that she has been having black, tarry stools for several weeks, which she thought started after she began taking iron supplements. She also shares with you that she has been having burning abdominal pain precipitated by eating food for the past 2 weeks. Blood work reveals the following:

Complete Blood Count
   WBC: 4,500 (normal, 5,000 to 10,000)
   Hemoglobin: 8.2 (normal, 12 to 15 g/dL [females])
   Hematocrit: 26.6 (normal, 36 to 46 percent [females])
   Platelets: 276,000 (normal, 150,000 to 400,000)
Coagulation studies are all within normal limits.

Arterial Blood Gas
   pH: 7.37
   Paco$_2$:   47 mm Hg
   Pao$_2$:   70 mm Hg
   Sao$_2$:   96 percent (on 4 L of oxygen per nasal cannula)

Vital Signs

	Lying	Sitting
Blood pressure:	130/70	110/50
Heart rate:	110	130
Respiration:	24	28
Temperature:	98.5°F (37°C)	

The decision was made to admit Mrs. H. to the hospital for further evaluation and management. She was admitted to a step-down unit and placed on continuous cardiac monitoring because of her age and complaints of chest pain. An upper endoscopy is performed on Mrs. H., which reveals a large gastric ulcer. The ulcer appears to be oozing blood. This finding is compatible with her reports of pain following eating, her "tarry" stools, and her low hematocrit. She is diagnosed with peptic ulcer disease: gastric ulcer.

QUESTION

How do the clinical features of a gastric peptic ulcer compare to those of a duodenal peptic ulcer?

ANSWER

Characteristics of Duodenal and Gastric Ulcers

INCIDENCE. The incidence ratio of duodenal and gastric ulcers is approximately 4:1. The most common age group affected is 25 to 50 year olds, with men being affected four times more than women.

PATHOGENESIS OF DUODENAL ULCERS. Hyperacidity is the most important factor in the pathogenesis of duodenal ulcers. Diseases associated with hyperacidity include hyperparathyroidism, chronic pulmonary disease, chronic pancreatitis, alcoholism, and cirrhosis. Duodenal ulcers are also associated with tobacco use and high stress levels.

PATHOGENESIS OF GASTRIC ULCERS. Disruption of the GI mucosal barrier is the most important factor in the pathogenesis of duodenal ulcers. However, hydrochloric acid production is normal to low in most patients. Some drugs contribute to the development of gastric ulcers, such as alcohol, tobacco, and NSAIDs. *Helicobacter pylori* infection increases the risk of developing both gastric and duodenal ulcers.

LOCATION. The location of duodenal ulcers is within the duodenal bulb in 90 percent of cases. The location of gastric ulcers is in the antrum and lesser curvature of the stomach in 90 percent of cases.

CLINICAL FEATURES OF DUODENAL ULCERS. Duodenal ulcers exhibit a pain–food relief pattern (i.e., when food is eaten, the pain from a duodenal ulcer is relieved). Night pain is common. Weight loss seldom affects the occurrence of a duodenal ulcer.

CLINICAL FEATURES OF GASTRIC ULCERS. Eating may relieve or exacerbate the pain from a gastric ulcer. Night pain is less common than with a duodenal ulcer. Anorexia and weight loss are common with a gastric ulcer (Beers & Berkhow, 1999; Del Valle, 2001; Elliot, 2002).

QUESTION

What presenting symptoms influenced the decision to admit Mrs. H. to the hospital?

ANSWER

The symptoms that hastened her hospital admission were her complaints of dizziness, shortness of breath, and chest pain, and the fact that these symptoms have recently been occurring with increased frequency. These presenting symptoms combined with her advanced age indicate a potentially life-threatening situation. Furthermore, she demonstrated orthostatic hypotension when her blood pressure measurements were compared between lying (supine) and sitting (erect) positions. Significant orthostatic hypotension exists if the patient becomes dizzy, has a pulse increase of 20 beats per minute or greater, or has a systolic blood pressure decrease of 20 mm Hg or greater. Because Mrs. H.'s systolic blood pressure decreased from 130 to 110 and her heart rate increased from 110 to 130 when going from a sitting to a lying position, it can be concluded that she demonstrates orthostasis. This significant change in her vital signs indicates hypovolemia or dehydration. Furthermore, her hematocrit is low, and her stool is positive for blood. Her report of "tarry" stools lends support to a diagnosis of GI bleeding.

Based on the available data, you make the following nursing diagnoses and goals (Carpenito-Moyet, 2004):

- *Fluid volume deficit* related to gastric ulcer bleeding and fluid loss

  SUPPORTIVE DATA. Melena (tarry stools), abdominal pain (especially after eating), hyperactive bowel sounds, orthostasis, low Hct and Hgb, dizziness, weak pulse, and bleeding gastric ulcer per endoscopic evaluation.

  GOAL. The patient will regain fluid volume homeostasis AEB:

  1. Blood pressure within acceptable limits for patient, lying and sitting
  2. Strong, regular pulse
  3. No evidence of active bleeding
  4. Good skin turgor
  5. Moist mucous membranes
  6. Urine output greater than 30 mL per hour

- *Alteration in tissue perfusion* related to bleeding and fluid loss

  SUPPORTIVE DATA. Low Hct and Hgb, chest pain, shortness of breath, and increased heart rate.

  GOAL. The patient will have restored/maintained circulating blood volume AEB:

  1. Hct and Hbg improving or within acceptable limits
  2. Denies chest pain
  3. Denies shortness of breath
  4. No use of accessory respiratory muscles
  5. Heart rate within acceptable range for patient

- *Acute pain* related to peptic ulcer disease and GI bleeding

  SUPPORTIVE DATA. Abdominal and chest discomfort.

  GOAL. Patient will have minimal or no abdominal or chest discomfort AEB:

  1. Verbalizes minimal discomfort or absence of pain
  2. Absence of nonverbal behaviors suggesting discomfort

- *Imbalanced nutrition: Less than body requirements* related to GI bleeding, abdominal pain, and NPO status

  GOAL. Patient will have nutritional needs maintained AEB:

  1. Weight ± 2 pounds (4.4 kg) of baseline
  2. Serum electrolytes and protein levels improving or within acceptable limits

- *Anxiety/fear* related to emergent situation and hospitalization

  GOAL. Patient will have reduced or no anxiety or fear AEB:

  1. Verbalizes anxieties and fears
  2. Demonstrates progress toward positive coping behaviors

- *Knowledge deficit* regarding treatments, interventions, and home care needs

  GOAL. Patient and/or family will have adequate knowledge regarding treatments, interventions, and home care needs AEB:

  1. Demonstrates understanding of all interventions, treatments, medications, home care, and follow-up instructions.

QUESTION

From the history, what factors increase Mrs. H.'s risk for the development of peptic ulcer disease (PUD)?

ANSWER

Mrs. H. takes NSAIDs for her rheumatoid arthritis. Chronic use of NSAIDs can increase the risk for the development of ulcer disease by causing damage to the gastric mucosa. Overwhelming evidence associates chronic NSAID use with PUD, particularly gastric ulcers. NSAIDs and aspirin impair ulcer healing and induce ulcer formation through prostaglandin inhibition and directly irritate the gastric and duodenal mucosa. Prostaglandins, which are produced by the cells in the GI tract, play an important role in preventing injury to the gastroduodenal mucosa by inhibiting gastric acid secretion, maintaining blood flow, and stimulating mucus and bicarbonate production. Mrs. H. has smoked two packs of cigarettes a day for the past 60 years. Cigarette smoking causes decreased biliary bicarbonate secretion, thus causing duodenal gastric reflux, which contributes to ulcer formation. Furthermore, her advanced age is in itself a risk factor for ulcer development. Other risk factors that may contribute to the development of PUD include chronic aspirin use and alcohol use, both of which cause damage to the gastric mucosa, and heredity, which may be responsible for an increased number of parietal cells, resulting in hypersecretion of gastric acid. *Helicobacter pylori* infection also has been implicated in the pathogenesis of peptic ulcers. The inflammatory response associated with *H. pylori* infection is thought to disrupt the mucosal resistance to injury from gastric acid. This disruption in the mucosal defense mechanism allows the gastric acid to contribute to ulcer formation.

QUESTION

What was the cause of Mrs. H.'s chest pain?

ANSWER

This patient has a history of coronary artery disease, which, when combined with an impaired tissue perfusion secondary to blood loss from a gastric ulcer, could contribute to myocardial ischemia and chest pain. The blood loss and decreased Hct could be causing a decreased perfusion to the myocardium, resulting in ischemic chest pain. However, because her ECG was normal (without evidence of ischemia/infarction), her chest pain might be referred pain from her gastric ulcer.

QUESTION

What is the rationale for performing the upper endoscopy?

ANSWER

Because GI bleeding was suspected, the endoscopic procedure was needed to directly observe the GI tract mucosa for the source of the bleeding. After the bleeding ulcer was confirmed, a sclerosing agent was injected directly into the bleeding vessel to stop the bleeding. The sclerosing agent actually traumatizes the endothelium, causing necrosis and eventually sclerosis of the bleeding vessel. Her bleeding is stopped, and she is started on a clear liquid diet.

QUESTION

What possible complications should the nurse assess for in a patient who has undergone sclerotherapy of a bleeding gastric ulcer?

ANSWER

Several complications can result from endoscopic sclerotherapy, including ulcer perforation; strictures; bacteremia; increased bleeding (especially if coagulation abnormalities exist); aspiration; dysphagia; fever; venous thrombosis involving the mesentery; and systemic effects of sclerosis, such as acute respiratory distress syndrome (ARDS).

QUESTION

What pharmaceutical options exist for the control of gastric pH?

ANSWER

Pharmaceutical options include antacids (which provide a direct alkaline buffer to control the pH of the gastric mucosa), histamine blockers (which block parietal cell stimulation and secretion of hydrochloric acid), and proton pump inhibitors (which work within the parietal cells to decrease the acidity of the acid produced). Mucosal enhancers (e.g., sucralfate) act directly on the mucosa to reduce the effects of acid secretion (George-Gay, 2001).

Patient Outcome

Forty-eight hours following sclerotherapy of her bleeding gastric ulcer, Mrs. H.'s condition deteriorates. Her WBC rises dramatically to 21,000. She becomes hypotensive and difficult to arouse. Her blood pressure decreases to 70/52. She is transferred to the ICU, where intravenous vasopressor agents (e.g., dopamine) are started for blood pressure support. She is electively intubated and placed on mechanical ventilation. After 48 hours, her abdomen becomes distended and bowel sounds are absent. Blood cultures are positive for gram-negative rods, supporting a diagnosis of gram-negative septicemia and shock. Antibiotics are administered intravenously to treat or minimize septic complications. Dopamine and fluid resuscitation with normal saline is needed to support the blood pressure. Abdominal x-rays are taken and reveal distended bowel loops compatible with paralytic ileus. All oral foods and fluids are withheld, and an NG tube is inserted and attached to low wall suction in order to decompress the abdominal distention. The nurse monitors Mrs. H.'s electrolyte levels closely. She requires potassium replacement to treat hypokalemia.

QUESTION

What assessment findings support the diagnosis of acute paralytic ileus?

ANSWER

Abdominal distention, absent bowel sounds, and distended loops of bowel seen with radiological examination support the diagnosis of adynamic or paralytic ileus. Paralytic ileus is a complication of septic shock. The decreased blood pressure and vasodilation that accompanies septic shock produce hypoperfusion to the bowel. This "low flow" state causes a reduction in the normal peristaltic activity of the GI tract, resulting in an obstruction. It is common for bowel sounds to be decreased or absent on auscultation of the abdomen. Gas and fluid accumulate above the obstructed segment of bowel and result in the intestinal distention (George-Gay, 2001).

The physician orders gastric tonometry every hour. A special nasogastric tube is placed and a measurement is taken. This tube measures the gastric CO_2 levels ($Prco_2$). Also, a serum lactic acid and arterial blood gas, Hg, and Hct are ordered. The following are the results of these tests:

$Prco_2$:	Elevated
Lactic acid:	12
ABG:	pH: 7.26, $Paco_2$: 33, Po_2: 88, Sao_2: 90 percent, HCO_3: 18, base deficit: -9
Hgb, Hct:	8.4, 20

QUESTION

What interventions would be appropriate based on the data?

ANSWER

The new data suggest hypoperfusion and gut ischemia. The elevated $Prco_2$ level indicates ischemia to the gastric mucosa. The large base deficit indicates some degree of anaerobic metabolism, which is supported by the elevated serum lactic acid. The pH is decreased and the $Paco_2$ is increased slightly. Along with the large base deficit, a metabolic acidosis is in effect. This patient would benefit from volume expansion, oxygen administration, and packed red blood cell transfusions to increase oxygen-carrying capacity and improve tissue perfusion and oxygenation.

ANSWER

Maintain NPO status until bowel function returns. Until the patient can resume enteral feeding, an NG tube will need to be in place and attached to low wall suction in order to prevent gastric contents from entering the intestines and to rest the bowel. Hyperalimentation or total parenteral nutrition (TPN) may be required. As soon as bowel sounds return, the patient will need to be fed using her GI tract. It is very important that the nurse observe for signs and symptoms that reflect perforation, ischemia, or necrosis of the bowel. These symptoms include rebound tenderness of the abdomen, increased pain and distention, increased WBC, and fluid and electrolyte imbalances (George-Gay, 2001).

Pain and comfort relief measures are appropriate, as is frequent oral care.

Patient Outcome

Mrs. H. stabilizes hemodynamically. The dopamine is weaned off. Her bowel sounds return without any evidence of bowel necrosis. She is weaned off of mechanical ventilation and extubated. Oral feedings are reinitiated without any evidence of bowel obstruction. Her hematocrit remains stable, and her WBC count returns to normal. She is discharged to home to reside with her daughter, with follow-up.

QUESTION

What nursing interventions are necessary when caring for a patient who has developed an adynamic paralytic ileus?

REFERENCES

Arnell, T. (2002). Gastrointestinal bleeding. In F. S. Bongard & D. Y. Sue (Eds.), *Current critical care diagnosis and treatment* (2nd ed., p. 756). New York: Lange.

Beers, M. H., & Berkhow, R. (Eds.). (1999). *The Merck manual of diagnosis and therapy* (17th ed.). Whitehouse Station, NJ: Merck Research Laboratories.

Bucher, L. (2004). Nursing management: Critical care environment. In S. M. Lewis, M. M. Heitkemper, & S. R. Dirksen (Eds.), *Medical-surgical nursing: Assessment and management of clinical problems* (6th ed., pp. 1758–1793). St. Louis: C. V. Mosby.

Carpenito-Moyet, L. (2004). *Nursing diagnosis: Application to clinical practice* (11th ed.). Philadelphia: Lippincott Williams & Wilkins.

Del Valle, J. (2001). Peptic ulcer disease and related conditions. In E. Braunwald, A. Fauci, D. Kasper, S. Hauser, D. Longo, & J. L. Jameson (Eds.), *Harrison's principles of internal medicine* (15th ed.). CD-ROM version 1.0. New York: McGraw Hill

Elliot, D. (2002). The treatment of peptic ulcers. *Nursing Standard, 13*(22), 37–42.

George-Gay, B. (2001). Acute gastrointestinal bleeding. In J. H. Swearinger & J. Keen (Eds.). *Manual of critical care nursing: Nursing interventions and collaborative management* (4th ed., pp. 541–557). St. Louis: C. V. Mosby.

Kee, J. (2002). *Handbook of laboratory and diagnostic tests with nursing implications* (6th ed.). Upper Saddle River, NJ: Prentice Hall.

Urden, L. D., Stacy, K. M., Lougin, M. E. (2002). *Thelan's critical care nursing: Diagnosis and management.* St. Louis: Mosby.

Zhou, Y. Qiao, L., Wu, J., Hu, H., & Xu, C. (2002). Comparison of the efficacy of octreotide, vasopressin, and omeprazole in the control of acute bleeding in patients with portal hypertensive gastropathy: A controlled study. *Journal of Gastroenterology & Hepatology, 17*(9), 973–980.

PART

8

Injury

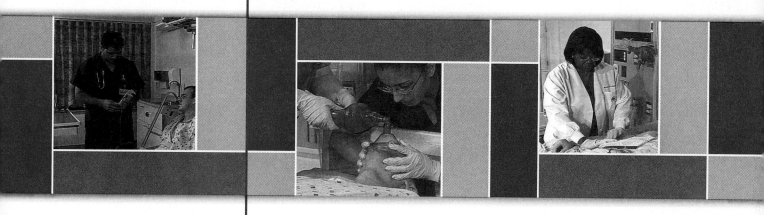

MODULE 34   Complex Wound Management

MODULE 35   Acute Burn Injury

MODULE 36   Trauma

MODULE 37   Nursing Care of the Patient with Multiple Injuries

34 Complex Wound Management

Catherine J. McDonald, Karen L. Johnson

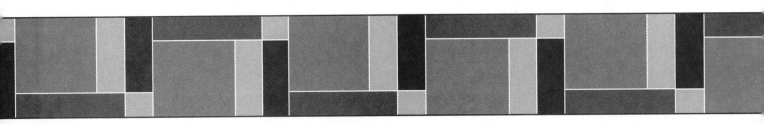

OBJECTIVES Following completion of this module, the learner will be able to

1. Identify anatomic structures and physiologic functions of the skin, and discuss age-related changes.
2. State the three phases of wound healing.
   - Describe the events that occur in each phase of wound healing.
   - Define three methods of wound closure.
3. State physiologic and environmental factors that affect wound healing.
4. Identify conditions that predispose a patient to developing a wound infection.
   - Identify criteria used to diagnose a wound infection.

- State interventions that can be used to prevent and treat wound infections.
5. Discuss the rationale for various treatment modalities used in wound management.
6. Identify the common clinical assessments made to evaluate wound healing.
7. Identify patients at risk for pressure ulcer development.
   - State interventions for the prevention of pressure ulcers.
8. Identify components of a pressure ulcer treatment program.

This self-study module describes the anatomic structures and physiologic functions of the skin (Section One), physiologic events that occur when an alteration in skin integrity occurs (Section Two), factors that affect wound healing (Section Three), principles of wound management (Sections Four and Five), nursing assessment of and interventions for the patient with an alteration in skin integrity (Section Six), and pressure ulcer prevention and treatment (Sections Seven and Eight).

To help determine your current level of understanding of this topic, the module begins with a pretest. Each section includes a set of review questions to help the learner evaluate his or her understanding of the section's content before moving on to the next section. All Section Reviews and the module Pretest and Posttest include answers. It is suggested that the learner review those concepts answered incorrectly in the review questions before proceeding to the next section.

 PRETEST

1. The layer of the skin that contains connective tissue, elastic fibers, blood vessels, and nerves is the
   A. epidermis
   B. dermis
   C. hypodermis
   D. subcutaneous tissue
2. Which of the following is not a function of the skin?
   A. regulation of body temperature
   B. production of vitamin D

C. protection from the external environment
D. production of calcium
3. Which of the following is not a major event that occurs during the proliferative phase of wound healing?
   A. hemostasis
   B. epithelialization
   C. granulation
   D. collagen cross-linking

4. The four cardinal signs of inflammation occur as a result of
   A. normal chemical and vascular events
   B. an infectious process
   C. bradykinins
   D. an increased number of white blood cells (WBCs)

5. Wounds that have significant contamination or significant tissue loss usually are not sutured. These wounds are left open to heal by the process of
   A. primary intention
   B. secondary intention
   C. delayed primary intention
   D. delayed secondary intention

6. Which of the following does NOT affect wound healing?
   A. age
   B. weight
   C. serum glucose of 450 mg/dL
   D. gender

7. Which of the following would not predispose a patient to developing a wound infection?
   A. susceptible host
   B. compromised wound
   C. infectious organism
   D. low hematocrit

8. A wound is considered to be infected when
   A. pus is present in the wound
   B. organisms elicit a host immune response
   C. the wound is found to be colonized
   D. yellow-green slough is present

9. Which of the following does NOT promote local wound healing?
   A. application of a heat lamp
   B. debridement with scissors
   C. irrigation with normal saline
   D. application of dressings

10. A solution used for wound irrigation that aids in mechanical debridement but does not damage granulation tissue is
    A. Betadine (povidone–iodine)
    B. normal saline
    C. acetic acid
    D. hydrogen peroxide

11. A patient has an abdominal wound that is healing by secondary intention. On assessment of this wound, seropurulent drainage is noted from granulating tissue, with some necrotic tissue present. Which type of dressing would you select to remove the debris and necrotic tissue without causing harm to the granulation tissue?
    A. dry sterile dressing
    B. alginate dressing
    C. synthetic dressing
    D. hydrocolloid dressing

12. Pressure ulcer risk assessments can be made using the
    A. Brazen scale
    B. Braden scale
    C. Newton scale
    D. Norris scale

13. A pressure ulcer is defined as
    A. a sore on the skin over a bony prominence
    B. reactive hyperemia
    C. full-thickness skin loss with damage to muscle
    D. any lesion caused by unrelieved pressure resulting in damage of underlying tissue

14. Which of the following is NOT a part of standard management of pressure ulcers?
    A. heat lamps
    B. management of tissue loads
    C. debridement
    D. operative repair

Pretest Answers: 1. B, 2. D, 3. A, 4. A, 5. B, 6. D, 7. D, 8. B, 9. A, 10. B, 11. B, 12. B, 13. D, 14. A

GLOSSARY

abrasion   Partial-thickness denudation of skin caused by friction or scraping.

autolytic debridement   Use of dressing materials that allow endogenous enzymes to liquefy necrotic tissue.

avulsion   Full-thickness skin loss; wound edges cannot be approximated.

chemical debridement   Use of topical enzymes applied to a wound to remove necrotic tissue.

collagen   Major component of new connective tissue that gives tensile strength to the wound.

compromised wound   Wound that contains devitalized tissue.

contraction   Wound margins begin to pull toward the center of the wound to decrease the wound surface area.

contusion   Injury to superficial tissues, with disruption of blood vessels with extravasation into the skin.

debridement   Removal of foreign material in wound.

dermis   Middle layer of skin, referred to as true skin.

endogenous   Arising from within the patient.

epidermis   Outermost layer of skin.

epithelialization   Migration of epithelial cells along the wound surface.

eschar   Hard, black, dehydrated tissue.

exogenous   Entering from the external environment.

exudate   Fluid produced by wounds.

granulation tissue   Tissue in wound with a characteristic pink-red color.

laceration   Open wound causing incision or abrupt disruption of tissue.

maceration   Situation in which drainage from the wound has prolonged contact with healthy skin tissue around the wound; periwound skin is white or pale.

mechanical debridement   Use of moist dressings, irrigation, or whirlpool to remove foreign material from a wound.

neovascularization   Formation of new blood vessels in order to reestablish perfusion to the wound bed.

pressure ulcer   Any lesion caused by unrelieved pressure resulting in damage of underlying tissue.

primary intention   Method of wound closure using sutures or tape.

proliferative phase   Phase of wound healing that lasts for several weeks after injury; wound is restored with a functional barrier.

puncture wound   Deep, narrow, open wound resulting from penetrating or sharp objects.

remodeling phase   Final wound repair process; lasts up to 2 years; final product is the scar.

rete ridges   Provide structural support for epidermis.

secondary intention   Method of wound closure in which the wound is allowed to heal gradually, using the biological phases of wound healing to fill in a cavity or defect.

sharp debridement   Removal of necrotic areas in wounds using scissors or a scapel.

slough   Moist, stringy, thick, yellow tissue that is dying.

susceptible host   Patient with some degree of local or systemic impairment of resistance to bacterial invasion.

tertiary intention   Method of wound closure in which a combination of primary and secondary intention is used.

tissue load   Distribution of shear, pressure, and friction on tissue.

ABBREVIATIONS

E. coli	Escherichia coli	**VAC**	Vacuum-assisted closure®
Psi	Pounds per square inch	**WBC**	White blood cell

SECTION ONE: Anatomy and Physiology of the Skin

At the completion of this section, the learner will be able to identify the anatomic structures and physiologic functions of the skin and discuss age-related changes.

The skin is a tough membrane covering the entire body surface. It is the largest organ of the body and is composed of three layers of tissue: the epidermis, the dermis, and the hypodermis or subcutaneous tissue. The **epidermis** is the outermost layer and contains epithelial cells. The middle layer, often referred to as the true skin, is the **dermis.** This layer contains connective tissue and elastic fibers, sensory and motor nerve endings, and a complex network of capillary and lymphatic vessels and muscles. From the dermis arise the appendages of the skin—hair, nails, and sebaceous and sweat glands—which then penetrate the epidermis. The dermis lacks exact boundaries and merges with subcutaneous tissues containing blood vessels, nerves, muscle, and adipose tissue. The anatomy of the skin is depicted in Figure 34–1.

The epidermis contains epithelial tissue that is responsible for regeneration of the skin. This tissue is composed of cells that rapidly reproduce and regenerate through the process of epithelialization.

The various components of the dermis provide elements to protect and combat foreign materials and regenerate itself after exposure to the external environment. Connective tissue and elastic fibers provide strength and pliability to protect the inter-nal environment. Nutrients are delivered to and cellular wastes are removed by the blood and lymphatic vessels. Nerve endings present within the dermis respond to cold, heat, touch, pain, and pressure.

The subcutaneous tissues store caloric energy in adipose tissue and assist in regulating the body temperature by acting as insulation, acting as a cushion against external forces, and providing the body with shape and substance. Table 34–1 provides a summary of the physiologic functions of the skin.

Age-related changes in skin physiology have numerous clinical applications. **Rete ridges,** found at the epidermal–dermal junction, provide structural support for the epidermis. With advancing age, the rete ridges flatten, increasing the likelihood of skin tears. Thermoregulation becomes more difficult because of a decreased number of sweat glands and a decreased

TABLE 34–1 Physiologic Functions of the Skin

Protection
Insulation
Sensation
Excretion
Communication
Preservation of internal fluids
Production of vitamin D
Storage for calories
Provision of shape and substance for the body

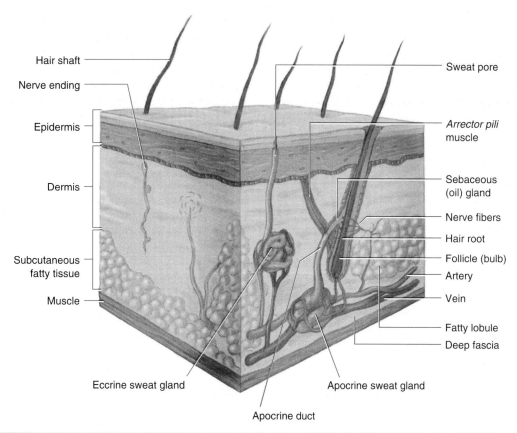

Figure 34–1 ■ Anatomy of the skin. The skin is composed of three layers of tissue: the epidermis, dermis, and hypodermis. *(Reprinted by permission of Prentice Hall.)*

thickness in the dermis and subdermis. The skin's immuno-competency decreases as a result of the declining number of Langerhan's cells, inhibiting the skin's ability to resist infection (Irion, 2002). The stratum corneum, or horny layer, has reduced water content and may inhibit the skin's ability to absorb topical medication (Zatz, 2001).

A **wound** creates an alteration and disruption of the anatomic and physiologic functions of the skin. A wound can be created intentionally, as with a surgeon's knife; by accidental trauma, such as occurs in a motor vehicle crash; or by chronic forces, such as that which occurs with pressure ulcer formation.

Terms used to describe injuries to the skin include **abrasion, avulsion, contusion, laceration,** and **puncture.**

Any wound interrupts normal skin and tissue integrity, thus interrupting the normal physiologic functions of the skin. Healing begins at the moment of injury. The healing process is discussed in Section Two.

In summary, the skin is composed of three layers. The outermost layer is the epidermis, which contains epithelial tissue. This tissue rapidly regenerates when injured through the process of epithelialization. The dermis is the middle layer and contains connective tissue, nerves, blood, and lymphatic vessels. The innermost layer is subcutaneous tissue containing adipose tissue that stores energy, regulates body heat, and acts as a cushion. The skin has several physiologic functions. A wound results in altered structure and function of the skin.

SECTION ONE REVIEW

1. Which of the following is NOT a layer of the skin?
   A. epithelial tissue
   B. epidermis
   C. dermis
   D. subcutaneous tissue

2. The components of the dermis are
   A. epithelial cells, subcutaneous tissue
   B. adipose tissue, subcutaneous tissue
   C. hair, nails, and sebaceous glands
   D. connective tissue, blood, and lymph vessels

3. The physiologic functions of the skin include
   A. secretion, production of vitamin C
   B. excretion, production of vitamin D
   C. storage of information, communication
   D. regulation of body temperature, storage of vitamin A

4. Wound healing begins
   A. within an hour after injury
   B. within 6 hours after injury
   C. at the moment of injury
   D. within 24 hours of injury

Answers: 1. A, 2. D, 3. B, 4. C

SECTION TWO: Wound Physiology

At the completion of this section, the learner will be able to state the three phases of wound healing, describe the events that occur in each phase of wound healing, and define the three methods of wound closure.

A wound disrupts the skin's integrity and its physiologic mechanisms. On injury, the body immediately begins the process of restoring its integrity and the physiologic functions of the skin. A basic understanding of the wound healing process helps to assess, diagnose, plan, and evaluate nursing interventions for the patient with altered skin integrity.

From the moment of injury, overlapping physiologic processes work to restore a functional barrier. Wound healing occurs by two methods: regeneration, when lost tissue is replaced with identical tissues, and connective tissue repair, when lost tissue is replaced by scar formation (Waldrop & Doughty, 2000). The method of repair depends on the layers of tissue involved and their ability to regenerate. Superficial dermal and epidermal wounds heal by regeneration. Wounds extending through the dermis heal by scar formation. There are three phases of wound healing: (1) the inflammatory phase, (2) the proliferative phase, and (3) the remodeling phase.

Inflammatory Phase

The inflammatory phase occurs immediately after injury and lasts several days. This is a critical phase because the wound environment is being prepared for subsequent tissue development. The major events that occur in this phase are hemostasis and removal of cellular debris and infectious agents.

Immediately on injury, vascular and cellular events are initiated. Thromboplastin is released from injured cells activating the clotting cascade. Platelets aggregate at the injury site to form a plug to seal a break in the vessel wall. The platelets also liberate growth factors essential in tissue development during the subsequent phase of healing (platelet-derived growth factor, epidermal growth factor, etc.). A great deal of research currently revolves around the activities of these factors and other cytokines. Once hemostasis is achieved, the blood vessels dilate to bring needed nutrients, chemical, and white blood cells (WBCs) to the injured area. WBCs quickly adhere to the endothelium

and begin to control any bacterial contamination that has gained entry into the wound. Macrophages appear and begin to engulf and remove dead tissue. The chemical and vascular events that occur during the reaction phase of wound healing produce the four cardinal signs of inflammation: heat, redness, swelling, and pain (Fig. 34–2).

Proliferative Phase

The **proliferative phase** begins several days after injury and continues for several weeks. Major processes that occur during this phase are focused on building new tissue to fill the wound space and restore a functional barrier. Major events that occur during this phase include neovascularization, epithelialization, collagen formation, granulation tissue formation, and contraction.

Neovascularization is the formation of new blood vessels in order to reestablish perfusion to the wound bed. The process is driven by growth factors, cytokines, and the hypoxic gradient that exists from the healthy tissue near the wound to the center of the wound (Kirsner & Bogensberger, 2002). Capillary buds arise from venules in close proximity to the wound bed. Capillary formation is then followed by the creation of arterioles, which grow to form a network across the wound and eventually undergo reanastamosis with preexisting vessels (Waldrop & Doughty, 2000).

Epithelialization involves the migration of epithelial cells across a wound's surface. The cells rapidly undergo mitotic divisions and migrate along fibrin strands to reestablish layers of epithelium in an attempt to cover the defect. A moist environment enhances epithelialization. Epithelial cells cannot spread on a surface laden with debris or bacteria. Therefore, the wound healing process will be inhibited by the presence of debris or bacteria. The process of epithelialization serves to provide a barrier against the external environment and further bacterial invasion. The epithelial wound will regenerate in about four days if the wound is kept moist, but if the wound dries out it will take six to seven days to regenerate (Kirsner & Bogensberger, 2002; Waldrop & Doughty, 2000).

The proliferative phase provides strength to the healing wound. The dominant cells of this phase are fibroblasts. Fibroblasts produce **collagen,** the major component of new connective tissue. Fluid collections, hematomas, dead tissue, and foreign materials act as physical barriers to prevent fibroblast

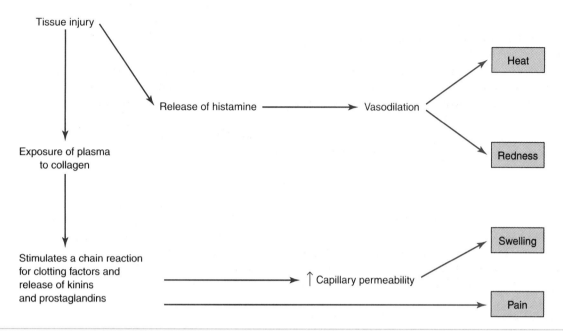

Figure 34–2 ■ Basic inflammatory response produces the four cardinal signs of inflammation. The chemical and vascular events that occur during the reaction phase of wound healing produce the four cardinal signs of inflammation.

penetration. Therefore, removal of these materials is one of the primary goals of wound management (Section Five). The wound space fills with fiber bundles that enlarge and form a dense collagenous structure (the scar) that binds the tissues firmly together.

As the population of fibroblasts decreases, collagen fibers become dominant in the wound. Collagen cross-linking provides tensile strength to the wound. Collagen requires several nutrients and minerals for its synthesis. Thus, the nutritional status of the patient becomes very important during wound healing. This is discussed in greater detail in Section Three.

At the same time that epithelialization is occurring and collagen is forming, the formation of **granulation tissue** continues. The vascular endothelium proliferates, and a great deal of capillary budding appears. These buds give the new granulation tissue its characteristic pink-red color and appearance. As new granulation tissue fills in the wound, the wound margins begin to contract or pull together, and the surface area of the wound decreases.

Contraction of a wound occurs when the wound margins begin to pull toward the center of the wound to decrease the wound surface area. Shrinkage of the wound progresses from the wound's edges to heal open defects.

Remodeling

Usually, by the third week after a disruption in skin integrity, the wound has closed and the remodeling phase begins. **Remodeling** is the final repair process. This phase can last months to years. Major events of this final phase include increased collagen reorganization and increased tensile strength. The final product of all

the events that occur during wound healing is the scar, which has covered the defect and restored the protective barrier against the external environment. Factors affecting the final appearance of the scar include wound tension, body location, and wound closure technique (Brinker et al., 2003).

Methods of Wound Closure

The rate of wound healing differs depending on the method used to close the wound. The method used depends on the amount of tissue damage or loss and the potential for wound infection. Methods of wound closure include primary intention, secondary intention, and tertiary intention (Fig. 34–3).

Primary intention refers to closing the wound by mechanical means. This method is used when there is minimal tissue loss and skin edges are well approximated. Clean lacerations and most surgical incisions are closed using primary intention.

Mechanical means to close wounds include tape, sutures, staples, or glue. Taping with microporous tape (steri-strips) is best used in areas that are not over hairy surfaces or joints (Brinker at al., 2003). However, these tapes cannot be exposed to water and frequently fall off. Benzoin placed on the skin prior to tape application may prevent the tape from falling off. Suturing is the most common technique to close wounds to heal by primary intention. Absorbable sutures are used to close dermal and subcutaneous layers and nonabsorbable sutures are used for external closure (Brinker et al., 2003). Staples allow for rapid closure and are typically used on the extremities, torso, or scalp. Tissue glue (Dermabond) is a glue that can be applied topically along the wound. Best results are achieved in simple lacerations

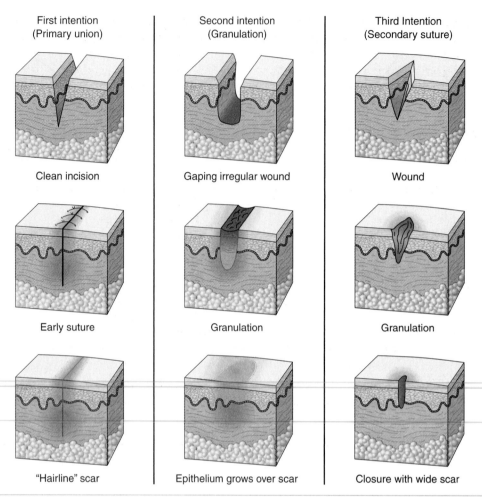

First intention
(Primary union)

Clean incision

Early suture

"Hairline" scar

Second intention
(Granulation)

Gaping irregular wound

Granulation

Epithelium grows over scar

Third Intention
(Secondary suture)

Wound

Granulation

Closure with wide scar

Figure 34–3 ■ Methods of wound closure. *(From Lynn-McHale, D. J., & Carlson, K. K. (Eds.). [2001].* AACN Procedure manual for critical care, *(4th ed., p. 852). Philadelphia: W. B. Saunders. With permission from Elsevier.*

with low skin tension because the tensile strength, at least initially, is only 15 percent that of a suture-repaired wound (Brinker et al., 2003).

Wounds that repair by primary intention progress through the normal phases of wound healing in an efficient fashion. Under normal conditions the incision line is resurfaced and impenetrable to bacterium within 72 hours (West & Gimbel, 2000). The wound lacks structural integrity because the underlying tissue repair requires more time. The proliferative phase may take up to 21 days, depending on the depth of the original wound. A healing ridge develops along the incision line between days 5 and 9 after repair. The healing ridge may be palpated as a firm swelling, or induration, and it extends about a centimeter along each side of the incision line. The healing ridge is considered a positive predictor of healing. If the healing ridge does not develop within the 5 to 9 day period, interventions to reduce mechanical stressors on the wound may be instituted (West & Gimbel, 2000).

Wounds that heal by **secondary intention** usually are large wounds in which there is significant tissue loss, damage, or bacterial contamination. These wound cavities heal gradually and use the biological phases of wound healing to fill in the cavity or

defect. Wounds healing by secondary intention include open abdominal wounds, dehisced sternal wounds, and stages III and IV pressure ulcers. These wounds require significantly more time to heal than do wounds healing by primary intention.

Tertiary intention is a method of wound closure that uses a combination of primary and secondary intention. The wound is left open for a short period of time, usually a few days, to allow edema and exudate to resolve. The wound is packed with dressings that are changed to remove any debris and is closed later by primary intention.

The expected outcome of the wound healing process is restoration of the skin and tissue integrity and its physiologic functions. The wound healing process depends on various factors that affect the efficiency and effectiveness of all events in the process. The next section discusses these factors.

In summary, wound healing is a complex process of events that begins at the moment of injury and continues for years after injury. The inflammatory phase in a clean acute wound lasts about 72 hours. Hemostasis and removal of cellular debris and infectious agents are the goals of this phase. The proliferative phase normally lasts 3 to 21 days. Major events include neovascularization, epithelialization, formation of granulation tissue and collagen, and wound contraction. The final phase of wound healing, the remodeling phase, can last up to 2 years. During the final phase, collagen reorganization and increased tensile strength of the scar occur. The three methods of wound closure are primary, secondary, and tertiary intention. The rate of wound healing differs depending on the method used to close the wound. An understanding of the wound healing process helps to assess, diagnose, plan, and evaluate nursing interventions to facilitate the wound healing process.

SECTION TWO REVIEW

1. Heat, redness, swelling, and pain occur during which of the following phases of wound healing?
   A. remodeling
   B. contraction
   C. proliferative
   D. inflammatory
2. Epithelialization
   A. is enhanced by a moist environment
   B. is enhanced by a dry, sterile environment
   C. occurs to remove debris
   D. spreads on surfaces laden with debris
3. Fluid collections, hematomas, and dead tissue act as
   A. scaffolds for fibroblast proliferation
   B. barriers for fibroblast proliferation
   C. protective covers for new epithelial cells
   D. a moist environment to enhance epithelialization

4. An incision for a cholecystectomy usually would be allowed to heal by
   A. tertiary intention
   B. secondary intention
   C. primary intention
   D. delayed secondary intention
5. Delayed primary (tertiary) intention allows
   A. immediate resolution of the inflammatory phase
   B. edema and exudate to resolve
   C. gradual healing of the wound
   D. reorganization and cell differentiation for remodeling

Answers: 1. D, 2. A, 3. B, 4. C, 5. B

SECTION THREE: Factors That Affect Wound Healing

At the completion of this section, the learner will be able to state physiologic and environmental factors that affect wound healing.

Acutely ill patients experience many risk factors that increase their vulnerability for wound complications. These include impaired oxygenation, compromised nutritional status, age, preexisting disease, medications, and obesity. These risk factors increase the risk of delayed wound healing, development of wound infections, and wound dehiscence. It is a nursing challenge to provide the optimal environment that supports the wound healing process.

Oxygenation/Tissue Perfusion

Many drugs and treatments have been investigated to accelerate healing. However, perfusion of injured tissue with well-oxygenated blood may be most important. Adequate oxygen supply to wounds is required by immune and inflammatory cells to produce proteins, reestablish vascular structure and epithelium, and provide resistance to bacterial invasion of the wound space (Whitney, 2003). Adequate oxygenation promotes neovas-cularization and optimizes collagen deposition, which increases the tensile strength of wound beds (Gordillo & Sen, 2003). Adequate levels of oxygen in wound beds also act as a major determinant of susceptibility to infection (Gordillo & Sen, 2003).

Availability of oxygen to tissue and wound beds depends on vascular supply, vasomotor tone, arterial oxygen tension, and the diffusion distance for molecular oxygen. Edema and necrotic debris increase the diffusion distance for oxygen to reach cells in the wound, which is why debridement is so important to wound healing (Gordillo & Sen, 2003). For optimal wound perfusion and oxygenation, patients must be warm, have adequate intravascular volume, and have adequate control of pain and anxiety.

Many conditions interfere with the delivery of oxygen to the wound (e.g., thrombosis, radiation, obesity, diabetes, cardiovascular disease, cigarette smoking, hypotension, hypothermia, and administration of vasoactive drugs). Adipose tissue has a poor blood supply; therefore, wounds that occur in areas of regional adipose tissue have poor oxygen delivery. Poor glycemic control and diabetic neuropathy place the diabetic patient at increased risk for traumatic injury, particularly to the feet, and subsequent poor healing. Smoking adversely affects wound healing. Toxins of greatest concern include carbon monoxide, nicotine, and hydrogen cyanide (Whiteford, 2003). Nicotine causes vasoconstriction and decreased tissue perfusion.

Carbon monoxide combines with hemoglobin, inhibits the binding with oxygen, and decreases the oxygen-carrying capacity of hemoglobin; all contribute to decreased oxygen delivery to wound beds. Hydrogen cyanide inhibits enzyme reaction necessary for aerobic metabolism and oxygen transport at the cellular level (Whiteford, 2003). Smoking also increases platelet adhesiveness, making them more "sticky," and sets up a situation of microclots in small vessels that decrease oxygen delivery. Significant blood loss, as frequently occurs in traumatically injured patients, results in hypovolemia, hypotension, and decreased tissue perfusion.

Hyperbaric oxygen therapy (HBOT) is gaining recognition as a treatment to improve oxygen delivery to wounds and promote wound healing. It is used in conjunction with standard wound care. HBOT delivers 100 percent oxygen at 2 to 3 atmospheres of pressure. This exposes tissues to greater concentrations of oxygen than would otherwise be possible and essentially "hypersaturates" the bloodstream with oxygen (Heyneman & Lawless-Liday, 2002). HBOT can increase arterial oxygen tension to 1,200 mm Hg (Gordillo & Sen, 2003). Patients typically require 10 to 30 treatments that last 60 to 120 minutes each and are performed in specialized chambers at facilities with a hyperbaric oxygen chamber (Gordillo & Sen, 2003). HBOT is useful for resolution of hypoxic conditions, such as gas gangrene, necrotizing fasciitis, traumatic crush injuries, and carbon monoxide poisoning (Heyneman & Lawless-Liday, 2002). The American Diabetes Association recommends HBOT as adjunctive therapy for severe and limb or life-threatening wounds unresponsive to other treatments, particularly if ischemia is present that cannot be corrected by vascular surgery (Cianci, 2000).

Evidence-Based Practice

- *In people with diabetic foot ulcer HBOT decreases the risk of major amputation and may improve long-term healing (Kranke et al., 2004).*

- *Supplemental postoperative activity (arm/leg exercises and walking protocol) does not improve oxygen delivery to wounds (Whitney & Parkman, 2004).*

- *Keeping patients normothermic and administering supplemental oxygen enhances wound oxygenation and decreases the rate of infection in surgical patients (Grief et al., 2000).*

- *Patients having cardiovascular surgery have low wound oxygen tensions secondary to decreased fluid supplementation, use of diuretics, and decreased core body temperature that produces peripheral vasoconstriction (Heiner et al., 2002).*

Nutrition

Adequate nutrition is a critical factor predisposing the acutely ill patient to immunocompetence and poor wound healing. It is essential to ensure that patients with wounds receive adequate nutritional support.

Metabolic processes involved in wound healing rely heavily on adequate nutritional substances. Physiologic and psychological stress, traumatic injury, and fever further increase the basal metabolic rate, demanding adequate nutritional reserves. Because of these demands, malnutrition in the acutely ill patient is common. During the wound healing process, the main components of energy requirements emanate from collagen synthesis. Large, complicated wounds or thermal injuries require a significant amount of energy to heal the wound (Williams & Barbul, 2003). A sufficient amount of protein is one of the most important nutritional substances for wound healing. Protein is required for collagen synthesis, immune responses, formation of granulation tissue, and fibroblast proliferation. Draining wounds lose vital nutrients and protein. Every reasonable effort is made to quantify the loss so that correctional measures are instituted. Frequently, amino acid supplementation is prescribed to enhance the functioning of growth factors and immune cells, and to support the collagen deposition (Himes, 2003). Serum albumin levels reflect the level of visceral protein stores. Because the half-life of albumin is 18 to 21 days, a prealbumin is ordered in a high-acuity setting. The half-life of prealbumin is only 1 to 2 days. This allows for a more accurate prescription of protein replacement (Williams & Barbul, 2003). Glycolysis contributes the majority of the energy needed for restoring tissue integrity and fighting infection. Fats serve as building blocks for prostaglandins, which regulate cell metabolism, inflammation, and circulation. Vitamins and trace elements are necessary for numerous events in the tissue healing and rebuilding process.

Age

Aging affects almost every stage of wound healing and the wound healing process is markedly slower as patients age. In addition to the physiologic effects of aging, the elderly are more likely to have nutritional deficiencies and pulmonary or cardiovascular diseases that further diminish local oxygenation to wounds and immunologic resistance.

Diabetes

Wound healing in the patient with diabetes is compromised as a result of macrovascular and microvascular changes, poor glycemic control, and loss of sensation. These disease-associated changes result in impaired oxygenation and perfusion, slowed epithelialization and wound contraction, and impaired phagocytosis. Glucose levels have direct effects on several phases of wound healing, and the importance of glycemic control cannot be overstated. The nurse caring for the acutely ill diabetic patient with a wound can achieve a significant, positive impact on wound healing through scrupulous glucose monitoring and maximizing glycemic control (Waldrop & Doughty, 2000; Williams & Barbul, 2003).

Medications

Steroid therapy, used to block the inflammatory component of many diseases, has a well-known inhibitory effect on wound healing. Decreased protein synthesis, delayed development of granulation tissue, inhibition of fibroblast proliferation, and reduced epithelialization are effects of steroid administration. In addition, inhibition of the inflammatory response and the immunosuppressive actions of steroids make the patient more susceptible to developing a wound infection. Administration of vitamin A can counteract the effects of corticosteroid administration. Topical administration of vitamin A may be a safer route because there is less chance of reversing the therapeutic effects of the corticosteroids (Waldrop & Doughty, 2000). Nonsteroidal anti-inflammatory medications may have significant deleterious effects on soft tissue wound healing, which assumes greater significance to the acutely ill patient (Williams & Harding, 2003). Other medications that interfere with wound healing include chemotherapeutic agents, immunosuppressive drugs, and anticoagulants.

Obesity

The obese patient (weight greater than 20 percent ideal body weight) experiences an increased incidence of dehiscence, herniation, and infection. Adipose tissue is poorly vascularized, which increases the risk of ischemia. Adipose tissue is difficult to suture, which makes the obese patient at risk to develop a wound dehiscence. A binder or splint (pillow) to the incision provides support during straining or coughing and takes excess tension off the incision.

Blood Chemistries

Normal serum electrolytes enhance wound repair. Potassium is necessary for building proteins for wound repair. Phagocytosis is inhibited by elevated sodium and glucose levels. Oxygen is released more rapidly from oxyhemoglobin in slightly acidic environments. Wounds may heal more effectively in this type of local environment.

Moisture

The rate of epithelialization is enhanced in a moist, not dry, local wound environment. A wound bed is kept moist through the use of appropriate dressings. Ideally, the dressing will keep the wound surface moist without accumulation of excessive fluids that macerate the skin and allow bacterial proliferation.

Antibiotics and Infection

Traumatic wounds tend to be contaminated by the external environment. The administration of antibiotics greatly affects the outcome of healing. These two factors are so important to wound healing that they are discussed in greater detail in Section Four.

In summary, there are no medications or treatments to accelerate wound healing; there are conditions and factors known to affect the wound healing process. Perfusion of well-oxygenated blood to the wound is considered the most important factor affecting wound healing. It is important for the nurse to assess patients for any factor that may alter wound healing. Appropriate plans and nursing interventions must be instituted to manipulate as many variables as possible to promote efficient and effective wound healing.

SECTION THREE REVIEW

1. Small-vessel changes occur that impair tissue perfusion/oxygenation with
   A. malnutrition
   B. elevated sodium levels
   C. diabetes
   D. steroid therapy
2. The most important nutritional substance for wound healing is
   A. glucose
   B. fat
   C. vitamins
   D. protein
3. Which of the following is NOT an effect of steroid therapy on wound healing?
   A. decreased protein synthesis
   B. proliferation of fibroblasts
   C. delayed development of granulation tissue
   D. reduced epithelialization
4. The most important factor that affects wound healing is
   A. preventing infection
   B. total parenteral nutrition
   C. perfusion of injured tissues with well-oxygenated blood
   D. potassium replacements
5. A moist wound environment
   A. enhances epithelialization
   B. macerates the skin
   C. promotes bacterial proliferation
   D. impedes epithelialization

Answers: 1. C, 2. D, 3. B, 4. C, 5. A

SECTION FOUR: Etiology, Diagnosis, and Prevention of Wound Infections

At the completion of this section, the learner will be able to identify conditions that predispose a patient to developing a wound infection, identify criteria used to diagnose a wound infection, and state interventions that can be used to prevent and treat wound infections.

Infection is a common deterrent to effective wound healing. A disruption or compromise in skin integrity can increase the risk of a wound becoming infected. The skin normally has many microorganisms on its surface. These normal skin microorganisms can enter a wound bed, proliferate, and colonize a wound within 72 hours (Sjöberg et al., 2003). A wound is considered to be infected when it contains 1×10^5 microorganisms per gram (Conner-Kerr & Sullivan, 2003). A wound infection occurs when microorganisms overcome host defenses and invade healthy tissue. Cardinal signs of a wound infection include purulent drainage, erythema, induration, warmth, edema, increased pain, and sometimes fever (Conner-Kerr & Sullivan, 2003). Three elements predispose the patient to developing a wound infection: (1) a susceptible host, (2) a compromised wound, and (3) an infectious organism.

Susceptible Host

One of the major determinants of a subsequent infection after surgery or trauma is the patient's own ability to use defense mechanisms to resist the threat of infection. The patient who is a **susceptible host** has some degree of local or systemic impairment of resistance to bacterial invasion. Local impairment may be the result of dead, foreign material or hematomas directly in the wound or some interference in blood supply to the area as a result of vascular disease. Systemic impairment of the patient's resistance may include diabetes, acute or chronic use of steroids, renal disease, malnutrition, cardiovascular disease, extremes of age, obesity, cancer, or the use of immunosuppressive therapies. These patients usually have some impairment in the acute inflammatory response or phagocytic mechanisms. Any patient with altered skin integrity has lost the major mechanical barrier blocking invasion by pathologic organisms and, thus, is a susceptible host.

Compromised Wound

A **compromised wound** is one that contains devitalized tissue. Devitalized tissue is tissue that has been separated from the circulation and the body's antimicrobial defenses. Bacteria proliferate on wounds that contain dead tissue, hematomas, or foreign material. Debridement of these materials is essential to prevent an environment conducive to bacterial growth.

Infectious Organism

Many different organisms are capable of initiating a wound infection. Organisms come from endogenous or exogenous sources. **Endogenous** sources arise from within the patient. Many organisms exist on and in the human body—on the skin, in the respiratory tract, and in the gastrointestinal and genitourinary tracts. Organisms in these areas are not pathogenic until they are released from their normal inhabitant sites and allowed to proliferate in a sterile area of the body. **Exogenous** organisms enter the body from the external environment when the skin barrier has been broken. The external environment may be the accident scene (for trauma patients) or the health care setting.

Infection

A differentiation in wound bacterial colonization and infection is necessary. Colonization of wounds refers to a large number of organisms loosely attached to the wound surface, but there is no movement of bacteria into viable tissue and no host immune response. Infection is defined as the process by which organisms bind to tissue, multiply, invade viable tissue, and elicit a host immune response. Wound infection alters all three phases of wound healing.

Diagnosis of Wound Infections

Wound infections range from superficial cases of cellulitis to deep-seated abscesses. The cardinal signs of inflammation are present in a wound infection (redness, warmth, pain, and edema). The nurse may note a change in the drainage from serosanguinous in consistency to purulent and often malodorous. Wounds that have signs of inflammation that last longer than 5 days may be infected (Stotts, 2000). Fever and elevated WBCs indicate a more invasive infection. Wound cultures are often misleading because it is very difficult to avoid contamination from surface microorganisms. Culture and sensitivity reports take at least 72 hours. The results guide the appropriate administration of systemic antibiotics.

Bacteria contaminating wounds must be sensitive to the antibiotic administered. However, as previously stated, it may take up to 3 days to obtain bacterial information. Thus, a knowledge of the likely wound contaminants and their established sensitivities is helpful in instituting prompt treatment. For example, organisms in the colon that have leaked into the peritoneum and are likely to cause infections in wounds in the abdomen are anaerobic organisms (*Bacteroides, Clostridium, Escherichia coli*), which respond to aminoglycosides.

Wound infections may not be apparent for several days postoperatively or after traumatic injury. When a wound infection is suspected, prompt and appropriate treatment is instituted.

Prevention of Wound Infections

One of the greatest priorities in wound care is prevention of infection. Prevention of wound infections begins with recognition of the three elements that predispose the patient to a wound infection (susceptible host, compromised wound, and infectious organism).

For elective surgical procedures, prevention begins preoperatively through skin preparation, mechanical and antibiotic bowel preparations, prophylactic administration of antibiotics, and sterile operative site draping. Intraoperatively, careful surgical technique minimizes injury, and aseptic technique prevents endogenous and exogenous sources of bacterial contamination.

For patients with traumatically injured wounds, resuscitation and lifesaving measures often take priority over immediate treatment of wounds. Once the resuscitative phase is completed, prompt and proper management of the wounds decreases the likelihood of subsequent infection. It is not uncommon for traumatically incurred wounds to be contaminated with dirt, grass, glass, twigs, leaves, stool, schrapnel, or bullet or knife fragments. Management of these wounds begins with cleansing of the wounds using high-pressure irrigation and debridement to remove bacteria and foreign debris.

The importance of hand washing to prevent the transmission of infectious organisms was determined more than a century ago. Hand washing is still considered one of the most important methods of preventing wound infections. This is especially important in high-acuity settings where susceptible hosts, compromised wounds, and infectious organisms are in close proximity to each other.

In summary, it is imperative that the nurse recognize the importance of preventing wound infections and preventing further bacterial proliferation in already infected wounds. Nursing plans and interventions optimize the environment to promote wound healing. Each patient is assessed as a susceptible host for pathogenic organisms, and interventions must be instituted to promote and safeguard the patient's ability to resist infection. Astute nursing assessments identify a compromised wound. Measures are taken to prevent the wound from becoming an ideal environment for bacterial invasion and proliferation. Plans for prophylactic interventions to reduce the infective risk are made. Ongoing nursing assessments detect signs of infection so that prompt and appropriate treatment can be instituted.

SECTION FOUR REVIEW

1. Which of the following would NOT predispose the development of a wound infection?
   A. susceptible host
   B. exogenous organisms
   C. compromised wound
   D. infectious organism
2. Local impairment of resistance to bacterial invasion may be the result of
   A. foreign material
   B. malnutrition
   C. cancer
   D. immunosuppressive drugs

3. Organisms from endogenous sources may come from
   A. debris in the wound
   B. the accident scene
   C. the gastrointestinal tract
   D. the hospital setting
4. Which of the following conditions is NOT a criteria for the diagnosis of a wound infection?
   A. purulent drainage from a wound
   B. culture and sensitivity testing
   C. the four cardinal signs of inflammation
   D. elevated temperature

Answers: 1. B, 2. A, 3. C, 4. B

SECTION FIVE: Principles of Wound Management

The purpose of this section is to assist the learner in understanding treatment modalities and principles of wound management. At the completion of this section, the learner will be able to discuss the rationale for wound cleansing, wound debridement, and dressing changes. Additionally the learner will be able to identify tube and drain placement and their indications for use in wound management.

Nursing has a major influence on the outcome of wound healing. Nurses have the opportunity to favorably manipulate certain environmental factors that promote wound healing. This includes local wound care, which includes cleansing, debridement, and selection of appropriate wound dressing materials.

Wound Cleansing

Wound cleansing involves the use of nontoxic fluids to remove debris, microorganisms, contaminants, exudate, and devitalized tissue, usually by flushing the surface of the wound with an irrigating solution. This is a form of debridement that breaks the bond between wound contaminants and healthy tissue

(Barr, 2003). The size and condition of the wound determines the method of wound cleansing. A large wound with a significant amount of necrosis requires high-pressure (8 to 15 pounds per square inch [psi]) irrigation, using enough solution to adequately remove the debris. Several devices can be used to accomplish a high-pressure irrigation, and there are numerous commercially available irrigation kits. Conversely, a 30 mL syringe used with a 19-gauge angiocath delivers about 8 psi to the wound. The fluid should be warmed to body temperature because cool fluid inhibits phagocytic and cellular growth in the wound (Fernandez et al., 2003). The goal of cleansing proliferative, granulating wounds is to remove inorganic debris from the wound using a gentle flushing technique. Wounds are not scrubbed because this can cause trauma to healthy tissue. The use of pressures higher than 15 psi actually forces bacteria deeper into the tissue (Ovington, 2001). Whirlpool, as a method of wound cleansing, has significant limitations, including infection control, patient comfort, and the number of staff needed to perform the procedure. Pulsatile lavage with suction effectively irrigates the wound and removes fluid and debris with suction (Loehne, 2002).

Sterile normal saline is the solution of choice. In addition to using it as an irrigant, saline can be soaked in gauze and gently swiped around the wound, working from the least contaminated to the most contaminated portion of the wound. Tap water is a safe and effective alternative to sterile saline as a cleansing solution for chronic wounds without increased incidence of infection. Skin disinfectants (povidine–iodine, hydrogen peroxide, acetic acid, etc.) are not used because of toxicity to cells and potential systemic absorption of these chemicals. In particular, iodine absorbs through tissues and elevates serum levels. Diluted solutions of acetic acid and sodium hypochloride may be used. However, the concentrations needed to eliminate bacteria are often toxic to granulating cells (Lionelli & Lawrence, 2003; Loehne, 2002).

Debridement

Debridement is important to healing because the presence of foreign material fosters bacterial growth and inhibits formation of granulation tissue. Wound healing cannot take place until nonviable tissue is removed. Various methods of debridement exist: sharp, mechanical, chemical, and autolytic. **Sharp debridement** is the removal of necrotic areas using a scapel or scissors. This is usually done following a physician's order. **Mechanical debridement** is accomplished with moist dressing changes, irrigation, or whirlpool. **Chemical debridement** involves the use of topical enzymes that are applied to necrotic areas. **Autolytic debridement** involves the use of dressing materials (hydrocolloid wafer, Carrington gel gauze, etc.). When they are applied, these dressings allow endogenous enzymes in the wound to selectively liquefy necrotic tissue. Clinicians select a debridement method most appropriate for the type of

wound, the amount of necrotic tissue, the condition of the patient, the setting, and the clinician and the caregiver's experience.

Dressings

Dressings are placed over wounds for multiple purposes, including debridement; protection from the external environment; provision of a physiological environment conducive to wound healing; and to provide immobilization, support, comfort, information regarding quality and quantity of drainage, pressure, and absorption. The goal of using dressings in wound management is to provide a moist environment at the wound surface to optimize wound healing, prevent infection, control wound drainage, and minimize scarring.

The purpose of the dressing and condition of the wound bed determine the type of dressing used. As a wound changes, the dressing care is modified. It is essential that the nurse continues to assess the patient's wound throughout the wound healing process to evaluate the effectiveness of the wound management plan.

Specific types of dressings and their care are summarized in Table 34–2. Wounds healing by primary intention require dressings that absorb exudate and protect the wound from trauma and contamination. Dry, sterile gauze dressings remain the gold standard for wounds healing by primary intention. The length of time a dressing is required for wounds healing by primary intention varies greatly (usually less than 3 days).

Wounds healing by secondary or tertiary intention require dressing materials that provide a warm, moist, local wound environment conducive to wound healing; debride necrotic tissue; absorb exudate; and protect the wound from further trauma and contamination. As noted in Table 34–2, a variety of dressings can be used, including alginates, hydrocolloids, and traditional moist gauze dressings. Solutions frequently used when dressing wounds are listed in Table 34–3.

Vacuum-assisted closure® (VAC) (Kinetic Concepts Inc., San Antonio, Texas) can be used as a wound management system. The system uses polyurethane foam that is placed into the wound, then the dressing and the suction tubing is sealed to the skin with transparent film dressing and connected to a canister that collects the wound exudate. The VAC provides subatmospheric pressure to the wound bed (-125 mm Hg). In some wounds the pressures may be lower, such as in split-thickness skin grafts (Lionelli & Lawrence, 2003). Once the amount of drainage has decreased, the VAC therapy may be changed to intermittent suction, which further improves granulation rates (Copson, 2003). The VAC improves local wound perfusion by decreasing edema and bacterial contamination and improves neovascularization, granulation, and wound contraction (Baharestani, 2003). The VAC allows for accurate measurement of wound drainage and decreases the time spent doing dressing changes. The system is changed every couple of days.

TABLE 34–2 Wound Dressings

TYPE	INDICATIONS	CONSIDERATIONS
Wet-to-dry gauze: Apply wet; remove dry	Use with wounds healing by secondary intention Removes debris and necrotic materials from wounds; use as a debriding alternative for yellow wounds	No solution should be visibly dripping from the dressing as it is placed into the wound; this retards wound closure, increases bacteria, and macerates periwound skin Gauze touching wound surfaces should be a single layer Wounds with large amounts of exudate should be dressed using gauze with large interstices; as exudate decreases, gauze with small interstices should be used
Wet-to-damp gauze: Apply moist; remove moist	Use with wounds healing by secondary intention Use for mechanical debridement of red or yellow wounds Provides moist wound environment	As above Packing material is soaked in a solution, wrung out until moist, and packed into the wound If packing sticks to tissue as it is removed, remoisten it with normal saline before removing it; this will preserve regenerating tissue Continuous moist dressings can be used for protection of red wounds, for delivery of topical medications, or for autolytic debridement of yellow or black wounds May macerate periwound skin if drainage or moisture is allowed to remain in contact
Dry dressings: Apply dry; remove dry	Use with wounds healing by primary intention Protects the wound during epithelialization Can be used with heavily exudating red wounds	Carefully remove dressing to avoid reopening of incision
Polyurethane films	Cutaneous wounds Minor burns Abrasions Donor sites Protects partial-thickness red wounds Protects granulation and epithelial tissue Occlusive Autolytic debridement of small, noninfected yellow wounds	Do not use with draining or infected wounds Change only if dressing leaks
Hydrocolloid	Use on moderate to heavily exudating wounds; normally used as a wound filler; most require secondary dressing	Gel-like substance becomes puslike in appearance and may even become odiferous; this should not become confused with the development of a wound infection Is water resistant and can adhere to uneven surfaces Do not use on documented or suspected infected wounds Change when leakage or dislodgment becomes apparent
Alginates	Highly absorbant secondary cover for wounds with packing	Alginates absorb secretions to form a gel that provides humidity and temperature conducive to wound healing Use gentle irrigation with normal saline to remove the dressing
Foams	Use for moderate to heavily exuding wounds Pressure ulcers Skin tears and abrasions Skin graft donor sites	Some forms have adherent border, provide thermal insulation, and absorb light to heavy amounts of exudates Effective for wounds with dry eschar May not be used around tubes

Tubes and Drains

Various surgical tubes and drains are used whenever there is an actual or potential accumulation of fluid in naturally occurring or surgically created spaces. Drainage tubes are classified into one of three categories: simple drains, closed-suction drains, or sump drains. The categories and uses of drainage tubes are summarized in Table 34–4. It is the nurse's responsibility to maintain the security, integrity, and patency of all tubes and drains.

TABLE 34–3   Solutions for Dressings

Normal saline	Most commonly used solution
	Aids in mechanical debridement
	Does not damage granulation tissue
0.5 percent acetic acid	Used to treat *Pseudomonas* infections
	Toxic to fibroblasts
0.25 percent Dakin's solution	Chlorine bleach compound; use in a weak solution
	Antiseptic that slightly dissolves necrotic tissue
	Can be used in dirty, malodorous wounds
	Can inhibit growth of granulation tissue
Antibiotic solutions	Antibiotics in a solution that are applied topically
	Commonly used solutions include neomycin or bacitracin

In summary, nursing has a major influence on the outcome of wound healing through assessing the effectiveness of the wound management regimen. A wound management regimen may include wound cleansing, debridement, dressing changes, and placement of tubes and drains. Dressings are used in wound management for a multitude of purposes. The method of wound closure plays a large role in determining the type of dressing to be used in the regimen. Consideration must be made as to the solution to be used to irrigate, debride, or dress the wound. Various tubes and drains are used in wound management whenever there is an actual or potential accumulation of fluid.

TABLE 34–4   Categories and Uses of Drainage Tubes

CATEGORY	PURPOSE	EXAMPLES
Simple drains	Provide pathway to allow fluid to drain by gravity	Penrose, T-tube, gastrostomy tube, jejunostomy tube
Closed-suction drains	Collapsible device attached to tube creates a negative pressure, allowing for continual removal of fluids	Jackson Pratt, Hemovac, Davol
Sump drains	Double-lumen drains; air enters drainage area and breaks the vacuum, displacing air and fluid into the outflow lumen; used in conjunction with wall suction	Salem Sump, Shirley sump, Axion

SECTION FIVE REVIEW

1. What size syringe would you select to irrigate a wound?
   A. 30-mL
   B. 50-mL
   C. 60-mL
   D. 100-mL
2. What type of dressing would be indicated to cover a wound healing by primary intention?
   A. dry
   B. wet-to-wet
   C. wet-to-dry
   D. polyurethane
3. The layer next to the wound in wet-to-dry dressings
   A. should adhere to the wound to prevent disruption of epithelial layers
   B. provides protection and strength in immobilizing the wound
   C. debrides the wound
   D. should be put on wet so the wound remains soupy

4. A solution used to treat *Pseudomonas* wound infections is
   A. Dakin's solution
   B. acetic acid
   C. Betadine (povidone–iodine)
   D. half-strength hydrogen peroxide
5. An example of a closed-suction drain would be a
   A. gastrostomy tube
   B. Salem sump
   C. Penrose
   D. Hemovac

Answers: 1. A, 2. A, 3. C, 4. B, 5. D

SECTION SIX: Clinical Assessment of Wound Healing

At the completion of this section, the learner will be able to identify the common clinical assessments to evaluate wound healing.

In assessing wound healing, it is important to assess the patient's preexisting health problems; perform a physical assessment of the wound using inspection and palpation; and collect and evaluate objective data to assess the patient's tissue perfusion/oxygenation, immunologic, and nutritional status. Systematic assessment and comprehensive evaluation of both patient and wound provide a consistent method for assessing wound healing.

Preexisting Health Problems

In collecting the initial nursing database, it is important to assess the patient for diseases, conditions, and medications or treatments that may impair the healing process. This will assist in identifying patients at risk for delayed wound healing. It is important to assess for conditions that alter tissue perfusion/oxygenation and impair the body's resistance to infection.

Inspection

Wounds, suture lines, casts, pins, and surrounding skin integrity are inspected for signs of infection, breakdown, and irritation. Inspect wounds to assess and evaluate the healing process and the effectiveness of wound care. Inspection includes at least the following components.

Measurement of the Wound

Measure and record the length, width, and depth of the wound. A diagram is made for ongoing comparison of the healing process. The amount and depth of tissue loss and tunneling is assessed because this greatly influences the choice of treatment for wound management. Depth can be determined by inserting a sterile, cotton-tipped applicator into the deepest part of the wound and grasping the applicator where it meets the wound's edge. Irregular wound beds are difficult to measure accurately, so it is important to take measurements of depth and length from the same point each time. The same method of measurement is used each time, as well as a consistent approach to documentation of such information.

Presence of Exudate or Drainage

Estimating the amount of blood and fluid loss allows for appropriate fluid and electrolyte replacement. The fluid produced by wounds is called **exudate;** it can consist of blood, serum, serosanguineous fluid, and leukocytes. Exudate bathes the wound continuously, keeping it moist, supplying nutrients, and providing the best conditions for migration and mitosis of epithelial cells and control of bacteria at the wound surface. Documentation of all wound drainage includes color, amount, consistency, and odor. The amount of drainage is estimated as "mild," "moderate," or "heavy," and the presence or absence of odor is documented. In some cases, wound drainage can be measured more accurately if a wound manager is used or if a VAC device is used with a canister to collect the drainage.

Appearance of Wound Tissue

Wound color depends on the balance between granulation and necrotic tissue. Healing wounds are pink or red, characteristic of granulation tissue. In the presence of moisture and bacteria, exudate and devitalized tissue are yellow or cream-colored and puslike in consistency. This is **slough tissue.** Black or dark-brown color indicates the presence of **eschar,** which is thick, nonpliable necrotic tissue. Slough and necrotic tissue have a negative effect on wound healing because they prevent granulation and epithelialization. The ideal local wound environment should be free from slough and eschar and be moist with red-pink budding granulation tissue.

Inspection of Wound Edges

Inspect the wound for contraction (gradual healing from the edges to the center of the wound), and assess for gradual healing from the interior to the surfaces of deep wounds. Wound margins should not be erythematous or tender; nor should the wound margins have evidence of **maceration.** Maceration is evident when the periwound skin is white or pale. This occurs when drainage from the wound has prolonged contact with healthy skin tissue around the wound. If not stopped, macerated skin leads to altered skin integrity and further wound compromise. The periwound skin integrity can also be altered by frequent tape removal. Impaired periwound skin integrity compromises and complicates wound healing and contracture. Simple measures to protect the periwound area include the use of skin barriers before application of tape or other adhesives or the use of other protectant agents (petroleum jelly) prior to covering the wound.

Skin Color

Using a bright light, observe the surrounding tissues for color. Compare the color with similar, uninjured areas. Distinguish erythema from ecchymosis by blanching the area. Areas of erythema will blanch, but areas of ecchymosis will not.

Palpation

Palpation of the wound and surrounding areas assists in recognizing changes in size, consistency, moisture, and texture. If bone is visible or palpable, it is highly probable that osteomyelitis exists and needs to be reported to the physician. To assess circulation into and from the wound, assess the proximal and distal pulses by palpation or by doppler. Proximal pulses demonstrate adequate circulation to the area. Distal pulses indicate that the wound is not interfering with distal circulation. Capillary refill time is assessed. Compare the skin temperature bilaterally. Sensorimotor assessment distal to the wound is done by testing for discrimination between sharp and dull pressures.

Assessment of Tissue Perfusion/ Oxygenation Status

Adequate tissue perfusion/oxygenation is the most important factor to assess for in wound healing. Local and systemic factors that alter tissue perfusion and oxygenation are assessed. Necrotic areas, debris, and foreign materials in the wound do not allow adequate local tissue perfusion/oxygenation. Adequate systemic tissue perfusion/oxygenation depends on a full blood volume, adequate arterial oxygen content, and an adequate cardiac output. Tissue perfusion/oxygenation is assessed using invasive and noninvasive techniques. Noninvasive techniques include transcutaneous oximetry, assessment of capillary refill, skin temperature, and the presence of proximal and distal pulses around the wound. Invasive techniques include hemodynamic readings, such as right atrial pressure, cardiac output/cardiac index, arterial blood pressure, mean arterial pressure, pulmonary artery wedge pressure, and systemic vascular resistance. In addition, serum blood tests, including hematocrit and hemoglobin levels, are monitored and assessed.

Assessment of Immunologic Status

An intact immunologic response to injury, regardless of the cause of injury, is a key factor in proper wound healing. The patient is assessed for the three elements that predispose the patient to a wound infection: susceptible host, compromised wound, and infectious organism. Factors that cause local and systemic resistance of infection (Section Four) are assessed. Compromised wounds containing devitalized tissue, hematomas, and debris are debrided to prevent an environment conducive to bacterial proliferation. The patient is assessed for sources of pathogenic organisms.

Assessment of immunologic status includes WBC, fibrinogen, body temperature, wound cultures, and serum antimicrobial levels. The inflammatory phase of wound healing releases WBCs. It is not uncommon for patients with wounds to have elevated WBC counts during the initial phase of wound healing. Elevated WBCs in later phases of wound healing are more indicative of an infectious process.

Neutrophils are the primary cells involved in phagocytosis. Elevated neutrophil counts are indicative of an acute infection as mature and immature neutrophils are released in response to an increased need for phagocytosis. Neutrophils are essential in the presence of infection if wound healing is to occur. Adequate amounts of fibrinogen are needed to convert to fibrin. This aids in localizing the infectious process by providing a matrix for phagocytosis.

Increased body temperature is triggered by microorganisms, bacterial toxins and antigens, and the inflammatory process. Because fever is a manifestation of the inflammatory process and the infectious process, it is important to assess the patient's overall clinical picture for etiologic factors of the fever. Patients in a hypothermic state experience decreased tissue perfusion/oxygenation and decreased leukocyte activity.

Monitoring concentrations of antimicrobial agents in the blood confirms therapeutic drug levels and determines toxicity. The best assessment of this can be made by drawing serum peak and trough samples, depending on the antimicrobial administered. The nurse must be aware of these protocols so that accurate therapeutic concentrations and toxicity can be assessed.

Assessment of Nutritional Status

The metabolic processes involved in wound healing rely on an adequate nutritional supply. Malnutrition affects the patient's ability to defend against pathogenic microorganisms. A complete and thorough nutritional assessment for all patients with altered skin and tissue integrity is made. Nutritional assessment is discussed in detail in Module 23.

In summary, when assessing wound healing, it is important to assess the patient's preexisting health problems, oxygenation/perfusion, immunologic and nutrition status, and to perform a physical assessment of the wound.

SECTION SIX REVIEW

1. In assessing wound healing, it is important to assess the patient's
   A. past medical history
   B. renal status
   C. mental status
   D. fluid and electrolyte balance

2. Which of the following is not a part of a physical examination of wounds?
   A. inspection
   B. palpation
   C. auscultation
   D. documentation

3. A noninvasive technique to assess tissue perfusion would be
  A. mean arterial pressure
  B. presence of proximal/distal pulses
  C. systemic vascular resistance
  D. hemoglobin levels

4. If a wound is suspected as being infected
  A. the WBC and core temperature will be high
  B. there will be exudate in the wound
  C. antimicrobial levels should be drawn
  D. wound cultures should be taken

Answers: 1. A, 2. C, 3. B, 4. D

SECTION SEVEN: Pressure Ulcers: Prediction and Prevention

At the completion of this section, the learner will be able to identify patients at risk for pressure ulcer development and to state interventions for the prevention of pressure ulcers.

Staging of Pressure Ulcers

The Panel for the Prediction and Prevention of Pressure Ulcers in Adults (1992) defined **pressure ulcer** as any lesion caused by unrelieved pressure resulting in damage of underlying tissue. Pressure ulcers most frequently occur over bony prominences and are staged to classify the degree of tissue damage observed. The staging of pressure ulcers as defined by the Panel for the Prediction and Prevention of Pressure Ulcers in Adults (1992) is summarized in Table 34–5. Three important assessment limitations must be considered during the staging of pressure ulcers:

1. For patients with darkly pigmented skin, identification of stage I pressure ulcers may be difficult.
2. When eschar is present in a pressure ulcer, staging is not possible. Accurate staging cannot be made until the eschar has sloughed or the wound has been debrided.
3. It may be difficult to assess patients with orthopedic devices (casts) or support hose. Nursing assessments may fail to de-

tect pressure ulcers. For patients with these devices, assess the skin under the edges of casts, determine whether casts should be altered to relieve pressure, remove support stockings to assess skin conditions, and be alert to patient complaints of pressure-induced pain.

Risk Assessment Tools and Risk Factors

High acuity ill patients are at high risk for developing a pressure ulcer because they have decreased activity and are immobile as a result of surgical and diagnostic procedures, the need to maintain various catheters and the critical nature of their illness. These risk factors are compounded by altered sensation because of neurologic dysfunction or administration of drugs (sedatives, neuromuscular blocking agents, etc.).

Patients are assessed for factors that increase the risk for developing pressure ulcers. These factors include immobility, incontinence, nutritional factors (inadequate dietary intake or impaired nutritional status), and altered level of consciousness. Patient risk factors are assessed using a validated risk assessment tool, such as the Braden Scale (Braden, 1989) or the Norton Scale (Norton, 1989). The Braden Scale is widely used throughout North America (Bergstrom & Braden, 2002). The Braden Scale is a summated rating scale comprised of six subscales (sensory perception, mobility, activity, moisture, nutrition, and friction and shear). Each subscale is scored from 1 to 4 (except friction, which is scored from 1 to 3), with total possible points ranging from 6 to 23.

Because of multiple disease processes and the instability of patients in the high-acuity setting, pressure ulcer risk assessment should be done on a daily basis (Arnold, 2003). These risk predictor tools improve the ability to predict which patients will develop pressure ulcers so that preventive measures can be promptly instituted.

TABLE 34–5 Staging of Pressure Ulcers

Stage I	Area of persistent redness in lightly pigmented skin; area of persistent red, blue, or purple in darker skin tones.
Stage II	Partial-thickness skin loss involving epidermis and/or dermis. The ulcer is superficial and presents clinically as an abrasion, blister, or shallow crater.
Stage III	Full-thickness skin loss involving damage or necrosis of subcutaneous tissue that may extend down to, but not through, underlying fascia. The ulcer presents clinically as a deep crater with or without undermining of adjacent tissue.
Stage IV	Full-thickness skin loss with extensive destruction, tissue necrosis, or damage to muscle, bone, or supporting structures (e.g., tendon or joint capsule). *Note:* Undermining and sinus tracts may also be associated with stage IV pressure ulcers.

Prevention

The Panel for the Prediction and Prevention of Pressure Ulcers in Adults (1992) identified nine interventions that can be used to maintain and improve tissue tolerance to pressure in order to prevent injury. These interventions are listed in Table 34–6.

TABLE 34–6 Nursing Interventions to Maintain and Improve Tissue Tolerance to Pressure in Order to Prevent Injury

1. Complete a skin assessment daily on all individuals at risk, with particular attention given to bony prominences. Document findings.
2. Cleanse skin at time of soiling and as needed. Frequency of skin cleansing should be individualized according to need or patient preference. Avoid hot water, and use a mild cleansing agent that minimizes irritation and dryness of the skin. During the cleansing process, use care to minimize the force and friction applied to the skin.
3. Minimize environmental factors leading to skin drying, such as low humidity (less than 40 percent) and exposure to cold. Treat dry skin with moisturizers.
4. Avoid massage over bony prominences, as this may be harmful.
5. Minimize skin exposure to moisture as a result of incontinence, perspiration, or wound drainage. Underpads or briefs can be used.
6. Minimize skin injury secondary to friction and shear forces through proper positioning, transferring, and turning techniques. Friction injuries may be reduced by the use of lubricants (corn starch and creams), protective films (transparent film dressings and skin sealants), protective dressings (hydrocolloids), and protective padding.
7. Ensure adequate dietary intake of protein and calories. Nutritional supplements or support may be needed. If dietary intake remains inadequate and if consistent with overall goals of therapy, more aggressive nutritional intervention, such as enteral or parenteral feedings, should be considered.
8. Institute rehabilitation efforts aimed at mobility and activity, if consistent with the overall goals of therapy. Maintaining current activity level, mobility, and range of motion is an appropriate goal for most patients.
9. Monitor and document interventions and outcomes.

TABLE 34–7 Nursing Interventions to Protect Against the Adverse Effects of External Mechanical Forces

1. Any bedridden patient assessed to be at risk for developing pressure ulcers should be repositioned at least every 2 hours if consistent with overall patient goals. Use a written schedule for systematic turning and repositioning.
2. Use positioning devices (pillows, foam wedges) for bedridden patients to keep bony prominences from direct contact with one another.
3. Completely immobile bedridden patients should have a care plan that includes the use of devices that totally relieve pressure on the heels (raising the heels off the bed). Do not use donut-type devices.
4. When the side-lying position is used, avoid positioning directly on the trochanter.
5. Limit the amount of time the head of the bed is elevated and maintain the head of the bed at the lowest degree of elevation consistent with medical conditions and other restrictions.
6. Use lifting devices (trapeze or bed linen) to move (rather than drag) patients in bed who cannot assist during transfers and position changes.
7. Any patient assessed to be at risk for developing pressure ulcers should have a bed with a pressure-reducing device (foam, static air, alternating air, gel, or water mattresses).
8. Avoid uninterrupted sitting for any patient at risk for developing pressure ulcers. Reposition the patient, shifting the points under pressure at least hourly.
9. For chair-bound patients, the use of a pressure-reducing device (made of foam, gel, air, or a combination) is indicated. Do not use donut-type devices.
10. Positioning of chair-bound individuals should include consideration of postural alignment, distribution of weight, balance and stability, and pressure relief.
11. Include in the written care plan all positioning devices and schedules.

Mechanical Loading and Support Surfaces

The Panel for the Prediction and Prevention of Pressure Ulcers in Adults (1992) identified 11 interventions that can be used to protect against the adverse effects of external mechanical forces, such as pressure, friction, and shear. These interventions are listed in Table 34–7.

In summary, pressure ulcers most frequently occur over bony prominences and can be staged to classify the degree of tissue damage observed. Patients are assessed on admission for their risk for pressure ulcer development using the Norton Scale or the Braden Scale. Patients at risk for pressure ulcer development require prompt preventive interventions. Skin care and early treatment are instituted to maintain and improve tissue tolerance to pressure in order to prevent injury. Interventions include measures to protect against the adverse effects of external mechanical forces.

SECTION SEVEN REVIEW

1. Nonblanchable erythema of intact skin could be staged as
   A. stage I
   B. stage II
   C. stage III
   D. stage IV
2. Which of the following is NOT a nursing intervention that can be used to maintain and improve tissue tolerance to pressure?
   A. treat dry skin with moisturizers
   B. massage over bony prominences
   C. minimize skin exposure to moisture by using underpads
   D. use hydrocolloid dressings to reduce friction injuries

3. Pressure ulcer risk assessments should be made on
   A. patients who are immobile
   B. patients who have altered levels of consciousness
   C. patients who are incontinent
   D. all patients
4. Which of the following interventions can be used to protect against the adverse effects of mechanical forces?
   A. elevate the head of the bed continuously
   B. reposition patients who are sitting at least every 4 hours
   C. use lifting devices to move patients in bed
   D. use donut-type foam devices for bedridden patients

Answers: 1. A, 2. B, 3. D, 4. C

SECTION EIGHT: Management of Pressure Ulcers

At the completion of this section, the learner will be able to identify the components of a pressure ulcer treatment program, including assessment of the patient and the pressure ulcer, management of tissue loads, ulcer wound management, management of bacterial colonization and infection, and operative repair of the pressure. Figure 34–4 provides an overview of these activities related to pressure ulcer treatment.

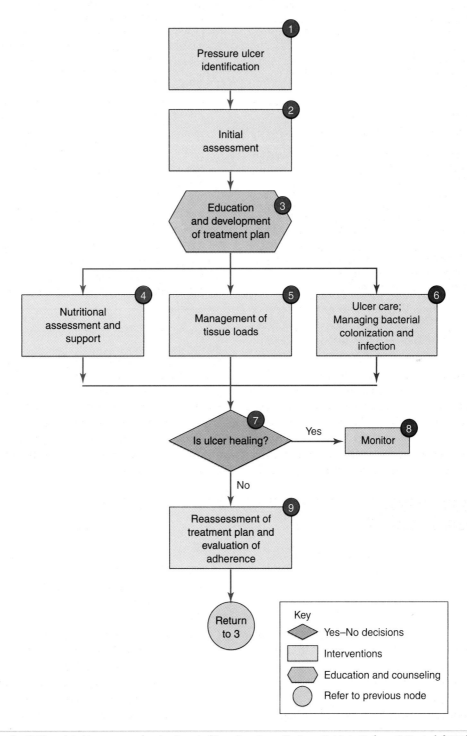

Figure 34–4 ■ Overview of activities related to pressure ulcer treatment. *(From Bergstrom, N., Bennett, M. A. Carlson, C. E., et al. [1994]. Pressure ulcer treatment Clinical practice guidelines. In Quick reference guide for clinicians, No. 15. Rockville, MD: U.S. Department of Health and Human Services, AHCPR Pub. No. 95–0653.)*

TABLE 34–8 Nursing Assessment of a Pressure Ulcer

1. Initial assessment of the pressure ulcer should include location, stage, size, sinus tracts, undermining, tunneling, exudate, necrotic tissue, and the presence or absence of granulation tissue and epithelialization.
2. Pressure ulcers should be reassessed at least weekly. If the patient's condition or the pressure ulcer's condition deteriorates, immediately reevaluate the treatment program.
3. Some evidence of pressure ulcer healing should be noted within 2 to 4 weeks. If no progress has been noted, reevaluate the treatment plan as well as adherence to the treatment plan and modify as needed.

Assessment

A systematic nursing assessment of the patient with a pressure ulcer provides the basis for planning and evaluating pressure ulcer treatment. This assessment includes psychosocial status, pain level, nutritional status, and physical health. Table 34–8 summarizes the assessment guidelines recommended for use with pressure ulcers (Arnold, 2003).

Management of Tissue Loads

Tissue load refers to the distribution of shear, pressure, and friction on tissue. Nursing interventions are instituted that reduce tissue loads in an effort to create an environment that promotes healing of the pressure ulcer and enhances soft tissue viability. The algorithm in Figure 34–5 can be used to guide clinical decisions on the management of tissue loads.

Management of tissue load begins with proper positioning techniques and support surfaces for patients while in bed. Avoid positioning patients on the pressure ulcer because this can delay healing. Positioning devices can be used to raise the pressure ulcer off the bed; however, few studies have documented the effects of ring cushions (donuts), and they should not be used. The care plan includes repositioning of the patient plan that is designed to protect uninvolved areas. Patients placed on a pressure-reducing support surface must be regularly repositioned because ulcers can still develop.

When selecting a support surface for a patient, the nurse considers the performance characteristics of the various products. A variety of support surfaces are available; however, research to date demonstrates that one support device is no better than the others. Table 34–9 summarizes the various classes of support surfaces and their abilities to counteract forces that contribute to pressure ulcer development. After determining which forces might be increasing a patient's risk for pressure ulcer development, the nurse can use this table to select an appropriate support surface. There is an increasing amount of research that shows air-loss beds may not reduce the incidence of pressure ulcers, but their use may improve healing rates (Cullum et al.,

2004). Certain patient conditions warrant specific support surfaces. Patient characteristics to consider when selecting a support surface are summarized in Table 34–10.

Ulcer Wound Management

Management of pressure ulcers includes debridement, wound cleansing, and dressing changes. Recommended management of ulcer care is summarized in Figure 34–6.

The following guidelines have been recommended for the debridement of pressure ulcers (Bergstrom et al., 1994):

1. When the need for removal of devitalized tissue is not urgent, sharp mechanical debridement, or enzymatic or autolytic techniques can be used. If the need for debridement is urgent (progressive cellulitis or sepsis), sharp debridement should be used.
2. Use clean, dry dressings for 8 to 24 hours after sharp debridement associated with bleeding, then reinstitute moist dressings. Clean dressings may be used in conjunction with mechanical or enzymatic debridement techniques.
3. Heel ulcers with dry eschar need not be debrided if they do not have edema, erythema, fluctuance, or drainage. Assess these wounds daily to monitor for pressure ulcer complications requiring further debridement.
4. Prevent or manage pain associated with debridement as needed.

The process of cleaning a wound involves selection of a solution and the appropriate mechanical means to deliver the solution to the wound. Current guidelines recommend the following (Bergstrom et al., 1994):

1. Wounds should be cleaned at each dressing change, using minimal mechanical force when cleaning the ulcer with gauze, cloth, or sponges.
2. Normal saline is recommended for cleaning wounds.
3. Use enough irrigation pressure to cleanse the wound without causing trauma to the wound.
4. Whirlpool treatments are effective in cleansing pressure ulcers that contain thick exudate, slough, or necrotic tissue; the treatments should be discontinued when the ulcer is clean.

The condition of the pressure ulcer and the desired dressing function determine the type of dressing that should be used for a pressure ulcer. The cardinal rule is to keep the ulcer tissue moist and the surrounding skin dry, which can be accomplished by the following (Bergstrom et al., 1994):

1. Wet-to-dry dressings should be used only for debridement.
2. Use clinical judgment to select a type of moist dressing; current research demonstrates no difference in pressure ulcer healing outcomes related to type of moist wound dressing used.

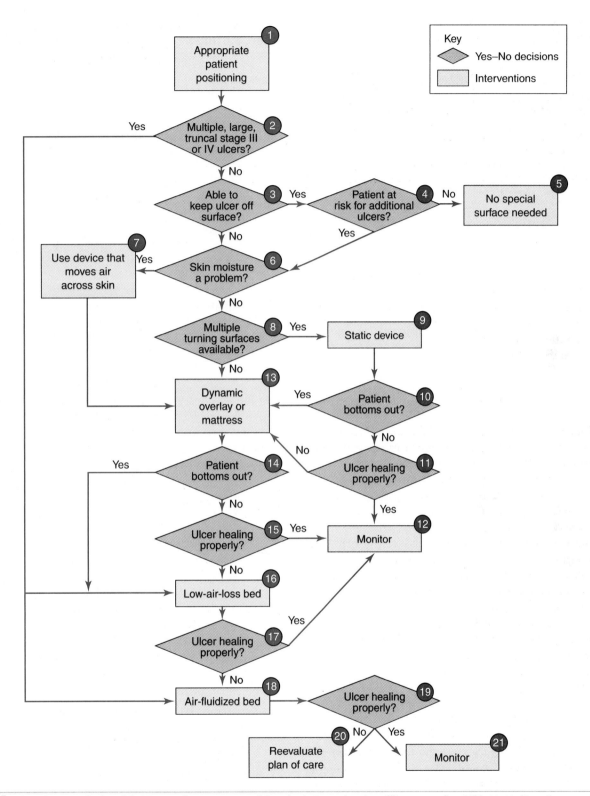

Figure 34–5 ■ Algorithm to guide clinical decisions on the management of tissue loads. For explanation of "bottoms out" see Table 34–10. *(From Bergstrom, N., Bennett, M. A., Carlson, C. E., et al. [1994]. Pressure ulcer treatment: Clinical practice guideline. In Quick reference guide for clinicians, No. 15. Rockville, MD: U.S. Department of Health and Human Services, A-CPR Pub. No. 95–0653.)*

TABLE 34–9 Selected Characteristics for Classes of Support Surfaces

PERFORMANCE CHARACTERISTICS	AIR-FLUIDIZED	LOW-AIR-LOSS	ALTERNATING AIR	STATIC FLOTATION (AIR OR WATER)	FOAM	STANDARD MATTRESS
Increased support area	Yes	Yes	Yes	Yes	Yes	No
Low moisture retention	Yes	Yes	No	No	No	No
Reduced heat accumulation	Yes	Yes	No	No	No	No
Shear reduction	Yes	Yes	Yes	Yes	No	No
Pressure reduction	Yes	Yes	Yes	Yes	Yes	No
Dynamic	Yes	Yes	Yes	No	No	No
Cost per day	High	High	Moderate	Low	Low	Low

From Bergstrom, N., Bennett, M. A., Carlson, C. E., et al. (1994). Pressure ulcer treatment: Clinical practice guideline. In Quick reference guide for clinicians, No. 15. Rockville, MD: U.S. Department of Health and Human Services, AHCPR Pub. No. 95–0653.

TABLE 34–10 Matching Patient Characteristics with Support Surfaces

TYPE OF SUPPORT SURFACE	INDICATIONS FOR USE
Pressure-reducing	Use if patient is at risk for further pressure ulcer development.
Static	Use if the patient can assume a variety of positions without bearing weight on a pressure ulcer and without *"bottoming out."* To assess for bottoming out, place outstretched hand with palms up under the overlay below the pressure ulcer or below the part of the body at risk for pressure ulcer development. If less than an inch of support material is felt, the patient has bottomed out and the support surface is inadequate.
Dynamic	Patient cannot assume a variety of positions without bearing weight on a pressure ulcer. Patient fully compresses the static support surface. Pressure ulcer does not show evidence of healing within 2 to 4 weeks.
Low-air-loss and air-fluidized beds.	Patient has stage III or IV pressure ulcers on multiple turning surfaces. Patient bottoms out or fails to heal on a dynamic overlay or mattress. To control excess moisture on intact skin (follow manufacturer's instructions for the use of linens and pads so as to not obstruct air flow).

3. Choose a dressing that controls exudate but does not desiccate the ulcer bed.
4. Eliminate wound dead space by loosely filling all cavities with dressing material and avoid overpacking the wound.
5. Monitor dressings applied near the anus because they are difficult to keep intact.

Managing Bacterial Colonization and Infection

Stage II, III, and IV pressure ulcers are likely to be infected. Adequate cleansing and debridement can prevent bacterial colonization from progressing into a clinical infection. The following guidelines are recommended (Bergstrom et al., 1994):

1. If purulence or a foul odor is detected, more frequent cleansing and debridement may be required.
2. Proper technique must be followed when obtaining a wound culture: (a) thoroughly cleanse the wound with normal saline, (b) access the deepest wound compartment, and (c) roll the culturette swab a full rotation to the part of the wound with the most visible signs of infection (Arnold, 2003).
3. Topical antibiotics used should be effective against gram-positive, gram-negative, and anaerobic organisms. If the ulcer does not respond to topical antibiotic therapy after 2 weeks, soft tissue cultures should be performed and the potential for osteomyelitis should be evaluated. Systemic antibiotics are indicated in the event of bacteremia, advancing cellulitis, or osteomyelitis.
4. Topical antiseptics should not be used to reduce bacteria in wound tissue.
5. Pressure ulcers should be protected from exogenous sources of contamination.

Operative Repair

Operative repair of pressure ulcers may be indicated when clean stage III or IV pressure ulcers do not respond to conventional guidelines (Bergstrom et al., 1994). Operative repair of pressure

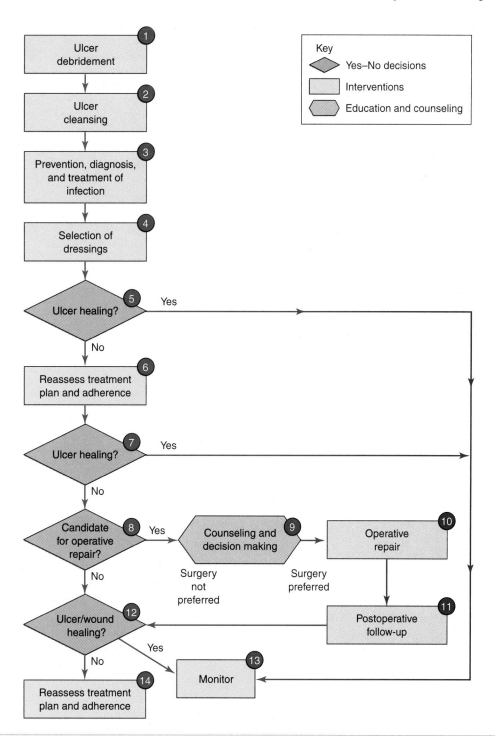

Figure 34–6 ■ Management of ulcer care. *(From Bergstrom, N., Bennett, M. A., Carlson, C. E., et al. [1994]. Pressure ulcer treatment: Clinical practice guidelines.* In Quick reference guide for clinicians, *No. 15. Rockville, MD: U.S. Department of Health and Human Services, AHCPR Pub. No. 95–0653.)*

ulcer wounds may include direct closure, skin grafting, skin flaps, musculocutaneous flaps, or free flaps. Nursing care postoperatively must include interventions to promote wound healing. Pressure to the operative site should be minimized through the use of an air-fluidized, low-air-loss bed for at least 2 weeks (Bergstrom et al., 1994).

In summary, management of pressure ulcers begins with a systematic nursing assessment; management of tissue load through the use of proper positioning techniques and support surfaces for the patient in bed; ulcer wound management using debridement, wound cleansing and dressing changes; managing bacterial colonization and infection; and possible operative repair.

SECTION EIGHT REVIEW

1. Pressure ulcer healing is usually evidenced
   A. in less than a week
   B. within 1 to 2 weeks
   C. within 2 to 4 weeks
   D. within 4 to 6 weeks
2. Which support surface should be used if a patient is at risk for further pressure ulcer development?
   A. a pressure-reducing surface
   B. a static support surface
   C. a dynamic support surface
   D. a low-air-loss surface
3. Which of the following treatments is recommended for cleansing pressure ulcers containing thick exudate, slough, and necrotic tissue?
   A. wet-to-dry dressing changes
   B. enzymatic debridement

C. normal saline irrigation
D. whirlpool treatments

4. Bacterial colonization can be prevented from progressing to a clinical infection by
   A. adequate wound cleansing
   B. adequate wound debridement
   C. adequate wound cleansing and debridement
   D. systemic antibiotics
5. Which of the following interventions is recommended if a pressure ulcer wound develops purulent drainage?
   A. swab the drainage for culture
   B. institute systemic antibiotics
   C. increase the frequency of wound cleansing and debriding
   D. institute topical antiseptics

Answers: 1. C, 2. A, 3. D, 4. C, 5. C

POSTTEST

1. Skin tears are more likely to occur with advancing age because
   A. sweat glands decrease in number
   B. there is increased thickness in the dermis
   C. rete ridges flatten
   D. thermoregulation is lost
2. Epithelialization
   A. occurs even in the presence of debris
   B. spreads on surfaces laden with bacteria
   C. occurs only in healthy tissue
   D. occurs within moments after injury
3. A patient has undergone an appendectomy. Most likely, his incision would be allowed to heal by
   A. primary intention
   B. secondary intention
   C. delayed primary (tertiary) intention
   D. delayed secondary intention
4. Of the factors that affect wound healing, which of the following has been found to be the most important?
   A. age
   B. normal serum potassium levels
   C. moisture
   D. adequate tissue perfusion

5. Which of the following interventions would NOT help to prevent a wound infection?
   A. hand washing
   B. skin preparation
   C. mechanical bowel preparation
   D. use of acetic acid dressings
6. Topical enzymes applied to necrotic wounds is
   A. contraindicated
   B. a form of mechanical debridement
   C. a form of autolytic debridement
   D. a form of chemical debridement
7. Which of the following dressing materials should NOT be used for documented or suspected wound infections?
   A. wet-to-dry dressings
   B. hydrocolloid dressings
   C. wet-to-damp dressings
   D. wet-to-wet dressings
8. Acetic acid is a solution used with wet-to-dry dressings that may be used
   A. to promote vasodilation in the wound
   B. to treat *Pseudomonas* infection in the wound
   C. to slightly dissolve necrotic debris in the wound
   D. as a fast-acting broad-spectrum antimicrobial

9. Red-pink tissue with a budding appearance is characteristic of
   A. granulation tissue
   B. imminent wound infections
   C. poor tissue perfusion
   D. the inflammatory process
10. Moist, yellow, stringy tissue in a wound is
   A. a sign of epithelialization
   B. eschar
   C. slough
   D. granulation tissue
11. Friction injuries may be reduced by
   A. massaging over bony prominences
   B. use of donut foam devices

C. protective dressings (hydrocolloids)
D. vigorous cleansing of soiled skin
12. Pressure ulcer wounds should be reassessed
   A. daily
   B. at least twice a day
   C. at least twice a week
   D. weekly
13. Which of the following repositioning schedules would be used for a patient placed on a pressure-reducing support surface?
   A. reposition until the patient "bottoms out"
   B. reposition the patient regularly
   C. turn no more frequently than needed
   D. the patient will not require repositioning

POSTTEST ANSWERS

Question	Answer	Section		Question	Answer	Section
1	C	One		8	B	Five
2	C	Two		9	A	Six
3	A	Two		10	C	Six
4	D	Three		11	C	Seven
5	D	Four		12	D	Eight
6	D	Five		13	B	Eight
7	B	Five				

REFERENCES

Arnold, M. C. (2003). Pressure ulcer prevention and management. *AACN Clinical Issues, 14,* 411–428.

Baharestani, M. M. (2003). Negative-pressure wound therapy. In C. T. Milne, L. Q. Corbett, & D. L. Dubuc (Eds.), *Wound, ostomy, and continence nursing secrets* (pp. 125–131). Philadelphia: Hanley & Belfus.

Barr, J. E. (2003). Wound cleansing. In C. T. Milne, L. Q. Corbett, & D. L. Dubuc (Eds.), *Wound, ostomy, and continence nursing secrets* (pp. 49–53). Philadelphia: Hanley & Belfus.

Bergstrom, N., Bennett, M. A., Carlson, C. E., et al. (1994). Pressure ulcer treatment: Clinical practice guidelines. In *Quick reference for clinicians,* No. 15. Rockville, MD: U.S. Department of Health and Human Services, AHCPR Publication 95–0653.

Bergstrom, N., & Braden, B. J. (2002). Predictive validity of the Braden Scale among black and white subjects. *Nursing Research, 51,* 398–403.

Braden, B. J. (1989). Clinical utility of the Braden Scale for predicting pressure sore risk. *Decubitus, 2*(3), 44–46, 50–51.

Brinker, D., Hancox, J. D., & Bernardon, S. O. (2003). Assessment and initial treatment of lacerations, mammalian bites, and insect stings. *AACN Clinical Issues, 14,* 401–410.

Cianci, P. (2000). Consensus development conference on diabetic foot wound care: A randomized controlled trial does exist supporting use of adjunctive hyperbaric therapy. *Diabetes Care, 23,* 873–874.

Conner-Kerr, T. A., & Sullivan, P. K. (2003). Diagnosing wound infections. In C. T. Milne, L. Q. Corbett, & D. L. Dubuc (Eds.), *Wound, ostomy, and continence nursing secrets* (pp. 74–75). Philadelphia: Hanley & Belfus.

Copson, D. (2003). Topical negative pressure and necrotosing fasciitis. *Nursing Stand, 18*(6), 71–80.

Cullum, N., McInness, E., Bell-Syer, S. E. M., & Legood, R. (2004). Support surfaces for pressure ulcer prevention. *The Cochrane Database Systemic Reviews 3.* Art. No.: CD001735.DOI:10.1002/14651858.CD001735.pubz.

Fernandez, R., Griffiths, R., & Ussia, C. (2003). Water for wound cleansing. *The Cochrane Database for Systemic Reviews, 3.*

Gordillo, G. M., & Sen, C. K. (2003). Revisiting the essential role of oxygen in wound healing. *American Journal of Surgery, 186,* 259–263.

Grief, R., Akca, O., Horn, E. P., et al. (2000). Supplemental perioperative oxygen to decrease the incidence of surgical wound infection. *New England Journal of Medicine, 342,* 161–167.

Heiner, S., Whitney, J. D., Wood, C., et al. (2002). Effects of an augmented postoperative fluid protocol to wound healing in cardiac surgery patients. *American Journal of Critical Care, 11,* 554–566.

Heyneman, C. A., & Lawless-Liday, C. (2002). Using hyperbaric oxygen to treat diabetic foot ulcers: Safety and effectiveness. *Critical Care Nursing, 22*(6), 52–60.

Himes, D. M. (2003). Nutrition and wound healing. In C. T. Milne, L. Q. Corbett, & D. L. Dubuc (Eds.), *Wound, ostomy, and continence nursing secrets* (pp. 32–36). Philadelphia: Hanley & Belfus.

Irion, G. L. (2002). *Comprehensive wound management.* Thorofare, NJ: Slack, Inc.

Kirsner, R. S., & Bogensberger, G. (2002). The normal process of healing. In L. C. Kloth & J. M. McCulloch (Eds.), *Wound healing: Alternatives in management* (3rd ed., pp. 1–34). Philadelphia: F. A. Davis.

Kranke, P., Bennett, M., Toeckl-Wiedman, I., et al. (2004). Hyperbaric oxygen therapy for chronic wounds. *Cochrane Database Syst Rev 2.* Art No.: CD004954.DOI: 10.1002/14651858.CD004954.

Lionelli, G. T., & Lawrence, W. T. (2003). Wound dressings. *Surgical Clinics of North America, 82,* 617–638.

Loehne, H. B. (2002). The normal process of healing. In L. C. Kloth & J. M. McCulloch (Eds.), *Wound healing: Alternatives in management* (3rd ed., pp. 1–34). Philadelphia: F. A. Davis.

Norton, D. (1989). Calculating the risk: Reflections on the Norton Scale. *Decubitus, 2*(3), 24–31.

Ovington, L. G. (2001). Battling bacteria in wound care. *Home Healthcare Nurse, 19,* 662–630.

Panel for the Prediction and Prevention of Pressure Ulcers in Adults. (1992). *Pressure Ulcers in Adults: Prediction and Prevention. Clinical Practice Guideline,* Number 3. AHCPR Publication No. 92. Rockville, MD: Agency for Health Care Policy and Research, Public Health Service, U.S. Department of Health and Human Services.

Sjöberg, T., Mzezewa, S., Jönsson, K., Robertson, V., & Salemark, L. (2003). Comparison of surface swab cultures and quantitative tissue biopsy culture to predict sepsis in burn patients: A prospective study. *Journal of Burn Care and Rehabilitation, 24,* 365–370.

Stotts, N. A. (2000). Wound infection: Diagnosis and management. In R. A. Bryant (Ed.), *Acute and chronic wounds* (2nd ed., pp. 180–188). St. Louis: C. V. Mosby.

Waldrop, J. D., & Doughty, D. B. (2000). Wound-healing physiology. In R. A. Bryant (Ed.), *Acute and chronic wounds* (2nd ed., pp. 17–37). St. Louis: C. V. Mosby.

West, J. M., & Gimbel, M. L. (2000). Acute surgical and traumatic wound healing. In R. A. Bryant (Ed.), *Acute and chronic wounds* (2nd ed, pp. 189–196). St. Louis: C. V. Mosby.

Whiteford L. (2003). Nicotine, CO, and HCN: The detrimental effects of smoking on wound healing. *Wound Care* (December), 522–526.

Whitney, J. D. (2003). Supplemental perioperative oxygen and fluids to improve surgical wound outcomes: Translating research into practice. *Wound Repair and Regeneration, 11,* 462–467.

Whitney, J. D., & Parkman, S. (2004). The effect of early postoperative physical training in tissue oxygen and wound healing. *Biological Research for Nursing, 6*(2), 79–89.

Williams, D. T., & Harding, K. (2003). Healing responses of skin and muscles in critical illness. *Critical Care Medicine, 31,* S547–557.

Williams, J. Z., & Barbul, A. (2003). Nutrition and wound healing. *Surgical Clinics of North America, 83,* 571–596.

Zatz, J. L. (2001). The quality of skin care products and their ingredients. *Ostomy Wound Management, 47*(2), 22–33.

Acute Burn Injury

Dayna Gary

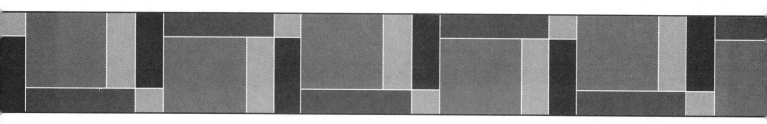

OBJECTIVES Following completion of this module, the learner will be able to

1. List the risk factors that place people at a greater risk for burn injury and have greater morbidity and mortality as a result of burn injury.

   ■ Discuss five mechanisms of burn injury.

2. Differentiate burn wound descriptors based on level of dermis and tissue involved in the injury.

   ■ Calculate the extent of total body surface area involved.

3. Discuss criteria for transfer of a patient to a burn center.

   ■ Describe the unique structures, processes, and personnel that make up a burn center.

4. Discuss priority cardiovascular and pulmonary assessments and interventions during the resuscitative phase for the patient with a burn injury.

5. Discuss priority assessments and interventions during the resuscitative phase for neurological effects and pain management for patients with burn injuries.

   ■ Identify stages of psychological adaptation following burn injury and state an appropriate nursing intervention for each stage.

6. Discuss priority nursing assessments and interventions during the resuscitative phase for metabolic and renal effects of burn injury.

7. Compare burn wound healing and wound healing from other injuries.

   ■ State the wound care priorities during the resuscitative phase.

8. Describe burn wound management in the acute rehabilitative phase.

9. Describe expected behaviors, emotional status, and levels of pain for burn patients during the acute rehabilitative phase, and their related nursing actions.

10. Describe the goals, interventions, and health professionals involved with promoting physical mobility during the acute rehabilitative phase of burn care.

11. Discuss nursing interventions related to physical conditioning, protection of new skin, scar management, and psychosocial adjustment during the long-term rehabilitative phase of burn care.

This self-study module focuses on the three phases of burn injury: the resuscitative, acute rehabilitative, and long-term rehabilitative phases. The module is composed of 11 sections. Sections One through Three discuss the mechanisms of burn injury, assessment and classification of burns, and burn centers. Sections Four through Six describe the cardiovascular, pulmonary, neurologic, cognitive, metabolic, and renal effects of burn injury during the resuscitative phase. Section Seven provides an overview of burn wound healing and describes initial wound care during the resuscitative phase. Section Eight de-

scribes burn wound management in the acute rehabilitative phase. Sections Nine and Ten describe the acute rehabilitative phase of burn injury. Section Eleven discusses the long-term rehabilitative phase of burn care. Each section includes a set of review questions to help the learner evaluate his or her understanding of the section's content before moving on to the next section. All Section Reviews and the module Pretest and Posttest include answers. It is suggested that the learner review those concepts answered incorrectly in the review questions before proceeding to the next section.

PRETEST

1. Of the following demographic groups, which is at highest risk for burn injury/death?
   A. Caucasians
   B. suburbanites
   C. women
   D. children

2. Which of the following mechanisms of burn injury causes protein liquification producing a soupy wound that allows for continued tissue damage into deeper structures?
   A. acid burn
   B. alkali burn
   C. electrical burn
   D. radiation burn

3. A sunburn is an example of a
   A. superficial burn
   B. superficial partial-thickness burn
   C. deep partial-thickness burn
   D. subdermal burn

4. A patient arrives at the emergency department with burns to bilateral anterior lower limbs and perineum. Calculate the extent of total body surface area (TBSA) of this injury using the rule of nines.
   A. 10 percent
   B. 18 percent
   C. 19 percent
   D. 36 percent

5. Single rooms with positive airflow are ideal in a burn unit because this arrangement promotes
   A. privacy
   B. noise reduction
   C. infection control
   D. adequate ventilation

6. Current guidelines recommend that an escharotomy should be performed when compartment pressures are
   A. greater than 20 mm Hg
   B. 25 to 40 mm Hg
   C. greater than 40 mm Hg
   D. greater than 75 mm Hg

7. Upper airway edema usually peaks during which time period postinhalation injury?
   A. 24 to 48 hours
   B. 1 to 2 hours
   C. 4 to 8 hours
   D. 12 to 24 hours

8. Fluid resuscitation should be calculated for patients with _____ total body surface area burned.
   A. 10 percent
   B. 15 percent
   C. 20 percent
   D. 30 percent

9. The most effective method for delivering pain medication during the resuscitative phase is
   A. orally
   B. subcutaneously
   C. intramuscularly
   D. intravenously

10. During the initial stage of psychological adaptation after burn injury (survival anxiety) the nurse should
    A. praise attempts for autonomous functioning
    B. give reality-based responses
    C. acknowledge reality-based responses
    D. force the staff's expectations on the patient

11. Enteral nutrition should be initiated
    A. within 24 hours postburn injury
    B. when bowel sounds return
    C. at 72 hours postburn
    D. after parenteral nutrition is completed

12. A red-brown color in the urine that appears after an electrical burn may indicate
    A. a urinary tract infection
    B. renal tubular acidosis
    C. renal hypoperfusion
    D. myoglobinuria

13. The major consequence of hypertrophic scar formation is
    A. contractures
    B. muscle atrophy
    C. that epithelialization cannot occur
    D. wound healing is delayed

14. Ointments and creams should not be applied during initial care of burn wounds because they
    A. induce the inflammatory process
    B. make wounds soupy and susceptible to infection
    C. interfere with burn wound evaluation
    D. interfere with an escharotomy

15. Bullae larger than 2 cm may be
    A. left intact
    B. drained by aspiration
    C. opened with the loose skin removed
    D. all of the above

16. Monitoring the patient after a tangential excision includes monitoring the patient for
    A. infection
    B. bleeding
    C. bullae
    D. soupy drainage

17. Which of the following organizations or groups might be MOST helpful in helping the patient with burn injuries through psychosocial issues in the acute rehabilitative phase?
    A. Tucson Society
    B. Phoenix Society
    C. American Burn Association
    D. the patient's visitors

18. Failure to apply compression wraps to recently grafted lower extremities prior to ambulation could result in
    A. extreme pain
    B. contracture formation
    C. graft loss
    D. bullae formation
19. Pressure garments are worn
    A. only at night
    B. continuously
    C. to help regain muscle stability
    D. until hospital discharge

Pretest Answers: 1. D, 2. B, 3. A, 4. C, 5. C, 6. C, 7. A, 8. C, 9. D, 10. B, 11. A, 12. D, 13. A, 14. C, 15. D, 16. B, 17. B, 18. C, 19. B

GLOSSARY

allograft   Biologic dressings obtained from human donor; usually a cadaver.

autografting   Transplanting tissue from one part of the patient's body to another part of the patient's body.

bulla   A large blister or skin vesicle filled with fluid (plural, bullae).

burn shock   Hypovolemic shock that develops secondary to fluid shifts occurring with burn injury.

carboxyhemoglobin   A compound formed by carbon monoxide and hemoglobin.

compartment syndrome   Pressure within a muscle compartment rises and exceeds microvascular pressure, thereby interfering with cellular perfusion.

debridement   The removal of foreign material and nonviable tissue from a wound.

deep partial-thickness burn   Burn that involves the epidermis and deep layers of the dermis.

eschar   A tough, dry inelastic wound indicative of a full-thickness burn.

escharotomy   Surgical incision of the eschar and superficial fascia of a circumferentially burned limb or trunk in order to restore blood flow distal to the affected area.

full-thickness burn   Burn that destroys epidermis, dermis, and portions of subcutaneous tissues (formerly known as third- and fourth-degree burns).

heterograft   Biological dressings obtained from animals; also referred to as xenografts.

homograft   Tissue transplanted from another individual to be used as a biological dressing.

myoglobin   Substance released from damaged muscle tissue.

myoglobinuria   The presence of myoglobin in the urine.

resuscitative phase   Lasts from time of burn injury to 48 to 72 hours postinjury.

subdermal burn   Burn that destroys all layers of the skin and may include injury to muscle, tendons, or bone.

superficial burn   Burn that destroys the epidermis only.

superficial partial-thickness burn   Burn that destroys the epidermis and superficial layer of the dermis.

xenograft   Biological dressings obtained from animals; also referred to as heterografts.

ABBREVIATIONS

AC	Alternating current		MAP	Mean arterial pressure
CO	Carbon monoxide		OT	Occupational therapist
DC	Direct current		PT	Physical therapist
GI	Gastrointestinal		TBSA	Total body surface area

SECTION ONE: Mechanisms of Burn Injury

At the completion of this section, the learner will be able to list the risk factors that place people at a greater risk for burn injury and have greater morbidity and mortality as a result of burn injury; and discuss five mechanisms of burn injury.

Incidence and Risk Factors

More than 1 million people are burned each year, resulting in approximately 4,500 deaths per year (American Burn Association, 2000). The economic costs from burn injury recovery rise into the billions of dollars per year as do the social costs from days lost from work and physical and vocational rehabilitation. Most burn injuries occur in the home. Children and the elderly are most prone to burn injuries. The elderly have impaired senses and reaction times, and tend to incorrectly assess risk. They commonly have chronic diseases requiring polymedicines. The elderly have thinner skin, with decreased microcirculation and an increased susceptibility to infection. All of these factors not only put the elderly at a greater risk for burn injuries but also lead to a greater morbidity and mortality (Redlick et al., 2002). People with diabetes are at higher risk of sustaining burn injuries with an associated increase in morbidity and mortality. Diabetics commonly have decreased sensation leading to an increased risk of injury as well as delayed recognition of the injury. A poor blood supply decreases the ability of oxygen to reach the wound leading to an anaerobic environment. Other associated complications with diabetes, such as blindness, limb amputation, and end-stage renal disease, place these people at further risk. Diabetic patients with burn injuries have an increased length of hospital stay and number of surgeries as well as higher rates of infection when compared to nondiabetic patients (McCampbell et al., 2002).

Mechanisms of Injury

Burn injury may occur from exposure to heat (flames, hot objects), caustic chemicals, electrical current, radiation, or extreme cold. The severity of the injury depends on the length of exposure, temperature of the offending substance, and tissue conductance (Kagan & Smith, 2000).

Thermal burns caused by exposure to flame or a hot object produce microvascular and inflammatory responses within minutes of the injury (Fig. 35–1). The effects from these two responses can last from 2 to 3 days. Substances released by damaged cells increase vascular permeability, causing fluid, electrolytes, and proteins to leak into the interstitial space. The

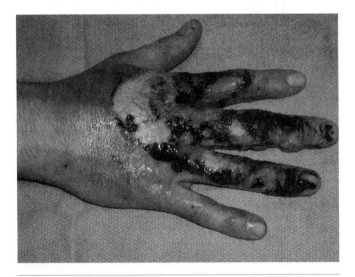

Figure 35–1 ▪ Thermal burn: Tar burn.

various inflammatory mediators also contribute to cell wall changes that permit intravascular fluid and proteins to leak into the interstitial spaces. Both of these responses contribute to burn edema formation. Burn edema is usually limited to the injured tissues with smaller size burns. In larger size burns edema occurs in noninjured tissues also. The fluid shift from intravascular to interstitial spaces may cause a hypovolemic shock state. Fluid loss by evaporation from the burn wound also contributes to the volume deficit. This hypovolemic shock state is frequently referred to as **burn shock.**

Chemical burns are the result of exposure to acid, alkali, or organic substances. The extent of injury depends on the concentration of the substance, the amount, the length of exposure, and the mechanism of chemical action. An acid substance will cause an eschar type of wound resulting from a coagulation necrosis. The eschar prevents continued tissue damage beneath the layer of eschar. An alkali substance usually causes more tissue damage than an acid substance (given the same volume) because an alkali causes protein liquefaction producing a soupy wound, which allows continued tissue damage into deeper structures. Damage occurs rapidly and will continue until the pH level returns to a normal physiologic level (Andrews et al., 2003). Organic substances produce a thermal component and may be absorbed systemically, producing renal and hepatic toxicity. Inhalation of chemical substances can cause direct parenchymal lung injury. Absorption of a chemical through either the pulmonary system or through direct skin contact can cause systemic effects involving the pulmonary, cardiovascular, renal, or hepatic systems.

Electrical burns result from the conversion of electrical energy into heat. The extent of thermal injury depends on the type of current, the pathway of current flow, local tissue resistance, and the duration of contact. All tissues are conductive to some extent but there are differences in the resistance to the current flow. Externally, the skin is the primary resistor to electrical current. Its ability to resist depends on its thickness and amount of moisture. Internally, nerves and blood vessels are the best electrical conductors (Koumbourlis, 2002). Because of the internal damage that can be caused by electrical injuries, the severity of an electrical burn is difficult to determine on initial exam.

Electrical contact injuries can be caused by low-voltage lines. These lines, most commonly found in homes and offices, are usually in the form of alternating current (AC). Because AC produces a current that flows back and forth in a cyclical manner, the former terminology of describing an entrance and exit wound is incorrect. AC, as opposed to direct current (DC), causes a more severe injury because it produces tetanic muscle contractions that do not allow disengagement from the current source. DC causes the person to be cast away from the current source. These differences between AC and DC are only significant with low voltages. Electrical burns can be caused by high-voltage lines. High-voltage injuries are caused by a current that is sent from the electrical source in an arc, either into the person or over the person. The arc can generate temperatures up to 5,000°C causing thermal injuries (Koumbourlis, 2002). Another type of electrical burn is termed *electrical flash* burn because the injury involves no electrical contact and it is a true thermal injury. Delineating among the different types of electrical burns is important because it will lead the health care practitioner to determine depth of injury as well as other possible associated injuries.

Radiation burns result from radiant energy being transferred to the body resulting in production of cellular toxins. The effect is most rapidly evident on those cells that reproduce rapidly, such as skin, blood vessels, intestinal lining, and bone marrow. The greater the exposure, the more significant the damage and the more types of cells that are affected. A radiation victim's injury usually results from radiation therapy or from an industrial or laboratory incident.

Exposure to severe cold temperatures can cause *frostbite injuries* (Fig. 35–2). Conditions that increase a person's susceptibility to this type of injury include amount of muscle and fat to provide insulation, nutrition status, amount of exertion required to generate heat, and alcohol and drugs affecting judgment, as well as the ability to shiver. The elderly are at greater risk for this type of injury because of their decreased ability for heat generation and vasoconstriction. Frostbite injuries are treated conservatively because it may take weeks before there is a clear demarcation between viable and nonviable tissue (Biem et al., 2003).

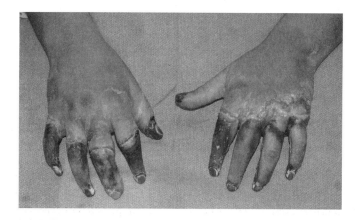

Figure 35–2 ■ Frostbite injury.

In summary, more than 1 million Americans are burned every year, resulting in 4,500 fatalities. Children, the elderly, and diabetics are at higher risk for burn injuries and a greater morbidity and mortality from these injuries. Mechanisms of injury include exposure to heat (flames, hot objects), extreme cold, caustic chemicals, radiation, and electrical current. Each injury produces a characteristic burn and sequelae.

SECTION ONE REVIEW

1. Which of the following patient groups are NOT at an increased risk for burn injuries?
   A. African Americans
   B. elderly
   C. children
   D. diabetics
2. The type of burn where tissues are deeply penetrated and necrosis may continue to occur for several hours after injury is MOST likely a(n)
   A. acidic burn
   B. alkaline burn
   C. electrical burn
   D. flash burn

3. Electrical contact injuries can be caused by low-voltage lines in the form of
   A. alternating current
   B. direct current
   C. current source
   D. a reflex arc
4. Which of the following burn injuries are treated conservatively because it takes weeks before there is a demarcation of viable and nonviable tissue?
   A. thermal burns
   B. electrical burns
   C. radiation burns
   D. frostbite

Answers: 1. A, 2. B, 3. A, 4. D

SECTION TWO: Burn Wound Assessment

At the completion of this section, the learner will be able to differentiate burn wound descriptors based on level of dermis and tissue involved in the injury and calculate the extent of total body surface area involved.

Burns are classified according to depth of injury and extent of body surface area involved. Burn depth has been traditionally described as first-, second-, or third-degree (Fig. 35–3). Currently, burn wounds are more specifically differentiated, depending on the level of dermis and subcutaneous tissue involved. Descriptors of burn depths include superficial, superficial partial thickness, deep partial thickness, full thickness, and

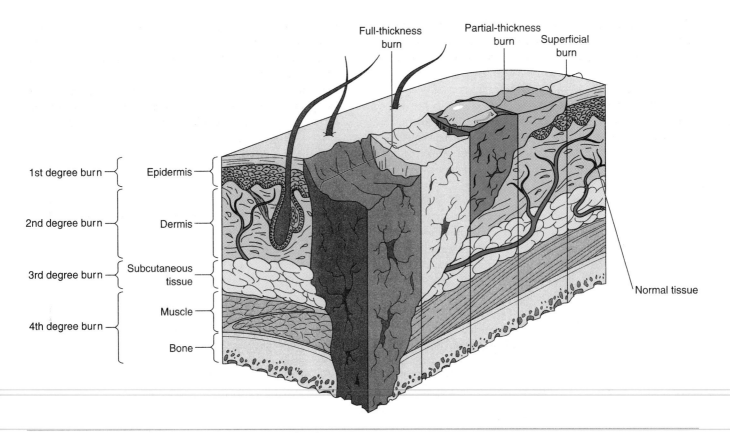

Figure 35–3 ■ Burn injury classification according to the depth of the burn.

subdermal burns (Table 35–1). **Superficial burns** involve the epidermis only. An example is a sunburn. **Superficial partial-thickness** burns involve the epidermis and superficial layer of the dermis. These burns may occur with brief contact with hot objects. **Deep partial-thickness burns** involve the epidermis and deep layer of the dermis. An example is a tar burn. **Full-thickness burns** involve the epidermis, dermis, and subcutaneous layer. Exposure to flames, electricity, or chemicals can cause these severe burns. **Subdermal burns** usually involve all layers of skin and may include injury to muscle, tendons, or bone as a result of prolonged contact with flames, hot objects, or electricity.

The depth of the burn is often difficult to assess initially. Calculation of the extent of injury should be reevaluated after the initial wound debridement and over the course of the ensuing 72 hours to accurately describe the wound. Wound conversion sometimes occurs when viable tissue becomes nonviable, thereby increasing the depth of the wound. Thermal burns consist of three zones. The outermost area is termed the *zone of hyperemia;* it blanches with pressure and will heal in 7 to 10 days. The innermost area is termed the *zone of coagulation;* it is an area of immediately nonviable tissue. Surrounding this central zone is the *zone of stasis.* This area can easily convert to nonvi-

able tissue if the restoration of blood flow is not adequately achieved. Proper fluid resuscitation is essential in preventing this from occurring (Kim et al., 2001; Merz et al., 2003). Other causes of wound conversion include infection, hypothermia, and external pressure.

The extent of injury is expressed by the percentage of total body surface area (TBSA) burned. When determining TBSA, superficial burns are not involved in the calculation. The most accurate guide in determining the extent of injury is the Lund and Browder Chart, which adjusts TBSA for age (Fig. 35–4). This is important because various pediatric patients' body parts are disproportionate to adults'. For example, a child's head is allowed a greater TBSA percentage than an adult's. To use the guide, one assesses all partial- and full-thickness burns and shades the figure accordingly. The percentage of each anatomic area involved is calculated, then all are totaled. For example, if an adult were to sustain a scald injury to the right lower arm and hand, his or her TBSA burned wound would be 5.5 percent.

Another guide used to calculate TBSA is the rule of nines (Fig. 35–5). This estimation divides the body into areas of 9 percent or multiples of 9 percent. The head is 9 percent, each upper extremity is 9 percent, each lower extremity is 18 percent, the back is 18 percent, the trunk (front) is 18 percent, and the genitalia is 1 percent, with the sum total equaling 100 percent. This method is quick and easy, but less accurate than the Lund and Browder method. This is especially true for children (Johnson & Richard, 2003).

Another method of evaluating burn injuries, especially those that are irregularly shaped or occur in patches, is to use the palmar surface of the patient's hand which represents approximately 1 percent of the patient's body surface area. Just the palm accounts for 0.5 percent TBSA. For example, if a patchy burn to the torso includes four burned areas, each approximately the size of the patient's palm, the TBSA involved would be 2 percent.

In summary, burns are classified according to the extent of body surface area injured and their depth. Various charts and formulas are used to guide the estimation of the extent of injury.

TABLE 35–1 Descriptions of Burn Depths

DEPTH OF BURN	DESCRIPTION
Superficial burn	Involves epidermis only
	May be caused by the sun, or brief exposure to hot liquids
	Erythema, pain, minimal edema
	No blisters, dry skin
	Heals in 3 to 5 days via sloughing of the epidermal layer, no scarring
Superficial partial-thickness burn	Involves the epidermis and the papillary layer of the dermis (superficial layer)
	May be caused by hot liquids, brief contact with hot objects, or flash flame
	Erythema, brisk capillary refill, blisters, moist
	Moderate edema, very painful
	Heals in 10 to 14 days via reepithelialization
	No scarring, potential for hypo/hyperpigmentation
Deep partial-thickness burn	Involves the epidermis and the reticular layer of the dermis (deep layer)
	May be caused by flame, hot liquids, radiation, tar, or hot objects
	Erythematous or pale, sluggish or absent capillary refill
	Moist or dry, no blisters
	Significant edema and altered sensation
	Heals in 2 to 3 weeks or longer
	Potential for scarring and hypo/hyperpigmentation
	May require skin grafting for optimal function or appearance
Full-thickness burn	Involves the epidermis, dermis, and subcutaneous layer
	May be caused by flame, electricity, or chemicals
	Dry, leathery, white
	Absent capillary refill
	Generally requires skin grafting
	Healing via contraction and granulation tissue formation
	Scarring and hypo/hyperpigmentation
Subdermal burn	Involves the epidermis, dermis, subcutaneous layer, and muscle, tendon, or bone
	May be from electricity, prolonged contact with flame or a hot object
	Charred, dry
	Requires skin grafting, flap, or amputation

Data from Carrougher, G. I. (1998). Burn wound assessment and topical treatment. In G. J. Carrougher (Ed.), Burn therapy and care *(pp. 133–165). St. Louis: C. V. Mosby; Kagan, R. C., & Smith, S. C. (2000). Evaluation and treatment of thermal injuries. Dermatology Nurses 12, 334–350; Johnson, R. M., & Richard, R. (2003). Partial-thickness burns: Identification and management. Skin & Wound Care, 16, 178–186.*

Area	Age (years)					% 1°	% 2°	% 3°	% Total
	0–1	1–4	5–9	10–15	Adult				
Head	19	17	13	10	7				
Neck	2	2	2	2	2				
Ant. trunk	13	13	13	13	13				
Post. trunk	13	13	13	13	13				
R. buttock	2½	2½	2½	2½	2½				
L. buttock	2½	2½	2½	2½	2½				
Genitalia	1	1	1	1	1				
R.U. arm	4	4	4	4	4				
L.U. arm	4	4	4	4	4				
R.L. arm	3	3	3	3	3				
L.L. arm	3	3	3	3	3				
R. hand	2½	2½	2½	2½	2½				
L. hand	2½	2½	2½	2½	2½				
R. thigh	5½	6½	8½	8½	9½				
L. thigh	5½	6½	8½	8½	9½				
R. leg	5	5	5½	6	7				
L. leg	5	5	5½	6	7				
R. foot	3½	3½	3½	3½	3½				
L. foot	3½	3½	3½	3½	3½				
					Total				

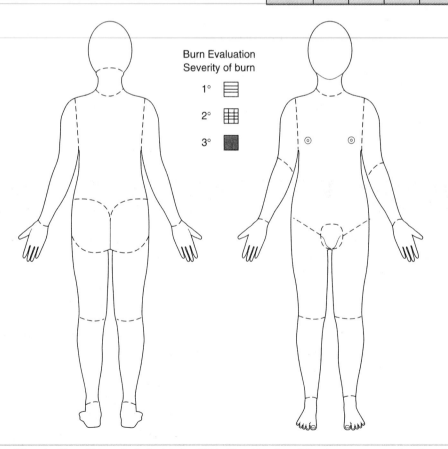

Burn Evaluation
Severity of burn

1°
2°
3°

Figure 35–4 ■ The Lund and Browder Chart. This method of estimating TBSA affected by a burn injury is more accurate than the rule of nines because it accounts for changes in body surface area across the life span.

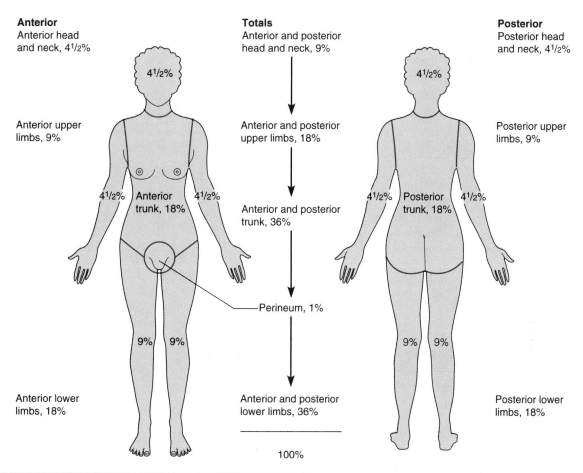

Anterior
Anterior head
and neck, 4$\frac{1}{2}$%

Anterior upper
limbs, 9%

4$\frac{1}{2}$%   Anterior
trunk, 18%   4$\frac{1}{2}$%

Anterior lower
limbs, 18%

Totals
Anterior and posterior
head and neck, 9%

Anterior and posterior
upper limbs, 18%

Anterior and posterior
trunk, 36%

Perineum, 1%

Anterior and posterior
lower limbs, 36%

100%

Posterior
Posterior head
and neck, 4$\frac{1}{2}$%

Posterior upper
limbs, 9%

4$\frac{1}{2}$%   Posterior
trunk, 18%   4$\frac{1}{2}$%

Posterior lower
limbs, 18%

4$\frac{1}{2}$%   4$\frac{1}{2}$%

9%   9%   9%   9%

Figure 35–5 ■ The rule of nines is a method of quickly estimating the percentage of TBSA affected by a burn injury. Although useful in emergency care situations, the rule of nines is not accurate for estimating TBSA for adults who are short, obese, or very thin.

SECTION TWO REVIEW

1. An adult patient received partial-thickness flash burns to his head and neck. The estimated extent of his injury according to the Lund and Browder Chart would be
   A. 21 percent
   B. 19 percent
   C. 9 percent
   D. 7 percent

2. Using the rule of nines, calculate the extent of burn for a patient with burns to the posterior head and posterior trunk.
   A. 22.5 percent
   B. 18 percent
   C. 20 percent
   D. 13 percent

3. White, charred, leathery-textured wounds are the result of
   A. full-thickness burns
   B. superficial burns
   C. deep partial-thickness burns
   D. superficial partial-thickness burns

4. Which of the following terms describes a burn that involves the epidermis and deep layer of the dermis and has sluggish or absent capillary refill?
   A. superficial partial-thickness burn
   B. deep partial-thickness burn
   C. full-thickness burn
   D. subdermal burns

Answers: 1. C, 2. A, 3. A, 4. B

SECTION THREE: Burn Centers

At the completion of this section, the learner will be able to discuss criteria for transfer of a patient to a burn center and to describe the unique structures, processes, and personnel that make up a burn center.

Burn Center Referral Criteria

Once the extent and depth of the burn injury has been classified, the severity of the injury is evaluated. Patients with complex burn injuries have complex physiological and psychosocial needs. These needs require specialized resources and personnel and these patients are referred to a burn center. The American Burn Association (1999) has established criteria that, when present, indicate the need to transfer a patient to a burn center (Table 35–2). Burn centers treat adults and/or children.

TABLE 35–2 Burn Center Referral Criteria

- Partial-thickness burns greater than 10 percent TBSA
- Burns involving face, hands, feet, genitalia, perineum, or over major joints
- Full-thickness and subdermal burns in any age group
- Electrical burns, including lightning injuries
- Chemical burns
- Inhalation injuries
- Burn injury in patients with preexisting medical disorders that complicate management, prolong recovery, or affect mortality
- Any patient with burns and concomitant trauma
- Burned children in hospitals unqualified to take care of this type of patient
- Burn injury in patients that may require special social, emotional, or long-term rehabilitation

From American Burn Association. (1999). Burn unit referral criteria. Available at: www.ameriburn.org. Accessed June 5, 2004.

Structure of the Burn Unit

Patients in the burn unit are susceptible to infection because of altered resistance to microorganisms as a result of the presence of open wounds and immunosuppression. A model burn unit provides an environment that promotes isolation from pathogens and prevents infection. In the ideal unit each patient occupies a single room that provides positive airflow and the unit is access restricted. Techniques such as strict hand washing and the proper use of masks, gowns, gloves, and caps during dressing changes are strictly followed (Thompson et al., 2002). These techniques decrease the patient's risk for infection. Each patient room should contain individual controls for temperature and humidity and have ample space for equipment and supplies.

The typical burn unit is equipped to provide standard invasive monitoring and ventilatory support. Hydrotherapy or whirlpool facilities are often located in burn units because patients may require hydrotherapy to promote wound healing. Operating room suites may also be located within the burn unit.

Burn Team Members

Care of the critically injured burn patient is complex and requires a multidisciplinary approach. Burn team members include nurses, physicians (plastic and general surgeons), physical therapists (PTs), occupational therapists (OTs), pharmacists, dietitians, discharge planners, social workers, chaplains, and psychologists. Additional services may be needed.

In summary, patients with burn injuries require specialized care, often in a burn center. Burn centers are designed to treat patients with burns using a multidisciplinary approach. Burn units are equipped to provide standard hemodynamic monitoring, ventilatory support, hydrotherapy, and reverse isolation for those recovering from critical burn injury.

SECTION THREE REVIEW

1. Which of the following criteria indicate a burn center referral should be made?
   A. partial-thickness burn greater than 10 percent
   B. chemical burns
   C. any patient with burns and trauma
   D. all of the above

2. In the ideal burn unit
   A. patients are in semiprivate rooms with positive airflow
   B. patients are in private rooms with positive airflow
   C. patients are in private rooms with negative airflow
   D. access is not restricted

Answers: 1. D, 2. B

SECTION FOUR: Resuscitative Phase: Cardio-vascular and Pulmonary Effects

At the completion of this section, the learner will be able to discuss priority cardiovascular and pulmonary assessments and interventions during the resuscitation phase for the patient with a burn injury.

The **resuscitative phase** lasts from the time of burn injury to 48 to 72 hours postinjury. Burn shock with cardiovascular collapse can occur during this time period. Traumatic injuries, such as head trauma, internal injuries, and fractures that may occur concurrently with burn injuries, are identified and treated early in this phase. Primary and secondary assessments for traumatic injury are completed on all burn patients (see Module 36 for these assessments).

Cardiovascular

Adults with large burns are frequently tachycardic (heart rate 110 and 125 beats per minute). Burns of more than 40 percent TBSA produce significant myocardial dysfunction. A decrease in myocardial contractility occurs and cardiac output falls within the first few minutes of injury, even prior to a decreased plasma volume. During the initial few hours, plasma volume drops contributing to the decreased cardiac output. An increased peripheral vascular resistance accompanies decreased cardiac output. The causes of myocardial dysfunction in burn patients are not well understood; however, there are several theories as to the causes including those that propound the release of a substance from the burn wound itself called myocardial depressant factor and the release of oxygen free radicals from the ischemic myocardial tissues.

Administration of fluids dramatically improves the outcome of the burn patient. Fluid resuscitation will usually be initiated in adult patients with greater than 20 percent TBSA involvement, in the elderly with greater than 5 to 15 percent TBSA involvement, and in children with greater than 10 to 15 percent TBSA involvement (Gordon & Winfree, 1998). Children and the elderly are less able to tolerate the stress of injury. Volume replacement must be implemented very carefully in children and the elderly because they are very sensitive to volume. Children usually require more fluid than adults, averaging about 5.8 mL/kg percent TBSA burn (American Burn Association, 2001a). A pulmonary artery catheter may be used to monitor fluid status in the elderly.

Patients with thermal burns that involve a TBSA of greater than 40 percent may experience hypovolemic shock or burn shock. Chemical and vasoactive mediators produced as a result of burn injury cause arterial constriction initially, followed by vasodilation and increased capillary permeability. Vasodilation in combination with increased capillary permeability is referred to as a loss of capillary seal. The loss of capillary seal leads to

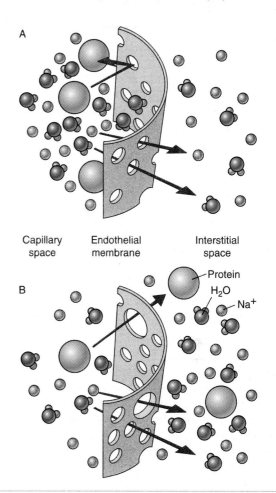

Figure 35–6 ■ Changes in capillary permeability determine extravascular fluid levels. *A.* Under normal conditions large molecules, such as proteins, are held in the capillary. When permeability of the capillary changes, such as in sepsis and ARDS, capillary permeability increases *B.* This allows proteins and other substances that normally control fluid movement to move into the interstitial space. The result is an increase in fluid outside the blood vessel. *(From Ahrens & Rutherford.* Essentials of oxygenation. *Copyright 1993. Jones and Bartlett Publishers, Sudbury, MA. www.jbpub.com. Reprinted with permission.)*

massive fluid and electrolyte shifts from intravascular spaces to the interstitium. Figure 35–6 illustrates fluid and protein loss as a result of increased capillary permeability. Hypovolemic shock is a complication of loss of capillary seal and other factors. Although the exact mechanisms for vascular and fluid changes are not well understood, the capillary seal is usually restored within 36 hours postinjury.

Restoration of intravascular volume by fluid resuscitation is a critical intervention for burn shock. The goal is to maintain vital organ perfusion without exacerbating tissue edema. A minimal mean arterial pressure (MAP) for the adult is 70 mm Hg (Kim et al., 2001). The patient's physiologic responses, such as urine output, adequate vital signs, appropriate mentation, capillary refill, and peripheral pulses, will guide fluid administration efforts. The best determinant of adequate fluid resuscitation (in the first 24 to 48 hours) is urine output as long as the patient is not receiving a medication that will cause diuresis (e.g., diuretics or mannitol) and does not have glucosuria (glucose in the urine causes an osmotic diuresis). After the initial resuscitation, urine output is not the best predictor of fluid status. Generally, in adults a urine output of 30 to 50 mL per hour must be maintained (Kim et al., 2001). For children, a urine output of 1 to 2 mL/kg per hour for children weighing less than 30 kg should be maintained (Merz et al., 2003). Laboratory values such as serum sodium concentration, serum and urine glucose concentrations, as well as body weight changes, clinical examination, and intake and output records are followed to best determine fluid replacement (American Burn Association, 2001a).

Fluids are infused at a steady rate by two large-bore (14 to 16 gauge) intravenous (IV) catheters placed through unburned skin if possible. If an IV catheter must be inserted into a burned area, the cannula is threaded in a long vein so that edema does not push the hub out and cause an infiltration (Weibelhaus & Hansen, 2001).

There are a number of formulas used to guide crystalloid fluid administration during the first 24 hours. Each formula will have to be modified according to the patient's response. One of the most frequent formulas used is the Parkland formula:

$$4 \text{ mL Ringer's lactate} \times \text{TBSA \% burned} \times \text{patient weight (kg)}$$

With the Parkland formula, one half of the amount is infused during the first 8 hours postinjury. This is followed by the last half during the next 16 hours. For example, using the Parkland formula, a patient weighing 68 kilograms who experiences a 50 percent TBSA burn would require 6,800 mL of IV fluids during the first 8 hours postinjury with a subsequent infusion of 6,800 mL during the next 16 hours. Urinary output trends are monitored to determine the adequacy of fluid replacement.

Fluid administration requirements are altered under certain circumstances. Patients with inhalation injuries in conjunction with thermal burns require increased amounts of fluid initially (up to 40 to 50 percent more) (Gordon & Winfree, 1998). Patients with electrical burns and associated trauma, extensive deep thermal burns, alcohol intoxication, those receiving delayed resuscitation (greater than 2 hours after the time of injury), or those with preexisting medical conditions (e.g., patients receiving diuretic therapy) may require increased amounts of fluid according to their physiological responses.

Isotonic crystalloid fluid are used for patients with less than 40 percent TBSA and no pulmonary injury (American Burn Association, 2001a). For patients with greater than 40 percent TBSA or pulmonary injuries, hypertonic saline can be used in the initial 8 hours, followed by lactated Ringer's solution. Although hypertonic saline is currently recommended (American Burn Association, 2001a), considerable controversy over its efficacy exists. Some studies have noted clinically important outcomes (Brown, 2002). For pediatric and elderly patients, a lower hypertonic concentration is used to prevent excessive sodium retention and hypernatremia. A combination of fluids are used for patients with major burns, young chil-dren, and those with burns combined with a severe inhalation injury. Dextrose solutions are not to be given because these solutions can cause osmotic diuresis, complicating fluid resuscitation (Weibelhaus & Hansen, 2001). All resuscitative formulas should be considered guidelines and should be individualized according to patient assessments. Burn resuscitation fluids should be used until the volume infused is maintaining proper urine output and is equal to the maintenance rate, which consists of the normal maintenance volume plus considerations for evaporative water loss.

Patients who have been exposed to electrical currents may have necrosis of the myocardium and may be predisposed to cardiac dysrhythmias, including sinus tachycardia, nonspecific *ST* or *T* wave changes, *QT* segment prolongation, ventricular ectopy, atrial fibrillation, a bundle branch block, ventricular fibrillation, varying degrees of heart blocks, supraventricular tachycardia, and asystole (Koumbourlis, 2002). Patients who experience lethal dysrhythmias (ventricular fibrillation or asystole) from electrical or lightning contact receive aggressive resuscitation because of the frequency with which these patients can be successfully resuscitated. Cardiac monitoring continues for at least 24 hours postinjury, even for patients having electrical contact who do not seem to have any obvious injury.

Peripheral Vascular

Peripheral vascular assessment of each extremity occurs in the initial assessment and is repeated every hour thereafter throughout the resuscitative phase. Each extremity is evaluated for color, temperature, pulses, capillary refill, sensation, pain, and motor movement. A doppler may be required to make a better assessment of peripheral pulses because edema can interfere with palpation. Increased pressure within the limb from edema can cause tissue ischemia. Elevating burned extremities above the level of the heart helps decrease edema. Jewelry and constricting clothing is removed as soon as possible. **Compartment syndrome** occurs when the tissue pressure within a muscle compartment exceeds microvascular pressure causing an interruption in perfusion at the cellular level.

Signs and symptoms of compartment syndrome include pain on passive stretching of the muscle, decreased sensation, weakness, swelling, and pain beyond that expected for the injury sustained. Current guidelines recommend that escharotomies be performed (1) when compartmental pressures are greater than 40 mm Hg (however, pressures between 25 and 40 mm Hg may cause muscle and nerve ischemia leading to consideration of escharotomies at lower pressures) and (2) if doppler pulses are absent in the major distal arteries or in the palmar or plantar arches (however, the presence of doppler pulses does not confirm adequate perfusion of the underlying structures) (American Burn Association, 2001b) as shown in Figure 35–7. Escharotomies are performed in a longitudinal fashion midlateral or midmedial in the supinated extremity

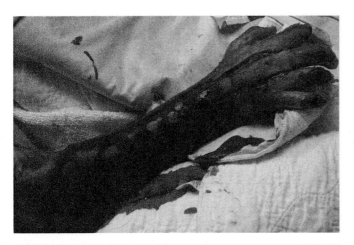

Figure 35–7 ▪ Escharotomy of the hand.

TABLE 35–3 Clinical Indicators of Inhalation Injury

- Facial burns with charred lips and tongue
- Carbonaceous sputum
- Wheezing or rhonchi on auscultation
- Stridor
- Cough
- Tachypnea
- Singed nasal hair
- Altered level of consciousness
- Injury in enclosed space
- History of flash burn
- Elevated carboxyhemoglobin levels
- Abnormal arterial blood gases

through the entire involved area (American Burn Association, 2001b). Continued close monitoring is necessary to ensure that the area was adequately released and that elevated pressures have not recurred.

Pulmonary

Alterations in pulmonary function can occur as part of the systemic response to burn injury or from direct inhalation injury. The systemic response to burn injury results in an increased systemic vascular resistance with a corresponding increase in pulmonary vascular resistance. This results in pulmonary edema from the increased capillary pressure and vasoconstriction of microcirculation. A decrease in pulmonary perfusion results in decreased diffusion of oxygen at the capillary level. Respiratory insufficiency can occur at two points postinjury: immediately during the resuscitation phase and 10 days to 2 weeks postinjury during the acute rehabilitation phase. Respiratory failure during the resuscitative phase is usually a result of inhalation injury, and failure in the acute rehabilitation phase is usually a result of infection.

Circumferential (or near circumferential) full-thickness burns to the chest can also cause alterations in pulmonary function. Full-thickness burns result in **eschar** formation, which is a tough, dry, inelastic wound that does not allow for adequate expansion of the chest. If these eschar chest wounds are circumferential, the patient cannot adequately expand the chest to ventilate effectively and respiratory distress will develop. **Escharotomy** incisions may be performed at the bedside to allow movement of the chest wall and to restore adequate ventilation.

An inhalation injury is suspected in the patient who presents with an altered level of consciousness or one from within a confined space in a burning environment. It is imperative to obtain information regarding the circumstances of the fire during the initial assessment. Inhalation injury occurs from chem-

ical and thermal mechanisms, such as gases, toxic fumes, or steam. The clinical indicators of inhalation injury are listed in Table 35–3. The composition and amount of the inhaled substance correlates with the severity of the injury. Inhalation injury will be discussed in reference to upper-airway injury (above the glottis, supraglottic), lower-airway injury (below the glottis, infraglottic), and carbon monoxide injury.

Upper-Airway Injury

Upper-airway injury refers to an injury that is supraglottic, resulting from either heat or chemicals dissolved in water. Heat causes an immediate injury to the mucosa. Thermal burns from hot air are usually isolated to the supraglottic (as opposed to the infraglottic) area because of the ability of the nasopharynx to absorb the heat and a reflex closure of the glottic opening when exposed to heat. Evaluation of patients with upper-airway burns may reveal facial burns, singed nasal hairs, erythema, swelling, tachypnea, dyspnea, hoarseness, a brassy cough or stridor, and ulceration, especially of the nasopharynx. Initial treatment for upper-airway injury is humidified 100 percent oxygen by a snugly fitting nonrebreather mask. Careful observation is necessary to identify impending airway obstruction. Once the tissues start to swell, patients can rapidly experience an airway occlusion. Patients with hoarseness, stridor, or pharyngeal burns are intubated and transferred to a burn center. Upper-airway edema peaks at 24 to 48 hours postinjury (Cioffi, 1998). If it is not contraindicated by concurrent trauma, the head of the bed is elevated to help reduce edema. Circumferential burns to the neck can also cause airway obstruction as a result of edema. These patients also require intubation.

Lower-Airway Injury

There is an increased mortality in patients who have an inhalation component to their injury. Lower-airway injury (infraglottic) is usually the result of toxic gases and chemicals contained in inhaled smoke. The inhaled smoke contains gaseous and chemical by-products of combustion. When these products come into contact with the pulmonary mucosa, a variety of things happen, such as irritation, an inflammatory reaction, or alkali or acid burns. The result is an ulceration of mucous membranes, edema, excessive secretions, decreased ciliary action, bronchospasms, inactivation of surfactant, and atelectasis, among other things. The end result is an airflow obstruction causing hypoxemia and pulmonary dysfunction. These patients develop respiratory failure and are prone to the development of pulmonary infections.

The onset of symptoms of lower-airway injury is unpredictable. Patients with lower-airway injury may present without symptoms to the emergency department. However, they also may present with the signs and symptoms for upper-airway injury, in addition to a cough, carbonaceous (sooty) sputum, signs of hypoxemia (agitation, anxiety, cyanosis, impaired mental status), chest tightness, flaring nostrils, grunting, crackles, rhonchi, or wheezing. If the potential for inhalation injury exists, the patient is monitored closely for at least 24 hours postinjury. Parenchymal lung injuries may take longer to evolve. Diagnostic tests for determining the effects and extent of inhalation injury include physical examination, arterial blood gases (partial pressure of oxygen may be normal initially), serial chest radiographs, fiber-optic bronchoscopy (to visualize tracheobronchial injuries), ventilation–perfusion scan (to identify small airway and parenchymal injuries), carboxyhemoglobin levels, and cyanide levels (American Burn Association, 2001c).

Treatment for lower-airway injury is supportive. Any patient with the potential for inhalation injury must receive high-flow humidified oxygen (100 percent by nonrebreather mask). Patients with severe inhalation injuries or impending respiratory failure must receive high-flow humidified oxygen while preparations for endotracheal intubation are made. Intubation is not performed prophylactically; however, there must be a low threshold for intubation if there is concern about progressive edema (American Burn Association, 2001d). Mechanical ventilation provides positive pressure ventilation, peak inspiratory pressures to below 40 cm H_2O, and allows for permissive hypercapnia (although this is contraindicated in the presence of closed-head injury) (American Burn Association, 2001d).

One of the major goals of nursing care is meticulous pulmonary toilet. Ensuring that the patient does the coughing and deep breathing exercises, turning the patient, suctioning, chest physiotherapy, and pharmacologic interventions will help achieve this goal. Repeated assessments of respiratory status and accurate documentation for other caregivers is necessary. Ventilatory support is tailored to each patient's needs, with the ultimate goal of improvement to a point such that support is no longer needed. Ensuring that the endotracheal tube is secured appropriately is very important, especially in children under the age of 8 because the endotracheal tube does not have a cuff. Accidental displacement of an endotracheal tube in a patient with airway edema can have catastrophic results. A fine balance must be made between tightly securing the airway and preventing pressure ulcers from the straps, which are especially difficult with facial burns and the resulting edema.

Carbon Monoxide Poisoning

Carbon monoxide (CO) poisoning is a chemical inhalation injury that has an action different from other inhaled chemicals. Carbon monoxide is a colorless, odorless gas that is a by-product of the combustion of organic material. CO is more than 200 times more likely to bind to hemoglobin than oxygen. In the presence of CO, hemoglobin becomes saturated with CO rather than oxygen. This results in hypoxemia. The diagnosis of CO poisoning is made by obtaining a history of exposure to by-products of combustion, especially in an enclosed space, and by drawing a serum **carboxyhemoglobin** level (percentage of CO bound to hemoglobin). CO poisoning represents a transport shock state (refer to Module 15).

Symptoms caused by CO poisoning are the result of exposure to low levels of CO for prolonged periods or from exposure to higher levels for a shorter duration. The severity of poisoning depends on several factors, including underlying health. The most common symptoms of carbon monoxide poisoning are headache, malaise, nausea, difficulties with memory, and personality changes, as well as gross neurologic dysfunction (Weaver, 1999). An elevated carboxyhemoglobin level confirms CO poisoning. Whereas carboxyhemoglobin levels may be greater than 70 percent, the carboxyhemoglobin level is not indicative of the level of neurological injury (Weaver, 1999).

The treatment for CO poisoning consists of the administration of high fractional concentrations of supplemental oxygen. Data indicate that early, aggressive hyperbaric oxygen therapy may decrease the negative sequelae of CO poisoning (Hampson et al., 2001). Serial carboxyhemoglobin levels are monitored to evaluate patient response to treatment. Pulse oximetry does not differentiate between hemoglobin saturated with oxygen and hemoglobin saturated with CO, so readings may be misleading.

In summary, the resuscitative phase lasts into 72 hours postburn. Cardiovascular and pulmonary complications that can occur after burn injury include myocardial dysfunction, hypovolemic shock, cardiac dysrhythmias, and compartment syndrome. Pulmonary complications include pulmonary edema, respiratory insufficiency, respiratory failure, inhalation injuries (upper and lower airways), and carbon monoxide toxicity. Astute nursing assessments help determine fluid requirements during this phase. Guidelines are individualized to meet patient needs. Nursing assessments are required for early detection of pulmonary compromise.

SECTION FOUR REVIEW

1. The resuscitative phase of burn injury occurs from the time of injury to
   A. 24 to 48 hours after injury
   B. 36 to 60 hours after injury
   C. 48 to 72 hours after injury
   D. 60 to 84 hours after injury

2. Critically burned patients are at high risk for which of the following complications during the resuscitative phase?
   A. burn shock
   B. neurogenic shock
   C. contractures
   D. myocardial infarction

3. Calculate the fluid resuscitation requirements for Mr. C using the Parkland formula. Mr. C has a 55 percent TBSA burn and weighs 75 kilograms. His requirements for the first 8 hours are
   A. 8,250 mL
   B. 16,500 mL
   C. 4,125 mL
   D. 12,375 mL

4. Patients exposed to electrical injuries are at risk for developing
   A. nonspecific *ST* wave changes
   B. *QT* segment prolongation
   C. ventricular ectopy
   D. all of the above

5. To detect compartmental syndrome in those with critical burns, assess for
   A. pain in extremity with exercise
   B. pain in extremity with passive movement
   C. contractures
   D. pallor in extremity

6. Treatment for carbon monoxide poisoning includes
   A. 100 percent O_2
   B. hypertonic saline
   C. keeping peak inspiratory pressure less than 40 cm H_2O
   D. pulmonary hygiene

Answers: 1. C, 2. A, 3. A, 4. D, 5. B, 6. A

SECTION FIVE: Resuscitative Phase: Neurological and Cognitive Effects

At the completion of this section, the learner will be able to discuss priority assessments and interventions during the resuscitative phase for the neurological effects and pain management for patients with burn injuries, identify stages of psychological adaptation following burn injury, and state an appropriate nursing intervention for each stage.

Neurological effects are common with electrical and lightning injuries. Neurological tissue offers low resistance to electrical currents and is easily damaged. The skull is a common entry site for electrical current. Respiratory paralysis can occur and loss of consciousness is frequent, especially with high-voltage injury, although it is usually transient. Patients may experience confusion, exhibit a flat affect, be unable to concentrate, or have short-term memory problems. Seizures, headaches, peripheral nerve damage, and loss of muscle strength may be seen. Long-term or permanent numbness, prickling, tingling, heightened sensitivity, or paralysis may also occur. Spinal cord injuries can occur with high-voltage injuries. The onset of clinical manifestations may be acute or delayed.

Pain

Burn injury cannot be discussed without considering the pain that accompanies the injury. Full-thickness burns are usually insensate, except for the edge of the wound where partial-thickness injury exists. Partial-thickness burns are exceptionally sensitive and painful even to an air current passing over them. Pain and anxiety can hinder a patient's recovery, so the relief of pain and anxiety are critical. Patients typically experience two types of physical pain after burn injury: (1) chronic pain from damaged tissue and (2) acute pain as a result of procedures, such as wound care, occupational therapy, and physical therapy. There are many analgesics that may be given; however, morphine and fentanyl are two of the most commonly used agents (Weibelhaus & Hansen, 2001). The intravenous route is preferred during the resuscitative phase because absorption from muscle is unpredictable as a result of vasoconstriction and edema. A self-report pain scale should be used to evaluate pain when possible, and medication should be given on a schedule, not as an intermittent dose.

Psychological Adaptation

Watkins and associates (1988) describe seven stages of psychological adaptation to burn injury. Patients move forward and backward through the stages of adaptation, and the stages frequently overlap. Stages of psychological adaptation, patient response, and nursing interventions appropriate for patients and families are outlined in Table 35–4.

Coping with a burn injury is complex and requires a multifaceted approach. Emotional support from family and friends can be very helpful to the patient. Distraction, imagery, self-hypnosis, information, and relaxation techniques can also help a patient to cope with the stress, pain, and anxiety that occur. Crisis intervention counseling immediately following an event may have positive long-term effects for some patients. Frequently, patients will need counseling into the long-term rehabilitation phase.

In summary, neurological difficulties experienced by burn patients during the emergent phase include altered levels of consciousness, acute pain, and suboptimal psychological adaptation. Nursing interventions to relieve pain and promote adaptation are important components of the nursing care plan.

TABLE 35–4 Stages of Psychological Adaptation Following Burn Injury

ADAPTIVE STAGE	PATIENT RESPONSE	NURSING INTERVENTIONS
Stage 1: Survival anxiety Patient is concerned about survival; fear of death prevails	Tremulousness, easy startle response, difficulty concentrating or following instructions, tearfulness, poor cooperation with treatments, social withdrawal, silence	Educate patient regarding extent of burn injury and most likely course for recuperation. Allow time for verbalization of fears, give reality-based responses.
Stage 2: The problem of pain Burn injuries can be extremely painful; patients focus on pain relief in this stage	Increased reports of pain, frequent requests for analgesia, poor cooperation with treatments, demanding and dependent behaviors	Assess and treat pain with pharmacologic and nonpharmacologic interventions.
Stage 3: The search for meaning During this stage the patient searches for a logical, understandable explanation for the injury	Repeated recounts of events preceding and during injury	Provide nonjudgmental listening and discussion to assist patient with finding acceptable answers. This is called "validation." If the patient does not successfully complete stage 3, posttraumatic stress disorder can occur.
Stage 4: Investment in recuperation Patients in this stage focus on understanding and participating in treatments necessary for obtaining daily life skills, such as walking, self-feeding, and grooming	Open interest in treatments; asks many questions; desires to complete tasks without assistance; high motivation; hostility if unsuccessful with tasks	Praise attempts for autonomous functioning. Orient to physical phenomena related to healing such as itching and decreased activity tolerance. Continue education on expected course of recovery.
Stage 5: Acceptance of losses Comprehension of long-term losses occur cognitively and emotionally	Sadness over losses exhibited by tearfulness, decreased appetite, social withdrawal, sleep disturbance, or anger	Allow time for discussion of feelings. Legitimize patient feelings (reassure that feelings are appropriate for loss). Encourage interactions with family and friends to provide evidence of worth despite injury. Depression can occur if acceptance does not take place.
Stage 6: Investment in rehabilitation Patients work on resuming own unique lifestyle	Interest in treatments; increased motivation; trial-and-error attempts to return to preburn functioning	Praise patient's efforts to adapt to injuries and manipulate environment to provide new ways of functioning.
Stage 7: Reintegration of identity Assessment of the cumulative effects of burn injury helps the patient cognitively and affectively define postburn "self"	Verbalizes perceptions of how functioning has changed from preburn norm	Acknowledge patient's view of self. Refrain from forcing the staff's expectations for those recovering from burn injury on patients.

Data from Watkins, P. N., Cook, E. L., May, S. R., & Ehleben, C. M. (1988). Psychological stages in adaptation following burn injury: A method for facilitating psychological recovery of burn victims. Journal of Burn Care & Rehabilitation, 9(4), 376–384.

SECTION FIVE REVIEW

1. In general, full-thickness burns are
   A. not painful
   B. mildly painful
   C. moderately painful
   D. extremely painful

2. During the survival-anxiety stage of psychological adaptation to burn injury (stage 1), patients typically
   A. recount events preceding the injury
   B. ask many questions
   C. fear death
   D. are highly motivated

3. During the resuscitative phase, patients with burn injuries experience which of the following types of pain?
   A. chronic pain from damaged tissue
   B. acute pain from wound care
   C. acute pain from occupational and physical therapy
   D. all of the above

Answers: 1. A, 2. C, 3. D

SECTION SIX: Resuscitative Phase: Metabolic and Renal Effects

At the completion of this section, the learner will be able to discuss priority nursing assessments and interventions during the resuscitative phase for gastrointestinal (GI), metabolic, and renal effects of burn injury.

Metabolic Effects

The metabolic changes that occur in the burn patient are related to the extent of injury. Initially, metabolism is depressed. Within a few days, when capillary wall integrity is restored and the patient becomes hemodynamically stable, marked hormonal changes occur resulting in a hypermetabolic state. Patients experience an increase in cardiac output, oxygen consumption, carbon dioxide production, caloric requirements, energy consumption, heart rate, respiratory rate, and body temperature. This hypermetabolic state will remain until the wounds close.

Nutritional requirements are strongly influenced by the metabolic response to stress. Adequate caloric intake is imperative for wound healing and maintaining the immune system. Multiple formulas exist for estimating caloric needs of burn patients. Energy requirements are assessed and formulas that calculate both energy and protein needs are used. Increased protein intake is needed to counteract the use of lean body mass and viscera as sources of protein in this hypermetabolic state.

Enteral nutrition is initiated early (within 24 hours post-injury) (American Burn Association, 2001e). Early nutrition reduces cumulative caloric deficits, stimulates insulin secretion, and conserves lean body mass (Gottschlich et al., 2002). Enteral nutrition is preferred over parenteral support when possible and should provide a calorie-to-nitrogen ratio of 110:1 for burns 20 percent or greater TBSA (American Burn Association, 2001e). Enteral feedings that are placed postpyloric can continue throughout the pre-, intra-, and postoperative periods. Nutritional status is closely monitored via clinical examination of wound healing, serial weights, prealbumin levels, and indirect calorimetry.

Evidence-Based Practice

- *Early wound excision and wound closure coupled with aggressive enteral nutritional support with high protein formulas do not prevent marked hypermetabolism that accompanies thermal injury (Noordenbos et al., 2000).*

- *Patient controlled analgesia (PCA) with fentanyl can be used for management of pain during dressing changes. The optimal PCA–fentanyl demand dose for adults with greater than 20 percent TBSA burn is 30 mcg after an initial loading dose of 1 mcg/kg and a lockout interval of 5 minutes (Prakash et al., 2004).*

- *Enteral glutamine supplements in adult burn patients reduces blood infections, prevents P. aeruginosa, and may decrease mortality rate (Garrel et al., 2003).*

- *The degree of muscle tissue damage in electrical burns corresponds with the initial excess of serum creatinine kinase levels (Kopp et al., 2004).*

Renal Effects

If a patient has experienced muscle damage from exposure to an electrical current or a crush-type injury, the urine may be a red to reddish-brown color. This discoloration is because of **myoglobin** in the urine. Myoglobin is released from damaged muscle tissue and can clog the renal tubules, causing renal failure, especially in the face of inadequate fluid resuscitation, shock, or acidosis (refer to Module 28). If myoglobin is present in the urine (**myoglobinuria**), adequate urine output (75 to 100 mL per hour in an adult) must be maintained (through IV fluid administration) to prevent myoglobinuric renal failure. This rate of urine output is maintained as long as the pigment is present. In addition to increasing the amount of fluids administered, alkalinization of the urine also prevents myoglobin from crystallizing in the tubules and causing an obstruction. The solubility of myoglobin increases in an alkaline environment, so maintaining alkaline urine will increase the rate of myoglobin clearance. By adding 50 mEq of sodium bicarbonate to each liter of intravenous fluids, a slight alkalinization of the blood is maintained (pH 7.45), ensuring that the urine is also alkaline (Cooper, 1998). An osmotic diuretic, such as mannitol, may be used to increase diuresis and promote the clearance of myoglobin.

In addition to myoglobin causing discoloration of the urine, hemoglobin released from damaged red blood cells can also cause red to reddish-brown urine. It is difficult to distinguish myoglobin from hemoglobin by looking at the urine, so until laboratory tests confirm the presence of one or both of these substances, treat all red to reddish-brown discoloration of the urine as if it were myoglobin. Both myoglobin and hemoglobin are excreted more readily if the urine pH is alkaline.

In summary, patients with burns require early initiation of nutrition, preferably enteral nutrition started within 24 hours postinjury. These patients are in a hypermetabolic state for a variety of reasons. Patients who have experienced muscle damage from exposure to an electrical current or a crush-type injury are at risk for developing myoglobinuria and renal failure. Fluid administration, diuretics, and administration of sodium bicarbonate IV solution help prevent this complication.

SECTION SEVEN: Overview of Burn Wound Healing and Initial Wound Care

At the completion of this section, the learner will be able to compare burn wound healing and wound healing from other injuries, and state the wound care priorities during the resuscitative phase. Before reading this section, it may be helpful to review normal wound healing as discussed in Module 34.

Wound Healing

The cellular and biochemical events that occur during the healing of burn injuries are similar to those that occur in the healing of other wounds. The major difference is that the phases of wound healing in the burn occur more slowly and last longer. Wound healing begins immediately after the injury occurs with the inflammatory response. The inflammatory phase lasts approximately 2 weeks, extending into the acute rehabilitative phase; thus, overall wound repair is delayed. Once the inflammatory phase is finished, the proliferative phase of healing begins, which lasts up to 1 month. During this phase, collagen synthesis, revascularization, and reepithelialization occur although at a slower rate than in wounds from other injuries. Collagen layers are not as organized as they are in other wounds,

which contributes to excessive scar tissue (Fig. 35–8). The maturation phase of wound healing follows the proliferative phase and can last 6 to 18 months or longer depending on the wound. New collagen layers are placed, strengthening the wound, whereas old collagen layers are broken down. Excessive deposits of collagen during this time will produce hypertrophic scars that are characteristic of deep partial- and full-thickness burns. Hypertrophic scars contract while maturing, which can lead to contractures. Wound contraction can produce both cosmetic and functional deformities.

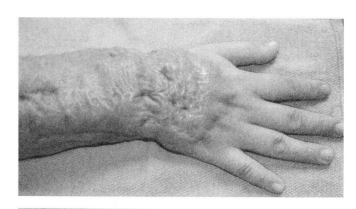

Figure 35–8 ■ Disorganized collagen layers lead to excessive scar tissue.

Initial Wound Care During the Resuscitative Phase

The first step in caring for the burn wound is to ensure the burning process has stopped. The longer the patient's skin is in contact with the burning agent and the higher the temperature, the deeper the cellular damage (Weibelhaus & Hansen, 2001). Clothing, jewelry, belts, or anything containing heat is removed from the patient (adhered clothing or tar is left in place and cooled with water because removing it will cause further damage to the skin). Dry chemicals are brushed from the patient (taking care not to contaminate the caregiver) and continuous water lavage is initiated.

The initial assessment of the burn wound takes place in the secondary assessment after the head-to-toe evaluation has been completed. Burned extremities are elevated above the level of the heart to decrease edema formation. The head of the bed is also elevated to reduce upper body and head edema if not contraindicated by trauma. Tetanus prophylaxis is administered.

Initial care of the burn wound depends on the severity of the burn. If the patient meets criteria for transfer to a burn cen-ter, the patient is covered with a clean, dry sheet. Care is taken to avoid hypothermia. If time permits, the wound is gently cleansed with sterile saline or a mild soap. Creams or ointments are not applied as removal of the substance is necessary on arrival to the burn center to evaluate the wound. This is a painful procedure, so unless directed to do so by the receiving physician, leave the wound clean and cover with a sheet. An escharotomy may be required for a circumferential burn. Definitive care of the wound begins once the patient has been admitted to the hospital, whether that is a burn center or a hospital with the ability to care for the burn injury effectively.

In summary, the cellular and biochemical events that occur during healing of burn wounds are similar to those that occur in the healing of other wounds except that the phases of burn wound healing occur more slowly and last longer. The burn wound assessment begins in the secondary assessment. Initial wound care includes removing clothing and chemicals. Initial wound management depends on the severity of the burn. Care is taken to prevent hypothermia. Creams and ointments are not applied during this phase. Wounds are cleaned and covered with a sheet until definitive care is rendered by a burn center.

SECTION SEVEN REVIEW

1. Initial evaluation of burn wounds takes place
   A. immediately on arrival
   B. at the end of the primary assessment
   C. at the end of the head-to-toe evaluation during the secondary assessment
   D. on admission to the burn center
2. You are the nurse in the emergency department caring for a patient with 60 percent TBSA burns. The helicopter is 20 minutes away, and the patient is to be transferred to a regional burn center. What is the

appropriate initial wound care management at this time?
   A. cleanse the wounds and cover the patient with a sheet
   B. place Neosporin ointment on all open burn wounds
   C. put antibiotic cream on all wounds
   D. cleanse the wounds and leave them open to air to dry out

Answers: 1. C, 2. A

SECTION EIGHT: Acute Rehabilitative Phase: Burn Wound Management

At the completion of this section, the learner will be able to describe burn wound management in the acute rehabilitative phase.

The acute rehabilitative phase of burn care occurs after the resuscitative phase, beginning 2 to 3 days postinjury and lasting until wound closure. The goals of burn wound management include prevention and control of infection, preservation of viable tissue, and promotion of wound closure with minimal side effects. Interventions aimed at supporting these goals include wound cleansing, debridement, topical antimicrobial therapy, and wound closure. Wound care must be performed in a warm environment to prevent hypothermia. Ideally, wound care is performed with the patient in isolation using aseptic technique.

In addition, appropriate analgesia must be given prior to initiation of the wound care. The analgesia must be given time to take effect.

Wound Cleansing

In-patient burn care begins with wounds being initially cleansed with water, known as hydrotherapy, and a mild soap to remove exudate and devitalized tissue. This can be accomplished (1) by showering if the patient is able, (2) by immersion in a tub if the burn is moderate in size, (3) by placing the patient on a table where the wounds are washed and rinsed with running water from spray hoses, or, if these methods are contraindicated, (4) wounds can be cleaned while the patient is in bed. Body hair within 2.5 cm of the wound is shaved. Once the wound has been cleaned, it must be debrided.

Wound Debridement

Wound **debridement** is the removal of debris and nonviable tissue from a wound. Wound debridement can be achieved mechanically, biologically, chemically, or surgically (refer to Module 34). Mechanical debridement includes hydrotherapy, or wound irrigation. With all methods of mechanical debridement, care is taken to avoid disrupting newly formed granulation tissue or epithelial buds in the healing wound. Wound irrigation and pulse lavage are easier to control than hydrotherapy, but all can cause disruption of newly formed tissue. The use of wet-to-dry dressings is no longer recommended because this is a nonselective form of debridement and causes harm to newly formed tissue and is also very painful. Biological debridement is the use of maggot therapy. This type of debridement is very beneficial because it only affects dead tissue.

Treatment of burn blisters, or **bullae,** is controversial. Fluid-filled blisters less than 2 cm in diameter are usually left intact. Blisters larger than 2 cm in diameter may be left intact, drained by aspiration using sterile technique, or opened and the loose skin removed.

Chemical debridement involves the application of an enzymatic or fibrinolytic preparation to the burn wound to digest necrotic tissue and hasten eschar separation. These products work best in a moist environment within a specific pH range, and they have no antimicrobial properties.

Surgical debridement is accomplished under anesthesia in the operating room and usually takes place within the resuscitative phase or within the first week postburn. There are two methods of burn wound excision: tangential excision and fascial excision. The method used depends on the depth and extent of burn. Tangential excision involves the shaving away of thin layers of eschar until viable tissue is exposed (Fig. 35–9). This method gives a better cosmetic result than fascial excision; however, significant blood loss may occur causing hypovolemia. Fascial excision involves removing nonviable tissue down to the fascial or subcutaneous planes. This method is often used for patients with a large component of full-thickness burns because it is less stressful. Fascial excision does not produce as good a cosmetic result as tangential excision; however, if the injury is such that the patient will not survive the stress of tangential excision, fascial excision is used.

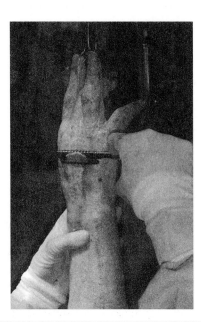

Figure 35–9 ▪ Tangential excision.

Topical Antimicrobial Therapy

Initially, the burn wound surface is colonized by gram-positive bacteria. After the first week, the surface becomes colonized by gram-negative bacteria. Burn wounds are typically treated with a topical antimicrobial to control bacterial proliferation. Systemic antibiotics are not used prophylactically but are initiated when there is clinical evidence of an infection and culture confirmation. To prevent the formation of antibiotic-resistant strains of bacteria, the physician chooses an antibiotic based on sensitivity results.

Application of the topical agent is performed using aseptic technique once or twice daily. Table 35–5 lists the topical agents most frequently used, and the advantages and disadvantages of each. The most frequently used topical antimicrobial is silver sulfadiazine, 1 percent (Silvadene).

Once the antimicrobial has been applied, an open- or closed-dressing technique is used. The open method leaves the antimicrobial-covered wound open to air. This method is primarily used for burns to the face and ears. The closed method involves the application of gauze dressings over the antimicrobial agent. Proponents of this method argue its superiority because it assists with debridement and protects granulation tissue and fragile epithelial buds, while also decreasing the evaporative fluid loss from the wounds. It is crucial that the dressings are applied with function in mind. The dressings should not be so tight as to restrict motion but tight enough to stay in place with motion. Disadvantages to the closed method include fewer opportunities to evaluate the wound.

Biological, synthetic, and biosynthetic materials act as skin substitutes and are used to temporarily cover a burn. The type used depends on the depth of the wound and the goal of therapy. Biological dressings obtained from animals (frequently pigs) are referred to as **xenografts** or **heterografts.** Biological dressings obtained from humans are called **allografts** or **homografts.** These grafts are used to cover clean, superficial partial-thickness burns; maintain a moist wound environment; protect the ungrafted wound; and test the receptivity of a wound to autografting (Carrougher, 1998). If an infection or necrotic tissue is present in the wound, the biological dressing will not adhere to the wound. If the biological dressing will not adhere, it is termed a failure and it is better to have failure of a biological dressing than failure of a valuable donor site autograft (Carrougher, 1998). Biological dressings are occlusive, so they also

TABLE 35-5 Topical Antimicrobials

MEDICATIONS	ADVANTAGES	DISADVANTAGES
1 percent silver sulfadiazine (Silvadene, SSD)	Bacteriostatic Broad spectrum Soothing Painless on application	Poor penetration through eschar Transient leukopenia Poor cartilage penetration Questionable use with sulfa allergy Delays partial-thickness wound healing
Mafenide acetate cream (Sulfamylon cream)	Bacteriostatic Broad spectrum Effective against *Pseudomonas* species Penetrates eschar Penetrates cartilage	Limited fungal coverage Painful on partial-thickness burns Metabolic acidosis
Mafenide acetate solution (5 percent Sulfamylon solution)	Same properties as above Used as an irrigant after debridement and postgraft Less painful on application than Sulfamylon cream Less incidence of metabolic acidosis than Sulfamylon cream	Same as above
0.5 percent silver nitrate solution	Broad spectrum, yeast and fungus No known bacterial resistance No pain	Poor penetration of eschar Staining Messy Leeching of electrolytes

Antimicrobial ointments (e.g., Bacitracin, Bactroban)	Bactericidal for a variety of gram-positive and
	    gram-negative organisms (exact coverage
	    depends on type of ointment)
		Poor eschar penetration
		Rash

Acticoat (Smith & Nephew)	Broad spectrum, fungus
	Can be left on wound up to 7 days
	When used over mesh grafts, found to increase
	    reepithelialization
		May be difficult to remove
		If minimal wound exudate, must be moistened with
		    water to release silver
		Unable to visualize wound daily

Aquacel Ag (Convatec)	Broad spectrum Can be left on wound up to 14 days Absorbent	Unable to visualize wound daily Shrinks and may expose burn

help to reduce pain. The functions of temporary wound coverings are listed in Table 35–6.

Synthetic materials such as thin film dressings are used to cover donor sites and to protect clean, small superficial wounds. These dressings are waterproof, transparent, reduce pain, and maintain moisture in the wound to promote healing. Examples include Opsite and Tegaderm (from 3M Medical Surgical Division, St. Paul, Minnesota).

Biosynthetic dressings may be used to cover clean, superficial partial-thickness burns, meshed autografts, donor sites, and exudative wounds (Carrougher, 1998). An example is Biobrane (from Dow Hickam Pharmaceuticals, Inc., Sugar Land, Texas). TransCyte (Smith & Nephew, Largo, Florida) is a human fibroblast-derived temporary skin. This product can be used on middermal to indeterminate-depth partial-thickness burns as well as middermal burns after debridement.

Nonbiologic dressings can be used on superficial and superficial partial-thickness burns to provide a moist wound healing environment (Johnson & Richard, 2003). Examples of nonbiologic dressings include Mepitel (from Molnlycke Health Care, Newton, Pennsylvania) and Xeroform (from Kendall Healthcare, Mansfield, Massachusetts) (Johnson & Richard, 2003).

TABLE 35-6 Functions of Temporary Wound Coverings

- Decrease bacterial proliferation
- Prevent desiccation
- Control heat loss
- Decrease protein loss in wound exudate
- Increase patient comfort
- Protect underlying structures
- Stimulate healing
- Prepare and test wound bed for autografting

VAC therapy (see Module 34) provides negative-pressure wound therapy to promote wound healing. The VAC promotes the formation of granulation tissue, decreases wound size, removes exudate, and provides an environment for moist wound healing. This treatment device is typically used postdebridement and the goals are to decrease the wound size prior to grafting or to promote graft take by placing it on top of skin grafts.

The use of growth factors is another type of topical wound covering that can be used on burn injuries to stimulate wound healing. This is a current area of great interest, but few studies have been performed to determine its efficacy.

Nursing care related to temporary wound coverings include the periodic application and removal of the dressing material. It is imperative that dressings and the surrounding tissues be inspected for dislodgment, suppuration, fluid accumulation, and cellulitis. Most of these complications can be prevented by stabilizing the temporary covering with gauze, keeping it dry, keeping out contamination, and preventing wound shearing. It is important to note that wounds are dynamic and the wound management choices should be based on the state of the wound at a particular time. Wounds are evaluated at regular intervals, and wound dressings are changed as indicated by the wound state.

Wound Closure

Superficial partial-thickness burns heal by spontaneous reepithelialization within 7 to 10 days. Small full-thickness burns may be allowed to heal on their own by granulation tissue formation and contraction. Full-thickness burns are typically grafted for several reasons, including better cosmetic appearance, improved function, decreased risk of infection, and for a faster return to before-burn lifestyle. A large TBSA or a deep partial-thickness burn will also be grafted because healing usually takes more than 14 days and because otherwise significant scarring will usually occur.

Early excision and closure of burn wounds have several advantages, including improved survival rates, reduction in the incidence of infection, reduced in-hospital stays, less grafting required, improved cosmetic results, and better functional outcome. Once the wound has been excised, steps are taken to close the wound. Small wounds are closed via primary wound closure. Larger wounds are closed via skin grafts, flaps, or skin substitutes. **Autografting** is the process of transplanting skin from one part of the body to fill in another part that has been injured, as in a burn wound. It is a method of permanent burn wound closure and uses either full-thickness or split-thickness skin grafts.

When the skin is removed down to the subcutaneous layer for grafting, it is termed a full-thickness skin graft (Fig. 35–10). Full-thickness skin grafts are used to cover areas that need the extra thickness and the durability it provides, such as the palm of the hand, or to cover a point that will be exposed to pressure, such as the elbow or the scapula. When removing skin for a full-thickness graft, the donor site becomes a full-thickness skin

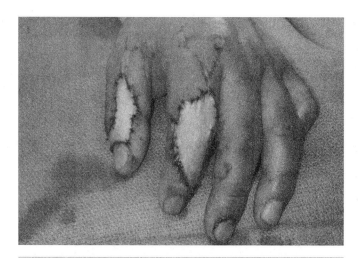

Figure 35–10 ■ Full-thickness skin grafts on fingers.

defect. This defect is closed by either suturing or by using a split-thickness skin graft. Full-thickness grafting is used for small areas only.

Split-thickness skin grafts (0.2 to 0.3 mm thick) are not as thick as full-thickness grafts (0.64 to 0.76 mm thick). The donor site is a partial-thickness skin defect that will heal within 10 to 14 days. A split-thickness skin graft can be used as a sheet graft or as a meshed graft. Skin is harvested from a donor site using an instrument called a dermatome. The sheet graft is taken from the donor site and placed on the recipient wound (Fig. 35–11). To make a meshed graft, the skin is taken from the donor site, then expanded using a mesh dermatome (Fig. 35–12). The mesh dermatome makes multiple small slits in the skin, giving it a netting type of appearance. A meshed graft is expanded to cover a larger area; however, the wider the mesh is spread, the

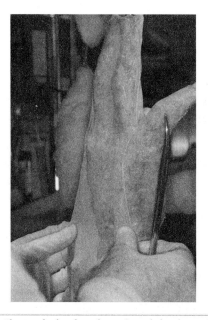

Figure 35–11 ■ Sheet graft taken from donor site and placed on recipient's wounds.

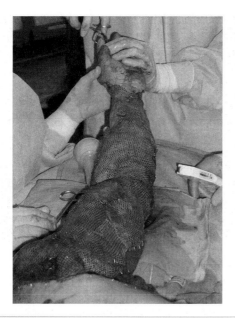

Figure 35–12 ■ Placement of mesh graft on arm.

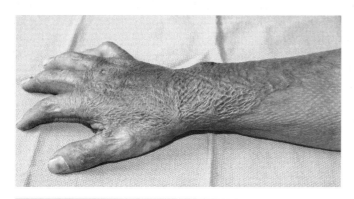

Figure 35–13 ■ Mature mesh graft on hand.

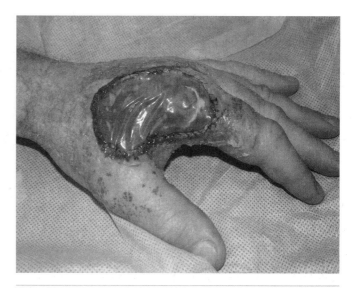

Figure 35–14 ■ Integra artificial skin.

longer it takes for wound closure which causes an increase in scar formation (Fig. 35–13). Sheet grafts usually provide a better cosmetic appearance than meshed grafts, so they are usually used for conspicuous sites such as the face and hands and are the most optimal coverage for burns less than 40 percent TBSA (Kagan & Smith, 2000).

Skin grafts adhere to the recipient site by the presence of serum between the two layers. Soon, a fibrin matrix forms, which better secures the graft to the donor site. Within 48 hours, the wound will take on a pink or red color, indicating graft vascularization has taken place.

Flaps are another choice for burn wound coverage. Flaps are typically chosen for full-thickness burns over tendons and subdermal burns where the wound either will not support skin graft coverage or would benefit from a thicker and more stable covering (Stefanacci et al., 2003).

Integra Artificial Skin (from Integra Lifesciences, Plainsboro, New Jersey) is composed of a dermal replacement layer consist-

ing of cross-linked bovine tendon collagen and chondroitin-6-sulfate covered with a silicone layer. Typically, Integra is applied to an excised full-thickness burn wound and it provides a structure for a more organized neodermis to form (Fig. 35–14). Approximately 2 to 3 weeks after placement, the silicone layer is removed and a thin epidermal autograft is placed. This product allows for early coverage of extensive full-thickness burns. Integra also has been used in conjunction with cultured skin substitutes. Further applications include the use of Integra for burn wound reconstruction (Heimbach et al., 2003).

Nursing care of the burn wound includes monitoring for infection. Signs of noninvasive wound infection include reddened wound edges, generalized wound discoloration, change in the color of the wound exudate, foul-smelling exudate, loss of a healed skin graft, and an increase in wound pain. Signs of more severe invasive infection include conversion of a partial-thickness injury to a full-thickness injury, early separation of eschar, small necrotic subcutaneous vessels, tenderness at the wound edges, and edema. Burn wounds are not always easy to evaluate, so surface wound culture and sensitivity tests are frequently done. A burn wound biopsy will be done if an infection is suspected.

The goals of burn wound management in the acute rehabilitative phase include prevention and control of infection, preservation of viable tissue, and promotion of wound closure. Interventions to achieve these goals include wound cleansing and debridement, topical antimicrobial therapy, and wound closure. Several methods of hydrotherapy can be used to clean wounds. Wound debridement may include mechanical, biological, chemical, or surgical techniques. Each has its own advantages and limitations. Burn wounds are treated with topical antibiotics based on culture and sensitivity results. Biological, synthetic, and biosynthetic materials act as skin substitutes and are used to cover a burn. Small wounds are closed via primary wound closure. Larger wounds are closed via skin grafts, flaps, or skin substitutes.

SECTION EIGHT REVIEW

1. Which of the following harms newly formed tissue and is, therefore, not recommended for burn wound care?
   A. sharp debridement
   B. biological debridement
   C. chemical debridement
   D. wet-to-dry dressings
2. Which topical antimicrobial is the most frequently used?
   A. Neomycin ointment
   B. silver nitrate
   C. silver sulfadiazine (Silvadene)
   D. mafenide acetate (Sulfamylon)
3. Biological dressings (allografts, homografts) are used to
   A. determine if the wound bed is adequate to accept an autograft
   B. maintain a moist environment
   C. protect the ungrafted wound
   D. all of the above

4. The process of transplanting skin from one part of the body to fill in another part that has been injured is known as
   A. xenograft
   B. autograft
   C. heterograft
   D. allograft
5. Nursing care related to temporary wound coverings includes inspection for
   A. dislodgement
   B. suppuration
   C. cellulits
   D. all of the above

Answers: 1. D, 2. C, 3. D, 4. B, 5. D

SECTION NINE: Acute Rehabilitative Phase: Psychosocial Needs

At the completion of this section, the learner will be able to describe expected behaviors, emotional status, and levels of pain for burn patients during the acute rehabilitative phase, as well as their related nursing actions.

Behavioral Changes

In addition to the physical recovery during the rehabilitative phase, emotional recovery also must continue. The ramifications of the injury begin to be apparent to the patient and the response by the patient is varied. The patient's ability to cope with the injury will, in part, depend on past coping mechanisms the patient has learned. These mechanisms may be healthy or they may be dysfunctional. Problems most frequently experienced by burn patients include anxiety, fear, grief, depression, sleep problems, acute stress disorder, and aggressive or regressive behavior.

Psychological and emotional problems can be minimized by involving the patient in self-care activities soon after the injury is sustained. Patients should participate in wound care, feeding, exercising, and administering medications as soon as they are physically and emotionally able to improve their self-concept. Fear and anxiety as a result of burn injury can be reduced with repeated and consistent explanations in appropriate terms. Visitors can help encourage a depressed burn patient. Visits by recovered burn patients allow patients to discuss their concerns with nonmedical personnel who can offer practical advice on coping with burns. This can be arranged by contacting the national office of the Phoenix Society, a support group for burn survivors. Contact information is as follows.

Phoenix Society for Burn Survivors

2153 Wealthy Street, SE, 215

East Grand Rapids, MI 49506

E-mail: info@phoenix-society.org

Phone: 800-888-2876; 616-458-2773

Fax: 616-458-2831

Pain

Pain experienced in the acute rehabilitative phase may be different from pain experienced in the resuscitative phase (Section Five). During the acute rehabilitative phase of burn injury, patients generally experience decreasing levels of pain. However, pain continues to occur as chronic or background pain and as procedural pain. Procedures, surgery, or infection delay the easement of pain. Interventions vary depending on the duration and severity of the pain. Patients achieve better pain control when they are given opportunities to choose interventions that work best for them. As the patient stabilizes and pain levels begin to decrease, oral analgesics are used with greater frequency. Nonpharmacologic interventions for pain control include, but are not limited to, biofeedback, hypnosis, relaxation therapy, and guided imagery. Thorough pain assessments are conducted on a regular basis throughout the patient's recovery and the plan of care adjusted accordingly.

In summary, behavioral changes and pain are common concerns during the acute rehabilitative phase of burn injury. Continued education and support coupled with a combination of psychological and pharmacological support assists the patient in coping with the effects of the burn injury. Thorough assessment coupled with consistent intervention diminish these complications.

SECTION NINE REVIEW

1. Members of the Phoenix Society are
   A. burn nurses
   B. safety educators
   C. social workers
   D. burn survivors
2. Which of the following statements is true about pain that burn patients experience?
   A. burn wounds are ischemic so burn patients do not experience pain
   B. pain generally increases during the acute rehabilitative phase
   C. patients achieve better pain control when they can chose the interventions that work best for them
   D. nonpharmacologic interventions have been tried in burn patients, but they do not work

Answers: 1. D, 2. C

SECTION TEN: Acute Rehabilitative Phase: Physical Mobility

At the completion of this section, the learner will be able to describe the goals, interventions, and health care professionals involved with promoting physical mobility during the acute rehabilitative phase of burn care.

Physical mobility problems during the acute rehabilitative phase of burn care are directly related to the healing wound itself and the therapeutic interventions necessary to maintain life and close the wound. During the resuscitative phase, excessive edema develops in the extremities, and mobility is restricted by edema and pain. Later, this problem is compounded by the limitations placed on mobility in an effort to protect healing grafts from shearing. As the wound heals, mobility is restricted by scar formation and contraction, and the desire to assume a position of comfort, which is typically flexed. Therefore, the treatment goals related to physical mobility during the acute rehabilitative phase include

- Return to preinjury level of functioning
- Maintenance of musculoskeletal, cardiopulmonary, and respiratory function
- Promotion of wound healing
- Protection of healing skin grafts
- Prevention of contractures and soft tissue deformity
- Preserving and strengthening extremity function
- Scar management
- Achievement of maximum functional recovery
- Education of patient and family

The burn team members most involved in this process are the physical therapist (PT), occupational therapist (OT), and nursing staff. The OT and PT develop a treatment plan, fashion appliances, and perform daily treatments. The role of the nursing staff is to integrate the treatment plan into their delivery of care and to provide assessment feedback to the OT and PT. In addition, nurses play a pivotal role in gaining patient compliance because they have continuous contact with the patient and many opportunities to support the patient toward these rehabilitation goals.

Interventions to promote physical mobility during the acute phase of burn care employ many techniques and devices. Antideformity positioning begins at the time of admission unless contraindicated by a complicating condition. Its use is imperative during the acute phase because it decreases scar contracture across flexor surfaces, which often compromises joint mobility and functional capacity (Table 35–7).

Joint function is also preserved by active and passive range of motion exercises. Mobility outcomes may actually be improved by the administration of analgesics prior to therapy and is discussed with the patient.

Early total body mobilization is important because of the impact that upright positioning has on cardiopulmonary functioning. Patients are assisted out of bed and ambulated early in the acute phase after hemodynamic stabilization. It is important to apply compression wraps on lower extremities before getting the patient out of bed, in order to prevent venous stasis. If extremities are not wrapped, the patient is at risk for capillary bed bleeding, which could cause autograft failure or delay donor-site healing. Venous pooling coupled with prolonged immobility also predisposes the patient to deep-vein thromboses. Wrapping the extremities continues until all wounds are healed and pressure garments are available.

In summary, the physical mobility needs of burn patients in the acute phase of burn injury are managed by an interdisciplinary team. Goals are focused on returning to preinjury level of functioning. Methods used include antideformity positioning, range of motion, and total body mobilization.

TABLE 35–7 Antideformity Positioning

BODY PART	SUPINE POSITION	PRONE POSITION
Head and neck	There should be no pillow allowed under the head to maintain at least a neutral head position. Slight extension of the neck is preferred.	A pillow is placed under the upper chest with a small roll under the forehead to maintain the neck position for ease of breathing.
Shoulders	Upper extremities should be placed so there is no more than 90 degrees of abduction at the shoulders in neutral horizontal abduction. This position will assist in preventing anterior and posterior axillary banding.	Upper extremities should be placed in no more than 90 degrees abduction.
Elbows	Elbows should be fully extended. Patients will experience decreased personal independence in activities of daily living if the elbow is allowed to tighten in a flexed position. Flexion is easier to regain than extension owing to the greater strength of the flexor muscle groups.	Elbows may be moved from full extension to 40 degrees flexion for brief periods of time as a position change.
Ankles	Neutral position of dorsiflexion/plantar flexion and inversion/eversion should be maintained. Heels should be kept free from pressure.	A space should be maintained between the foot of the bed and the end of the mattress so that the feet may hang off the end of the bed in a neutral position at the ankle.

SPECIAL CARE AREAS	
Wrist and hand	In supine or prone positions the hands should be splinted with 90 degrees flexion at the MCP joints with the fingers in full extension. The thumb web space should be preserved and the wrist held at 30 to 40 degrees extension. This functional positioning will prevent deformities which are difficult to treat and limit patient activities.
Hips	In both supine and prone positions, the hips should be maintained in neutral or slight extension. Fifteen degrees of abduction is advisable. Prevention of hip flexion contractures is important to facilitate early ambulation.

Adapted from Harden, N. G., & Luster, S. H. (1991). Rehabilitation considerations in the care of the acute burn patient. Critical Care Nursing Clinic in North America, *3(2), 245–253, with permission from Elsevier.*

SECTION TEN REVIEW

1. Antideformity positioning should begin
   A. after skin grafting
   B. after the patient can walk again
   C. at the time of admission
   D. on discharge from the high-acuity area
2. Which nursing action is MOST important in the prevention of autograft failure secondary to capillary bed bleeding?
   A. applying compression wraps to extremities
   B. encouraging high vitamin K intake
   C. monitoring prothrombin time/partial thromboplastin time (PT/PTT) and INR lab values
   D. maintaining the patient on bedrest
3. Treatment goals related to physical mobility during the acute rehabilitative phase include
   A. return to preinjury functioning
   B. promotion of wound healing
   C. scar management
   D. all of the above

Answers: 1. C, 2. A, 3. D

SECTION ELEVEN: Long-Term Rehabilitative Phase

At the completion of this section, the learner will be able to discuss nursing interventions related to physical conditioning, protection of new skin, scar management, and psychosocial adjustment during the long-term rehabilitative phase of burn care.

Traditionally, the rehabilitative phase of burn care was thought to begin at the time that all wounds were healed and continue throughout the patient's life span. From this paradigm it would seem that the rehabilitative phase would not fall into the realm of high-acuity nursing. However, it is important to recognize that preventive rehabilitative interventions actually begin during the resuscitative phase—which directly involves high-acuity nurses.

Physical Conditioning

Interventions during the rehabilitative phase are focused on physical conditioning, care of healing skin, and support of psychosocial adjustment. Physical conditioning during the rehabilitative phase moves beyond range of motion exercises and begins to address aerobic endurance and muscle strength. This process begins in the burn unit but is mainly accomplished after discharge.

Care of Healing Skin

Interventions related to the care of healing skin include protection of newly formed epithelium, scar management, and prevention of joint contractures. The epithelium over healing burn wounds is extremely fragile. Daily skin care includes cleansing with a mild soap and generous application of a high-quality emollient. Patients are instructed to apply this emollient several times a day because their sebaceous glands have been destroyed in the burning and grafting process. The skin is protected from mechanical traumas, such as shearing and pressure. Finally, patients are instructed to protect their scar from sun exposure for 1 year or until the scar turns silvery white. Otherwise, the scar will "tan" and remain permanently pigmented, leaving the patient with a less satisfactory cosmetic result.

Scar management is achieved by the wearing of compression garments (Fig. 35–15). These garments are custom made and costly. The constant pressure from the garment assists in the remodeling of irregular collagen into a more parallel pattern to improve both function and appearance. Because hypertrophic scars are also hypervascular, pressure therapy also may help to reduce local blood supply, thereby improving the scars' appearance. Patient compliance is difficult to obtain because the garments are hot, difficult to put on, and require continuous wearing (except when bathing). Compression garments are worn until scars are mature as evidenced by a flat, white, and avascular appearance, which is usually achieved in 12 to 18 months.

Patients with burn wounds over a joint are at risk for future joint contracture. Preventive measures include compression garments, night splinting, silicone, serial splinting/casting, and range of motion exercises. Should a contracture and functional deficit occur, surgical intervention may be necessary to regain full mobility.

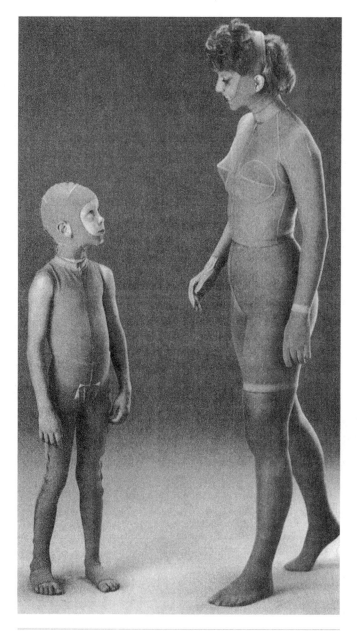

Figure 35–15 ■ Jobst compression garments.

Psychosocial Adjustment

Psychosocial adjustment is a major task of the rehabilitative phase. During this time, patients begin to renew their interests in the outside world, invest in their rehabilitation, and reintegrate their identities. Burn unit nurses may witness some of these behaviors, but the majority of the behaviors occur after discharge. The burn team is challenged to find appropriate community resources for discharged patients as they adapt to postburn alterations in appearance, level of physical functioning, and role concept. For example, patients with facial burns often struggle with their altered body images and have difficulty resuming preburn lifestyle. Therefore, it may be helpful to refer

these patients to a licensed aesthetitian familiar with scar therapy and camouflage makeup techniques. The Phoenix Society maintains a registry of these professionals and can assist with appropriate referrals.

In summary, the rehabilitative phase of burn care begins during the resuscitative phase and continues for a lifetime. Nursing care during this phase is focused on physical conditioning, care of healing skin, and support of psychosocial adjustment. The high-acuity nurse may not witness the resolution of these issues because they often occur after discharge. However, it is the nurse's responsibility to provide patients with resources to facilitate their reentry into society.

SECTION ELEVEN REVIEW

1. Rehabilitative interventions begin during which phase of burn care?
   A. resuscitative
   B. acute rehabilitative
   C. long-term rehabilitative
   D. transitional
2. Pressure garments improve immature scars by
   A. thinning hypertrophic epithelium
   B. remodeling irregular collagen
   C. reducing skin friction
   D. increasing arterial blood flow

3. In relation to psychological adjustment, which behavior is MOST likely to occur in the long-term rehabilitative phase?
   A. survival anxiety
   B. searching for meaning
   C. adaptation to severe pain
   D. reintegration of identity

Answers: 1. A, 2. B, 3. D

 POSTTEST

1. The elderly are prone to burn injuries because they
   A. have impaired senses
   B. have decreased reaction times
   C. tend to incorrectly assess risk
   D. all of the above
2. Which of the following structures is the most resistant to electrical current?
   A. skin
   B. nerves
   C. blood vessels
   D. muscles
3. Using the Lund and Browder Chart, what is the percentage of burn to an adult patient with burns to his anterior head, neck, and trunk?
   A. 13 percent
   B. 22 percent
   C. 15 1/2 percent
   D. 18 1/2 percent
4. Painful wounds that blanch on palpation and have large blisters are classified as
   A. full-thickness burns
   B. superficial partial-thickness burns
   C. deep partial-thickness burns
   D. first-degree burns
5. Using the American Burn Association's criteria, which of the following conditions would warrant admission to a burn center?
   A. full-thickness burn, less than 5 percent TBSA
   B. first-degree burn, 90 percent TBSA
   C. deep partial-thickness burn, entire face
   D. superficial partial-thickness burn, 10 percent

6. Which pulmonary tests are indicated to assess inhalation injury?
   A. electrocardiogram, thallium
   B. arterial blood gases, bronchoscopy
   C. serum potassium, sodium levels
   D. pulmonary angiograms, hemoglobin levels
7. Patients experiencing full-thickness burns involving the entire circumference of an extremity require frequent peripheral vascular checks to detect
   A. ischemia
   B. adequate wound healing
   C. arteriosclerotic changes
   D. hypothermia
8. Top treatment priorities during the resuscitative phase of care include
   A. obtaining lab work to assess pulmonary status
   B. flushing the skin with cool water for 60 minutes
   C. maintaining airway, breathing, and circulation
   D. starting intravenous fluids
9. Which of the following is the most important to monitor during fluid resuscitation?
   A. hemoglobin
   B. blood pressure
   C. thirst
   D. urine output
10. The medication given most frequently for relief of pain to the burn patient is
    A. midazolam
    B. meperidine
    C. methadone
    D. morphine sulfate

11. The first stage of psychological adaptation following burn injury is
    A. survival anxiety
    B. search for meaning
    C. investment in recuperation
    D. anger
12. The hypermetabolic state of burn injury is characterized by
    A. decreased cardiac output, tachycardia
    B. increased cardiac output, increased oxygen consumption
    C. decreased caloric requirement, tachycardia
    D. increased heart rate, decreased carbon dioxide production
13. Myoglobinuria can be treated with
    A. increasing amount of IV fluids
    B. slight alkalinization of the blood
    C. osmotic diuresis
    D. all of the above
14. The major difference between burn wound healing and wound healing from other injuries is that burn wounds
    A. do not go through an inflammatory phase
    B. do not go through a proliferative phase
    C. do not mature
    D. have the same phases, but occur more slowly and last longer
15. Until a transfer to a burn center, the nurse should
    A. debride all wounds as soon as possible
    B. place ointment on the wounds as soon as possible
    C. clean all wounds with sterile saline
    D. prepare for an escharotomy
16. The surgical procedure used to shave thin layers of eschar until viable tissue is exposed is called
    A. tangential excision
    B. fascial excision
    C. eschar excision
    D. escharotomy
17. Which of the following topical antimicrobials have poor penetration through eschar?
    A. Silvadene
    B. 0.5 percent silver nitrate
    C. Bacitracin
    D. all of the above
18. Psychological and emotional problems that occur during the acute rehabilitative phase can be minimized by
    A. involving the patient in self-care activities soon after injury
    B. giving the patient sedatives
    C. keeping the patient from negative interactions
    D. not letting the patient see himself or herself in a mirror
19. Antideformity positioning
    A. decreases deep vein thrombosis formation
    B. decreases scar contractures across flexor surfaces
    C. increases deep vein thrombosis formation
    D. increases scar contractures across flexor surfaces
20. Patients require emollient application several times a day to
    A. prevent wound infection
    B. keep skin moist because sebaceous glands are destroyed
    C. protect the skin from sheering injuries when moving in bed
    D. protect the skin from sun exposure

POSTTEST ANSWERS

Question	Answer	Section
1	D	One
2	A	One
3	B	Two
4	B	Two
5	C	Three
6	B	Four
7	A	Four
8	C	Four
9	D	Four
10	D	Five

Question	Answer	Section
11	A	Five
12	B	Six
13	D	Six
14	D	Seven
15	C	Seven
16	A	Eight
17	D	Eight
18	A	Nine
19	B	Ten
20	B	Eleven

REFERENCES

American Burn Association. (1999). Burn unit referral criteria. Available at: *http://www.ameriburn.org*. Accessed June 5, 2004.

American Burn Association. (2000, August 7). Burn incidence and treatment in the US: 2000 Fact Sheet. Available at: *http://www.ameriburn.org/pub/BurnIncidenceFactSheet.htm*. Accessed May 30, 2004.

American Burn Association. (2001a). Burn shock resuscitation: Initial management and overview. *Journal of Burn Care & Rehabilitation, 22* (suppl), 27S–37S.

American Burn Association. (2001b). Escharotomy. *Journal of Burn Care & Rehabilitation, 22* (suppl), 53S–58S.

American Burn Association. (2001c). Inhalation injury: Diagnosis. *Journal of Burn Care & Rehabilitation, 22* (suppl), 19S–22S.

American Burn Association. (2001d). Inhalation injury: Initial management. *Journal of Burn Care & Rehabilitation, 22* (suppl), 23S–26S.

American Burn Association. (2001e). Initial nutritional support of burn patients. *Journal of Burn Care & Rehabilitation, 22* (suppl), 59S–66S.

Andrews, K., Mowlavi, A., & Milner, S. (2003). The treatment of alkaline burns of the skin. *Plastic & Reconstructive Surgery, 111*, 1918–1921.

Biem, J., Koehncke, N., Classen, D., & Dosman, J. (2003). Out of the cold: Management of hypothermia and frostbite. *Canadian Medical Association Journal, 168*, 305–311.

Brown, M. D. (2002). Hypertonic versus isotonic crystalloid for fluid resuscitation in critically ill patients. *Annals of Emergency Medicine, 40*, 113–114.

Carrougher, G. I. (1998). Burn wound assessment and topical treatment. In G. J. Carrougher (Ed.), *Burn therapy and care* (pp. 133–165). St. Louis: C. V. Mosby.

Cioffi, W. G. (1998). Inhalation injury. In G. J. Carrougher (Ed.), *Burn therapy and care* (pp. 35–60). St. Louis: C. V. Mosby.

Cooper, M. A. (1998). Electrical and lightning injuries. In P. Rosen & R. Barker (Eds.), *Emergency medicine concepts and clinical practice* (4th ed., pp. 1010–1022). St. Louis: C. V. Mosby.

Garrel, D., Patenaude, J., Nedelec, B., et al. (2003). Decreased mortality and infectious morbidity in adult burn patients given enteral glutamine supplements: A prospective, controlled, randomized clinical trial. *Critical Care Medicine, 31*, 2555–2560.

Gordon, M. D., & Winfree, J. H. (1998). Resuscitation after a major burn. In G. J. Carrougher (Ed.), *Burn therapy and care* (pp. 107–132). St. Louis: C. V. Mosby.

Gottschlich, M. M., Jenkins, M. E., Mayes, T., Khoury, J., Kagan, R. J., & Warden, G. D. (2002). An evaluation of the safety of early vs. delayed enteral support and effects on clinical, nutritional, and endocrine outcomes after severe burns. *Journal of Burn Care & Rehabilitation, 23*, 401–415.

Hampson, N. B., Mathieu, D., Piantadosi, C. A., Thom, S. R., & Weaver, L. K. (2001). Carbon monoxide poisoning: Interpretation of randomized clinical trials and unresolved treatment issues. *Undersea and Hyperbaric Medicines, 28*, 157–164.

Heimbach, D. M., Warden, G. D., Luterman, A., et al. (2003). Multicenter postapproval clinical trial of Integra dermal regeneration template for burn treatment. *Journal of Burn Care & Rehabilitation, 24*, 43–48.

Johnson, R. M., & Richard, R. (2003). Partial-thickness burns: Identification and management. *Skin & Wound Care, 16*, 178–186.

Kagan, R. C., & Smith, S. C. (2000). Evaluation and treatment of thermal injuries. *Derm Nursing, 12*, 334–350.

Kim, D. E., Phillips, T. M., Jeng, J. C., et al. (2001). Microvascular assessment of burn depth conversion during varying resuscitation conditions. *Journal of Burn Care & Rehabilitation, 22*, 406–416.

Kopp, J., Loos, B., Spilker, G., et al. (2004). Correlation between serum creatinine kinase levels and extent of muscle damage in electrical burns. *Burns, 30*, 680–683.

Koumbourlis, A. C. (2002). Electrical injuries. *Critical Care Medicine, 30* (suppl), S424–S430.

McCampbell, B., Wasif, N., Rabbitts, A., Staiano-Coico, L., Yurt, R. W., & Schwartz, S. (2002). Diabetes and burns: Retrospective cohort study. *Journal of Burn Care & Rehabilitation, 23*, 157–166.

Merz, J., Schrand, C., Mertens, D., Foote, C., Porter, K., & Regnold, L. (2003). Wound care of the pediatric burn patient. *AACN Clinical Issues, 14*, 429–441.

Noordenbos, J., Hansbrough, J. F., Gutmacher, H., Dore, C., & Hansbrough, W. B. (2000). Enteral nutritional support and wound excision and closure do not prevent postburn hypermetabolism as measured by continuous metabolic monitoring. *Journal of Trauma, 49*, 667–671.

Prakash, S., Fatima, T., & Pawar, M. (2004). Patient controlled analgesia with fentanyl for burn dressing changes. *Anesthesia & Analgesia, 99*, 552–555.

Redlick, F., Cooke, A., Gomez, M., Banfield, J., Cartotto, R. C., & Fish, J. S. (2002). A survey of risk factors for burns in the elderly and prevention strategies. *Journal of Burn Care & Rehabilitation, 23*, 351–356.

Stefanacci, H. A., Vandevender, D. K., & Gamelli, R. L. (2003). The use of free tissue transfers in acute thermal and electrical extremity injuries. *Journal of Trauma, Infection & Critical Care, 55*, 707–712.

Thompson, J. T., Meredith, J. W., & Molnar, J. A. (2002). The effect of burn nursing units on burn wound infections. *Journal of Burn Care & Rehabilitation, 23*, 281–286.

Watkins, P. N., Cook, E. L., May, S. R., & Ehleben, C. M. (1988). Psychological stages in adaptation following burn injury: A method for facilitating psychological recovery of burn victims. *Journal of Burn Care & Rehabilitation, 9*, 376–384.

Weaver, K. L. (1999). Carbon monoxide poisoning. *Critical Care Clinics, 15*, 297–317.

Weibelhaus, P., & Hansen, S. L. (2001). Managing burn injuries. *Dimensions of Critical Care Nursing, 20*(4), 2–9.

Trauma

Michelle Willis

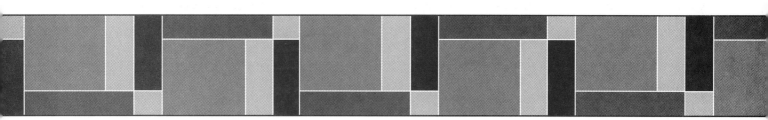

1. Define injury, potential mechanisms of injury, and risk factors that influence injury patterns.

2. Define the forces associated with blunt trauma and apply these concepts to the clinical assessment of a patient with blunt trauma.

3. Define the forces associated with penetrating trauma and apply these concepts to the clinical assessment of a patient with penetrating trauma.

4. Translate the mechanism of injury into potential injury patterns manifested by the patient for both blunt and penetrating injuries.

5. State clinical conditions that mediate a patient's response to injury, including underlying medical conditions, substance abuse, and physiological alterations including pregnancy and advancing age.

6. Identify the clinical assessment format used to identify life-threatening injuries during the primary survey.

7. Discuss the components of the secondary survey and the suggested format for conducting the secondary survey.

8. Describe the trimodal distribution of trauma-related mortalities and how this is integrated into clinical assessment.

   ■ Discuss important nursing responsibilities during the trauma resuscitation phase.

   ■ Compare and contrast various end points of traumatic shock resuscitation.

9. Describe basic principles of collaborative management for injuries to the chest, abdomen, and pelvis.

10. Cluster patient symptoms and derive nursing diagnoses appropriate for the patient with traumatic injuries.

11. Link posttrauma complications with physiology of a traumatic injury and preexisting risk factors.

   ■ Discuss interventions to prevent complications of traumatic injury.

This self-study module is intended to facilitate the learner's understanding of trauma. Focused attention is given to mechanism of injury for both blunt and penetrating trauma as an assessment factor to raise the learner's index of suspicion for certain injuries. The module is composed of 11 sections. Sections One through Four focus on mechanism of injury and kinematics of trauma. Section Five presents specific clinical and age-related variances that may mediate injury response. Sections Six and Seven focus on the trauma assessment and resuscitative principles based on primary and secondary assessments. Section Eight summarizes key points in the mediation of life-

threatening injury related to trauma with a brief discussion on traumatic shock. Section Nine discusses the management of the patient with traumatic injuries to the chest, abdomen, and pelvis. Section Ten examines nursing care of the trauma patient, and Section Eleven addresses trauma sequelae. Each section includes a set of review questions to help the learner evaluate his or her understanding of the section's content before moving on to the next section. All Section Reviews and the module Pretest and Posttest include answers. It is suggested that the learner review those concepts answered incorrectly in the review questions before proceeding to the next section.

PRETEST

1. The most common cause of injury is
   A. falling
   B. motor vehicle crashes
   C. gunshot wounds
   D. near drowning
2. The typical profile of a trauma victim would be
   A. male, 15 to 24 years of age, intoxicated
   B. female, 15 to 24 years of age, intoxicated
   C. female, 24 to 32 years of age, intoxicated
   D. male, 24 to 32 years of age, not intoxicated
3. The most common force associated with blunt trauma is
   A. acceleration/deceleration
   B. compression
   C. shearing
   D. axial loading
4. The best definition of tensile forces is
   A. forces opposing one another across a plane
   B. the squeezing or compartmentalization of tissue
   C. forces precipitating laceration, avulsion
   D. forces causing tissues to stress and extend
5. The process of temporary displacement of tissue forward and laterally by a penetrating missile is called
   A. tensile forces
   B. cavitation
   C. yaw
   D. tumbling
6. The extent of cavitation and tissue deformation produced by a missile is determined by
   A. yaw
   B. tumbling
   C. missile caliber and velocity
   D. all of the above
7. Secondary missiles often are created with penetrating trauma involving
   A. teeth and bone
   B. brain and soft tissue
   C. abdominal organs and vessels
   D. great vessels and brain
8. The most frequently seen pattern of injury for a pedestrian child hit by an automobile is
   A. fractures of femur, tibia, and fibula on side of impact
   B. fracture of femur, chest injury, and injury to contralateral skull
   C. pelvic fractures, compression fractures
   D. fractured spleen or liver, upper extremity fractures
9. An unrestrained driver is likely to have injuries to the
   A. head
   B. ribs
   C. small bowel
   D. all the above
10. Cocaine is a
    A. central nervous system depressant
    B. sympathomimetic
    C. hallucinogenic
    D. antidepressant
11. Which of the following statements is true about trauma and the elderly?
    A. they have a high incidence of rib fractures
    B. head injuries are common
    C. shock is difficult to assess
    D. all of the above
12. The immediate nursing intervention for the hypotensive pregnant trauma patient should be
    A. turning the patient to the right lateral decubitus position
    B. turning the patient to the left lateral decubitus position
    C. administering high-flow oxygen
    D. positioning the patient in Trendelenburg position
13. Ordered priorities in the primary survey are
    A. disability, airway, breathing
    B. cervical spine immobilization, circulation, breathing
    C. hemorrhage, fractures, chest trauma
    D. airway, breathing, circulation, disability, and exposure
14. During the primary survey, when assessing the "D" component, you would assess
    A. ability to move extremities
    B. neurologic status
    C. breath sounds
    D. dyspnea
15. The goal of airway management during the primary survey is optimization of ventilation and oxygenation while also
    A. protecting the cervical spine
    B. establishing IV access
    C. inserting an oral airway
    D. controlling bleeding
16. Key assessment techniques used in the secondary survey include all of the following except:
    A. palpation
    B. inspection
    C. x-rays
    D. auscultation
17. The distribution of trauma-related mortalities is
    A. modal
    B. bimodal
    C. trimodal
    D. quasimodal
18. After loss of up to 15 percent of circulating blood volume, a patient would most likely demonstrate
    A. hypotension
    B. tachycardia
    C. tachypnea
    D. none of the above

19. Interventions that may be completed during the resuscitative phase include
    A. insertion of a Foley catheter
    B. cutting clothes off for better exposure
    C. turning the patient to examine for injuries to the back
    D. assessing the airway
20. Trachea diplaced from midline, absent breath sounds, and respiratory distress are signs of
    A. pulmonary contusions
    B. flail chest
    C. tension pneumothorax
    D. open pneumothorax
21. The most frequently injured organ in the abdomen is the
    A. liver
    B. spleen
    C. pelvis
    D. small intestine
22. Perianal ecchymosis, pain with palpation to the iliac crests, and hematuria are signs of
    A. bladder rupture
    B. liver laceration
    C. splenic laceration
    D. pelvic fracture

23. Which of the following data suggests the presence of life-threatening injury?
    A. absent breath sounds
    B. paradoxical chest wall movement
    C. deviated trachea
    D. all of the above
24. Which of the following is a key assessment finding that helps to differentiate spinal shock from hypovolemia?
    A. bradycardia
    B. tachycardia
    C. hypotension
    D. pulmonary edema
25. Which of the following contributes the greatest to the development of posttrauma complications?
    A. hypoperfusion
    B. delay in supporting nutrition
    C. infection
    D. vasoconstriction

Pretest Answers: 1. B, 2. A, 3. A, 4. D, 5. B, 6. D, 7. A, 8. B, 9. D, 10. B, 11. D, 12. B, 13. D, 14. B, 15. A, 16. C, 17. C, 18. D, 19. A, 20. C, 21. B, 22. D, 23. D, 24. A, 25. A

GLOSSARY

acceleration   An increase in the rate of velocity or speed of a moving body.

blunt trauma   Injury without interruption of skin integrity.

cavitation   Creation of a temporary cavity as tissues are stretched, compressed, and displaced forward and laterally, creating a tract from a penetrating missile.

compression   The process of being pressed or squeezed together with a resulting reduction in size or volume.

cricothyroidotomy   A surgical airway created by division and cannulation of the trachea between the cricoid and thyroid cartilage.

deceleration   A decrease in the rate of velocity or speed of a moving body.

exsanguination   The most extreme form of hemorrhage, with an initial loss of blood volume of 40 percent and a rate of hemorrhage exceeding 250 mL per minute.

penetrating trauma   The result of the transmission of energy from a moving object into the body tissue as the object disrupts the integrity of the skin and the underlying structures.

shearing   Structures sliding in opposite directions causing a tearing or degloving type of injury.

tensile forces   Forces that cause tissues to stretch or extend.

tracheostomy   A surgical airway created by cutting into the trachea below the cricothyroid membrane.

ABBREVIATIONS

ARDS	Acute respiratory distress syndrome	**DIC**	Disseminated intravascular coagulation
ATP	Adenosine triphosphate	**ETOH level**	Ethanol level
BAC	Blood alcohol concentration	**FIO$_2$**	Fraction of inspired oxygen
CO	Cardiac output	**GCS**	Glasgow Coma Scale
COPD	Chronic obstructive pulmonary disease	**MAP**	Mean arterial pressure
CT	Computed tomography	**MODS**	Multiple organ dysfunction syndrome
CVP	Central venous pressure	**Mph**	Miles per hour

MVC	Motor vehicle crash	Spo$_2$	Arterial oxygen saturation measured by pulse oximetry
Pao$_2$	Partial arterial pressure of oxygen	SVR	Systemic vascular resistance
PEEP	Positive end-expiratory pressure	Svo$_2$	Mixed venous oxygen saturation
RAP	Right atrial pressure		

SECTION ONE: Overview of the Injured Patient

At the completion of this section, the learner will be able to define injury, potential mechanisms of injury, and personal and environmental factors that influence injury patterns.

Injury

Understanding trauma enables the nurse to approach a patient in crisis with a level-headed, systematic plan based on a body of nursing knowledge surrounding the concept. Historically, injuries or accidents were viewed as the result of random chance beyond human control. Now, injury is viewed as an event with an identifiable cause via the interaction of energy and force with a recipient. The recipient may be an inanimate object, such as a car, or may be a human being.

Injury results from acute exposure to energy, such as kinetic (for example, a motor vehicle crash [MVC], fall, or bullet), chemical, thermal, electrical, and ionizing radiation, or from a lack of essential agents, such as oxygen and heat (drowning and frostbite). Motor vehicle crashes are the most common cause of injury, followed by falls. The injury occurs because of the body's inability to tolerate excessive exposure to the energy source. Effects of injury on the human body vary depending on the injuring agent. For the purposes of this module, the focus will be on two major categories of injury—blunt and penetrating.

Mechanism of Injury

Blunt trauma is considered injury without interruption of skin integrity. Blunt trauma may be life threatening because the extent of the injury may be covert, making diagnosis difficult. Blunt forces transfer energy causing tissue deformation. The nature of the injury is related to both the transfer of energy and the anatomic structure involved.

Penetrating trauma refers to injury sustained by the transmission of energy to body tissues from a moving object that interrupts skin integrity, whereas blunt trauma produces tissue deformation by the transfer of energy. Penetrating trauma produces actual tissue penetration and may also cause surrounding tissue deformation based on the energy transferred by the penetrating object.

Because the transfer of energy occurs with both blunt and penetrating injury, deformation and displacement of body tissue and organs occurs with both forms of injury. Injury takes place as the structural limits of the organ are exceeded. Damage may be localized, such as hematoma formation, or systemic, as in shock states. The local response of the patient varies according to the organ involved. Additional examples are bone fractures, bleeding vessels, or tissue edema.

Injuries, like other diseases, do not occur at random. Identifiable risk factors are present that predispose individuals to certain injury patterns. A brief discussion of a few of these risk factors is presented.

Age

Injury is the leading cause of death in all Americans ages 1 through 44. The death rate from injury is highest for patients more than 75 years old. The highest injury rate is for patients ages 15 through 24 because of their exposure to high-risk activities (including poor judgment with the use of alcohol, drugs, and driving practices). The highest homicide rate occurs among people between 20 and 29 years of age.

The elderly are predisposed to trauma because of age-related changes in reaction time, balance and coordination, and sensory motor function. Trauma in the elderly is associated with higher mortality and morbidity with less severe injury. A 79-year-old with multiple rib fractures will have a very different clinical course than an 18-year-old with multiple rib fractures. The higher morbidity and mortality rates are attributed to a decreased ability to compensate for severe injury (or a "limited physiological reserve") and preexisting medical conditions (Victorino et al., 2003). Limited physiological reserve is a concept of limited organ function in the face of a physiologic challenge. Organ dysfunction may not appear in the resting state, but in a physiological stress situation (such as traumatic injury), the ability of the organs to augment function is compromised (Jacobs, 2003).

Gender

Injury rates are highest for 15- to 24-year-old males. The risk for males is 2.5 times that of females, possibly because of male involvement in hazardous activities.

Alcohol

The use and abuse of alcoholic beverages influence the likelihood of virtually all types of injury, even among young teenagers. An alcohol-related MVC kills someone every 30 minutes, and every 2 minutes, a nonfatal crash occurs (Blincoe et al., 2002). Alcohol-related trauma is a major public health problem. Communities have enacted programs to decrease alcohol-related MVCs, including reducing legal blood alcohol levels to 0.08 percent and initiating sobriety checkpoints (Shults et al., 2002).

Race, Income, Geography

Native Americans have the highest death rates from unintentional injury, African Americans have the highest homicide rates, and Caucasians and Native Americans have the highest suicide rates. An inverse relationship between income levels and death rates exists for African Americans and whites. There is a higher unintentional injury rate in rural areas and a higher intentional injury rate in urban areas. Mechanisms of rural unintentional injuries commonly are MVCs, lightning, and chemical exposure. Urban intentional injuries usually are related to homicide attempts.

In summary, there are two major categories of injury: penetrating and blunt. Risk factors for trauma include increasing age, gender, alcohol, race, income, and geography. Trauma is not an accident; there is always an identifiable cause.

SECTION ONE REVIEW

1. The two major categories of injury are
   A. chemical and thermal
   B. fractures and burns
   C. blunt and penetrating
   D. MVCs and gunshot wounds
2. The death rate from injury is highest for patients
   A. 24 to 42 years old
   B. 15 to 24 years old
   C. 5 to 14 years old
   D. more than 75 years old
3. The elderly have higher mortality and morbidity with traumatic injury because they
   A. have limited physiological reserve
   B. are exposed to high-risk activities
   C. drink more alcohol
   D. have poor judgment

4. The risk for males versus females for injury is
   A. 2.5 times lower
   B. 2.5 times higher
   C. 5 times higher
   D. equal
5. Reducing blood alcohol levels to _____ has been shown to decrease alcohol-related MVCs.
   A. 0.10 percent
   B. 0.05 percent
   C. 0.08 percent
   D. 0.04 percent

Answers: 1. C, 2. D, 3. A, 4. B, 5. C

SECTION TWO: Mechanism of Injury: Blunt Trauma

At the completion of this section, the learner will be able to define the forces associated with blunt trauma and be able to apply these concepts to the clinical assessment of a patient with blunt trauma.

Blunt trauma is most commonly seen with MVCs, motor vehicles striking pedestrians, and falls from significant heights. One of the most basic principles of physics is used to explain trauma: the law of conservation of energy. Energy can neither be created or destroyed; it is only changed from one form to another. Blunt trauma is this translation of energy between forms via force.

Forces Associated with Blunt Trauma

Force is a physical factor, the push or pull that changes the state of an object that is either at rest or already in motion. Injury resulting from force is related to the amount and speed (velocity) of energy transmission, the surface area to which the energy is applied, and the elasticity of the tissues affected. The more slowly the force is applied, the more slowly energy is released, with less subsequent tissue deformation. The forces most often applied are acceleration, deceleration, shearing, and compression (ACSCT, 1997).

Acceleration is an increase in the rate of velocity or speed of a moving body. The most significant determinant of the amount of injury sustained is velocity. As velocity increases, so does tissue damage because of the greater amount of energy present. The following example illustrates the concept of acceleration. On impact with a solid object (e.g., another car, a brick wall, or a telephone pole), the driver is suddenly propelled forward. He experiences a sudden acceleration of body mass determined by the rate of speed at which he was traveling and his body mass. This relationship is reflected in the following formula.

Body weight × mph = pounds per square inch of impact

A person weighing 100 pounds, traveling at 35 miles per hour (mph), will hit at 3,500 pounds per square inch. This is equivalent to jumping head-first from a three-story building!

Deceleration is a decrease in the rate of velocity of a moving object. The same driver in the preceding example who is moving forward after hitting a solid object will experience a sudden deceleration after he comes into contact with the mass that impedes his forward (or backward) progression (e.g., the steering wheel, a tree, the road, or another passenger).

Shearing refers to injury resulting from two structures or two parts of the same structure, sliding in opposite directions causing a tearing or degloving type of injury. For example, shearing forces are frequently the cause of spinal injury at the C7–T1 juncture because the mobile cervical spine attaches at that point to the relatively immobile thoracic spine. Shearing forces are often the cause of aortic tears; splenic and renal injuries; and liver, brain, or heart injuries. These structures have a relatively immobile section connected to a relatively mobile section and, therefore, are subject to shearing forces.

Compression is the process of being pressed or squeezed together with a resulting reduction in volume or size. For example, sudden acceleration or deceleration during an MVC can cause compression of the heart and lung parenchyma between the posterior and anterior chest wall. The small bowel may be compressed between the vertebral column and the lower part of the steering wheel or an improperly placed seat belt. The bowel may rupture. The same mechanism can cause compression of the liver causing it to burst.

Acceleration and deceleration injuries are most common with blunt trauma. An example of this mechanism of injury is injury to the thoracic aorta. Typically, MVCs and falls from 20 feet or higher precipitate stretching, bowing, and shearing in major vessels, such as the aorta. Aortic damage may occur to any or all layers of the vessel wall. The aortic vessel wall can tear, dissect, rupture, or form an aneurysm immediately or at any time postinjury.

Shearing damage occurs in the vessels when deceleration occurs at a different rate than that occurring in other internal structures. For example, the relatively mobile ascending aorta continues to move after the relatively stationary descending aorta has stopped moving. A shearing injury occurs from the two sections of the aorta moving at different speeds. One is still moving (ascending aorta), whereas the other has stopped (descending aorta).

Injuries Associated with Blunt Trauma

Injuries associated with blunt trauma forces include head injuries (think about the movement of the brain inside the skull with acceleration, deceleration, and shearing coup injury), spinal cord injuries (the cervical spine is predisposed to shearing and acceleration/deceleration because of its instability and poor support), fractures (from shearing and compression), and abdominal injuries (especially the spleen and liver).

Tissue responsiveness to applied forces varies, creating characteristic limits of the tissues' abilities to withstand the forces of acceleration, deceleration, compression, and shearing. Tissue deformation is generally the result of tensile forces or shear forces. **Tensile forces** cause tissues to stretch and extend. Tensile strength of a specific tissue is the greatest longitudinal stretch or stress it can withstand without tearing apart. Joint dislocations, muscle sprains, and strains are frequently the result of tensile forces. Tensile forces are also the cause of contrecoup brain injuries. Brain tissue is pulled away from the skull with the initial alteration in motion as a result of acceleration or deceleration.

Tissue, organ, and systemic responses to the forces applied with blunt trauma often present a complex interrelationship of potential injury manifestation. Trauma patients with similar mechanisms of injury typically have different combinations of organ and systemic injury based on individual variances in ability to withstand the forces applied. A myriad of potential injury combinations, manifestations, and outcomes exist, prompting the clinician to approach the patient in a systematic fashion.

In summary, different types of forces are related to blunt injury. Forces associated with blunt trauma include acceleration, deceleration, shearing, and compression. Tissue, organ, and systemic responses to the forces applied with blunt trauma often present a complex interrelationship of potential injury manifestation.

SECTION TWO REVIEW

1. Acceleration is a change in the rate of velocity or speed of a moving body. As velocity increases, tissue damage
   A. decreases
   B. increases
   C. remains constant
   D. cannot be determined

2. A decrease in the velocity of a moving object is
   A. acceleration
   B. deceleration
   C. compression
   D. shearing

3. Structures slipping in opposite directions to each other is a force known as
  A. acceleration
  B. deceleration
  C. compression
  D. shearing

4. The process of being pressed or squeezed is known as
  A. acceleration
  B. deceleration

  C. compression
  D. shearing

5. Forces that cause tissues to stretch are known as
  A. tensile
  B. shearing
  C. mass
  D. compression

Answers: 1. B, 2. B, 3. D, 4. C, 5. A

SECTION THREE: Mechanism of Injury: Penetrating Trauma

At the completion of this section, the learner will be able to define the forces associated with penetrating trauma and apply these concepts to the clinical assessment of a patient with penetrating trauma.

Forces Associated with Penetrating Trauma

Penetrating trauma is the result of the transmission of energy from a moving object into body tissues as the object disrupts the integrity of the skin and the underlying structures. The amount of kinetic energy transmitted by the object has a direct relationship to the amount of tissue damage. With tissue or organ penetration, the severity of the injury depends on the structures damaged by the transmission of the energy. A penetrating object can be almost anything—a knife, a bullet, shrapnel, an arrow, a stick, a metal rod, a fork, a gear shift, and so on.

The amount of kinetic energy available to be transmitted to tissues depends on the surface area of the point of impact, the density of the tissue, and the velocity of the projectile at the time of impact (ACSCT, 1997). Weapons are usually classified by the amount of energy they are capable of producing: Low-energy weapons include knives, arrows, or any type of hand missile; medium-energy weapons include handguns and some rifles; and high-energy weapons include hunting rifles and shotguns.

Low- to Medium-Energy Missiles

Low- to medium-energy missiles travel less than 2,000 feet per second. The injury sustained usually results from the missile contacting the tissue. Typically, damage is localized to those structures directly in the missile's path. However, special consideration must be given when injury occurs where body cavities lie in close proximity to one another. This principle is of critical importance when considering the close proximity of the thoracic and abdominal cavities, especially with injuries occurring near the diaphragm, which offers very little resistance to the penetrating agent. Penetrating injuries to the chest below the nipple line, the sixth rib, or the scapula may involve both intrathoracic and abdominal structures.

If the offending weapon is impaled in the body, it is critical that the object be left in place and protected from further movement until definitive surgical intervention is available. Protective padding can be placed around the object, such as gauze rolls or abdominal pads, or a protective device, such as a plastic cup, can be secured around the protruding handle of objects such as knives or the end of a stick or metal rod. Impaled objects may actually be controlling hemorrhage from damaged structures and removal may precipitate exsanguination.

High-Energy Missiles

High-energy missiles are those traveling more than 2,000 feet per second. At higher velocities, a tremendous amount of tissue destruction can occur as a result of forces transmitted to the tissues by the missile. High-energy missiles (also referred to as high-velocity missiles) transmit more kinetic energy, creating an intense blast result within the tissues. As the missile penetrates the tissue, the transmission of kinetic energy displaces tissues forward and laterally to form a temporary cavity. The process of cavity formation is called **cavitation** (Fig. 36–1). The degree of cavitation is directly related to the amount of kinetic energy transmitted to the tissues, which in turn is determined by the velocity of the missile. The size of the cavity may be up to 30 times the diameter of the missile (ACSCT, 1997). Tissue surrounding the missile tract is exposed to tensile (stretching), compressing, and shearing forces, which produce damage outside the direct path of the missile. Vessels, nerves, and other structures that were not directly damaged by the missile may be affected. The phenomenon of structure injury outside the direct missile path is referred to as a blast effect. Higher-velocity missiles produce more serious injury because of the destructive process of cavitation and blast effect to surrounding tissue and organs.

Another concept to consider when evaluating the forces that can injure a patient is the missile's trajectory. Consider a missile moving in stable flight toward the host (for our purposes, the patient). The missile passes from air into human tissue, which is several hundred times denser than air. As the missile passes into the tissue, the surrounding environment changes, precipitating instability of the missile. The unstable missile may yaw, tumble, deform, fragment, or any combination of these actions.

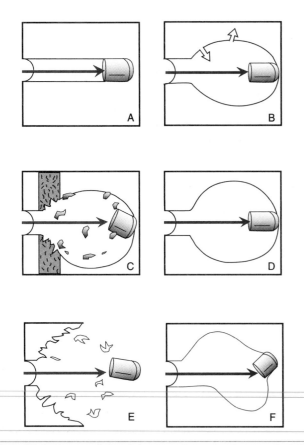

Figure 36–1 ■ Patterns of tissue injury secondary to gunshot wounds. *A.* Low velocity, small entrance, and exit wounds. *B.* Higher velocity, cavitation present with energy dispersion outward from missile path (blast effect). *C.* Same velocity as in *B* but with penetration of bone and greater blast effect because of projections of bone being spread through tissue. *D.* Higher velocity than in *B* or *C* with greater cavitation effect, small entrance and exit wounds. *E.* Same velocity as in *D*, but person or extremity hit is thinner resulting in large exit wound. *F.* Asymmetrical cavitation as bullet begins to yaw and tumble.

Yaw is the deviation of a missile either horizontally or vertically about its axis. *Tumble* is the action of forward rotation around the center of a mass (somersaulting) (Fig. 36–1F). The action of yawing or tumbling increases the surface area of the missile as it impacts the body (side of the missile versus the point of the missile). This creates a larger entrance wound. It also allows for increased energy transfer to the surrounding tissues, creating a larger area of tissue destruction. Higher-velocity missiles have a greater propensity for yaw and tumble.

Secondary Missiles

Another principle to consider when analyzing the effects of penetrating injury is the creation of secondary missiles by the penetrating object. A missile or its fragments may impart sufficient kinetic injury to dense tissue, such as bone or teeth, to create highly destructive secondary missiles. These secondary missiles may take erratic, unpredictable courses, resulting in additional injury. Secondary missiles also may be created by fragmentation of the primary missile. Thus, the anticipated missile path may be compounded, complicated, or enhanced by tissue damage precipitated by a secondary missile.

Injuries Associated with Penetrating Trauma

An evaluation of the wounds caused by the missile is necessary, noting the location; size; shape; if there is any foreign substance on the surrounding tissue, such as a black powder; and if the wound is actively bleeding. If there are two wounds, noting the location of each only gives the clinician a hint of the trajectory the missile may have taken if the same missile caused both wounds. Missiles usually take the path of least resistance, so the path the missile followed may not be a straight line between the two wounds. Entrance wounds are usually smaller than exit wounds. However, the characteristics of a wound depend on the forces causing the injury such as velocity, cavitation, and blast effect. A summary of the effects of these forces on a wound are depicted in Figure 36–1. Identifying which is the entrance wound and which is the exit wound is not necessary and should be left to experienced personnel. Identifying the wounds as wound 1 and wound 2 will suffice. The presence of two wounds does not necessarily mean one is an entrance and one is an exit wound. They may be two entrance wounds from two separate missiles. Not all medium- and high-energy penetrating injuries have a resulting exit wound because the missile may remain inside the body.

In summary, kinematics influence penetrating injury. Velocity, cavitation, yaw, and tumbling were reviewed for their influence on ultimate injury of structures. Critical application of these concepts will maximize the clinician's ability to evaluate penetrating traumatic injury based on mechanism.

2. Cavitation demonstrates a(n) _____ relationship with the amount of kinetic energy transmitted to tissue.
  A. inverse
  B. direct
  C. insignificant
  D. diagonal

3. The phenomenon of structure injury outside the direct missile path is referred to as
  A. cavitation
  B. blast effect
  C. yaw
  D. tumbling

4. Yaw and tumble will _____ the area of tissue destruction precipitated by a missile.
  A. decrease
  B. increase

  C. minimize
  D. not affect

5. A patient has an impaled knife in the upper abdomen. You should immediately
  A. remove the knife and apply pressure
  B. manipulate the knife to facilitate assessment of injured organs
  C. stabilize the knife without removal and minimal manipulation
  D. leave the knife alone

Answers: 1. D, 2. B, 3. B, 4. B, 5. C

SECTION FOUR: Mechanism of Injury Patterns

At the completion of this section, the learner will be able to translate mechanism of injury into potential injury patterns manifested by the patient for both blunt and penetrating injuries.

Certain mechanisms result in predictable injury patterns. Thus, the history of the event preceding the injury should elicit an increased index of suspicion for certain combinations of injured structures. Some commonly seen injuries resulting from blunt and penetrating trauma and their injury mechanisms are listed in Table 36–1. This table addresses pedestrian/motor

TABLE 36–1 Commonly Seen Injuries

MECHANISM OF INJURY	POTENTIAL STRUCTURE INJURY
Pedestrian hit by automobile	
Adult	Fractures of femur, tibia, and fibula on side of impact; ligamental damage to impacted knee; mild contralateral head injury
Child	Fractures of femur, chest injury, contralateral head injury
Unrestrained driver (Fig. 36–2)	Head and/or facial injury, rib fractures, sternum with underlying myocardial or pulmonary contusion, cervical spine fractures, laryngotracheal injuries, spleen injuries, liver injuries, small bowel injuries, posterior fracture–dislocation of hip, femur fractures
Unrestrained front seat passenger	Head and/or facial injuries, laryngotracheal injuries, posterior fracture–dislocation of femoral head, femur/patellar fractures
Restrained driver (lap and shoulder harness)	Contusions of structures underlying harness (i.e., pulmonary contusion, contusion of small bowel)
Restrained passenger (lap belt only)	Flexion/distraction fractures, especially lumbar vertebrae (L1–L4), duodenal injuries, cervical spine injuries
Fall injuries	Compression fractures of lumbosacral spine and calcaneus fractures; fractures of radius/ulna, patella if victim falls forward
Vehicular ejection	Multiple injuries, especially head and cervical spine injuries; injury risk increases by 300 percent when ejection occurs
Low-velocity impalement	Local tissue/organ disruption, little or no cavitation
High-velocity missile, short missile path	Entrance wound larger than missile caliber; large ragged exit wound with cavitation
High-velocity missile, long missile path	Entrance wound larger than missile caliber; exit wound slightly larger than or equal to missile caliber; extensive cavitation (blast effect to deep structures absorbing lost kinetic energy)
High-velocity missile hitting bone or teeth	Entry wound larger than missile caliber; possibly no exit wound with missile fragmentation; secondary missile injury in unpredictable, erratic pattern

vehicle injuries, motor vehicle driver and passenger injuries, fall injuries, and missile injuries.

An example illustrating the importance of the application of mechanism of injury follows. A 21-year-old male, unrestrained driver hits another vehicle head-on (Fig. 36–2). Travel-ing speed was in excess of 95 mph. Both the steering wheel and windshield were broken. A high index of suspicion must be maintained for the following injuries:

1. Potential intracranial injury because of the high rate of speed and shattered windshield
2. Potential cervical vertebrae injury because of suspected acceleration/deceleration at a high rate of speed and the broken windshield
3. Potential intrathoracic injuries because of the broken steer-ing wheel—suspect rib fractures, myocardial and pul-monary contusions, and great vessel injury
4. Potential intra-abdominal injuries because of the broken steering wheel and acceleration/deceleration mechanism; injuries could include splenic/liver lacerations, small bowel injuries, and great vessel injuries
5. Potential long-bone fractures, especially femur fractures or posterior hip fracture–dislocation, because of impact of knees with dashboard
6. Potential multiple skin lacerations, avulsions, punctures from the patient impacting various parts of the vehicle interior

In summary, mechanisms of injury can help anticipate an injury pattern. Both blunt and penetrating injuries were ad-dressed.

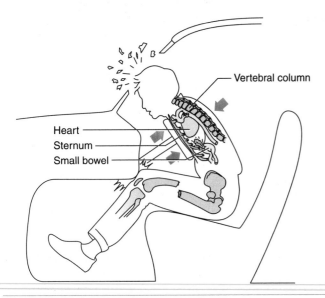

Figure 36–2 ■ Typical injuries of an unrestrained driver.

Labels: Vertebral column, Heart, Sternum, Small bowel

SECTION FOUR REVIEW

1. A restrained passenger (lap belt only) may exhibit flexion/distraction fractures in which area of the vertebral column?
   A. cervical
   B. lumbar
   C. thoracic
   D. sacral
2. A restrained (lap and shoulder harness) occupant involved in an MVC can receive what types of injuries from the restraints?
   A. pulmonary contusions
   B. lumbar fractures
   C. femur fractures
   D. facial injuries
3. Which of the following is true?
   A. vehicular ejection increases the risk for potential injury
   B. vehicular ejection decreases the risk for potential injury
   C. vehicular ejection is not related to the risk for potential injury
   D. vehicular ejection is associated with seat belt use

Answers: 1. B, 2. A, 3. A

SECTION FIVE: Mediators of Injury Response

At the completion of this section, the learner will be able to state clinical conditions that mediate a patient's response to injury, in-cluding underlying medical conditions, substance abuse, and physiological alterations, including pregnancy and advancing age.

Comorbidities

Comorbidities, or underlying medical conditions, are ex-tremely important to identify when considering the patient's physiological and hemodynamic response to trauma. The most commonly encountered conditions include chronic obstructive pulmonary disease (**COPD**), heart disease, and underlying cerebral insufficiency, as with brain attacks (stroke). These conditions or the medication used to control their effects may alter the physiological response to trauma. The patient with COPD who sustains a minor pulmonary contusion related to blunt trauma may require prompt, life-saving intubation because of the alteration in the ventilation–perfusion ratio and effects on the resilience of affected lung tissue. Beta blockade used for coronary artery disease to minimize oxygen demands by the heart could prevent a normal response to hypovolemia (i.e., tachycardia). The patient with a head injury who has had a stroke in the past may experience an altered level of consciousness, difficulty in communication, or sensorimotor dysfunction as a result of the stroke and not the acute head injury. Eliciting a complete medical history is crucial during the initial assessment.

Substance Abuse

Substance abuse is characterized by recurrent and clinically significant adverse consequences related to the repeated use of substances. Adverse consequences include failing to meet major role obligations, use of drugs in physically hazardous situations, substance-abuse related legal problems, and persistent or recurrent social or interpersonal problems as a result of continued drug use (Cami & Farre, 2003).

The high incidence of alcohol as a contributing factor to injury has already been demonstrated. How is injury affected by alcohol ingestion? The most common effect is the inability to establish clearly a baseline level of consciousness. As a central nervous system (CNS) depressant, the effects of alcohol on the brain are concentration dependent. The most sensitive tool for evaluation of brain injury is level of consciousness. Therefore, alcohol involvement is a critical consideration.

Blood alcohol concentration (BAC) is a measurement of intoxication. Measurement is conducted in milligrams per deciliter (mg/dL) or grams per deciliter (g/dL), varying from institution to institution. Legal intoxication in most states is 100 mg/dL or 0.100 g/dL. However, impaired judgment occurs at a level of 50 mg/dL or 0.05 g/dL. A history of alcohol use should be obtained because a degree of tolerance ensues with frequent alcohol ingestion. As plasma levels increase, sedation, motor incoordination, ataxia, and impaired psychomotor performance become apparent. States that have adopted the legal limit of 0.08 have noticed decreased MVCs (Shults et al., 2002).

The concomitant use of alcohol and other CNS depressants (e.g., barbiturates, opiates, sedative–hypnotics) may result in potentiation of each drug's effects, creating a synergistic effect. CNS stimulants, such as cocaine, also can alter the level of consciousness in the injured patient. Cocaine use mimics and intensifies a sympathetic stimulation or the fight-or-flight response in the patient. Notably, increase in heart rate and blood pressure occur along with vasoconstriction, dilated

pupils, tremors, excitability, and restlessness. Cocaine can induce myocardial ischemia as well as many dysrhythmias, including heart block, tachydysrhythmias, ventricular fibrillation, asystole, and bundle branch block (Lange & Hillis, 2001). Neurologically, mental status changes range from anxiety to acute paranoid psychosis. For the high-acuity nurse, it is very difficult to obtain a baseline level of consciousness when the patient is intoxicated with alcohol or other drugs that cloud his or her sensorium.

The Pregnant Patient

The pregnant trauma patient presents unique aspects of care that must be considered carefully. Major trauma affects up to 8 percent of pregnant patients (Myriam et al., 2000). Familiarity with trauma assessment and management during pregnancy is important for the nurse in the high-acuity setting.

Anatomic Changes

Anatomic rearrangement as pregnancy progresses is inevitable and may cause confusion in physical diagnosis. Depending on the gestational size of the uterus, different patterns of injury may occur to the mother as well as to the fetus. Blunt abdominal trauma in the pregnant patient is associated with different injuries from those in the nonpregnant patient.

Hemodynamic Changes

After the tenth week of pregnancy, cardiac output is increased by 1.0 L to 1.5 L per minute. A high-output, low-resistance hemodynamic state is characteristic in pregnancy. Maternal heart rate increases by 10 to 15 beats per minute throughout pregnancy, with a slight increase in stroke volume. Blood pressure decreases during pregnancy by 15 to 20 percent (Van Hook, 2002). An important fact to remember is that some women experience profound hypotension when placed in the supine position (especially during the third trimester). This is known as the *vena cava syndrome* and is caused by the enlarged uterus compressing the inferior vena cava against the spinal column, decreasing venous return and preload. The hypotension can be relieved by turning the patient to the left lateral decubitus position.

Blood Volume and Composition

During pregnancy maternal plasma volume expands 40 to 50 percent by the end of the third trimester with maximal volume expansion by 28 to 32 weeks gestation (Van Hook, 2002). Therefore, mild blood loss as a result of traumatic injury is usually well tolerated. The pregnant trauma patient responds very differently to physiological stress than the nonpregnant patient. Because of the hypervolemic state associated with pregnancy, a 30 to 35 percent (1,200 to 1,500 mL) blood loss may occur in a pregnant patient before signs and symptoms of hypovolemia occur. A physiological anemia results in pregnancy as plasma volume increases by 50 percent and red blood cell volume increases by only 35 percent. Late in pregnancy, the hemoglobin may have fallen to 10.5 to 11 g and the hematocrit to 31 to 35 percent. The white blood cell count increases during pregnancy (15,000 to 18,000/mm^3) and during labor may be as high as 25,000/mm^3. White blood cell counts are valuable when evaluating abdominal trauma (ACSCT, 1997).

The Elderly Patient

Physiological changes associated with aging (ages 65 and older), such as delayed reaction times, disturbances of gait and balance, diminished visual acuity, and hearing loss, predispose the elderly to traumatic injury. Also, age-related deterioration in body systems alters the elderly trauma victim's response to injury and increases the susceptibility to complications. Respectively, falls, motor vehicle crashes, pedestrian versus automobile crashes, and penetrating trauma are the four most common mechanisms of injury in this age group.

Chronic Disease States

Chronic disease states exacerbate or compound traumatic injury. Common underlying medical conditions include COPD, coronary artery disease, diabetes mellitus, congestive heart failure, hypertension, and conditions leading to diminished neurological acuity (e.g., stroke and carotid insufficiency). The patient not only may have a chronic medical condition but also could be treated with a polypharmaceutical regimen that may affect the response to a traumatic injury.

Limited Physiologic Reserve

The higher morbidity and mortality rates associated with trauma in the elderly can be attributed to limited physiological reserve (as discussed in Section One). The limited physiological reserve is most often in the cardiorespiratory, neurological, and musculoskeletal systems. Cardiorespiratory effects include decreased distensibility of blood vessels, increased systolic blood pressure and systemic vascular resistance, increased vascular resistance, decreased coronary blood flow, decreased cardiac output, decreased respiratory muscle strength, limited chest expansion, and decreased number of functioning alveoli. These alterations combine to reduce greatly the ability to sustain adequate tissue perfusion and oxygenation. Mild anemia is also common in this age group and potentiates alterations in oxygenation by limiting oxygen transport capabilities.

Neurological changes associated with aging include short-term memory loss and reduced cerebral blood flow. Preexisting neurological conditions, such as senility, dementia, and Alzheimer's disease, may significantly affect evaluation of the patient's neurological status. Head injuries are common in the elderly. A high index of suspicion, awareness of the patient's preexisting neurological status, and frequent, thorough neurological assessments are necessary to avoid detrimental delays in diagnosis and intervention.

Osteoporosis and decreasing muscle mass contribute to the high incidence of fractures in the elderly. The incidence of rib fractures with blunt trauma in the elderly is 60 percent and they have twice the mortality and morbidity of younger patients with these same injuries (Bulger et al., 2000). Normal aging processes diminish blood supply to the skin and result in delayed healing of soft tissue injuries. This reduction of blood supply also predisposes the elderly trauma patient to the development of decubitus ulcers.

Difficulties during the initial assessment related to normal aging may present themselves to the clinician. Shock is difficult to diagnose secondary to age-related changes that affect the patient's response to trauma, including decreased cardiac output, decreased maximal heart rate, and increased peripheral vascular resistance (Schulman & Caridge, 2002). Because of the decline in gag and cough reflexes, airway integrity may be difficult to maintain. Detection of shock may be difficult because of the propensity toward hypertension. Thus, normal blood pressures actually may indicate low perfusion states in the elderly.

In summary, clinical conditions that mediate the patient's response to injury include comorbidities, substance abuse, and physiological alterations including pregnancy and advancing age. Comorbidities and the medications used to treat these conditions alter the physiological response to traumatic injury. Substance abuse, particularly alcohol intoxication, impairs neurological assessment. The pregnant patient's response to traumatic injury is mediated by anatomic changes, hemodynamic changes, and changes in blood volume and composition that occur as a result of the pregnancy. The elderly patient's response to injury is mediated by chronic disease states and limited physiologic reserve. Multiple factors affecting evaluation of the elderly trauma patient have been discussed. The following example illustrates these concepts. A 72-year-old male is involved in an MVC. He has a previous history that includes myocardial infarction and hypertension and currently is taking Inderal. A syncopal episode precipitated the MVC. The patient arrives with a blood pressure of 105/60, heart rate 65, and initial hematocrit 25 percent. A computed tomography (CT) scan of the abdomen reveals a complex splenic laceration. Although the patient was in hypovolemic shock, the tachycardia usually associated with the shock state was prevented by the beta blockade and the diminished cardiorespiratory responsiveness.

SECTION FIVE REVIEW

1. Alcohol use in the trauma patient acts as a CNS
   - A. stimulant
   - B. depressant
   - C. vasoconstrictive agent
   - D. vasodilator
2. Cocaine use in the trauma patient acts as a CNS
   - A. stimulant
   - B. depressant
   - C. vasodilator
   - D. vasoconstrictor
3. The immediate nursing intervention for a pregnant woman in her third trimester who is hypotensive after an MVC is
   - A. administering vasopressors
   - B. colloid transfusion
   - C. turning the patient to the left lateral decubitus position, maintaining immobilization
   - D. placing the patient in the Trendelenburg position
4. Increasing progesterone levels causing smooth muscle relaxation may elicit esophageal reflux in the pregnant woman. Thus, a predisposition to _____ may occur.
   - A. aspiration
   - B. increased gastric motility
   - C. difficulty in intubation
   - D. gastritis
5. After the tenth week of pregnancy, cardiac output is increased by _____ L per minute.
   - A. 0.5 to 1.0
   - B. 1.0 to 1.5
   - C. 1.5 to 2.0
   - D. 2.0 to 2.5

6. A 24-year-old female, 7-month pregnant victim of an MVC has arrived. Her initial hematocrit is 31 percent. You should
   - A. check fetal heart tones
   - B. check for vaginal bleeding
   - C. anticipate transfusion
   - D. consider this normal
7. Hypotension may not be a reliable sign of shock in the elderly because
   - A. the elderly patient may be taking vasodilators for hypertension
   - B. coronary blood flow increases with aging
   - C. reflux tachycardia occurs
   - D. systemic vascular resistance decreases in aging
8. The incidence of rib fractures associated with blunt injury in the elderly patient has been established to be
   - A. 10 percent
   - B. 25 percent
   - C. 60 percent
   - D. 75 percent
9. Shock is difficult to assess in elderly trauma patients, secondary to which of the following age-related changes?
   - A. decrease in cardiac output
   - B. decrease in heart rate
   - C. increase in peripheral vascular rate
   - D. all of the above

Answers: 1. B, 2. A, 3. C, 4. A, 5. B, 6. D, 7. A, 8. C, 9. D

SECTION SIX: Primary Survey

At the completion of this section, the learner will be able to identify the clinical assessment format used to identify life-threatening injuries during the primary survey.

Because of the unpredictable effects of trauma-related injury on the patient, the nurse must develop a rapid, systematic approach to assessing each patient to ensure that no effects of injury are overlooked. Remember, trauma should never be approached as a unisystem disease but rather as a multisystem disease. Thus, a rapid systematic approach to assessment with establishment of management priorities is essential.

Trauma presents a myriad of potentially life-threatening injuries. The life-threatening injuries must be evaluated

quickly, with immediate intervention. The trauma assessment is divided into three phases: primary survey, resuscitation, and secondary survey.

The primary survey is the focus of this section. The purpose of the primary survey is to identify and treat life-threatening conditions and intervene appropriately. Primary survey is done using the A, B, C, D, and E approach, as outlined here:

- **A—Airway (with cervical spine immobilization).** Ensure that the patient has an open airway.
- **B—Breathing.** Is the patient breathing? Are respirations effective? Does the patient need assistance via bag-valve-mask or mechanical ventilation?
- **C—Circulation.** The trauma patient is at very high risk of hypovolemic shock from acute blood loss and third spacing

of fluid with soft tissue damage. Identify hypovolemia quickly and search for the etiology.

■ **D—Disability.** Perform a quick neuroexamination of the patient's level of consciousness and motor function.

■ **E—Exposure and evacuation.** Completely undress the patient to provide for visualization of external causes of injury. If the severity of the patient's injury exceeds the capability of the hospital, consider transport of the patient to a definitive care facility.

Each of the components of the primary survey is explored in detail to ensure that you have all the information necessary to approach the multiple-injured patient using critical thinking and problem-solving strategies.

Airway and Cervical Spine

The goal of airway management is optimization of ventilation and oxygenation, with cervical spine protection. The first step in the primary survey is assessment of patency of the patient's airway. An injury to the cervical spine should always be assumed in the patient with multisystem trauma, especially in the patient with an injury above the clavicle. Excessive manipulation of the head, face, or neck, precipitating hyperextension or hyperflexion of the cervical spine, may convert a fracture without neurological manifestations into a fracture–dislocation with spinal cord contusion, laceration, compression, or transection. Therefore, cervical immobilization is imperative during airway assessment.

Potential causes of airway obstruction include the tongue falling back into the oropharynx, obstructing the airway; blood, vomitus, secretions, or foreign objects obstructing the airway; fractures of the facial bony structures; or crushing injuries of the laryngotracheal tree. Actual or potential airway obstruction may be present with the following symptoms:

■ Dyspnea
■ Diminished breath sounds despite respiratory effort
■ Dysphonia (hoarseness, stridor)
■ Dysphagia
■ Drooling

Airway management techniques range from simple positional maneuvers to complex surgical procedures. During all maneuvers, it is critical that the cervical spine be maintained by in-line immobilization with the head in the neutral position. Cervical spine immobilization can be achieved best by manual in-line axial traction by a caregiver or by a hard cervical collar, disposable head blocks, or towel rolls placed on both sides of the patient's head, with tape across the patient's forehead. These actions prevent forward flexion, hyperextension, and lateral rotation of the cervical spine. Sandbags are no longer an acceptable means of lateral cervical immobilization because of the increased lateral pressure to the cervical spine that occurs with turning or tilting of the backboard.

The first, and most simple, maneuver to open the airway is a chin lift or modified jaw thrust. This maneuver may open the airway adequately and allow ventilation to take place. The airway can be suctioned for debris, secretions, blood, or vomitus. An oropharyngeal or nasopharyngeal airway may be used to facilitate airway maintenance. The oropharyngeal airway should be used only in patients who are unconscious and have no gag reflex. Using this airway in a conscious patient may precipitate gagging, vomiting, and potential aspiration. Improper placement of the oropharyngeal airway may cause airway obstruction. The nasopharyngeal airway can be used to facilitate airway integrity in the conscious victim with an intact gag reflex.

If the aforementioned procedures are inadequate in establishing an airway, more aggressive measures must be taken. The patient is hyperventilated with a bag-valve-mask with 100 percent oxygen. A frequent complication of hyperventilation with this technique is gastric distention. Increased risks secondary to the distention include vomiting, aspiration, and diaphragmatic impingement. After a definitive airway has been secured, placement of a gastric tube decompresses the stomach.

Endotracheal intubation is achieved either orally or nasally. Nasotracheal intubation is often performed in the injured patient because hyperextension of the neck is minimized. With the nasotracheal method, the tube is advanced during the inspiratory effort when the epiglottis is open. Orotracheal intubation is necessary when the patient is apneic or a cribriform plate fracture is suspected, as with basilar skull fractures. With fractures of the cribriform plate, the nasally inserted endotracheal tube could pass into the cranial vault, injuring brain tissue. If orotracheal intubation is necessary, absolute and vigilant care must be taken to avoid hyperextension of the cervical spine.

After intubation is achieved, breath sounds are auscultated to confirm tracheal intubation. The clinician also should auscultate over the epigastrium for gurgling sounds to help rule out an esophageal intubation. Repeated assessment of breath sounds in any intubated patient is a crucial nursing action.

The indication for a surgical airway is the inability to intubate the trachea. Inability to intubate the trachea may result from edema of the glottis, larynx fracture, severe oropharyngeal hemorrhage, or gross instability of the midface. A surgical airway can be achieved by a needle cricothyroidotomy, surgical cricothyroidotomy, or tracheostomy. Surgical cricothyroidotomy is performed by making an incision through the cricothyroid membrane and into the trachea. Tracheostomy must be considered in the patient with suspected laryngeal trauma. Symptoms of laryngeal injury include tenderness, hoarseness, subcutaneous emphysema, and intolerance of the supine position. The supine position is poorly tolerated by these patients because, on assuming the position, the airway will collapse where the laryngeal injury has occurred. With the patient sitting upright, an open airway is maintained even though the larynx is injured.

Aggressive airway management is critical. Assurance of airway integrity is the priority in the primary survey. Remember, however, that airway integrity does not ensure adequate ventilation. The airway must be opened and secured before ventilation is assessed.

Breathing

The next step in the primary survey is to assess adequacy of ventilation. The primary goal of ventilation is to achieve maximum cellular oxygenation by providing an oxygen-rich environment. Thus, all trauma patients should receive high-flow oxygen during the initial evaluation.

Breathing is evaluated by the look, listen, and feel parameters. Look to detect the presence of respiratory excursion, listen for breath sounds, and feel for breathing. Positive pressure ventilation may be required in some patients and is provided in a number of ways: mouth-to-mask, bag-valve-mask, or positive pressure ventilator.

Confirmation of the adequacy of ventilation is best achieved by obtaining an arterial blood gas (ABG) or continuous monitoring of end-tidal carbon dioxide and arterial oxygen saturation using noninvasive measures. If arterial blood gases are inadequate, the airway is reevaluated, and the patient is evaluated for the presence of pneumothorax, hemothorax, hemopneumothorax, or tension pneumothorax. Tube thoracostomy is indicated for any of these conditions because they are all life threatening injuries.

Circulation

The third step in the primary survey is assessment of circulation. Inadequate circulation is manifested as shock. Shock is a clinical state characterized by inadequate organ perfusion and tissue oxygenation (Module 15).

Assessment for adequate circulation includes palpating for strength, rate, rhythm, and symmetry of carotid, radial, femoral, and pedal pulses. Skin temperature is evaluated, as is capillary refill. Adequacy of tissue perfusion is reflected by the patient's level of consciousness.

Successful treatment of shock depends on early recognition, controlling obvious hemorrhage, and aggressive fluid resuscitation to prevent the development of hypotension. Intravenous (IV) access is critical for volume infusion. Two large-bore IVs are established (16 gauge or larger in adults), and crystalloids are administered. Warm lactated Ringer's solution is the solution of choice. Lactated Ringer's solution can be infused at a wide-open rate. If there are no signs of improvement after 2 L, crystalloid infusion continues along with administration of blood products. Failure to respond to crystalloid and blood infusions indicates a rapid surgical intervention is required (ACSCT, 1997).

Recognition of the source of blood loss is critical. Blood volume loss in quantities large enough to produce a shock state can occur in one or more of the following five areas:

1. **Chest.** In the adult, 2.5 L of blood can be lost in each hemothorax. Thus, a total of 5 L can be lost inside the chest, which would be the total blood volume of a 70-kg person.
2. **Abdomen.** As much as 6 L of blood can be lost via intraperitoneal bleeding from damaged organs or vessels.
3. **Pelvis and retroperitoneum.** Unstable pelvic fractures, especially those involving the posterior elements of the pelvis, can precipitate liters of blood loss. A patient actually may exsanguinate from an unstable pelvic fracture involving posterior bony elements.
4. **Femur fractures.** For each femur fracture, 500 to 1,000 mL of blood can be lost.
5. **External hemorrhage.** Bleeding wounds are a consideration. A scalp laceration, particularly, requires proper hemostasis because a significant amount of blood can be lost with this injury.

Of the causes of early postinjury deaths in the hospital that are amenable to effective treatment, hemorrhage is predominant. The most common cause of shock in the injured patient is hypovolemia resulting from acute blood loss. Fluid resuscitation is the fundamental treatment for hypovolemic shock until definitive surgical intervention is available to treat the site (or sites) of injury.

Disability

After airway, breathing, and circulation are assessed and adequately managed, the fourth step in the primary survey is assessment of neurological disability. The purpose of the neurological examination in the primary survey is to establish quickly the patient's level of consciousness and pupillary size and reaction.

The patient's level of consciousness is quickly determined using the AVPU method.

- A—Alert
- V—Responds to verbal stimulation
- P—Responds to painful stimulation
- U—Unresponsive

A more detailed neurological examination is included in the secondary survey.

Exposure

At this point in the primary survey, the patient is completely disrobed in preparation for the secondary survey. Exposure to cold ambient temperatures of resuscitation areas, large volumes of room temperature IV fluids and cold blood products, and wet clothing all predispose the trauma patient to hypothermia. Careful attention to heat conservation measures cannot be overemphasized.

In summary, the purpose of the primary survey is to identify and treat life-threatening injuries. The primary survey is done using the A, B, C, D, E approach. A is for airway. The airway patency is assessed. Actual or potential airway obstruction is treated with a secure airway which may include chin lift, oropharyngeal or nasopharyngeal airway, endotracheal intubation, or placement of a surgical airway. Cervical spine immobilization is required during airway placement. B is for breathing which is assessed by look, listen, and feel parameters. C is for circulation. Signs of impaired circulation indicate a shock state. Aggressive fluid administration is required. Recognition of the source of blood loss is critical. D is for disability. During this step a rapid neurological assessment is made using the AVPU method. The final step is E, which stands for exposure. The patient is disrobed and kept warm so as to prevent hypothermia.

SECTION SIX REVIEW

1. Life-threatening injuries are detected during
   A. the primary survey
   B. resuscitation
   C. the secondary survey
   D. the tertiary survey
2. The primary survey is done using the A, B, C, D, E approach. The D stands for assessment of
   A. dyspnea
   B. diminished breath sounds
   C. dysphagia
   D. disability
3. Assessment of ventilation can be made using
   A. ABG determination
   B. continuous end-tidal CO_2
   C. listening to all breath sounds
   D. all of the above
4. Assessment for circulation should include
   A. palpation of all pulses
   B. capillary refill
   C. level of consciousness
   D. all of the above
5. Which of the following assessments is done during the "E" component of the primary survey?
   A. expel all gastric contents
   B. extricate the patient from harm
   C. apply external pressure to hemorrhage
   D. assess for external causes of injury

Answers: 1. A, 2. D, 3. D, 4. D, 5. D

TABLE 36–2 Key Points in the Secondary Survey

SURVEYED SYSTEM	EVALUATED CRITERIA
Head	Complete neurological examination using a tool such as the Glasgow Coma Scale (GCS); reevaluation of pupillary size and reactivity; inspection and palpation of cranium for lacerations, fractures, contusions, hemotympanium, cerebrospinal fluid leakage and edema
Maxillofacial	Assessment for facial fractures via inspection, palpation for open fractures, lacerations, and mobility or instability of facial structures
Cervical spine/neck	Inspection and palpation of neck anteriorly (maintaining cervical spine immobilization) and palpation anteriorly and posteriorly for pain, crepitus, bony stepoffs indicating fracture–dislocation, neck vein distention, and tracheal deviation
Chest	Inspection for paradoxical movement, flail segments, open chest wounds, and ecchymosis; palpation for rib fractures, subcutaneous emphysema, respiratory excursion, and sternal fractures; auscultation for quality, equality of breath sounds, and presence of adventitious sounds; auscultation of heart sounds for quality, extra heart sounds, murmurs, or pericardial friction rubs possibly indicating pericardial effusion
Abdomen	Inspection and auscultation before palpation to prevent precipitation of misleading bowel sounds by manual manipulation; abdomen inspection for abrasions, contusions, lacerations, and distention; auscultation for bowel sounds in four quadrants, bruits, and breath sounds; light and deep palpation precipitating a painful response may indicate intraperitoneal bleeding and should be quickly attended
Pelvis, perineum, genitalia	Pelvis inspection for deformation and palpation for stability; perineum and genitalia inspection for bleeding at the meatus, hematoma, vaginal bleeding, and lacerations; rectal examination to evaluate rectal wall integrity, presence of blood, position of prostate, presence of palpable pelvic fractures, and quality of sphincter tone
Musculoskeletal	Visual evaluation of extremities for contusions or deformities; palpation of all extremities for tenderness, crepitation, or abnormal range of motion, which may raise index of suspicion for fracture; all peripheral pulses should be evaluated, and capillary refill, skin color, temperature rechecked
Back	All patients should be log rolled with careful attention to spinal immobilization to afford the clinician a full view of the patient's posterior surfaces, including neck, back, buttocks, and lower extremities; these areas should be carefully inspected and palpated to detect any area of injury
Complete neurologic examination	Motor and sensory evaluation of the extremities and reevaluation of the patient's GCS score and pupils; any evidence of paralysis or paresis should prompt immediate immobilization of the entire patient if not already done

SECTION SEVEN: Secondary Survey

This section outlines the components of the secondary assessment during the initial trauma evaluation. At the completion of this section, the learner will be able to discuss the components and the suggested format for conducting the secondary survey.

The secondary survey begins after the primary survey is completed and all immediately life-threatening injuries have been addressed. A head-to-toe approach is used, with a thorough examination of each body system. A critical point to remember is that if the patient becomes hemodynamically unstable at any point during the secondary survey, immediately return to the primary survey format (A, B, C, D, and E) to trou-

bleshoot the problem. A summary of key points in the secondary survey has been adapted in Table 36–2 from the American College of Surgeons Committee on Trauma's *Advanced Trauma Life Support Course Manual* (ACSCT, 1997).

At the completion of the secondary survey, remember that the trauma patient demands repeated reevaluation so that any new signs or symptoms are not overlooked. Other life-threatening problems may appear, or exacerbation of previously treated injuries may occur (such as tension pneumothorax, pericardial tamponade, or intracranial bleeding). Continuous monitoring of vital signs is critical.

In summary, secondary survey should be conducted during initial assessment and resuscitation of the trauma patient. Key criteria for evaluation were identified in each area to facilitate assessment parameters.

SECTION SEVEN REVIEW

1. During the secondary assessment, the patient becomes hemodynamically unstable. You should immediately
   A. stop the secondary survey and reinstitute the primary assessment
   B. finish the secondary survey, looking for potential etiologies of instability
   C. start at the beginning of the secondary survey
   D. reevaluate patency and flow rates of IVs
2. The purpose of the secondary survey is to
   A. identify and intervene with life-threatening injuries
   B. identify the existence of all injuries
   C. facilitate treatment of airway and breathing
   D. assess response of resuscitative interventions
3. The complete and immediate immobilization of the entire patient should take place with the following findings during secondary survey
   A. inability to establish airway

B. tense, distended abdomen
C. Glasgow Coma Scale score less than 8
D. evidence of paralysis or paresis
4. Presence of abdominal pain on light or deep palpation in the injured patient usually indicates
   A. gastritis
   B. presence of intraperitoneal blood
   C. pelvic fracture
   D. intracerebral pathology
5. Rectal examination should be done to evaluate all of the following EXCEPT
   A. rectal wall integrity
   B. presence of blood
   C. bladder injury
   D. palpable pelvic fractures

Answers: 1. A, 2. B, 3. D, 4. B, 5. C

SECTION EIGHT: Trauma Resuscitation

At the completion of this section, the learner will be able to describe the trimodal distribution of trauma-related mortalities and how this is integrated into clinical assessment, discuss important nursing responsibilities during the trauma resuscitation phase, and compare and contrast various end points of traumatic shock resuscitation.

The primary survey and resuscitation occur simultaneously. As this is occurring, other therapies are also initiated. For example, a Foley catheter is inserted during resuscitation (unless contraindicated). A gastric tube also is placed to prevent aspiration.

Trauma Deaths

When plotted on a graph, trauma-related mortalities exhibit a trimodal distribution; that is, death from trauma has three peak periods of occurrence. The first peak occurs within minutes of the injury. These deaths usually result from injuries to the brain, upper spinal cord, heart, aorta, or other major blood vessel. The second peak occurs within 2 hours of injury, and death usually is related to subdural or epidural hematomas, hemopneumothorax, ruptured spleen, lacerated liver, fractured femurs, or other injuries resulting in significant blood loss. The third peak occurs days to weeks after the injury and usually results from complications of sepsis or multiple organ failure (ACSCT, 1997).

How does the knowledge of this distribution affect clinical practice? This knowledge can empower the nurse to anticipate the needs of the patient based on time from injury and physiological manifestation of the injury. If a patient is received within minutes of injury, what are the life-threatening injuries that may cause death in this time frame? Has the patient experienced brainstem compression or laceration resulting in respiratory center dysfunction? What assessment and intervention must be performed to mediate these injuries?

If an unstable female patient arrives within 30 minutes of injury, what conditions must be appreciated clinically to anticipate a life-threatening situation? Conditions might include hemopneumothorax (What is her respiratory effort? How are her lung sounds? Will a chest tube be necessary?), ruptured spleen or lacerated liver (Does she have a tense and painful abdomen? Is she hypotensive with no signs of obvious blood loss?), or fractured femur (Is her leg painful, with an obvious fracture?).

The high-acuity nurse caring for a patient 3 days postinjury anticipates a much different scenario. If the patient is experiencing multiple organ dysfunction syndrome or sepsis, what could be the precipitating factors or contributing factors to his condition? Was he overhydrated during the first 24 to 48 hours and acute respiratory distress syndrome (ARDS) has ensued? Did he have a missed intra-abdominal injury predisposing him to sepsis?

Shock from Trauma

Mortality from trauma may result from what is considered a preventable cause. One of the most frequently encountered clinical states in the injured patient is traumatic shock. Because of the frequency of traumatic shock, a brief discussion of hemorrhagic shock ensues (refer to Module 15 for an in-depth examination of the cellular tissue, organ, and system response to shock).

Shock has been defined as the consequence of insufficient tissue perfusion that results in inadequate cellular oxygenation and accumulation of metabolic wastes (ACSCT, 1997). The most common cause of shock in the injured patient is hypovolemia resulting from acute blood loss. Acute blood loss can occur externally, as with lacerations, open fractures, avulsion injuries, or amputations, or internally within a body cavity, as with bleeding into the chest cavity, abdominal cavity, retroperitoneum, or soft tissue.

Exsanguination is the most extreme form of hemorrhage. There is an initial loss of 40 percent of the patient's blood volume, with a rate of blood loss, or a rate of hemorrhage, exceeding 250 mL per minute. If uncontrolled, the patient may lose 50 percent of the entire blood volume within a very few minutes. Loss of up to 15 percent of circulating volume (700 to 750 mL for a 70-kg patient) may produce little in terms of obvious symptoms, whereas loss of up to 30 percent of circulating vol-

ume (1.5 mL) may result in mild tachycardia, tachypnea, and anxiety. Hypotension, marked tachycardia (pulse 110 to 120 beats per minute) and confusion may not be evident until more than 30 percent of blood volume has been lost. Loss of 40 percent of circulating volume (2 L) is immediately life threatening. Most injuries precipitating exsanguination are from penetrating trauma. Regardless of the mechanism, exsanguinations will lead to hypovolemic shock.

Resuscitation of the patient who is exsanguinating rests on the intensified basic principles of circulation management. IV access is established quickly with adequate, large-bore catheters. Because the underlying source of the hypotension is hypovolemic shock, administering fluids is crucial in shock management. Vasopressors are not given to treat the hypotension until fluid volume has been restored. Blood and blood products may be given in addition to IV fluids. Type specific blood should be given, but in an emergency situation low-titer O-positive blood may be given to men and O-negative to women of childbearing age.

Other adjuncts are available in the acute phase of resuscitation of the patient with exsanguination. Rapid infusion devices are available and can deliver large amounts of crystalloid and colloid quickly. The use of autotransfusion devices facilitates resuscitative efforts. Emergency department open resuscitative thoracotomy also may be used to manage the exsanguinating patient, especially if exsanguination is suspected to be related to injury to the great vessels (i.e., aorta) or the heart.

Critical analysis during the primary assessment and quick recognition of traumatic shock are essential skills in the resuscitative phase of trauma. Twenty percent of preventable trauma-related mortalities can be mediated with improved prehospital and hospital care under the provision of highly skilled clinicians who can evaluate the injured patient rapidly and effectively.

End Points of Resuscitation

How is it determined that the patient has been adequately resuscitated? The goal of the resuscitation is to treat shock so it does not progress to an irreversible state.

Recall from earlier in this section that shock has been defined as the consequence of insufficient tissue perfusion that results in inadequate cellular oxygenation and accumulation of metabolic wastes (ACSCT, 1997). The patient who is in shock, therefore, would have signs and symptoms of inadequate tissue perfusion and cellular oxygenation and accumulation of metabolic wastes. The patient who is not in shock would have signs of adequate tissue perfusion that results in adequate cellular oxygenation and no evidence of accumulation of metabolic wastes. Knowing when tissue perfusion has been restored is a challenge. Unfortunately, traditional signs of sufficient tissue perfusion (normal blood pressure, heart rate, and urine output) cannot be used in shock states because normal vital signs and urine output may be the result of compensatory mechanisms (renin–angiotensin–aldosterone and the sympathetic nervous system; see Module 15). The best clinical indicator of sufficient tissue perfusion is not currently available. Current indicators include traditional hemodynamic parameters, global parameters, and organ specific parameters as summarized by Schulman (2002) (Table 36–3).

The high-acuity nurse should not be lured into a false sense of security when vital signs and basic hemodynamic parameters have been restored to normal values during resuscitation (Shulman, 2002). During resuscitation from traumatic hemorrhagic shock, normalization of blood pressure, heart rate, and urine output are not adequate (EAST, 2003a). Optimizing hemodynamic variables to improve cardiac output/index, oxygen delivery, and oxygen consumption may be beneficial, especially if initated early in the resuscitation process (Kern & Shoemaker, 2002). A right ventricular end diastolic volume index using a special right ventricular ejection fraction oximetry catheter has been advocated as being more reflective of preload in trauma patients than pulmonary artery wedge pressure or right atrial pressure (RAP) (Chang & Meredith, 1996). Current guidelines recommend the use of base deficit, lactate, and gastric pH_i as end points, with the goal of correcting all of these within 24 hours of injury (EAST, 2003a).

In summary, the process of trauma assessment can be refined and polished with the knowledge of clinical conditions that cause deaths in the trauma population. Nursing can play a key role in mediating the preventable deaths from trauma that continue to plague modern society.

TABLE 36–3 End Points in Trauma Resuscitation

Traditional Hemodynamic Parameters

PARAMETER	END-POINT VALUE
Blood pressure	Systolic blood pressure greater than 90 mm Hg; mean arterial pressure (MAP) greater than 70 mm Hg
Heart rate	Less than 100 beats per minute
Urine output	Greater than 30 mL per hour
Skin	Warm, dry

Global Parameters

PARAMETER	END-POINT VALUE
Oxygen delivery index	Greater than 500 mL/min/m^2
Oxygen consumption index	125 mL/min/m^2
Systemic mixed venous oxygen saturation	65 to 80 percent
Lactate	Less than 2.2 mMol/L
Base deficit	± 3.0 mMol/L
Tissue arteriovenous carbon dioxide gradient	Less than 11 mm Hg
Sublingual capnography	Less than 70
Gastric pH_i	pH_i greater than 7.35

SECTION EIGHT REVIEW

1. Trauma-related mortalities exhibit a _____ distribution.
   A. modal
   B. bimodal
   C. trimodal
   D. bell-shaped
2. The most common shock state in the injured patient is
   A. hypovolemic
   B. cardiogenic
   C. neurogenic
   D. septic
3. Hypotension, marked tachycardia, and confusion may not be evident until _____ of blood volume is lost?
   A. 15 percent
   B. 30 percent
   C. 50 percent
   D. 75 percent
4. Which of the following parameters is the BEST reflection that resuscitation efforts have improved the shock state?
   A. MAP greater than 70 mm Hg
   B. heart rate 80 beats per minute
   C. urine output 30 mL per hour
   D. lactate less than 2.2 mMol
5. Current guidelines recommend which of the following parameters should be corrected within 24 hours of injury?
   A. base deficit
   B. lactate
   C. gastric pH_i
   D. all of the above

Answers: 1. C, 2. A, 3. B, 4. D, 5. D

SECTION NINE: Management of Selected Injuries

At the completion of this section, the learner will be able to describe basic principles of collaborative management for injuries to the chest, abdomin, and pelvis. Care of the patient with traumatic brain injury is discussed in Module 20 and care of the patient with spinal cord injury is reviewed in Module 21. Management of chest, abdominal, and pelvic injuries were selected for this section because they are injuries commonly seen in high-acuity units. As with any emergent condition, these systems are not addressed until the airway, breathing, and circulation are stabilized as described in Section Six.

Chest Injuries

Injuries to the chest are usually a result of an MVC or a violent crime. Chest injuries cause one in every four deaths in North America. Injuries to the chest involve trauma to the chest wall, lungs, and heart.

Chest Wall

Rib Fractures. Rib fractures are typically caused by blunt trauma. Multiple ribs can be fractured. Rib fractures are very painful and the pain is aggravated by movement of the chest wall, even with breathing. Therefore, the patient with rib fractures often takes shallow breaths. Ateleactsis can develop and the patient is at risk for developing pneumonia. Pain management, including nonsteriodal anti-inflammatory agents, intercostal nerve block, thoracic epidural analgesia, and narcotics, may be used to optimize pain management (Wanek & Mayberry, 2004). There is no treatment for rib fractures other than to let the fractures heal naturally with time.

Flail Chest. Flail chest occurs when two or more rib fractures occur in two or more places (Fig. 36–3). The chest wall does not have bony support and normal chest wall movement is disrupted. Complications ensue as a result of extreme pain with inspiration and expiration, and hypoxemia often results from inadequate respiratory effort. Signs of a flail chest include uncoordinated, asymmetrical movement of the chest wall, crepitus, and hypoxemia on blood gas. Treatment goals are directed at preventing and treating hypoxemia. Mechanical ventilation may be required.

Pulmonary Injuries

Pulmonary Contusions. Blunt trauma to lung parenchyma can result in a unilateral or bilateral pulmonary contusion (a bruising of lung parenchyma). These injuries can be quite serious because the bruising can lead to alveolar hemorrhage, edema, and inflammation within the lung. A large pulmonary contusion can result in respiratory failure. Clinical manifestations of pulmonary contusion may not be present for several days. The chest x-ray may reveal pulmonary infiltrates. Crackles may be auscultated. The patient is at risk for impaired gas exchange. Therefore, nursing care must focus on improving gas exchange through deep breathing exercises, ambulation, and removal of secretions. As with rib fractures, pain management is paramount. The patient is monitored for worsening respiratory status. Intubation and mechanical ventilation may be required if signs of respiratory failure are present. The major complication of pulmonary contusions include pneumonia and ARDS (refer to Module 5).

Tension Pneumothorax. A tension pneumothorax occurs when air leaks from the lung or through the chest wall, gets trapped in the thoracic cavity without means of escape, and col-

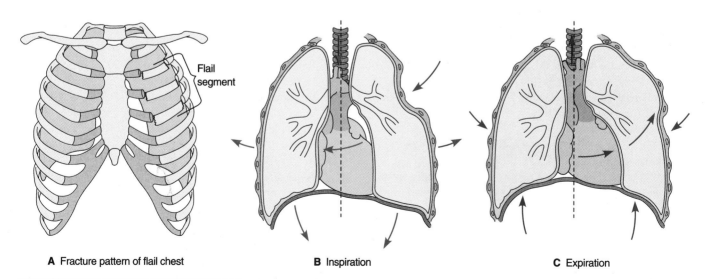

A Fracture pattern of flail chest   **B** Inspiration   **C** Expiration

Figure 36–3 ■ Flail chest. Physiologic function of the chest wall is impaired as the flail segment (*A*) is sucked inward during inspiration (*B*) and moves outward with expiration (*C*).

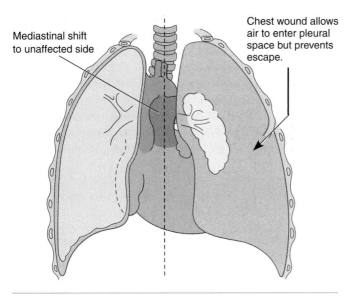

Figure 36–4 ■ Tension pneumothorax.

lapses the affected lung (Fig. 36–4). As intrathoracic pressure continues to increase, this pressure is transmitted to the heart, causing decreased venous return and cardiac output. Tension pneumothorax is characterized by chest pain, air hunger, respiratory distress, tachycardia, neck vein distention, trachea displaced from midline, and absent breath sounds on the affected side. In an emergent situation, the increased intrathoracic pressure is relieved by a large-bore (14-gauge) needle or immediate placement of a chest tube.

Open Pneumothorax. An open pneumothorax is a penetrating chest wall injury that sucks air, causing intrathoracic pressure and atmospheric pressure to equilibrate (Fig. 36–5). The clinical manifestations are the same as for a tension pneumothorax. Ini-

tial treatment includes temporizing the wound by taping an occlusive dressing over three edges of the wound, creating an occlusion with inspiration (the dressing is sucked into the wound as the patient breathes in), with an outlet through the lower edge for expiration. A chest tube is placed as soon as possible and surgery may be required.

Massive Hemothorax. Massive hemothorax is defined as the accumulation of more than 1,500 mL of blood in the chest cavity (ACSCT, 1997). Usually, the cause is a penetrating wound that disrupts the vessels. Assessment findings may include decreased breath sounds or dullness to percussion on the affected side and hypotension. Management is aimed at restoring blood volume and decompression of the chest cavity with a chest tube. An autotransfusion device may be attached to the chest tube collection chamber. Surgery may be required for patients who have continued bleeding, defined as more than 200 mL per hour for 2 to 4 hours (ACSCT, 1997).

Cardiac Injuries

Cardiac Tamponade. Whether from penetrating or blunt trauma, cardiac tamponade causes the pericardium (the sac around the heart) to fill with blood. This restricts the heart's ability to pump and also impedes venous return. Signs and symptoms include Beck's triad, (elevated right atrial pressure with neck vein distention, hypotension, and muffled heart sounds). Pulsus paradoxus (an increase of greater than 10 mm Hg systolic blood pressure on inspiration) is also a classic sign of cardiac tamponade. Pulseless electrical activity (PEA) may be present (refer to Module 10). Treatment is initially directed at volume resuscitation until pericardiocentesis can be performed (Fig. 36–6).

Blunt Cardiac Injury. Blunt cardiac injury, formerly called cardiac contusion, is a bruising of the myocardium. Chest discomfort,

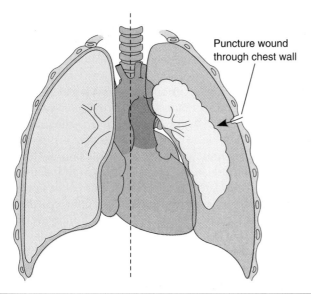

Figure 36–5 ■ Open pneumothorax.

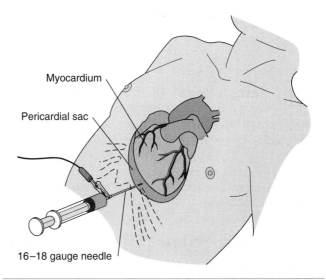

Figure 36–6 ■ Pericardiocentesis.

sinus tachycardia, and hypotension are suggestive of this injury. Electrocardiogram (ECG) changes may also be present and may include *ST* changes, dysrhythmias, or heart block. If the admission ECG is abnormal on admission, the patient is admitted to the high-acuity unit for continuous ECG monitoring for 24 to 48 hours (EAST, 1998). An echocardiogram may be done to evaluate cardiac function.

Abdominal Injuries

Blunt trauma creates devastating injury to the abdomen. In a motor vehicle crash, a compression injury from a steering wheel may rupture solid organs (Fig. 36–2). Shearing injury from a seat belt can result in similar injuries. Deceleration may cause lacerations to the spleen and liver because these organs are movable from the fixed structures surrounding them. The incidence of injury to the spleen is the highest (40 to 50 percent) followed by that to the liver (35 to 45 percent) (ACSCT, 1997). Penetrating trauma from stab wounds most commonly involve the liver, small bowel, diaphragm, or colon. Gunshot wounds have a greater kinetic energy and more often involve the small bowel, colon, liver, and abdominal vascular structures.

Spleen Injuries

The spleen is located in the left upper quadrant of the abdomen and is the most common organ injured in blunt trauma to the abdomen. The spleen has important immunologic functions; therefore, steps are taken to let the spleen wound heal after injury instead of removing it. Diagnosis of injury to the spleen is made by CT scan. Patients with splenic injury are admitted to a high-acuity unit for serial monitoring of vital signs and hematocrit. It is crucial to monitor vital signs for evidence of continued bleeding in or around the spleen. Continued hemodynamic instability may indicate the need for surgical intervention (EAST, 2003c). Patients who do have a splenectomy will be at risk for streptococcal infections and, therefore, require a pneumococcal vaccine (Pneumovax) prior to discharge from the hospital.

Liver Injuries

Though anterior and lateral portions of the liver are protected by the lower rib cage, the liver remains vulnerable to injury in blunt or penetrating trauma. The majority of liver injuries are minor and do not require surgery. However, the mortality may be greater than 50 percent in a complex liver injury, and death is usually the result of hemorrhage. Diagnosis of liver injury is made by CT scan. Liver injuries are graded using a liver injury scale. A grade of 1 to 6 is given, with 6 being a complete hepatic avulsion and the worst injury possible. Medical management may include hepatic arteriography to embolize any bleeding in the liver or the bleeding may require an operation to stop it. However, most liver injuries up to grade 4 are successfully managed nonoperatively (EAST, 2003c). Bleeding is the most common complication associated with liver injury, and patients must be monitored for changes in vital signs and continued decline in hematocrit values.

Patients with liver injuries are usually admitted to a high-acuity unit for serial monitoring of vital signs and hematocrit. In the event the patient becomes hemodynamically unstable from continued bleeding and hypovolemic shock, the high-acuity nurse must be prepared to implement volume resuscitation as ordered. This may include crystalloids and blood or blood products. Coagulopathies may be corrected with fresh-frozen plasma, platelets, or cryoprecipitate. It is crucial that the nurse monitors the patient's response to these interventions. Continued hemodynamic instability may require surgical interventions to find and control the source of hemorrhage within the liver.

Damage Control Surgery

Patients with abdominal injuries that need an operative procedure may require a technique referred to as *damage control surgery*. There are three phases to this surgical technique: initial operation, resuscitation, and definitive restoration. During the *initial operation*, time in the operating room (OR) is kept to a minimum. The goal is to quickly locate and control sources of hemorrhage. The longer this takes, the greater the risk of three conditions: hypothermia, continued bleeding, and systemic acidosis. The triad of hypothermia, coagulopathy, and acidosis creates a self-propagating cycle that can eventually lead to an irreversible physiological insult (Screiber, 2004). Therefore, the goal of this initial operation is to quickly control hemorrhage, which may be done by simply packing the abdomen with sterile dressing to control the bleeding.

After this initial phase, the patient is taken to the ICU for *resuscitation*. The goal is to correct hypothermia, acidosis, and coagulopathies. Warmed IV solutions are given. Serial measurements of lactate and base deficit are assessed for signs of improving metabolic acidosis. Coagulopathies are corrected with blood and blood products. During this time, the patient is assessed for abdominal compartment syndrome (Refer to Module 30). Abdominal compartment syndrome is essentially intra-abdominal hypertension, or too much pressure buildup within the abdominal cavity. It is caused by continued bleeding or visceral edema. Signs and symptoms include a taut distended abdomen, decreased cardiac output, increased peak pulmonary pressures, and decreased urine output (McNeilis et al., 2003). Intra-abdominal pressures may be directly measured by instilling 50 to 100 mL of sterile normal saline into the bladder via a Foley catheter. A transducer interprets the pressure. These pressures can be monitored intermittently or continuously as ordered. Abdominal pressures greater than 20 to 25 mm Hg are considered high and may indicate that the patient's abdomen needs to be opened to relieve the pressure (McNeilis et al., 2003).

Once the hypothermia, acidosis, and coagulopathies are corrected (usually within 72 hours of the initial operation), the patient is taken back to the OR for definitive repair of injuries.

Pelvic Injuries

Pelvic fractures can be life-threatening injuries. They are associated with blunt trauma—an MVC or a crushing injury to the pelvic region. Because the pelvis protects major blood vessels, patients with pelvic fractures are at high risk for hemorrhage. Signs of a pelvic fracture include perianal ecchymosis, pain on palpation or "rocking" of the iliac crests, hematuria, and lower extremity rotation or paresis (Mirza & Ellis, 2004). Confirmation of pelvic fractures is made by CT scan.

Initial management includes the prevention or treatment of life-threatening hemorrhage. This may require surgical intervention. Patients who are hemodynamically stable are treated conservatively with bedrest and orthopedic stablization within 3 days (Scalea & Burgess, 2004). Stablization may be temporary with an external fixation device for patients who are unstable. If the patient is stable, definitive management includes internal fixation (Mirza & Ellis, 2004).

Nursing management centers around monitoring for signs of continued hemorrhage and resuscitation with fluids. Before the patient can be moved or turned, the nurse must find out if the physician has determined whether the pelvic fracture is stable or unstable. A stable pelvic fracture implies that no further pathologic displacement of the pelvis can occur with turning. An unstable pelvic fracture means that further pathologic displacement can occur with turning (Walls, 2002). The nurse should monitor color, motion, and sensitivity of the bilateral lower extremities for signs of neurological or vascular compromise.

In summary, oftentimes patients in high-acuity units involved in trauma have injuries to the chest, abdomen, or pelvis. Injuries to the chest involve trauma to the chest wall, lungs, and heart. Chest wall injuries include rib fractures and flail chest. Pain management is key in patients with these injuries. Pulmonary injuries include pulmonary contusion, tension pneumothorax, open pneumothorax, and massive hemothorax. These injuries can be life threatening. Cardiac injuries include cardiac tamponade and blunt cardiac injuries. Beck's triad and pulses paradoxus are signs of cardiac tamponade. ECG changes are signs of blunt cardiac trauma. The spleen and liver are the most commonly injured organs in the abdomen. Patients with these injuries must be monitored for hemorrhage and may require surgical repair. Damage control surgery may be required. Injuries to the pelvis can be life-threatening. Prior to moving a patient with these injuries, the nurse must know if the pelvic fractures are unstable.

SECTION NINE REVIEW

1. A major complication of pulmonary contusions is
   A. ARDS
   B. pneumothorax
   C. hemothorax
   D. tension pneumothorax
2. Which of the following are important interventions for the patient with multiple rib fractures?
   A. chest tube placement
   B. needle aspiration
   C. pain management and pulmonary hygiene
   D. placing a gauze dressing over the wound
3. You are the nurse caring for a patient with a hemothorax. You note that 200 mL has drained from the chest tube in 2 hours. What should you do?
   A. nothing; this is a normal amount
   B. notify the physician
   C. empty the collection chamber
   D. recheck the drainage in 2 hours
4. Patients with injuries to the spleen or liver may require operative repair if
   A. their abdominal girths increase
   B. they have a change in level of consciousness
   C. the hematocrit increases
   D. they become hemodynamically unstable
5. During damage control surgery, the initial operation time is restricted to prevent
   A. hypothermia
   B. coagulopathy
   C. metabolic acidosis
   D. all of the above
6. You are the nurse caring for a patient with a pelvic fracture. Before turning the patient you must first
   A. medicate the patient
   B. ask the physician if the fracture is stable or unstable
   C. remove the fixation device
   D. assess color, motion, and sensitivity of the legs

Answers: 1. A, 2. C, 3. B, 4. D, 5. D, 6. B

Nursing Diagnoses Associated with Traumatic Injury

At the completion of this section, the learner will be able to cluster patient symptoms and derive appropriate nursing diagnoses for the patient with traumatic injuries.

If a traumatic injury is suspected, the nurse focuses on assessing the symptoms most commonly associated with life-threatening conditions. These symptoms include ineffective breathing, altered blood pH, hypotension, distended neck veins, decreased urine output, and a change in level of consciousness. The nursing diagnoses associated with these symptoms include altered airway clearance, ineffective breathing patterns, impaired gas exchange, fluid volume deficit, altered urinary elimination, and altered cerebral tissue perfusion.

Ineffective Airway Clearance, Ineffective Breathing Pattern, and Impaired Gas Exchange

In the trauma patient, the airway is always assessed first and necessary interventions made. The airway may be compromised if the patient has a depressed mental status. The gag reflex may be absent, and foreign bodies may be present in the oropharynx. A partially obstructed airway will be noisy. Snoring, gargling, or wheezing may be present. If the airway is obstructed, it is re-opened using a manual maneuver (chin lift maneuver if cervical spine injury has not been ruled out), immediately suctioned, and an oral or nasopharyngeal artificial airway placed. Oral or nasotracheal intubation is another method of securing a patent airway. Facial trauma may produce copious amounts of bleeding, and skeletal integrity of the face may be disrupted. The performance of a **cricothyroidotomy** (surgical airway) is preferred to obtain a patent airway in a patient with massive facial injuries. Direct trauma to the airway may occur from blunt larnygotracheal injuries. These patients are unable to tolerate a supine position, are hoarse, have subcutaneous emphysema, and are tender over the tracheal area. A **tracheostomy** is the best method of securing an airway in these patients.

Ineffective breathing patterns are associated with tracheobronchial and thoracic injuries. The chest is observed for bruising, open wounds, and symmetry of chest wall movement. Open wounds are evaluated further by log rolling the patient and inspecting the posterior surface. No chest wall movement and the presence of abdominal breathing may indicate a cervical cord lesion. The patient's respiratory rate is noted, as is the degree of breathing effort. Paradoxical movement of the chest (inward motion of a segment of the chest during inhalation and outward motion of the same segment with expiration) indicates multiple rib fractures and a flail segment. The patient with a large flail segment may require intubation and mechanical ventilation or pain control therapy to prevent respiratory compromise and to

promote tissue oxygenation. The chest area is palpated to detect the presence of subcutaneous emphysema, rib/sternum tenderness, or defects. Auscultation detects the presence of breath sounds bilaterally in the primary survey. Gross differences in breath sounds are an important finding because it usually indicates a pneumothorax or hemothorax. A more detailed pulmonary assessment is performed during the secondary assessment. High-flow oxygen is administered to trauma patients before obtaining arterial blood gas results. A nonrebreathing mask or a bag-valve-mask device with an oxygen reservoir may be used depending on the patient's responsiveness level. Pulse oximetry and end-tidal carbon dioxide measurement (if the patient is intubated) provide additional data regarding oxygenation.

Fluid Volume Deficit

Peripheral vasoconstriction may artificially elevate blood pressure readings even though central arterial pressures are low. This is a short-acting compensatory mechanism. The value of clustering assessment data is to prevent misdiagnosis by focusing on one symptom while ignoring others. It is important to monitor the trauma patient's blood pressure and at the same time assess neck veins, level of consciousness, and urine output.

Hypotension in the trauma patient usually is related to hypovolemia. Hypovolemia may result from internal bleeding or uncontrolled external bleeding. Fractures and lacerations of abdominal organs are frequent sources of bleeding in the trauma patient. However, hypotension may be related to factors that inhibit cardiac output (CO) or the loss of peripheral vascular resistance. The two most frequently encountered conditions associated with restriction of CO are cardiac tamponade and tension pneumothorax. In cardiac tamponade, hypotension occurs in response to decreased CO. A tear in the pericardium produces bleeding into the pericardial sac. The increased pressure prohibits filling of the ventricles and decreases stroke volume. The increased pericardium pressure also impedes coronary blood flow. Myocardial ischemia results and further decreases CO. Lung parenchymal injury from chest trauma may produce a tension pneumothorax. As atmospheric air enters the pleural cavity through the injury site, the lung on the affected side collapses while mediastinal contents and the trachea are pushed away from the injury site. The pressure placed on the great vessels inhibits venous return. Thus, the neck veins become distended.

Both cardiac tamponade and tension pneumothorax are life-threatening conditions that require immediate treatment. Blood in the pericardial sac is removed by pericardiocentesis. Insertion of a chest tube and covering the open chest wound (if present) with an impermeable dressing are appropriate interventions for the patient with a tension pneumothorax.

Hypotension also may occur in patients with spinal cord injuries who develop spinal shock. In spinal shock, the patient's blood pressure may be less than 70 mm Hg as a result of a loss of sympathetic tone that occurs secondary to transection of the spinal cord. The parasympathetic nervous system is unopposed, so peripheral vasodilation and bradycardia occur. Bradycardia is the key assessment finding that helps to differentiate spinal shock from hypovolemic shock. However, the patient also may be hemorrhaging but unable to compensate by increasing the heart rate. Atropine or intravenous fluids are administered to increase the heart rate high enough to perfuse core organs. Fluid resuscitation is appropriate for a patient with spinal cord injury who is hypotensive because internal trauma cannot be ruled out initially. However, caution must be taken to avoid causing pulmonary edema. For the patient with an isolated spinal cord injury, if a fluid challenge does not resolve the hypotension, careful administration of a vasopressor may be considered (ACSCT, 1997).

The presence of a radial pulse indicates an arterial pressure of 80 mm Hg. A pressure of at least 70 mm Hg is required for palpation of a femoral or brachial pulse. If a cartoid pulse can be palpated, the pressure is at least 60 mm Hg (ACSCT, 1997). The nurse can discriminate hypotension resulting from hypovolemia from that associated with increased pericardial pressure by assessing for the presence of a paradoxical pulse. The systolic blood pressure will fall more during inspiration if tension pneumothorax or cardiac tamponade exists. In these conditions, the increased thoracic pressure from inspiration further decreases left ventricle filling and results in blood backing up into the right heart, compromising CO. If a right atrial pressure (RAP) catheter or pulmonary arterial catheter is in place, the RAP reading is elevated because of increased right atrial filling with decreased emptying. A RAP reading of greater than 15 cm H_2O is significant. Jugular venous distention will be present. Hypotension resulting from hypovolemia is associated with flat neck veins. Decreased pedal pulses and pale or mottled skin also may be present.

Altered Urinary Elimination

The kidneys receive 20 percent of the CO, and the kidneys may reflect decreased CO earlier than other organs. In most circumstances, decreased or absent urine output in the trauma patient indicates decreased core perfusion from an extrarenal cause. The adult trauma patient should maintain an hourly urine output of at least 25 to 30 mL to ensure adequate core circulation.

Altered Cerebral Tissue Perfusion

A change in consciousness in the trauma patient may be related to numerous factors. In the presence of hypovolemia, cerebral blood flow decreases, resulting in stupor, unconsciousness, and eventually failure of subconscious mental processes, including vasomotor control and respiration. The more highly specialized the tissue, the more vulnerable it is to hypoxemia. Cortical functions are lost first with cerebral hypoxia. Cerebral hypoperfusion is present when the systolic blood pressure is below 60 mm

Hg. Hypoxia, hypoglycemia, and drug use also may impair responsiveness. Because a change in responsiveness may be present from cerebral injury or from systemic causes, clustering of assessment data is helpful. Responsiveness generally is evaluated at the same time that pupillary size and reaction and motor responses are assessed. If a spinal cord injury is present, the patient may not be able to respond to commands even if the patient comprehends. It is important to document the stimulus used to elicit a motor response, the exact response, and bilateral differences. The use of a standardized scale, such as the Glasgow Coma Scale (refer to Module 19), can facilitate monitoring of neurological status and improve communication among multiple health care providers.

Airway protection is of major concern in a patient with decreased responsiveness. An oral or nasopharyngeal airway is inserted to maintain airway patency. Unconscious patients should be intubated endotracheally. Oxygen administration is necessary in a patient with decreased responsiveness to promote cerebral oxygenation.

Focused Assessment Findings and Nursing Diagnoses

Life-threatening conditions produce characteristic symptoms that the nurse can identify. The following cluster of data strongly suggests the presence of a life-threatening injury:

- Noisy airway
- Absent breath sounds
- Deviated trachea
- Flat or distended neck veins
- Paradoxical chest movement
- Open chest wound
- Subcutaneous emphysema
- Hypotension
- Decreased responsiveness
- Decreased urine output

Nursing diagnoses that pertain to the trauma patient can be clustered in the same manner as the assessment data. Clustering around the ABCs of airway, breathing, and circulation will assist the nurse in prioritizing nursing care.

- *Ineffective airway clearance* related to obstruction or cognitive impairment
- *Ineffective breathing pattern* related to tracheobronchial or chest wall injury, decreased area for gas exchange or pain
- *Impaired gas exchange* related to ventilation–perfusion imbalance or decreased hemoglobin
- *Decreased cardiac output* related to impairment of venous return or myocardial injury
- *Altered tissue perfusion* related to an imbalance between cellular oxygen demands and supply
- *Fluid volume deficit* related to hemorrhage or extravasation (i.e., burns)

Evidence-Based Practice

- *Variables associated with the development of renal failure in patients with rhabdomyolyis include age greater than 55 years, peak creatine kinase greater than 5,000 U/L, male gender, and body mass index greater than 30 kg/m² (Brown et al., 2004).*

- *Early hyperglycemia (glucose greater than 200 mg/dL) is associated with significantly higher infection and mortality rates in trauma patients independent of injury severity or shock (Laird et al., 2004).*

- *Older patients (between 60 and 69 years of age) with traumatic injury have higher risks for developing ARDS when compared with younger patients (Johnston et al., 2003).*

- *Major in-hospital complications contribute significantly to the long-term reduction in quality of life after serious injury (Holbrook et al., 2001).*

In summary, nursing diagnoses associated with life-threatening injuries include ineffective airway clearance, ineffective breathing patterns, impaired gas exchange, fluid volume deficit, altered urinary elimination, and altered cerebral tissue perfusion. These diagnoses require astute nursing assessments of the pulmonary, cardiovascular, and neurologic systems, and frequent monitoring of vital signs and urine output. The high acuity nurse must be able to recognize life-threatening injuries, cluster data from a focused assessment, and identify nursing diagnoses pertinent to these injuries.

SECTION TEN REVIEW

Mary is admitted into the emergency department following an assault where she was beaten in the face and head. She has a large amount of facial edema, and both eyes are swollen shut. She has broken teeth and blood in her mouth. Mary follows commands but does not verbalize a response to questions. Breathing pattern is rapid and noisy.

1. Based on Mary's history, which of the following interventions should be performed first?
   A. open the airway and clear the oral pharynx
   B. apply 100 percent oxygen by mask
   C. obtain arterial blood gases
   D. insert an intravenous catheter

2. Mary's arterial blood gases reflect respiratory acidosis. The acidosis is MOST likely related to
   A. ineffective breathing pattern
   B. pain
   C. partially obstructed airway
   D. head injury

3. Mary loses consciousness. The nurse should prepare for which of the following first?
   A. CT scan of the head
   B. endotracheal intubation or surgical airway placement
   C. placement of a second IV line
   D. placement of a nasogastric tube

Answers: 1. A, 2. C, 3. B

SECTION ELEVEN: Complications of Traumatic Injury

At the completion of this section, the learner will be able to link posttrauma complications with the physiology of a traumatic injury and preexisting risk factors, and discuss interventions to prevent complications of traumatic injury.

As discussed in Section Eight, trauma deaths occur in three peaks. The first peak is within the first hour postinjury, and the major causes of death are massive bleeding secondary to great vessel tears and head injuries. The second peak occurs during the initial hours postinjury during the resuscitation phase. Deaths in this phase generally are attributed to internal bleeding. The final peak of trauma-related deaths occurs days to weeks after the injury event.

The primary responsibilities of the nurse caring for a trauma patient in the final phase are prevention and surveillance. Treatment of trauma sequelae is controversial and primitive because research in this area is still in its infancy as compared with trauma resuscitation research. Therefore, the goal of nursing care is to prevent complications. Patients with traumatic injuries are at a greater risk of complications than patients with other injuries for a variety of reasons. Patients with traumatic injuries are at risk for undernutrition, ARDS, disseminated intravascular coagulation (DIC), acute renal failure, and multiple organ dysfunction syndrome (MODS). Many of these complications have been discussed in detail throughout this book, but they will be reviewed here briefly specifically as they relate to the patient with traumatic injuries. The reader is referred to the following modules for additional information: undernutrition (Module 23), ARDS (Module 4),

TABLE 36–4 Traumatic Injuries and Associated Sequelae

CONDITION	PATHOPHYSIOLOGY	COMPLICATION
Thoracic Trauma		
Great vessel tears	Hemorrhage	DIC, ARF
Hemothorax	Decreased gas exchange	ARDS
Tension pneumothorax	Decreased gas exchange	ARDS
Open pneumothorax	Disruption in skin integrity	Sepsis
Abdominal Trauma		
Perforation of intestine	Extravasation of GI contents into peritoneum	Sepsis
Liver/splenic laceration	Hemorrhage	DIC, ACS, ARF
Orthopedic Trauma		
Femur/pelvis fracture	Hemorrhage	DIC, ARF
Long-bone fractures	Disruption of fat-containing tissue, increased flow of fat globules in microcirculation	ARDS, ARF

Note: DIC = disseminated intravascular coagulation; ARF = acute renal failure; ARDS = acute respiratory distress syndrome; ACS = abdominal compartment syndrome

DIC (Module 24), acute renal failure (Module 28), and MODS (Module 16).

Risks for Complications

Several types of injuries predispose the trauma patient to complications. Table 36–4 summarizes traumatic injuries and their associated sequelae. Thoracic trauma may produce massive hemorrhage in addition to disruption in the lung parenchyma. Thus, the thoracic trauma patient is at high risk for DIC and ARDS. Abdominal trauma increases the likelihood of hemorrhage, abdominal compartment syndrome, and infection. Orthopedic trauma predisposes the patient to pulmonary emboli and prolonged immobility, which may compound the effect on gas exchange. The physiological complications of trauma are intimately related. It is common for a patient to have a combination of these disorders. Although the etiologies of these conditions may differ slightly, the result is the same: inadequate oxygen delivery to the tissue. For this reason, it is important to keep in mind when reviewing Table 36–4 that the patient may be at higher risk for one of these disorders because of the initial injury, but, in reality, any one of and more than one of these conditions may occur.

Metabolic Response to Injury: Risk for Undernutrition

Two phases occur in the metabolic response after injury: ebb phase and flow phase. The ebb phase occurs in the first 3 days during acute resuscitation. Characteristics of the ebb phase, as described by Orr and colleagues (2002), are summarized in Table 36–5. The body requires a large amount of glucose during this

TABLE 36–5 Metabolic Response to Trauma

METABOLIC PHASE	CHARACTERISTICS PRESENT
Ebb phase (first 72 hours after injury)	Hypometabolism
	Decreased body temperature
	Decreased energy expenditure
	Normal glucose production with insulin resistance
	Mild protein catabolism
	Increased catecholamines
	Increased glucocorticoids
	Decreased cardiac output
	Decreased oxygen consumption
	Vasoconstriction
Flow phase (72 hours after injury)	Hypermetabolism
	Increased energy expenditure
	Increased glucose production
	Increased oxygen consumption
	Profound protein catabolism
	Increased glucocorticoids
	Increased catecholamines
	Increased potassium and sodium losses
	Loss of serum proteins through wounds, exudates, drains, and hemorrhage

time, which is achieved by breakdown of glycogen stores through gluconeogenesis. Prolonged gluconeogenesis depletes skeletal muscle protein and can lead to wasting. This phase typically ends after the resuscitative phase, about 72 hours after injury.

The next phase is the flow phase, which is characterized by a hypermetabolic response (Table 36–5). This hypermetabolic phase results in catabolism of lean body mass, negative nitrogen balance, and altered glucose metabolism.

Nutritional support is required for amino acids and adequate energy for protein synthesis as new tissues are synthesized and wounds are repaired. Current guidelines recommend enteral feedings be initiated within 72 hours for patients with severe head injuries and patients with blunt and penetrating abdominal injuries (EAST, 2003b). Because access to the stomach can be obtained more quickly than in the duodenum, early gastric feeding is recommended (EAST, 2003b). However, patients who are at risk for pulmonary aspiration or who have gastric retention or gastroesophageal reflux should receive enteral feedings through the jejunum (EAST, 2003b). If enteral feedings are not successful, total parenteral nutrition should by instituted by day 7 (EAST, 2003b).

Sepsis

Sepsis is the presence of microorganisms in the blood. Septic shock is the physiologic response to microorganisms in the blood that results in hemodynamic instability (refer to Module 15). A pathogen is identified in the body from cultures. The pathogens may be part of the patient's normal flora or may be present in the external environment. Gram-negative and gram-positive bacteria, viruses, and fungi can produce sepsis. There are several portals of entry for these microorganisms.

The patient with traumatic injuries is particularly at risk for infection and sepsis because of so many potential ports of entry, including urinary catheters, endotracheal tubes, surgical wounds, invasive hemodynamic monitoring catheters, and IV catheters. Foreign devices in the nose represent a major risk factor for the development of nosocomial sinusitis, which itself is a risk factor for the development of pneumonia. Nasotracheal intubation should be avoided (Eggimann & Pittet, 2001). Additional risk factors for infection are summarized in Table 36–6.

TABLE 36–6 Risk Factors for Infection in the Patient with Traumatic Injury

- High injury severity
- Shock on admission
- Prolonged ICU length of stay
- Age greater than 60 years
- Size of ICU (more than 10 beds)
- Parenteral nutrition
- Days with arterial catheter
- Days with mechanical ventilation
- Days with central venous catheters
- Tracheostomy
- Neurological failure at day 3
- ICP monitor

Acute Respiratory Distress Syndrome

ARDS is characterized by the presence of bilateral pulmonary infiltrates, a pulmonary capillary wedge pressure of 18 mm Hg (in the absence of left ventricular dysfunction), and a PaO_2/FIO_2 ratio less than 200, regardless of the amount of positive end-expiratory pressure (PEEP) (Bernard et al., 1994). The trauma patient is at risk for ARDS as a result of direct and indirect lung injury. Primary lung injury includes direct blunt or penetrating injury to the lungs, aspiration, or inhalation. Indirect injuries include sepsis, fat embolism, ischemia/reperfusion, and missed injuries (Micheals, 2004).

Disseminated Intravascular Coagulation

DIC is an exaggeration of a normal response. Normal clotting is a localized reaction to injury, whereas DIC is a systemic response. The healthy individual maintains a balance between clot formation and lysis. In trauma, both the extrinsic and intrinsic pathways of coagulation may be stimulated. Head injury can precipitate the release of tissue thromboplastin (extrinsic pathway). Hypoxia and acidosis also stimulate the extrinsic pathway. Crush injuries, burns, and sepsis result in blood cell injury as well as platelet aggregation (intrinsic pathway). For more information, refer to Module 24.

Acute Renal Failure

In the trauma patient, renal failure rarely occurs as a result of direct trauma to the kidneys. More often it is the result of renal hypoperfusion, gradual acute tubular necrosis, or toxin-mediated damage to the tubules (contrast dyes, medications, myoglobin). Toxin-mediated renal failure is caused by many of the drugs trauma patients frequently receive, including aminoglycosides, nonsteroidal anti-inflammatory agents, and radiologic contrast dyes used for CT scanning. Myoglobin from crushed skeletal muscle can accumulate in the tubules and cause obstruction and renal failure.

Assessment and Nursing Diagnosis

Complications may occur at any time in the postinjury phase. It should be clear from this discussion why baseline laboratory and diagnostic data are so important in the trauma patient. With these data, the nurse is able to monitor for subtle changes that indicate that a complication is occurring. The following assessment data would indicate the presence of a posttrauma complication:

- Elevation of white blood cell count
- Fever
- Change in characteristics of wound drainage (foul odor, thick, and colored)
- Inability to tolerate movement or nursing procedures (e.g., decreasing SpO_2, PaO_2)
- Decreasing level of responsiveness (related to decreased oxygenation or increased serum ammonia levels)

- Decreased urine output
- Diaphoresis
- Cool, mottled skin
- Presence of bleeding (melena, hemoptysis, hematemesis, petechiae, or hematuria)
- Changing trends in vital signs/hemodynamic readings (e.g., elevated CO, decreased systemic vascular resistance, SVR)

Nursing diagnoses that pertain to the trauma patient can be clustered mainly into the two broad areas of ventilation and perfusion.

Ventilation

- *Impaired gas exchange* related to increased capillary permeability and decreased surface area for gas exchange, or obstruction in pulmonary capillary perfusion
- *Ineffective breathing patterns* related to decreased skeletal muscle mass and denervation
- *Ineffective airway clearance* related to fatigue and artificial airway placement with mechanical ventilation

Perfusion

- *Fluid volume deficit* related to vasodilation, bleeding, or interstitial fluid shift
- *Decreased tissue perfusion* related to capillary obstruction and vasodilation
- *Increased cardiac output* related to catecholamine excretion and decreased systemic vascular resistance
- *Decreased cardiac output* related to decreased vascular volume

Additional nursing diagnoses would include

- *Altered urinary elimination patterns* related to obstruction (microemboli and myoglobin) of renal blood flow and tissue necrosis
- *Altered nutrition: less than body requirements* related to catecholamine release, activation of inflammatory response resulting in a hypermetabolic state, and decreased or absent oral intake
- *Risk of infection* related to open wounds, invasive procedures, surgical incisions, debilitated state, and altered nutrition

Although this section has emphasized physical manifestations of posttrauma complications, psychosocial aspects should not be ignored. The reader is referred to Module 1 for additional information. Patients who have complications posttrauma remain in the critical care unit for prolonged periods and are susceptible to sensory disturbances. Quality-of-life issues need to be considered by the patient and the family. Extensive rehabilitation may be necessary to regain skeletal muscle mass and neurological function. The family's standard of living may decrease because of financial factors related to change in the role of the patient as well as health care costs.

In summary, the patient with traumatic injury is susceptible to undernutrition, ARDS, DIC, acute renal failure, and multiple organ dysfunction syndrome. Multiple risk factors for each of these complications is present in every trauma patient. The primary responsibility of the nurse caring for a trauma patient in the days to weeks postinjury is to monitor for and prevent these complications.

SECTION ELEVEN REVIEW

SW was pinned underneath his tractor for 1 hour before being extricated and transported to the hospital for treatment. He has open fractures of both legs and abdominal tenderness. Questions 1 through 3 pertain to SW.

1. What risk is associated with this delay in treatment?
   A. he will not be able to produce the same number of immunoglobulins
   B. he will have a higher microorganism count because of delay in wound debridement
   C. he is at higher risk for antibiotic resistance
   D. he will be unable to mount a local inflammatory response

2. Because of his crush injury, DIC may occur as a result of
   A. activation of the intrinsic pathway via platelet aggregation
   B. activation of the extrinsic pathway via thromboplastic release
   C. a high microorganism count
   D. long-bone injury

3. All of the following nursing diagnoses would be appropriate for SW EXCEPT
   A. risk for infection
   B. decreased peripheral tissue perfusion
   C. risk for fluid volume deficit
   D. risk for trauma

4. Which of the following statements best describes the relationship between ARDS and MODS?
   A. decreased ventilation leads to decreased tissue oxygenation and cellular death
   B. pulmonary edema produces a fluid volume deficit and hypoperfusion of tissues
   C. organ death releases endotoxins that kill pulmonary epithelial cells
   D. increased carbon dioxide retention stimulates peripheral vasodilation and hypoperfusion of tissue

Answers: 1. B, 2. A, 3. D, 4. A

POSTTEST

1. Typically, a trauma patient has which demographic profile?
   A. 15 to 24 years, male, using alcohol, lower-income level
   B. 24 to 32 years, male, using alcohol, upper-income level
   C. 15 to 24 years, female, using alcohol, lower-income level
   D. 15 to 24 years, male, no alcohol involvement, lower-income level

2. Diminished physiological reserve occurs in response to trauma in
   A. Native Americans
   B. the elderly
   C. women
   D. the very young

3. What are the four forces that must be considered in assessment of injury?
   A. acceleration, mass, axial loading, deceleration
   B. shearing, compression, impact, axial loading
   C. acceleration, deceleration, shearing, synergistic
   D. acceleration, deceleration, shearing, compression

4. The coup and contrecoup injury is an example of application of _____ and _____ forces, respectively.
   A. shear, tensile
   B. tensile, shear
   C. compression, axial loading
   D. acceleration, tensile

5. The extent of cavitation and tissue deformation is most determined by
   A. yaw
   B. velocity
   C. blast effect
   D. tissue density

6. A patient is admitted to your unit with a stab injury to the right sternal border, fifth intercostal space. Injury must be considered to the abdomen as well as to the thorax because
   A. the left diaphragm can rise as high as the fourth intercostal space during maximum expiration
   B. the right diaphragm can rise as high as the fourth intercostal space during maximum expiration
   C. the diaphragm recedes to the eighth intercostal space during maximum inspiration at the midclavicular line
   D. the diaphragm recedes to the sixth intercostal space during maximum inspiration at the midaxillary line

7. Which of the following statements is true about high-velocity missiles and potential structural injury?
   A. the entrance wound is smaller than missile caliber
   B. there is little or no cavitation
   C. there is no exit wound
   D. the exit wound is usually large

8. Fall injuries are typically associated with
   A. cervical spine fractures
   B. multiple injuries to long bones
   C. compression fractures of lumbosacral spine
   D. contusions to underlying structures

9. Trauma victims who have ingested cocaine may exhibit
   A. tachycardia, dilated pupils, tremors, elevated blood pressure
   B. tachycardia, constricted pupils, tremors, elevated blood pressure
   C. bradycardia, hypotension
   D. dilated pupils, hypotension, bradycardia

10. The metabolic derangement typically seen in the pregnant trauma patient is
    A. respiratory alkalosis
    B. respiratory acidosis
    C. metabolic alkalosis
    D. metabolic acidosis

11. In the elderly, each additional rib fracture increases mortality by
    A. 5 percent
    B. 11 percent
    C. 25 percent
    D. 30 percent

12. The first three components of the primary assessment are
    A. airway, circulation, cervical spine control
    B. airway, breathing, circulation
    C. circulation, cervical spine control, breathing
    D. breathing, disability, circulation

13. Actual or potential airway obstruction may be evidenced by
    A. dyspnea
    B. diminished breath sounds
    C. dysphonia
    D. all of the above

14. IV access and administration of fluids is achieved during the "C" component of the primary survey. Which of the following scenarios is recommended for this intervention?
    A. two 19-gauge IVs with lactated Ringer's solution
    B. two 22-gauge IVs with lactated Ringer's solution
    C. an 18-gauge IV with normal saline
    D. a 22-gauge IV with normal saline

15. The purpose of the secondary assessment is to
    A. identify and intervene with life-threatening injuries
    B. identify the existence of all injuries
    C. facilitate treatment of airway and breathing
    D. assess response to resuscitative interventions

16. Any injured patient in a shock state should be evaluated for the most common etiology of traumatic shock, which is
    A. hypovolemic
    B. cardiogenic
    C. neurogenic
    D. sepsis

17. The third peak of death after trauma occurs
   A. after discharge from ICU
   B. in the OR
   C. days to weeks after surgery
   D. a year after injury
18. Which of the following may be an indicator of a continued shock state?
   A. Svo_2 65 to 80 percent
   B. lactate 10.4 mMol
   C. oxygen delivery index greater than 500 mL/min/m^2
   D. gastric pH_i greater than 7.35
19. An occlusive dressing should be placed over a(n)
   A. open pneumothorax
   B. tension pnemothorax
   C. flail chest
   D. pulmonary contusion
20. Which of the following bladder pressures is consistent with intra-abdominal hypertension and abdominal compartment syndrome?
   A. 100 mm Hg
   B. 75 mm Hg
   C. 50 mm Hg
   D. 25 mm Hg
21. Which of the following assessments is important for the nurse to perform for a patient with an unstable pelvic fracture?
   A. assess color and motion of extremities
   B. assess for signs of bleeding

C. assess urine for hematuria
   D. all of the above
22. Which of the following symptoms are most commonly associated with life-threatening injuries?
   A. ineffective breathing
   B. altered pH
   C. distended neck veins
   D. all of the above
23. A paradoxical pulse is associated with
   A. cardiac tamponade
   B. spinal shock
   C. hypovolemic shock
   D. hemothorax
24. The initial metabolic response in the first 24 hours postinjury is associated with
   A. hypermetabolism
   B. hypometabolism
   C. increased O_2 consumption
   D. increased energy expenditure
25. Which of the following is a risk factor for the development of acute renal failure in the trauma patient?
   A. hypoperfusion
   B. radiologic contrast dye
   C. myoglobinuria
   D. all of the above

POSTTEST ANSWERS

Question	Answer	Section	Question	Answer	Section
1	A	One	14	A	Six
2	B	One	15	B	Seven
3	D	Two	16	A	Eight
4	A	Two	17	C	Eight
5	B	Three	18	B	Eight
6	B	Three	19	A	Nine
7	D	Four	20	D	Nine
8	C	Four	21	D	Nine
9	A	Five	22	D	Ten
10	A	Five	23	A	Ten
11	B	Five	24	B	Eleven
12	B	Six	25	D	Eleven
13	D	Six			

REFERENCES

ACSCT [American College of Surgeons Committee on Trauma]. (1997). *Advanced trauma life support course manual.* Chicago: American College of Surgeons.

Bernard, G. R., Artigas, A., Brigham, K. L., et al. (1994). The American European Consensus Conference on ARDS: Definitions, mechanisms, relevant outcomes and clinical trial coordination. *American Journal of Respiratory and Critical Care Medicine, 149,* 818–824.

Blincoe, L., Seay, A., Zaloshnja, E., et al. (2002). The economic impact of motor vehicle crashes, 2000. NHTSA, Department of Transportation, Washington DC Available at *www.NHTSA.dot.gov/people/economic/econimpact2000.* Accessed July 8, 2004.

Brown, C. V., Rhee, P., & Chan, L. (2004). Preventing renal failure in patients with rhabdomyolysis: Do bicarbonate and mannitol make a difference? *Journal of Trauma, 56,* 1191–1196.

Bulger, E. M., Arneson, M. S., Mock, C. N., et al. (2000). Rib fractures in the elderly. *Journal of Trauma, 48,* 1040–1046.

Cami, J., & Farre, M. (2003). Drug addiction. *New England Journal of Medicine, 349,* 975–986.

Chang, M. C., & Meredith, J. W. (1996). Occult hypovolemia and subsequent splanchnic ischemia in globally resuscitated trauma patients in association with multiple organ failure and mortality. *Journal of Trauma, 41,* 192–198.

EAST. (1998). *Practice management guidelines for screening of blunt cardiac trauma.* Eastern Association for the Surgery of Trauma.

EAST. (2003a). *Clinical practice guidelines: End points of resuscitation.* Eastern Association for the Surgery of Trauma.

EAST. (2003b). *Practice management guidelines for nutrition.* Eastern Association for the Surgery of Trauma.

EAST. (2003c). *Practice management guidelines for the non-operative management of blunt injury to the liver and spleen.* Eastern Association for the Surgery of Trauma.

Eggimann, P., & Pittet, D. (2001). Nonantibiotic measures for the prevention of gram-positive infections. *Clinical Microbiology & Infection, 7* (Suppl. 4), 91–99.

Holbrook, T. L., Hoyt, D. B., & Anderson, J. P. (2001). The impact of major in-hospital complications on functional outcome and quality of life after trauma. *Journal of Trauma, 50,* 91–95.

Jacobs, D. G. (2003). Special considerations in geriatric trauma. *Current Opinion in Critical Care, 9,* 535–539.

Johnston, C. J., Rubenfeld, G. D., & Hudson, L. D. (2003). Effect of age on the development of ARDS in trauma patients. *Chest, 124,* 653–659.

Kern, J. W., & Shoemaker, W. (2002). Meta-analysis of hemodynamic optimization in high risk patients. *Critical Care Medicine, 30,* 1686–1696.

Laird, A. M., Miller P. R., & Kilgo, P. D., et al. (2004). Relationship of early hyperglycemia to mortality in trauma patients. *Journal of Trauma, 56,* 1058–1062.

Lange, R. A., & Hillis, D. (2001). Cardiovascular complications of cocaine use. *New England Journal of Medicine, 345,* 351–358.

McNeilis, J., Marini, C. P., & Simm, H. H. (2003). Abdominal compartment syndrome: Clinical manifestations and predictive factors. *Current Opinion in Critical Care, 9,* 133–136.

Micheals, A. J. (2004) Management of post traumatic respiratory failure. *Critical Care Clinics, 20,* 83–99.

Mirza, M. M., & Ellis, J. R. (2004). Initial management of pelvic and femoral fractures in the multiply injured patient. *Critical Care Clinics, 20,* 158–170.

Myriam, C., Schermer, C., Demarest, G. B., et al. (2000). Predictors of outcome in trauma during pregnancy: Identification of patients who can be monitored for less than 6 hours. *Journal of Trauma, 49,* 18–25.

Orr, P. A., Keiko, C., & Stevenson, J. (2002). Metabolic response and parenteral nutrition in trauma, sepsis, and burns. *Journal of Infusion Nursing, 25*(1), 45–53.

Scalea, T. M., & Burgess, A. R. (2004). Pelvic fractures. In E. E. Moore, D. V. Feliciano, & K. L. Mattox, (Eds.), *Trauma* (5th ed). New York: McGraw Hill.

Screiber, M. A .(2004). Damage control surgery. *Critical Care Clinics, 20,* 119–134.

Schulman, A. M., & Caridge, J. S. (2002). Young versus old: Factors affecting mortality after blunt traumatic injury. *Annals of Surge, 68,* 942–947.

Schulman, C. (2002). End points of resuscitation: Choosing the right parameters to monitor. *Dimensions of Critical Care Nursing, 21*(1), 2–14.

Shults, R. A., Sleet, P. A., Elder, R. W., et al. (2002). Association between state level drinking and driving countermeasures and self-reported alcohol impaired driving. *Injury Prevention, 8,* 106–110.

Van Hook, J. (2002). Trauma in pregnancy. *Clinical Obstetrics and Gynecology, 45,* 414–424.

Victorino, G., Chong, T. G., & Pal, J. D. (2003). Trauma in the elderly. *Archives of Surgery, 138,* 1093–1098.

Walls, M. (2002). *Orthopedic trauma, RN, 65*(7), 52–58.

Wanek, S., & Mayberry, J. C. (2004). Blunt thoracic trauma: Flail chest, pulmonary contusion, and blast injury. *Critical Care Clinics, 20,* 71–81.

Nursing Care of the Patient with Multiple Injuries

Karen L. Johnson

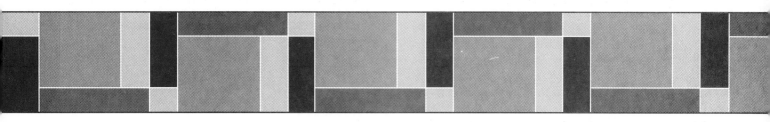

OBJECTIVES Following completion of this module, the learner will be able to

1. Identify relationships among traumatic injury patterns, trauma assessment, and resuscitation issues.

2. Cluster assessment data to formulate nursing diagnoses associated with traumatic injury.

3. Appraise a traumatically injured patient's status based on a nursing assessment.

4. Identify priorities in nursing care for a patient with traumatic injuries.

5. Explain the relationship between trauma resuscitation and complications following traumatic injury.

6. Explain rationale for nursing actions that prevent complications associated with traumatic injuries.

This module is designed to integrate the major points discussed in Modules 34 to 36. It summarizes relationships between key concepts and assists the learner in clustering information to facilitate clinical application. Content is applied in an interactive learning style. The learner is encouraged to identify nursing actions based on the assessment of a patient in a case study format. Consequences of selecting a particular action are discussed, and the rationale for correct actions is presented. The first part of the module addresses assessment of the trauma patient and interpretation of laboratory data. Development of nursing diagnoses and supporting data follows next.

ABBREVIATIONS

ABG	Arterial blood gas	**IV**	Intravenous
Bpm	Beats per minute	**mm Hg**	Millimeters mercury
CBC	Complete blood count	**O$_2$**	Oxygen
CT	Computed tomography	**PERRLA**	Pupils equal round reactive to light accommodation
ED	Emergency department	**Spo$_2$**	Arterial oxygen saturation measured by pulse oximetry
GCS	Glasgow Coma Scale		

Case Study

MR. B, A PATIENT WITH MULTIPLE TRAUMATIC INJURIES

Mr. B, an 86-year-old male, unrestrained driver, hit another vehicle head on while driving at 45 miles per hour. He was brought to the emergency department (ED) via helicopter. On arrival to the ED his vital signs were blood pressure: 125/85, heart rate: 110 beats per minute (bpm), respiration rate: 34, temperature: 98.6°F (37°C), Glasgow Coma Scale (GCS):15. His workup revealed the following injuries: multiple rib fractures (right fifth to eighth), pulmonary contusions, and a right lower lobe pneumothorax. A chest tube was placed. Past medical history revealed previous myocardial infarction and hypertension. Mr. B is transferred to the high-acuity unit and you are the nurse receiving Mr. B from the ED.

QUESTION

Because of Mr. B's advanced age, he is at a greater risk for mortality and morbidity because he
   A. has limited physiological reserve
   B. cannot get out of bed as easily as younger patients
   C. drinks more alcohol
   D. has a lifetime of neglect of his health

ANSWER

The correct answer is A. Trauma in the elderly is associated with higher mortality and morbidity rates with less severe injuries. The higher mortality and morbidity rates are attributed to a decreased ability to compensate for severe injury because of limited physiological reserves. Limited physiological reserves is a concept of limited organ function in the face of physiological change (Jacobs, 2003). Organ dysfunction may not appear in the resting state, but in a physiological stress situation, such as trauma, the ability of organs to augment function is compromised.

QUESTION

Mr. B was the unrestrained driver of the car. He hit another vehicle head on. Both the steering wheel and the windshield were broken. A high index of suspicion must be maintained for certain injuries. Name four injuries commonly associated with this mechanism of injury.

ANSWER

A high index of suspicion must be maintained for the following injuries:
   1. Potential intracranial injury as a result of the high rate of speed and shattered windshield
   2. Potential cervical vertebrae injury as a result of suspected acceleration/deceleration at a high rate of speed and the broken windshield
   3. Potential intrathoracic injuries as a result of the broken steering wheel—suspect rib fractures, myocardial and pulmonary contusions, and great vessel injury

   4. Potential intra-abdominal injuries as a result of the broken steering wheel and acceleration/deceleration mechanism; injuries could include spleen/liver lacerations, small bowel injuries, and great vessel injuries
   5. Potential long-bone fractures, especially femur fractures or posterior hip fracture-dislocation, because of impact of knees with dashboard
   6. Potential multiple skin lacerations, avulsions, and punctures from the patient impacting various parts of the vehicle interior

QUESTION

Because of Mr. B's past medical history of myocardial infarction and hypertension, what additional information do you need?

ANSWER

It would be helpful to know what medications he was taking at home and when he last took these drugs. Patients with chronic conditions may have polypharmaceutical regimens that may affect their responses to injury. Also the nurse should question the patient as to when he last ate in case the need for surgery arises.

Initial Appraisal: Primary Survey

Because of the unpredictable effects of trauma-related injury on the patient, you must develop a rapid, systematic approach to assessing each patient to ensure that no effects of injury will be overlooked. Remember, trauma should never be approached as a unisystem disease, but rather it should be approached as a multisystem disease. If one body system is injured, you must ensure that no other body system has been adversely affected. Thus, a rapid systematic approach to assessment with establishment of management priorities is essential. Primary assessment and resuscitation are the focus of this section. The purpose of the primary survey is to identify life-threatening conditions and intervene appropriately. Primary assessment is done via the A, B, C, D, E approach.

GENERAL APPEARANCE. On entry to his room, you introduce yourself to Mr. B. He responds appropriately. He appears to be a "healthy," well-nourished man. He is lying in bed with the head of bed elevated 30 degrees. His hair is gray and he is wearing glasses. He has oxygen (O_2) by nasal cannula. You note a chest tube on his right side. There is a small amount of serosanguineous drainage in the collection chamber.

SIGNS OF DISTRESS. Mr. B is grimacing. He is taking short, panting breaths. He is not diaphoretic. He states that he has pain in his right chest when he breathes in and it hurts to take a deep breath.

AIRWAY. Mr. B's airway is open and he is breathing spontaneously. There is no need for cervical spine immobilization because a cervical spine injury was ruled out in the ED.

BREATHING. Respiratory rate is 28 and shallow. Respiratory excursion is equal bilaterally. Breath sounds are present in all lobes bilaterally, although they are diminished in the right lower lobe and you note crackles in the right middle lobe. Currently, Mr. B is receiving oxygen at 2 L by nasal cannula. No arterial blood gases (ABGs) are available at the present time.

CIRCULATION. Mr. B's blood pressure is 135/85 mm Hg; his heart rate is 90 bpm. Pulses are 4+ in all extremities. His skin is warm and dry. Capillary refill is less than 2 seconds. Mucous membranes are pink. He is alert and oriented to person, place, and time. There is an 18-gauge intravenous (IV) tube in the right antecubital vein with lactated Ringer's solution running at 100 mL per hour. Spo$_2$ is 88 percent.

DISABILITY. Mr. B is alert; he responds to verbal stimulation by moving all extremities and following commands. PERRLA are at 4 mm.

QUESTION

During the primary survey, you noted that breath sounds were present bilaterally although diminished in the right lower lobe. What additional data could help you assess the adequacy of ventilation?

ANSWER

Confirmation of the adequacy of ventilation is best achieved by obtaining an arterial blood gas determination to assess Paco$_2$. Noninvasive measures include end-tidal carbon dioxide (CO$_2$) monitoring and pulse oximetry.

Focused Respiratory Assessment

The data from Mr. B's primary survey reveal an abnormal assessment of breathing. You proceed to perform a focused respiratory assessment. You note the O$_2$ is on and connected properly to the outlet and the flow meter is on. You assess the chest tube dressing and note it is dry and intact, without drainage. You palpate around the dressing and note there is no evidence of subcutaneous air. You check all chest tube connections and note they all are intact. The chest tube is connected to suction at −20 cm H$_2$O and a water seal of 2 cm. There is about 50 mL serosanguinous drainage in the collection chamber and you mark the drainage on the chamber. You observe the water seal chamber and see no evidence of an air leak. The pulse oximeter probe is on his right middle finger. You note a good waveform. On a scale of 1 to 10, he states his pain in his right chest is an 8 with inspiration and a 5 when he breathes out.

Development of Nursing Diagnoses

CLUSTERING DATA. Mr. B's primary survey reveals breathing abnormalities. At this point you cannot proceed with the secondary survey until his breathing improves.

Subjective.   On a scale of 1 to 10, he states his pain in his right chest is an 8 with inspiration and a 5 when he breathes out.

Objective.   Mr. B is grimacing. He is taking short, panting breaths with shallow respirations at a rate of 28. His injuries include multiple rib fractures, pnemothorax, and pulmonary contusions. Spo$_2$ is 88 percent.

At this point your nursing diagnosis is *ineffective breathing patterns* related to pain with inspiration secondary to multiple rib fractures. Mr. B has an order for morphine sulfate 3 mg intravenous IV prn pain.

QUESTION

Would you administer the morphine to Mr. B at this point? State the rationale for your answer.

ANSWER

Yes. Mr. B's vital signs have been stable. Morphine can cause vasodilation and hypotension. You should assess his vital signs within 20 minutes after administration of the morphine. Also, the pain is interfering with Mr. B's breathing. Recall from Module 36 that rib fractures are very painful and the pain is aggravated by movement of the chest wall, even with breathing. Therefore, the patient with rib fractures often takes shallow breaths. Atelectasis can develop and the patient is at risk for developing pneumonia. Pain management in patients with pulmonary contusions and rib fractures is paramount.

RESUSCITATIVE PHASE After the primary survey, the resuscitative phase begins. Twenty minutes after administration of the morphine, Mr. B's vital signs remain stable: blood pressure: 132/80 mm Hg, heart rate 88 bpm, respiration rate: 22, Spo$_2$ 92 percent. He states that he is much more comfortable although it still hurts to take a deep breath in. He rates his pain now as a 2 out of 10. Mr. B's vital signs remain stable; his skin is warm and dry. A Foley catheter was inserted and his urine output has been 35 mL per hour. His IV is infusing at 100 mL per hour.

QUESTION

Do you think Mr. B has been adequately resuscitated?

ANSWER

Actually, you cannot determine from these data whether Mr. B has been adequately resuscitated. Traditional signs of sufficient tissue perfusion cannot be used in shock states because they may be the result of compensatory mechanisms (renin–angiotensin–aldosterone, sympathetic nervous system). Recall that the high-acuity nurse should not be lured into a false sense of security when vital signs and basic hemodynamic parameters have been restored to normal values during resuscitation (Schulman, 2002).

QUESTION

What additional data may be more helpful in determining whether Mr. B has been adequately resuscitated? (Mr. B does not have a pulmonary artery catheter.)

ANSWER

Base deficit, lactate, and gastric pH$_i$ would help determine whether Mr. B has been adequately resuscitated. Current guidelines recommend the use of these three parameters as end points with the goal of correcting all three within 24 hours after injury (EAST, 2003). Normal values are as follows: lactate less than 2.2 mMol/L, base deficit ± 2, and gastric pH$_i$ greater than 7.35.

Secondary Survey

HEAD AND NECK. Neck veins are full but not distended. Oxygen is flowing via nasal cannula. His eyes are open. GCS remains at 15.

CHEST. Chest tube dressing is in place. No lacerations, redness, or other signs of injury are noted. Chest expansion equal bilaterally. Electrocardiogram (EKG) reveals normal sinus rhythm.

ABDOMEN. There are no signs of ecchymosis. Positive bowel sounds are heard in all four quadrants. There is no tenderness on palpation.

PELVIS. The urinary catheter is intact. Urine output has been 50 mL per hour for the past hour; the urine is clear.

EXTREMITIES. There are no signs of external bleeding, no lacerations, and no drainage. The right antecubital IV catheter is in place, patent, and the dressing is dry and intact. No erythema is noted at the insertion site. The patient denies pain at the site.

POSTERIOR. Posterior breath sounds are auscultated. Breath sounds are equal bilaterally, although somewhat diminished in the right lower lobe. No abrasions, lacerations, or signs of ecchymosis on the back, flank, or buttocks are evident.

The following laboratory studies were performed in the emergency department:

- Arterial blood gas (ABG)
- Complete blood count (CBC)
- Serum electrolyte profile with glucose
- Type and screen
- Serum ethanol
- Lactate
- Prothrombin and partial thromboplastin times (PT and PTT)

The following radiographic studies were performed:

- Cervical spine films
- Chest X-rays
- Computed tomography (CT) scan of the head and abdomen

Quick Review

What is the rationale for ordering these tests in a trauma patient?

ABG. (normal values: pH, 7.35 to 7.45; P_{CO_2}, 35 to 45; P_{O_2}, 75 to 100; HCO_3, 24 to 28; base excess, +2 to −2). Baseline ABGs assist in the assessment of ventilatory status (P_{CO_2}), oxygenation status (P_{O_2}, Sa_{O_2}), and adequacy of tissues perfusion (base deficit, pH). In hypovolemic shock, metabolic acidosis results (for assistance in interpreting arterial blood gases, refer to Module 4). Results: pH, 7.30; P_{CO_2}, 30; P_{O_2}, 92; HCO_3, 25; S_{O_2} 88 percent.

CBC. (normal values: male: hemoglobin, 13 to 17 g/dL; hematocrit, 40 to 54 percent; white blood cell (WBC) count 5,000 to 10,000 mL; platelets, 150,000 to 400,000 mL). The CBC provides a baseline measurement of fluid loss. The hemoglobin will decrease after hemorrhage. The hematocrit will increase, indicating hemoconcentration. The WBC count may be slightly elevated because of tissue damage. A decreased platelet count will prolong clotting. Mr. B's hemoglobin is 12 g/dL; hematocrit is 40 percent. His WBC count is 9,000, and platelets are 300,000. These values may be indicative of hypovolemia, or they may be related to a chronic anemia.

SERUM ELECTROLYTE PROFILE. (normal values: potassium (K), 3.5 to 5.3 mEq/L; sodium (Na), 135 to 145 mEq/L; calcium (Ca), 9 to 11 mg/dL; chloride (Cl), 95 to 105 mEq/L; glucose, 80 to 120 mg/dL). Potassium levels may increase in the trauma patient as a result of tissue injury and hypoxia. Hyponatremia may be present if a large amount of cellular damage has occurred because sodium moves into the cell as potassium moves out. Calcium may accumulate at the injury site, producing hypocalcemia. Chloride will usually decrease because it combines with sodium. Hyperglycemia (blood sugar is usually greater than 100 and less than 200 mg/dL) is associated with traumatic injury as a result of the release of corticosteroids and catecholamines. All of Mr. B's electrolyte values are within normal limits.

TYPE AND SCREEN. The type and screen test is used to determine blood compatibility in case blood volume replacement is needed. Mr. B's blood type is O.

SERUM ETHANOL LEVEL. Alcohol can produce vasodilation and hypotension. A change in responsiveness may be associated with ethanol use. Mr. B's level is 0.

LACTATE. (normal value: less than 2.2 mMol/L). Lactic acid accumulation is directly related to cellular hypoxia. An elevated lactic acid level indicates acidosis. Mr. B's level is normal.

PT/PTT. (normal values: PT, 11 to 15 seconds; PTT, 60 to 70 seconds). These tests are ordered to provide baseline data on the patient's ability to clot in case hemorrhaging occurs. Mr. B's clotting times are normal.

CERVICAL SPINE FILMS. Mr. B has the potential for cervical vertebrae injury as a result of suspected acceleration/deceleration and the broken windshield. To rule out a cervical spine fracture, all seven cervical and T1 vertebrae must be visualized on the film. Mr. B's spinal films were negative.

CHEST FILMS. Chest films can be useful to diagnose rib fractures and pulmonary status. Mr. B's chest film reveals fractured ribs on the right side (fifth to eighth). Patchy pulmonary infiltrates are evident in the right middle lobe and there is a right lower lobe pneumothorax. The patchy infiltrates may be consistent with pulmonary contusions.

HEAD CT SCAN. Because of the rate of speed and shattered windshield, Mr. B is at risk for an intracranial injury. Head CT results were normal; there is no evidence of hematoma. If, however, he exhibits any change in neurological status, a head CT will be obtained again.

CHEST CT. Because Mr. B was the unbelted driver, he was thrown against the steering wheel; therefore, potential intrathoracic injuries may include rib fractures, pulmonary contusions, great vessel injury, and blunt cardiac trauma. These can be life-threatening injuries and must be ruled out. Mr. B's chest CT revealed fractured ribs and a pneumothorax.

ABDOMINAL CT. Because Mr. B was the unbelted driver, he was thrown against the steering wheel; therefore, potential intra-abdominal injuries could include spleen/liver lacerations, small bowel injuries, and great vessel injuries. Mr. B's abdominal CT was negative.

Based on the data obtained, the following nursing diagnoses are appropriate for Mr. B.

- Pain
- Ineffective airway clearance related to pain with coughing
- Ineffective breathing patterns related to chest wall injury and pain
- Impaired gas exchange related to ventilation–perfusion imbalance

QUESTION

List at least six desired patient outcomes for Mr. B that would be appropriate for these diagnoses.

1.
2.
3.
4.
5.
6.

ANSWER

1. Normal respiratory rate, depth, and rhythm
2. Improved or clear breath sounds
3. Improving or no dypsnea
4. Usual mental status
5. Mucous membranes pink
6. ABGs within acceptable limits

Developing the Plan of Care

Mr. B's injuries are life threatening. Treatment goals include (1) relief of pain, (2) optimizing his oxygenation status, (3) promoting airway clearance, and (4) promoting effective pulmonary gas exchange. These general goals are reflected in the nursing diagnoses and desired patient outcomes on the nursing care plan. Nursing interventions are based on activities to help Mr. B meet these outcomes. They consist of collaborative interventions, which are activities ordered by the physician, but that require some actions by the nurse, and independent interventions, which are activities that are within the nursing scope of practice to write and carry out as nursing orders.

Collaborative Interventions Related to Pulmonary Status

1. **Pain management.** Pain management may include nonsteriodal anti-inflammatory agents, intercostal nerve blocks, thoracic epidural analgesia, and narcotics.
2. **Pulmonary drug therapy.** Mr. B will receive oxygen therapy to treat his mild hypoxemia.
3. **Chest tube management.** The chest tube will remain in place until a chest film reveals that the pneumothorax has resolved. Once the film reveals this, the chest tube is left in place but taken off wall suction. Four hours later, another film is taken. If the lung is still inflated, the chest tube may be removed.

4. **Laboratory and x-ray testing.** Laboratory and x-ray tests may be ordered intermittently. It will be important to monitor for an elevation in WBC counts because this may indicate a developing pneumonia. Of particular interest will be ABGs and the chest x-ray.
5. **Intravenous fluids.** IV fluids are ordered to hydrate secretions, which is crucial in loosening secretions for improved airway clearance. An IV access site is also necessary for IV antibiotic therapy, if ordered. However, given Mr B's history of myocardia infarction and hypertension, the nurse must monitor him for signs of heart failure.

Independent Nursing Interventions

1. Assess for decreased respiratory function (report abnormal):
   - Respirations less than 8 per minute or greater than 30 per minute
   - Increasingly shallow, labored breathing
   - Increasing dyspnea or central cyanosis
   - Change in mental status, including increased restlessness or lethargy
   - Increasingly abnormal ABGs
   - Increasingly abnormal breath sounds, adventitious sounds
   - Change in sputum
   - Accessory muscle use
2. Turn, cough, deep breathing exercises every 2 hours
3. Position head of bed at least 30 degrees
4. Monitor lab report results (report abnormals)
5. Instruct patient/family regarding condition, procedures, medications, treatment
6. Encourage self-care as tolerated
7. Encourage ambulation
8. Assess for pain; administer analgesics as ordered.

Plan Evaluation and Revision

Mr. B's plan of care is now developed and implemented. His progress is monitored at regular intervals to evaluate the effectiveness of the various therapeutic actions. If progress is not being noted toward attainment of his various desired patient outcomes, his plan may need revisions. Alternative interventions that may be more effective should be explored. His ventilatory status should be monitored in particular. Patients with his type of injuries must be monitored for worsening respiratory status. Intubation and mechanical ventilation may be required if respiratory failure is present. The major complication of pulmonary contusions and rib fractures are pneumonia and acute respiratory distress syndrome.

REFERENCES

EAST. (2003). *Clinical practice guidelines: End points of resuscitation.* Eastern Association for the Surgery of Trauma. Available at: *www.east.org.* Accessed July 31, 2004.

Jacobs, D. G. (2003). Special considerations in geriatric trauma. *Current Opinion in Critical Care, 9,* 535–539.

Schulman, C. (2002). End points of resuscitation: Choosing the right parameters to monitor. *Dimensions of Critical Care Nursing, 21*(1), 2–14.

Index

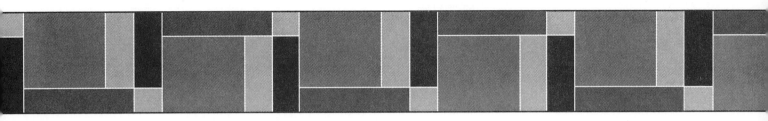

Page numbers followed by italic *f* indicate figures and those followed by italic *t* indicate tables or boxes.

A

a/A ratio. *See* Arterial/Alveolar ratio
A beta fibers, 27
A delta fibers, 27
A waves, 417, 417*f*
A–a gradient. *See* Alveolar–arterial pressure gradient
Abdominal compartment syndrome (ACS), 696, 725. *See also* Intra-abdominal hypertension
Abdominal injury, 870–871
ABGs. *See* Arterial blood gases
Ablation, 520
ABO incompatibility
    donor-recipient, 599, 600*t*
    hemolytic anemia caused by, 532
Abrasion, 793
Absolute neutrophil count (ANC), 535, 535*t*
Absolute refractory period, 265, 266–267
Absolute shunt, 81, 95. *See also* Pulmonary shunt(s)
AC. *See* Assist-control mode
Academy of Medical Surgical Nurses (AMSN), on nurse-patient ratios in high-acuity units, 15
Accelerated junctional rhythm, 279, 279*f*
Acceleration
    definition, 851, 854–855
    injury caused by, 450
Accessory muscles
    definition, 81
    in dyspnea, 105
ACCM. *See* American College of Critical Care Medicine
ACE inhibitors. *See* Angiotensin-converting enzyme (ACE) inhibitors
Acetic acid, as dressing solution, 806*t*
Acetoacetic acid, 621, 625, 626*f*
Acetone, 621, 625, 626*f*
Acetyl-CoA. *See* Acetylcoenzyme A
Acetylcoenzyme A (acetyl-CoA), 625
Acetylsalicylic acid (ASA)
    for acute coronary syndromes, 313
    for ischemic stroke, 436
Acid–base balance. *See also* Arterial blood gases
    buffer systems, 100, 100*f*
    compensation, 100, 100*t*
        algorithm for determining degree of, 113*f*

metabolic (renal) mechanism, 101
    respiratory mechanism, 101
    definition, 650
    determinants, 110
Acid–base disturbances. *See also* Arterial blood gases
    in acute ventilatory failure, 169
    algorithms for interpreting, 112*f*, 113*f*
    metabolic
        lactic acidosis, 102, 102*t*
        acidosis. *See* Metabolic acidosis
        alkalosis, 102–103, 103*t*
    mixed
        clinical problems associated with, 116, 116*t*
        comparison, 117*t*
        identification
            expected compensatory response, 117–118
            initial recognition, 116
            systemic evaluation, 116, 117*t*
    respiratory
        respiratory acidosis, 101, 101*t*
        respiratory alkalosis, 101–102, 102*t*
Acid–base physiology, 99–100
Acidosis, 650. *See also* Metabolic acidosis; Respiratory acidosis
Acids, 81, 99
Acinus, 762, 763*f*, 764*f*
ACMV. *See* Assist-control mode
Acquired immunity
    active, 556, 560
    characteristics, 560*t*
    passive, 556, 560
Acquired immunodeficiency disease syndrome (AIDS). *See also* Human immunodeficiency virus (HIV) disease
    in children, 577
    clinical manifestations, 577
    diagnosis, 577
    opportunistic infections, 578
    treatment, 577–578
    in women, 577
ACS. *See* Abdominal compartment syndrome; Acute coronary syndromes
ACTH. *See* Adrenocorticotropic hormone
Acticoat, 839*t*
Action potential
    definition, 265
    phases, 266–267, 266*f*, 267*f*
Activated partial thromboplastin time (APTT), 742
Activated protein C

in multiple organ dysfunction syndrome, 389
    in septic shock, 380
Active transport, 650, 652
Acute brain attack. *See* Stroke
Acute coronary syndromes (ACS). *See also* ST elevation myocardial infarction
    characteristics, 312
    collaborative management, 312–313
    diagnosis, 312
    nursing diagnoses, 312, 312*t*
Acute hepatitis, 736, 744. *See also* Hepatitis
Acute illness
    coping with, 9–10
    environmental stressors, 10–11
    stages, 6, 8, 8*t*
    transfer to higher care levels, 7*f*
Acute lung injury (ALI), 128–129, 134–135. *See also* Acute respiratory distress syndrome
Acute lymphocytic leukemia (ALL), 536. *See also* Leukemia
Acute myelogenous leukemia (AML), 536. *See also* Leukemia
Acute pain. *See also* Pain
    assessment
        alternative tools, 33, 34*f*, 35–36, 35*f*
        evidence-based practice, 37*t*
        multidimensional tools
            advantages and disadvantages, 33*t*
            characteristics, 31
            McGill Pain Questionnaire, 33
            short-form McGill Pain Questionnaire, 33
        unidimensional tools
            adaptation for severely ill patient, 32–33
            advantages and disadvantages, 33*t*
            characteristics, 31
            faces scale, 32, 32*f*
            numeric rating scale, 32, 32*f*
            verbal descriptor scales, 32
            visual analog scale, 32, 32*f*
    definition, 25, 28
    effects on body, 30
    history, 31
    management
        cultural considerations, 44*t*
        nonpharmacologic, 38, 39*t*
        nursing approach
            preventive, 42
            titration, 42, 42*t*
        in older adults, 43, 45*f*

Acute pain—(continued)
    in patients with concurrent medical
        disorders, 44
    pharmacologic
        adjuvant, 37
        administration routes, 37–38
        local anesthetics, 38, 39t
        nonopioid, 37, 39t
        opioid, 37, 39t
    in substance abuser, 44–46, 46t, 47t, 48
    World Health Organization ladder approach,
        36, 36f
    potential sources, 30
    undertreatment reasons, 40–41
Acute rejection, 587, 603. See also Rejection
Acute renal failure
    assessment
        diagnostic procedures, 666
        electrolyte imbalances, 665–666
        laboratory tests, 665, 665t
        nursing history, 663
        physical assessment, 663, 664f
            cardiovascular and pulmonary effects, 663
            gastrointestinal effects, 663
            hematologic effects, 665
            integumentary effects, 665
            neurologic effects, 663
            skeletal effects, 665
    in burn injury, 835–836
    collaborative management
        catabolic processes, 668
            nursing diagnoses, 668
            nursing implications, 668
        dialysis. See Dialysis
        electrolyte imbalances, 668
        fluid overload, 667–668
            nursing diagnoses, 668
            nursing interventions, 668
        infections
            nursing diagnoses, 669
            nursing implications, 669
        metabolic acidosis
            nursing diagnoses, 669
            nursing interventions, 669
    definition, 650, 656
    drug-induced, 657
    electrolyte balance in
        calcium and phosphate imbalances, 662
        magnesium imbalance, 662
        potassium imbalance, 661
        sodium imbalance, 661
    balance in, 661
    intrinsic
        acute tubular necrosis, 658
        definition, 650, 657
        incidence, 658
    metabolic acidosis in, 662
    mortality rate, 656
    nutritional/metabolic alterations, 506
    phases
        maintenance, 660, 660t
        onset, 659, 660t
        recovery, 660, 660t
    postrenal
        causes, 650, 657t
        definition, 650, 658

prerenal
    causes, 657t
    decreased cardiac output and, 656–657
    definition, 656
    in traumatic injury, 876
    vascular obstruction and, 657
Acute respiratory distress syndrome (ARDS)
    case study, 395–400
    chemotherapy-induced, 539
    clinical presentation, 137–138, 138t
    definition, 81, 129, 134–135
    diagnosis, 135–136, 135t
    vs. edema of congestive heart failure, 135
    etiologic factors, 135, 135t
    exudative phase, 138t
    fibroproliferative phase, 138t
    mortality rate, 141
    in multiple organ dysfunction syndrome,
        389–390, 398–399
    pathogenesis, 136–137, 137f
    prognosis, 141
    pulmonary shunts in, 95
    in traumatic injury, 876
    treatment
        drug therapy
            corticosteroids, 140–141
            inhaled nitric oxide, 141
            partial liquid ventilation, 141
            surfactant replacement therapy, 141
        mechanical ventilation, 139, 140t
        nursing role, 138–139
        patient positioning strategies, 139–140, 140f
        positive end expiratory pressure, 139
        supportive care, 139t
Acute respiratory failure. See Respiratory failure
Acute tubular necrosis (ATN)
    case study, 689–690
    causes
        intratubular obstruction, 658
        nephrotoxicity, 658
        renal tubular ischemia, 658
    definition, 650
    in pancreatitis, 773
    risk factors, 658
Acute ventilatory failure (AVF), 166, 169, 170t. See
    also Ventilatory failure
Addiction. See Psychologic dependence
Adenosine
    as antiarrhythmic agent, 289t
    for supraventricular tachycardia, 276
ADH. See Antidiuretic hormone
Adjective rating scale (ARS), 35f
Adrenocorticotropic hormone (ACTH)
    in body fluid regulation, 59
    in shock, 374, 374f
Adventitia, 302, 303f
Aerobic metabolism
    vs. anaerobic metabolism, 361t
    definition, 355
    physiology, 360–361, 361f, 496, 496f
Affinity
    definition, 355
    of oxygen to hemoglobin, 361
African Americans, pain expression, 44t
Afterload
    blood pressure and, 223–224, 223f

definition, 219, 238, 245
    factors affecting, 222, 226
    pathophysiology, 245
Agency for Health Care Policy and Research
    (AHCPR), pain definition, 28
Aging. See Older adults
Agnosia
    definition, 428, 442
    nursing care, 442
    types, 442t
AHA. See American Heart Association
AHCPR. See Agency for Health Care Policy and
    Research
AIDS. See Acquired immunodeficiency disease
    syndrome
Air embolism, in total parenteral nutrition, 515
Airway, artificial, 172, 172f. See also Mechanical
    ventilation
Airway clearance, ineffective
    in mechanical ventilation, 190–192
    standard plan of care, 158
    in traumatic injury, 872
Airway protection
    in injured patient, 862
    during mechanical ventilation, 192
Airway resistance (R_{AW})
    definition, 166
    increased, pressure support ventilation for, 178
Akinesis, 300, 311
Alanine aminotransferase (ALT), 736, 741, 741t
Albumin
    in hepatic dysfunction, 743
    in nutritional/metabolic assessment, 498, 499t
Alcohol abuse
    erosive gastritis and, 715
    pancreatitis and, 766
    traumatic injury and, 859
    withdrawal onset and manifestations, 48t
Aldolase, 650, 658
Aldosterone
    characteristics, 650
    kidney function and, 654
    in shock, 374, 374f
ALG. See Antilymphocyte globulin
Alginates, for wound dressing, 805t
ALI. See Acute lung injury
Alkaline phosphatase (ALP), 736, 741, 741t
ALL. See Acute lymphocytic leukemia
Allergic response, 556, 568–569, 568f. See also
    Hypersensitivity reactions
Allograft
    cadaver donor, 590
    definition, 587, 590, 821
    live donor, 590
ALP. See Alkaline phosphatase
Alpha-fetoprotein (AFP), 556, 561–562
Alpha-interferon, for chronic leukemia, 539
Alpha receptors, 360t
ALT. See Alanine aminotransferase
Alveolar ventilation ($\dot{V}A$), 166, 167, 168f
Alveolar–arterial pressure gradient (A–a gradient)
    aging effects, 122
    calculation, 121, 122t
Alveolar–capillary membrane, 89–90
American College of Cardiologists, heart failure
    management guidelines, 334

American College of Critical Care Medicine (ACCM)
   definition of intensive care unit levels of care, 6t
   prioritization model for intensive care units, 5, 5t
American Heart Association (AHA)
   atherosclerosis classification, 302
   heart failure management guidelines, 334
American Indians, pain expression, 44t
American Nurses Association (ANA), *Standards of Clinical Nursing Practice*, 19
American Pain Society (APS), pain assessment position, 31
American Society of Pain Management Nurses (ASPMN), on pain treatment in substance abusers, 45, 47t
American Spinal Association (ASIA), classification of spinal cord injury, 467, 468f
Aminoacidemia, 621
Amitriptyline, for dysesthetic pain, 477
AML. *See* Acute myelogenous leukemia
Ammonia
   in hepatic dysfunction, 743
   reduction, in hepatic encephalopathy treatment, 751
Amniotic embolism, 143. *See also* Pulmonary embolism
Amphetamines, 48t
Ampulla of Vater, 762, 763
Amrinone, for contractility enhancement, 256
AMSN. *See* Academy of Medical Surgical Nurses
Amylase
   functions, 765t
   in pancreatitis, 768, 768t
Amylolytic, 762, 765
ANA. *See* American Nurses Association
Anabolism, 492, 496
Anaerobic metabolism
   vs. aerobic metabolism, 361t
   definition, 355
   physiology, 361, 361f, 496, 497f
Anal wink reflex, 469
Anaphylactic shock
   clinical manifestations, 376
   pathophysiology, 371–372
   treatment, 379, 569
Anaphylaxis
   pathophysiology, 569, 570f
   treatment, 569
Anastomosis
   complications, 603
   definition, 587
Anatomic shunt, 81, 95, 96f
ANC. *See* Absolute neutrophil count
Anemia
   categories, 528, 531, 531f
      blood loss, 533
      decreased red blood cell production
         acquired aplastic, 532
         iron-deficiency, 531
         megaloblastic, 531–532
      hemolytic, 532–533
      polycythemia, 533–534
   clinical manifestations, 530
   definition, 520, 530
   red cell distribution width in, 529
   severity based on hemoglobin levels, 528t

Anergy, 492
Anergy screen, 499
Aneurysm
   cerebral
      hemorrhagic stroke and, 429
      surgical management, 436
   definition, 428, 429
Angina pectoris
   assessment, 307–308
   definition, 300
   grading, 307t
   pathophysiology, 307
   types, 307–308
   in women, evidence-based practice, 308
Anginal equivalents, 300, 307
Angio-seal device, 317
Angiodysplasia. *See* Arteriovenous malformation
Angiography
   cerebral, in neurological assessment, 418–419
   coronary. *See* Percutaneous coronary intervention
   gastrointestinal
      diagnostic, 708
      for intervention in hemorrhage, 721t
Angioplasty
   cerebral, 436
   coronary. *See* Percutaneous coronary intervention
Angiotensin-converting enzyme (ACE) inhibitors
   for afterload reduction, 256
   common, 332t
   cough caused by, 337
   for heart failure, 334, 336, 336f
   for hypertension, 340
   for valvular heart disease, 332
Angiotensin II, 59
Angiotensin receptor blockers (ARBs)
   common, 332t
   for heart failure, 336, 336f
Anicteric hepatitis, 736, 745. *See also* Hepatitis
Anion gap, 621, 632
Anions, 55, 66, 650
Anorexia, in heart failure, 507
Anosognosia, 428, 442
ANP. *See* Atrial natriuretic peptide
Antacids, for gastrointestinal bleeding, 721t
Antiarrhythmic agents
   characteristics, 288–289, 289t
   nursing considerations, 289
Antibiotics
   for bacterial endocarditis, 331
   macrolide, 607
   for severe acute respiratory distress syndrome, 150
Antibody titer, 560, 566
Anticoagulants
   for ischemic stroke, 436
   for pulmonary embolism, 147t
   for valvular heart disease, 332–333
Anticonvulsants, 480
Antidiuretic hormone (ADH)
   in body fluid regulation, 59
   definition, 650
   kidney function and, 654
   in shock, 374, 374f
Antigen-antibody reaction, 563

Antigenic determinant site, 556, 562–563
Antigens. *See also* Human leukocyte antigens
   definition, 556, 561, 587, 599
   entry site, 563
   immune system response, 562–563, 562f
   types, 561
Antilymphocyte globulin (ALG), posttransplantation, 607
Antimetabolites. *See* Cytotoxic agents
Antimicrobial ointments, 839t
Antiplatelet therapy, for ischemic stroke, 436, 436t
Antiretroviral therapy, 577–578
Antithymocyte globulin (ATG)
   for aplastic anemia, 532
   posttransplantation, 607
Antiviral therapy, for severe acute respiratory distress syndrome, 150
Anuria, 650, 660
Anxiety, during mechanical ventilation, 193–194
Aortic regurgitation (AR)
   assessment and diagnosis, 331–332, 331t
   causes, 330
   collaborative management, 332
   definition, 325
   nursing management, 332–333
   pathophysiology, 330, 330f
   risk factors, 328t
Aortic stenosis (AS)
   assessment and diagnosis, 331–332, 331t
   causes, 328
   collaborative management, 332
   definition, 325
   nursing management, 332–333
   pathophysiology, 328, 329f
Aphasia
   definition, 428, 443
   types, 404, 413
Apical-radial pulse deficit, 219, 230
Aplastic anemia, 532
Apnea test, 456
Apoptosis
   definition, 385, 386
   in multiple organ dysfunction syndrome, 389
Apraxia
   assessment, 442
   definition, 428, 442
   treatment, 442
   types, 442t
APS. *See* American Pain Society
APTT. *See* Activated partial thromboplastin time
Aquacel Ag, 839t
AR. *See* Aortic regurgitation
Arab Americans, pain expression, 44t
ARBs. *See* Angiotensin receptor blockers
ARDS. *See* Acute respiratory distress syndrome
Aromatherapy, 4, 9
Around-the-clock schedule (ATC), 42
Arousal
   assessment, 411–412, 412f, 412t
   definition, 404, 411
   impaired, causes, 411
ARS. *See* Adjective rating scale
Arterial/Alveolar ratio (a/A ratio), 122, 123t
Arterial blood gases (ABGs)
   acid–base status determinants, 110
   in acute respiratory distress, 205

Arterial blood gases (ABGs)—(continued)
in acute respiratory failure, 133*t*
in chronic respiratory insufficiency, 132
in gastrointestinal dysfunction, 707, 707*t*
interpretation, 111, 111*t*, 112*f*, 113*f*, 114, 117*t*
in mixed acid–base disorders, 116–118, 116*t*, 117*t*
normal values, 111, 111*t*, 114*t*
oxygenation status determinants, 110
in pulmonary embolism, 146
Arteriogram, renal, 666
Arteriovenous malformation
lower gastrointestinal, 717, 717*t*
upper gastrointestinal, 716
Artery, anatomy, 302, 303*f*
Arthus vasculitis reaction, 556, 571
AS. *See* Aortic stenosis
As-needed schedule (PRN), 42
ASA. *See* Acetylsalicylic acid
Ascites, 736, 749
ASIA. *See* American Spinal Association
Aspartate aminotransferase (AST)
definition, 736
in gastrointestinal dysfunction, 706
in liver dysfunction, 741, 741*t*
Aspiration, postextubation failure and, 199
Aspiration biopsy, in pancreatitis, 769
Aspirin. *See* Acetylsalicylic acid
ASPMN. *See* American Society of Pain
Management Nurses
Assist-control mode (AC), 166, 178
AST. *See* Aspartate aminotransferase
Astereognosia, 442
Asterixis, 755
Asthma, allergic, 569
Ataxia, 428
Ataxic breathing, 415
ATC. *See* Around-the-clock schedule
ATG. *See* Antithymocyte globulin
Atheroma, 300, 302
Atherosclerosis
cerebral, 429, 431
coronary
American Heart Association classification, 302
definition, 300, 302
pathophysiology, 302
risk factors
collaborative management, 305, 305*t*
modifiable, 304, 304*t*
nonmodifiable, 304, 304*f*
definition, 621, 643
Atrial fibrillation
characteristics, 276–277, 278*f*, 278*t*
treatment, 278*t*
Atrial flutter
characteristics, 276, 277*f*, 278*t*
treatment, 278*t*
Atrial gallop, 219, 229
Atrial natriuretic peptide (ANP)
definition, 55
in heart failure, 334
increased, in hypovolemia, 61
Atrioventricular (AV) blocks
characteristics and treatment, 287*t*
first-degree, 284–285, 285*f*
second-degree, 285, 286*f*
third-degree, 285, 287*f*

Atropine
for AV blocks, 287*t*
for junctional rhythm, 279
for sinus bradycardia, 274, 275*f*
Auscultation
cardiac
in cardiac output assessment, 228–229
murmurs, 229, 229*t*
peripheral vasculature system, 229
pulmonary, 107, 107*t*
Auto-PEEP, 166
Autodigestion, 762, 765
Autograft
in burn injury, 840
definition, 587, 590, 821
Autoimmune disorders, 571*t*
Autoimmunity, 556, 571
Autolytic debridement, 793, 804
Automaticity, 265, 267
Autonomic dysreflexia
definition, 461
after spinal cord injury, 475, 475*t*
Autonomic nervous system
gastrointestinal tract, 702, 702*f*
in oxygen delivery, 359, 360*t*
Autoregulation
cerebral blood flow, 406
definition, 355, 404, 650
in kidney function, 654
physiology, 359
AV blocks. *See* Atrioventricular (AV) blocks
AVF. *See* Acute ventilatory failure
AVPU method, 863
Avulsion, 793
AZA. *See* Azathioprine
Azathioprine (AZA)
development, 589
posttransplantation, 606
Azotemia
in acute renal failure, 660, 660*t*
definition, 650

B

B cells, 556, 564
B lymphocytes. *See* B cells
B-type natriuretic peptide (BNP), 229
B waves, 417, 417*f*
Bacteria, gastrointestinal, 704–705
Bacteroides fragilis, 704–705
Balloon angioplasty, 317, 317*f*. *See also*
Percutaneous coronary intervention
Bandemia, 520, 529
Bands, 520, 529. *See also* Neutrophils
Barbiturates
for increased intracranial pressure, 422
street names, 48*t*
withdrawal onset and manifestations, 48*t*
Baroreceptors
definition, 55
functions, 59
kidney function and, 654
Barotrauma
clinical signs, 186
definition, 166
pathophysiology, 177

Base deficit, 365, 376
Base excess (BE)
definition, 81, 110
interpretation, 110
in metabolic acidosis, 102, 102*t*
in metabolic alkalosis, 102–103, 103*t*
normal values, 114*t*
Bases, 81, 99
Basilar skull fracture, 450–451. *See also* Closed-
head injury (CHI)
Basiliximab, posttransplantation, 606
Basophils
causes of abnormal results, 523*t*, 529
evaluation, 529
functions, 525
reference values, 523*t*
Batista procedure, 337
Battle's sign, 450
BE. *See* Base excess
Beck's triad, 301, 320
Behavioral observation scale, 35–36, 35*f*
Beta 1 receptors, 360*t*
Beta 2 receptors, 360*t*
Beta-blockers
for acute coronary syndromes, 313
as antiarrhythmic agents, 288, 289*t*
common, 332*t*
for heart failure, 334, 336
for hypertension, 340
Beta-endorphin, 27, 27*t*
Beta-hydroxybutyric acid, 621, 625, 626*f*
Bicarbonate (HCO₃)
definition, 110
for diabetic ketoacidosis, 633
interpretation, 111*t*, 112*f*, 113*f*
in metabolic acidosis, 102, 102*t*
in metabolic alkalosis, 102–103, 103*t*
in mixed acid–base disorders, 116–118, 117*t*
normal values, 114*t*
Bigeminy, 265, 281*f*
Bile, 736, 737
Bile acid sequestrants, 305
Bilirubin
definition, 736
testing, 742, 742*t*
types, 741–742
Biopsy
bone marrow, 529
heart, 611, 611*f*
renal, 666
Bisphosphonates, for hypercalcemia, 541
Bladder dysfunction
after spinal cord injury, 474, 477
after stroke, 440–441, 441*t*
Blast crisis, 537
Bleb, 129, 151
Bleomycin, pulmonary toxicity, 539
Blood
components, 521–522, 521*f*, 522*f*
erythrocytes. *See* Red blood cells
leukocytes. *See* White blood cells
platelets. *See* Platelets
laboratory results, 523*t*
Blood loss
anemia caused by, 533
posttransplantation, 603

Blood pressure (BP). *See also* Hypertension
    afterload and, 223–224, 223*f*
    direct monitoring. *See* Systemic arterial pressure
        measurement, 340
Blood urea nitrogen (BUN)
    in acute renal failure, 665, 665*t*
    in gastrointestinal dysfunction, 706, 707*t*
    in serum osmolality calculation, 57
Blood–brain barrier, 404, 407
Blunt trauma
    cardiac, 869–870
    characteristics, 852
    definition, 851
    forces associated with, 853–854
    injuries associated with, 854
    pulmonary, 868
Body fluid(s)
    age effects on content, 55–56
    compartments, 56, 56*f*, 56*t*
    distribution, 55
    imbalances
        edema. *See* Edema
        fluid volume deficit. *See* Fluid volume deficit
        fluid volume excess. *See* Fluid volume excess
        intravenous fluids for
            hypertonic, 65, 65*f*, 65*t*
            hypotonic, 64, 65*f*, 65*t*
            isotonic, 64, 65*f*, 65*t*
        third spacing, 61
    intercompartmental movement, 57–58, 57*f*
    regulation
        nervous system, 58–59
        renal and endocrine, 59
Body surface area (BSA), 219. *See also* Total body
    surface area
Bone marrow biopsy, 529
Bone marrow transplant, 539
Bowel sounds, feeding initiation and, 510
Bowman's capsule, 650, 651
Braces, for spinal cord injury, 471–472
Bradycardia. *See* Dysrhythmias
Brain
    arterial circulation, 405, 406*f*
    nutrient needs, 493
    oxygenation, 406. *See also* Cerebral tissue
        perfusion
    venous circulation, 405
Brain attack. *See* Stroke
Brain death
    after closed-head injury, 456
    definition, 446
    diagnosis, 456
        cerebral blood flow, 593
        clinical examination, 593
        electroencephalogram, 593
        pretest conditions, 592
    family support, 456
    organ donation and, 590, 593, 593*t*
Brain natriuretic peptide (BNP), 334
Breath sounds, 107, 107*t*
Breathing. *See* Ventilation
Breathing pattern, ineffective
    in brain function deterioration, 414–415, 415*t*
    during mechanical ventilation, 192
    standard plan of care, 157
    in traumatic injury, 872

Broca's aphasia, 443
Bronchioles, 85
Bronchitis, chronic. *See* Chronic bronchitis
Bronchoalveolar lavage (BAL) fluid, 135
Brush border, 696, 698
BSA. *See* Body surface area
Buffer
    definition, 81, 99
    systems, 100, 100*f*
Bulbocavernosus reflex, 469
Bulla, 821, 838
BUN. *See* Blood urea nitrogen (BUN)
Bundle branch block (BBB), 287
Burn centers
    referral criteria, 828, 828*t*
    team members, 828
    unit structure, 828
Burn injury
    acute rehabilitative phase
        behavioral changes, 842
        goals, 837
        pain, 842
        physical mobility, 843, 844*t*
        skin substitutes, 838–839, 839*t*
        topical antimicrobial therapy, 838, 839*t*
        wound cleansing, 837
        wound closure, 840–841, 840*f*, 841*f*
        wound debridement, 838, 838*f*
    classification, 823–824, 824*f*
    depth, 824, 824*t*
    evidence-based practice, 835*t*
    incidence, 821–822
    long-term rehabilitative phase
        care of healing skin, 845, 845*f*
        physical conditioning, 844–845
        psychosocial adjustment, 845
    mechanisms, 822–823
    nutritional/metabolic alterations, 508
    resuscitative phase
        cardiovascular effects, 829–830, 829*f*
        fluid administration, 829–830
        initial wound care, 837
        metabolic effects, 835
        neurological effects, 833
        pain, 833–834
        peripheral vascular effects, 830–831
        psychological adaptation, 833–834, 834*t*
        pulmonary effects
            carbon monoxide poisoning, 832
            inhalation injury, 831, 831*f*
            lower-airway injury, 831–832
            pulmonary function alterations, 831
            upper-airway injury, 831
        renal effects, 835–836
    risk factors, 821–822
Burn shock, 821, 822
Burnout, 4, 16, 16*t*
Bursa equivalent, 556, 559

C

C fibers, 27
C-reactive protein (CRP), 219, 229
C waves, 417, 417*f*
Ca. *See* Calcium

CABG. *See* Coronary artery bypass graft
Cachexia, 492, 507
Cadaver donor, 587, 590
Calcitonin, for hypercalcemia, 541
Calcium (Ca)
    contractility and, 224
    elevated intracellular, 466
    functions, 69
    imbalances, 69–70, 70*t*
    measurements, 69
    normal ranges and critical abnormal values, 66*t*
    regulation, 69
Calcium channel blockers
    as antiarrhythmic agents, 288–289, 289*t*
    common, 332*t*
Calorimetry, 500–501
Capillary colloidal osmotic pressure, 58, 60
Capillary hemoglobin saturation. *See* Pulse
    oximetry
Capillary hydrostatic pressure, 58, 60
Capillary permeability, 60
Capillary shunt
    causes, 95
    definition, 81, 95
    types, 96*f*
Capnogram
    definition, 81, 119
    interpretation, 120
Capnometry
    definition, 81, 119
    sublingual, 710
Capoten. *See* Captopril
Captopril, for afterload reduction, 256
Carbamazepine, for dysesthetic pain, 477
Carbohydrates
    definition, 621, 623
    functions, 494*t*
    metabolism, 493
        insulin and, 623
        insulin deficit and, 625
        liver's role, 739
Carbon dioxide
    narcosis, 129
    partial pressure
        alveolar. *See* P_{ACO_2}
        arterial. *See* Pa_{CO_2}
        venous. *See* Pv_{CO_2}
Carbon monoxide toxicity
    clinical manifestations, 376–377, 832
    in inhalation injury, 832
    pathophysiology, 372
    treatment, 380, 832
Carboxyhemoglobin, 821, 832
Carcinoembryonic antigen (CEA), 556, 561
Cardiac catheterization. *See* Percutaneous coronary
    intervention
Cardiac conduction
    abnormalities. *See* Atrioventricular (AV) blocks
    pathway, 268–269, 268*f*
Cardiac death, organ donation and, 590
Cardiac failure. *See* Heart failure
Cardiac glands, 696, 698
Cardiac index (CI)
    calculation, 244, 245, 258
    definition, 219, 238, 245
    normal values, 239

Cardiac markers
    definition, 301
    in myocardial ischemia assessment, 310, 310t
Cardiac output (CO)
    alterations
        in acute renal failure, 656–657
        after coronary artery bypass graft surgery, 320
        in heart failure, 336
        during mechanical ventilation, 192–193, 193t
    body size effects, 245
    calculation, 92–93, 220
    components, 245f
        afterload
            assessment, 230
            factors affecting, 226
        contractility
            assessment, 230, 245
            factors affecting, 221–222, 224, 226
        heart rate
            assessment, 225
            factors affecting, 230
        preload
            assessment, 230, 230t
            factors affecting, 221, 225–226
    definition, 92, 219, 238, 244, 355, 650
    diagnostic laboratory tests, 229–230
    measurement
        continuous, 246
        normal curve, 246, 246f
        thermodilution method, 245–246
            conditions affecting, 245
            equipment preparation, 245
            fluid bolus, 245
            fluid temperature, 245
            injection method, 246
            injection timing, 245
    normal values, 92, 239
    nursing assessment
        nursing history, 227
        nursing physical assessment, 227–228, 227t, 228f, 229t
        present illness and past medical history, 227
    oxygen delivery and, 359
Cardiac tamponade
    clinical manifestations, 377
    after coronary artery bypass surgery, 320
    definition, 301
    obstructive shock state and, 373
    pulmonary artery wedge pressure in, 255
    right atrial pressure in, 249
    SvO₂ pattern, 366f
    in trauma patient, 869
    treatment, 869, 869f
Cardiac valves, 326, 327f. See also Valvular heart disease
Cardiogenic shock states
    clinical manifestations, 377
    etiology, 371t, 373
    pathophysiology, 371t, 373
    treatment, 381
Cardiomyopathy
    classifications, 337, 338t
    definition, 325
    patient and family education, 337
    treatment, 337
Cardiomyoplasty, 337

Cardiopulmonary bypass (CPB), 318, 318f
Cardiopulmonary circuit, 88, 88f
Cardiopulmonary resuscitation (CPR), family presence during, 14
Cardiovascular diagnostic procedures, nursing responsibilities, 231–234
Cardioversion, 265, 289. See also Implantable cardioverter/defibrillator
Carina, 81, 84–85
Carotid endarterectomy, 437, 437f, 437t
CARS. See Compensatory anti-inflammatory response syndrome
Case studies
    acute respiratory distress syndrome, 395–400
    acute tubular necrosis, 689–690
    diabetes mellitus, 686–692
    fluid volume deficit, 344–348
    fluid volume excess, 348–352
    gastrointestinal bleeding, 782–787, 787–790
    impaired cerebral tissue perfusion, 485–488
    impaired oxygenation, 395–400
    mechanical ventilation, 213–215
    multiple organ dysfunction syndrome, 395–400
    myocardial ischemia, 348–352
    obstructive pulmonary disease, 208–213
    peptic ulcer disease, 787–790
    pneumonia, 204–208
    restrictive pulmonary disease, 204–208
    stroke, 485–488
    traumatic injury, 882–885
CAT. See Complementary and alternative therapies
Catabolism, 492, 496, 621
Catheter-related sepsis (CRS), 492, 514
Cations, 55, 66, 650
CAVH. See Continuous arteriovenous hemofiltration
CAVH-D. See Continuous arteriovenous hemofiltration-dialysis
Cavitation, 851, 855, 856f
CBF. See Cerebral blood flow
CD markers, 556, 564
CEA. See Carcinoembryonic antigen
Cell differentiation, 520
Cell-mediated immunity, 556–567
CellCept. See Mycophenolate mofetil
Central herniation
    characteristics, 409t, 410f
    after closed-head injury, 456, 456f
CEO₂. See Cerebral oxygen extraction
Cerebral angiography, 418–419
Cerebral blood flow (CBF)
    autoregulation, 406
    definition, 404
    factors affecting, 407t
Cerebral blood volume
    definition, 404
    factors affecting, 407t
    increased intracranial pressure and, 410
Cerebral edema, 409
Cerebral hematoma
    definition, 449
    types, 451–452, 452f
Cerebral oxygen extraction (CEO₂), 417–418
Cerebral perfusion pressure (CPP)
    calculation, 408–409
    in closed-head injury, 453–454

    definition, 404, 408
    in mechanical ventilation, 187
    normal values, 408
    optimization, 420–421
    pathophysiology, 409
Cerebral salt wasting (CSW), 455–456, 456t
Cerebral tissue oxygen content (PbtO₂), 453–454
Cerebral tissue perfusion
    assessment
        diagnostic procedures
            cerebral angiography, 419
            computed tomography, 418
            electroencephalography, 419
            evoked potentials, 419
            lumbar puncture, 419
            magnetic resonance angiography, 419
            magnetic resonance imaging, 418
            positron emission tomography, 418
            single photon emission computed tomography, 418
            transcranial Doppler, 418–419
        intracranial pressure monitoring
            devices, 416–417, 416f
            evidence-based practice, 418t
            indications, 415–416
            jugular bulb oximetry, 417–418
            nursing care, 422–423, 423t
            sites, 416t
            waveform patterns, 417, 417f
        level of consciousness
            arousal, 411–412, 412f, 412t
            content, 412–413
            oculomotor responses, 413–414, 414f
            pupillary reactions, 413, 413f
            vital signs, 414–415, 415f
    components
        arterial circulation, 406f, 506
        oxygenation, 406
        venous circulation, 405
    impaired
        case study, 485–488
        causes, 411
        management
            optimization of cerebral oxygenation, 421
            optimization of cerebral perfusion pressure, 420–421
            pharmacologic therapy, 421–422
            ventilation support, 421
        manifestations, 415t
        in traumatic injury, 873
    measurement, 453–454
Cerebrospinal fluid (CSF)
    drainage
        complications, 422
        indications, 422
        in skull fracture, 451
    increased, 410, 410t
    normal pressure, 408
    physiology, 408
Cervical collars, 472t
Cervical spine injury, 465. See also Spinal cord injury
Cervical traction, 471, 471f, 472t
Chemical burns, 822. See also Burn injury
Chemical debridement, 793, 804
Chemoreceptors, kidney function and, 654

Chemotaxis, 520, 525, 525*f*, 556, 567
Chemotherapy
    for leukemia, 538–539
    treatment crises. *See* Oncologic emergencies
Chest drainage
    definition, 151
    indications, 151–152
    systems, 154, 154*f*
    tube insertion
        assessment, 154–155, 155*t*
        nursing considerations, 153*t*
        nursing diagnoses, 155
        procedure, 152–153, 153*f*
Chest injury
    cardiac
        blunt injury, 869–870
        tamponade, 869, 869*f*
    chest wall
        flail chest, 868, 868*f*
        rib fractures, 868
    pulmonary
        contusions, 868
        massive hemothorax, 869
        open pneumothorax, 869, 869*f*
        tension pneumothorax, 868–869, 869*f*
Chest pain. *See also* Angina pectoris
    in acute coronary syndromes, 312
    initial management, 313
    nursing assessment, 105
Chest physiotherapy, in spinal cord injury, 473
Chest radiography
    in acute respiratory distress syndrome, 135
    nursing responsibilities, 231–232
    in pancreatitis, 769
    in pulmonary embolism, 146
Chest tube. *See* Chest drainage
Cheyne-Stokes respiration, 414
CHI. *See* Closed-head injury
Chief cells, 696, 698
Chinese Americans, pain expression, 44*t*
Chloride (Cl)
    functions, 68
    imbalances, 68–69, 68*t*
    normal ranges and critical abnormal values, 66*t*
Cholecystokinin (CCK)
    definition, 696
    gastric functions, 698, 699*t*
Cholestatic hepatitis, 736, 745. *See also* Hepatitis
Cholesterol, classification of levels, 304*t*
Chronic airflow limitation, 130. *See also* Chronic
    obstructive pulmonary disease
Chronic bronchitis, 129
Chronic lymphocytic leukemia (CLL), 536–537.
    See also Leukemia
Chronic myelogenous leukemia (CML), 537. *See
    also* Leukemia
Chronic obstructive pulmonary disease (COPD)
    acute ventilatory failure in, 169
    case study, 208–213
    definition, 129, 130
Chronic rejection, 587, 603. *See also* Rejection
Chronic renal failure (CRF)
    definition, 650, 677
    evidence-based practice, 677
    incidence, 677, 677*t*
    nursing considerations, 678–679

nutritional/metabolic alterations, 506–507
    stages, 678*t*
        diminished renal reserve, 677
        end-stage renal disease, 678
        renal failure, 678
        renal insufficiency, 677–678
    survival rate, 677
Chvostek's sign, 771
Chyme, 696, 762, 764
Chymotrypsin, 762, 765*t*
CI. *See* Cardiac index
Cingulate herniation
    characteristics, 409*t*, 410*f*
    after closed-head injury, 456, 456*f*
Circle of Willis, 404, 405, 406*f*
CISD. *See* Critical incident stress debriefing
CK. *See* Creatine kinase
CK-MB. *See* Creatine kinase-myocardial band
Cl. *See* Chloride
C_L. *See* Compliance
CLL. *See* Chronic lymphocytic leukemia
Clopidogrel, for acute coronary syndromes, 313
Closed-head injury (CHI)
    complications
        brain death, 456
        cerebral salt wasting, 455–456, 456*t*
        diabetes insipidus, 455, 456*t*
        herniation, 456, 456*f*
        syndrome of inappropriate antidiuretic
            hormone, 455, 456*t*
    diffuse
        concussion, 452
        diffuse axonal injury, 452–453
    focal
        epidural hematoma, 451–452, 452*f*
        subarachnoid hematoma, 452
        subdural hematoma, 452, 452*f*
    mechanisms, 450, 450*f*
    nutritional/metabolic alterations, 508
    secondary injury
        causes, 453
        medical interventions, 454, 454*f*
        nursing interventions, 454
        prevention, 453–454, 454*t*
    skull fractures
        medical management, 451
        nursing priorities, 451
        types, 450–451
Closed-suction drains, 806*t*
CLRT. *See* Continuous lateral rotation therapy
Cluster breathing, 414–415
CML. *See* Chronic myelogenous leukemia
CO. *See* Cardiac output
CO_2. *See* Carbon dioxide
Coagulation cascade
    in disseminated intravascular coagulation,
        545, 546*f*
    in septic shock, 380
Coagulation tests, 742
Coagulopathy, microvascular, 389
Cocaine, 48*t*
Codeine, equianalgesic doses, 42*t*
Collagen, 793, 796
Colloids, for shock, 378
Colonoscopy, 708, 709*t*
Colony-stimulating factors, 565

Committed stem cell, 520, 522, 522*f*
Communication
    impairment, in stroke, 443
    with mechanically ventilated patients, 11
    nonverbal, 11
Compartment syndrome
    abdominal. *See* Abdominal compartment
        syndrome
    in burn injury, 830
    definition, 821
Compensated acid–base state. *See also* Acid–base
        disturbances
    algorithms for determining, 112*f*, 113*f*
    characteristics, 100*t*
    definition, 81, 100
Compensation, 100, 100*t*
Compensatory anti-inflammatory response
        syndrome (CARS), 387
Compensatory pause, 280
Complement system, 556, 567
Complementary and alternative therapies (CAT)
    in acute illness, 9
    definition, 4
Complete blood count (CBC), 523*t*
Complete spinal cord injury, 461, 464. *See also*
        Spinal cord injury
Compliance (C_L)
    definition, 81, 86, 129, 166
    pathophysiology, 86–87
Compression, 851, 854
Compression garments, 845, 845*f*
Compression injury
    characteristics, 854
    spinal cord, 464–465, 465*f*
Compromised wound, 793, 802
Computed tomography (CT)
    in acute renal failure, 666
    in gastrointestinal dysfunction, 708
    in neurological assessment, 418
    in pancreatitis, 769
    in spinal cord injury, 467
    in stroke assessment, 435
Concussion. *See also* Closed-head injury
    clinical manifestations, 452
    definition, 449, 452
    nursing care, 452
Conduction abnormalities. *See* Atrioventricular
        (AV) blocks
Congestive heart failure. *See* Heart failure
Conjugated bilirubin, 736, 742, 752*t*
Consciousness
    assessment
        arousal, 411–412
        AVPU method, 863
        content, 412–413
        Glasgow Coma Scale, 411–412, 412*t*
    definition, 404
    impaired
        causes, 411
        manifestations of progressive
            deterioration, 415*t*
Consolidation chemotherapy, 538
Constipation
    after spinal cord injury, 474
    after stroke, 441
Constrictive cardiomyopathy, 325, 337, 338*t*

Constructional apraxia, 442, 442t
Content
    in consciousness assessment, 412
    definition, 404
Continuous arteriovenous hemofiltration (CAVH).
        See also Dialysis
    characteristics, 671f, 672–673, 673f
    definition, 394
Continuous arteriovenous hemofiltration-dialysis
        (CAVH-D), 673. See also Dialysis
Continuous lateral rotation therapy (CLRT),
        139–140, 140f
Continuous positive airway pressure (CPAP)
    characteristics, 183
    complications, 183
    definition, 166
    indications, 183
    in mechanical ventilation, 179
Continuous renal replacement therapy (CRRT),
        672–673, 673f. See also Dialysis
Continuous venovenous hemofiltration (CVVH),
        673. See also Dialysis
Continuous venovenous hemofiltration-dialysis
        (CVVH-D), 673. See also Dialysis
Contractility
    assessment, 230, 245
    calcium levels and, 224
    definition, 219, 221, 245, 265
    factors affecting, 221–222, 224, 226
Contraction, wound, 793, 797
Contrast dye
    allergy, 316
    renal effects, 316
Contusion, 793
COPD. See Chronic obstructive pulmonary disease
Cor pulmonale
    definition, 81, 97, 129
    pathophysiology, 97–98, 98f
Coronary arteries, 306, 306f
Coronary artery bypass graft (CABG)
    indications, 318
    nursing diagnoses, 319t
    postsurgical care, 319–321
    procedure, 318–319, 319f
Coronary artery disease (CAD). See Atherosclerosis
Coronary perfusion. See Myocardial tissue
        perfusion
Coronary perfusion pressure (CPP), 306
Coronavirus, SARS-associated, 149. See also Severe
        acute respiratory syndrome
Corrected acid–base state, 81, 100, 100t. See also
        Acid–base disturbances
Corticospinal tract, 463
Corticosteroids
    for acute respiratory distress syndrome, 140–141
    for hypercalcemia, 541
    posttransplantation, 606
    for severe acute respiratory distress syndrome, 150
    for spinal cord compression, 541
    wound healing and, 801
Cortisol, in glucose metabolism, 622
Cough
    assisted, 473
    nursing assessment, 105–106
Coup–contrecoup injury, 450, 450f. See also
        Closed-head injury

CPB. See Cardiopulmonary bypass
CPP. See Cerebral perfusion pressure; Coronary
        perfusion pressure
CPR. See Cardiopulmonary resuscitation
Crackles, 81, 107
Cranial nerve reflexes, 413–414, 414f, 415
Craniotomy, 454, 454f
Creatine kinase (CK), 310t
Creatine kinase-myocardial band (CK-MB),
        229, 310t
Creatinine, 665, 665t
Cricothyroidotomy, 851, 872
Critical incident stress debriefing (CISD), 17
Crossmatching, 599
CRP. See C-reactive protein
CRRT. See Continuous renal replacement therapy
CRS. See Catheter-related sepsis; Cytokine release
        syndrome
Crystalloid solutions, for shock, 378
CsA. See Cyclosporine
CSW. See Cerebral salt wasting
CT. See Computed tomography
CT$_n$. See Troponins
Cuirass, 173–174
Cullen's sign, 771
Cultural considerations, pain management, 44t
Cushing's triad, 404, 415
CVVH. See Continuous venovenous
        hemofiltration
CVVH-D. See Continuous venovenous
        hemofiltration-dialysis
CyA. See Cyclosporine
Cycle
    definition, 166, 175
    types, 175–176
Cyclosporine (CyA or CsA), posttransplantation,
        605–606
Cystitis, hemorrhagic, 542
Cytokine release syndrome (CRS), 542, 587, 606–607
Cytokines, 556, 565
Cytopathic hypoxia, 385, 388
Cytotoxic agents, 587, 606
Cytoxan, cardiac toxicity, 539

D

D-dimer
    definition, 520
    in disseminated intravascular coagulation,
        546, 547t
    in pulmonary embolism, 146
Daclizumab, posttransplantation, 606
DAI. See Diffuse axonal injury
Dakin's solution, 806t
DASH. See Dietary approaches to stop
        hypertension
dBA. See Decibels
DDAVP. See Desmopressin acetate
Deadspace ventilation (V̇D), 166, 167, 168f
Death. See also Brain death; Cardiac death
    determination, 592–593
    legal definition, 591, 592
Debridement, 793, 804
    in burn injury, 838, 838f
    definition, 821
Deceleration

definition, 851, 854
    injury caused by, 450
Decerebrate posturing, 404, 412, 412f
Decibels, in hospitals, 10–11
Decorticate posturing, 404, 412, 412f
Decoupling, 594
Deep partial-thickness burn, 821, 824, 825t. See
        also Burn injury
Deep tendon reflexes
    neural source of origin, 469t
    in spinal cord injury, 469
Deep-vein thrombosis (DVT). See also
        Thromboembolism
    predisposing factors, 143–144
    prophylaxis after spinal cord injury, 475
    prophylaxis after stroke, 438
Defibrillation. See also Implantable
        cardioverter/defibrillator
    automatic external, 295
    characteristics, 383
    definition, 265
    procedure, 289–290, 290f
Dehydration, stroke risk and, 432
Demerol. See Meperidine
Depolarization, 266, 267f, 267t
Depressed skull fracture, 450. See also Closed-head
        injury (CHI)
Dermatome, 461, 467, 469f
Dermis, 793, 794, 795f
Desmopressin acetate (DDAVP), for diabetes
        insipidus, 597
Detrusor
    hyperreflexia, 441, 441t
    hyporeflexia, 440–441, 441t
Detrusor–sphincter dyssynergy, 440, 441t
Diabetes insipidus
    clinical manifestations, 455
    after closed-head injury, 455, 456t
    in organ donor, 597
Diabetes mellitus
    acute complications
        case study, 686–692
        diabetic ketoacidosis. See Diabetic
                ketoacidosis
        hyperglycemic hyperosmolar state. See
                Hyperglycemic hyperosmolar state
        hypoglycemic coma, 629–630
        nursing history, 628
    burn injuries and, 822
    chronic complications
        glucose control and, 642
        infection risk, 644
        macrovascular disease, 643
        microvascular disease, 643
        neuropathy, 643
        peripheral neuropathy, 642–643
        peripheral vascular disease, 643
        retinopathy, 643
    definition, 621
    insulin therapy. See Insulin therapy
    type 1, 627, 628t
    type 2, 627–628, 628t
    wound healing and, 800
Diabetic ketoacidosis (DKA)
    assessment, 631, 686–687
    case study, 686–692

causes, 632–633
definition, 621
vs. hyperglycemic hyperosmolar state, 636*t*
management
    collaborative interventions, 633–634, 634*f*
    nursing interventions, 634–635
    plan of care, 687–688
pathophysiology, 631–632
signs and symptoms, 631*t*
stress and, 632–633
Dialysis
continuous renal replacement therapy,
    672–673, 673*f*
    nursing considerations, 675*t*
definition, 650, 671
dialysate solutions, 675, 675*t*
drug therapy and, 675–676, 676*t*
hemodialysis
    nursing considerations, 675*t*
    nutritional/metabolic alterations, 506–507
    parenteral nutrition during, 507
    system, 672, 672*f*
    venous access, 671, 671*f*
peritoneal, 673, 673*f*, 674*f*, 675
    nursing considerations, 675*t*
types, 670*t*
Diapedesis, 520, 525
Diastolic dysfunction, 325, 333. *See also* Heart
    failure
Dietary approaches to stop hypertension
    (DASH), 340
Diffuse axonal injury (DAI)
definition, 449, 452
diagnosis, 453
management, 453
mechanisms, 452–453
Diffuse head injury, 449, 451. *See also*
    Closed-head injury
Diffusion
aging effects, 91
definition, 81, 89, 355, 650, 652
factors affecting
    length of exposure, 90
    partial pressures and gradient, 89–90, 89*f*,
      90*f*, 357
    surface area of lung, 90, 357
    thickness of alveolar–capillary membrane,
      90, 357
impaired, 358*t*
Digestion, 495
Digoxin
as antiarrhythmic agent, 289*t*
for contractility enhancement, 256
Dilated cardiomyopathy, 325, 337, 338*t*
Dilaudid. *See* Hydromorphone
Dilutional effect, 55, 67
Dimethyl ketone. *See* Acetone
Diprivan. *See* Propofol
Direct bilirubin, 742, 742*t*
Direct calorimetry, 492, 500
Disseminated intravascular coagulation (DIC)
clinical manifestations, 545, 547*t*
laboratory studies, 546, 547*t*
in pancreatitis, 773
pathophysiology, 545, 546*f*
risk factors, 544–545, 545*t*

in traumatic injury, 876
treatment, 546–547
Diuretics
for acute renal failure, 668
definition, 650
for heart failure, 334, 336
for increased intracranial pressure, 421
Diverticula, bleeding, 717, 717*t*
DKA. *See* Diabetic ketoacidosis
DNR orders. *See* Do not resuscitate (DNR) orders
DO₂. *See* Oxygen delivery
Do not resuscitate (DNR) orders, 18
Dobutamine
for contractility enhancement, 256
for exercise stress tests, 311
for shock, 378
Doll's eye movements, 404, 413–414, 414*f*
Donor
cadaver, 590
consent issues, 594
definition, 587
legal aspects, 590–591
live, 590
management, 596*t*
    endocrine function loss, 597
    fluid and electrolyte instability, 597
    hematopoietic dysfunction, 597
    hemodynamic instability, 596–597
    pulmonary dysfunction, 597
    thermoregulation loss, 597
recipient compatibility testing, 599–600, 600*t*
referral to organ procurement organization,
    593, 593*t*
suitability evaluation, 594, 594*t*
testing, 594–595
Dopamine, for shock, 378, 380
Dopaminergic receptors, 360*t*
Drains, for wounds, 806*t*
Dressing apraxia, 442, 442*t*
Drotrecogin alfa
for multiple organ dysfunction syndrome, 389
for septic shock, 380
Drug allergy, 325, 337
Drug-seeking behavior, 45–46, 46*t*
Drug side effects, 325, 337
Duct of Santorini, 762, 763
Duct of Wirsung, 762
Duodenal ulcer, 788. *See also* Peptic ulcer disease
Duragesic. *See* Fentanyl
Dynorphins, 27, 27*t*
Dysarthria, 428, 443
Dysesthetic pain, 461, 477
Dyskinesis, 301, 311
Dysoxia, 355, 362
Dysphagia, 428, 440
Dysphasia, 428, 443
Dyspnea, 81, 105
Dysrhythmias
atrial, 276–277, 277*f*, 278*f*, 278*t*
junctional, 279, 279*f*, 279*t*
risk factors for, 273–274
sinus, 274–275, 275*f*, 275*t*
treatment
    antiarrhythmic agents, 288–289, 289*t*
    cardioversion, 289
    defibrillation, 289–290, 290*f*

implantable cardioverter/defibrillator,
    294–295, 295*t*
pacemakers. *See* Pacemakers
ventricular, 282–283, 283*f*, 284*t*

E

Ebb phase, metabolic stress response, 492, 503
Ecchymosis, in skull fracture, 450
ECF. *See* Extracellular fluid
ECG. *See* Electrocardiogram
Echocardiogram
definition, 301, 325
in heart failure assessment, 334
in myocardial ischemia assessment, 311
nursing responsibilities, 232
in valvular heart disease assessment, 331–332
Edema
assessment, 63, 63*f*, 228
clinical manifestations, 62–63
in kwashiorkor, 503
mechanisms
    lymphatic obstruction, 60–61
    Starling forces problems, 60
pathophysiology, 228
in perfusion disorders, 228
in spinal cord injury, 466
EDH. *See* Epidural hematoma
Educational needs, patients and families,
    12–13, 12*t*
EEG. *See* Electroencephalogram
EF. *See* Ejection fraction
Ejection fraction (EF)
definition, 219, 222, 265, 301
in myocardial infarction, 314
Elastase
definition, 762
functions, 765*t*
in pancreatitis, 767
Elavil. *See* Amitriptyline
Elderly patients. *See* Older adults
Electrical burn injury. *See also* Burn injury
cardiovascular effects, 830
characteristics, 822–823
Electrocardiogram (ECG)
in acute coronary syndromes, 312
exercise. *See* Exercise stress test
interpretation guidelines, 271–272, 271*f*, 272*f*
lead placement, 270
in myocardial ischemia assessment, 309,
    309*f*, 310*t*
normal waveforms and intervals, 268–269,
    268*f*, 269*f*
nursing care of patient requiring, 269–270, 270*f*
in pulmonary embolism, 146
Electroencephalogram (EEG)
in brain death assessment, 593
in neurological assessment, 418–419
Electrolytes.
in acute renal failure, 661–662
definition, 66, 650
in diabetic ketoacidosis, 633, 634*f*
in gastrointestinal dysfunction, 706, 707*t*
membrane permeability and, 266–267, 267*f*
normal ranges and critical abnormal values, 66*t*

Electrophysiology study (EPS), nursing responsibilities, 234
ELISA. *See* Enzyme-linked immunosorbent assay
Embolectomy, 147*t*
Embolic stroke, 429, 430*t. See also* Stroke
Emphysema, 129
Empyema, 129
Encephalopathy, hepatic. *See* Hepatic encephalopathy
End-stage renal disease (ESRD), 678, 678*t*
End-tidal carbon dioxide (PETCO$_2$)
    definition, 81, 119
    interpretation, 120
    measurement, 119–120
Endocrine system, response to shock, 374*f*
Endogenous, 793, 802
Endoscopic retrograde cholangiopancreatography (ERCP), 762, 769
Endoscopy
    in diagnosis of gastrointestinal dysfunction, 708, 709*t*
    for intervention in gastrointestinal hemorrhage, 722*t*
Endothelial cells, 386, 386*t*
Endothelin-1, in hypertension, 339
Endothelium, 301, 303
Endotracheal tubes, 170–171, 171*f*, 171*t. See also* Mechanical ventilation
Energy
    definition, 492, 496
    measurement, 496–497
Energy expenditure
    in burn patients, 508
    calculation
        calorimetry, 500–501
        Harris-Benedict equation, 500, 500*t*
    in closed-head injury, 508
    in hepatic failure, 505–506
Enkephalins, 27, 27*t*
Enoxaparin, for acute coronary syndromes, 313
Enteral nutrition
    benefits, 510
    in burn injury, 835
    complications, 511, 512*t*
    contraindications, 510
    definition, 492
    evidence-based practice, 509*t*
    feeding tube placement, 511
    gastric vs. postpyloric, 511
    selection criteria
        gastrointestinal integrity and function, 509
        illness severity and possible duration, 509–510
        timing, 510
    in traumatic injury, 876
Enteric nervous system, 702
Enzyme-linked immunosorbent assay (ELISA), 576
Enzymes
    definition, 736
    gastric, 698
    liver, 740–741, 741*t*
    pancreatic, 765, 765*t*
Eosinophils
    causes of abnormal results, 529
    evaluation, 529
    functions, 525
Epidermis, 793, 794, 795*f*

Epidural, 25, 38
Epidural hematoma (EDH)
    characteristics, 452*f*
    clinical manifestations, 451–452
    definition, 449
    medical management, 452
    pathophysiology, 451
Epidural probe, 416, 416*f*, 416*t*
Epilepsy, 461, 479. *See also* Seizure(s)
Epinephrine
    for anaphylactic shock, 379
    in glucose metabolism, 622
    in hypoglycemic coma, 629–630
Epistaxis, in thrombocytopenia, 543
Epithelialization, 793, 796
EPS. *See* Electrophysiology study
ERCP. *See* Endoscopic retrograde cholangiopancreatography
Erythrocyte sedimentation rate (ESR), 529
Erythrocytes. *See* Red blood cells (RBCs)
Erythrocytosis, 532–533
Erythropoietin, 524
Eschar
    characteristics, 807
    chest, 831
    definition, 793, 821
Escharotomy
    characteristics, 831*f*
    chest, 831
    definition, 821
    indications, 830–831
Escherichia coli, 705
Esophageal varices
    case study, 782–787
    management, 752, 753*f*, 753*t*
    portal hypertension and, 748–749
Esophagogastroduodenoscopy (EGD), 708, 709*t*
ESR. *See* Erythrocyte sedimentation rate
ESRD. *See* End-stage renal disease
EST. *See* Exercise stress test
ETCO$_2$. *See* End-tidal carbon dioxide
Evidence-based practice
    burn injury, 835*t*
    cardiac output assessment, 227*t*
    coronary artery disease in women, 308*t*
    enteral nutrition, 509*t*
    head injury, 454*t*
    heart failure management, 337*t*
    hepatic dysfunction, 743*t*
    immunocompromised patient, 579–580*t*
    implantable cardioverter/defibrillator, 295*t*
    injury, 874*t*
    insulin therapy, 638*t*
    intracranial pressure monitoring, 418*t*
    mechanical ventilation, 190*t*
    multiple organ dysfunction syndrome, 391*t*
    music therapy, 11*t*
    organ procurement, 592*t*
    oxygenation assessment, 365*t*
    pain assessment, 37*t*
    pancreatitis, 774*t*
    respiratory care, 157*t*
    septic shock, 380*t*
    spinal cord injury, 477*t*
    stroke, 440*t*
    wound healing, 800*t*

Evoked potentials, 418–419
Excitability, 265
Exercise stress test (EST)
    in myocardial ischemia assessment, 310–311
    nursing responsibilities, 232
Exogenous, 793, 802
Expressive aphasia, 404, 413
Exsanguination, 851
External respiration, 81, 88, 88*f. See also* Respiration
Extracellular, 55
Extracellular fluid (ECF), 56. *See also* Fluid volume deficit; Fluid volume excess
Extracorporeal membrane oxygenation (ECMO), 394
Extubation, 166, 199. *See also* Mechanical ventilation, weaning
Exudate, 793, 807

F

Faces scale, 32, 32*f*
Family-centered care
    definition, 14
    during mechanical ventilation, 194
Fast sodium channel blockers, 288, 289*t*
Fat embolism, 143. *See also* Pulmonary embolism
Fat metabolism
    insulin and, 624
    insulin deficit and, 625, 626*f*
    liver's role, 739
Fatigue, in heart failure, 336
Fatty streaks, 301, 302, 303*f*
Fentanyl, equianalgesic doses, 42*t*
FEV. *See* Forced expiratory volume
FHF. *See* Fulminant hepatic failure
Fibrous atheromatous plaque, 301, 302, 303*f*
Fick equation, 501, 501*t*
FIO$_2$. *See* Fraction of inspired oxygen
FK 506. *See* Tacrolimus
Flaccid paralysis, 461
Flaccidity, 428
Flagyl. *See* Metronidazole
Flail chest, 868, 868*f*
Flow-cycled ventilation, 176. *See also* Mechanical ventilation
Flow-directed thermodilution catheter. *See* Pulmonary artery catheter
Flow phase, metabolic stress response, 492, 503–504
Fludarabine, for chronic leukemia, 539
Fluid volume deficit. *See also* Hypovolemia
    case study, 344–348
    nursing assessment, 63, 63*f*
    nursing interventions, 64, 634
    pathophysiology, 61, 61*t*
    right atrial pressure in, 250
    SvO$_2$ pattern, 366*f*
    in traumatic injury, 872–873
Fluid volume excess. *See also* Hypervolemia
    in acute renal failure, 667–668
    case study, 348–352
    nursing assessment, 64, 64*t*
    nursing interventions, 64
    pathophysiology, 61, 61*t*
Fluids. *See* Body fluid(s)
Foams, for wound dressing, 805*t*

Focal head injury, 449, 451. *See also* Closed-head injury
Folic acid
    deficiency, 531–532
    role in erythrocytes, 524
Forced expiratory volume (FEV)
    definition, 81, 109, 129
    in obstructive pulmonary disorders, 131, 131*t*
Four poster brace, 472*t*
Fraction of inspired oxygen (FIO₂), 166, 177–178
Frank-Starling law, 222, 223*f*
FRC. *See* Functional residual capacity
Frostbite injury, 823, 823*f*
Full-thickness burn, 821, 824, 825*t*. *See also* Burn injury
Fulminant hepatic failure (FHF), 736, 746, 746*t*, 752. *See also* Hepatic failure
Functional residual capacity (FRC), 108, 109*f*
Fundic glands, 696, 698
Furosemide, for heart failure, 334

G

G-CSF. *See* Granulocyte-colony stimulating factor
Gabapentin, for dysesthetic pain, 477
Gallstones, 766
GALT. *See* Gut-associated lymphoid tissue
Gamma glutamyl transferase (GGT), 741, 741*t*
Gardner-Wells tongs, 471, 471*f*, 472*t*
Gas exchange
    calculations
        Alveolar-arterial pressure gradient, 121, 122*t*
        arterial/Alveolar ratio, 122, 123*t*
        ideal alveolar gas equation, 121, 121*t*
        Pao₂/Fio₂ ratio, 122, 123*t*
    impaired
        during mechanical ventilation, nursing management, 192
        nutritional/metabolic alterations, 506
        standard plan of care, 157–158
        in traumatic injury, 872
    mechanical ventilation for, 139, 140*t*
    noninvasive monitoring
        end-table carbon dioxide monitoring, 119–120
        pulse oximetry. *See* Pulse oximetry
Gastric enzymes, 698
Gastric feeding, vs. postpyloric, 511
Gastric inhibitory peptide (GIP), 696, 699, 699*t*
Gastric tonometry
    definition, 696
    interpretation, 710*t*
    technique, 708, 709*f*
Gastric ulcer, 788. *See also* Peptic ulcer disease
Gastrin, 696, 698
Gastritis
    alcoholic, 715
    NSAID-related, 714–715
    prevention, 715
    stress-related, 715
    treatment, 715
Gastrointestinal tract
    anatomy and physiology, 697, 697*f*
        arterial blood supply, 701, 701*f*, 701*t*
        gastric enzymes, 698

gastrointestinal wall, 696–697
    innervation, 702, 703*f*
    large intestine, 699–700
    small intestine, 698–699, 699*f*, 699*t*
    venous drainage, 702, 702*t*
bacterial translocation, 507
bleeding
    case studies, 782–787, 787–790
    lower tract
        arteriovenous malformations, 717
        causes, 717, 717*t*
        diverticular, 717
        inflammatory bowel disease, 718
        ischemic bowel disease, 717–718
        neoplasms, 718
    management
        arterial angiotherapy interventions, 720, 721*t*
        diagnostic approach, 719–720, 719*f*
        endoscopy interventions, 722*t*
        initial assessment, 720
        pharmacologic interventions, 721*t*
        resuscitation, 720
        severe hemorrhage, 721*t*
        specific lesions, 720–722
    nursing diagnoses, 729, 729*t*
    nursing interventions, 730, 730*t*
    upper tract
        arteriovenous malformation, 716
        causes, 712, 712*t*
        clinical manifestations, 711
        erosive gastritis, 715–715
        incidence, 711
        Mallory-Weiss tears, 715
        peptic ulcer disease, 713–714, 713*f*, 714*f*
        varices. *See* Esophageal varices
cellular layers, 495
defense mechanisms
    immunologic, 705
    mucosal integrity, 705, 705*f*
    nonimmunologic, 704–705
dysfunction
    abdominal compartment syndrome. *See* Abdominal compartment syndrome
    acute paralytic ileus. *See* Paralytic ileus
    acute small-bowel obstruction, 723–724
    diagnostic studies, 708
    intra-abdominal hypertension. *See* Intra-abdominal hypertension
    laboratory tests, 706–707, 707*t*
    nursing considerations, 708–710
    nursing diagnoses, 729–730, 729*t*
immune function, 495
ischemia, 507
metabolic alterations, 502
Gauze dressings, 804, 805*t*
GCS. *See* Glasgow Coma Scale
Generalized seizure, 461, 479. *See also* Seizure(s)
GIP. *See* Gastric inhibitory peptide
Glasgow Coma Scale (GCS), 411–412, 412*t*
Gleevec. *See* Imatinib mesylate
Global aphasia
    definition, 404, 413
    nursing care, 443
Glomerular filtration, 650, 652
Glomerular filtration rate (GFR), 650, 652

Glomerulus, 650, 651
Glucagon, 493, 621, 623
Gluconeogenesis, 492, 493, 621
Glucose metabolism
    altered. *See* Diabetes mellitus
    definition, 493
    normal, 622–623
Glycogen, 621
Glycogenolysis, 492, 493, 621
Glycoprotein (GP) IIb/IIIa inhibitors, 313
Glycosuria, 621–622
Glycosylated hemoglobin (Hb A₁c), 621, 642
GM-CSF. *See* Granulocyte macrophage-colony stimulating factor
GP IIb/IIIa inhibitors. *See* Glycoprotein (GP) IIb/IIIa inhibitors
Graft
    definition, 587, 590
    rejection, 603
Granulation tissue, 793, 797
Granulocyte, 520, 524
Granulocyte-colony stimulating factor (G-CSF), 535
Granulocyte macrophage-colony stimulating factor (GM-CSF), 535
Gray matter, spinal cord, 463
Grey Turner's sign, 771
Growth hormone, in glucose metabolism, 622
Gut, 696. *See also* Gastrointestinal tract
Gut-associated lymphoid tissue (GALT), 705

H

Halo device, 471, 471*f*, 471*t*, 472*t*
Hardiness, 4, 17
Harris-Benedict equation, 492, 500, 500*t*
Haustral churning, 700
Hb. *See* Hemoglobin
Hb A₁c. *See* Glycosylated hemoglobin
HCO₃. *See* Bicarbonate
Hct. *See* Hematocrit
HDL. *See* High-density lipoprotein
Head halter, 172, 172*f*
Head injury, closed. *See* Closed-head injury
Heart and heart-lung transplantation
    history, 609
    indications, 609, 609*t*
    organ function evaluation, 611
    postoperative management, 610–611
    posttransplantation biopsy, 611, 611*f*
    recipient preparation, 610, 610*f*
Heart biopsy, 611, 611*f*
Heart failure (HF)
    assessment and diagnosis, 334
    cachexia in, 507
    causes, 334, 334*t*
    classes, 333
    clinical manifestations, 333, 377
    collaborative management, 334, 336, 381
    definition, 325, 333
    diastolic dysfunction, 333
    end-stage, 337, 338*t*
    evidence-based practice, 337*t*
    multisystem effects, 335*f*
    nursing management, 336–337
    nutritional/metabolic alterations in, 507

Heart failure (HF)—(continued)
  pulmonary artery diastolic pressure in, 253
  pulmonary edema in
    vs. acute respiratory distress syndrome, 135
    pathogenesis, 136
  right atrial pressure in, 249
  systolic dysfunction, 333
Heart murmurs, 331, 331t. *See also* Valvular heart
  disease
Heart rate (HR)
  assessment, 230
  cardiac output and, 221
  factors affecting, 225
  measurement on ECG, 271, 271f
  in mitral stenosis, 328
Heart valves, 326–327, 327f. *See also* Valvular heart
  disease
Helicobacter pylori, 713–714, 714f
Hematemesis, 696, 711
Hematochezia, 696, 711
Hematocrit (Hct)
  causes of abnormal results, 523t, 528
  definition, 528
  in gastrointestinal bleeding, 706–707, 707t
  reference values, 523t
Hematologic dysfunction.
  nursing assessment, 549
  nursing history, 548–549
  nursing plan of care, 549–550
Hemianopia, 428
Hemineglect syndrome, 442
Hemiparesis, 428
Hemiparetic posture, 438f, 439
Hemiplegia, 428
Hemodialysis. *See* Dialysis
Hemodynamic monitoring. *See also specific*
    parameters
  data interpretation, 243
  educational resources, 243t
  equipment, 242, 242f
  nursing care of patient requiring, 347–348
  patient positioning, 243
  provider competency, 243
  readings at end expiration, 244
Hemodynamic parameters, 239. *See also specific*
    parameters
Hemoglobin (Hgb)
  capillary saturation. *See* Pulse oximetry
  characteristics, 524
  evaluation, 528
    in anemia, 528t
    causes of abnormal results, 523t
    interpretation, 111t
    normal values, 110, 114t
    reference values, 523t
  functions, 110
  in gastrointestinal bleeding, 706–707, 707t
  in oxygen delivery, 359
  oxygen saturation. *See* Oxyhemoglobin
    dissociation curve
  structure, 110
Hemolytic anemia
  categories
    immune disorders, 532
    infectious agents, 532

    microangiopathic, 533
    physical agents, 533
  definition, 520
Hemopneumothorax, 129, 151
Hemoptysis, 81, 106
Hemorrhage
  anemia caused by, 533
  posttransplantation, 603
Hemorrhagic stroke. *See also* Stroke
  characteristics, 429, 430t
  during thrombolytic therapy, 315
Hemostasis
  definition, 520
  disorders. *See* Disseminated intravascular
    coagulation; Thrombocytopenia
  platelets and, 526
Hemothorax, 129, 151, 869
Henry's law, 89
Heparin
  for acute coronary syndromes, 313
  for DVT prophylaxis in stroke, 438
  for ischemic stroke, 436
  for pulmonary embolism, 147t
Heparin-induced thrombocytopenia (HIT), 544
Hepatic coma. *See* Hepatic encephalopathy
Hepatic encephalopathy
  contributing factors, 748
  definition, 736
  management, 751
  precipitating factors, 751t
  stages, 747, 747t
Hepatic failure
  causes, 745–746
  clinical manifestations, 746–747, 747t
  as complication of chronic liver disease, 746
  complications, 748t
    esophageal varices, 748–749
    hepatic encephalopathy. *See* Hepatic
      encephalopathy
    hepatorenal syndrome, 749, 749t
    portal hypertension. *See* Portal hypertension
    sepsis, 749
    spontaneous bacterial peritonitis, 749
  definition, 736
  management, 750–752, 751t, 752t
  in multiple organ failure, 746
  nursing considerations
    general goals, 754
    nursing assessment, 755–756
    nursing care plan, 756
    nursing history, 755
  nutritional/metabolic alterations, 505, 747
  as primary disease, 746, 746t
Hepatitis
  clinical manifestations, 745, 745t
  epidemiology, 744
  medical management, 750, 750t
  pathophysiology, 744
  types, 744
Hepatitis B. *See also* Hepatitis
  at-risk populations, 744t
  epidemiology, 744t
Hepatorenal syndrome (HRS), 736, 749, 749t
Herniation
  after closed-head injury, 456, 456f

  definition, 404
  syndromes, 409t, 410f
Herniation picture, 597
Heterograft
  definition, 587, 590, 821
  uses, 590
HF. *See* Heart failure
Hgb. *See* Hemoglobin
HHS. *See* Hyperglycemic hyperosmolar state
High-acuity patients
  educational needs, 12–13, 12t
  nurses' values and care of, 19–20, 20f
  resource allocations for, 17–18
  technology and caring interface, 15–16
High-acuity unit. *See also* Intensive care unit (ICU)
  nurses' stress factors, 16–17, 16t
  resource allocations and, 17–18
High-density lipoprotein (HDL), 301, 304
Highly active retroviral therapy, 578
Histamine receptor antagonists, 715, 721t
Histocompatibility
  antigens. *See* Human leukocyte antigens
  definition, 587, 598–599
HIT. *See* Heparin-induced thrombocytopenia
HIV. *See* Human immunodeficiency virus (HIV)
  disease
HLA. *See* Human leukocyte antigens
Homeostasis, 650
Homograft, 821
Hormone-sensitive lipase, 621
Hormones, small intestine, 698–699, 699t
HR. *See* Heart rate
HRS. *See* Hepatorenal syndrome
Human immunodeficiency virus (HIV) disease.
    See also Acquired immunodeficiency disease
    syndrome
  cellular manifestations, 574
  in children, 577
  epidemiology, 575
  fetal transmission, 577
  incubation period, 577
  occupational exposure prophylaxis, 578
  opportunistic infections, 578
  phases, 576, 576t
  screening, 576–577
  treatment, 577–578
  viral invasion, 575, 575f
  in women, 577
Human leukocyte antigens (HLA)
  characteristics, 561
  class I, 599
  class II, 599
  definition, 556, 587
  donor-recipient compatibility, 599
Humoral immunity
  definition, 556
  mechanisms, 565–566
  response patterns, 566, 567f
Hyalinization, 621
Hydrocephalus, 404, 410
Hydrochloric acid, 696, 698
Hydrocolloid dressings, 805t
Hydromorphone
  in acute pancreatitis, 775
  equianalgesic doses, 42t

Hyperacute rejection, 588, 603. *See also* Rejection
Hyperbaric oxygen therapy, 800
Hypercalcemia
  during cancer treatment, 541
  clinical manifestations, 70, 70*f*
  definition, 69
  pathophysiology, 69–70
Hypercatabolism, 492, 502, 503
Hyperchloremia, 68, 68*t*
Hypercholesterolemia
  definition, 301
  stroke risk and, 432
Hypercoagulability, 144
Hyperemia, 404, 406
Hyperextension injury, spinal cord, 464, 465*f*
Hyperglycemia
  definition, 622, 628
  in hepatic failure, 505
  in metabolic stress response, 503–504
  pathophysiology, 631
Hyperglycemic hyperosmolar state (HHS)
  clinical presentation, 636
  definition, 622, 635
  vs. diabetic ketoacidosis, 636*t*
  medical interventions, 636, 637*f*
  pathophysiology, 635–636
Hyperkalemia
  in acute renal failure, 661, 668
  clinical manifestations, 72*f*
  definition, 71, 650
  pathophysiology, 71
Hyperlipidemia, 219, 230
Hypermagnesemia
  in acute renal failure, 662
  clinical manifestations, 73*t*
  definition, 72
  pathophysiology, 72
Hypermetabolism
  characteristics, 503
  in closed-head injury, 508
  definition, 492, 502
  vs. starvation, 504*t*
Hypernatremia
  in acute renal failure, 661, 668
  clinical manifestations, 67, 67*t*
  definition, 67
  pathophysiology, 67
Hyperphosphatemia
  in acute renal failure, 662
  clinical manifestations, 74*t*
  definition, 74
  pathophysiology, 74*t*
Hyperreflexion injury, spinal cord, 464, 465*f*
Hypersensitivity reactions
  anaphylaxis, 569
  chemotherapy and, 542
  definition, 556
  type I, 568–569, 568*f*
  type II, 569–570
  type III, 570–571
  type IV, 571
Hypertension
  assessment and diagnosis, 340
  causes, 339
  classification, 339*t*

collaborative management, 340
  definition, 650
  intra-abdominal. *See* Intra-abdominal
    hypertension
  intracranial. *See* Intracranial pressure
  in kidney transplant patient, 609
  nursing management, 340
  pulmonary. *See* Pulmonary hypertension
  risk factors, 339*t*
  stroke risk and, 432
Hypertonic, 55, 65
Hypertonic solutions
  characteristics, 65*f*, 65*t*
  for fluid volume imbalances, 65
  in head injury, 454
Hypertrophic cardiomyopathy, 325, 337, 338*t*
Hyperventilation
  central neurogenic, 414
  respiratory alkalosis and, 101–102, 102*t*
Hypervolemia
  in acute renal failure, 661
  case study, 348–352
  definition, 55, 650
  nursing assessment, 64, 64*t*
  nursing interventions, 64
  pathophysiology, 61, 61*t*
Hypocalcemia
  in acute renal failure, 662
  clinical manifestations, 70, 70*f*
  definition, 70
  pathophysiology, 70
Hypochloremia, 68, 68*t*
Hypochromic, 520, 528
Hypoglycemia
  causes, 629
  definition, 622, 629
  in hepatic failure, 751
Hypoglycemic coma
  catecholamine effects, 629–630
  central nervous system effects, 629
  clinical presentation, 629
  medical interventions, 630
  in older patients, 630
  rapid onset, 630
  slow onset, 630
Hypokalemia, 71, 72*f*
Hypokinesis, 301, 311
Hypomagnesemia, 73, 73*f*
Hypometabolism, 502
Hyponatremia, 67, 67*t*
Hypophosphatemia
  clinical manifestations, 74*t*
  definition, 74
  pathophysiology, 74*t*
  in refeeding syndrome, 504
Hypotension
  definition, 650
  orthostatic, after spinal cord injury, 477
  in pregnancy, 859
  stroke risk and, 432
  in traumatic injury, 872–873
Hypothalamus, 58–59
Hypotonic, 55, 64
Hypotonic solutions
  characteristics, 65*f*, 65*t*
  for fluid volume imbalances, 64

Hypoventilation, respiratory acidosis and,
  101, 101*t*
Hypovolemia
  case study, 344
  definition, 55
  nursing assessment, 63, 63*f*
  nursing interventions, 64
  pathophysiology, 61, 61*f*
  right atrial pressure in, 250
Hypovolemic shock states
  in burn injury, 822, 829–830
  clinical manifestations, 376
  etiology, 371–372, 371*t*
  in pancreatitis, 773
  pathophysiology, 371, 371*t*
  treatment, 379–380
Hypoxemia
  cytopathic, 385, 388
  definition, 355, 362
  as indication for mechanical ventilation,
    169, 170*t*
  PaO_2 levels in, 111
Hypoxia
  definition, 355, 362
  in multiple organ dysfunction syndrome, 388

I

IAH. *See* Intra-abdominal hypertension
IC. *See* Inspiratory capacity
ICD. *See* Implantable cardioverter/defibrillator
ICF. *See* Intracellular fluid
ICH. *See* Intracerebral hematoma
ICU. *See* Intensive care unit
Ideal alveolar gas equation, 121, 121*t*
Ideational apraxia, 442, 442*t*
Ideomotor apraxia, 442, 442*t*
Idiopathic thrombocytopenic purpura (ITP), 544
IE. *See* Infective endocarditis
IF. *See* Intrinsic factor
Ig. *See* Immunoglobulin(s)
Ileus. *See* Paralytic ileus
Imagery, in acute illness, 9
Imatinib mesylate, for chronic leukemia, 539
IMC. *See* Intermediate care unit
Immune system
  aging effects, 572
  cells, 564–565, 564*f*
  characteristics, 560
  organs and tissues, 558–559, 558*f*
  response to antigens, 562–563, 562*f*
  stress and, 573
  trauma and, 573
  types, 560, 560*t*
Immunity
  definition, 556, 560
  mechanisms
    nonspecific, 567
    specific, 565–566, 566*t*
  types, 560*t*
Immunocompromised patient
  nursing assessment, 579
    evidence-based practice, 579–580*t*
    laboratory findings, 580
    nursing history, 579

Immunocompromised patient—(continued)
  nursing management
    collaborative interventions, 580
    nursing interventions, 580–581
Immunodeficiency. See also Human
    immunodeficiency virus (HIV) disease;
    Immunocompromised patient
  primary, 557, 574
  secondary, 557, 574
Immunodeficiency state, 556, 574
Immunogenicity, 557, 561
Immunoglobulin A (Ig A), 566
Immunoglobulin G (IgG), 566
Immunoglobulin M (Ig M), 566
Immunoglobulin(s) (Ig)
  classes, 566, 566t
  definition, 557
  hypersensitivity. See Hypersensitivity reactions
Immunosuppressants
  complications
    infections, 603–604, 604f
    malignancy, 604
    organ dysfunction, 604
    steroid-induced, 606
  definition, 588
  history of development, 589
  types
    antibodies, 606–607
    corticosteroids, 606
    cyclosporine, 605–606
    cytotoxic agents, 606
    macrolide antibiotics, 607
Impaled objects, 855. See also Penetrating trauma
Implantable cardioverter/defibrillator (ICD),
  294–295
Imuran. See Azathioprine
IMV. See Intermittent mandatory ventilation
Incomplete spinal cord injury, 461, 464, 464t. See
  also Spinal cord injury
Indirect bilirubin, 742, 742t
Indirect calorimetry, 492, 500
Induction chemotherapy, for leukemia, 538
Infarction, 622
Infection
  diabetes and, 644, 688
  posttransplantation, 603–604, 604f
  wound, 802–803
Infection control, in severe acute respiratory
  distress syndrome, 150
Infective endocarditis (IE)
  causes, 330
  definition, 325
  pathophysiology, 330
  risk factors, 330–331
  treatment, 331
Inflammation
  physiology, 796f
  uncontrolled systemic, 388
  in wound infection, 802
Inflammatory bowel disease, 718
Inflammatory phase. See Wound healing
Inflammatory response, 386, 796f
Inhalation injury, 831–832, 831t. See also Burn
  injury
Inhaled nitric oxide (iNO), for acute respiratory
  distress syndrome, 141

Injury
  abdominal. See Abdominal injury
  assessment
    diagnostic tests, 884
    primary survey, 861–862, 882–883
      airway and cervical spine, 862
      breathing, 863
      circulation, 863
      disability, 863
      exposure, 863
    secondary survey, 864t, 865
  from blunt trauma, 854
  case study, 882–885
  causes, 852
  chest. See Chest injury
  complications
    acute renal failure, 876
    acute respiratory distress syndrome, 876
    assessment, 876–877
    disseminated intravascular coagulation, 876
    nursing diagnoses, 877
    risks for, 875, 875t
    sepsis, 876, 876t
    undernutrition, 875–876
  evidence-based practice, 874
  exsanguination from, 866
  head. See Closed-head injury
  immune system effects, 573
  mechanisms, 852, 857–858, 857t, 858f. See also
    Blunt trauma; Penetrating trauma
  metabolic response, 875–876, 875t
  mortality pattern, 865–866
  nursing assessment, 873
  nursing diagnoses, 872–873
  nursing responsibilities, 874
  patterns, 857t
  pelvic, 871
  from penetrating trauma, 856
  response mediators
    age, 860
    comorbidities, 858–859
    pregnancy, 859–860
    substance abuse, 859
  resuscitation, 865–867, 867t
  risk factors
    age, 852
    alcohol, 853
    gender, 852
    race, income, geography, 853
  shock and, 866
  spinal cord. See Spinal cord injury
Innate immunity, 557, 560
iNO. See Inhaled nitric oxide
Inotropes, 219, 224
Inspiratory capacity (IC), 108, 109f
Insulin
  carbohydrate metabolism and, 623, 625
  characteristics, 622
  deficit, consequences of, 625–627, 625t, 626f. See
    also Diabetic ketoacidosis
  definition, 622
  fat metabolism and, 624, 625–626
  fluid/electrolyte balance and, 626–627
  functions, 622
  glucose metabolism and, 622–624
  liver and, 623–624

  muscle tissue and, 624
  protein metabolism and, 624, 626
Insulin-dependent cells, 622
Insulin therapy
  continuous low-dose intravenous infusion,
    639–640
  evidence-based practice, 638t
  factors affecting dosage, 638t
  intensive, 640, 641t
  side effects, 639
  sliding-scale administration, 640, 640t
  Somogyi effect, 640–641, 641f
  sources, 638
  types, 638–639, 639f, 639t
Integra artificial skin, 841, 841f
Intensive care unit (ICU). See also High-acuity
  unit
  levels of care, 5, 6t, 7f
  nursing staffing issues, 14–15
  prioritization model, 5, 5t
  reasons for development, 5
  transfer anxiety, 13
  visitation policies, 13–14
Interferons, 557, 567
Interleukin 2, cardiac toxicity, 539
Interleukins, 557, 565
Intermediate care unit (IMC), 5
Intermittent mandatory ventilation (IMV)
  characteristics, 178
  definition, 166
  for ventilator weaning, 198–199, 198t
Internal respiration, 81, 88, 88f. See also
  Respiration
International normalized ratio (INR), 742
Interstitial fluid pressure, 58
Intestinal strangulation, 696, 723
Intestine transplantation
  history, 613–614
  indications, 609t, 614
  organ function evaluation, 614
  postoperative management, 614
  recipient preparation, 614
  types, 614
Intima, 302, 303f
Intra-abdominal hypertension (IAH)
  vs. abdominal compartment syndrome, 725
  causes, 725
  complications, 728
  multisystem effects, 725–726, 726t
  nursing implications, 728
  pressure measurement, 726–727, 727f
  risk factors, 725
  treatment, 727–728
Intra-aortic balloon pump (IABP), for cardiogenic
  shock, 381
Intracellular, 55
Intracellular fluid (ICF), 56
Intracerebral hematoma (ICH)
  characteristics, 452, 452f
  clinical manifestations, 452
  definition, 449
  medical management, 452
Intracranial hemorrhage. See also Stroke
  characteristics, 429, 430t
  during thrombolytic therapy, 315

Intracranial hypertension, 404, 409. *See also* Intracranial pressure, elevated
Intracranial pressure (ICP)
    components
        brain volume, 407
        cerebral blood volume, 407, 407*t*
        cerebrospinal fluid, 408
    definition, 404
    elevated
        causes
            increased brain volume, 409, 410*t*
            increased cerebral blood volume, 409, 410*t*
            increased cerebrospinal fluid, 410, 410*t*
            herniation caused by, 409, 409*t*, 410*f*
        management
            optimization of cerebral oxygenation, 420–421
            optimization of cerebral perfusion pressure, 420–421
            pharmacologic therapy, 421–422
            ventilation support, 420–421
    in mechanical ventilation, 187
    monitoring
        devices, 416–417, 416*f*, 423*t*
        evidence-based practice, 418*t*
        indications, 415–416
        jugular bulb oximetry, 417–418
        nursing care, 422–423, 423*t*
        sites, 416*t*
        waveform patterns, 417, 417*f*
    Monro-Kellie hypothesis, 404, 407
    normal values, 408
    physiology, 408
Intraparenchymal catheter, 416*t*, 417
Intrapulmonary shunt (Qs/Qt), 364
Intrathecal, 25, 38
Intravascular, 55, 56
Intravenous immune globulin (IVIG), 544
Intravenous pyelogram (IVP), 666
Intraventricular catheter, 416, 416*f*, 416*t*
Intrinsic factor (IF)
    definition, 696
    gastric functions, 698
    loss of, 531
Intrinsic factor (IF)–cobalamin complex, 531
Intrinsic renal failure, 650. *See also* Acute renal failure
Iron, liver storage, 739
Iron-deficiency anemia, 531
Iron lung, 173–174
Ischemic bowel disease, 717–718, 717*f*, 729*t*
Ischemic stroke, 429, 430*t*. *See also* Stroke
Isoelectric, 265
Isoenzymes
    definition, 736
    in liver dysfunction, 741, 741*t*
Isograft, 588
Isosthenuria, 677
Isotonic, 55, 64
Isotonic solutions
    characteristics, 65*f*, 65*t*
    for fluid volume imbalances, 64
ITP. *See* Idiopathic thrombocytopenic purpura
IVIG. *See* Intravenous immune globulin
IVP. *See* Intravenous pyelogram

J

Jaundice
    definition, 736, 742
    in hepatitis, 745
Jugular bulb oximetry
    calculations, 417–418
    nursing care, 422–423, 423*t*
    procedure, 418
Jugular venous distention, 228, 228*f*
Junctional rhythm, 279, 279*f*, 279*t*
Junctional tachycardia, 279, 279*t*

K

K. *See* Potassium
Kallikrein, 762, 767
Ketone bodies, 503
Ketonuria, 622
Ketosis, 622
Kidney(s)
    anatomy, 651–652, 651*f*, 652*f*
    failure. *See* Acute renal failure; Chronic renal failure
    function
        aging effects, 652
        cardiovascular influences, 654
        compensatory mechanisms, 654, 654*f*
        endocrine system influences, 654
        nervous system influences, 654
    physiology, 652, 653*f*
    transplantation. *See* Renal transplantation
Kupffer's cells, 736, 739
Kussmaul breathing, 632
Kwashiorkor
    causes, 502–503
    definition, 492
    symptoms, 503

L

Laceration, 794
Lactate levels, increased, 364, 376
Lactic acidosis, 102, 102*t*
Lactic dehydrogenase (LDH)
    in gastrointestinal dysfunction, 706
    in liver dysfunction, 741, 741*t*
Lactulose, for hepatic encephalopathy, 751
Lacunar infarcts, 429
LAD. *See* Left anterior descending artery
Large intestine, 697*f*, 699–700. *See also* Gastrointestinal tract
Lasix. *See* Furosemide
Latency period, 576
Lateral transtentorial herniation, 409*t*, 410*f*
LCX. *See* Left circumflex artery
LDH. *See* Lactic dehydrogenase
LDL. *See* Low-density lipoprotein
Left anterior descending artery (LAD)
    anatomy, 306, 306*f*
    ECG leads, 310*t*
Left circumflex artery (LCX)
    anatomy, 306, 306*f*
    ECG leads, 310*t*
Left main coronary artery (LMCA), 306
Left ventricular assist device (LVAD), 381

Left ventricular failure, 377. *See also* Heart failure
Left ventricular stroke work index (LVSWI)
    calculation, 259–260
    low, 260
    normal values, 239, 260
    in ventricular function curve, 260*f*
Leukemia
    causes, 536
    classification, 538*t*
    clinical manifestations, 537–538, 537*t*
    diagnosis, 538
    pathophysiology, 535–536
    treatment, 538–539
    types
        acute lymphocytic, 536
        acute myelogenous, 536
        chronic lymphocytic, 536–537
        chronic myelogenous, 537
Leukocytes. *See* White blood cells
Leukostasis, 538
Linear skull fracture, 450. *See also* Closed-head injury (CHI)
Lipase
    definition, 762
    functions, 765*t*
    in pancreatitis, 768, 768*t*
Lipids, 494, 494*t*
Lipogenesis, 494, 622, 625
Lipolysis, 622, 625
Lipolytic, 762
Lipoproteins, 301
Liquid ventilation, 141
Liver
    anatomy, 737–738, 737*f*, 738*f*
    failure. *See* Hepatic failure
    functions, 740*t*
        blood clotting factors, 739
        blood filter, 739
        blood volume reservoir, 739
        drug metabolism and detoxification, 740
        metabolic, 505, 623–624, 739
    injury, 870
    laboratory tests
        coagulation studies, 742
        serum albumin, 743
        serum ammonia, 743
        serum enzymes, 740–741, 741*t*
Liver failure. *See* Hepatic failure
Liver flap, 755
Liver transplantation
    alternative approaches, 612
    history, 611
    indications, 611
    organ function evaluation, 612
    postoperative management, 612
    recipient preparation, 611–612
LMCA. *See* Left main coronary artery
Lobule, liver, 736, 737, 737*f*, 738*f*
Loop diuretics
    common, 332*t*
    for heart failure, 334
Low-density lipoprotein (LDL)
    classification of values, 304*t*
    definition, 301, 304
    reduction, 305, 305*t*
LP. *See* Lumbar puncture

Lumbar puncture (LP), 418–419
Lumbar spine injury, 465. *See also* Spinal cord injury
Lund and Browder chart, 826*f*
Lung
  collapsed, 152. *See also* Chest drainage
  testing. *See* Pulmonary function evaluation
Lung transplantation
  history, 609
  indications, 609, 609*t*
  organ function evaluation, 611
  postoperative management, 610–611
  posttransplantation biopsy, 611
  recipient preparation, 610
LVAD. *See* Left ventricular assist device
LVSWI. *See* Left ventricular stroke work index
Lymph system, 558*f*, 559
Lymphatics, obstruction, 60–61
Lymphocytes, 523*t*
Lymphokines, 557, 565

M

mAb. *See* Monoclonal antibodies
Maceration, 794, 807
Macroangiopathy, 622, 643. *See also* Atherosclerosis
Macrocytic, 520, 528
Macrolide antibiotics, posttransplantation, 607
Macronutrients, 492, 493
Macrophages
  definition, 520, 557
  functions, 525, 565
Macrovascular disease, diabetic, 643. *See also* Atherosclerosis
Mafenide acetate, 839*t*
Magnesium (Mg)
  functions, 72
  imbalances, 72–73, 73*t*
  normal ranges and critical abnormal values, 66*t*
Magnet hospital program, 15
Magnetic resonance angiography (MRA), 418–419
Magnetic resonance cholangiopancreatography (MRCP), 762, 769
Magnetic resonance imaging (MRI)
  in gastrointestinal dysfunction, 708
  in neurological assessment, 418
  nursing responsibilities, 232
  in spinal cord injury, 467
Maintenance chemotherapy, for leukemia, 538–539
Major histocompatibility complex (MHC), 557, 561. *See also* Human leukocyte antigens
Mallory-Weiss tears, 715, 722
Malnutrition
  definition, 492, 502
  in hospitalized patients, 502
  immune system effects, 572
Mandatory minute ventilation (MMV), 198*t*, 199
Mannitol, for increased intracranial pressure, 421
MAP. *See* Mean arterial pressure
Marasmus, 492, 502
Margination, 520, 525
MARS. *See* Mixed antagonistic response syndrome
Mast cells, 557, 569
Maximum inspiratory force (MIF). *See* Negative inspiratory force
McGill Pain Questionnaire (MPQ), 33
MCH. *See* Mean corpuscular hemoglobin (MCH)

MCHC. *See* Mean corpuscular hemoglobin concentration (MCHC)
MDF. *See* Myocardial depressant factor
Mean arterial pressure (MAP). *See also* Systemic arterial pressure
  calculation, 93, 258
  definition, 238
  normal values, 93, 239, 256
Mean corpuscular hemoglobin concentration (MCHC)
  causes of abnormal results, 523*t*
  definition, 520, 527*t*, 528
  reference values, 523*t*
Mean corpuscular hemoglobin (MCH)
  causes of abnormal results, 523*t*
  definition, 520, 527*t*, 528
  reference values, 523*t*
Mean corpuscular volume (MCV)
  causes of abnormal results, 523*t*
  definition, 520, 527*t*, 528
  descriptions, 527*t*
  reference values, 523*t*
Mechanical debridement, 794, 804
Mechanical ventilation. *See also* Ventilator(s)
  in acute respiratory distress syndrome, 139, 140*t*
  artificial airway complications
    cuff trauma, 188–189, 189*f*
    nasal damage, 188
  case study, 213–215
  complications
    cardiovascular, 185
    gastrointestinal, 187
    neurovascular, 187
    pulmonary
      altered ventilation and perfusion, 185–186
      barotrauma/volutrauma, 186
      nosocomial infection, 186
      oxygen toxicity, 186
    renal, 187
  equipment
    endotracheal tubes, 170–171, 171*f*, 171*t*
    securing airway, 172, 172*f*
    supportive, 172–173
    tracheostomy, 171–172
  indications
    acute ventilatory failure, 169
    critical values, 170*t*, 214
    hypoxemia, 169
    pulmonary mechanics, 169
    special considerations in elderly patients, 169
  in injured patient, 862
  intragastric tube feeding and, 511
  multisystem effects, 185*t*, 193*t*
  nursing management of physiologic needs
    airway protection, 192
    alteration in cardiac output, 192–193, 193*t*
    alteration in nutrition, 193
    impaired gas exchange, 192
    ineffective airway clearance, 190–191
      excessive secretions, 191
      pooled secretions, 191–192
      thick secretions, 191
    ineffective breathing patterns, 192
  nursing management of psychosocial needs
    anxiety and pain, 193–194
    communication and sensation, 194
    evidence-based practice, 190*t*

    family support, 194
    sleep pattern disturbance, 194
  patient care goals, 190
  postintubation assessment, 173
  special considerations in the elderly, 199
  weaning
    definition, 195
    determination of patient readiness, 195, 196*t*, 197
    methods
      manual weaning/spontaneous breathing trial, 197–198
      ventilator weaning, 198–199, 198*t*
    patient categories, 195
    postextubation follow-up, 199
    rapid, 197, 197*f*
    slow, 197
Media, 302, 303*f*
Mediators, 385, 386
Medicare, organ transplantation conditions, 591
Megaloblastic anemias, 531–532
Melena, 696, 711
Membrane permeability, in cardiac cells, 266–267, 267*f*
Meperidine
  in acute pancreatitis, 774–775
  equianalgesic doses, 42*t*
  in patients with concurrent medical disorders, 44
Mesenteric circulation, 696, 700, 700*f*, 700*t*
Mesentery, 696, 698
Metabolic acidosis. *See also* Acid–base disturbances; Arterial blood gases
  in acute renal failure, 662
  acute vs. chronic, 102*t*
  anion gap in, 632
  causes, 102
  definition, 102, 622
  in diabetic ketoacidosis, 635
  in hepatic failure, 751
  in hyperglycemia, 631–632
Metabolic acids. *See* Nonvolatile acids
Metabolic alkalosis. *See also* Acid–base disturbances; Arterial blood gases
  acute vs. chronic, 103*t*
  causes, 103
  definition, 102
Metabolic stress response
  definition, 492
  ebb phase, 503
  flow phase, 503–504
Metabolism. *See also* Nutrition
  aerobic. *See* Aerobic metabolism
  alterations
    after burn injury, 835
    gastrointestinal tract, 502
    in hepatic failure, 747
    metabolic stress response
      ebb phase, 503, 875, 875*t*
      flow phase, 503–504, 875, 875*t*
      hypermetabolism, 503, 504*t*
    nutritional, 502
      malnutrition, 502
      starvation, 502–503, 504*t*
    refeeding syndrome, 504
    after traumatic injury, 875–876
  anaerobic. *See* Anaerobic metabolism
  assessment

energy expenditure, 500–501, 500t
oxygen consumption, 499–501, 501t
insulin and, 623–624
Methylprednisolone, for spinal cord injury, 472
Metolazone, for heart failure, 334
Metronidazole, for hepatic encephalopathy, 751
Mexican Americans, pain expression, 44t
Mg. See Magnesium
Microangiopathy, 622
Microcytic, 520, 528
Micronutrients, 492, 493
Microvascular disease, 622, 643
Microvilli, 696, 698
Mild traumatic brain injury (MTBI). See
    Concussion
Milliosmoles (mOsm), 57
Milrinone, for shock, 378
Minute ventilation. See V̇E
Misoprostol, for gastrointestinal bleeding,
    715, 721t
Mitral regurgitation (MR)
    assessment and diagnosis, 331–332, 331t
    collaborative management, 332
    definition, 325
    nursing management, 332–333
    pathophysiology, 329, 329f
    risk factors, 328t
Mitral stenosis (MS)
    assessment and diagnosis, 331–332, 331t
    collaborative management, 332
    definition, 325
    nursing management, 332–333
    pathophysiology, 327–328, 328f
    risk factors, 328t
Mitral valve prolapse, 325, 329–330, 330f
Mixed acid–base disorders. See also Acid–base
    disturbances
    clinical problems associated with, 116, 116t
    comparison, 117t
    identification
        expected compensatory response, 117–118
        initial recognition, 116
        systemic evaluation, 116, 117t
Mixed antagonistic response syndrome (MARS),
    387
Mixed venous oxygen saturation (Svo₂)
    for assessment of oxygen consumption, 365, 366f
    decreased, 366t
    increased, 366t
MMF. See Mycophenolate mofetil
MMV. See Mandatory minute ventilation
Mobitz type I heart block, 285, 286f, 287t
Mobitz type II heart block, 285, 286f, 287t
Modifiable risk factors, 301, 304
MODS. See Multiple organ dysfunction syndrome
    (MODS)
Monoclonal antibodies (mAb)
    definition, 588
    posttransplantation, 606–607
Monocyte-macrophage system. See
    Reticuloendothelial system
Monocytes
    causes of abnormal results, 523t, 529
    evaluation, 529
    functions, 525
    reference values, 523t
Monro-Kellie hypothesis, 404, 407

Morphine
    for acute coronary syndromes, 313
    equianalgesic doses, 42t
mOsm. See Milliosmoles
Motor apraxia, 442, 442t
Motor assessment, in spinal cord injury, 467, 468f
MPI. See Myocardial perfusion imaging (MPI)
MPQ. See McGill Pain Questionnaire
MR. See Mitral regurgitation
MRA. See Magnetic resonance angiography
MRCP. See Magnetic resonance
    cholangiopancreatography
MRI. See Magnetic resonance imaging
MS. See Mitral stenosis
Mucomyst. See N-acetylcysteine
Mucosa
    definition, 696
    gastrointestinal, 495, 698, 698f
Multiple organ dysfunction syndrome (MODS).
    See also Systemic inflammatory response
    syndrome
    case study, 395–400
    characteristics, 388
    definition, 385
    evidence-based practice, 391
    nursing management, 391, 399–400
    in older adults, 388t
    organ involvement and failure, 389–390
    pathologic changes
        microvascular coagulopathy, 389
        systemic inflammation, 388
        tissue hypoxia, 388
        unregulated apoptosis, 389
    pathways, 388
    primary, 385, 388
    secondary, 385, 388
Murmurs, 229, 229t
Muromonab-CD3 (OKT3), posttransplantation,
    606
Muscle tissue, glucose metabolism and, 624
Muscularis externa, 696, 697, 698f
Muscularis propria, 495
Music therapy, 11t
Mycophenolate mofetil (MMF),
    posttransplantation, 606
Myocardial depressant factor (MDF)
    in burn injury, 829
    in pancreatitis, 773
Myocardial infarction. See Acute coronary
    syndromes
    non-ST elevation. See Non-ST elevation
        myocardial infarction
    ST elevation. See ST elevation myocardial
        infarction
Myocardial ischemia. See also Acute coronary
    syndromes
    case study, 348–352
    collaborative assessment
        cardiac markers, 310, 310t
        echocardiography, 311
        electrocardiogram, 309, 309f, 310t
        exercise stress test, 310–311
        myocardial perfusion imaging, 311
    physical assessment, 308
    signs and symptoms, 307–308, 307t
Myocardial perfusion imaging (MPI), 311

Myocardial tissue perfusion
    impaired. See Myocardial ischemia
    regulation of, 306
Myocardium, 310t
Myoglobin
    in burn injury, 835
    definition, 650, 821
    in rhabdomyolysis, 658
Myoglobinuria, 821, 835

N

N-acetylcysteine, 316
Na. See Sodium
NaHCO₃. See Bicarbonate; Sodium bicarbonate
Nasotracheal tube, 171, 172, 172f
National Institutes of Health (NIH), Stroke Scale,
    434t
National Organ Transplant Act, 591
Native Americans, pain expression, 44t
Natrecor. See Nesiritide
Natural immunity, 557, 560, 560t
Natural killer (NK) cells, 557
Negative inspiratory force (NIF)
    definition, 166
    as indication for mechanical ventilation,
        169, 170t
Negative pressure ventilators, 173–175, 174f
Neomycin, for hepatic encephalopathy, 751
Neovascularization, 794, 796
Nephron
    anatomy, 651, 652f
    definition, 650
    physiology, 652, 653f
Nephropathy, diabetic, 643
Nesiritide, for cardiomyopathy, 337
Neurogenic bladder, in acute stroke, 440–441, 441t
Neurogenic shock
    clinical manifestations, 376
    definition, 461
    pathophysiology, 371
    in spinal cord injury, 470
    treatment, 379
Neurological assessment. See Cerebral tissue
    perfusion, assessment
Neuromuscular blocking agents, for shock, 379
Neurontin. See Gabapentin
Neutropenia
    causes, 535
    clinical manifestations, 535
    definition, 520, 535
    enterocolitis and, 541–542
    grading scale, 535t
    nursing interventions, 581
    sepsis in, 541
    treatment, 535
Neutrophils
    characteristics, 524
    definition, 520
    evaluation, 529
        causes of abnormal results, 523t, 529
        reference values, 523t
    functions, 524–525, 525f
New York Heart Association (NYHA), heart failure
    classes, 333
NIF. See Negative inspiratory force

NIH. *See* National Institutes of Health
NIPPV. *See* Noninvasive intermittent positive
      pressure ventilation
Nipride. *See* Nitroprusside
Nitric oxide
      inhaled. *See* Inhaled nitric oxide
      inhibition in hypertension, 339
Nitrogen, 492
Nitrogen balance, 498–499, 499*t*
Nitroglycerin
      for acute coronary syndromes, 313
      for esophageal varices, 753
Nitroprusside, for afterload reduction, 256
NK cells. *See* Natural killer (NK) cells
Nociception, 25, 29
Nociceptor, 25, 29
Noise levels, in high-acuity units, 10–11
Non-*ST* elevation myocardial infarction
      (NSTEMI), 312. *See also* Acute coronary
      syndromes
Noncompensatory pause, 280
Noninvasive intermittent positive pressure
      ventilation (NIPPV)
      complications, 183
      contraindications, 183
      definition, 166, 182
      indications, 182–183
      masks/interfaces, 182
      mechanical ventilators, 182
      nursing considerations, 183–184
Nonmodifiable risk factors, 301, 304
Nonsteroidal anti-inflammatory drugs (NSAIDs)
      erosive gastritis and, 714–715
      glomerular effects, 657
      mechanism of action, 36
Nonverbal communication, 11
Nonvolatile acids, 81, 100
Norcuron. *See* Vecuronium
Normochromic, 520, 528
Normocytic, 520, 528
Noxious stimuli, 28
NRS. *See* Numeric rating scale
NSAIDs. *See* Nonsteroidal anti-inflammatory
      drugs
NSTEMI. *See* Non-*ST* elevation myocardial
      infarction
Nuchal rigidity, 428, 429
Numeric rating scale (NRS), 32, 32*f*
Numorphan. *See* Oxymorphone
Nurse(s)
      burnout in high-acuity units, 16–17, 16*t*
      personal value assessment, 19–20, 20*f*
Nursing staffing issues, in high-acuity units, 14–15
Nutrients
      definition, 492
      as energy source, 493–494, 494*t*
      as immune function support, 495
Nutrition. *See also* Metabolism
      altered. *See also* Metabolism, alterations
            in burns, 508
            in cardiac failure, 507
            in diabetic ketoacidosis, 634
            in gut failure, 507–508
            in hepatic failure, 505–506
            during mechanical ventilation, 193
            in pulmonary failure, 506

      in renal failure, 506–507, 668
      after spinal cord injury, 474
      after stroke, 440
      after traumatic brain injury, 508
      assessment
            anergy screen, 499
            history, 498
            laboratory data
                  albumin, 498
                  normal values, 499*t*
                  prealbumin, 498
                  transferrin, 498
            nitrogen balance, 498–499, 499*t*
            total lymphocyte count, 499
      definition, 492
      nutrients as energy source
            carbohydrates, 493, 494*t*
            lipids, 494, 494*t*
            proteins, 493–494, 494*t*
      nutrients as immune function support, 495
      wound healing and, 800
Nutritional support. *See also* Enteral nutrition;
      Total parenteral nutrition
      selection criteria
            baseline nutritional status, 510
            gastrointestinal function, 510
            present catabolic state and possible duration,
                  510–511
NYHA. *See* New York Heart Association
Nystagmus, 404, 414

O

Obesity, wound healing and, 801
Obstructive pulmonary disorders. *See* Pulmonary
      disorders, obstructive
Obstructive shock states
      clinical manifestations, 377
      etiology, 371*t*, 372–373
      pathophysiology, 371*t*
      treatment, 380
Octreotide, for gastrointestinal hemorrhage, 721*t*
Oculocephalic reflex, 413–414, 414*f*
Oculomotor responses, 413–414, 414*f*, 415*t*
Oculovestibular reflex, 414
Ogilvie's syndrome, 723
Ohm's law, 223
OKT3. *See* Muromonab-CD3
Older adults
      alveolar–arterial pressure gradient, 122
      burn injury risk, 822
      diffusion changes, 91
      fluid volume deficits, 64
      hypoglycemia in, 630
      immune system, 572
      mechanical ventilation issues, 169, 199
      multiple organ dysfunction syndrome
            risk, 388*t*
      pain management issues, 43
      renal function, 652
      resource allocations for, 18
      trauma effects, 852, 860
      ventilation changes, 87
      wound healing in, 800
Oligoanalgesia, 25, 40–41
Oliguria, 650, 660

Oncologic emergencies
      clinical manifestations, 540*t*
      hemorrhagic cystitis, 542
      hypercalcemia, 541
      hypersensitivity reactions, 542
      neutropenic enterocolitis, 541–542
      organ toxicity
            cardiac, 539
            liver, 540–541
            pulmonary, 539
      risk factors, 540*t*
      sepsis, 541
      spinal cord compression, 541
      superior vena cava syndrome, 541
      tumor lysis syndrome, 541
Open skull fracture, 450. *See also* Closed-head
      injury (CHI)
Opioids
      equianalgesic doses, 42*t*
      in older adults, 43
      in patients with concurrent medical disorders, 44
      pseudoaddiction, 25, 40
      street names, 48*t*
      withdrawal onset and manifestations, 48*t*
Opiophobia, 25, 41
Opsonins, 557, 567
OPTN. *See* Organ Procurement and
      Transplantation Network
Organ donor. *See* Donor
Organ Procurement and Transplantation Network
      (OPTN), 591
Organ recipient. *See* Recipient
Organ transplantation. *See* Transplantation
Orthopnea
      definition, 105, 325
      in heart failure, 334
Orthostatic hypotension, after spinal cord
      injury, 477
Osmolality
      in acute renal failure, 665
      definition, 55, 57
      formula, 57
Osmolarity, 57
Osmoreceptors, kidney function and, 654
Osmosis, 55, 57, 57*f*
Osmotic diuresis
      definition, 622
      in hyperglycemia, 632
      management, 633
OTC preparations. *See* Over-the-counter (OTC)
      preparations
Otorrhea
      definition, 404, 449
      in skull fracture, 451
Over-the-counter (OTC) preparations, in pain
      management, 43
Oxycodone, equianalgesic doses, 42*t*
Oxygen
      partial pressure
            alveolar. *See* P_{AO_2}
            arterial. *See* P_{aO_2}
            venous. *See* P_{vO_2}
            tension. *See* P_{O_2}
Oxygen consumption ($\dot{V}O_2$)
      assessment, 364–365
      brain, 508

decreasing, in shock, 379
definition, 355, 370
factors affecting, 361t, 362t, 499
Fick equation, 501, 501t
increased, S$v o_2$ pattern, 366f
measurement, 501, 501t
normal levels, 501t
physiology, 360–362
Oxygen delivery (DO$_2$)
assessment, 364
definition, 355
factors affecting, 359
physiology, 359, 360t
in shock states
increased, 374, 374f
optimization, 378–379
Oxygen extraction, 355, 361
Oxygen toxicity, 186
Oxygenation
assessment
evidence-based practice, 365t
oxygen consumption, 364–365
oxygen delivery, 364
pulmonary gas exchange, 363–364, 363t
failure
clinical manifestations, 133t
definition, 129, 133, 133t
pathophysiology, 133
impaired, 362–363
case study, 395–400
physiology, 356–357, 356f
status, 111, 111t. See also Arterial blood gases
wound healing and, 799–800, 808
Oxyhemoglobin dissociation curve
characteristics, 90–91, 91f
definition, 81, 90
shifts in, 91, 91f, 91t
Oxymorphone, equianalgesic doses, 42t

P

P$_{50}$, 91f
p24 antigen, in HIV infection, 576
P wave, 271–272
Pacemakers
classification, 294, 294t
components, 291
endocardial, 291, 291f
epicardial, 291, 291f
external, 291
failure to capture, 293, 294f
failure to sense, 292, 293f
programming, 291–293, 292f, 293f
Paclitaxel, cardiac toxicity, 539
Paco_2
definition, 89
in $\dot{V}Q$ ratio, 93–94
Paco_2
in acute respiratory failure, 133t
definition, 89, 110, 166
interpretation, 111t, 112f, 113f
in mixed acid–base disorders, 116–118, 117t
normal values, 110, 114t
in respiratory acidosis, 101, 101t
in respiratory alkalosis, 101–102, 101t

in restrictive and obstructive pulmonary
disorders, 131t
in ventilatory failure, 133t, 169
PAD pressure. See Pulmonary artery diastolic
(PAD) pressure
PAG. See Periaqueductal gray (PAG) areas
Pain. See also Acute pain
in burn injury, 833, 842
definition, 25–26, 28
effects on body, 30
during mechanical ventilation, 193–194
multifaceted model, 28–29
physiology
endogenous analgesia system, 27, 27t
pain nerve fibers, 27
pain transmission, 27
sensory receptors, 26, 26t
statis-related complications, 30
Pain behavior, 26, 29
Palpitations, 219, 227
Pancreas
anatomy, 762–763, 763f
enzymes, 765, 765t
exocrine functions, 764–765
Pancreas and pancreas-kidney transplantation
history, 612
indications, 609t, 612
organ function evaluation, 613
postoperative management, 612–613
recipient preparation, 612
surgical technique, 613f
types, 612
Pancreatitis
causes, 766, 767t
characteristics, 766, 766t
complications
local, 772
systemic, 772–773, 773t
definition, 762
diagnosis
laboratory tests, 768–769, 768t
procedures, 769
medical management
curative therapy, 775
evidence-based practice, 774t
supportive therapy, 774–775, 775t
mortality prediction, 769, 770t
nursing assessment, 770–772
nursing care plan
collaborative problems, 776
nausea and vomiting, 777
nursing diagnoses, 776–777
pain, 777
pathophysiology, 766–767
Pancuronium, for shock, 379
Pao_2
in alveolar-arterial pressure gradient, 121, 122t
calculation, 121, 121t
definition, 89
in $\dot{V}Q$ ratio, 93–94
Pao_2
in acute respiratory failure, 133t
in alveolar-arterial pressure gradient, 121, 122t
definition, 89, 110, 166
in hypoxemia, 111, 169
interpretation, 111t, 113f, 114f

normal values, 114t
in oxygenation failure, 133t
in oxyhemoglobin dissociation curve, 90–91, 91f
in restrictive pulmonary disorders, 130, 130t, 131t
Pao_2/Fio_2 ratio, 122, 123t, 364
PAP. See Peak airway pressure
PAR. See Pressure adjusted heart rate
Paralytic ileus
assessment, 723, 789
clinical manifestations, 723
management, 724, 790
nursing diagnoses, 729t
nursing interventions, 790
pathophysiology, 723
Paraplegia, 461, 464. See also Spinal cord injury
Parasympathetic nervous system, 463, 702, 702f
Parenteral nutrition, intradialytic, 507
Paresthesias, 428, 441
Parietal cells, 696, 698
Parietal pleura, 81, 86
Parkland formula, 830
Paroxysmal nocturnal dyspnea (PND)
clinical manifestations, 105
definition, 81
in heart failure, 334
Partial liquid ventilation, for acute respiratory
distress syndrome, 141
Partial pressures
atmosphere and alveoli, 89, 90f
carbon dioxide
alveolar. See Paco_2
arterial. See Paco_2
gastric. See Prco_2
venous. See Pvco_2
definition, 81, 89
gas distribution during diffusion and, 89, 89f
gradient. See Pressure gradient
oxygen
alveolar. See Pao_2
arterial. See Pao_2
venous. See Pvo_2
Partial seizure, 461, 479. See also Seizure(s)
Partial thromboplastin time (PTT), 736, 742
Partially compensated acid–base state
algorithms for determining, 112f, 113f
characteristics, 100t
definition, 81, 100
PAS pressure. See Pulmonary artery systolic (PAS)
pressure
Passive transport. See Diffusion
Pathogens, 557, 561
Patient care areas
intensive care unit. See Intensive care unit
intermediate care unit, 5
Patient-controlled analgesia (PCA), 37
Pavulon. See Pancuronium
PAWP. See Pulmonary artery wedge pressure
Pbto_2. See Cerebral tissue oxygen content
PCA. See Patient-controlled analgesia
PCI. See Percutaneous coronary intervention
Pco_2, 89
PCP. See Pneumocystis carinii pneumonia
Peak airway pressure (PAP)
definition, 166
in mechanical ventilation, 180
normal values, 239

PEEP. *See* Positive end expiratory pressure
Pelvic injury, 871
Penetrating trauma
    characteristics, 852
    definition, 851
    forces associated with, 855
    high-energy missiles, 855–856, 856*f*
    injuries associated with, 450, 856, 856*f*
    low-to-medium energy missiles, 855
    secondary missiles, 856
Penumbra, 428, 431, 431*f*
Pepsinogen, 696, 698
Peptic ulcer disease (PUD)
    case study, 787–790
    causes, 713, 714*f*
    diagnosis, 714
    gastric vs. duodenal, 788
    pathophysiology, 713, 713*f*
    risk factors, 789
    sites, 713, 713*f*
    treatment, 714
Perclose device, 317
Percocet. *See* Oxycodone
Percodan. *See* Oxycodone
Percutaneous coronary intervention (PCI)
    for cardiogenic shock, 381
    definition, 301
    guidelines, 315
    nursing responsibilities, 232–234
    patient preparation, 315–316
    postprocedure management, 233–234, 317–318
    preprocedure medications, 315
    procedure, 233, 233*f*, 316–317, 316*f*, 317*f*
Percutaneous transluminal coronary angioplasty
    (PTCA), 381. *See also* Percutaneous coronary
    intervention
Perfusion
    definition, 81, 92
    factors affecting
        affinity of oxygen to hemoglobin, 358
        cardiac output, 92–93
        gravity
            pulmonary shunt, 95, 96*f*, 97*f*
            ventilation-perfusion relationship, 93–94,
                93*f*, 94*f*, 95*t*
        hemoglobin concentration, 358
        pulmonary vascular resistance, 95, 97*t*, 358
            cor pulmonale, 97–98, 98*f*
            vessel radius, 96–97
    impaired, 358*t*
    pulmonary system, 92, 93*f*
    systemic system, 92, 93*f*
Perfusionist, 301, 318
Periaqueductal gray (PAG) areas, 27, 27*t*
Pericardiocentesis, 869*f*
Peripheral nerve block, 38
Peripheral neuropathy, diabetic, 642–643
Peripheral vascular disease, in diabetes, 643
Peristalsis, 704
Peritoneal dialysis. *See also* Dialysis
    characteristics, 673, 673*f*, 675
    cycler-assisted, 674*f*
    nursing considerations, 675*t*
    venous access, 671*f*
Peritoneal space, 698
Peritoneum, 696, 698

Peritonitis, 698, 749
Permeability, 650
PET. *See* Positron emission tomography
PETCO₂. *See* End-tidal carbon dioxide
Petit mal seizure, 461, 479. *See also* Seizure(s)
Peyer's patches, 696, 705
pH
    blood
        definition, 81, 99
        factors affecting, 110
        interpretation, 111*t*, 112*f*, 113*f*
        in metabolic acidosis, 102, 102*t*
        in metabolic alkalosis, 102–103, 103*t*
        in mixed acid–base disorders, 116–118, 117*t*
        normal, 100, 100*f*, 110, 114*f*
        in respiratory acidosis, 101, 101*t*
        in respiratory alkalosis, 101–102, 101*t*
    gastric mucosa, 507
Phagocytosis, 567
Phantom pain. *See* Dysesthetic pain
Phlebostatic axis, 238, 242
Phosphate (PO₄)
    functions, 74
    imbalances, 74, 74*t*
    normal ranges and critical abnormal values, 66*t*
    regulation, 74
Phospholipase A
    definition, 762
    functions, 765, 765*t*
    in pancreatitis, 767
Phosphorus, 74. *See also* Phosphate
Physical dependence
    definition, 26, 40
    fear of, 41
    as pain management consideration, 46
Pitting edema, 63, 63*f*. *See also* Edema
Plasma cells, 557, 565–566
Plateau phase, repolarization, 265, 266, 267*f*, 267*t*
Platelet factor 4, 520, 544
Platelets
    causes for abnormal results, 523*t*
    characteristics, 525–526
    hemostatic functions, 526
    reference values, 523*t*
Pleura, 86
Pleural effusion, 129
Pleural infusion, 38
Pleural rub, 81, 107
Pleurisy, 81, 105
Pleuritis. *See* Pleurisy
Pluripotential hematopoietic stem cells (PHSC),
    520, 522
PMNs. *See* Polymorphonuclear neutrophils
PND. *See* Paroxysmal nocturnal dyspnea
Pneumocystis carinii pneumonia (PCP), 578
Pneumonia
    case study, 204–208
    ventilator-associated, 186
Pneumothorax
    classification, 152
    clinical findings, 152, 152*t*
    definition, 129, 151
    open, 869, 869*f*
    origins, 152*t*
    pathogenesis, 152
    tension. *See* Tension pneumothorax
    in total parenteral nutrition, 514

PO₂, 89
PO₄. *See* Phosphorus
Poikilothermia, 461, 474
Polyclonal antibodies, 588, 607
Polycythemia, 520, 533–534
Polycythemia vera, 533
Polydipsia, 622, 627
Polymorphonuclear, 520
Polymorphonuclear neutrophils (PMNs), 524. *See
    also* Neutrophils
Polys, 524
Polyurethane films, for wound dressing, 805*t*
Polyuria
    in chronic renal failure, 677–678
    definition, 622
Portal hypertension
    causes, 738, 738*f*
    definition, 736
Portal vein, 702, 702*t*
Portosystemic encephalopathy. *See* Hepatic
    encephalopathy
Positioning, antideformity, 844*t*
Positive end expiratory pressure (PEEP)
    in acute respiratory distress syndrome, 139
    definition, 166
    in mechanical ventilation, 179–180, 179*f*
    mechanisms, 139
    suctioning during, 191
Positive pressure ventilators
    characteristics, 174*f*, 175, 175*f*
    flow-cycled, 176
    pressure-cycled, 175
    time-cycled, 175
    volume-cycled, 175
Positron emission tomography (PET), 418
Postictal period, 461, 480
Postpyloric feeding, vs. gastric feeding, 511
Postrenal failure, 650. *See also* Acute renal failure
Posturing, abnormal, 412, 412*f*
Potassium channel blockers, 288, 289*t*
Potassium (K)
    functions, 71
    imbalances. *See* Hyperkalemia; Hypokalemia
    normal ranges and critical abnormal values, 66*t*
PQRST mnemonic
    in assessment of angina, 307
    in assessment of pain, 227
PR interval
    in first-degree AV block, 284–285, 285*f*
    interpretation on ECG, 272
    in second-degree AV block, 285, 286*f*
PrCO₂, 708, 710*t*
PrCO₂–PaCO₂ gap, 708, 710*t*
Prealbumin, 498, 499*t*
Precordium
    auscultation, 229
    palpation, 228
Precursor lesions, 301, 302
Pregnancy, trauma in, 859–860
Prehypertension, 325, 339, 339*t*
Preload
    assessment, 230, 230*t*
    definition, 219, 239, 244, 254
    factors affecting, 221, 225–226
    measurement, 254
    pathophysiology, 244
    stroke volume and, 222, 223*f*

Premature atrial contractions (PACs)
    characteristics, 280, 280f, 282t
    treatment, 282t
Premature ventricular contractions (PVCs)
    characteristics, 280–281, 280f, 281f, 282t
    treatment, 282, 282t
Prerenal azotemia, in total parenteral nutrition, 514
Prerenal failure, 650. See also Acute renal failure
Pressure adjusted heart rate (PAR), 390
Pressure-cycled ventilation, 175. See also Mechanical
    ventilation
Pressure gradient, 81, 89
Pressure support ventilation (PSV)
    characteristics, 178
    definition, 166
    indications, 178
    for ventilator weaning, 198t, 199
Pressure ulcers
    definition, 794
    management
        algorithm, 811f
        infection control, 814
        operative repair, 814–815
        support surfaces, 812, 814t
        tissue loads, 812, 813f
        wound care, 812, 815f
    nursing assessment, 812, 812t
    nursing interventions, 810t
    prevention, 809–810
    risk assessment and risk factors, 809
    staging, 809, 809t
    in stroke patients, 441–442
Priapism, 461, 469
Primary immunodeficiency. See Immunodeficiency
Primary injury
    brain, 449. See also Closed-head injury
    spinal cord, 461. See also Spinal cord injury
Primary intention, 794, 797–798
Primary MODS, 385, 388. See also Multiple organ
    dysfunction syndrome
Primary response, 557, 566, 567f
Prinzmetal's angina, 301, 308
PRN. See As-needed schedule
Prograf. See Tacrolimus
Proliferative phase. See Wound healing
Prone position therapy, 140
Proplatelets, 526
Propofol
    for increased intracranial pressure, 421
    for shock, 379
Proprioception
    definition, 428, 461, 467
    testing, 467, 469t
Prostaglandins. for gastrointestinal bleeding, 721t
Protein metabolism
    insulin and, 624
    insulin deficiency and, 626
    liver's role, 739
Protein–energy malnutrition, 507. See also Cachexia
Proteins
    categories, 494
    functions, 493–494, 494t
    metabolism, 494
        in starvation, 503
    structure, 493
    in wound healing, 800

Proteolytic, 762
Prothrombin time (PT), 742
Proton pump inhibitors, for gastrointestinal
    bleeding, 715, 721t
Pseudoaddiction, opioid. See Opioids,
    pseudoaddiction
Pseudopods, 525
PSV. See Pressure support ventilation
Psychologic dependence
    definition, 26, 40
    fear of, 41
    pain management considerations, 46
PT. See Prothrombin time
PTCA. See Percutaneous transluminal coronary
    angioplasty
PTT. See Partial thromboplastin time
Pulmonary angiography, in pulmonary
    embolism, 146
Pulmonary artery catheter. See also specific
    parameters
    components, 240–242, 241f
    insertion
        nursing responsibilities, 243
        procedure, 242–243
        right ventricular waveforms during, 251
    nursing care of patient requiring, 347–348
    purpose, 240
    specialized, 240
Pulmonary artery diastolic (PAD) pressure
    definition, 239
    elevated, 253
    low, 253
    measurement, 252–253
    normal values, 239, 252
    waveform, 252f
Pulmonary artery systolic (PAS) pressure
    definition, 239
    elevated, 253
    measurement, 252–253
    normal values, 239, 252
    waveform, 252f
Pulmonary artery wedge pressure (PAWP)
    in acute respiratory distress syndrome,
        135, 135t
    definition, 239
    elevated, 255–256
    low, 256
    measurement, 244–245, 254–255
    normal values, 239
    in ventricular function curve, 260f
    waveform, 254f, 255
Pulmonary disorders
    evidence-based practice, 157t
    obstructive. See also Chronic obstructive
        pulmonary disease (COPD)
        case study, 208–213
        definition, 129
        examples, 130
        vs. restrictive, 131t
    restrictive
        case study, 204–208
        causes, 130
        clinical manifestations, 131t
        definition, 129
        examples, 130t
        nursing interventions, 208

    vs. obstructive, 131t
    pathophysiology, 130
    signs and symptoms, 130t
    standard plans of care
        airway clearance, ineffective, 158
        breathing pattern, ineffective, 157
        gas exchange, impaired, 157–158
Pulmonary embolism
    in abdominal compartment syndrome, 728
    definition, 129, 143
    diagnosis, 146
    nursing considerations, 146–147
    obstructive shock state and, 372
    pathophysiology, 145
    signs and symptoms, 145, 145t, 377
    syndromes, 145t
    treatment, 146, 147t, 380
    types, 143
Pulmonary failure. See Gas exchange, impaired
Pulmonary function evaluation
    bedside measurements, 108–109
    forced expiratory volumes, 109
    lung volumes and capacities, 109t
    normal values, 109t
    tests, 108, 108t
    total lung capacity, 108
Pulmonary gas exchange
    assessment, 363–364, 363t
    definition, 355
    impaired, 358t. See also Pulmonary disorders
    physiology, 357, 358f
Pulmonary hypertension
    cor pulmonale and, 97–98, 98f
    pulmonary artery systolic pressure in, 253
    right atrial pressure in, 249
Pulmonary shunt(s)
    definition, 81, 95
    as indication for mechanical ventilation, 169
    types, 95, 96f
Pulmonary vascular resistance index (PVRI),
    239, 259
Pulmonary vascular resistance (PVR)
    calculation, 97, 97t, 259
    definition, 81, 95, 239
    factors affecting
        cor pulmonale, 97–98, 98f
        vessel radius, 96–97
    normal values, 239, 259
    physiology, 95
Pulmonic valve stenosis, 249
Pulse oximetry (Spo₂)
    definition, 81, 119
    factors affecting, 119
    mechanisms, 119
Pulse pressure, 219, 230–231
Pulsus alternans, 219, 228
Pulsus paradoxus
    in cardiac tamponade, 377
    after coronary artery bypass surgery, 320
    definition, 301, 370
Puncture wound, 794
Pupillary reactions, 413, 413f, 415t
Pvco₂, 89
PVCs. See Premature ventricular contractions
Pvo₂, 89
PVR. See Pulmonary vascular resistance

Q

QRS complex
    interpretation on ECG, 272
    normal configurations, 268, 269*f*
    in second-degree AV block, 285, 286*f*
Qs/Qt. *See* Intrapulmonary shunt
QT interval, 268*f*, 269
Quad coughing, 473
Quadriplegia, 461, 464. *See also* Spinal cord injury

R

R-R interval, 271
Raccoon eyes, 450
Radiation burns, 823
Radiation therapy, pulmonary complications, 539
Radiographs
    in pancreatitis, 769
    in spinal cord injury, 467
Rales. *See* Crackles
Ranson criteria, 769, 770
Rapamune. *See* Sirolimus
Rapid eye movement (REM) sleep, promoting, 11
R$_{AW}$. *See* Airway resistance
RBC. *See* Red blood cell
RCA. *See* Right coronary artery
RDW. *See* Red blood cell distribution width
Receptive aphasia, 404, 413
Recipient
    definition, 588
    donor compatibility testing, 599–600, 600*t*
    evaluation, 601–602, 601*t*
    need determination, 600–601
    posttransplant complications
        graft rejection, 603
        immunosuppressant-related, 603–605, 604*t*
        technical, 603
Red blood cell distribution width (RDW)
    causes of abnormal results, 523*t*, 527*t*, 529
    definition, 527, 529
    reference values, 523*t*
Red blood cells (RBCs)
    causes for abnormal results, 523*t*
    definition, 520
    disorders. *See* Anemia; Polycythemia
    evaluation
        causes of abnormal results, 523*t*
        color, 528
        hematocrit, 528
        hemoglobin, 528
        indices, 527*t*
        mean corpuscular volume, 528
        red cell mass, 528
        reference values, 523*t*
        reticulocyte count, 527
        sedimentation rate, 529
        total count, 528
    hemoglobin in, 524
    indices, 527*t*
    production feedback loop, 524
    reference values, 523*t*
    total count, 528
Red cell mass, 528
REE. *See* Resting energy expenditure
Refeeding syndrome, 504
Regurgitation, 325. *See also* Valvular heart disease

Rejection
    definition, 557, 588
    laboratory tests, 612
    T cells in, 567
    types, 603
Relative refractory period, 265, 267
Relaxation techniques, for pain management, 39*t*
REM sleep. *See* Rapid eye movement (REM) sleep
Remodeling phase. *See* Wound healing
Renal arteriogram, 666
Renal biopsy, 666
Renal failure
    acute. *See* Acute renal failure
    chronic. *See* Chronic renal failure
    intrinsic. *See* Acute renal failure, intrinsic
    postrenal. *See* Acute renal failure, postrenal
    prerenal. *See* Acute renal failure, prerenal
Renal transplantation
    complications, 609
    indications, 608
    postoperative management, 609
    recipient preparation, 608, 608*f*
    renal function evaluation, 609
Renal ultrasound, 666
Renin-angiotensin system
    in body fluid regulation, 59
    kidney function and, 654, 655*f*
    response to shock, 374, 375*f*
Repolarization
    characteristics, 266, 266*f*, 267*t*
    definition, 265
Respiration
    abnormal patterns, 414–415, 414*f*, 415*t*
    definition, 81, 88, 166, 167
    external, 88, 88*f*
    internal, 88, 88*f*
Respirator, vs. ventilator, 167
Respiratory acidosis. *See also* Acid–base
    disturbances; Arterial blood gases
    acute vs. chronic, 101*t*
    causes, 101*t*
    chronic, 101, 101*t*
    definition, 101
    pathophysiology, 101
Respiratory alkalosis. *See also* Acid–base
    disturbances; Arterial blood gases
    causes, 102*t*
    definition, 101
    pathophysiology, 101–102
Respiratory depression, fear of, 41
Respiratory distress
    nursing assessment
        common complaints
            chest pain, 105
            cough, 105–106
            dyspnea, 105
            hemoptysis, 106
            sputum, 106, 106*t*
        focused respiratory assessment, 107, 204–205,
            209, 214
        nursing history
            cardiopulmonary history, 104
            elimination history, 104–105
            focused, 206, 209
            nutritional history, 104
            sleep–rest history, 105
            social history, 104

respiratory physical assessment
    auscultation, 107, 107*f*
    inspection and palpation, 106–107
    percussion, 107
    vital signs and hemodynamic values, 106
    nursing diagnoses, 206–207, 211
    nursing interventions, 208, 213
Respiratory failure
    cardiopulmonary system and, 132
    complications, 133
    components, 133, 133*t*
    definition, 129, 132
    pathogenesis, 133–134
Respiratory insufficiency, 129, 132
Respiratory plans of care
    airway clearance, ineffective, 158
    breathing pattern, ineffective, 157
    gas exchange, impaired, 157–158
Respiratory quotient (RQ), 492, 501
Respiratory rate
    as indication for mechanical ventilation,
        169, 170*t*
    mechanical ventilation settings, 178–179
Respiratory system, 84–85, 85*f*
Responsiveness, 404
Resting energy expenditure (REE), 500–501, 500*t*.
    See also Energy expenditure
Resting membrane potential, 265, 266, 267*f*, 267*t*
Restrictive pulmonary disorders. *See* Pulmonary
    disorders, restrictive
Resuscitative phase, 821. *See also* Burn injury
Rete edges, 794
Rete ridges, 794
Reticular activating system, 404, 411
Reticulocytes, 520, 527
Reticuloendothelial system, 520, 532, 557, 564–565
Retinopathy, diabetic, 643
Rh incompatibility, 520, 532
Rhabdomyolysis
    acute tubular necrosis and, 658
    definition, 650
    pathophysiology, 658
    risk factors, 658
Rhinitis, allergic, 569
Rhinorrhea, 449, 451
Rhonchi, 81, 107
Rib fractures, 868, 868*f*
Ribavirin, for severe acute respiratory distress
    syndrome, 150
Right atrial pressure (RAP)
    decreased
        causes, 248–249, 249–250
        clinical findings, 249, 250
        interventions, 249, 250
    definition, 239, 247–248, 248*f*
    measurement, 248
    in mechanical ventilation, 248, 249*f*
    normal values, 239
    waveform, 248*f*, 249*f*
Right coronary artery (RCA)
    anatomy, 306, 306*f*
    ECG leads, 310*t*
Right heart catheter. *See* Pulmonary artery catheter
Right ventricular end-diastolic pressure (RVEDP),
    248. *See also* Right atrial pressure
Right ventricular failure, 377. *See also* Heart
    failure (HF)

Right ventricular (RV) pressure, 251, 251*f*
Right ventricular stroke work index (RVSWI), 239, 260
Risk factors
   modifiable, 301, 304
   nonmodifiable, 301, 304
Rotational injury, 450
RQ. *See* Respiratory quotient
rtPA. *See* Tissue plasminogen activator
Rule of nines, 827*f*
RV pressure. *See* Right ventricular (RV) pressure
RVSWI. *See* Right ventricular stroke work index

S

SAH. *See* Subarachnoid hematoma
Saline, for wound cleaning, 804
SaO₂
   definition, 90, 110
   interpretation, 110, 111*t*
   normal values, 114*t*
   in oxyhemoglobin dissociation curve, 90–91, 91*f*
Sarcolemma, 265
SARS. *See* Severe acute respiratory syndrome
Saturation
   arterial capillary hemoglobin. *See* Pulse oximetry
   arterial oxygen. *See* SaO₂
Scar management, 845, 845*f*
Schistocytes, 533
Sclerotherapy, nursing interventions, 785
SDH. *See* Subdural hematoma
Secondary immunodeficiency. *See* Immunodeficiency
Secondary injury
   brain, 449, 453–454, 454*f*, 454*t*. *See also* Closed-head injury
   spinal cord, 461, 465–466. *See also* Spinal cord injury
Secondary intention, 794, 798, 798*f*
Secondary MODS, 385, 388. *See also* Multiple organ dysfunction syndrome
Secondary response, 557, 566, 567*f*
Secretin
   definition, 696, 762
   gastric functions, 698–699, 699*t*, 764–765
Secretions, in mechanical ventilation, 191–192
Sed rate. *See* Erythrocyte sedimentation rate
Sedation, 26, 41
Sedimentation rate. *See* Erythrocyte sedimentation rate
Segmented cells, 520, 529. *See also* Neutrophils
Segs. *See* Segmented cells
Seizure(s)
   definition, 461
   generalized, 479–480
   nursing management, 480, 480*t*
   partial, 479
   pharmacologic management, 480
   tonic-clonic, 479–480, 479*f*
   types, 461
Sengstaken-Blakemore tube, 753
Sensory assessment, 467, 468*f*, 469*f*, 469*t*
Sensory overload, 10
Sensory perceptual alteration (SPA)
   causes, 10
   definition, 4
   delirium and, 11

Sensory receptors, 26, 26*t*. *See also* Pain
Sepsis
   during cancer treatment, 541
   definition, 129, 377*t*, 385
   hepatic failure and, 749
   in traumatic injury, 876, 876*t*
Septic shock
   definition, 377*t*
   evidence-based practice, 380*t*
   pathophysiology, 372, 372*f*
   treatment, 379–380
Seroconversion, 576
Serosa, gastrointestinal, 495, 696, 697, 698*f*
Serous cavity
   definition, 55
   third spacing, 61
Severe acute respiratory syndrome (SARS)
   clinical features, 149
   clinical presentation and course, 149
   definition, 129
   diagnosis, 149
   history, 148–149
   infection control, 150
   transmission, 149
   treatment, 150
SF-MPQ. *See* Short-form McGill Pain Questionnaire
SGOT. *See* Aspartate aminotransferase
SGPT. *See* Alanine aminotransferase
Sharp debridement, 794, 804
Shearing, 851, 854
Shock states
   cardiogenic
      clinical manifestations, 377
      etiology, 371*t*, 373
      pathophysiology, 371*t*, 373
      treatment, 380
   clinical manifestations, 376
   compensatory mechanisms, 374
      endocrine system, 374*f*
      renin–angiotensin–aldosterone cycle, 375*f*
      sympathetic nervous system, 374*t*
   hepatic failure in, 746
   hypovolemic
      clinical manifestations, 376
      etiology, 371–372, 371*t*
      pathophysiology, 371, 371*t*
      treatment, 379–380
   obstructive
      clinical manifestations, 377
      etiology, 371*t*, 372–373
      pathophysiology, 371*t*
      treatment, 380
   progression, 374–375
   in spinal cord injury, 470
   transport
      clinical manifestations, 376–377
      etiology, 371*t*
      pathophysiology, 371*t*, 372
      treatment, 380
   in trauma, 866
   treatment
      decreasing oxygen consumption, 379
      optimizing oxygen delivery, 378–379
Short-form McGill Pain Questionnaire (SF-MPQ), 33
Shunting, 166, 169. *See also* Pulmonary shunt(s)

Shuntlike effect
   causes, 95
   definition, 81, 95
   types, 96*f*
SIADH. *See* Syndrome of inappropriate diuretic hormone
Sigh, 166, 177
Silvadene. *See* Silver sulfadiazine
Silver nitrate solution, 839*t*
Silver sulfadiazine, 839*t*
Simulect. *See* Basiliximab
SIMV. *See* Synchronous intermittent mandatory ventilation
Single photon emission computed tomography (SPECT), 418
Sinus bradycardia, 274, 275*f*, 275*t*
Sinus tachycardia, 274–275, 275*f*, 275*t*
Sirolimus, posttransplantation, 607
SIRS. *See* Systemic inflammatory response syndrome
SjO₂. *See* Jugular bulb oximetry
Skin
   anatomy and physiology, 794–795, 794*t*, 795*f*
   grafts, 840–841, 840*f*, 841*f*
   substitutes, 838–839, 839*t*, 841, 841*f*
Skull fractures. *See also* Closed-head injury (CHI)
   medical management, 451
   nursing priorities, 451
   types, 450–451
Skull tongs, 471, 471*f*, 472*t*
Sleep pattern disturbance
   in heart failure, 336
   during mechanical ventilation, 194
Sliding-scale insulin coverage, 640, 640*t*
Slough, 794, 807
Slow response action potential, 265
Small intestine. *See also* Gastrointestinal tract
   anatomy and physiology, 697*f*, 698–699, 699*f*
   hormone secretion, 698–699, 699*t*
   obstruction, 723–724
   transplantation. *See* Intestine transplantation
Smoking
   stroke risk and, 432
   wound healing and, 799–800
Sodium bicarbonate (NaHCO₃), 633. *See also* Bicarbonate
Sodium (Na)
   dietary intake, 67
   functions, 66
   imbalances
      hypernatremia. *See* Hypernatremia
      hyponatremia. *See* Hyponatremia
      normal ranges and critical abnormal values, 66*t*
   water balance and, 66–67
Somatosensory-evoked potentials (SEPs), 461, 467
Somatostatin
   for esophageal varices, 753
   for gastrointestinal hemorrhage, 721*t*
Somogyi effect, 622, 640–641, 641*f*
SPA. *See* Sensory perceptual alteration
Spastic paralysis, 461
Spasticity, 428, 439, 439*f*
SPECT. *See* Single photon emission computed tomography
Speech, in consciousness assessment, 413
Sphincter of Oddi, 762, 763

Spinal cord
  anatomy, 462–463
  compression, in malignant disease, 541
  neuronal function, 463
Spinal cord injury
  causes, 463
  complete, 464
  diagnosis
    history, 466–467
    radiographs, 467
    somatosensory-evoked potentials, 467
  incidence, 463
  incomplete, 464, 464t
  lower motor neuron injuries, 464
  mechanisms
    cervical, 465
    compression, 464–465, 465f
    hyperextension, 464, 465f
    hyperreflexion, 464, 465f
    lumbar, 465
    nontraumatic, 465
    primary injuries, 464–465, 465f
    secondary
      elevated intracellular calcium, 466
      inflammatory processes, 466
      ischemia, 466
    thoracic, 465
  methylprednisolone for, 472
  nursing care, 478t
    complication prevention
      autonomic dysreflexia, 475, 475t
      bladder dysfunction, 477
      bowel dysfunction, 477
      decreased joint mobility, 475
      deep vein thrombosis, 475
      orthostatic hypotension, 477
      sexual dysfunction, 477
      skin integrity, 474–475, 478t
    decreased cardiac output, 474, 478t
    elimination dysfunction, 474, 478t
    evidence-based practice, 477
    gas exchange impairment, 473, 478t
    ineffective breathing patterns, 473, 478t
    nutritional imbalances, 474
    psychosocial issues, 477
    self-care deficits, 474, 475t
    thermoregulation, 474
  physical assessment
    motor assessment, 467, 468f
    sensory assessment, 467, 468f, 469f, 469t
  physical effects, 476f
  shock states in, 470
  stabilization
    braces, 471–472
    manual
      halo device, 471, 471f, 471t
      skull tongs, 471, 471f
    surgical, 471
    techniques, 472t
  types, 463
  upper motor neuron injuries, 464
Spinal shock, 461, 470
Spine
  anatomy, 462–463, 462f
  unstable injury, 462. See also Spinal cord injury

Spinothalamic tract, 463
Spirituality, 4, 9
Splanchnic circulation, 696, 700, 736, 737, 738f
Spleen
  anatomy, 558f
  functions, 559
  injury, 870
Split-liver transplant, 612
SpO2. See Pulse oximetry
Spontaneous breaths, 166
Sputum
  nursing assessment, 106, 106t
  specimen collection, 106
ST elevation myocardial infarction (STEMI), 312.
    See also Acute coronary syndromes
  collaborative interventions
    coronary artery bypass graft surgery
      indications, 318
      nursing diagnoses, 319t
      postsurgical care, 319–321
      procedure, 318–319, 319f
    percutaneous coronary intervention
      guidelines, 315
      patient preparation, 315–316
      postprocedure management, 317–318
      preprocedure medications, 315
      procedure, 316–317, 316f, 317f
    thrombolytic therapy, 314–315
      contraindications, 315t
ST segment
  in myocardial ischemia assessment, 309
  normal configurations, 268f, 269
Stable angina, 301, 307–308
Stabs, 520, 529. See also Neutrophils
Staphylococcus aureus, 331
Starling forces, 57–58, 57f, 60
Starvation
  characteristics, 502–503
  definition, 502
  vs. hypermetabolism, 504t
  types, 502–503
Statins, 305
Status epilepticus, 461, 480
STEMI. See ST elevation myocardial infarction
Stenosis, 325. See also Valvular heart disease
Stents, intracoronary, 317, 317f
Stiff lungs, 87
Stomatitis, 581
Streptococci viridans, 331
Stress
  diabetic ketoacidosis and, 632–633
  gastritis and, 715
  immune system effects, 573
  for nurses in high-acuity units, 16–17, 16t
  pain and, 30
Stress factors, in energy expenditure, 500, 500t
Stroke
  assessment, 433–434
  case study, 485–488
  clinical manifestations, 433, 433t
  definition, 428
  diagnostic procedures, 435
  hemorrhagic, 429, 430t
  ischemic, 429, 430t
  medical management, 435–436, 436t

  National Institutes of Health scale, 434t
  nursing care, acute phase
    ambulation, 440
    case study, 485–488
    communication impairment, 443
    elimination alteration, 440–441, 441t
    evidence-based practice, 440t
    nutrition alteration, 440
    patient and family coping, 443–444
    physical mobility impairment, 438–440,
      438f, 439f
    sensory alterations, 441–442, 442t
    tissue perfusion alteration, 438
  nursing diagnoses, 435
  pathophysiology, 431, 431f
  risk factors, 432, 432f
  surgical management, 436–437, 437t
Stroke volume index (SVI)
  calculation, 258
  definition, 239, 245
  normal values, 239
Stroke volume (SV)
  calculation, 220, 221, 258
  components, 221
  definition, 219, 239, 265
  normal values, 239
  preload and, 222, 223f
Subarachnoid hematoma (SAH), 449, 452
Subarachnoid hemorrhage, 429, 430t. See also Stroke
Subarachnoid screw, 416f, 416t, 417
Subdermal burn, 821, 824, 825t. See also Burn injury
Subdural hematoma (SDH), 449, 452, 452f
Sublimaze. See Fentanyl
Subluxation, 428
Submucosa, 495, 696–697, 697f
Substance abuse
  common substances and withdrawal
    manifestations, 48t
  traumatic injury and, 859
Substance abuser, pain management for, 44–46, 46t,
    47t, 48
Suchman's stages of illness, 8t
Sucralfate, for gastrointestinal bleeding, 715, 721t
Suctioning, airway secretions, 191–192
Sulfamylon. See Mafenide acetate
Summation gallop, 220, 229
Sump drains, 806t
Sundowner's syndrome, 4, 11
Superficial burn, 821, 824, 825t. See also Burn injury
Superficial partial-thickness burn, 821, 824, 825t. See
    also Burn injury
Superior vena cava syndrome, 541
Support surfaces, 812, 814t
Supranormal period, 265
Supraventricular tachycardia (SVT), 276, 277f, 278t
Surface area
  body. See Body surface area; Total body surface
    area
  lung, 90
Surfactant, 81, 86, 129
Surfactant replacement therapy, 141
Susceptible host, 794, 802
SV. See Stroke volume
SVI. See Stroke volume index
SvO2. See Mixed venous oxygen saturation

SVR. *See* Systemic vascular resistance
SVRI. *See* Systemic vascular resistance index
SVT. *See* Supraventricular tachycardia
Swallowing, evaluation after stroke, 440
Swan–Ganz catheter. *See* Pulmonary artery catheter
Sympathetic nervous system, shock and, 374t
Synchronous intermittent mandatory ventilation (SIMV)
  characteristics, 178
  definition, 166
  for ventilator weaning, 198–199, 198t
Syncope, 220, 227
Syndrome of inappropriate diuretic hormone (SIADH)
  clinical manifestations, 455
  after closed-head injury, 455, 456t
  serum osmolality in, 57
Syngraft. *See* Isograft
Synthesis, 622
Systemic arterial pressure
  advantages of monitoring, 256
  measurement, 257
  patient assessment, 257
  waveform, 257, 257f
Systemic inflammatory response syndrome (SIRS). *See also* Multiple organ dysfunction syndrome
  definition, 385, 387, 387t
  hepatic failure in, 746
  pathophysiology, 387
Systemic vascular resistance index (SVRI), 239, 259
Systemic vascular resistance (SVR)
  calculation, 259
  definition, 239
  elevated, 259
  low, 259
  normal values, 239
Systolic dysfunction, 325, 333. *See also* Heart failure

T

T cells
  aging effects, 572
  definition, 557
  in HIV/AIDS, 574, 575f
  production, 558
  types, 564
T lymphocytes. *See* T cells
Tachycardia. *See* Dysrhythmias
Tacrolimus, posttransplantation, 607
Tamponade
  cardiac. *See* Cardiac tamponade
  for gastrointestinal hemorrhage, 721t
Target organ damage, 325, 340
TBSA. *See* Total body surface area
TCD. *See* Transcranial Doppler
Tegretol. *See* Carbamazepine
Tenckhoff catheter, 671f
TENS. *See* Transcutaneous electrical nerve stimulation
Tensile forces, 851, 854
Tension pneumothorax
  pathophysiology, 373
  in trauma patient, 868–869, 869f
  treatment, 380

Tertiary intention, 794, 798, 798f
Tetraplegia, 461, 464. *See also* Spinal cord injury
Thermal burns, 822, 822f, 824. *See also* Burn injury
Thermodilution, 239, 245–247
Thermoregulation, after spinal cord injury, 474
Thiazide diuretics
  common, 332t
  for heart failure, 334
  for hypertension, 340
Thienopyridines, 313. *See also* Clopidogrel
Third spacing, 61, 63
Thirst, regulation, 59, 654
Thoracic spine injury, 465. *See also* Spinal cord injury
Thorax, role in ventilation, 86, 86f
Thrombocytopenia
  causes, 544
  clinical manifestations, 543
  definition, 543
  heparin-induced, 544
Thromboembolism
  in heparin-induced thrombocytopenia, 544
  pathophysiology, 144f
  predisposing factors, 143–144, 144t
Thrombolytic therapy
  for cardiogenic shock, 381
  for myocardial infarction, 314–315, 315t
  for pulmonary embolism, 147t
Thrombosis, 520
Thrombotic stroke, 429, 430t. *See also* Stroke
Thymus, 557, 558, 558f
TIAs. *See* Transient ischemic attacks
Tidal volume (TV)
  definition, 81, 109, 129, 166, 176
  in mechanical ventilation
    high, adverse effects, 177
    high vs. low, 139
  normal values, 109t
  in restrictive pulmonary disorders, 130, 130t, 131t
Time-cycled ventilation, 175. *See also* Mechanical ventilation
TIPS. *See* Transjugular intrahepatic shunt
Tissue gel, 56
Tissue glue, 797–798
Tissue hydrostatic pressure, 58
Tissue load, 794, 812, 812f
Tissue plasminogen activator (rtPA), for ischemic stroke, 436
Tissue typing, 588, 59
Titration, in pain management, 42, 42t
TLC. *See* Total lung capacity
Tolerance, 26, 40, 41
Tonic-clonic seizure, 461, 479, 479f
Tonicity
  definition, 55, 64
  intravenous solutions classified by, 65f, 65t
Tonsillar herniation, 409f
Total body surface area (TBSA)
  calculation, 824–825
  Lund and Browder chart, 826f
  rule of nines, 827f
Total cholesterol
  classification of values, 304t
  reduction, 305, 305t

Total lung capacity (TLC)
  components, 108
  definition, 81, 108, 129
  in restrictive pulmonary disorders, 131t
Total lymphocyte count (TLC), 499
Total parenteral nutrition (TPN)
  complications
    infectious, 514
    mechanical, 514–515
    metabolic, 514
  contraindications, 514
  definition, 492, 513
  indications, 514
TPN. *See* Total parenteral nutrition
Tracheostomy
  definition, 851
  indications, 171–172
  in traumatic injury, 872
Transcellular fluid, 56
Transcranial Doppler (TCD), 418–419
Transcutaneous electrical nerve stimulation (TENS), 39t
Transesophageal echocardiogram (TEE), 232
Transferrin, 498, 499t
Transfusion reaction, 569–570
Transient ischemic attacks (TIAs), 428, 429
Transjugular intrahepatic shunt (TIPS), 753
Transplantation
  complications
    graft rejection, 603
    immunosuppressant-related, 603–605, 604t
    technical, 603
  donor management, 596t
    endocrine function loss, 597
    fluid and electrolyte instability, 597
    hematopoietic dysfunction, 597
    hemodynamic instability, 596–597
    pulmonary dysfunction, 597
    thermoregulation loss, 597
  heart and heart lung. *See* Heart and heart-lung transplantation
  history, 588–589
  indications, 609t
  intestine. *See* Intestine transplantation
  kidney. *See* Renal transplantation
  legal aspects, 590–591
  liver. *See* Liver transplantation
  lung. *See* Lung transplantation
  Medicare conditions of participation, 591
  need determination, 600–601
  organ preservation, 597–598, 598t
  pancreas and pancreas-kidney. *See* Pancreas and pancreas-kidney transplantation
  procurement process
    consent, 594
    donor suitability, 594, 594t
    donor testing, 594–595
    establishing death, 592–593
    evidence-based practice, 592–593
    non-heart-beating, 595
    referral to organ procurement organization, 593, 593t
  recipient evaluation, 601–602, 601t
  renal. *See* Renal transplantation
  small bowel. *See* Intestine transplantation

Transport shock states
  clinical manifestations, 376–377
  etiology, 371t
  pathophysiology, 371t, 372
  treatment, 380
Transtentorial herniation, 409t, 410f
Transthoracic echocardiogram, 232
Trauma. See Injury
Traumatic brain injury. See Closed-head injury
Trendelenburg's position, 379
Tricuspid regurgitation, 331t
Tricuspid stenosis, 331t
Trigeminy, 265, 281f
Triple H therapy, 436
Troponins (cT$_n$)
  characteristics, 229
  definition, 220
  in myocardial ischemia, 310t
Trousseau's sign, 771
True shunt, 81, 95
Trypsin, 762, 765, 765t
Tubular reabsorption, 652
Tubular secretion, 650, 652
Tumble, 856, 856f
Tumor-associated antigen, 557, 561–562
Tumor lysis syndrome, 541
TV. See Tidal volume

U

UA. See Unstable angina
UAGA. See Uniform Anatomical Gift Act
Ultrasound
  in deep venous thrombosis, 146
  in gastrointestinal dysfunction, 708
  in pancreatitis, 769
  renal, 666
Uncal herniation, 409t
Uncompensated acid–base state, 82, 100, 100t. See also Acid–base disturbances
Unconjugated bilirubin, 736, 742, 742t
Uniform Anatomical Gift Act (UAGA), 590–591
Uniform Determination of Death Act, 591
Unlicensed assistive personnel (UAP), 15
Unstable angina (UA), 301, 308. See also Acute coronary syndromes
Unstable spinal injury, 461, 462
UPA. See Unlicensed assistive personnel
Uptake, 622
Urea, 736, 739
Uremia. See also Acute renal failure; Chronic renal failure
  definition, 650, 678
  effects, 663, 664f, 665, 678
Urinary tract infection (UTI), in spinal cord injury, 477
Urine output, cardiac output and, 228
Urine urea nitrogen (UUN), 499, 499t
Urobilinogen, 736, 742, 742t
Urticaria, in anaphylaxis, 569
UUN. See Urine urea nitrogen

V

$\dot{V}Q$ ratio
  definition, 82, 93, 129, 166
  high vs. low, 94, 95t
  low, as indication for mechanical ventilation, 169
  in obstructive pulmonary disorders, 131
  physiology, 93–94
  positioning effects, 94, 94f
  in restrictive pulmonary disorders, 130
$\dot{V}Q$ scan
  in pulmonary embolism, 146
$\dot{V}A$. See Alveolar ventilation
VAC. See Vacuum-assisted closure
Vacuum-assisted closure (VAC), 804, 840
VAE. See Venous air embolism
Valvular heart disease
  assessment and diagnosis, 331–332, 331t
  collaborative management, 332
  nursing management, 332–333
  regurgitation
    aortic, 330, 330f, 331t
    characteristics, 329, 329f
    mitral, 329–330, 329f, 331t
    risk factors, 328t
    tricuspid, 331t
  stenosis
    aortic, 328, 328t, 329f, 331t
    characteristics, 326–327, 328f
    mitral, 327–328, 328f, 328t, 331t
    risk factors, 328t
    tricuspid, 331t
VAP. See Ventilator-associated pneumonia
Variant angina, 301, 308
Varices, 736. See also Esophageal varices
VAS. See Visual analog scale
Vascular thrombosis, 588, 603
Vasodilating drugs, for shock, 378–379
Vasopressin
  for diabetes insipidus, 597
  for esophageal varices, 753
  for gastrointestinal hemorrhage, 721t
  nursing considerations, 785
  for ventricular fibrillation, 283
Vasopressors, for shock, 37, 380
VC. See Vital capacity
$\dot{V}D$. See Deadspace ventilation
$\dot{V}_E$
  calculation, 179
  definition, 81, 109
  as indication for mechanical ventilation, 170t
  in mechanical ventilation, 178–179
  normal values, 109t
Vecuronium, for shock, 379
Venous admixture, 82, 95, 97f
Venous air embolism (VAE), 143. See also Pulmonary embolism
Venous stasis, 143
Ventilation
  aging effects, 87
  components, 167, 168f, 358
  definition, 82, 86, 166, 167, 355

  elastic forces, 86, 86f
  impaired, 358t
  lung compliance, 86–87
  mechanical. See Mechanical ventilation; Ventilator(s)
  mechanics, 174f
  movements, 86
Ventilation–perfusion relationship. See $\dot{V}Q$ ratio
Ventilator-associated pneumonia (VAP), 186
Ventilator breath, 166
Ventilator(s). See also Mechanical ventilation
  vs. respirator, 167
  settings, 177f
    alarms, 180
    continuous positive airway pressure, 179
    fraction of inspired oxygen, 177–178
    initial, 180–181
    peak airway pressure, 180
    positive end-expiratory pressure, 179–180, 179f
    respiratory rate, 178–179
    tidal volume, 139, 176–177
    ventilation modes
      assist-control, 178
      intermittent mandatory, 178
      pressure support, 178
  types
    negative pressure, 173–175, 174f
    positive pressure, 174f, 175, 175f
      flow-cycled, 176
      pressure-cycled, 175
      time-cycled, 175
      volume-cycled, 175
Ventilatory failure
  acute, 166, 169, 170t
  clinical manifestations, 133, 133t
  definition, 129, 133, 133t
  as indication for mechanical ventilation, 169
Ventricular fibrillation
  characteristics, 283, 283f, 284t
  treatment, 283, 284t
Ventricular gallop, 220, 229
Ventricular stroke work index, 239, 245
Ventricular tachycardia (VT)
  characteristics, 282–283, 283f, 284t
  treatment, 283, 284t
Verbal descriptor scales, 32
Vertebrae, 462, 462f. See also Spinal cord; Spinal cord injury
Vessel radius, 96–97
Villi, 696, 698
Virchow's triad, 143–144
Viscera, 700
Visceral pleura, 82, 86
Visitation policies, in high-acuity units, 13–14
Visual analog scale (VAS), 32, 32f
Vital capacity (VC)
  definition, 82, 109, 166
  as indication for mechanical ventilation, 169, 170t
  normal values, 109f, 109t
Vitamin A, for wound healing, 801

Vitamin B$_{12}$
    deficiency, 531–532
    role in erythrocytes, 524
Vitamin D, metabolism in liver, 739
V̇O$_2$. *See* Oxygen consumption
Volatile acids, 82, 99
Volume-cycled ventilation, 175. *See also*
    Mechanical ventilation
Volutrauma
    clinical signs, 186
    definition, 166
    pathophysiology, 177
Vowel-TIPPS mnemonic, for causes of impaired
    consciousness, 411
VT. *See* Tidal volume

W

Warfarin, for pulmonary embolism, 147t
Water, distribution in adult body, 56f, 56t. *See also*
    Body fluid(s)
Weaning, 166. *See also* Mechanical ventilation,
    weaning
Weight, ideal, 500
Wenckebach heart block. *See* Mobitz type I heart
    block
Wernicke's aphasia, 443
Western blot test, 576–577
Wheeze, 82, 107
White blood cells (WBCs). *See also specific cells*
    causes for abnormal results, 523t
    disorders
        leukemia. *See* Leukemia

        neutropenia. *See* Neutropenia
    evaluation, 529
    in gastrointestinal dysfunction, 707, 707t
    reference values, 523t
    types, 524–525
White matter, spinal cord, 463
WHO. *See* World Health Organization
Wong-Baker Faces Scale, 32, 32f
World Health Organization (WHO), ladder
    approach to pain management, 36, 36f
Wound healing
    assessment
        immunologic status, 808
        inspection, 807
        nutritional status, 808
        palpation, 807–808
        preexisting health problems, 807
        tissue perfusion/oxygenation status, 808
    in burn injury, 836, 836f
    closure methods, 797–799, 798f
    in diabetes, 644
    evidence-based practice, 800t
    factors affecting
        age, 800
        blood chemistry, 801
        diabetes, 800
        medications, 801
        moisture, 801
        nutrition, 800
        obesity, 801
        oxygenation/tissue perfusion, 799–800
    inflammatory phase, 796, 797f
    methods, 796

    proliferative phase, 796–797
    remodeling phase, 797
Wound infections
    diagnosis, 802
    prevention, 803
    risk factors, 802
    signs, 802
Wound management. *See also* Burn injury;
    Pressure ulcers
    cleaning, 803–804
    debridement, 804, 838, 838f
    dressings, 804, 805t, 806t
    skin grafts, 840–841, 840f, 841f
    tubes and drains, 805, 806t

X

Xanthoma, 301, 308
Xenograft, 821. *See also* Heterograft

Y

Yale brace, 472t
Yaw, 856, 856f

Z

Zaroxolyn. *See* Metolazone
Zenapax. *See* Daclizumab
Zinc, immune system effects, 572